Nelson Pediatrics Board Review

Nelson Pediatrics Board Review

Certification and Recertification

Terry Dean, Jr., MD, PhD

UCSF Benioff Children's Hospitals
Division of Critical Care Medicine
Department of Pediatrics
San Francisco, California

Louis M. Bell, MD

Chief, Division of General Pediatrics
Children's Hospital of Philadelphia
Professor of Pediatrics
Perelman School of Medicine at the University of Pennsylvania
Philadelphia, Pennsylvania

ELSEVIER

ELSEVIER

1600 John F. Kennedy Blvd.
Ste 1600
Philadelphia, PA 19103-2899

Content Strategist: Sarah Barth
Content Development Specialist: Jennifer Ehlers
Publishing Services Manager: Deepthi Unni
Project Manager: Srividhya Vidhyashankar
Design Direction: Margaret Reid

Printed in the United States of America

Last digit is the print number: 9 8 7 6 5 4

Preface

We are proud to add to the Nelson family of books with this volume, the inaugural edition of *Nelson Pediatrics Board Review*. With the specific purpose of focusing on content covered by the American Board of Pediatrics Certifying Examination in General Pediatrics, this book is divided by specialty and written by contributors with in-depth knowledge of their topics. It was imperative that the depth and breadth be appropriate for the general pediatrician and that the information be presented in a manner that aided in review. We hope that the reader finds helpful the comparative tables of similar disorders, the algorithms of medical decision making, and the review questions that emphasize key points tested by the actual board exam.

We feel that preparation for boards is an essential milestone in each pediatrician's career, whether he or she is recertifying or taking the exam for the first time after residency. It is a time to reflect on our practices and refresh our knowledge base to ensure that we are delivering the utmost excellence in care to our patients, a challenging task given the inexorable advances in science and technology that occur every day. To this end, we hope that this book becomes a vital component of your board review toolkit and that it serves as a foundation upon which to build a lifetime of learning.

We would like to acknowledge all of our contributors for generously offering their efforts and expertise, as they developed original chapters for this first edition. We thank Sarah Barth, Jennifer Ehlers, Vidhya Shankar, Beula Christopher King, and all the members of the Elsevier team who have shepherded this book into reality. Finally, we thank our families, as we recognize that this project would not have been possible without their patient support and encouragement.

Terry Dean, Jr.
Louis M. Bell

To my wife, Gina, for her strength and selflessness.
TD

To my parents, Louis and DeaSue, and my mentors,
Tom, Stanley, and Steve.
LMB

Contributors

Angela T. Anderson, MD
Post Pediatric Portal Fellow, Department of Child and Adolescent Psychiatry and Behavioral Sciences, Children's Hospital of Philadelphia, Philadelphia, Pennsylvania

Gabriela M. Andrade, MD
Attending Physician, Department of Child and Adolescent Psychiatry and Behavioral Sciences, Children's Hospital of Philadelphia, Philadelphia, Pennsylvania

Casandra Arevalo-Marcano, MD
Pediatric Pulmonary Fellow, Pulmonary Medicine, Children's Hospital of Philadelphia, Philadelphia, Pennsylvania

Fran Balamuth, MD, PhD
Associate Director of Research, Department of Pediatric Emergency Medicine, The Children's Hospital of Philadelphia, Philadelphia, Pennsylvania

Diana Bartenstein, MD
Research Fellow, Dermatology, Harvard Medical School, Massachusetts General Hospital, Boston, Massachusetts

Dionne Blackman, MD
Associate Professor of Medicine, Department of Medicine, The University of Chicago, Chicago, Illinois

Mercedes M. Blackstone, MD
Attending Physician, Division of Emergency Medicine, Children's Hospital of Philadelphia; Associate Professor of Clinical Pediatrics, Perelman School of Medicine, University of Pennsylvania, Philadelphia, Pennsylvania

Eric M. Bomberg, MD, MAS
Assistant Professor, Division of Pediatric Endocrinology, University of Minnesota, Minneapolis, Minnesota

Adam Bonnington, MD
Resident Physician, Department of Obstetrics, Gynecology & Reproductive Sciences, University of California, San Francisco, San Francisco, California

Diana K. Bowen, MD
Assistant Professor of Urology, Northwestern University, Feinberg School of Medicine; Ann & Robert H. Lurie Children's Hospital of Chicago, Chicago, Illinois

Kim Braly, MD
Clinical Pediatric Dietitian, Pediatric Gastroenterology and Hepatoloy, Seattle Children's Hospital, Seattle, Washington

Jason Z. Bronstein, MD
Fellow Physician, Division of Pulmonary Medicine, The Children's Hospital of Philadelphia, Philadelphia, Pennsylvania

J. Naylor Brownell, MD
Fellow, Gastroenterology and Clinical Nutrition, Gastroenterology, Hepatology, and Nutrition, Children's Hospital of Philadelphia, Philadelphia, Pennsylvania

Celina Brunson, BS, MD
Fellow Physician, Nephrology, Children's Hospital of Philadelphia, Philadelphia, Pennsylvania

Douglas A. Canning, MD
Professor, Surgery (Urology), Perelman School of Medicine, University of Pennsylvania; Chief, Division of Urology, Children's Hospital of Philadelphia, Philadelphia, Pennsylvania

Ricki S. Carroll, MD, MBE
Clinical Assistant Professor of Pediatrics, Division of General Pediatrics, Sidney Kimmel Medical College at Thomas Jefferson University, Nemours A. I. duPont Hospital for Children, Wilmington, Delaware

Alice Chan, MD, PhD
Assistant Professor, Division of Pediatric Allergy, Immunology, and Bone Marrow Transplant, Division of Pediatric Rheumatology, University of California, San Francisco, San Francisco, California

Joyce Chun-Ling Chang, MD
Division of Rheumatology, Children's Hospital of Philadelphia, Philadelphia, Pennsylvania

Pi Chun Cheng, MD, MS
Fellow Physician, Pediatric Pulmonology, Children's Hospital of Philadelphia, Philadelphia, Pennsylvania

Catherine S. Choi, MD
Assistant Professor, Ophthalmology, Tufts Medical Center, Boston, Massachusetts

Jennifer H. Chuang, MD, MS
Assistant Professor of Pediatrics, Craig-Dalsimer Division of Adolescent Medicine, Children's Hospital of Philadelphia, Philadelphia, Pennsylvania

Gwynne Church, MD
Associate Professor of Pediatrics, Division of Pediatric Pulmonary Medicine, University of California, San Francisco, San Francisco, California

Stephanie Clark, MD, MPH, MSHP
Assistant Professor of Pediatrics, Division of Nephrology, Children's Hospital of Philadelphia, Perelman School of Medicine, University of Pennsylvania, Philadelphia, Pennsylvania

Maire Conrad, MD, MS
Assistant Professor of Pediatrics, Perelman School of Medicine at the University of Pennsylvania, Division of Gastroenterology, Hepatology, and Nutrition, The Children's Hospital of Philadelphia, Philadelphia, Pennsylvania

Jonathan Bryan Cooper-Sood, MD
Fellow, Pediatric Emergency Medicine, Emergency Medicine, UCSF Benioff Children's Hospital Oakland and Mission Bay, Oakland and San Francisco, California

Lawrence A. Copelovitch, MD
Assistant Professor of Pediatrics, Nephrology, Children's Hospital of Philadelphia, Philadelphia, Pennsylvania

Danielle Cullen, MD, MPH, MSHP
Clinical Instructor, Pediatric Emergency Medicine, Children's Hospital of Philadelphia, Philadelphia, Pennsylvania

Terry Dean, Jr., MD, PhD
Clinical Fellow, Division of Pediatric Critical Care Medicine, UCSF Benioff Children's Hospitals, San Francisco, California

Sanyukta Desai, MD
Clinical Fellow, Hospital Medicine, Cincinnati Children's Hospital Medical Center, Cincinnati, Ohio

Conor M. Devine, MD
Fellow/Junior Attending, Pediatric Otolaryngology - Head and Neck Surgery, Children's Hospital of Philadelphia, Philadelphia, Pennsylvania

Erin Pete Devon, MD
Assistant Professor of Clinical Pediatrics, Pediatrics, Children's Hospital of Philadelphia, Philadelphia, Pennsylvania

Leah Dowsett, MD
Clinical Genetics Fellow, Division of Genetics and Metabolism, Children's Hospital of Philadelphia, Philadelphia, Pennsylvania

Matthew Drago, MD, MBE
Assistant Professor, Division of Neonatology, Department of Pediatrics, Yale University School of Medicine, New Haven, Connecticut

Fei Jamie Dy, MD
Assistant Professor of Pediatrics, Division of Pediatric Pulmonary Medicine, University of California, San Francisco, San Francisco, California

Abdulla Ehlayel, MD
Fellow, Nephrology, Children's Hospital of Philadelphia, Philadelphia, Pennsylvania

Marina Eisenberg, MD
Associate Staff, Ophthalmology, Cole Eye Institute, Cleveland Clinic; Clinical Assistant Professor of Surgery, Case Western Reserve University, Lerner College of Medicine, Cleveland, Ohio

Leslie Anne Enane, MD
Assistant Professor of Pediatrics, Ryan White Center for Pediatric Infectious Disease and Global Health, Indiana University School of Medicine, Indianapolis, Indiana

Ayca Erkin-Cakmak, MD, MPH
Pediatric Endocrinology, Clinical Fellow, Division of Endocrinology, University of California, San Francisco, San Francisco, California

Eileen M. Everly, MD
General Pediatrics, Children's Hospital of Philadelphia, Philadelphia, Pennsylvania

Lisa Fahey, MD
Attending Physician, Division of Gastroenterology, Hepatology and Nutrition, Children's Hospital of Philadelphia; Faculty, Department of Pediatrics, The Perelman School of Medicine, University of Pennsylvania, Philadelphia, Pennsylvania

Julie Fierro, MD, MPH
Fellow, Pediatric Pulmonology, Children's Hospital of Philadelphia, Philadelphia, Pennsylvania

Jessica Foster, MD
Division of Oncology, Children's Hospital of Philadelphia, Philadelphia, Pennsylvania

Nicholas L. Friedman, DO
Fellow Physician, Division of Pulmonary Medicine, The Children's Hospital of Philadelphia, Philadelphia, Pennsylvania

Radha Gajjar, MD, MSCE
Assistant Professor of Pediatrics, Department of Pediatrics, Division of Nephrology, Weill Cornell Medical College, New York, New York

Andrew Gambone, MD
Department of Orthopaedic Surgery, Bayhealth Medical Center, Dover, Delaware

Rebecca D. Ganetzky, MD
Assistant Professor of Pediatrics, Division of Human Genetics, Children's Hospital of Philadelphia, Philadelphia, Pennsylvania

Elizabeth Gibb, MD
Assistant Professor of Pediatrics, Division of Pediatric Pulmonary Medicine, University of California, San Francisco, San Francisco, California

Caroline Gluck, MD, MTR
Attending Physician, Division of Pediatric Nephrology, Nemours/AI Dupont Hospital for Children, Wilmington, Delaware

Bridget Godwin, MD
Assistant Professor of Pediatrics, Perelman School of Medicine, University of Pennsylvania; Attending Physician, Division of Gastroenterology, Hepatology and Nutrition, Children's Hospital of Philadelphia, Philadelphia, Pennsylvania

Rachel Gottlieb-Smith, MD
Clinical Assistant Professor, Division of Pediatric Neurology, C.S. Mott Children's Hospital, University of Michigan, Ann Arbor, Michigan

Rosheen Grady, BHSc, MD
Adolescent Medicine Fellow, Division of Adolescent Medicine, Children's Hospital of Philadelphia, Philadelphia, Pennsylvania

Arun Gurunathan, MD
Fellow, Hematology/Oncology, Cincinnati Children's Hospital Medical Center, Cincinnati, Ohio

Nicole Hames, MD, FAAP
Assistant Professor of Pediatrics, Pediatric Hospital Medicine, Emory University, Atlanta, Georgia

Lori Kestenbaum Handy, MD, MSCE
Assistant Professor of Clinical Pediatrics, Perelman School of Medicine at the University of Pennsylvania, Attending Physician, Infectious Diseases, Children's Hospital of Philadelphia, Philadelphia, Pennsylvania

Jessica Hart, MD
Assistant Professor of Pediatrics, Division of General Pediatrics, Children's Hospital of Philadelphia, Philadelphia, Pennsylvania

Erum Aftab Hartung, MD, MTR
Assistant Professor of Pediatrics, Division of Nephrology, Children's Hospital of Philadelphia, Perelman School of Medicine, University of Pennsylvania, Philadelphia, Pennsylvania

Elena B. Hawryluk, MD, PhD
Assistant Professor of Dermatology, Department of Dermatology, Harvard Medical School, Massachusetts General Hospital, Boston, Massachusetts

Noah Hoffman, MD, MSHP
Assistant Clinical Professor of Pediatrics, Tufts University School of Medicine, Boston, Massachusetts; Attending Physician, Pediatric Gastroenterology, Maine Medical Center, Portland, Maine

Alyssa Huang, MD
Clinical Fellow, Division of Pediatric Endocrinology, University of California, San Francisco, San Francisco, California

Raegan Hunt, MD, PhD
Assistant Professor of Pediatrics and Dermatology, Texas Children's Hospital, Baylor College of Medicine, Houston, Texas

Kensho Iwanaga, MD, MS
Assistant Professor of Pediatrics, Division of Pediatric Pulmonary Medicine, University of California, San Francisco, San Francisco, California

Aadil Kakajiwala, MBBS
Assistant Professor, Department of Pediatrics, Division of Nephrology, Washington University in St. Louis School of Medicine, St. Louis, Missouri

Shruti Kant, MBBS
Assistant Professor, Emergency Medicine and Pediatrics, University of California, San Francisco, San Francisco, California

Brandi Kenner-Bell, MD
Assistant Professor of Pediatrics and Dermatology, Northwestern University Feinberg School of Medicine, Ann and Robert H. Lurie Children's Hospital of Chicago, Chicago, Illinois

Eleanor Pitz Kiell, MD
Assistant Professor, Department of Otolaryngology, Wake Forest University School of Medicine, Winston Salem, North Carolina

Amy Kim, MD
Assistant Professor of Clinical Psychiatry, Department of Child and Adolescent Psychiatry and Behavioral Sciences, The Children's Hospital of Philadelphia, Philadelphia, Pennsylvania

Grace Kim, MD, FAAP
Attending Physician, Division of Pediatric Hospital Medicine, Rainbow Babies and Children's Hospital, Assistant Professor, Department of Pediatrics, Case Western Reserve University School of Medicine, Cleveland, Ohio

Alaina K. Kipps, MD, MS
Clinical Assistant Professor, Pediatric Cardiology, Lucile Packard Children's Hospital, Stanford University, Palo Alto, California

Lacey Kruse, MD
Assistant Professor of Pediatrics and Dermatology, Feinburg School of Medicine, Northwestern University, Ann and Robert H. Lurie Children's Hospital of Chicago, Chicago, Illinois

Evelyn J. Lai, RN, MSN, PNP-BC
Pediatric Nurse Practitioner, Infectious Diseases, Children's Hospital of Los Angeles, Los Angeles, California

Erin R. Lane, MD
Fellow, Pediatric Gastroenterology, University of Washington, Seattle, Washington

Beatriz Larru, MD, PhD
Assistant Professor, Pediatrics, Children's Hospital of Los
Angeles, Los Angeles, California

John Lawrence, MD, PhD
Assistant Professor, Orthopaedics, Children's Hospital
of Philadelphia; Orthopaedics, Perelman School of
Medicine, University of Pennsylvania, Philadelphia,
Pennsylvania

Janet Y. Lee, MD, MPH
Clinical Fellow, Medicine and Pediatrics, Division of
Endocrinology and Metabolism, University of California,
San Francisco, San Francisco, California

Dale Young Lee, MD, MSCE
Assistant Professor of Pediatrics, Pediatric
Gastroenterology and Hepatoloy, Seattle Children's
Hospital, Seattle, Washington

Daniella Levy Erez, MD
Attending Physician, Division of Nephrology, Children's
Hospital of Philadelphia, Philadelphia, Pennsylvania

Brock D. Libby, MD
Fellow Physician, Children's Hospital of Philadelphia,
Craig-Dalsimer Division of Adolescent Medicine,
Philadelphia, Pennsylvania

Nan Lin, MD
Pediatric Epilepsy Fellow, Cincinnati Children's Hospital,
Cincinnati, Ohio

Tiffany F. Lin, MD
Assistant Professor, Adjunct Instructor, Pediatric
Hematology/Oncology, University of California, San
Francisco, San Francisco, California

Christopher Liu, MD
Assistant Professor, Department of Otolaryngology - Head
and Neck Surgery, University of Texas at Southwestern
Medical Center, Dallas, Texas

Katharine C. Long, MD
Attending Physician, Pediatric Emergency Medicine, Mary
Bridge Children's Hospital, Tacoma, Washington

Patrick Donald Lee Mabray, MD, PhD
Director of Childhood Movement Disorders Program,
Pediatric Neurology, Boston Medical Center, Boston,
Massachusetts

Pradipta Majumder, MD
Attending Physician, Child and Adolescent Psychiatry,
WellSpan-Philhaven Meadowlands, York,
Pennsylvania

Elizabeth Clabby Maxwell, MD
Assistant Professor of Pediatrics, Perelman School of
Medicine at the University of Pennsylvania, Division
of Gastroenterology, Hepatology, and Nutrition, The
Children's Hospital of Philadelphia, Philadelphia,
Pennsylvania

Melissa R. Meyers, MD
Fellow, Division of Pediatric Nephrology, Children's
Hospital of Philadelphia, Philadelphia, Pennsylvania

Kevin Edward Meyers, MBBCh
Professor of Pediatrics, Nephrology/Pediatrics, Children's
Hospital of Philadelphia and University of Pennsylvania,
Philadelphia, Pennsylvania

Daniel James Miller, MD
Pediatric Orthopaedic Surgeon, Gillette Children's
Specialty Healthcare, St Paul, Minnesota

Courtney E. Nelson, MD
Attending Physician, Division of Emergency Medicine,
Nemours A. I. duPont Hospital for Children; Clinical
Assistant Professor of Pediatrics, Sidney Kimmel College
of Medicine at Thomas Jefferson University, Wilmington,
Delaware

Susan E. Nelson, MD, MPH
Assistant Professor of Orthopaedic Surgery, University of
Rochester Medical Center, Golisano Children's Hospital,
Rochester, New York

Carol Nhan, MD, FRCSC
Fellow/Junior Attending, Pediatric Otolaryngology - Head
and Neck Surgery, Children's Hospital of Philadelphia,
Philadelphia, Pennsylvania

Kevin C. Osterhoudt, MD, MS
Professor, Pediatrics, Perelman School of Medicine,
University of Pennsylvania; Medical Director, Poison
Control Center, Children's Hospital of Philadelphia,
Philadelphia, Pennsylvania

Kiran P. Patel, MD, MS
Assistant Professor, Pediatrics and Medicine, Emory
University, Attending Physician; Allergy and
Immunology, Children's Healthcare of Atlanta, Atlanta,
Georgia

Liat Perl, MD
Pediatric Endocrinology, University of California, San
Francisco, San Francisco, California

Craig Pollack, MD
Co-Director, General Internal Medicine Fellowship
Program, Associate Professor of Medicine, Children's
Hospital of Philadelphia, Philadelphia, Pennsylvania

Madhura Pradhan, MD
Associate Professor of Pediatric Nephrology, Children's
Hospital of Philadelphia, Philadelphia, Pennsylvania

Neha Joshi Purkey, MD
Clinical Assistant Professor, Pediatric Cardiology, Lucile
Packard Children's Hospital, Stanford University, Palo
Alto, California

Sneha Ramakrishna, MD
Pediatric Hematology-Oncology Clinical Fellow, Johns
Hopkins Hospital, Baltimore, Maryland

Charitha D. Reddy, MD
Clinical Assistant Professor, Pediatric Cardiology, Lucile Packard Children's Hospital, Stanford University, Palo Alto, California

Maria Esther Rivera, MD, MPH, FAAP
Resident Physician, General Preventive Medicine Program, Johns Hopkins Bloomberg School of Public Health, Baltimore, Maryland

Barbara Robles-Ramamurthy, MD
Forensic Psychiatry Fellow, Department of Psychiatry, University of Pennsylvania, Philadelphia, Pennsylvania

Michal Rebeka Rozenfeld Bar Lev, MD
Gastroenterology, Nutrition and Liver Diseases, Schneider Children's Medical Center, Petah Tikva, Israel

Nina N. Sainath, MD
Attending Physician, Division of Gastroenterology, Hepatology and Nutrition, Children's Hospital of Philadelphia, Philadelphia, Pennsylvania

Mamata V. Senthil, MD, MSEd
Fellow, Pediatric Emergency Medicine, Children's Hospital of Philadelphia, Philadelphia, Pennsylvania

Neil S. Shah, MD
Orthopaedic and Hand Surgeon, Parkview Physicians Group, Bryan, Ohio

Sheena Sharma, MD
Pediatric Nephrologist, Phoenix Children's Hospital, Phoenix, Arizona

Betty Shum, MD
Pediatric Resident Physician, UCSF Benioff Children's Hospital Oakland and Mission Bay, Oakland and San Francisco, California

Eric Shute, MD
Post Pediatric Portal Fellow, Department of Child and Adolescent Psychiatry and Behavioral Sciences, Children's Hospital of Philadelphia, Philadelphia, Pennsylvania

Douglas M. Smith, MD
Pediatric Epileptologist, Minnesota Epilepsy Group, St. Paul, Minnesota

Preeti Soi, MD
Attending Physician, Department of Child and Adolescent Psychiatry and Behavioral Sciences, Children's Hospital of Philadelphia, Philadelphia, Pennsylvania

Johanna S. Song, MD, MS
Dermatology Resident, Department of Dermatology, Harvard Combined Dermatology Residency Training Program, Boston, Massachusetts

Alanna Strong, MD, PhD
Medical Genetics and Genomics Fellow, Human Genetics, Children's Hospital of Philadelphia, Philadelphia, Pennsylvania

Salwa Sulieman, DO
Attending Physician, Pediatric Infectious Diseases, Nemours/Alfred I. duPont Hospital for Children, Wilmington, Delaware

Mala K. Talekar, MD
Director, Clinical Development-Oncology, GlaxoSmithKline, Collegeville, Pennsylvania; Division of Oncology, Children's Hospital of Philadelphia, Philadelphia, Pennsylvania

Sara Taub, MD, MBE
Assistant Professor, Pediatrics and Palliative Medicine, Oregon Health and Science University, Portland, Oregon

Catharyn Turner II, MEd, MD
Attending Physician, Department of Child and Adolescent Psychiatry and Behavioral Sciences, Children's Hospital of Philadelphia, Philadelphia, Pennsylvania

Jason Van Batavia, MD
Clinical Instructor, Surgery (Urology), Perelman School of Medicine, University of Pennsylvania; Division of Urology, Children's Hospital of Philadelphia, Philadelphia, Pennsylvania

Orith Waisbourd-Zinman, MD
Schneider Children's Medical Center, Petach-Tiqva, Israel; Sackler faculty of medicine, Tel-Aviv University, University of Pennsylvania, Philadelphia, Pennsylvania

Jennifer Webster, DO
Assistant Professor of Pediatrics, Perelman School of Medicine, University of Pennsylvania, Attending Physician, Division of Gastroenterology, Hepatology & Nutrition, Children's Hospital of Philadelphia, Philadelphia, Pennsylvania

Anna Weiss, MD, MSEd
Assistant Professor of Clinical Pediatrics, Department of Pediatrics, Perelman School of Medicine, University of Pennsylvania; Attending Physician, Division of Pediatric Emergency Medicine, Children's Hospital of Philadelphia, Philadelphia, Pennsylvania

Jeein Yoon, MD
Attending Physician, St. Christopher's Pediatric Associates, Philadelphia, Pennsylvania

Duri Yun, MD, MPH
Instructor of Pediatrics and Dermatology, Northwestern University Feinberg School of Medicine, Ann and Robert H. Lurie Children's Hospital of Chicago, Chicago, Illinois

Julie Ziobro, MD, PhD
Clinical Lecturer, Pediatric Neurology, University of Michigan, Ann Arbor, Michigan

Contents

1 Maximizing Test Performance: Effective Study and Test-Taking Strategies

DIONNE BLACKMAN, AB, MD

Research has identified a number of factors that affect test performance:

- Study skills
- Content knowledge
- Practice of questions in the same format as the test
- Test-taking skills
- Anxiety
- Fatigue and sleep deprivation

By reading this book, the examination taker will improve content knowledge and have the opportunity to test this knowledge with many case-based practice questions. This chapter, however, addresses the three topics not related to content knowledge: study skills, test-taking skills, and anxiety. The strategies provided will make studying for the Board Examination more effective and will optimize test performance on the exam.

Strategies for More Effective Studying

ANTICIPATE TEST CONTENT

A strategic approach to studying has been found to lead to better performance on examinations:

- Review the examination blueprint to understand the percentage of questions derived from each content area (available on the website for the American Board of Pediatrics [ABP] at https://www.abp.org)
- Complete the tutorial on taking the computer-based examination on the ABP website. The tutorial sample questions will explain how to use examination functions and provide a practice test to help you familiarize yourself with the different types of examination questions and format. Specifically, you will preview how to:
  - Answer questions
  - Change answers
  - Make notes electronically
  - Access the table of normal laboratory values, calculator, and electronic calipers
  - View figures
  - Mark questions for review

- Use the Progress Indicator and Time Remaining functions to keep track of item completion and time remaining for the test session
- Use the Navigation button or Review screen to view item completion status, items you have marked for review, or items with an electronic note, and to move quickly to items within the test
- Board Examination questions are derived using the following criteria and will:
  - Be focused on patient care
  - Address important clinical problems for which medical intervention has a significant effect on patient outcomes
  - Address commonly overlooked or mismanaged clinical problems
  - Pose a challenging management decision
  - Assess ability to make optimal clinical decisions
- Clinical decision-making can be broken down into different tasks; the Board Examination is meant to test your ability to perform these tasks:
  - Identify characteristic clinical features of diseases
  - Identify characteristic pathophysiologic features of diseases
  - Choose the most appropriate diagnostic tests
  - Determine the diagnosis
  - Determine the prognosis or natural history of diseases
  - Select the best treatment or management strategy
  - Choose risk-appropriate prevention strategies
- Board Examination questions will never address an area in which there is no consensus of opinion among experts in the field
- Carefully review visual information because this is frequently used in Board Examination questions regarding disorders with characteristic skin lesions or findings on blood smear, bone marrow, electrocardiogram, radiograph, and other visual diagnostic tests

TIME MANAGEMENT

- Use the Residency In-Training Examination or a full-length practice test to identify your areas of weakness
- Use a "question drill-to-content" review ratio of 2:1 or greater to review subjects because this has been shown to be more successful than traditional review using the reverse ratio

- After addressing your weaker subjects, conduct a focused review of other subjects as discussed earlier
- Create a realistic study schedule and stick to it
- Using the examination blueprint to budget your study time to cover all of the examination content areas without last-minute cramming
- Plan to complete your study several days before the examination
- Plan a question drill period for the last few days before the examination; use answers to incorrectly answered practice questions for targeted content review

Effective Approaches to Studying

- The Survey, Question, Read, Recite, Review (SQ3R) study method has proven effective in improving reading efficiency, comprehension, and material retention
- It provides a useful way to study for the Board Examination, regardless of the study resource used
- Steps in the method are outlined in Table 1.1
- Similar to the SQ3R method, students performing repeated cycles of studying, followed by writing down as much as they can recall, then restudying material and recalling again improved learning and retention of material and test performance
- Studying with a small group can enhance study effectiveness by providing social support and increased confidence because individuals assume responsibility to review and teach particular areas to the group

Strategies for More Effective Test-Taking

The following strategies will be effective only if practiced, so plan to practice them in your question drill sessions; the website accompanying this book allows examination takers to practice answering questions in a timed test format.

STRATEGIES FOR TIME USE

- Know the examination schedule for the computer-based examination (see http://www.abp.org)
- Return from breaks early; you must check in after breaks, and the examination clock restarts at the end of the break regardless of your return time
- Know the time allotted per examination question (i.e., examination time in minutes divided by number of examination questions)

Table 1.1. SQ3R Study Method

Step	Description
Survey	Survey section headings and summaries first.
Question	Convert headings, legends, and Board Examination tasks into "questions."
Read	Read to answer your "questions."
Recite	Recite answers and write down key phrases and cues.
Review	Review notes, paraphrase major points, draw diagrams, and make flashcards for material that is difficult to recall.

- Budget your time; unfinished questions are lost scoring opportunities
- Keep track of your use of time by checking time targets at each quarter of the total examination time
- To fully use other test-taking strategies, use less than the allotted time per question (we suggest 15–30 seconds less per question)
- To focus on pertinent data, read the question and answer options before reading the question stem; the stem is the part of the test item that precedes the question and answer options and is usually case-based
- Answer questions you know first and quickly guess on those you do not know

STRATEGIES FOR GUESSING AND REASONING

- Identify key words or phrases that affect the question's intent (e.g., *at this time, now, initially, most, always, never, except, usually, least*)
- Determine whether the following factors limit your thinking to certain disease categories:
  - Patient factors
  - Age, sex, race, or ethnicity
  - Exposures caused by occupation, travel, or residence
  - Immune status
  - Factors related to illness presentation
  - Time course of illness (i.e., acute, subacute, or chronic)
  - Symptoms or findings present or stated to be absent
  - Pattern of diagnostic data (e.g., presence of a known symptom triad, pathognomonic finding)
- Eliminate answer options likely to be incorrect. Remember that incorrect options are usually written to be plausible or even partially correct.
- Examine similarities and differences between answer options (e.g., mutually exclusive options)
- Answer questions based on established standards of care, not anecdotal experiences
- Do not be afraid to use partial knowledge to eliminate answers
- When unsure of an answer, enter your best guess (research shows it is often correct) and flag the question on the computer for later review
- Answer all questions—there is no penalty for wrong answers
- Please note that once you click the End Session button, you cannot go back to review or change responses for that test session
- Check that you have completed any answer review of changes and have entered a response for all questions before you click the End Session button

STRATEGIES FOR CHANGING ANSWERS

- Spending less than the allotted time per examination question allows you to finish examinations early; this extra time allows you to benefit from answer changing
- Despite conventional wisdom, research shows that most test takers benefit from answer changing
- You are more likely to change from a wrong to a right answer if you:
  - Reread and better understand the test item

- Rethink and conceptualize a better answer
- Gain information from another test item
- Remember more information
- Correct a clerical error (e.g., the intended answer was not the entered answer)

STRATEGIES FOR ERROR AVOIDANCE

- Read each question and all answer options carefully; be certain you understand the intent of the question before answering (e.g., questions stating "all of the following are correct except ...")
- Do not "read into a question" information or interpretations that are not there
- Check that the answer entered is the answer you intended

STRATEGIES FOR ANXIETY REDUCTION

- Anxiety is a natural part of taking an examination, but high test anxiety will adversely affect test performance
- Consider formal counseling if you have had problems with high test anxiety in the past
- Consider writing about your negative thoughts and worries about the examination for 10 minutes on the day of the test; this has been found to significantly improve test performance for those with high test anxiety
- Actively manage anxiety by decreasing the effect of unknowns on your anxiety level. Use the following methods:
  - Review the "Exam Day: What to Expect" section of the ABP's guide to the certification examination (see http://www.abp.org)
  - Test-drive the travel route and determine time to the test site; locate parking and the site itself if it is in a building with other businesses
  - Bring a sweater or dress in layers to prepare for examination room temperature variations
  - Bring a snack for unexpected hunger and medications for potential illness symptoms
  - Allow a minimum of 30 minutes before your test appointment for check-in procedures
  - Avoid overly anxious test takers; they heighten your anxiety level, which can hurt your test performance
- Use relaxation techniques:
  - Deep muscle relaxation is an effective relaxation technique; it involves tensing and relaxing each muscle group until all muscles are relaxed
  - To reduce anxiety further, engage in exercise during the period when you are preparing for the examination
- Being well rested is imperative

Suggested Readings

1. Frierson HT, Hoband D. Effect of test anxiety on performance on the NBME Part I Examination. *J Med Educ*. 1987;62:431–433.
2. Frierson HT, Malone B, Shelton P. Enhancing NCLEX-RN performance: assessing a three-pronged intervention approach. *J Nurs Educ*. 1993;32:222–224.
3. Harvill LM, Davis III G. Test-taking behaviors and their impact on performance: medical students' reasons for changing answers on multiple choice tests. *Acad Med*. 1997;72:S97–S99.
4. Hembree R. Correlates, causes, effects, and treatment of test anxiety. *Rev Educ Res*. 1988;58:47–77.
5. Karpicke JD, Blunt JR. Retrieval practice produces more learning than elaborative studying with concept mapping. *Science*. 2011;331:772–775.
6. McDowell BM. KATTS: a framework for maximizing NCLEX-RN performance. *J Nurs Educ*. 2008;47:183–186.
7. McManus IC, Richards P, Winder BC, Sproston KA. Clinical experience, performance in final examinations, and learning style in medical students: prospective study. *BMJ*. 1998;316:345–350.
8. Ramirez G, Beilock SL. Writing about testing worries boosts exam performance in classroom. *Science*. 2011;331:211–213.
9. Robinson FP, ed. *Effective Study*. New York: Harper & Row; 1961. Rev ed.
10. Seipp B. Anxiety and academic performance: a meta-analysis of findings. *Anxiety Res*. 1991;4:27–41.
11. Waddell DL, Blankenship JC. Answer changing: a meta-analysis of the prevalence and patterns. *J Cont Educ Nurs*. 1994;25:155–158.
12. Ward PJ. First year medical students' approaches to study and their outcomes in a gross anatomy course. *Clin Anat*. 2011;24:120–127.

Allergy

2 *Atopic Syndrome*

KIRAN P. PATEL, MD, MS

Atopic Syndrome

BASIC INFORMATION

- Consists of several allergic diseases: atopic dermatitis, food allergies, allergic rhinitis, and asthma
- "Atopic march" or "allergic march" refers to the natural progression and presentation of those diseases in that same order listed from infancy to childhood
  - Up to 50% of patients with atopic dermatitis will develop asthma
- Causes
  - Complex interaction between genetic risk factors with environmental influence
    - Parental history of atopic disease is most significant risk factor
    - Filaggrin gene mutations are another risk factor
    - Maternal diet and breastfeeding do not play a role in the development of atopy
    - Delaying introduction of solid foods past 4 to 6 months does *not* prevent development of food allergies; however, early introduction of peanut butter in infants with egg allergy or moderate to severe eczema *prevents* development of peanut allergy

Atopic Dermatitis

BASIC INFORMATION

- One of several forms of eczema
  - Others: nummular eczema, hand eczema, contact dermatitis
- Up to 20% prevalence in children
- See also Nelson Textbook of Pediatrics, Chapter 145, "Atopic Dermatitis."

CLINICAL PRESENTATION

- Presentation is 2 to 6 months of age, 90% present by age 5 years
- Chronic or relapsing course of red macules and papules with intense pruritus and lichenification of the flexural areas
  - <2 years: distribution is face and extensor aspects of extremities
  - >2 years: distribution is flexural areas of extremities
- Exacerbated by infections, heat, or chemical irritants
- Up to one-third of patients may have foods that exacerbate the atopic dermatitis
  - Food elimination is not recommended due to:
    - Negative impact on nutrition
    - Increased risk of food allergy development

DIAGNOSIS AND EVALUATION

- Clinical diagnosis is based on presentation
- Immunoglobulin E (IgE) levels are elevated during acute flares
- Biopsy of skin is not needed unless refractory case
- Differential diagnosis:
  - Allergic or irritant contact dermatitis from plants (e.g., poison ivy), metals (nickel-plated jewelry), and chemical products
  - Immunodeficiency (HIV, Wiskott-Aldrich syndrome, severe combined immunodeficiency, hyper IgE syndrome)
  - Metabolic disorders (zinc deficiency, vitamin B_6 or niacin deficiency)

TREATMENT

- Rehydration of skin with daily baths (soak 15–20 minutes)
  - Unscented bar soap as needed
- Using emollients and moisturizers several times a day
- Wet wrap therapy for severe eczema
- Topical corticosteroids are mainstay therapy, followed by topical calcineurin inhibitors
- Superinfection complications:
  - *Staphylococcus aureus* infections of eczema are common
  - Eczema herpeticum: herpes simplex virus infection; treatment with acyclovir

Food Allergies

- Please refer to Chapter 3 for more information

Allergic Rhinitis

BASIC INFORMATION

- Seasonal allergies are related to pollens: trees (spring), grass (summer), weeds (fall)
- Perennial allergies are related to indoor allergens like dust mites, pet or rodent dander, cockroaches, and/or molds
- Uncommon in children younger than 2 years of age
  - Seasonal allergies are rare in those younger than 2 years of age due to lack of seasonal exposure
- Average age of onset is 10 years of age; prevalence is up to 25%
- 80% of asthmatics have aeroallergen sensitization

CLINICAL PRESENTATION

- Nasal symptoms of congestion, rhinorrhea, sneezing, pale mucosa, cobblestoning of nasopharynx, turbinate hypertrophy, and nasal crease ("allergic salute")
- Ocular symptoms of itchy, watery swollen eyes, Dennie-Morgan lines, and lower eyelid edema ("allergic shiners")
- Increased sinus and acute otitis media infections

DIAGNOSIS AND EVALUATION

- Clinical diagnosis based on presentation
- Allergy testing can confirm perennial, seasonal, or mixed picture (see Chapter 3 for further details)
- Differential diagnosis
  - Vasomotor rhinitis: triggered by cold or dry air, temperature shifts, strong scents (perfumes or cleaning products), or humidity changes
  - Infectious (e.g. viral): common in younger children who are worse in winter
  - Nonallergic rhinitis with eosinophils: eosinophils on nasal smear but negative allergy testing
  - Rhinitis medicamentosa: rebound reaction due to overuse of adrenergic nasal sprays
  - For all of the above, clinical history and timing are the most important to distinguish between the entities; however, allergy testing can be helpful for those patients who have mixed histories and/or poorly controlled symptoms
  - The consistency or color of nasal discharge does not distinguish any of the diagnoses

TREATMENT

- First-line therapy: intranasal steroid sprays
  - Second-generation oral antihistamines can be used in conjunction with intranasal steroid sprays
- Additional agents:
  - Intranasal antihistamines
    - Antileukotriene therapy
    - Allergen immunotherapy can be curative option
  - Allergen exposure control
    - Dust mite allergy
      - Allergen covers for mattress and pillow
      - Weekly dusting, vacuuming, and bed sheet laundering (hot water)
      - Maintain humidity below 50% (very hard to do in practice)
      - HEPA and Ionic Breeze air units are not beneficial for dust mite allergy
    - Pet allergy
      - Pet removal is ideal, but effect can take up to 6 months post removal to be beneficial due to persistence of allergen
      - If pet cannot be removed (common scenario), pet should be kept out of patient's room
      - Washing clothes and showering are beneficial after contact with pet
    - Pollen allergy
      - Avoid going out on high-pollen-count days

Asthma

- Please refer to Chapter 76 for more information

Review Questions

For review questions, please go to ExpertConsult.com.

Suggested Readings

1. Lyons JJ, Milner JD, Stone KD. Atopic dermatitis in children: clinical features, pathophysiology, and treatment. *Immunol Allergy Clin North Am.* 2015;35(1):161–183.
2. Spergel JM. From atopic dermatitis to asthma: the atopic march. *Ann Allergy Asthma Immunol.* 2010;105(2):99–106; quiz 107-9, 117.
3. Tharpe CA, Kemp SF. Pediatric allergic rhinitis. *Immunol Allergy Clin North Am.* 2015;35(1):185–198.

Allergies, Immunotherapy, and Anaphylaxis

KIRAN P. PATEL, MD, MS

Allergy Testing

BASIC INFORMATION

- Allergy testing shows only sensitization; it is not a confirmation of a disease diagnosis
- Only clinical history and allergen challenges can confirm the diagnosis of disease
- Two forms of allergy testing—both have similar sensitivity and specificity:
  - Skin prick testing: cutaneous prick of skin with allergen extract measuring the wheal (3 mm above negative control is positive)
  - Serum IgE testing: ELISA-based assays measure serum IgE binding of fixed protein antigens; radioallergosorbent test (RAST) is an older method that is no longer used
- Serum testing can be performed on any patient, but skin testing cannot be performed if severe eczema is present or if recent use of any of the following types of medications that might interfere with the test:
  - H1 blockers: tricyclic antidepressants, first-generation H1 blockers (e.g., diphenhydramine, hydroxyzine, cyproheptadine), second-generation H1 blockers (e.g., cetirizine, loratadine, fexofenadine)
  - H2 blockers (e.g., ranitidine)
  - Muscle relaxants
  - Intranasal antihistamines
- The following do not interfere with skin testing and should not be stopped: asthma inhalers, intranasal corticosteroids, leukotriene inhibitors, proton pump inhibitors (PPIs), nonsteroidal antiinflammatory drugs (NSAIDs), selective serotonin reuptake inhibitors (SSRIs), and serotonin–norepinephrine reuptake inhibitors (SNRIs)

Food Allergy

BASIC INFORMATION

- Adverse food reaction is a reproducible reaction to a food, based on two large categories:
  - Immune mediated (focus of subsequent sections)
    - IgE mediated:
      Food allergy: IgE sensitization to food proteins that leads to mast cell activation when a food is ingested
      - Contact urticaria can also occur but does not lead to anaphylaxis or systemic symptoms
        90% of all cases are due to the following: cow's milk, eggs, soy, wheat, peanuts, tree nuts, fish, or shellfish

      Prevention with early introduction of peanuts at 4 to 6 months in patients with egg allergy or moderate to severe eczema
      Oral allergy syndrome: IgE sensitization to pollens that leads to cross-reactivity of homologous, usually heat-labile plant proteins
      Latex-fruit syndrome: avocado, banana, chestnut, melon, mango, kiwi, pineapple, peach, tomato
      Ragweed: melon
      Birch tree: apple, peach, pear, carrot
    - Mixed IgE/Non-IgE mediated:
      Eosinophilic esophagitis: it is unclear what the exact mechanism is that leads to eosinophil activation in response to a food protein allergen
      Atopic dermatitis: the exact mechanism is unclear, but it is thought to be related to food-specific T cells
    - Non-IgE mediated:
      Food protein–induced enterocolitis: cell-mediated inflammatory process confined to the gastrointestinal tract
      Cow's milk protein proctocolitis: cell-mediated inflammation of rectum
  - Atopic dermatitis and IgE-mediated food allergy are listed in two separate categories. The clinician should make the distinction between the two and not call both a generic "food allergy," because they are very different
    - Atopic dermatitis can be *exacerbated* by foods (up to 33% of patients) but is *not caused* by foods
    - Non-life-threatening reaction
    - The majority of these patients can still consume the offending food as long as good skin care is practiced and topical steroids are judiciously used to treat atopic dermatitis
    - If food-elimination diets are carried out and food is avoided for greater than 3 months, the patients are at high risk of developing an IgE-mediated food allergy
    - IgE-mediated food allergy patients are at risk for life-threatening allergic reactions
    - A history of atopic dermatitis is a major risk factor for the development of food allergy
  - Non–immune mediated (e.g., lactose intolerance, galactosemia)
  - See also Nelson Textbook of Pediatrics, Chapter 151, "Food Allergy and Adverse Reactions to Foods."

CLINICAL PRESENTATION

- IgE mediated:
  - Food allergy symptoms: hives, angioedema, emesis, diarrhea, wheezing, rhinitis, anaphylaxis within 2 hours of ingestion of food

- Delayed reactions (>2 hours) are seen in α-gal allergy (reaction to pork, lamb, or beef) or food-associated, exercise-induced anaphylaxis (reaction after consumption of food followed by exercise)
- Oral allergy syndrome symptoms: throat or tongue itching, lip swelling
  - Symptoms only with raw fruits, vegetables, spices, peanuts, or nuts; cooked forms are tolerated
  - Latex-fruit syndrome seen in patients with history of bladder exstrophy or spina bifida (exposure to latex)
- Mixed IgE/non-IgE mediated:
  - Eosinophilic esophagitis symptoms: dysphagia, odynophagia, weight loss, food impaction, emesis, abdominal pain
  - Atopic dermatitis symptoms: erythematous macules and papules; distinct from hives or angioedema
- Non-IgE mediated:
  - Food protein–induced enterocolitis occurs primarily in infants, usually after being solely breastfed and introduced to either solid foods or soy/cow's milk formula
    - Chronic exposure: emesis, diarrhea, poor growth, or lethargy
    - Acute exposure (after restriction): emesis, diarrhea, or hypotension within 2 to 6 hours after ingestion
  - Cow's milk protein proctocolitis: mucus and/or bloody stools

DIAGNOSIS AND EVALUATION

- IgG testing to foods has no known clinical utility in any food adverse reaction
- IgE mediated:
  - Tests are very sensitive but not specific
    - 40% of the general population will have at least one positive test to foods, leading to a high false-positive rate
  - Test values (millimeters for skin or kU/L for serum) predict only the probability of a clinical reaction to a food
  - Allergy testing (serum or skin) is helpful only in suspected foods causing IgE-mediated symptoms or in persistent eczema, despite optimized management and topical corticosteroid therapy (and testing only for foods in the diet)
  - Panel testing is not recommended in any situation
  - Oral allergy syndrome is confirmed by pollen sensitization and clinical history
- Mixed IgE/non-IgE mediated:
  - Eosinophilic esophagitis
    - Serum or skin allergy testing has no clinical utility
    - Elimination diets and food introductions with intermittent esophagogastroduodenoscopies (EGDs) are the only diagnostic tests to evaluate for causative food allergens
  - Atopic dermatitis
    - Skin or serum allergy may have clinical utility in only refractory cases
- Non-IgE mediated:
  - Food protein–induced enterocolitis is based on clinical history and response to elimination diet; skin or serum allergy testing has no clinical utility
    - May develop anemia, hypoalbuminemia, leukocytosis, acidosis, and methemoglobinemia during acute episodes

- Cow's milk protein proctocolitis is based on clinical history and response to elimination diet; skin or serum allergy testing has no clinical utility

TREATMENT

- IgE mediated:
  - Food allergy:
    - Avoidance of food; oral immunotherapy may play a role in the future
    - Peanut allergy has little cross-reactivity with other legumes
    - Hot-pressed peanut oils typically do not contain sufficient proteins and therefore are safe to consume
    - The majority of patients with cow's milk or egg allergy tolerate baked foods, including those with these allergens
    - Cow's milk allergy cross-reacts with the majority of mammalian milks; in IgE-mediated cow's milk allergy, soy milk may be an alternative with little cross-reactivity
    - No cross-reactivity exists between fish and shellfish
  - Natural history:
    - Cow's milk, egg, soy, and wheat allergies resolve in the majority of patients during childhood.
    - Peanut, tree nut, fish, and shellfish allergies are lifelong in the majority of patients
    - A small minority will outgrow it; therefore periodic reassessment with allergy testing and possible food challenges is warranted
- Mixed IgE/non-IgE mediated:
  - Eosinophilic esophagitis: elimination diet and elemental or swallowed steroids are options; periodic EGDs are needed to monitor
    - A subset of patients resolves with high-dose PPI therapy
  - Atopic dermatitis
    - Can consider elimination diet but can lead to poor nutrition and increased risk of IgE-mediated food allergy
- Non-IgE mediated:
  - Food protein–induced enterocolitis: elimination diet and referral to specialist for plan for food challenges around early childhood (2–5 years) because the majority self-resolve
    - Cow's milk and soy *are* cross-reactive in this disease
    - Acute episodes are treated with intravenous (IV) fluids and IV ondansetron
    - Epinephrine, H1 blockers, H2 blockers, and corticosteroids have no role in treatment
  - Cow's milk protein proctocolitis: elemental formula and avoidance of both soy and cow's milk
    - Challenge at 1 year

Hymenoptera Allergy

BASIC INFORMATION

- Hymenoptera stings are due to honeybees and vespids (yellow jacket, hornet, wasp) and can cause anaphylaxis
- Fire ant stings can cause anaphylaxis

CLINICAL PRESENTATION

- Cutaneous symptoms are common and present in 60% of stung children
  - Large local reactions at sting site do not put patient at increased risk for systemic reactions nor do full body hives without other symtpoms
- The presence of cutaneous, respiratory, or gastrointestinal symptoms or hypotension/syncope is concerning for anaphylaxis

DIAGNOSIS AND EVALUATION

- Patients with anaphylaxis need the following testing done:
  - ~ 4 to 6 weeks after initial episode: skin testing by a specialist (false-negative if done earlier)
  - ~1 to 2 weeks after initial episode: check a tryptase level. If persistently elevated (>11.4 ng/mL), then need referral to allergy/immunology or hematologist for possible bone marrow biopsy due to association with underlying mastocytosis or clonal mast cell disorder (up to 10%)

TREATMENT

- After anaphylaxis or systemic symptoms, there is a 20% to 60% risk of similar symptoms per future sting
  - Epinephrine autoinjector for all patients
  - Consider venom immunotherapy to reduce the risk to 5% to 10%

Drug Allergy

BASIC INFORMATION

- Only 10% of drug adverse reactions are drug allergy (immune mediated)
- Penicillin is the most commonly reported medication allergy
  - Self-reported by 10% of patients, but 85% to 90% of these are not found to be allergic
  - Patients may be allergic to the beta-lactam ring common to all penicillins or to the R-group side chain that are antibiotic specific
  - There is no increased risk of penicillin allergy in patients with a family history of penicillin allergy
- Vaccination allergy
  - Rare event (less than 1 per 1 million doses)
  - Immediate hypersensitivity reactions are usually caused by components of the vaccine (e.g., gelatin, yeast, neomycin)
  - There is no longer a contraindication for influenza vaccine in any egg-allergic patients.
- Multiple immune-mediated drug allergies
  - Most common is IgE mediated (immediate) (focused on here)
  - Others: drug rash with eosinophilia and systemic symptoms (DRESS), Stevens-Johnson syndrome, fixed drug eruption

CLINICAL PRESENTATION

- Symptoms: hives, angioedema, emesis, diarrhea, wheezing, rhinitis, anaphylaxis within 2 hours of medication or vaccine administration

DIAGNOSIS AND EVALUATION

- Penicillin skin testing has a high negative predictive value
  - Distinguish beta-lactam ring from R-group side chain

TREATMENT

- Desensitization is available treatment for immediate hypersensitivity reactions and some delayed reactions
- 50% of patients with immediate hypersensitivity reactions to penicillin after 5 years tolerate penicillin again; 80% after 10 years
- Cross-reactivity for cephalosporin in penicillin allergy is rare (2%)

Radiocontrast Media Allergy

BASIC INFORMATION

- An "anaphylactoid" reaction, the majority are non-IgE mediated, rather, due to the osmolarity of the solution destabilizing mast cell membranes
- The risk of cross-reaction between shellfish and radiocontrast material is a myth
- Up to 10% of individuals receiving radiocontrast media have reactions
- Presents with hives, angioedema, anaphylaxis with injection of media; remains a clinical diagnosis
- Treated prophylactically with corticosteroids starting at approximately 12 hours before contrast injection and IV diphenhydramine immcdiately before contrast injection
- No "desensitization" procedure exists

Immunotherapy

BASIC INFORMATION

- Used for treatment of allergic asthma, allergic rhinitis, allergic conjunctivitis, and stinging insect hypersensitivity
- There is risk of anaphylaxis with subcutaneous allergen immunotherapy, so it must be given in a physician's office
  - Increased likelihood with asthma history

Anaphylaxis

BASIC INFORMATION

- Acute, life-threatening systemic reaction due to mediator release from mast cells and basophils
- Food and medications are the most common causes
  - Rare causes are exercise-induced anaphylaxis and idiopathic anaphylaxis

CLINICAL PRESENTATION

- Wheezing, respiratory distress, urticaria, general discomfort, "sense of doom," angioedema of the lips and eyelids, syncope, vomiting, diarrhea, stridor
- Differential diagnosis:
  - Vasovagal/neurogenic syncope
  - Vocal cord dysfunction
  - Asthma exacerbation
  - Panic attack
  - Food poisoning (fish or shellfish)
- Food poisoning is commonly caused by fish or shellfish that have toxins or histamine precursors (histidine) that, when consumed, cause similar symptoms due to common biologically active substrates, but it is not immune mediated

DIAGNOSIS AND EVALUATION

- One of three criteria is satisfied within minutes to hours:
  1. Acute onset of illness with involvement of skin, mucosal surface, or both, and at least one of the following: respiratory compromise, hypotension, or end-organ dysfunction
  2. Two or more of the following occur rapidly after exposure to a likely allergen: involvement of skin or mucosal surface, respiratory compromise, hypotension, or persistent gastrointestinal symptoms
  3. Hypotension develops after exposure to a known allergen for that patient: age-specific low blood pressure or decreased systolic blood pressure more than 30% compared with baseline
- Can draw serum tryptase within 6 hours of a suspected reaction
  - May not be elevated in all causes

TREATMENT

- First-line therapy:
  - 0.01 mg/kg epinephrine (1:1000) given intramuscularly (IM) every 5 to 15 minutes as needed
    - Home: autoinjector if <30 kg: 0.15 mg; otherwise, the dose is 0.3 mg
- Second-line therapy:
  - 1–2 mg/kg diphenhydramine IV/IM
  - 1–2 mg/kg ranitidine IV/IM
  - Inhaled beta-agonist for bronchospasm/wheeze
  - Corticosteroids for long-term therapy
- Biphasic reaction can occur and be delayed up to 72 hours
- Protracted reactions require vasopressor infusions

Review Questions

For review questions, please go to ExpertConsult.com.

Suggested Readings

1. Bernstein IL, Li JT, Bernstein DI, et al. Allergy diagnostic testing: an updated practice parameter. *Ann Allergy Asthma Immunol.* 2008;100(3 suppl 3):S1–S148.
2. Golden DB, Demain J, Freeman T, et al. Stinging insect hypersensitivity: a practice parameter update 2016. *Ann Allergy Asthma Immunol.* 2017;118(1):28–54.
3. Joint Task Force on Practice Parameters, American Academy of Allergy, Asthma and Immunology, American College of Allergy, Asthma and Immunology, Joint Council of Allergy, Asthma and Immunology. Drug allergy: an updated practice parameter. *Ann Allergy Asthma Immunol.* 2010;105(4):259–273.
4. Kelso JM, Greenhawt MJ, Li JT, et al. Adverse reactions to vaccines practice parameter 2012 update. *J Allergy Clin Immunol.* 2012;130(1):25–43.
5. Lieberman P, Nicklas RA, Randolph C, et al. Anaphylaxis–a practice parameter update 2015. *Ann Allergy Asthma Immunol.* 2015;115(5):341–384.
6. Moore LE, Kemp AM, Kemp SF. Recognition, treatment, and prevention of anaphylaxis. *Immunol Allergy Clin North Am.* 2015;35(2):363–374.
7. Sicherer SH, Sampson HA. Food allergy: epidemiology, pathogenesis, diagnosis, and treatment. *J Allergy Clin Immunol.* 2014;133(2):291–307.
8. Wallace DV, Dykewicz MS, Bernstein DI, et al. The diagnosis and management of rhinitis: an updated practice parameter. *J Allergy Clin Immunol.* 2008;122(suppl 2):S1–S84.

4 *Selected Topics in Allergy*

KIRAN P. PATEL, MD, MS

Hypersensitivity Reactions

BASIC INFORMATION

See Table 4.1 for a comparison of the different types of hypersensitivity disorders.

Urticaria

BASIC INFORMATION

- Acute urticaria can occur due to a variety of triggers:
  - Infectious diseases (viruses are the most common cause of acute urticaria in children)
  - Aeroallergens (pollen, animal dander), foods, medications, insects
  - Physical factors (cold, pressure, heat, light)
- Chronic urticaria
  - Urticaria for >6 weeks
  - Idiopathic in the majority of cases
    - If other disease-specific symptoms are present, evaluate for underlying disorders:
      - Thyroid disease
      - Rheumatologic diseases
      - Malignancy
  - Food is not a cause of *chronic* urticaria
  - Up to 50% of patients may have autoantibody that can activate mast cells
  - See also Nelson Textbook of Pediatrics, Chapter 148, "Physical Urticaria."

CLINICAL PRESENTATION

- Urticaria
  - Pruritic, blanching, erythematous, circumscribed, often coalescent wheals
  - Lesions typically migrate and do not stay in any location for >24 hours
  - The presence of arthralgia, scarring, or bruising raises concern for urticarial vasculitis

DIAGNOSIS AND EVALUATION

- Acute urticaria is diagnosed based on clinical history and possible allergy testing based on concern for a specific trigger
- Chronic urticaria
  - Rule out underlying disorders based on history and examination
  - Allergy testing for food, pollens, animal dander, or molds is not necessary in chronic cases because this is not the etiology, and presence of these allergens would not cause persistent symptoms (e.g., eating dairy at one meal in a day would not lead to >6 weeks of hive symptoms despite eliminating the dairy from other meals in that time frame)
  - Empiric food elimination diets are not warranted in chronic urticaria because the food allergens are not the cause
  - If concerned for underlying disorder, additional testing may be warranted:
    - Thyroid disease: thyroid-stimulating hormone (TSH)
    - Rheumatologic diseases: complete blood count (CBC) with differential, ESR, CRP, C3, C4, LFT, Cr
    - Malignancy: CBC with differential
  - Can consider sending for autoantibody levels: Chronic Urticaria Index
    - Helps only in etiology and has no bearing on treatment or prognosis
- Differential diagnosis of urticaria
  - Contact dermatitis
  - Erythema multiforme: targetoid appearance
  - Mast cell disorders (see below)
  - Papular urticaria: insect bite–induced delayed hypersensitivity
    - Chronic or recurrent eruptions of papules, vesicles, and wheals, especially on extensor surfaces (usually spares genital, perianal, and axilla); classically appearing as a linear cluster on exposed body surfaces
    - Palms and soles are often spared
    - Episodic nature (especially at nighttime)

TREATMENT

- Acute urticaria
  - Avoid triggers
  - Treat with second-generation antihistamines (e.g., cetirizine, fexofenadine, loratadine) as first-line approach
    - May consider first-generation antihistamines for breakthrough
    - Consider short course of corticosteroids with high burden or poor response to antihistamines
- Chronic urticaria
  - Similar to treatment of acute urticaria
  - First line: second-generation antihistamines (up to four times maximum daily dose for age, usually managed by specialist)
  - If poor response, consider H2 antagonist (ranitidine, cimetidine), leukotriene antagonist, or even a short course of corticosteroids

Table 4.1.   Different Types of Hypersensitivity Disorders

Type of Hyper-sensitivity Reaction	Name	Mechanism	Example(s)
I	Immediate	IgE-mediated activation of mast cells and basophils	IgE-mediated food allergy Anaphylaxis and "anaphylactoid" reactions Allergic rhinitis Asthma
II	Antibody mediated	IgG or IgM	Hemolytic anemia Graves' disease Myasthenia gravis
III	Immune complex mediated	IgG and complement deposition	Systemic lupus erythematosus Glomerulonephritis Serum sickness Arthus reaction Vasculitis
IV	Delayed	T cell activation	Contact dermatitis PPD testing

- If refractory to the above therapies, refer to specialist for omalizumab or immunosuppression therapies
- Prognosis is good with resolution in up to 50% by 1 year of onset

Hereditary Angioedema (HAE)

BASIC INFORMATION

- Most often an autosomal dominant disease due to a deficiency in C1-esterase inhibitor, leading to dysregulation of the complement pathway and intermittent episodes of swelling of various body parts
  - Type 1: 85% of patients, quantitative defect in C1-esterase inhibitor
  - Type 2: 15% of patients, qualitative defect in C1-esterase inhibitor

CLINICAL PRESENTATION

- Swelling of any body part without urticaria
  - Laryngeal swelling is one of the most feared episodes and can be fatal
  - Abdominal pain can refer to intestinal swelling
- Episodes may be preceded by trauma
- No pruritus and rarely with urticaria
- Symptoms can last for several days

DIAGNOSIS AND EVALUATION

- C4 level is a cost-effective initial screening test that is generally decreased when asymptomatic or absent during acute attacks
- C1 esterase inhibitor activity can be sent as a confirmatory test if the C4 level is low; can also be sent if, despite a normal C4 level, clinical suspicion for HAE is very high

TREATMENT

- Replacement of C1 esterase inhibitor

Mastocytosis

BASIC INFORMATION

- Two forms:
  - Cutaneous mastocytosis (predominantly children), three subcategories:
    - Maculopapular cutaneous mastocytosis (MPCM) or urticaria pigmentosa
    - Diffuse cutaneous mastocytosis (DCM)
    - Mastocytoma of the skin
  - Systemic mastocytosis (predominantly adults), four subcategories:
    - Indolent systemic mastocytosis
    - Aggressive systemic mastocytosis
    - Systemic mastocytosis with non-mast-cell lineage hematologic disease
    - Mast cell leukemia
    - Majority of patients in all four subcategories have cutaneous symptoms

CLINICAL PRESENTATION

- Cutaneous mastocytosis
  - 80% of patients will have brown or red skin lesions
  - Darier's sign is seen in most patients
    - Whealing or reddening of the skin with mechanical stroking or rubbing
  - Categorized based on skin findings into subcategory
  - <10% of patients develop systemic symptoms
- Systemic mastocytosis
  - Previously mentioned cutaneous symptoms
  - Systemic symptoms: idiopathic anaphylaxis, flushing, hives, angioedema, diarrhea, fatigue, bone pain, wheezing

DIAGNOSIS AND EVALUATION

- Cutaneous mastocytosis
  - No bone marrow biopsy needed in children
  - Confirmed clinically but can do skin biopsy if unclear
- Systemic mastocytosis
  - Bone marrow biopsy and biopsy of the affected organs
  - D816V mutation analysis
  - Tryptase level

TREATMENT

- Cutaneous mastocytosis
  - Topical corticosteroids for pruritic lesions
  - Oral second-generation antihistamines for pruritus
- Systemic mastocytosis
  - Depending on subcategory, management often by a hematologist

Hypereosinophilic Syndrome (HES)

BASIC INFORMATION

- Hypereosinophilia defined as absolute eosinophil counts (AEC) >500 cells/μL
  - Severity
    - Mild: AEC 500–1500 cells/μL
    - Moderate: AEC 1500–5000 cells/μL
    - Severe: >5000 cells/μL
- Primary causes:
  - Myeloproliferative variants HES
  - Lymphocytic HES
  - Familial HES (autosomal dominant)
- Secondary causes:
  - Infections:
    - Parasites (e.g., Ascaris, Strongyloides, Schistosoma, Toxocara)
    - Fungal infections
    - Mycobacterial infections
    - Human immunodeficiency virus
  - Malignancy-related (leukemia or lymphoma)
  - Eosinophilic gastrointestinal (GI) disease
  - Eosinophilic pneumonia
  - Allergic bronchopulmonary aspergillosis
  - Adrenal insufficiency
  - Vasculitis (e.g., eosinophilic granulomatosis with polyangiitis, formerly known as Churg-Strauss syndrome)
  - Atopic diseases (e.g., asthma, atopic dermatitis)
  - Primary immunodeficiency (Hyper IgE syndrome, Omenn syndrome)

CLINICAL PRESENTATION

- For primary causes of HES, it is usually insidious with rashes, respiratory, GI, and/or cardiac symptoms
- Others are symptoms of the secondary cause

Table 4.2. Disorders Associated with Elevated Serum Immunoglobulin E

Allergic disease
Atopic dermatitis (eczema)
Tissue-invasive helminthic infections
Hyperimmunoglobulin E syndromes
Allergic bronchopulmonary aspergillosis
Wiskott-Aldrich syndrome
Bone marrow transplantation
Hodgkin disease
Bullous pemphigoid
Idiopathic nephrotic syndrome

DIAGNOSIS AND EVALUATION

- Bone marrow biopsy to evaluate for primary HES
- Testing for secondary causes is disease specific and will depend on the history and physical examination
- IgE may be elevated for certain diseases (see Table 4.2)

TREATMENT

- Primary HES is treated only if there is end-organ involvement
- Secondary causes are treated for the underlying disorder

Review Questions

For review questions, please go to ExpertConsult.com.

Suggested Readings

1. Bernstein JA, Lang DM, Khan DA, et al. The diagnosis and management of acute and chronic urticaria: 2014 update. *J Allergy Clin Immunol.* 2014 may;133(5):1270–1277.
2. Klion A. Hypereosinophilic syndrome: current approach to diagnosis and treatment. *Annu Rev Med.* 2009;60:293–306.

Cardiology

5 | Clinical Approach to Common Cardiac Complaints

NEHA J. PURKEY, MD, CHARITHA D. REDDY, MD and ALAINA K. KIPPS, MD, MS

Hypertension

BASIC INFORMATION

- The American Academic of Pediatrics (AAP) revised blood pressure monitoring guidelines in 2017, including new normative BP tables (by age, sex, and height). See Suggested Readings.
- Current screening recommendation for otherwise healthy children is each annual visit, starting at three years of age.
- Children with risk factors for blood pressure issues (e.g. obesity, diabetes, history of aortic arch obstruction, renal disease) are recommended to have blood pressure checks at every healthcare encounter.
- Children at higher risk should be screened earlier:
  - Renal or urologic disease, including recurrent urinary tract infections
  - History of prematurity or low birth weight
  - Solid-organ transplant recipients
  - Oncologic disease
  - Systemic illnesses associated with hypertension (neurofibromatosis, tuberous sclerosis)
  - Increased intracranial pressure
  - Cardiac disease
- Lower dietary sodium intake is associated with lower blood pressure
- See also Nelson Textbook of Pediatrics, Chapter 445, "Systemic Hypertension."

CLINICAL PRESENTATION

- Most patients are asymptomatic
- Assess for stigmata of causes of secondary hypertension (see Table 5.1)
- Severe hypertension may present with encephalopathy, heart failure, or stroke

DIAGNOSIS AND EVALUATION

- Stages of hypertension:
  - Normal blood pressure: <90th percentile for age, height, and gender
  - Elevated blood pressure (formerly "prehypertension"): ≥90th percentile
  - Stage 1 hypertension: ≥95th percentile
  - Stage 2 hypertension: ≥95th percentile + 12 mm Hg
- To ensure blood pressure readings are accurate:
  - Measurements should be taken in the right arm, patient seated, feet flat on floor
  - The blood pressure cuff should have a bladder length of 80% to 100% of the arm circumference and a bladder width of at least two-thirds the length of the arm
- Evaluate for causes of secondary hypertension (see Table 5.1)

TREATMENT

- Elevated Blood Pressure
  - Recommend weight management and an active lifestyle for all ages
  - Recommend the CHILD-1 diet for patients over 12 years old
  - Repeat blood pressure in 6 months with upper and lower extremities. If the blood pressure remains elevated for a year (i.e. 3 checks), then may proceed with further diagnostic evaluation and treatment (see below).
- Stage 1 hypertension
  - If asymptomatic, then repeat measurement in 1-2 weeks (with upper and lower extremities). If persistent, repeat in 3 months. If elevated after three checks, proceed with diagnostic evaluation and treatment and consider referral.
  - Basic workup for etiology: medical history, family history, sleep history, physical examination, CBC, renal panel, urinalysis, renal and cardiac ultrasounds, lipid panel, glucose level
  - Focused studies if there is suspicion for a secondary cause of hypertension
  - Echocardiogram to assess for left ventricular hypertrophy (end-organ dysfunction)
  - Screen for other cardiovascular risk factors: hyperlipidemia, obesity, diabetes mellitus
- Stage 2 hypertension
  - Check upper and lower extremity blood pressures. Recheck blood pressure or refer to pediatric hypertension expert within 1 week
  - Workup is as above for Stage 1 hypertension.
  - Initiate blood pressure treatment (calcium channel blockers, angiotensin-converting enzyme inhibitors, angiotensin receptor blockers, beta-blockers, or diuretics may all be considered)
  - If patient is symptomatic or if the BP is >30 mm Hg above the 95th %ile (or (or >180/120 mm Hg in an adolescent), refer an emergency care center.

Table 5.1. Causes of Secondary Hypertension in Children and Adolescents

RENAL	CARDIAC
Pyelonephritis	Coarctation of the aorta
Glomerulonephritis	**GENETIC CAUSES**
Henoch-Schönlein purpura	Neurofibromatosis
Hemolytic uremic syndrome	Tuberous sclerosis
Hydronephrosis	Williams syndrome
Wilms tumor or other renal tumors	Turner syndrome
Renal trauma	**DRUG-INDUCED HYPERTENSION**
Systemic lupus erythematosus	Corticosteroids
Reflux nephropathy	Stimulants
Ureteral obstruction	Oral contraceptives
Renal artery stenosis or thrombosis	Drugs of abuse: cocaine, PCP, nicotine
Renal vein thrombosis	Caffeine
	Sympathomimetics
ENDOCRINE	Heavy metal poisoning
Diabetes mellitus	
Hyperthyroidism	**OTHER**
Cushing syndrome	White coat hypertension
Hyperparathyroidism	Preeclampsia
Congenital adrenal hyperplasia	Autonomic instability
Primary hyperaldosteronism	Intracranial mass
Pheochromocytoma	Arteriovenous shunt
Neuroblastoma	Liddle syndrome
	Hypercalcemia

Table 5.2. Causes of Chest Pain in Children and Adolescents

CARDIAC CAUSES	GI CAUSES
Left ventricular outflow tract obstruction	Reflux
■ Hypertrophic cardiomyopathy	Gastritis
■ Aortic stenosis	Peptic ulcer disease
■ Coarctation of the aorta	Cholecystitis
Coronary artery anomalies	Pancreatitis
■ Abnormal origin of a coronary artery	**MUSCULOSKELETAL CAUSES**
■ Kawasaki disease	Costochondritis/Tietze syndrome
■ Myocardial bridge	Slipped rib syndrome
■ Hyperlipidemia causing atherosclerosis	Precordial catch syndrome
Coronary vasospasm	Muscle strain
Pericarditis	Trauma
Myocarditis	**PULMONARY CAUSES**
Dilated cardiomyopathy	Pneumothorax
Arrhythmias	Pulmonary embolus
Aortic root dissection	Pneumonia
Ruptured sinus of Valsalva aneurysm	Acute chest syndrome in sickle cell disease
Pulmonary hypertension	Asthma
	Pleuritis
	OTHER
	Skin infections
	Breast disease
	Psychosomatic pain

Chest Pain

BASIC INFORMATION

- The differential diagnosis for pediatric chest pain is quite broad (see Table 5.2)
- Whereas cardiac chest pain is due to inappropriate oxygen supply to the myocardium, chest pain in children is most often of noncardiac origin and carries a low risk for mortality

CLINICAL PRESENTATION

- The presentation of chest pain varies with underlying etiology. Common presentations are covered in their respective chapters. Briefly:
  - Costochondritis: localized "sharp" chest pain, reproducible on examination with palpation of the ribs
  - Asthma: chest "tightness" during an exacerbation
  - Reflux: "burning" chest pain, usually correlated with eating
  - Mastalgia: common cause of chest pain in pubertal adolescent females
- "Red flags" for cardiac-related chest pain:
  - Chest pain described as "deep," "crushing," or "substernal"
  - Associated emesis, diaphoresis, altered mental status, or dyspnea
  - Chest pain, dizziness, or syncope with exertion
  - Palpitations
  - Symptoms of heart failure, including exercise intolerance, fatigue, tachypnea, difficulty with feeds, and peripheral edema (see Chapter 8 for additional details)
  - Personal history of congenital heart disease, heart transplant, Kawasaki disease, or substance abuse
  - Family history of cardiomyopathy, arrhythmia, sudden death, connective tissue disease, or hypercoagulable states

DIAGNOSIS AND EVALUATION

- History is the most important tool for identifying the etiology of chest pain
- Vital signs
- Electocardiogram (ECG): refer to a cardiologist if abnormal
- Chest x-ray
- Consider a trial of nonsteroidal antiinflammatory drugs (NSAIDs) if a musculoskeletal cause is suspected
- Cardiology consultation if there are red flags for a cardiac etiology of chest pain

TREATMENT

- Address the underlying cause of noncardiac chest pain
- If there is a concern for a cardiac cause of chest pain, the child should be restricted from exercise until seen by a cardiologist

Syncope

BASIC INFORMATION

- Syncope describes loss of consciousness for any reason
- The differential diagnosis for syncope is in Table 5.3
  - Most syncope in children and adolescents is benign and is usually neurocardiogenic syncope (vasovagal syncope)
  - Vasovagal syncope presents with prodromal symptoms before loss of consciousness, including dizziness, nausea, tachycardia, diaphoresis, and/or tunnel vision

CLINICAL PRESENTATION

- "Red flags" for cardiac-related syncope
  - Loss of consciousness without prodromal symptoms
  - Syncope in response to loud noise, surprise, or emotional distress is suspicious for long QT syndrome

- Syncope during exercise
- Syncope while lying flat
- Family history of sudden death
- Syncope with an abnormal ECG

DIAGNOSIS AND EVALUATION

- History, history, history!
- Vital signs should include orthostatic blood pressure and heart rate evaluation
- ECG: refer to a cardiologist if abnormal
- Consider a 24-hour ambulatory heart rate monitor or 30-day cardiac event monitor
- Consider a neurologic workup, such as with an electroencephalogram (EEG) or consultation with a neurologist

TREATMENT

- Depends on the etiology
- Patients with orthostasis should be encouraged to drink at least eight glasses of water per day and increase sodium intake
- If there is concern for syncope with exertion, the child should be restricted from exercise until seen by a cardiologist

Murmur

BASIC INFORMATION

- Murmurs are caused by turbulent blood flow
- The intensity of the murmur depends on the degree of turbulence and is affected by the size of the orifice or vessel through which blood flows, the pressure difference across the site of flow, and the volume of flow

CLINICAL PRESENTATION

- "Innocent murmurs" (see Table 5.4) share common features called "the seven S's":
  - Sensitive: varies with changes in position or respiration, loudest when supine
  - Short duration
  - Single: no associated clicks or gallops
  - Small: limited to a small area, nonradiating
  - Soft

Table 5.3. Causes of Syncope in Children and Adolescents

CARDIAC CAUSES	NONCARDIAC CAUSES
Arrhythmias	Neurocardiogenic (vasovagal) syncope
■ Long QT syndrome	Breath-holding spells
■ Complete heart block	Postural orthostatic tachycardia syndrome
■ Supraventricular tachycardia	Seizures
■ Ventricular tachycardia	Psychogenic
Left ventricular outflow tract obstruction	
Vasculitis	

Table 5.4. Innocent Murmurs of Childhood

	Age	Timing and Configuration	Intensity	Pitch	Quality	Location	Etiology
Still's murmur	2–6 years, may be audible from infancy to adulthood	Early systole	Grades 1–3	Low to medium	Vibratory "twang" or "musical" ↑when supine	LLSB, extends to apex	Ventricular false tendons
Pulmonary flow murmur	All ages	Early to mid-systolic, crescendo-decrescendo	Grades 2–3		Rough, dissonant ↑when supine	Second and third intercostal spaces	Audible flow across pulmonary outflow tract
Peripheral pulmonic stenosis	0–6 months	Ejection murmur beginning in mid-systole	Grades 1–2	Low to medium		LUSB, radiates to bilateral axillae and back	Acute takeoff of the branch PAs in neonates ↑with respiratory infections
Venous hum	~3–8 years	Continuous murmur, ↑in diastole	Grades 1–3		Whining, roaring, or whirring ↑when supine ↑with head turned away from examiner ↓with compression of jugular vein	Low anterior neck, extends to infraclavicular area, R>L	Turbulence at confluence of jugular and subclavian veins as they enter SVC, or angulation of IJV as it courses over transverse process of atlas
Supraclavicular or brachiocephalic systolic murmur	Children and teenagers	Brief, crescendo-decrescendo	Grades 1–3	Low to medium	Disappears with hyperextension of shoulders	Above clavicles, radiates to neck	Major brachiocephalic vessels arising from aorta
Aortic systolic murmur	Older children and adults	Ejection	Grades 1–3	Low to medium		RUSB	↑with anxiety, anemia, hyperthyroidism, or fear
Mammary artery soufflé	Teenagers and pregnant women	Systolic murmur, extends into diastole	Grades 1–3	High	Varies from day to day	Anterior chest wall over breast	Blood flow in arteries and veins leading to and from breasts

LLSB: left lower sternal border; LUSB: left upper sternal border; PAs: pulmonary arteries; SVC: superior vena cava, IJV: internal jugular vein; RUSB: right upper sternal border.

- Sweet: not harsh
- Systolic
- Features concerning for a pathologic murmur:
  - History concerning for cardiac disease
  - Systolic murmur that intensifies with standing
  - Presence of a holosystolic or diastolic murmur
  - Grade 3 or higher murmur
  - Abnormal S2 or audible click
  - Young age (neonates or young infants)

DIAGNOSIS AND EVALUATION

- History is key for accurate diagnosis of the murmur. Important questions include:
  - At what age was the murmur first detected?
  - Is there a family history of congenital heart disease?
- ECG
- Consider referral to a cardiologist and echocardiogram if there is concern for a pathologic murmur

Review Questions

For review questions, please go to ExpertConsult.com.

Suggested Readings

1. Daniels SR. Coronary risk factors in children. In: Allen HD, Shaddy RE, Penny DJ, Feltes TF, Cetta F, eds. *Moss and Adams' Heart Disease in Infants, Children, and Adolescents: Including the Fetus and Young Adults.* 9th ed. Philadelphia: Lippincott Williams & Wilkins; 2016:1633–1667.
2. Expert panel on integrated guidelines for cardiovascular health and risk reduction in children and adolescents: summary report. *Pediatrics.* 2011;128(suppl 5):S213–S256.
3. Frank JE, Jacobe KM. Evaluation and management of heart murmurs in children. *Am Fam Physician.* 2011;84(7):793–800.
4. Johnson JN, Driscoll DJ. Chest pain in children and adolescents. In: Allen HD, Driscoll DJ, Shaddy RE, Feltes TF, eds. *Moss and Adams' Heart Disease in Infants, Children, and Adolescents: Including the Fetus and Young Adults.* 8th ed. Philadelphia: Lippincott Williams & Wilkins; 2013:1509–1513.
5. Kocis KC. Chest pain in pediatrics. *Pediatr Clin North Am.* 1999; 46(2):189–203.
6. Lewis DA, Dhala A. Syncope in the pediatric patient. *Pediatr Clin North Am.* 1999;46(2):205–219.
7. Flynn JT, Kaelber DC, Baker-Smith CM, Blowey D, Carroll AE, Daniels SR, de Ferranti SD, Dionne JM, Falkner B, Flinn SK, Gidding SS, Goodwin C, Leu MG, Powers ME, Rea C, Samuels J, Simasek M, Thaker VV, Urbina EM, Subcommittee on Screening and Management of High Blood Pressure in Children. Clinical practice guideline for screening and management of high blood pressure in children and adolescents. *Pediatrics.* 2017:e20171904.

6 Structural Heart Disease: Acyanotic and Cyanotic Lesions

CHARITHA D. REDDY, MD, NEHA J. PURKEY, MD and
ALAINA K. KIPPS, MD, MS

Congenital heart disease is a fascinating topic with a diverse set of diagnoses, ranging from normal variants to severely debilitating defects. Although there are many ways to categorize these diagnoses, we have divided the chapter into acyanotic and cyanotic lesions. However, it is important to note that many lesions will have a spectrum of severity that allows them to present in either category. Additionally, patients may present with other complex cardiac abnormalities or combinations of abnormalities that are beyond the scope of this chapter.

General Approach to Congenital Heart Disease

BASIC INFORMATION

- The history, physical examination, and basic evaluation strategies can lead to a swift diagnosis and appropriate management, particularly in the ill neonate
- Elements of the history include:
  - Symptoms: feeding tolerance, tachypnea, cyanosis, fatigue, urine output, growth history
  - Family history of heart disease and other genetic syndromes, prenatal care, prenatal exposures and complications, and results of fetal imaging studies
- Elements of the physical examination include:
  - Murmurs (see Chapter 5)
  - Four-extremity blood pressures, brachial and femoral pulses
  - Pre- and postductal saturations
  - Clubbing
  - Cyanosis (central versus peripheral)
- Elements of the diagnostic evaluation include:
  - Chest x-ray: evaluation for pulmonary edema, dark lung fields from diminished pulmonary blood flow (i.e. oligemic lung fields), enlarged or abnormally shaped cardiac silhouette, dextrocardia, other respiratory or abdominal findings
  - ECG
  - Hyperoxia test for cyanotic newborns to determine whether cyanosis is due to lung disease or congenital heart disease
    - Arterial blood gas (ABG) is obtained while the infant is breathing room air and then repeated after the infant has been placed on 100% oxygen for 10 minutes
  - See Fig. 6.1 for schema of diagnostic approach
- Management
  - Management of cardiac diseases is dictated by underlying physiology of the cardiac defect

- In most cases of critical neonatal heart disease, oxygen and prostaglandins (PGE) are likely indicated; stable central access (e.g., umbilical vein catheter) is also often necessary
- See also Nelson Textbook of Pediatrics, Chapter 434, "General Principles of Treatment of Congenital Heart Disease."

Cyanosis

BASIC INFORMATION

- Cyanosis can present as central or peripheral cyanosis
  - Central cyanosis: caused by true arterial desaturation (low PaO_2)
    - Bluish discoloration of skin, mucous membranes (lips, gums), clubbing
    - Usually requires 5 g/dL of deoxyhemoglobin to appear cyanotic. In a patient with a normal hematocrit, this corresponds to ≤85% saturation. Anemic patients may have a significantly lower saturation before appearing cyanotic (~65%). Polycythemic patients may appear cyanotic earlier than those with a normal red blood count
    - Occurs in congenital heart disease with limited pulmonary blood flow or transposition
  - Peripheral cyanosis: normal arterial saturation (normal PaO_2)
    - Bluish discoloration of skin of extremities or perioral area
    - Acrocyanosis can be normal in neonates
    - Abnormal if patient has signs of poor perfusion or shock

ACYANOTIC LESIONS

Patent Ductus Arteriosus (PDA)

BASIC INFORMATION

- The ductus arteriosus is a connection between the aorta and the pulmonary artery that is a normal and essential structure in fetal life (see Fig. 6.2)
- In utero, blood pumped by the right ventricle mostly bypasses the lungs via the ductus into the descending aorta, allowing perfusion to the body and back to the placenta
- With the first breath after birth, the drop in pulmonary vascular resistance (PVR) and the increase in systemic vascular resistance (SVR) reverse the direction of ductal flow, causing blood to flow from the aorta into the pulmonary artery via the PDA. The more oxygenated blood now flowing through the PDA promotes closure of the ductus, usually within the first few days of life

ASD: atrial septal defect
CDH: congenital diaphragmatic
CXR: chest X-ray
HLHS: hypoplastic left heart syndrome
PH: pulmonary hypertension
PPHN: persistent pulmonary hypertension of the new born
RDS: respiratory distress syndrome
TAPVR: total anomaious pulmonany venous return
TGA: transposition of the great arteries

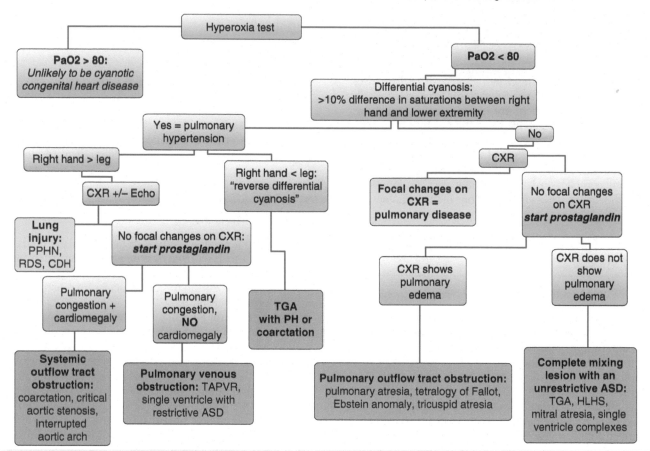

Fig. 6.1. Approach to the neonate with cyanosis.

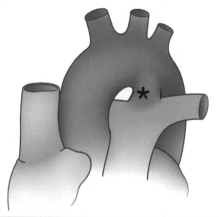

Fig. 6.2. The ductus arteriosus is a connection between the aorta and the pulmonary artery that is a normal and essential structure in fetal life. Illustration provided by Charitha D. Reddy, MD.

- A persistent PDA beyond the first few weeks of life causes a left-to-right shunt in a structurally normal heart
- Many forms of congenital heart disease have either limited pulmonary or systemic blood flow, leading to reliance on the PDA to be a key or sole source of blood flow to either the lungs or the body, making the lesion ductal dependent

CLINICAL PRESENTATION

- Small PDAs are generally asymptomatic. They may be first suspected as a systolic or continuous murmur
- Moderate to large PDAs are associated with:
  - Increased risk of respiratory tract infections
  - Congestive heart failure symptoms
  - Examination:
    - Grade I–IV/VI continuous murmur, often described as "machinery-like." Usually heard at the left upper sternal border (LUSB)
    - May have widened pulse pressure and associated bounding pulses
- In premature infants, PDAs can cause a hemodynamically significant left-to-right shunting severe enough to lead to systemic hypoperfusion
  - Diminished systemic blood flow can contribute to risk for Necrotizing enterocolitis, myocardial ischemia, renal injury, and so forth

- Meanwhile, Excessive pulmonary blood flow leads to pulmonary edema
- Murmur is less common
- Natural history:
  - After the first few weeks of life, spontaneous closure is rare, especially in full-term infants and children
  - Small PDAs may be asymptomatic into adulthood
  - A large PDA left untreated can lead to pulmonary hypertension. If pulmonary hypertension develops, the shunt will become right to left (Eisenmenger), resulting in differential cyanosis (normal saturation in upper extremities; lower saturation in lower extremities with clubbing developing in the toes)
  - A patent PDA allowing enough flow to create a murmur has a 1% per year risk of bacterial endarteritis

DIAGNOSIS AND EVALUATION

- Chest x-ray: pulmonary edema
- Echocardiogram confirms the diagnosis

TREATMENT

- Hemodynamically significant PDAs in premature infants:
  - Fluid restriction and diuretics
  - Indomethacin or NSAIDs to close the PDA
    - Contraindicated in infants with bleeding risks (e.g. NEC, thrombocytopenia, intracranial hypertension)
  - If medical management fails, the PDA can be ligated surgically
- Persistently patent PDAs in full-term infants and children:
  - Small PDAs
    - If a PDA is tiny on echocardiogram and no murmur is auscultated, no closure is recommended
    - If an audible murmur is present, catheterization closure is recommended due to a risk of infective endocarditis
  - Moderate or large PDAs
    - Should be closed via catheterization to treat congestive heart failure and prevent the development of pulmonary hypertension
- Options for closure
  - Device closure in the catheterization laboratory is standard for generally asymptomatic older infants and children
  - Surgical closure involves ligation and division; generally used for premature infants
    - Common complications:
      Vocal cord paralysis (injury to recurrent laryngeal nerve)/diaphragm paresis (injury to phrenic nerve)
      Chylothorax (injury to thoracic duct)
      Later-onset scoliosis related to thoracotomy

Atrial Septal Defects (ASD)

BASIC INFORMATION

- Accounts for 13% of congenital heart disease
- An ASD is an opening in the septum between the right and left atrium and is categorized by the location of the defect (see Fig. 6.3)

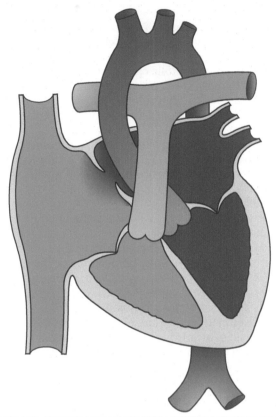

Fig. 6.3. An atrial septal defect is an opening in the septum between the right and left atrium. Illustration provided by Charitha D. Reddy, MD.

- Patent foramen ovale (PFO)
  - In utero, placental blood returns to the heart, and the majority crosses the PFO to the left atrium. This allows for the most oxygenated blood to reach the coronary arteries and the brain
  - ~30% of normal, healthy adults have a residual PFO
- Primum ASD (15%–20%)
  - Endocardial cushion defect
  - Comprises the atrial component of atrioventricular (AV) canal defects
- Secundum ASD (70%)
  - Defect in the septum primum
- Sinus venosus defect (5%–10%)
  - Majority of these defects occur in conjunction with partial anomalous pulmonary venous return (PAVPR)
- Coronary sinus defect (<1%)
- In severe cases, left atrial pressure rises due to increased pulmonary venous blood return. In PFOs, this usually helps the flap to close. In other forms of ASDs, this increases the left-to-right atrial shunting
- An atrial-level communication is required for survival in many other congenital cyanotic heart lesions to ensure adequate mixing of systemic and pulmonary blood flow

CLINICAL PRESENTATION

- Often asymptomatic until adolescence or adulthood
  - Symptoms may include exercise intolerance, shortness of breath, and fatigue
  - May have palpitations due to atrial arrhythmias (atrial flutter and/or atrial fibrillation) related to atrial stretch

- Examination
  - Wide, fixed splitting of S2 due to delayed closure of pulmonary valve from increased volume in the right ventricle
  - Can also have a systolic ejection murmur at the LUSB (due to increased flow across the pulmonary valve) and a diastolic rumble at lower left sternal border (LLSB) (due to increased flow across the tricuspid valve)
- Genetic syndromes associated with secundum-type ASDs
  - Holt-Oram syndrome (*TBX5* gene), Noonan syndrome, Treacher Collins, and thrombocytopenia with absent radius (TAR) syndrome
- Natural history
  - PFOs will generally close spontaneously in the first few weeks to months of life
  - Spontaneous closure of secundum defects can occur in younger patients (usually up to 8 years of age)
  - In 5% to 10% of patients, increased pulmonary blood flow over time will cause pulmonary hypertension, leading to Eisenmenger physiology:
    - In Eisenmenger physiology, the elevated PVR causes reversal of atrial shunting, with desaturated blood flowing from the right atrium to the left atrium, leading to cyanosis

DIAGNOSIS AND EVALUATION

- Often the physical examination is indicative of diagnosis
- On ECG, look for RSR′ pattern in V1
- Echocardiography confirms the diagnosis

TREATMENT

- PFO: no treatment recommended unless there is high risk for paradoxical embolism
- Catheter-based device closure can be performed for secundum ASDs that meet specific criteria for size and location
- Surgical closure is required for other types of ASDs and secundum defects not amenable to device closure
- Surgery is contraindicated in patients with Eisenmenger physiology

Ventricular Septal Defects (VSD)

BASIC INFORMATION

- Second most common congenital heart lesion
- A VSD is an opening between the right and left ventricles and is categorized by the location of the defect (see Fig. 6.4)
  - Membranous or perimembranous VSD (70%)
    - Located in the membranous portion of the septum and may extend to the entrance of the pulmonary or aortic valve
  - Muscular VSD (5%–20%)
    - Located in the muscular portion of the septum
  - Inlet VSD or AV canal–type VSD (5%–8%)
    - Complete AV canal defect: inlet VSD, primum ASD, common atrioventricular valve
    - Commonly associated with Down syndrome
  - Supracristal or infundibular VSD (5%–7%)

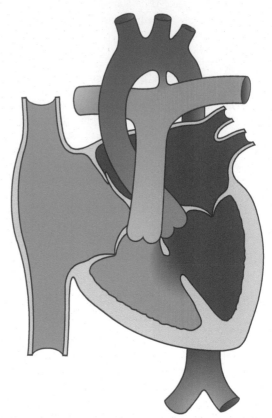

Fig. 6.4. A ventricular septal defect is an opening between the right and left ventricles. Illustration provided by Charitha D. Reddy, MD.

- Most VSDs result in shunting from the left ventricle to right ventricle, with increasing pulmonary blood flow. The amount of shunting is dictated by the size of the VSD and the relative downstream resistance of the pulmonary and systemic vasculature; if the defect is very large, there may be an equalization of pressures in the two ventricles

CLINICAL PRESENTATION

- Small muscular defects usually present with a holosystolic murmur heard best at the LLSB
- Defects that are close to valves can cause poor closure of valve leaflets, leading to tricuspid or aortic insufficiency and can have additional murmurs
- Large defects cause pulmonary overcirculation and symptoms of heart failure in the absence of pulmonary hypertension:
  - Failure to thrive, tachypnea, hepatomegaly
  - Cardiac examination: right ventricular (RV) heave; may not hear murmur due to equalization of pressures; thus there is a lack of turbulent flow across the defect
- Natural history
  - Small VSDs are usually asymptomatic, and the majority will close on their own: >90% close up by age 1 year, and they can take up to ages 8 to 10 years to close; thus they will not require intervention
  - Large VSDs cause increased pulmonary blood flow, which can progress to pulmonary hypertension and Eisenmenger physiology (see section on ASD, above)

DIAGNOSIS AND EVALUATION

- ECG may show RV hypertrophy (RVH)
- Chest x-ray (CXR) may show pulmonary edema in a large defect
- Echocardiography confirms the diagnosis

TREATMENT

- Hemodynamically significant VSDs:
  - Initial medical management is heart failure (diuretics, increasing caloric intake)
  - Surgical closure
    - Infants: before 1 year of age or if failure to thrive (before 6 months for patients with Down syndrome due to increased risk of pulmonary hypertension)
    - Surgery is contraindicated in patients with Eisenmenger physiology

Pulmonary Stenosis (PS)

BASIC INFORMATION

- 25% to 30% of all congenital heart disease; frequently associated with other lesions
- Pulmonary stenosis is characterized by obstruction to pulmonary blood flow. It can occur below the valve (subvalvar), at the level of the valve (valvar), above the valve (supravalvar), and in the branch pulmonary arteries. Valvar PS is the most common (80%–90%) (see Fig. 6.5)
- The valve can be abnormally formed and thickened, causing impaired flow, or the overall annulus size can be small
- Spectrum of disease from mild PS to critical PS
  - Critical pulmonary stenosis: very little blood can cross the pulmonary valve due to severe narrowing, preventing sufficient flow across the tricuspid valve and forcing deoxygenated from right atrium to left atrium across the PFO. The deoxygenated blood mixes with fully oxygenated blood in the left atrium and proceeds to the left ventricle and aorta. A portion of this mixed blood crosses the PDA to allow blood to enter the pulmonary arteries and become reoxygenated (left-to-right flow). Thus critical PS is a *ductal-dependent lesion*

CLINICAL PRESENTATION

- Presentation is dependent on degree of stenosis
  - Mild PS:
    - Usually asymptomatic
    - Systolic ejection murmur heard best at left upper sternal to midsternal border
  - Moderate to severe PS:
    - May be asymptomatic in early life
    - High-pitched systolic ejection murmur; may have midsystolic click
    - May have RV heave if RVH has developed
    - Exertional dyspnea and fatigue
    - May have cyanosis if there is a PFO or ASD allowing blood to flow right to left from elevated pressures in the right ventricle

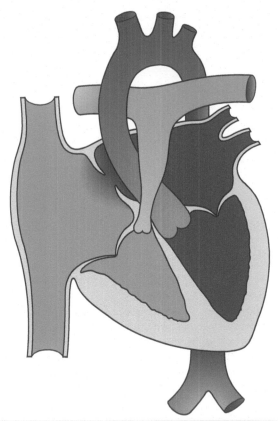

Fig. 6.5. Pulmonary stenosis is characterized by obstruction to pulmonary blood flow. It can occur below the valve (subvalvar), at the level of the valve (valvar), above the valve (supravalvar), and in the branch pulmonary arteries. Valvar pulmonary stenosis is the most common. Illustration provided by Charitha D. Reddy, MD.

- Critical PS:
  - Becomes symptomatic soon after birth
  - If the duct is open: cyanosis but can maintain cardiac output
  - If the duct is closed: severe cyanosis and hypoxia, acidosis, shock
  - Likely will not hear PS murmur (too little flow crossing to generate turbulence); may hear holodiastolic tricuspid regurgitation murmur

DIAGNOSIS AND EVALUATION

- CXR: may have dark lung fields from diminished pulmonary blood flow (severe PS)
- Echocardiography confirms diagnosis and characterizes specific type (valvar or sub- or supravalvar)

TREATMENT

- Mild PS may not require intervention and may even improve over time
- Moderate PS to severe PS may progress over time and require intervention by catheter or surgery
- Critical PS
  - Ductal-dependent lesion: PGE should be started immediately after birth to ensure ductal patency for pulmonary blood flow
  - Catheter balloon valvuloplasty may be attempted, but if this fails or valve is not amenable, surgery is recommended

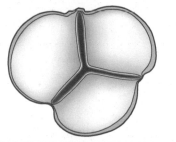
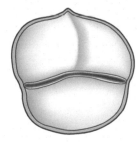

Fig. 6.6. Bicuspid aortic valve is defined by fusion of commissure between two of the three coronary cusps. Illustration provided by Charitha D. Reddy, MD.

Bicuspid Aortic Valve

BASIC INFORMATION

- 1% to 2% of general population; thus it is the most common congenital heart defect
- Defined by fusion of commissure between two of the three coronary cusps (see Fig. 6.6)
- Can be associated with aortic valvar stenosis and/or regurgitation, coarctation, or other left-sided obstructive lesions (including hypoplastic left heart syndrome [HLHS])
- There appears to be a genetic etiology because bicuspid aortic valves and other left-sided obstructive lesions often cluster in families

CLINICAL PRESENTATION

- May be asymptomatic for many years
- Examination: midsystolic ejection click; may have additional murmurs if aortic stenosis or insufficiency is present
- Natural history
  - Valvar calcification and sclerosis may begin in teenage years and progress to stenosis
  - As the valve degenerates, aortic insufficiency can develop as well
  - Aortic root dilation and dissection can be late sequelae

DIAGNOSIS AND EVALUATION

- Echocardiography confirms the diagnosis
- Requires serial echocardiograms to evaluate the size, dilation, stenosis, and insufficiency of the valve, as well as monitor for associated dilation of the ascending aorta

TREATMENT

- Requires strict hypertension control to avoid aortic dissection
- Need for intervention depends on the severity of aortic stenosis and/or regurgitation and on the size of the aortic root

Coarctation of the Aorta

BASIC INFORMATION

- 4% to 6% of all congenital heart disease; more common in males than in females

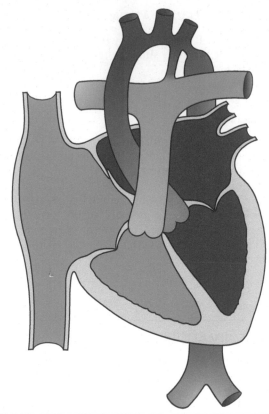

Fig. 6.7. Coarctation of the aorta is a narrowing of the descending aorta. Illustration provided by Charitha D. Reddy, MD.

- Coarctation of the aorta is a narrowing of the descending aorta, preventing adequate blood flow to downstream areas and leading to end-organ damage (see Fig. 6.7)
- The narrowing is usually located at the site of PDA insertion (juxtaductal). It can be discrete narrowing or long-segment narrowing. The most severe presentation can be complete interruption of the aortic arch
- Bimodal distribution: can present early or later in life depending on absence or presence of collaterals to aid in systemic blood flow. Bicuspid aortic valve is common in both types of patients
- Can be associated with more complex congenital heart disease (TGA, HLHS, posteriorly malaligned VSD, etc.)

CLINICAL PRESENTATION

- Neonatal/early presentation:
  - Critical coarctation/interrupted aortic arch: narrowing does not allow sufficient blood flow to the lower half of the body, or distal arch is completely disconnected from the proximal arch. The systemic blood flow is ductal dependent (right to left)
  - Infants present in shock and/or heart failure and can present as late as 6 weeks of life if the duct closes later. Cardiac examination features include:
    - Differential cyanosis: areas past the narrowing will be supplied by PDA flow. Lower-extremity saturation will be lower than upper-extremity saturation
    - May have diminished femoral pulses and decreased lower-extremity blood pressures

Table 6.1. Common Radiographic Associations with Congenital Heart Disease Lesions

Syndrome	Radiographic Finding	Anatomic Correlate for Radiographic Finding
Coarctation	"3" sign	Due to "infolding" at the junction of the ascending aorta and descending aorta
Tetralogy of Fallot	"Boot-shaped" heart	Due to right ventricular hypertrophy causing elevation of the apex
Transposition of the great arteries	"Egg-on-a-string" heart	Narrowed mediastinal silhouette because of the parallel position of the great vessels, and the heart is more globular, possibly due to increased pulmonary venous return to the left atrium
Truncus	Narrowed mediastinal silhouette	Single arterial trunk
Total anomalous pulmonary venous return (TAPVR)	"Snowman in a snowstorm"	Occurs in supracardiac TAPVR when the vertical vein, superior vena cava, and innominate vein create the "head" and a dilated right atrium creates the "body" of the snowman. In obstructed TAVPR, pulmonary venous blood flow cannot exit the lungs, causing diffuse pulmonary edema, or the "snowstorm."
Severe Ebstein anomaly	"Wall-to-wall" heart	Severe cardiomegaly due to an extremely enlarged right atrium

- Upon duct closure, there will be further systemic blood flow restriction, leading to decreased pulses, decreased urine output, tachypnea, acidosis, and shock
- Late presentation:
  - Majority have discrete coarctation but otherwise have normal arch size. To bypass the narrowing, collaterals develop in fetal life and continue as the child ages
  - Due to limited blood flow to lower extremities, may present with fatigue or pain with exercise. Cardiac examination features include:
    - Continuous murmur from collaterals
    - Diminished or delayed lower-extremity pulses
    - Four-extremity blood pressure differential (usually right arm hypertension)
- ~30% of patients with Turner syndrome have coarctation

DIAGNOSIS AND EVALUATION

- Critical coarctation:
  - Echocardiography confirms diagnosis
- Asymptomatic children:
  - Four-extremity blood pressures will show a differential between the upper and lower extremities
  - ECG: normal or may show left ventricular hypertrophy (LVH); in infants shows RVH
  - CXR: "3 sign" from aortic indentation, rib notching from collaterals
  - Magnetic resonance imaging (MRI): can also confirm diagnosis, identifies collateral supply; after surgical repair, good for monitoring for aneurysm development
  - Echocardiography confirms diagnosis and identifies associated anomalies

TREATMENT

- Critical coarctation:
  - Ductal-dependent lesion: initiate immediate PGE to maintain ductal patency; may need medical therapy for heart failure and inotropic support
  - Surgical repair urgently
- Asymptomatic children:

- Surgical repair better for first management; recoarctation can be addressed well with balloon angioplasty or stenting
- Risk of persistent hypertension if corrected too late

CYANOTIC LESIONS

This section covers a select portion of possible diagnoses for infants and children with cyanotic heart disease. It should be noted that extremes of some of the acyanotic lesions are mentioned earlier (e.g., critical PS, neonatal aortic coarctation) may also cause cyanosis. Although prenatal screening has improved significantly over the years, a large proportion of patients may not be diagnosed until after birth or later. The Neonatal Cyanosis Flowchart (see Fig. 6.1) is meant to serve as a guide for the infants that present with cyanosis within a few hours or days, but each entry later discusses the most likely time frame for presentation. In addition, many of these diagnoses are associated with classic radiographic findings, detailed in Table 6.1.

Tetralogy of Fallot (TOF)

BASIC INFORMATION

- Approximately 10% of cases of congenital heart disease; is the most common cause of cyanotic congenital heart disease
- TOF is made up of four components due to one developmental problem, the anterior deviation of the infundibular septum: pulmonary stenosis, RVH, aortic override, and a VSD (usually large). Many patients also have an ASD or PFO, but this is not required (see Fig. 6.8)
- Significant association with right-sided aortic arch, 22q11.2 deletion, Holt–Oram syndrome, Alagille syndrome, and trisomies 21, 18, and 13

CLINICAL PRESENTATION

- Clinical symptoms depend on degree of pulmonary stenosis and age of presentation.
  - Minimal obstruction:

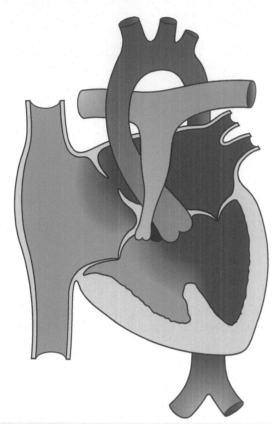

Fig. 6.8. Tetralogy of Fallot is made up of four components due to one developmental problem, the anterior deviation of the infundibular septum: pulmonary stenosis, right ventricular hypertrophy, aortic override, and a ventricular septal defect. Illustration provided by Charitha D. Reddy, MD.

- Neonates:
  May have normal saturations—"pink tet"—and behave more like large VSD with heart failure and poor growth by 4 to 6 weeks
- Severe obstruction:
  - Neonates:
    Cyanosis due to diminished pulmonary blood flow and increased right-to-left shunting across VSD—"blue tet"
    If very stenotic or atretic pulmonary valve, these are ductal dependent for pulmonary blood flow (left to right)
- Examination:
  - Normal first heart sound
  - Loud systolic ejection murmur heard best that can radiate to the back. The murmur is from pulmonary stenosis, not the VSD
  - If very severe PS, may have very soft or no murmur due to minimal flow across the pulmonary valve
  - In long-standing unrepaired TOF: progressive cyanosis, clubbing
  - Active precordium
- Natural history
  - If unrepaired, progressive stenosis and worsening RVH reduce pulmonary blood flow and increase right-to-left shunting across the VSD, resulting in worsening cyanosis

DIAGNOSIS AND EVALUATION

- Many patients are now diagnosed prenatally with fetal echocardiogram
- Chest x-ray: "boot-shaped" heart due to RVH
- Echocardiography confirms the diagnosis

TREATMENT

- Hypercyanotic episodes, or "tet spells," present as sudden onset or worsening of cyanosis, usually caused by acute increase in pulmonary obstruction and right-to-left shunting at the VSD in the setting of agitation/crying or dehydration
  - Management (in order of severity progression):
    - Comfort the patient and remove stressors
    - Flex knees or place in squatting position
    - Give fluid bolus
    - Morphine
    - IV propranolol
    - Phenylephrine to increase SVR and reverse shunting at VSD level back to left to right
    - Anesthesia with intubation and possible paralysis
  - Once a patient has had a hypercyanotic episode, surgery should be scheduled promptly
- Surgical repair: VSD and PFO/ASD closure and relief of pulmonary obstruction

Transposition of the Great Arteries (TGA)

BASIC INFORMATION

- ~3% of all congenital heart diseases and 20% of all cyanotic congenital heart diseases. There is a male predominance
- TGA is characterized by aorta arising from the right ventricle and the pulmonary artery arising from the left ventricle. Deoxygenated blood returning from the body is sent back to the aorta and to the body, and the oxygenated blood returning from the lungs is sent back through the pulmonary artery to the lungs. They are parallel circulations (see Fig. 6.9)
- To survive, there must be adequate mixing of the oxygenated and deoxygenated blood, which is best at the atrial level due to adequate atrial communication (PFO or ASD). Flow left to right at PDA can help mixing at the atrial level (more pulmonary venous return) but is not a key site of mixing
- Associated with maternal diabetes, certain chromosomal syndromes, dextrocardia and heterotaxy, and maternal hypervitaminosis A

CLINICAL PRESENTATION

- Cyanosis is present in all patients with transposition
- Examination:
  - Normal first heart sound, single second heart sound
  - Usually no murmur unless associated pulmonary stenosis
  - Inadequate mixing:
    - Hypoxemia and poor systemic perfusion, eventual hypotension and shock

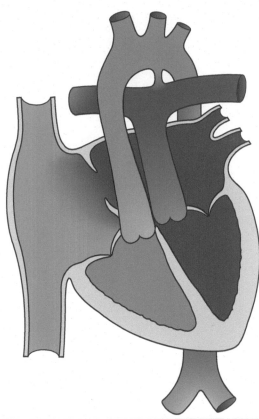

Fig. 6.9. Transposition of the great arteries is characterized by the aorta arising from the right ventricle and the pulmonary artery arising from the left ventricle. Deoxygenated blood returning from the body is sent back to the aorta and to the body, and the oxygenated blood returning from the lungs is sent back through the pulmonary artery to the lungs. They are parallel circulations. Illustration provided by Charitha D. Reddy, MD.

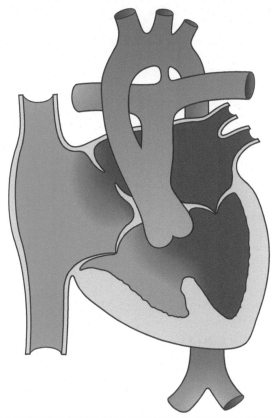

Fig. 6.10. Truncus is defined by having a single, common arterial trunk that supplies the systemic, coronary, and pulmonary blood flow. Illustration provided by Charitha D. Reddy, MD.

- Adequate mixing:
  - Cyanotic (saturations ~80%–90%)
  - Pre- and postductal saturations are similar
- Pulmonary hypertension or coarctation in TGA
  - Reverse differential cyanosis: blood from the pulmonary artery (oxygenated blood) crosses PDA into the aorta (deoxygenated blood). Lower-extremity saturations (postductal) are higher than upper-extremity saturations (preductal)
- Natural history
  - Untreated TGA is usually fatal within the first 2 weeks of life
  - Late presentation, seen more often in developing countries, is possible if ASD and VSD are present to provide adequate mixing

DIAGNOSIS AND EVALUATION

- Chest x-ray: "egg-on-a-string" appearance due to side-by-side orientation of aorta and pulmonary artery
- Echocardiography confirms the diagnosis

TREATMENT

- This is *not* a ductal-dependent lesion, although a patent duct can be helpful to increase mixing
- Definitive treatment is surgical repair

- Immediate postnatal medical management:
  - Central/umbilical access
  - PGE initiation to improve mixing
  - Mixing occurs predominantly at the atrial level. If ASD is small, there is still a risk of severe cyanosis
    - Progressively worsening cyanosis would necessitate a balloon atrial septostomy (BAS) to open the atrial septum
- Surgical repair—arterial switch operation (ASO):
  - Usually done in the first week of life
  - Transects both great arteries above the valves and switches and reattaches to the opposite valve
  - Coronaries need to be relocated to the root of neo-aorta!
- Long-term management:
  - Although most children can have fairly normal lives, neurodevelopmental aspects should be followed closely

Truncus Arteriosus

BASIC INFORMATION

- Rare defect in congenital heart disease
- Truncus is defined by having a single, common arterial trunk that supplies the systemic, coronary, and pulmonary blood flow; the truncal valve is often dysplastic (see Fig. 6.10)

- Must have a VSD to allow for both ventricles to empty into the common trunk, allowing for complete mixing of blood to enter the pulmonary arteries and the aorta
- Usually this is an isolated defect but is associated with 22q11 deletion

CLINICAL PRESENTATION

- Mild cyanosis at birth
- As PVR drops, blood flow through the truncal valve will preferentially go to the pulmonary arteries, leading to pulmonary overcirculation and heart failure. By this time, patients may not be cyanotic due to excessive pulmonary blood flow
- Examination:
  - Single loud S2 (only one valve!)
  - Tachypnea
  - Tachycardia, diaphoresis, poor feeding
- Natural history
  - If unrepaired, the majority will be fatal by 1 month of life due to pulmonary overcirculation and heart failure

DIAGNOSIS AND EVALUATION

- CXR: cardiomegaly and pulmonary edema; narrow mediastinal silhouette
- Echocardiography confirms the diagnosis

TREATMENT

- This is *not* a ductal-dependent lesion. Many do not have a PDA
- Medical management for heart failure while waiting for surgery
- Surgical repair is performed in the neonatal period (while awaiting surgery, diuretics, and heart failure management)

Total Anomalous Pulmonary Venous Return (TAPVR)

BASIC INFORMATION

- Accounts for approximately 1% of infants with congenital heart disease
- Total anomalous pulmonary venous return (TAPVR) is characterized by a lack of connection between all of the pulmonary veins and the left atrium (see Fig. 6.11)
- All the oxygenated blood returning from the lungs empties into the right-sided circulation, mixing with the deoxygenated blood. For this mixed blood to enter the left-sided circulation and provide systemic blood flow, there is an obligate right-to-left shunt at the atrial level (resulting in cyanosis)
  - TAPVR is usually classified into four groups depending on where the anomalous pulmonary veins drain: supracardiac, cardiac, infracardiac, and mixed
  - The presentation of TAPVR depends on whether the connection between the pulmonary venous confluence and drainage site (often a vertical vein) becomes obstructed by virtue of its anatomic course

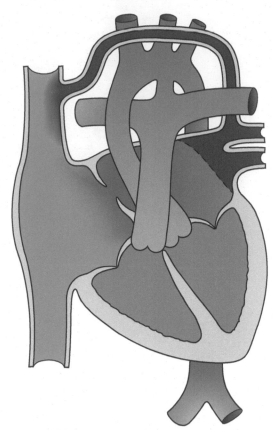

Fig. 6.11. Total anomalous pulmonary venous return is characterized by a lack of connection between all of the pulmonary veins and the left atrium. Illustration provided by Charitha D. Reddy, MD.

CLINICAL PRESENTATION

- TAPVR without pulmonary venous obstruction presents with cyanosis at birth (SpO_2 75%–85%); however, as PVR decreases, there is significant pulmonary overcirculation, leading to tachypnea, pulmonary edema, failure to thrive, and congestive heart failure
  - Examination: loud S1, fixed widely split S2, active precordium with RV lift, third heart sound always heard at the apex
- TAPVR with pulmonary venous obstruction presents with severe respiratory distress (due to inability of oxygenated blood to leave the lungs), cyanosis (due to lack of oxygenated blood), acidosis and shock (due to diminished blood flow entering the left ventricle and aorta). This is a surgical emergency!
  - Examination: split S2 with loud P2; diffuse rales at bilateral lung bases; hepatomegaly and peripheral edema are usually present
- Associations
  - TGA, Truncus arteriosus, TOF, HLHS
  - TAVPR is also associated with patients diagnosed with heterotaxy
- Natural history
  - TAPVR without obstruction will progress to congestive heart failure, usually in the first 6 months of life
  - TAPVR with obstruction will progress to neonatal death rapidly if not surgically managed

DIAGNOSIS AND EVALUATION

- CXR:
  - TAPVC without obstruction: "snowman" appearance in supracardiac type due to all the veins entering the superior vena cava (SVC)
  - TAPVC with obstruction: "whiteout" of the lung fields due to backup of blood flow into lungs. Can be difficult to differentiate from other severe neonatal lung disease
- Echocardiography confirms the diagnosis and is typically required before extracorporeal membrane oxygenation (ECMO) for severe neonatal respiratory distress

TREATMENT

- This is *not* a ductal-dependent lesion
- Medical management:
  - TAVPR without obstruction: diuretics and heart failure management until surgery
  - TAPVR with obstruction: none, proceed to surgery

Severe Pulmonary Stenosis

See earlier section on Pulmonary Stenosis

Hypoplastic Left Heart Syndrome (HLHS)

BASIC INFORMATION

- 1% to 3% of all congenital heart disease
- HLHS is characterized by diffuse hypoplasia of all left-sided structures, including the left atrium, mitral valve, left ventricle, aortic valve, and aorta. This is a single-ventricle lesion because the right ventricle is the sole functional ventricle (see Fig. 6.12)
- Because of the small size of the left-sided structures, systemic blood flow is compromised and is ductal dependent
- Oxygenated blood from the pulmonary veins enters the left atrium, and only a limited amount or no blood can cross the mitral valve to the left ventricle into the aorta
  - To allow egress of pulmonary venous return, an ASD must be present and open to allow oxygenated blood to pass from the left atrium to the right atrium. The oxygenated and deoxygenated blood mixes and enters the right-sided circulation
  - To perfuse the body, the PDA must remain patent, allowing mixed blood to pass from the pulmonary artery to the aorta—to perfuse the brain and heart, retrograde flow in the ascending aorta; the body gets antegrade right-to-left ductal flow
- Associations:
  - Turner syndrome; Jacobsen syndrome; trisomies 13, 18, and 21; Noonan syndrome; Holt–Oram syndrome; CHARGE syndrome; Smith-Lemli-Opitz syndrome
  - Some indication that there is a familial inheritance pattern (see Bicuspid Aortic Valve)
  - Can have extracardiac anomalies, including brain anomalies

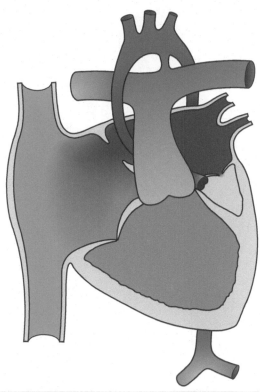

Fig. 6.12. Hypoplastic left heart syndrome is characterized by diffuse hypoplasia of all left-sided structures, including the left atrium, mitral valve, left ventricle, aortic valve, and aorta. This is a single-ventricle lesion because the right ventricle is the sole functional ventricle. Illustration provided by Charitha D. Reddy, MD.

CLINICAL PRESENTATION

- Presentation depends on size of ASD and patency of PDA
- Infants with HLHS have cyanosis
- Examination:
  - May have slight dusky appearance/cyanosis and occasionally may appear normal due to appropriate size of ASD and PDA, providing adequate systemic blood flow. If the ASD is restrictive, neonates will present in shock within a few hours of life
  - As PDA closes, systemic blood flow decreases and pulmonary blood flow increases, leading to:
    - Diminished peripheral pulses, tachypnea, hypotension, tachycardia, cool extremities, usually no murmur, shock, and death
- Natural history
  - Untreated, HLHS is almost always fatal within the first few weeks of life

DIAGNOSIS AND EVALUATION

- Echocardiography confirms the diagnosis

TREATMENT

- Medical management:
  - Ductal-dependent lesion: initiate PGE immediately after birth to maintain ductal patency
  - If ASD is restrictive, will need catheter-based atrial septostomy or stenting

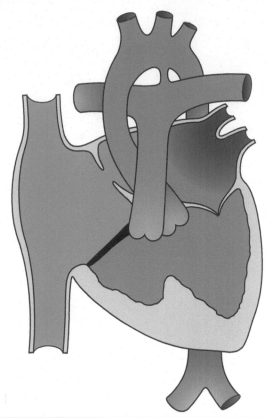

Fig. 6.13. Tricuspid atresia is defined by a lack of connection between the right atrium and the right ventricle due to agenesis of the tricuspid valve. Illustration provided by Charitha D. Reddy, MD.

- As PVR drops, may have to manage pulmonary over-circulation with diuretics
- Proceed to surgery within 1 week of life
- Surgical management: depending on the presence of other cardiac anomalies, there is generally a three-stage palliative approach to maximize the efficiency of the single viable ventricle by reconfiguring the heart's vascular connections such that blood flows from the heart to the systemic circulation and then passively to the lungs for reoxygenation before returning to the heart (known as Fontan circulation). Details of these surgeries beyond the scope of this chapter

Tricuspid Atresia

BASIC INFORMATION

- 2% to 3% of all congenital heart disease
- Tricuspid atresia is defined by a lack of connection between the right atrium and the right ventricle due to agenesis of the tricuspid valve (see Fig. 6.13)
- Must have an ASD or PFO to allow for blood to exit the right atrium, creating an obligate right-to-left shunt from the right to the left atrium; a PDA or VSD is necessary for survival

CLINICAL PRESENTATION

- Although the exact presentation of tricuspid atresia depends on the constellation of other associated cardiac anomalies (e.g., VSD, pulmonary stenosis, transposed

great vessels), neonates usually present with cyanosis and may be ductal dependent if pulmonary blood flow is compromised
- Examination:
  - May have VSD murmur, diminished RV impulse, loud S1
- Natural history
  - If there is pulmonary atresia or critical pulmonary stenosis, neonates will die within a few days without intervention. With mild pulmonary stenosis, there is a 90% mortality rate by 1 year of life. With unobstructed blood flow, patients will develop signs of overcirculation and eventual congestive heart failure

DIAGNOSIS AND EVALUATION

- CXR: enlarged right atrium; may have oligemic x-ray if restricted pulmonary blood flow
- ECG: "northwest" axis
- Echocardiography confirms the diagnosis

TREATMENT

- Medical management:
  - For cyanotic patients with restricted pulmonary blood flow, PGE should be initiated immediately
  - For patients with excessive pulmonary blood flow, diuretics and heart failure management
- Surgical:
  - For severely cyanotic patients, patients will undergo neonatal shunt placement for pulmonary blood flow
  - For patients with excessive pulmonary blood flow, a pulmonary artery band may be placed to control symptoms of overcirculation
  - Eventually both types of patients will proceed with steps toward establishing Fontan circulation (see HLHS, previous)

Ebstein Anomaly

BASIC INFORMATION

- Occurs in 1/10,000 to 2/10,000 live births
- Ebstein anomaly is defined by downward displacement of abnormal septal and inferior leaflets of the tricuspid valve, leading to tricuspid valve regurgitation and a larger right atrium and smaller right ventricle (see Fig. 6.14)
- There is a bimodal distribution of presentation in infancy and then in adolescence or adulthood. This is due to a wide spectrum of disease, largely dependent on the amount of displacement of the valve. If the valve is severely displaced, this can lead to an extremely small and nonfunctional right ventricle and severe tricuspid valve regurgitation, and can also be associated with pulmonary atresia. Alternatively, a mildly displaced tricuspid valve may remain undiagnosed for years

CLINICAL PRESENTATION

- May present in utero with fetal hydrops due to severe tricuspid regurgitation
- Severe Ebstein anomaly: presents in the neonatal period with cyanosis due to severe tricuspid regurgitation

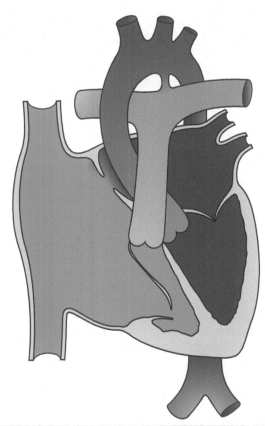

Fig. 6.14. Ebstein anomaly is defined by downward displacement of abnormal septal and inferior leaflets of the tricuspid valve, leading to tricuspid valve regurgitation and a larger right atrium and smaller right ventricle. Illustration provided by Charitha D. Reddy, MD.

and right-to-left flow at the level of the PFO. Respiratory failure can also occur due to associated lung hypoplasia
  - Examination: clicking heart sounds due to redundant valve leaflets, holosystolic tricuspid valve regurgitation murmur, cyanosis
- Mild Ebstein anomaly: may be asymptomatic, soft tricuspid regurgitation murmur. May have occasional cyanosis or exertional dyspnea if there is a small amount of right-to-left flow at PFO in adolescence or adulthood. First presentation may also be arrhythmia
- Associations
  - Wolff-Parkinson-White (WPW), left ventricular non-compaction, pulmonary atresia, mitral valve abnormalities
- Natural history
  - Severe Ebstein anomaly is fatal if left untreated. Patients with mild Ebstein anomaly may develop progressive exercise intolerance over time. All patients have varying levels of RV dysfunction

DIAGNOSIS AND EVALUATION

- CXR:
  - Severe Ebstein anomaly: "wall-to-wall" heart—extreme cardiomegaly due to severe right atrial dilation
  - Mild Ebstein anomaly: normal x-ray
- ECG: almost always abnormal—can have signs of right atrial enlargement, right bundle branch block, prolonged PR interval, or a delta wave consistent with WPW
- Echocardiography confirms the diagnosis

TREATMENT

- Medical management:
  - In severe Ebstein anomaly, patients may require PGE to sustain adequate pulmonary blood flow before surgical intervention. Often they require aggressive respiratory support due to associated lung hypoplasia from cardiomegaly
  - In mild Ebstein anomaly, patients may require only outpatient follow-up and arrhythmia management, unless there are signs of exercise intolerance, cyanosis, or worsening right ventricular function
- Surgical management varies, with severe cases requiring neonatal intervention to provide pulmonary blood flow followed by steps toward Fontan circulation (see HLHS), and less severe cases are able to undergo tricuspid valve repair/replacement and preservation of biventricular circulation.

Review Questions

For review questions, please go to ExpertConsult.com.

Suggested Readings

1. Beekman III RH. Coarctation of the aorta. In: Allen HD, Shaddy RE, Penny DJ, Feltes TF. Philadelphia: Lippincott Williams & Wilkins; 2016:1107–1123.
2. Gaca AM, Jaggers JJ, Dudley T, Bisset GS. Repair of congenital heart disease: a primer – Part 2. *Radiology.* 2008;248(1):54..
3. Park MK. *Park's pediatric cardiology for practitioners.* 6th ed. Philadelphia: Elsevier Saunders; 2014. Chapter 12: Left-to-Right Shunts; 168–174.
4. Park MK. *Park's Pediatric Cardiology For Practitioners.* 6th ed. Philadelphia: Elsevier Saunders; 2014. Chapter 13: Obstructive Lesions; 184–205.
5. Park MK. *Park's Pediatric Cardiology For Practitioners.* 6th ed. Philadelphia: Elsevier Saunders; 2014. Chapter 14: Cyanotic Congenital Heart Defects; 206–289.
6. Rubio AE, Lewin MB. Ventricular septal defects. In: Allen HD, Driscoll DJ, Shaddy RE. Philadelphia: Lippincott Williams & Wilkins; 2013: 713–721.

7 Acquired Heart Disease

NEHA J. PURKEY, MD, CHARITHA D. REDDY, MD and ALAINA K. KIPPS, MD, MS

Infective Endocarditis

BASIC INFORMATION

- Endocarditis is an infection of the endocardial surface of the heart, including native or prosthetic heart valves, septal defects, the mural endocardium, foreign devices or patches, surgical shunts, and indwelling central venous catheters
- Platelets, fibrin, and red blood cells deposit at sites of damaged endothelium. If bacteria adhere to this thrombus, a vegetation may form
- The most common pathogen is α-hemolytic (Viridans group) streptococci (see Table 7.1).
- In children, the annual incidence of infective endocarditis is between 0.05 and 0.12 cases per 1000 hospital admissions
- See also Nelson Textbook of Pediatrics, Chapter 437, "Infective Endocarditis."

CLINICAL PRESENTATION

- Patients typically present with unremitting fevers and vague constitutional symptoms, including fatigue, weight loss, and malaise
- Patients may have evidence of emboli from the vegetation:
  - Emboli in a major artery (e.g., stroke, renal infarct, splenic infarct) if the vegetation is on the mitral or aortic valves
  - Pulmonary embolism if the vegetation is on the tricuspid or pulmonic valves
  - Mycotic aneurysm (or infected aneurysm or microbial arteritis)
  - Intracranial hemorrhage
  - Conjunctival hemorrhages
  - Janeway lesions: microabscesses of the dermis, appearing as nontender, erythematous macules or nodules on the palms and soles
- Patients may have signs of immune complex deposition:
  - Glomerulonephritis
  - Osler nodes: painful, erythematous, raised lesions on the palms and soles
  - Roth spots: retinal hemorrhages with pale centers
  - Positive rheumatoid factor

DIAGNOSIS AND EVALUATION

- Infective endocarditis is diagnosed using the Modified Duke Criteria (see Table 7.2)
- Blood cultures (at least two cultures from different sites) should be drawn for patients with fever of unexplained origin, a pathologic heart murmur, a history of heart disease, or previous endocarditis

- Echocardiography has a sensitivity of >80% when the diagnosis is suspected, but it cannot be used to rule out the diagnosis. Transesophageal echocardiography is more sensitive than transthoracic imaging. However, persistently positive blood cultures are the gold standard for diagnosis!

TREATMENT

- Intravenous antibiotics for 2 to 8 weeks of therapy, depending on the infectious organism and the site of endocarditis (often broad spectrum, with narrowing based on sensitivities)
- Certain patient populations require prophylactic antibiotics against infective endocarditis (detailed in Table 7.3)

Rheumatic Fever

BASIC INFORMATION

- See Chapter 81 for details
- Streptococcal antigens cross-react with proteins in the heart, leading to immune-mediated damage and pancarditis
  - The endothelial surface of the valves is particularly affected, because recruited T cells and macrophages lead to the formation of Aschoff bodies, which are pathognomonic for rheumatic heart disease
  - On histology, they appear as a central clearing of collagen with multinucleated "owl eye" cells
- "Carditis" in the Jones Criteria (Table 81.1) includes any of the following:
  - Valvulitis: 1- to 2-mm verrucous vegetations form on the valve
    - Over time, fibrotic changes of the valve and subvalvular apparatus lead to thickening of valve leaflets and fusion of chordae

Table 7.1. Pathogens Causing Infective Endocarditis

Most Common	α-Hemolytic (Viridans group) streptococci
Second Most Common	*Staphylococcus aureus*
Uncommon	β-Hemolytic streptococci Coagulase-negative staphylococci Candida Other streptococcus species
Rare	Enterococci Pneumococci Gram-negative enteric bacteria *Pseudomonas* species *Neisseria* species HACEK organisms: *Haemophilus, Actinobacillus, Cardiobacterium, Eikenella, Kingella* Other fungi

Table 7.2. Modified Duke Criteria for Diagnosis of Infective Endocarditis

MAJOR CRITERIA

Positive blood culture for infective endocarditis

Typical microorganisms consistent with infective endocarditis from two separate blood cultures
OR
Persistently positive blood culture
OR
Single positive blood culture for *Coxiella burnetii* or phase I IgG antibody titer >1:800

Evidence of endocardial involvement:

Positive echo

Vegetation
OR
Abscess
OR
New partial dehiscence of a prosthetic valve

New valvular regurgitation on echo

MINOR CRITERIA

Predisposing factor: IV drug use or presence of a predisposing cardiac condition
Fever ≥38.0°C
Vascular phenomena
Immunologic phenomena
Microbiologic evidence: positive blood cultures that do not meet major criteria, or active infection with an organism consistent with infective endocarditis

DEFINITE INFECTIVE ENDOCARDITIS

Pathologic Criteria

Pathologic lesions: vegetation or intracardiac abscess demonstrating active endocarditis on histology
OR
Microorganism on culture, or histology of a vegetation or intracardiac abscess

Clinical Criteria

Two major clinical criteria
OR
One major and three minor clinical criteria
OR
Five minor clinical criteria

POSSIBLE INFECTIVE ENDOCARDITIS

Presence of one major and one minor clinical criteria
OR
Presence of three minor clinical criteria

REJECTED INFECTIVE ENDOCARDITIS

A firm alternate diagnosis is made
OR
Resolution of clinical manifestations occurs after ≤4 days of antibiotic therapy
OR
No pathologic evidence of infective endocarditis found at surgery or autopsy after ≤4 days of antibiotic therapy
OR
Clinical criteria for possible or definite infective endocarditis not met

- Mitral regurgitation occurs in 95% with acute rheumatic carditis
- Aortic regurgitation occurs in 20% to 25% with acute rheumatic carditis, usually in combination with mitral regurgitation
- Pericarditis
- Myocarditis
- Vasculitis of the coronaries and aorta

Table 7.3. Recommendations for Prophylaxis of Infective Endocarditis (2007)

- For dental procedures and perforation of the oral mucosa
- *No longer* recommended for patients undergoing gastrointestinal or genitourinary procedures
- In general, prophylaxis is recommended only for *high*-risk patients (not *moderate* risk)

Prosthetic cardiac valve or prosthetic material used for repair of a valve

Previous infective endocarditis

Congenital heart disease
- Unrepaired cyanotic CHD, including palliative shunts and conduits
- Completely repaired CHD with prosthetic material or device (placed surgically or by catheter) for the first 6 months after the procedure
- Repaired CHD with residual defects at the site or adjacent to the site of a prosthetic patch or prosthetic device (that could inhibit endothelialization)

Cardiac transplant recipients with cardiac valvulopathy

CHD, Congenital heart disease.

- Aschoff nodules
- Chronic rheumatic heart disease can develop if the initial cardiac disease was severe or if acute rheumatic fever recurs
  - Affected valves may be regurgitant after the initial illness, but over time the valve leaflets typically will thicken and the valve will become stenotic
  - Ventricular dysfunction will develop over time without intervention
  - Associated comorbidities include atrial fibrillation and thromboembolic events
- May require acute and/or chronic management of congestive heart failure due to valve disease; some may even require surgical intervention

Myocarditis

BASIC INFORMATION

- Myocarditis describes inflammation and damage to the myocardium or heart muscle
- Common etiologic agents of myocarditis are summarized in Table 7.4
- Many children will have normalization of ventricular function over time (53% at 3 years), but a proportion of patients (4%–18%) go on to require chronic heart failure management or heart transplantation

CLINICAL PRESENTATION

- Patients may present in a number of ways:
  - Fulminant myocarditis, with the sudden onset of heart failure with severe ventricular dysfunction, shock, and arrhythmias
  - Subacute disease, with the slow development of left ventricular dysfunction and a dilated cardiomyopathy
    - Less likely to demonstrate hypotensive shock; rather, subtle signs such as tachycardia, tachypnea, fatigue, and vague gastrointestinal complaints (abdominal pain, emesis)
  - Sudden death or aborted sudden cardiac death due to a ventricular arrhythmia
- Patients should be asked about a history of preceding illness, particularly viral upper respiratory tract infections

Table 7.4.   Etiologies of Myocarditis

VIRAL (MOST COMMON)

Enteroviruses (Coxsackieviruses A and B)	Cytomegalovirus
Adenovirus	Epstein-Barr virus
HHV6	Hepatitis C
Parvovirus B19	HIV
Influenza A and B	Respiratory syncytial virus

BACTERIAL

Mycoplasma pneumonia	Streptococcus
Chlamydia pneumonia	Lyme disease
Listeria monocytogenes	(*Borrelia burgdorferi*)
Staphylococcus	Tuberculosis
	Corynebacterium diphtheria

FUNGAL

Eosinophilic myocarditis

Toxins	Kawasaki disease
Hypersensitivity reactions Autoimmune disease (systemic lupus erythematosus, irritable bowel disease, sarcoid, etc.)	Parasites: Chagas disease (*Trypanosoma cruzi*)

Giant cell myocarditis

DIAGNOSIS AND EVALUATION

- Laboratory tests may reveal elevated inflammatory markers, elevated troponin T or I, or identification of an infectious agent
- An electrocardiogram (ECG) may show sinus tachycardia, tachyarrhythmias, low voltages, ST- and T-wave changes, conduction delays, or AV block (first to third degree)
- The chest x-ray is abnormal in about 50% of cases with cardiomegaly, pulmonary edema, and/or pleural effusions
- If the diagnosis is suspected, an echocardiogram should be ordered to assess left ventricular function and dilation and to rule out other etiologies of heart failure
- Cardiac MRI can suggest the diagnosis; delayed enhancement of contrast is evidence of myocardial injury and fibrosis
- Endomyocardial biopsy is the gold standard for diagnosis and may show an inflammatory cell infiltrate, cardiac myocyte injury, or an infectious agent

TREATMENT

- Treatment with intravenous immunoglobulin (IVIG) is associated with improved survival from myocarditis
- Heart failure and arrhythmias will require supportive care
- Some patients may require extracorporeal membrane oxygenation (ECMO) as a bridge to myocardial recovery

Pericarditis

BASIC INFORMATION

- Pericarditis refers to inflammation of the pericardial sac
- The most dangerous sequela of pericarditis is cardiac tamponade: compression of the heart by fluid in the pericardial sac
- See Table 7.5 for common etiologies of pericarditis

Table 7.5.   Etiologies of Pericarditis

		Treatment
VIRAL (MOST COMMON)		
Enteroviruses (Coxsackie B)	Cytomegalovirus	Supportive care
Adenovirus	Epstein-Barr virus	NSAIDs
Influenza A and B	Herpes simplex virus	Colchicine
Rubella	HIV	Steroids
Mumps	Respiratory syncytial virus	
Measles	Hepatitis B	
BACTERIAL (VIA HEMATOGENOUS SPREAD)		
Staphylococcus aureus (most common)		IV antibiotics for 3–4 weeks
Haemophilus influenzae	*Pseudomonas aeruginosa*	Drainage of the pericardial fluid via pericardiocentesis or surgical pericardial window
Streptococcus pneumoniae	*Mycoplasma species*	
Other streptococci	*Legionella*	
Neisseria species	*Chlamydia psittaci*	
	Tuberculosis	
Fungal		
Parasitic		
Protozoal		
Rickettsial		
Spirochetal		

ONCOLOGIC PROCESSES

Primary tumors
Metastatic disease
Complication of chemotherapy
Complication of mediastinal irradiation

OTHER

Renal failure
Kawasaki disease
Drug-induced
Hypothyroidism
Trauma
Autoimmune and connective tissue diseases

CLINICAL PRESENTATION

- Chest pain
  - Positional: the pain is usually relieved by sitting upright and leaning forward
  - Pleuritic: the pain is aggravated by movement or coughing
- A friction rub may be heard on examination and is pathognomonic for pericarditis
  - A friction rub will not be present if there is a large pericardial effusion; in these cases, the heart sounds will be muffled on examination
- Patients may have fever or abdominal pain from hepatic distention
- Cardiac tamponade
  - Fluid around the heart limits ventricular filling and therefore limits cardiac output
  - Patients will present with tachycardia, tachypnea, and a narrowed pulse pressure with pulsus paradoxus
  - Beck triad (more common in older children and adults): distant heart sounds, hypotension, jugular venous distention

DIAGNOSIS AND EVALUATION

- Chest x-ray may show cardiomegaly if an effusion is present

- ECG will show diffuse ST-segment elevation, PR depression in the limb leads, T-wave inversions, diffuse low voltages, or electrical alternans if a significant effusion is present
- Echocardiogram can diagnose a pericardial effusion
  - Tamponade is a clinical diagnosis and is *not* diagnosed by echocardiogram

TREATMENT

- See Table 7.5 for treatment of different etiologies of pericarditis
- Tamponade is treated with intravenous fluids and urgent pericardiocentesis

Kawasaki Disease

BASIC INFORMATION

- See Chapter 83 for more details
- Cardiac sequelae include coronary aneurysms:
  - Giant aneurysms carry the risk of sudden death due to thrombosis or rupture of the aneurysm
  - After the disease resolves, the coronary arteries may show evidence of scarring or stenosis at the sites of aneurysms
  - Pericarditis, valvulitis, conduction system disease, and fulminant myocarditis have also been reported

Review Questions

For review questions, please go to ExpertConsult.com.

Suggested Readings

1. Baltimore RS, Gewitz M, Baddour LM, et al. Infective endocarditis in childhood: 2015 update. A scientific statement from the American Heart Association. *Circulation.* 2015;132:1487–1515.
2. Gewitz MH, Baltimore RS, Tani LY, et al. Revision of the Jones criteria for the diagnosis of acute rheumatic fever in the era of Doppler echocardiography: a scientific statement from the American Heart Association. *Circulation.* 2015;131(20):1806–1818.
3. Johnson JN, Cetta F. Pericardial diseases. In: Allen HD, Shaddy RE, Penny DJ, Feltes TF, Cetta F, eds. *Moss and Adams' Heart Disease in Infants, Children, and Adolescents: Including the Fetus and Young Adult.* 9th ed. Philadelphia: Lippincott Williams & Wilkins; 2016:1427–1440.
4. Newburger JW, Takahashi M, Burns JC. Kawasaki disease. *JACC.* 2016;67(21):1738–1749.
5. Newburger JW, Takahashi M, Gerber MA, et al. Diagnosis, treatment and long-term management of Kawasaki disease: a statement for health professional from the committee on rheumatic fever, endocarditis and Kawasaki disease, Council on Cardiovascular Disease in the Young, American Heart Association. *Circulation.* 2004;110:2747–2771.
6. Simpson KE, Anwar S, Canter CE. Myocarditis. In: Allen HD, Shaddy RE, Penny DJ, Feltes TF, Cetta F, eds. *Moss and Adams' Heart Disease in Infants, Children, and Adolescents: Including the Fetus and Young Adult.* 9th ed. Philadelphia: Lippincott Williams & Wilkins; 2016:1313–1330.
7. Wilson W, Taubert KA, Gewitz M, et al. Prevention of infective endocarditis: guidelines from the American Heart Association. *Circulation.* 2007;116:1736–1754.

8 Selected Topics in Cardiology

CHARITHA D. REDDY, MD, NEHA J. PURKEY, MD and ALAINA KIPPS, MD, MS

Arrhythmias

BASIC INFORMATION

- Cardiac dysrhythmias are less common in children than in adults but can be seen in children with structurally normal hearts, and they frequently are seen in children with congenital heart disease or cardiomyopathy
- Arrhythmias can present in a variety of ways, with some children being asymptomatic and others presenting with an abrupt cardiac arrest. Although many arrhythmias may be benign or tolerated well, sustained abnormalities in the heart rate and rhythm can affect function and cause long-term complications
- Arrhythmias can be divided in two broad categories: bradycardias and tachycardias (Fig. 8.1 and Table 8.1)
- Abnormal bradycardic rhythms can be due to sinus node dysfunction or atrioventricular node (atrioventricular [AV] node) dysfunction and usually present with signs and symptoms of fatigue and syncope
- Abnormal tachycardic rhythms are categorized by the morphology of the QRS complex and are characterized as either narrow complex or wide complex tachycardias.
    - When the abnormal signal originates in the atria (supraventricular), conduction still occurs through the normal His-Purkinje system, rapidly depolarizing the ventricle; thus the QRS remains narrow.
    - If the abnormal signal arises from the ventricle, the signal must depolarize cell to cell, causing a wide QRS
- Narrow complex tachycardias can be due to extra conduction pathways that create a reentrant circuit or extra electrical signals in the atria
    - Wolff-Parkinson-White (WPW) is a diagnosis made when a patient has a slurred upstroke (delta wave) of his or her QRS complex on electrocardiography (ECG) in sinus rhythm (See Figure 8.4). This finding indicates the presence of an "accessory pathway." When the accessory pathway is engaged, it creates a rapid pathway for the electrical signal to travel between the atria and ventricles. This tachycardia has an abrupt onset and offset, and patients often complain of palpitations
        - Patients with "high-risk" WPW can have reentrant tachycardia that degenerates into atrial fibrillation, which can then cause ventricular fibrillation (via the accessory pathway transmitting the rapid atrial signal), causing sudden death
        - Only 25% of patients with a reentrant circuit tachycardia have the finding of WPW on their baseline ECG
    - Atrial flutter occurs because of reentrant circuit within the atria

- Atrial fibrillation is due to multiple foci of electrical signals within the atria
- Wide complex tachycardias are defined as rhythms in which the QRS complex is wider than normal for age and baseline (in case patient has a baseline bundle branch block)
    - Wide complex tachycardia is ventricular tachycardia until proven otherwise! Ventricular tachycardia is usually caused by a reentrant circuit within the ventricle (See Figure 8.6)
    - Some patients with supraventricular tachycardia (SVT) and a bundle branch block may also appear to have a wide complex tachycardia
    - Torsades de pointes is a form of ventricular tachycardia with a classic "twisting around a point" of the QRS complex and can progress to ventricular fibrillation and death. Can occur in the setting of hypokalemia or channelopathies like long QT syndrome or Brugada syndrome
    - Ventricular fibrillation is a disorganized rhythm that originates from the ventricle and that does not allow for appropriate filling or emptying of the heart, leading to sudden death
- There are many other rhythm abnormalities that do not contribute to a bradycardia or tachycardia; they may occur transiently or may be related to an underlying diagnosis
    - Premature atrial complexes occur because of early depolarization of a focus separate from the sinus node, causing an early beat (See FIgure 8.7). They are usually benign and found incidentally in children
    - Premature ventricular complexes occur because of an abnormal focus originating in the ventricle, causing the ventricle to depolarize before the next sinus beat and resulting in a wide QRS (See Figure 8.8). These are common in adolescence
- Channelopathies:
    - Genetic mutations in the ion channels critical for cardiac function; they can lead to sudden death
    - Examples of channelopathies include long QT syndrome, Brugada syndrome, and catecholaminergic polymorphic ventricular tachycardia
    - Long QT syndrome (LQTS): due to potassium or sodium channel gene mutations within the myocardium, causing abnormal ventricular repolarization and a prolonged QT interval. The QT interval is assessed by "correcting" for heart rate, giving a "QTc." The QTc is considered abnormal if >450 ms in males and >460 ms in females (See Figure 8.9). Patients may present with palpitations, syncope, or even sudden death as their first manifestation

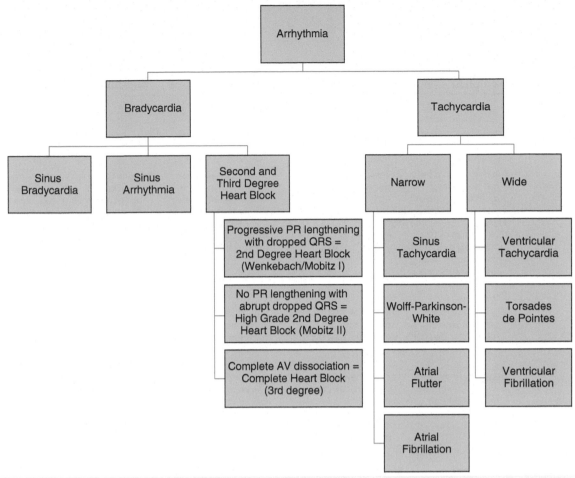

Fig. 8.1. Arrhythmia flow sheet.

Table 8.1. Common Arrhythmias

Arrhythmia	Description	Common Causes	Presentation	Diagnosis	Treatment
BRADYCARDIA					
Sinus Bradycardia	Regular, sinus, slower than normal heart rate for age	Sleep, athletic habitus, anorexia, breath-holding spells, hypothyroidism, medications, steroids, elevated intracranial pressure, severe hypoxia, sinus node dysfunction	■ Can be asymptomatic in athletic individuals ■ If significant, can have fatigue, exercise intolerance, and syncope	Auscultation and ECG	■ May not require treatment ■ Reversible causes should be treated individually ■ Bradycardic arrest: CPR and atropine ■ Sinus node dysfunction can be treated with pacemaker
Sinus Arrhythmia	Irregular, sinus, varying distance between QRS complexes (Fig. 8.2)	Respirophasic variation: heart rate increases with inspiration, decreases with expiration	■ Usually asymptomatic	Auscultation and ECG	■ No treatment required
Second-Degree Heart Block (Wenckebach/Mobitz I)	Gradual PR interval prolongation followed by dropped QRS complex	Occur during times of high vagal tone, often during sleep, athletic habitus, AV node dysfunction	■ Usually asymptomatic	ECG	■ Usually transient and does not require treatment
Second-Degree Heart Block (Mobitz II)	Constant PR interval with abrupt dropped QRS complex	Most common cause of myocarditis, postsurgical complications, AV node dysfunction, Lyme disease	■ Can be asymptomatic ■ Can also have fatigue	ECG	■ Always pathologic ■ Treat reversible cause if present ■ Pacemaker placement if no treatable cause
Third-Degree Heart Block or Complete Heart Block	AV dissociation with constant P wave faster than QRS rate (Fig. 8.3)	Congenital (maternal autoimmune disorders), structural heart disease, postsurgical, Lyme disease	■ Can be asymptomatic ■ Fatigue ■ Syncope	ECG, Holter, exercise test, echocardiogram	■ If reversible, can treat ■ If symptomatic or hemodynamic compromise, will need pacemaker

Continued

Table 8.1.   Common Arrhythmias—cont'd

Arrhythmia	Description	Common Causes	Presentation	Diagnosis	Treatment
TACHYCARDIA					
Narrow Complex					
Sinus Tachycardia	Regular, sinus, faster than normal heart rate for age	Anemia, dehydration, pain/agitation, hyperthyroidism	▪ Usually symptomatic from other causes ▪ May have "palpitations"	Auscultation and ECG	▪ Treat reversible causes, rare in isolation
Supraventricular Tachycardia (SVT) And Wolff-Parkinson-White (WPW)	*Baseline:* sinus, WPW has delta wave causing slurring of P wave into QRS (Fig. 8.4) *In SVT:* narrow QRS complex, much faster than normal heart rate, P waves may not be visible (Fig. 8.5)	Accessory conduction pathway	▪ At baseline, may not have any symptoms ▪ Will feel palpitations during tachycardia ▪ Can have syncope and sudden cardiac death (high-risk WPW)	Baseline ECG, Holter, Exercise test to determine if high risk for sudden death, SVT ECG	▪ *Acute treatment of SVT:* breath-holding, adenosine, direct cardioversion ▪ *Long-term treatment:* beta- blockers, catheter ablation
Atrial Flutter	Regular, "sawtooth pattern" with atrial rates faster than QRS waves	Uncommon in children, can be seen in neonates with no other associations	▪ Can be asymptomatic ▪ If rhythm is very fast, can show hemodynamic compromise	ECG, Holter, echocardiogram to rule out structural heart disease	▪ Direct synchronized cardioversion ▪ Usually neonates do not require further therapy
Atrial Fibrillation	Irregularly irregular, P waves are abnormal and different morphologies, QRS similar to sinus rhythm	Very uncommon in children, can occur in patients with WPW who have SVT that degenerates into atrial fibrillation, postsurgical	▪ Palpitations ▪ Can be at risk of stroke due to left atrial thrombus formation	ECG, Holter, echocardiogram to rule out structural heart disease	▪ Direct cardioversion (must be anticoagulated first due to risk of stroke)
Wide Complex					
Ventricular Tachycardia	Regular, wide complex, QRS different from baseline (Fig. 8.6)	Structural heart disease, postsurgical, myocarditis, long QT, medication overdose, cardiomyopathy	▪ May be asymptomatic ▪ Palpitations ▪ Fatigue ▪ Syncope ▪ <u>Sudden death</u>	ECG, Holter, exercise test, echocardiogram to rule out structural heart disease	▪ If asymptomatic, can consider medical management with beta-blockers ▪ If syncope or aborted sudden cardiac arrest, implantable cardiac defibrillator (ICD) placement
Torsades de Pointes	Irregular, fast, wide complex, sinusoidal pattern along baseline	Hypokalemia, hypomagnesemia Prolonged QTc, Brugada	▪ Palpitations ▪ Syncope ▪ <u>Sudden death</u>	ECG	▪ Correct if reversible cause ▪ If progresses to ventricular fibrillation, defibrillate! ▪ May respond to magnesium
Ventricular Fibrillation	Irregular, wide complex, can be disorganized	Electrolyte abnormalities, channelopathies, postsurgical	▪ Palpitations ▪ Syncope ▪ <u>Sudden death</u>	ECG	▪ Correct if reversible cause ▪ Defibrillate!
MISCELLANEOUS RHYTHM ABNORMALITIES					
Premature Atrial Complex (PAC)	Single, early, narrow complex beat (Fig. 8.7)	Abnormal focus in atria, electrolyte abnormalities, can be normal finding	▪ Likely asymptomatic if isolated	ECG, Holter, electrolytes, echocardiogram if frequent PACs	▪ No treatment necessary in isolation ▪ Can treat reversible causes
Premature Ventricular Complex (PVC)	Single, early, wide complex beat, different QRS than baseline (Fig. 8.8)	Abnormal focus in ventricle, electrolyte abnormalities, Long QT syndrome, myocarditis, HCM, structural heart disease, can be normal finding	▪ Likely asymptomatic if isolated	ECG, Holter, electrolytes, echocardiogram if frequent PVCs	▪ No treatment necessary in isolation ▪ Can treat reversible causes

Table 8.1. Common Arrhythmias—cont'd

Arrhythmia	Description	Common Causes	Presentation	Diagnosis	Treatment
First-Degree Heart Block	PR interval prolonged beyond normal for age	AV node dysfunction, increased vagal tone (e.g., sleep), rheumatic fever, Ebstein's anomaly, Atrial septal defect (ASDs), AV canal defects, hypocalcemia medications	▪ Likely asymptomatic	ECG, Holter, echo-cardiogram if persistent	▪ Usually benign and no treatment required
Prolonged QT	QT interval is corrected (QTc) for heart rate and is prolonged beyond normal for age (Fig. 8.9)	*Congenital:* familial or de novo genetic mutation *Acquired:* electrolyte abnormalities, medications, postsurgical, myocarditis, infections	▪ At baseline, likely asymptomatic ▪ Predisposes to ventricular fibrillation and can cause syncope or <u>sudden death</u>	ECG, Holter, exercise test, echocardio-gram to rule out structural heart disease, genetic testing	▪ Avoid QTc- prolong-ing medications ▪ Beta-blocker for genetic cause ▪ ICD if history of syncope or aborted sudden cardiac arrest

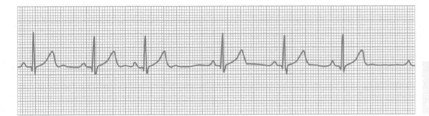

Fig. 8.2. Sinus arrhythmia. (From Beerman LB, Kreutzer J, Allada V. Cardiology. In: Zitelli BJ, McIntire SC, Nowalk AJ. Zitelli and Davis' Atlas of Pediatric Physical Diagnosis. 6th ed. Philadelphia, PA: Saunders; 2012:145–179.)

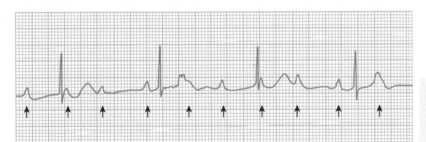

Fig. 8.3. Third-degree heart block/complete heart block. (From Beerman LB, Kreutzer J, Allada V. Cardiology. In: Zitelli BJ, McIntire SC, Nowalk AJ. Zitelli and Davis' Atlas of Pediatric Physical Diagnosis. 6th ed. Philadelphia, PA: Saunders; 2012:145–179.)

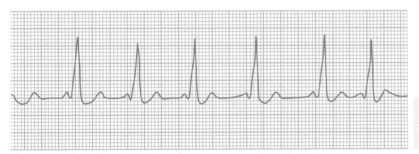

Fig. 8.4. Wolff-Parkinson-White. (From Beerman LB, Kreutzer J, Allada V. Cardiology. In: Zitelli BJ, McIntire SC, Nowalk AJ. Zitelli and Davis' Atlas of Pediatric Physical Diagnosis. 6th ed. Philadelphia, PA: Saunders; 2012:145–179.)

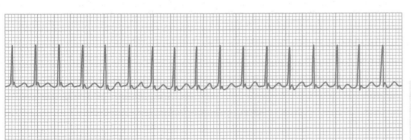

Fig. 8.5. Narrow complex tachycardia – reentrant tachycardia. (From Beerman LB, Kreutzer J, Allada V. Cardiology. In: Zitelli BJ, McIntire SC, Nowalk AJ. Zitelli and Davis' Atlas of Pediatric Physical Diagnosis. 6th ed. Philadelphia, PA: Saunders; 2012:145–179.)

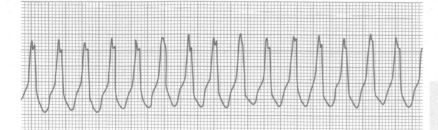

Fig. 8.6. Ventricular tachycardia. (From Beerman LB, Kreutzer J, Allada V. Cardiology. In: Zitelli BJ, McIntire SC, Nowalk AJ. Zitelli and Davis' Atlas of Pediatric Physical Diagnosis. 6th ed. Philadelphia, PA: Saunders; 2012:145–179.)

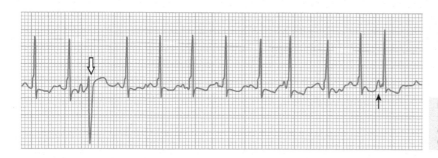

Fig. 8.7. Premature atrial complex. (From Beerman LB, Kreutzer J, Allada V. Cardiology. In: Zitelli BJ, McIntire SC, Nowalk AJ. Zitelli and Davis' Atlas of Pediatric Physical Diagnosis. 6th ed. Philadelphia, PA: Saunders; 2012:145–179.)

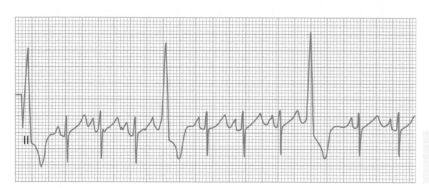

Fig. 8.8. Premature ventricular complex. (From Beerman LB, Kreutzer J, Allada V. Cardiology. In: Zitelli BJ, McIntire SC, Nowalk AJ. Zitelli and Davis' Atlas of Pediatric Physical Diagnosis. 6th ed. Philadelphia, PA: Saunders; 2012:145–179.)

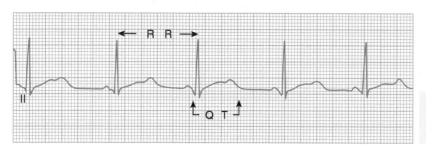

Fig. 8.9. Prolonged QT interval. (From Beerman LB, Kreutzer J, Allada V. Cardiology. In: Zitelli BJ, McIntire SC, Nowalk AJ. *Zitelli and Davis' Atlas of Pediatric Physical Diagnosis.* 6th ed. Philadelphia, PA: Saunders; 2012:145–179.)

- LQTS 1: usually has broad-based, peaked T waves. Triggers: exertion, particularly swimming
- LQTS 2: usually notched T waves. Triggers: auditory (e.g., horns, alarms) and postpartum
- LQTS 3: usually late-breaking but normal T wave. Triggers: events occur during sleep
- Multiple genes have been found to cause long QT syndrome. Autosomal dominant LQTS (Romano-Ward), autosomal recessive LQTS (Jervell and Lange-Nielsen), which is associated with congenital deafness, and multisystem or complex LQTS (Timothy syndrome and Andersen-Tawil) are all

examples. Of note, some patients may be genotype positive but have a normal resting QTc
- Treatment: beta-blockade is first-line therapy. Indications for implantable cardiac defibrillator (ICD) are history of aborted cardiac arrest, syncopal events despite beta-blockade, or noncompliance or intolerance of medication. All patients are recommended to follow exercise restriction, although those recommendations are evolving
- Brugada syndrome is typically associated with a sodium channel mutation causing altered repolarization. The classic ECG finding is a "cove-type" ST-segment

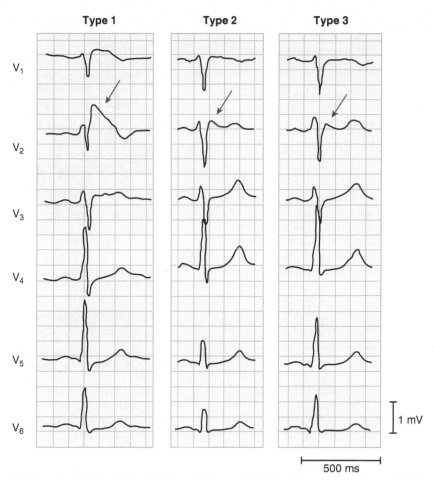

Fig. 8.10. Brugada syndrome. (Olgin JE, Tomaselli GF, Zipes DP. *Braunwald's Heart Disease: A textbook of Cardiovascular Medicine.* 10th ed. Philadelphia, PA: Elsevier/Saunders; 2015: 753–771.)

elevation (see Fig. 8.10). There is a male predominance, and often initial presentation is syncope or sudden cardiac death due to ventricular fibrillation
- See also Nelson Textbook of Pediatrics, Chapter 435, "Disturbances of Rate and Rhythm of the Heart."

CLINICAL PRESENTATION, DIAGNOSIS AND EVALUATION, TREATMENT

- The causes, presentation, diagnosis, and treatment for many of these arrhythmias are discussed in Table 8.1

Congestive Heart Failure

BASIC INFORMATION

- Congestive heart failure (CHF) is defined as an inability of the heart to fill or empty blood adequately
- There are many etiologies for CHF in pediatric patients, including the following: cardiomyopathies, myocarditis, myocardial ischemia, arrhythmia induced, drug induced, sepsis, congenital heart disease, volume overload, and pressure overload
- Symptoms depend on underlying etiology
  - If the systolic function of the ventricle is compromised, this leads to decreased cardiac output

- If the systolic function is preserved but there is volume overload (large left-to-right shunts), this leads to excessive pulmonary blood flow
- If the systolic function is preserved but there is a pressure load, there may be diminished cardiac output as well an inability to fill the heart
- B-type natriuretic peptide (BNP) is a cardiac biomarker used often in the assessment of heart failure. It is released from the ventricular myocardium in response to increased ventricular volume and myocardial stretch. Elevated numbers correlate with progression of heart failure and severity

CLINICAL PRESENTATION

- Most symptoms are related to inadequate cardiac output or pulmonary or systemic overload.
- Inadequate cardiac output: cool extremities, exercise intolerance, fatigue, gallop rhythm
- Pulmonary overload: tachypnea, coarse breath sounds, higher-than-expected saturations in patients with congenital heart disease, difficulty with feeding
- Systemic overload: edema and hepatomegaly
- Acute heart failure: hypotension, tachycardia, poor perfusion

DIAGNOSIS AND EVALUATION

- Chest x-ray (CXR): cardiomegaly, pulmonary edema
- ECG: sinus tachycardia, various findings depending on etiology
- Echocardiogram to evaluate possible etiologies and evaluate ventricular function
- BNP
- Staging of heart failure (see Table 8.2)

TREATMENT

- Depends heavily on etiology and symptoms
- If in acute heart failure: emergent admission to intensive care unit for pressor support, diuretics, fluid restriction
- If in chronic heart failure: diuretics, angiotensin converting enzyme inhibitors, increased caloric intake
- May need to progress to heart transplantation if underlying cause is not reversible

Cardiomyopathies

BASIC INFORMATION

- Cardiomyopathies are diseases that affect the myocardium, resulting in cardiac dysfunction
- There are four types: hypertrophic cardiomyopathy (HCM), dilated cardiomyopathy (DCM), restrictive cardiomyopathy, and arrhythmogenic right ventricular cardiomyopathy. Hypertrophic and DCM are more frequent in the pediatric population
  - **HCM** is disproportionate left ventricular hypertrophy (LVH) without dilation of the left ventricle. Approximately two-thirds of patients with HCM can develop left ventricular outflow obstruction, called **hypertrophic obstructive cardiomyopathy (HOCM).** HCM is the most common genetic heart disease
  - **DCM** is defined by progressive left ventricular dilation and dysfunction leading to decreased cardiac output and heart failure. Approximately 30% of patients with DCM have an underlying genetic disorder, but there are many other etiologies, including myocarditis, chemotherapy, congenital heart disease, myocardial ischemia, and excessive shunting

CLINICAL PRESENTATION

- HCM:
  - May be asymptomatic for a prolonged period of time
  - Common complaint is exercise intolerance, may have chest pain
  - *Without obstruction*: may have no murmur and may be asymptomatic. Can be at risk of arrhythmia and sudden death, unrelated to exercise
  - *With obstruction*: systolic ejection murmur, strong point of maximal impulse (PMI) with ventricular heave. Can be at risk for syncope and sudden death, particularly during exercise
  - Long-standing problems are related to left ventricular outflow obstruction, myocardial ischemia, and diastolic dysfunction

Table 8.2. Ross Classification of Heart Failure in Children

Class I	No limitations or symptoms
Class II	Mild tachypnea or diaphoresis with feeding in infants; dyspnea with exertion in older children
Class III	Marked tachypnea or diaphoresis with feeding in infants and prolonged feeding times with growth failure from congestive heart failure; marked dyspnea on exertion in older children
Class IV	Symptomatic at rest with symptoms such as tachypnea, retractions, grunting, or diaphoresis

Data from Ross RD. The Ross classification for heart failure in children after 25 years: a review and an age-stratified revision. *Pediatr Cardiol.* 2012;33:1295–1300.

- DCM:
  - May be asymptomatic, especially in patients with underlying diagnosis in which DCM develops over time
  - As the disease progresses, patients develop signs of heart failure (see "Congestive Heart Failure")

DIAGNOSIS AND EVALUATION

- ECG: can be variable, showing signs of right ventricular hypertrophy (RVH) or LVH, or arrhythmias
- CXR: pulmonary edema, cardiomegaly
- Echocardiography confirms the diagnosis and helps differentiate types

TREATMENT

- Confirmed diagnosis of HCM requires exercise restriction to allow only low-intensity sports. Medical therapy includes beta-blockade to relax myocardium. If history of syncope, sustained ventricular tachycardia, aborted cardiac arrest, or severe LVH and/or obstruction, an ICD is recommended
- DCM is treated with diuretics and blood-pressure-reducing medications
- As patients progress to failure, they will be referred for heart transplantation

Hyperlipidemia

BASIC INFORMATION

- Dyslipidemia is defined as high levels of total serum cholesterol and low-density lipoprotein (LDL), high levels of triglycerides, or low levels of high-density lipoprotein (HDL)
- It can be associated with cigarette smoking or exposure, obesity, family history of heart attacks or coronary artery disease, and genetic disorders of cholesterol metabolism (familial hypercholesterolemia, hyperbetalipoproteinemia, familial combined hyperlipidemia, etc.) (see Table 8.3)
- There is a higher risk for coronary artery disease in the setting of diabetes, heart transplant, nephrotic syndrome, chronic kidney disease, and Kawasaki disease with coronary aneurysms

Table 8.3.   Genetic Dyslipidemias

Disorder	Lipid Levels	Clinical Findings	Treatment	Genetics
Familial Hypercholesterol-emia (Heterozygous)	High total cholesterol (TC) (~300 mg/dL) High LDL-C (~240 mg/dL)	Asymptomatic in childhood, premature coronary artery disease (30–50 yo)	Statin ± cholesterol absorption inhibitors (e.g., ezetimibe)	Gene dosing response (homozygous more symptomatic than heterozygous)
Familial Hypercholesterol-emia (Homozygous)	High TC (600–1000 mg/dL) High LDL (450–800 mg/dL) Normal triglyceride (TG)	Xanthomas (usually by 5 yo), coronary artery disease in childhood (10–20 yo)	Statin, cholesterol absorption inhibitor, may require more aggressive therapy (apheresis, liver transplant)	Gene dosing response (homozygous more symptomatic than heterozygous)
Familial Hypertriglyceridemia	High TG	Obesity, usually asymptomatic, may have pancreatitis, less risk of premature coronary artery disease	Diet modification, fibric acid derivative (e.g., gemfibrozil)	Autosomal dominant
Hyperapobetalipoprotein-emia	High Apo-B Normal to mildly elevated LDL	Obesity in childhood, premature coronary heart disease	Statin, add fibrates or nicotinic acid if no reduction in Apo-B	May be dominant, recessive gene has not been ruled out
Familial Combined Hyperlipidemia	Elevated TC Mildly elevated LDL-C Elevated TG	Asymptomatic in child-hood, premature coronary	Diet modification, fibric acid derivative ± statin	Dominant

CLINICAL PRESENTATION

- May be asymptomatic and found on a general well-child check
- Examination:
  - Some conditions may cause xanthomas (yellow fatty deposits under the skin), typically around eyes

DIAGNOSIS AND EVALUATION

- Diet history, physical activity assessment, family history, and social history are important components to determine diagnosis as well as tailor management
- Assess associated problems: hypertension, diabetes, endocrine abnormalities
- Lipid screening recommended at ages 9 to 11 and 17 to 21, and more frequently if family history of dyslipidemias

TREATMENT

- Depends on etiology of dyslipidemia
- If related to weight and other reversible factors, recommend increased physical activity and healthy eating
- Inherited disorders may require treatment with statins or other lipid-lowering medications

Genetics and Cardiology

- See Table 8.4 for common genetic diseases and associated structural cardiac diagnoses

Review Questions

For review questions, please go to ExpertConsult.com.

Table 8.4.   Dysmorphology Syndromes and Trisomies with Associated Cardiovascular Abnormalities

Syndrome	Common Cardiac Defect
DiGeorge/velocardiofacial (22q11 deletion)	Aortic arch abnormalities: interrupted arch (type B), right aortic arch Conotruncal abnormalities: truncus arteriosus, tetralogy of Fallot, pulmonary atresia with ventricular septal defect
Ellis–van Creveld	Atrial septal defect or single atrium
Fetal alcohol	Ventricular septal defect
Holt–Oram	Atrial and ventricular septal defects, arrhythmias
Marfan	Dilation of ascending aorta/aortic sinus, aortic and mitral insufficiency
Noonan	Dysplastic pulmonic valve, atrial septal defect
Turner	Coarctation of the aorta, bicuspid aortic valve
Williams	Supravalvular aortic stenosis, pulmonary artery stenosis
Trisomy	
13	Patent ductus arteriosus, septal defects, pulmonic and aortic stenosis (atresia)
18	Ventricular septal defect, polyvalvular disease, coronary abnormalities
21 (Down)	Atrioventricular septal defects, ventricular septal defect, patent ductus arteriosus, anomalous subclavian artery

From Beerman LB, Kreutzer J, Allada V. Cardiology. In: Zitelli BJ, McIntire SC, Nowalk AJ. *Zitelli and Davis' Atlas of Pediatric Physical Diagnosis.* 6th ed. Philadelphia, PA: Saunders; 2012:145–179.

Suggested Readings

1. Al-Khatib SM, Yancy CW, Solis P, et al. 206 AHA/ACC Clinical performance and quality measures for prevention of sudden cardiac death: a report of the American college of cardiology/American heart association task force on performance measures. *Circ Cardiovasc Qual Outcomes.* 2017.

2. Cannon BC, Snyder CS. Disorders of cardiac rhythm and conduction. In: Allen HD, Shaddy RE, Penny DJ, Feltes TF, Cetta F, eds. *Moss and Adams' Heart Disease in Infants, Children, and Adolescents: Including the Fetus and Young Adult.* 9th ed. Philadelphia: Lippincott Williams & Wilkins; 2016:623–653.

3. Expert Panel on Integrated Guidelines for Cardiovascular Health and Risk Reduction in Children and Adolescents, National Heart, Lung, and Blood Institute. Expert panel on integrated guidelines for cardiovascular health and risk reduction in children and adolescents: summary report. *Pediatrics.* 2011;128(suppl 5):S213–S256.

4. Kirk R, Dipchand AI, Rosenthal DN, et al. The International Society for Heart and Lung Transplantation Guidelines for the management of pediatric heart failure: executive summary. [Corrected]. *J Heart Lung Transplant.* 2014;33:888.

5. Tester DJ, Ackerman MJ. Cardiac channelopathies, syncope, and sudden death. In: Allen HD, Shaddy RE, Penny DJ, Feltes TF, Cetta F, eds. *Moss and Adams' Heart Disease in Infants, Children, and Adolescents: Including the Fetus and Young Adult.* 9th ed. Philadelphia: Lippincott Williams & Wilkins; 2016:565–577.

Dermatology

Neonatal Skin Disorders

RAEGAN D. HUNT, MD, PhD

TRANSIENT NEWBORN SKIN ERUPTIONS

Many newborn skin eruptions are benign and self-resolving. Prompt diagnosis and an understanding of the natural history of these entities can often help alleviate parental concern.

Sebaceous Hyperplasia

CLINICAL PRESENTATION

- Physical signs
  - Pinpoint, yellow-hued papules on the forehead, nose, upper cutaneous lip, and cheeks of full-term neonates
- Natural history
  - Gradual disappearance within several weeks of life
  - See also section titled "Sebaceous Hyperplasia," on p. 3116 in Nelson Textbook of Pediatrics, Chapter 647, "Diseases of the Neonate."

Neonatal Cephalic Pustulosis (Neonatal Acne)

CLINICAL PRESENTATION

- Physical signs
  - Erythematous papules and pustules on the forehead, nose, and cheeks of newborns (see Fig. 9.1)
  - Typically develops in the first month of life
  - The lack of comedones (blackheads, whiteheads) and/or acne cysts distinguishes neonatal cephalic pustulosis from true infantile acne
- Natural history
  - Develops in approximately 50% of newborns
  - *Malassezia* spp. yeast contribute to eruption
  - Treatment is usually not needed because lesions spontaneously resolve; if treatment is desired, consider topical azole (antifungal) cream

Milia

CLINICAL PRESENTATION

- Physical signs
  - Superficial, small (~0.5–2 mm), round, white papules, most often on face, gingiva, or palate of neonates
    - Epstein pearls: milia on mucosal palate in neonate
    - Bohn nodules: milia on gingiva in neonate

- Natural history
  - Milia typically spontaneously rupture and resolve with no complications
- Disease associations
  - In rare genetic disorders, newborns may have numerous or persistent milia

Miliaria Crystallina

CLINICAL PRESENTATION

- Physical signs
  - Tiny 0.5- to 1-mm clear, fragile superficial vesicles (see Fig. 9.2)
  - No associated itch or pain
- Natural history
  - Superficial blockage of eccrine sweat ducts in the skin
  - Occurs in the context of overheating, often with swaddling
  - Resolves spontaneously once triggering conditions are corrected

Sucking Blisters

CLINICAL PRESENTATION

- Physical signs
  - One or few isolated blisters (bulla) or ovoid superficial erosions with no surrounding erythema on the upper extremities of healthy newborns
  - Common locations: thumb, radial forearm, first finger
- Natural history
  - Induced by infant sucking of an accessible body part *in utero*
  - Sucking blisters resolve quickly with no complications; supportive wound care is indicated

Transient Neonatal Pustular Melanosis

CLINICAL PRESENTATION

- Physical signs
  - Present at birth
  - Three different characteristic skin lesions:
    - Small, fragile superficial pustules with a nonerythematous base
    - Small collarettes of scale at sites of ruptured pustules

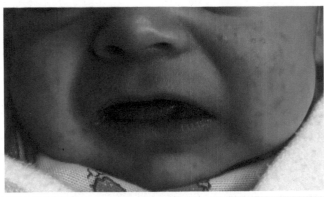

Fig. 9.1. Neonatal cephalic pustulosis. Erythematous papules and pustules scattered on the cheeks of a newborn. No open or closed comedones are present.

Fig. 9.2. Miliaria crystallina. Fragile, small clear superficial vesicles that result from superficial blockage of eccrine sweat ducts.

- Small, hyperpigmented macules at sites of former pustules
- Commonly involved anatomic sites include the forehead, chin, trunk, posterior scalp, and extremities. Palms and soles may be involved
- Expressed pustules show numerous neutrophils but no bacteria on Gram stain; cultures from pustules are sterile
- Natural history
    - More common in full-term versus premature neonates and in black (5%) versus white infants (<1%)
    - Pustules generally last 2 to 3 days, and hyperpigmented macules often persist for several weeks to months
    - No treatment is needed. Lesions self-resolve

Erythema Toxicum Neonatorum

CLINICAL PRESENTATION

- Physical signs
    - Scattered 1- to 2-mm white-to-yellow papules or pustules over splotchy, irregular erythematous macules, mostly on the trunk in term neonates
    - Spares palms and soles
    - Eruption is not present at birth; it typically appears within 2 days to a few weeks of life
- Expressed pustules demonstrate numerous eosinophils on Wright stain; cultures from pustules are sterile
- Natural history
    - Occurs in approximately 50% of full-term neonates; rare in premature infants
    - No treatment needed. Lesions self-resolve, generally in 5 to 14 days

Congenital Cutaneous Candidiasis (CCC)

CLINICAL PRESENTATION

- Physical signs
    - Eruption develops within first week after birth
    - In term infants, CCC presents with widespread erythematous macules, papules, and pustules with superfi-

cial scaling. Palms and soles may be involved. Nails may be thickened and yellowed
- In preterm and low-birthweight infants, CCC may present with erosive dermatitis and is often invasive with multiorgan disease
- Natural history
    - Ascending *Candida* infection; premature rupture of membranes may be subclinical

TREATMENT

- Consultation with infectious disease service is advised. In a healthy term neonate with CCC skin lesions but no other symptoms, watchful waiting or topical antifungal treatment may be reasonable. In a premature infant, systemic antifungals are generally recommended

Seborrheic Dermatitis (Cradle Cap)

CLINICAL PRESENTATION

- Physical signs
    - Greasy, yellow scales on scalp with no hair loss (see Fig. 9.3)
    - Pink erythematous patches in neck, axillary and inguinal folds
- Natural history
    - Most often develops by approximately 2 to 3 months of age
    - Tends to resolve by 12 months of age
    - *Malassezia* spp. yeasts contribute to eruption
- Disease associations
    - Infants with Langerhans cell histiocytosis (LCH) may present with seborrheic dermatitis–like features. Consider LCH as a diagnosis in infants with seborrheic dermatitis who fail to respond to topical treatment, have petechiae in the skinfolds, or demonstrate other concerning signs such as copious ear discharge or excessive urine output

TREATMENT

- Treatment of infantile seborrheic dermatitis is not necessary. Scales from scalp can be removed with mineral oil and soft toothbrush. Antifungal shampoo or cream may

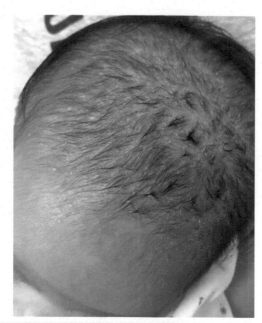

Fig. 9.3. Infantile seborrheic dermatitis of the scalp. Greasy, yellow scalp scaling with no hair loss.

be helpful if this mild eruption is bothersome. In more troubling or symptomatic cases, low-potency topical steroids in ointment or oil base may be a useful treatment addition
- Avoid use of olive oil because it may potentially worsen the eruption by fueling *Malassezia* spp. yeasts

Acropustulosis of Infancy (Infantile Acropustulosis)

CLINICAL PRESENTATION

- Physical signs
  - Cyclic eruptions of pruritic papules and vesicles on the palms, soles, and lateral aspects of palms, soles, and digits
- Natural history
  - Typical age of onset: 2 to 10 months of age
  - Episodes during which new lesions develop generally last 1 to 2 weeks
  - Recurrent cyclic episodes occur every 2 to 6 weeks. The time in between eruptions may gradually become longer as affected children grow older
  - Around age 2 years, episodes generally cease
- Disease associations
  - Possible association with preceding scabies infestation

TREATMENT

- High-potency topical corticosteroids and oral antihistamines help alleviate itch
- If there is concern for scabies infestation, consider therapeutic trial of topical scabicide

Diaper Dermatitis

CLINICAL PRESENTATION

- Physical signs
  - Irritant diaper dermatitis
    - Erythematous, moist patches and/or scale on convex surfaces of buttocks and genitalia
  - Candidal diaper dermatitis
    - Beefy-red erythematous, moist patches involving skinfolds as well as convex surfaces in diaper area
    - Satellite papules and pustules are common
- Natural history
  - Skin exposed to excessive moisture in the diaper area is prone to decreased skin barrier function, frictional damage, irritation from urine or feces, and yeast superinfection
- Disease associations
  - Skin eruptions that are not a direct result of diaper wearing may also occur in the diaper area. These include diaper or "napkin" psoriasis, seborrheic dermatitis, bullous impetigo, acrodermatitis enteropathica, scabies, herpes simplex infections, and LCH. If diaper rash does not improve with standard treatment or has unusual features, these alternative diagnoses should be considered

TREATMENT

- Diapers should be changed promptly when wet or soiled
- Diaper area should be cleansed promptly with gentle soap or cleanser
- Frequent application of barrier ointments or creams is recommended
- If candidal infection is suspected, treat with antiyeast/antifungal topical cream twice daily until clear

Cutis Marmorata

CLINICAL PRESENTATION

- Physical signs
  - Widespread lacy, reticulated, mottled red-blue skin discoloration in newborns
  - Eruption exacerbated by cold temperatures
- Natural history
  - Skin findings result from physiologic vasomotor reaction to cold in neonates. Vasomotor reactivity diminishes with age
- Disease associations
  - Although common in healthy newborns, pronounced cutis marmorata may occur in the following conditions:
    - Down syndrome
    - Trisomy 18 syndrome
    - Cornelia de Lange syndrome
    - Menkes disease
    - Familial dysautonomia

Cutis Marmorata Telangiectatica Congenita (CMTC)

CLINICAL PRESENTATION

- Physical signs
  - Fixed reticulated violaceous atrophic plaques, which are often limited to one or a few segmental areas on extremities (see Fig. 9.4)
  - Lesions do not improve upon exposure to warm temperature
  - Lesions may ulcerate
  - Lesions may be associated with hypoplasia or hyperplasia of the affected limb
- Natural history
  - Considered to be a type of sporadic congenital vascular malformation
  - Lesions tend to fade and improve with time; however, affected children should be monitored for limb asymmetry or other complications

BIRTHMARKS

Benign birthmarks are very common; however, it is critical to recognize birthmarks that may be associated with other medical conditions

Dermal Melanocytosis (Mongolian Spots)

CLINICAL PRESENTATION

- Physical signs
  - Blue-to-gray macules and patches that are most commonly on the presacral skin and buttocks but may occur on shoulders, back, posterior thighs, or extremities
- Natural history
  - Approximately 80% of black, Asian, and East Indian infants are born with cutaneous dermal melanocytosis, whereas the incidence is <10% in white infants
  - Dermal melanocytosis lesions located on the buttocks or presacral area tend to spontaneously fade in the first few years of life, whereas lesions in less typical areas, such as on extremities, may be more persistent
- Disease associations
  - Most commonly, dermal melanocytosis is uncomplicated. However, extensive dermal melanocytosis may be present in children affected by Hurler syndrome (mucopolysaccharidosis 1) and GM1 gangliosidosis

Nevus Simplex (Salmon Patch)

CLINICAL PRESENTATION

- Physical signs
  - Light-pink, blanching vascular patch(es), most often on the glabella, upper eyelids, occipital scalp, and/or nape of neck of healthy neonates

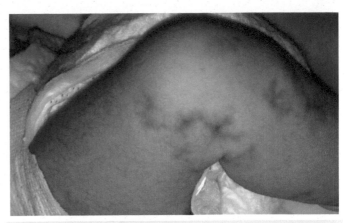

Fig. 9.4. Cutis marmorata telangiectatica congenita. Fixed atrophic reticulated violaceous plaques in the newborn that do not improve with warming of the extremity.

- Natural history
  - Pink discoloration is typically more notable with crying
  - Lesions on eyelids and glabella often disappear in a few years, but large lesions involving most of the central forehead and those on the posterior neck tend to persist

Capillary Malformation (Port-Wine Stain, Nevus Flammeus)

CLINICAL PRESENTATION

- Physical signs
  - Erythematous-to-violaceous nonblanching fixed patches
  - Present at birth
- Natural history
  - May occur on any skin site
  - Do not fade with time
  - May thicken or develop vascular blebs over time

DIAGNOSIS AND EVALUATION

- Although many capillary malformations are uncomplicated, special evaluation is indicated for the following situations:
  - Capillary malformation affecting the forehead and/or eyelid may be an indication of Sturge Weber syndrome (SWS), which is the constellation of a facial capillary stain affecting the forehead, ipsilateral glaucoma, and ipsilateral leptomeningeal angiomatosis. SWS can be associated with seizures and developmental delay. Affected individuals should have an eye examination to rule out glaucoma, and a careful history and neurologic examination should be conducted. Early MRI in the neonatal period is controversial because it does not rule out the condition or change short-term management
  - Isolated periocular capillary malformations can be associated with ipsilateral glaucoma. Ophthalmologic examination is warranted
  - Extensive capillary malformations on the extremities may indicate Klippel-Trenaunay syndrome (KTS). KTS

is characterized by capillary malformation, musculoskeletal overgrowth, and venous malformations. Clinical concerns include cellulitis, lymphedema, deep venous thrombosis, and leg length discrepancy

TREATMENT

- Capillary malformations can be lightened with a series of pulsed dye laser treatments. Referral to Dermatology is warranted

Infantile Hemangioma (IH)

CLINICAL PRESENTATION

- IH are uncommonly noted at birth; most lesions become apparent as they proliferate between 2 weeks and 3 months of life
- See Chapter 12 for details

Congenital Melanocytic Nevi (CMN)

CLINICAL PRESENTATION

- Presents with light brown to dark brown or black macules or barely elevated papules, which may have geographic, well-demarcated borders or speckled patterns interiorly
- See Chapter 12 for details

Nevus Depigmentosus

CLINICAL PRESENTATION

- Physical signs
  - Well-demarcated hypopigmented patch or macule, present since birth
- Natural history
  - Although a congenital lesion, a nevus depigmentosus may become apparent as the infant's pigment increases over first year of life
- Disease associations
  - Tuberous sclerosis should be considered when three or more hypopigmented lesions are observed in an infant

Nevus Anemicus (NA)

CLINICAL PRESENTATION

- Physical signs
  - NA is pale, hypopigmented patch in an infant, caused by local vasoconstriction in skin, which can be exaggerated by vigorously rubbing edges of lesion. Additionally, edges of an NA lesion can be blurred by pressure with glass slide
- Natural history
  - Catecholamine hypersensitivity of affected tissue causes local vasoconstriction, resulting in the pale appearance
- Disease associations
  - There is a high prevalence of NA in neurofibromatosis-1 (NF-1)

Café Au Lait Macules (CALMs)

CLINICAL PRESENTATION

- Physical signs
  - Well-demarcated tan macules or patches
- Natural history
  - Gradual, proportionate growth with the child
- Disease associations
  - Multiple CALMs may be associated with NF-1
  - Large "coast of Maine" CALMs may be associated with McCune-Albright syndrome

Review Questions

For review questions, please go to ExpertConsult.com.

Suggested Readings

1. Cohen B. Differential diagnosis of diaper dermatitis. *Clin Pediatr (Phila)*. 2017;56:22s–16s.
2. Hook KP. Cutaneous vascular anomalies in the neonatal period. *Semin Perinatol*. 2013;37:40–48.
3. Hulsmann AR, Oranje AP. Educational paper: neonatal skin lesions. *Eur J Pediatr*. 2014;173:557–566.
4. Rayala BZ, Morrell DS. Common skin conditions in children: neonatal skin lesions. *FP Essent*. 2017;453:1–17.

10 *Dermatologic Emergencies*

DIANA BARTENSTEIN, MD, JOHANNA S. SONG, MD, MS, and ELENA B. HAWRYLUK, MD, PhD

Most dermatologic conditions do not require immediate medical attention. But for a select few conditions, skin disease can lead to septicemia, shock, and fatal outcome. Early recognition and familiarity with these dermatologic emergencies are crucial for avoiding misdiagnosis and initiating appropriate treatment. For these diagnoses, if there is significant skin involvement, supportive care (maintenance of temperature, increased fluids and nutrition, pain control, wound care to prevent superinfection, dressings and emollients to protect blisters and bullae) is important, and the patient may warrant transfer to an intensive care or burn unit.

See also Nelson Textbook of Pediatrics, Chapter 654, "Vesiculobullous Disorders."

Erythema Multiforme (EM), Stevens-Johnson Syndrome (SJS)/ Toxic Epidermal Necrolysis (TEN)

BASIC INFORMATION

- Classification
  - EM spectrum is benign, self-limiting, and *not a dermatologic emergency*
  - SJS/TEN is distinct from EM but has historically been referred to as "EM major"
  - SJS/TEN occurs on a spectrum of severity and can be rapidly progressive and life-threatening
    - SJS involves <10% of total body surface area (BSA)
    - SJS/TEN overlap involves 10% to 30% BSA
    - TEN involves >30% BSA
- Causes and etiology
  - Delayed-type hypersensitivity reaction; most common causes include:
    - Medications: antiepileptics, sulfonamides, beta-lactams, quinolones, nonsteroidal antiinflammatory drugs (NSAIDs)
    - Infections: *Mycoplasma pneumoniae*, herpes simplex virus (HSV) 1 and 2
    - Less commonly, may be malignancy-related or idiopathic

CLINICAL PRESENTATION

- Physical signs
  - EM
    - Classically, target lesions with three distinct color zones, although other atypical morphologies may present

- SJS/TEN
  - Erythematous or purpuric macules or atypical target lesions progressing to flaccid bullae that desquamate and leave denuded skin
  - Palms and soles can be affected
  - Mucosal (oral, genital, ocular) involvement required for SJS/TEN diagnosis (note: there may also be oral lesions in EM minor, most commonly HSV ulcers)
- Natural history of EM
  - Lesions classically appear within 24 to 72 hours and may persist for up to 2 weeks
  - Recurrent eruptions can occur, especially with HSV infection
- Natural history of SJS/TEN
  - Prodromal symptoms such as fever, myalgias, sore throat, and headache
  - Eruption classically appears 1 to 3 weeks after drug initiation but may occur up to 2 months later
- Complications of SJS/TEN
  - Ophthalmic, pulmonary, gastrointestinal, and genitourinary involvement possible
  - Sepsis/shock
  - SCORTEN scale provides indication of severity and estimates of mortality risk; however, validated in adults may provide insights for pediatric patients (Table 10.1)

DIAGNOSIS AND EVALUATION

- History and physical examination with or without biopsy (clinical diagnosis is often achieved, but biopsy may be useful in challenging presentations)
  - Physical examination for SJS/TEN: positive Nikolsky sign (skin detachment with light pressure)
  - Histology for EM: keratinocyte degeneration, interface vacuolar change, lymphocytic infiltrate
  - Histology for SJS/TEN: full-thickness epidermal necrolysis
    - Urgent frozen tissue examination can differentiate TEN (full-thickness necrosis) vs. staphylococcal scalded skin syndrome (necrosis in granular layer only)
- Laboratory testing
  - EM: none routinely recommended
  - SJS/TEN: complete blood count (CBC), complete metabolic panel (CMP)
    - CBC for evidence of infection
    - CMP including liver enzymes may indicate additional organ involvement

TREATMENT

- Discontinue offending medication or treat underlying infection, and provide supportive care

- For SJS/TEN, in addition to dermatology consultation, consultations with ophthalmology, gynecology/urology, or otolaryngology should be guided by symptoms, to decrease risk of ocular damage and permanent mucosal scarring
- For SJS/TEN, no standard applies for use of active treatment
  - Some providers opt for supportive treatment only
  - The literature supports use of intravenous immunoglobulin (IVIG) or, historically, cyclosporine
  - Research on the efficacy of corticosteroids is mixed (may increase mortality)
  - Etanercept and infliximab are being studied as alternatives

Table 10.1. SCORTEN scale (SCORe of Toxic Epidermal Necrosis)

Risk Factor	Points 0	1
Age	<40 years	>40 years
Associated malignancy	No	Yes
Heart rate	<120 beats per minute	>120 beats per minute
Serum blood urea nitrogen	<28 mg/dL	>28 mg/dL
Body surface involvement	<10%	>10%
Serum glucose	<252 mg/dL	>252 mg/dL

Score	Mortality Rate
0–1	3.2%
2	12.1%
3	35.3%
4	58.3%
5 or more	>90%

Other Drug Reactions

BASIC INFORMATION

- There are various drug-related reactions, including acute generalized exanthematous pustulosis (AGEP) and drug reaction with eosinophilia and systemic symptoms (DRESS) (see Table 10.2)
- Causes and etiology
  - Delayed-type hypersensitivity reaction to medications; most common include:
    - AGEP: beta-lactams, tetracyclines, sulfonamides, antifungals, hydroxychloroquine
    - DRESS: antiepileptics (most commonly carbamazepine, though also caused by phenobarbital and phenytoin), sulfonamides, and allopurinol are common culprits, but various antibiotics, antivirals, and other medications have been implicated

CLINICAL PRESENTATION

- Physical signs
  - AGEP
    - Sterile, nonfollicular pustules on erythematous skin
    - Fever
  - DRESS
    - Erythematous, morbilliform eruption with or without pustules
    - Fever, centrofacial edema, lymphadenopathy
- Natural history and complications
  - AGEP
    - Symptoms occur 24 to 48 hours after start of offending medication
    - Spontaneous resolution in days after cessation of medication
    - Can develop hepatic, renal, pulmonary dysfunction

Table 10.2. Comparison of Pediatric Drug Reactions

	SJS/TEN	DRESS	AGEP	Anaphylactic	Exanthematous (nonemergent)
Skin findings	Mucocutaneous involvement, flaccid bullae, desquamation	Morbilliform with caudal spread with or without pustules	Pustules	Evanescent wheals	Coalescing macules and papules, less frequently urticarial
Systemic complications	Pulmonary, gastrointestinal, ophthalmology, genitourinary	Pulmonary, renal, cardiovascular, CNS, endocrine	Hepatic, renal, pulmonary	Pulmonary, GI, cardiovascular (hypotension)	Low-grade fever
Time to eruption after start of medication	1–3 weeks	2–6 weeks	1–2 days	Minutes to hours	4 to 21 days
Common medication triggers	Antiepileptics, sulfonamides, beta-lactams, quinolones, NSAIDs	Antiepileptics, sulfonamides, allopurinol	Beta-lactams, tetracyclines, sulfonamides, antifungals, hydroxychloroquine	Beta-lactams, aspirin, NSAIDs	Sulfonamides common, but can occur with any medication at any time in treatment course
Histology	Full-thickness epidermal necrolysis	Lymphocytic infiltrate	Subcorneal neutrophilic pustules	N/A	Nonspecific lymphocytic infiltrate with eosinophils
Treatment in addition to discontinuing offending medication and supportive care	With or without IVIG, systemic corticosteroids, and cyclosporine (used but controversial)	Antipruritics and topical corticosteroids with or without oral corticosteroids for organ dysfunction	Antipruritics and topical corticosteroids with or without oral corticosteroids for organ dysfunction	Epinephrine	Antipruritics and topical corticosteroids

AGEP, Acute generalized exanthematous pustulosis; *CNS,* central nervous system; *DRESS,* drug reaction with eosinophilia and systemic symptoms; *IVIG,* intravenous immunoglobulin; *NSAID,* nonsteroidal antiinflammatory drug; *SJS,* Stevens-Johnson syndrome; *TEN,* toxic epidermal necrolysis.

- DRESS
  - Symptoms occur 2 to 6 weeks after start of offending medication
  - Associated with reactivation of herpesvirus 6 (HHV6)
  - Liver involvement is most common (80%); manifestations of other organ dysfunction include pneumonitis, interstitial nephritis, myocarditis, encephalitis, and long-term thyroiditis with hypothyroidism

DIAGNOSIS AND EVALUATION

- History and physical with or without biopsy (clinical diagnosis is often achieved)
  - DRESS: RegiSCAR inclusion criteria (Table 10.3)
  - Histology for DRESS: lymphocytic infiltrate
  - Histology for AGEP: subcorneal neutrophilic pustules
  - Whereas mild mucocutaneous involvement is possible in AGEP and DRESS, SJS/TEN should be excluded whenever a child presents with this feature
- Laboratory testing
  - CBC with differential, basic metabolic panel (BMP), liver function tests (LFTs)
    - AGEP: leukocytosis and neutrophilia
    - DRESS: leukocytosis with atypical lymphocytes, eosinophilia, elevated liver enzymes, elevated kidney function tests
- 2 to 3 months after onset, thyroid function tests should be monitored

TREATMENT

- Discontinue offending medication, provide supportive care
- DRESS: systemic corticosteroids
- Antihistamine and topical corticosteroids for pruritus
- Consider alternative systemic therapy for refractory disease

Staphylococcal Scalded Skin Syndrome (SSSS)

BASIC INFORMATION

- Causes and etiology

Table 10.3. RegiSCAR Inclusion Criteria for DRESS Syndrome

CRITERIA
Hospital-level care
Drug-related presentation suspected
Acute dermatologic eruption*
Fever (temperature >38°C)*
Lymphadenopathy in at least two sites*
Internal organ involvement (at least one organ)
Blood count abnormality (lymphopenia*, lymphocytosis*, eosinophilia*, thrombocytopenia*)

*At least three starred criteria required for diagnosis. *DRESS*, drug reaction with eosinophilia and systemic symptoms.

- Exfoliative toxins A and B from toxigenic *Staphylococcus aureus* target desmoglein 1, found in desmosomes, and are most predominantly located in the superficial epidermis
- In children, focus of infection is usually upper respiratory tract infection; also consider sites of skin breakdown and other typical colonization sites
- Epidemiology
  - More common in infants due to decreased capacity for renal toxin excretion

CLINICAL PRESENTATION

- Physical signs
  - Exfoliative dermatitis with flaccid bullae, localized or generalized (Fig. 10.1)
- Natural history and complications
  - Prodrome of flulike symptoms and irritability
  - Sepsis/shock
  - After resolution, patients can expect no future scarring (epidermal process only) and no recurrence (antibodies protect against future disease)

DIAGNOSIS AND EVALUATION

- History and physical with or without biopsy (clinical diagnosis is often achieved)
  - Positive Nikolsky sign
  - Unlike with SJS/TEN, there are no mucocutaneous blisters or palm/sole involvement
  - Histology: intraepidermal detachment in the stratum granulosum

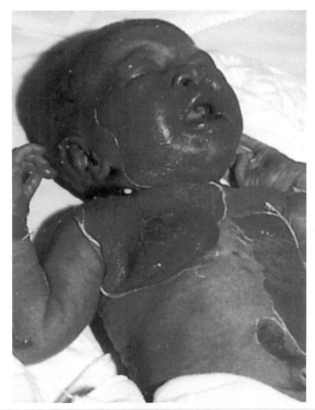

Fig. 10.1. Staphylococcal scalded skin syndrome. (From Kliegman R, Stanton B, St. Geme J, Schor N. *Nelson Textbook of Pediatrics.* 20th ed. Philadelphia, PA: Elsevier; 2016: Fig. 665-4.)

Table 10.4.   Comparison of Skin Findings in Dermatologic Emergencies Caused by Infectious Disease

	SSSS	TSS	Eczema Herpeticum	Necrotizing Fasciitis	Meningococcemia	RMSF
Skin findings	Exfoliative dermatitis with flaccid bullae	Erythroderma followed by desquamation	Monomorphic papulovesicles, crusting, punched-out monomorphic erosions, ulcers	Rubor, erythema, crepitus, ulceration	Morbilliform eruption, petechiae/purpura	Blanching macules and papules with progression to petechiae
Distribution	Localized or generalized	Diffuse; palms and soles may be affected	Overlying eczema	Localized with rapid spread	Trunk and distal extremities	Starts distally and spreads proximally

RMSF, Rocky Mountain spotted fever; *SSSS,* staphylococcal scalded skin syndrome; *TSS,* toxic shock syndrome.

- Urgent frozen tissue examination can differentiate SJS/TEN from SSSS (as described earlier)
- Laboratory testing
  - Bacterial cultures not required; fluid from bullae is typically sterile

TREATMENT

- Supportive care
- Oral or intravenous (IV) antistaphylococcal antibiotics (e.g., vancomycin in severe cases); some physicians may provide additional clindamycin due to inhibition of protein production and reduction of toxins
- Do not give systemic corticosteroids

Toxic Shock Syndrome (TSS)

BASIC INFORMATION

- Causes and etiology
  - Superantigen toxin from *S. aureus* or other bacteria (most commonly group A streptococcus) overstimulates the immune system with nonspecific T cell binding
    - Streptococcal TSS is most severe (mortality rate >50% vs. ~5% for other bacteria)
  - Although historically associated with retained tampon, TSS is now more commonly associated with nasal packing or other wound packing

CLINICAL PRESENTATION

- Physical signs (see Table 10.4 for comparison of skin findings in dermatologic emergencies caused by infectious disease)
  - Diffuse macular erythroderma (similar to sunburn) followed by desquamation 1 to 2 weeks after onset
    - Palms and soles may be affected
    - Streptococcal TSS is less likely to present with generalized eruption
  - High fever, hypotension
- Complications
  - Sepsis/shock
  - Streptococcal TSS may progress to necrotizing fasciitis

DIAGNOSIS AND EVALUATION

- Diagnostic criteria: In addition to hypotension, at least two (streptococcal TSS) or three (staphylococcal TSS) organ systems must be affected for diagnosis (Table 10.5)
- Laboratory testing
  - Perform bacterial cultures to identify source of infection

TREATMENT

- Source control (remove foreign body/debride infected wounds/drain abscesses)
- Supportive care
- Empiric antibiotics until culture results available
  - Suspected staphylococcus: vancomycin/linezolid + clindamycin
  - Suspected streptococcus: penicillin G + clindamycin
- For refractory and complicated cases, consider IVIG

Eczema Herpeticum

BASIC INFORMATION

- Causes and etiology
  - HSV infection of skin
  - Most commonly associated with compromised skin barrier such as atopic dermatitis, but may also present in patients with burns or other dermatitis
- Risk factors
  - Immunosuppression (e.g., cyclosporine for atopic dermatitis, chemotherapy)
  - Early-onset and severe atopic dermatitis

CLINICAL PRESENTATION

- Physical signs
  - Monomorphic papulovesicles overlying eczema with or without crusting; results in classic punched-out monomorphic erosions, ulcers; often painful (Fig. 10.2)
  - Fever, lymphadenopathy
- Natural history and complications
  - Herpes keratitis if periorbital involvement
  - Secondary bacterial infection

Table 10.5. Multisystem Involvement for TSS Diagnosis

Organ System	Streptococcal TSS	TSS Caused by Other Bacteria
Gastrointestinal	–	Vomiting/diarrhea at onset
Musculoskeletal/soft tissue	Necrotizing fasciitis, myositis, gangrene	Myalgia or creatine phosphokinase >2× upper limit of normal
Mucous membranes	–	Vaginal, oropharyngeal, or conjunctival hyperemia
Renal	Creatinine >2× upper limit of normal	Creatinine >2× upper limit of normal, blood urea nitrogen >2× upper limit of normal, or sterile pyuria
Hepatic	Total bilirubin, AST, or ALT >2× upper limit of normal	Total bilirubin, AST, or ALT >2× upper limit of normal
Hematology	Platelets <100,000/mm³	Platelets <100,000/mm³
Pulmonary	Acute respiratory distress syndrome	–
Dermatology	Eruption	*(Rash is often a presenting symptom, but it is not included for criteria.)*
Central nervous system	–	Disorientation/alterations in consciousness

TSS, Toxic shock syndrome.

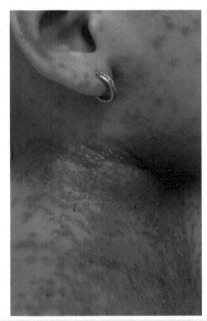

Fig. 10.2. Eczema herpeticum.

DIAGNOSIS AND EVALUATION

- History and physical examination with or without laboratory testing or biopsy (clinical diagnosis is often achieved)
- Laboratory testing
  - Viral culture is the gold standard, but results may take days
  - Tzanck smear is an appropriate rapid bedside test for HSV
  - Alternatives: polymerase chain reaction (PCR), direct fluorescent antibody, serologic testing
  - Skin and blood cultures to evaluate for concurrent secondary bacterial infection

TREATMENT

- Oral or IV acyclovir

- Mild cases, low-risk distribution; stable patient may be treated with oral antiviral medications in the outpatient setting
- Consider oral or IV antistaphylococcal antibiotics for possible secondary bacterial infection
- Immediate ophthalmology consultation if periorbital involvement
- Recurrence prevention
  - Optimize atopic dermatitis management
  - Consider suppressive antivirals if disease is recurrent

Necrotizing Fasciitis

BASIC INFORMATION

- Causes and etiology
  - Soft tissue infection with rapid spread along fascial planes
  - Result of skin barrier disruption
  - Blood vessel thrombosis results in soft tissue necrosis
  - Infection may be polymicrobial or monomicrobial:
    - Polymicrobial ("Type 1"):
      - Gram-positive cocci, Gram-negative rods, anaerobes
      - Mostly affects immunocompromised patients or those with diabetes
      - May occur after surgery or trauma
    - Monomicrobial ("Type 2"):
      - Group A streptococcus (but *S. aureus*/methicillin-resistant *S. aureus* [MRSA] have also been implicated)
      - Affects healthy children
  - Can occur as a consequence of omphalitis at the site of infected umbilical stump in newborns

CLINICAL PRESENTATION

- Physical signs
  - Early dermatologic signs:
    - Severe pain (out of proportion to examination)
    - Warm skin
    - With or without erythema
  - Late dermatologic signs:

- Loss of sensation (due to superficial nerve destruction)
  - Crepitus
  - Ulceration
- Fever, tachycardia
- Natural history
  - Rapid progression
  - May be associated with streptococcal TSS, compartment syndrome, or muscle infection/damage
  - Multiorgan failure possible

DIAGNOSIS AND EVALUATION

- History and physical with or without labs or imaging (clinical diagnosis is often achieved, and negative blood cultures do not rule out a diagnosis of necrotizing fasciitis)
- Laboratory testing
  - Leukocytosis
  - Elevated creatine kinase
  - Elevated lactate
- Imaging
  - Necrotizing fasciitis is a surgical emergency, and in the setting of high clinical suspicion, treatment should not be delayed for imaging or other workup
  - If imaging is performed, options include ultrasound, computed tomography (CT), and magnetic resonance imaging (MRI). MRI is generally recommended for care, but noncontrast CT has the highest sensitivity for detecting fascial plane gas

TREATMENT

- Surgery with repeated debridement until resolution
- IV antibiotics
  - Empirically, antibiotic coverage should cover Gram-positive, Gram-negative (including pseudomonas), and anaerobes. For instance, carbapenem or piperacillin-tazobactam with vancomycin will cover group A streptococcus and MRSA; alternatively, cefepime with Flagyl and vancomycin will provide similar coverage
  - For known group A streptococcus: penicillin and clindamycin

The following dermatologic conditions also require prompt recognition and treatment. Brief summaries of classic findings are provided later for quick comparison and reference:

Kawasaki Disease

BASIC INFORMATION

- See Chapter 83 for details
- The skin involvement in Kawasaki disease is variable, but it may present as an erythematous eruption with primary lesions, including maculopapular, evanescent, or targetoid lesions

Meningococcemia

BASIC INFORMATION

- See Chapter 44 for details.
- Patients presents as septic (from Gram-negative bacteria) with:
  - Early-onset blanching macular/morbilliform eruption
  - Petechiae/purpura on trunk and distal extremities

Rocky Mountain Spotted Fever (RMSF)

- See Chapter 44 for details
  - The skin involvement in RMSF presents as blanching macules and papules, beginning 2 to 5 days after the fever starts, with progression to petechiae
  - The eruption classically starts distally (ankles/wrists) and spreads proximally

Review Questions

For review questions, please go to ExpertConsult.com.

Suggested Readings

1. Bastuji-Garin S, Fouchard N, Bertocchi M, Roujeau JC, Revuz J, Wolkenstein P. SCORTEN: a severity-of-illness score for toxic epidermal necrolysis. *J Invest Dermatol.* 2000;115(2):149–153.
2. Dodiuk-Gad RP, Chung WH, Valeyrie-Allanore L, Shear NH. Stevens-Johnson syndrome and toxic epidermal necrolysis: an update. *Am J Clin Dermatol.* 2015;16(6):475–493.
3. Husain Z, Reddy BY, Schwartz RA. DRESS syndrome: part I. Clinical perspectives. *J Am Acad Dermatol.* 2013;68(5): 693.e1–e14; quiz 706–708.
4. Jamal N, Teach SJ. Necrotizing fasciitis. *Pediatr Emerg Care.* 2011;27(12): 1195–1199; quiz 200–202.
5. Stern RS. Clinical practice. Exanthematous drug eruptions. *N Engl J Med.* 2012;366(26):2492–2501.

11 Infectious Dermatology

LACEY KRUSE, MD

Many common bacterial and viral infections present with dermatologic manifestations. This allows for clinical diagnosis based on history and physical examination, with microbiology to confirm diagnostic suspicions. This chapter focuses on the cutaneous manifestations of infectious diseases; see Chapters 44, 45, and 46 for more details regarding additional manifestations, diagnosis, and treatment of these infectious diseases.

BACTERIAL INFECTIONS

See also Nelson Textbook of Pediatrics, Chapter 665, "Cutaneous Bacterial Infections."

Impetigo

BASIC INFORMATION

- Nonbullous impetigo is most commonly caused by *Staphylococcus aureus*, but it can also be caused by group A streptococcus
- Bullous impetigo is caused only by *S. aureus*
  - *S. aureus* produces an epidermolytic toxin, which cleaves the epidermis, leading to bullae formation

CLINICAL PRESENTATION

- Nonbullous impetigo:
  - Presents as superficial vesicles and/or pustules with honey-colored crust
  - Most often seen on the face and around the nose
- Bullous impetigo:
  - Initial presentation: thin walled, flaccid bullae
  - These quickly rupture, leaving tender, shallow erosions surrounded by a remnant of blister roof
  - Common locations: face, diaper area, extremities

DIAGNOSIS AND EVALUATION

- Diagnosis is typically made clinically; bacterial culture confirms diagnosis

TREATMENT

- If eruption is localized and caused by *S. aureus*, topical antibiotics may be considered
  - Bacitracin, mupirocin, polymixin, gentamycin, erythromycin all effective in mild cases
- For more extensive disease, treatment of choice is oral antibiotics with coverage for both strep and staph (with consideration for personal and community colonization rates of methicillin-resistant *S. aureus* [MRSA] – see later)
  - Examples include penicillinase-resistant penicillin derivatives (dicloxacillin), first (cephalexin) or second

(cefprozil) generation cephalosporins, and clindamycin; MRSA coverage is detailed later
  - Ampicillin/amoxicillin is inappropriate for coverage of staphylococcus
  - Severe infections may warrant intravenous (IV) antibiotics, including those with MRSA coverage (e.g., vancomycin)

Staphylococcal Scalded Skin Syndrome (SSSS)

BASIC INFORMATION

- Causative organism: *S. aureus*, phage group II
  - *S. aureus* produces exfoliative (or epidermolytic) toxins A and B, which cleave epidermal adhesion molecule desmoglein 1
- Most commonly affects children <5 years
  - Decreased renal function in young children impairs ability to excrete the toxin
- See Chapter 10 for details

Community-Acquired MRSA Skin Infections

BASIC INFORMATION

- MRSA is resistant to all beta-lactam antibiotics
  - Methicillin resistance gene, *mecA* (most commonly SCC-mec type IV), encodes an altered penicillin-binding protein
  - Many strains also produce exotoxins, most commonly Panton-Valentine leukocidin (PVL, which kills neutrophils)

CLINICAL PRESENTATION

- MRSA causes skin and soft tissue infections, including abscesses, folliculitis, and cellulitis
- More common in children, young adults, ethnic minorities, and groups with low socioeconomic status

DIAGNOSIS AND EVALUATION

- Bacterial culture is diagnostic
- Many strains also exhibit inducible clindamycin resistance
  - Consider when testing reveals clindamycin susceptibility but erythromycin resistance
  - Inducible clindamycin resistance can be determined by performing a "D test"

TREATMENT

- For abscesses, incise and drain

- Consider adding systemic antibiotics if abscess is recurrent or complicated (i.e., associated cellulitis, multiple sites of involvement, immunosuppressed patient, or symptoms of systemic illness)
- Antibiotic choice is based on local resistance patterns
  - Trimethoprim-sulfamethoxazole, clindamycin, doxycycline, linezolid, vancomycin, rifampin, and fluoroquinolones are often effective
- Consider MRSA decolonization if severe/recurrent infections
  - Intranasal mupirocin, bleach baths, chlorhexidine soap
  - Close contacts are also often colonized

Erysipelas

BASIC INFORMATION

- Superficial cellulitis with involvement of lymphatics
- Most cases are caused by group A streptococcus (less commonly, *S. aureus*)

CLINICAL PRESENTATION

- Presents as warm, painful, bright-red plaques with a well-demarcated border
- Most common sites: face, hands, scalp

DIAGNOSIS AND EVALUATION

- Typically diagnosed clinically; cultures are low yield
- No laboratory workup required, but leukocytosis and elevated in erythrocyte sedimentation rate (ESR) and C-reactive protein (CRP) are common

TREATMENT

- Antibiotic therapy directed at strep (often penicillins, or if penicillin-allergic, macrolides or clindamycin)

Scarlet Fever

BASIC INFORMATION

- Toxin-mediated exanthem caused by group A streptococcus
- More commonly associated with strep pharyngitis than strep skin infections

CLINICAL PRESENTATION

- Begins as fever, throat pain, headache, and chills, along with characteristic exanthem
- Skin eruption: diffuse maculopapular erythema with "sandpaper" or "goosebumps" texture
- Accentuated in skin folds, sometimes with petechial component (Pastia lines)
- In days 1 to 3, tongue appears to have a white coating, with red, edematous papillae
  - At day 4 to 5, the white coating peels off, leaving a red tongue with prominent papillae
- Tender anterior cervical lymphadenopathy is common

- Complications include pneumonia, pericarditis, meningitis, hepatitis, glomerulonephritis, and rheumatic fever
  - Antibiotic therapy for scarlet fever should be started within 9 days of onset to prevent rheumatic fever

DIAGNOSIS AND EVALUATION

- Clinical diagnosis; culture throat for group A streptococcus

Treatment

- Penicillin is first-line; if allergic, consider macrolides or clindamycin

Perianal Streptococcal Dermatitis

BASIC INFORMATION

- Perianal erythema caused by group A streptococcus (or occasionally, *S. aureus*)
- Often overlooked or mistaken for diaper dermatitis or candidiasis

CLINICAL PRESENTATION

- Presents as bright-red, sharply demarcated perianal erythema

DIAGNOSIS AND EVALUATION

- Bacterial culture for *S. aureus* or group A streptococcus
  - Notify laboratory of causative organisms because laboratories often use media selective for enteric pathogens on rectal swabs

TREATMENT

- Penicillin, macrolides, or cephalosporins

Lyme Disease

BASIC INFORMATION

- See Chapter 44 for additional details
- Caused by *Borrelia burgdorferi* (usually transmitted by *Ixodes scapularis*) and is the most common tick-borne illness in the United States
  - Most common in coastal Northeast, mid-Atlantic, and northern central United States

CLINICAL PRESENTATION

- Clinical findings are divided into three stages: early localized, early disseminated, and late
  - Early localized (Stage I)
    - Single lesion of erythema migrans
      Expanding erythematous annular patch, often with a central red papule (at site of tick bite)
    - Constitutional symptoms
      Headache, fatigue, arthralgias, myalgias, fever
      Lymphadenopathy

- Early disseminated (Stage II)
  - Multiple lesions of erythema migrans
  - Lymphadenopathy and constitutional symptoms
  - Neurologic features
    - Facial palsy, meningitis, neuropathy
  - Cardiac features
    - Atrioventricular conduction defects, congestive heart failure, myocarditis
  - Rheumatologic features
    - Arthritis
- Late (Stage III)
  - Neurologic: encephalopathy, encephalomyelitis, peripheral neuropathy
  - Rheumatologic: arthritis

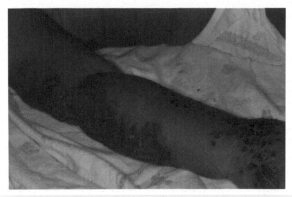

Fig. 11.1. Eczema herpeticum. Note the punched-out, crusted erosions overlying plaques of dermatitis.

DIAGNOSIS AND EVALUATION

- Diagnosis is made by clinical findings in combination with laboratory testing
- Enzyme-linked immunosorbent assay (ELISA) for IgM and IgG antibodies to *Borrelia*
  - Often negative in patients with early localized Lyme disease, which is therefore a clinical diagnosis
  - ELISA for *Borrelia* also limited by high rate of false positives
    - May cross-react with other spirochetes
    - False positive in patients with systemic lupus
    - High rate of positivity in asymptomatic patients from endemic areas
  - Western blot is more specific and can be used to confirm a positive ELISA

TREATMENT

- Early localized Lyme disease: 14 to 21 days of doxycycline in children older than age 8 years
  - Amoxicillin or cefuroxime (erythromycin or azithromycin if penicillin-allergic) for 14 to 21 days in children younger than 8 years
- Early disseminated or late Lyme disease: same regimen; treat for 21 days
- For persistent arthritis, carditis, meningitis, encephalitis: 14 to 21 days of IV penicillin or ceftriaxone

VIRAL INFECTIONS

Cutaneous Herpes

BASIC INFORMATION

- Double-stranded DNA viruses that most commonly infect the epidermis or mucosal surfaces
- After acute infection, the virus establishes latent infection in local nerve ganglia, allowing eventual reactivation
- See Chapter 45 for details regarding diagnosis and treatment

CLINICAL PRESENTATIONS

- Herpetic gingivostomatitis
  - Most commonly affects children ages 1 to 5 years
  - Begins as small vesicles on erythematous bases, which rupture, leaving shallow erosions and ulceration

  - Most common sites: palate, tongue gingivae
  - Often associated with fever, difficulty maintaining oral intake, and irritability
  - Self-limited, but complications include dehydration and secondary infection (staph or strep)
- Herpes labialis
  - Herpetic infection of the lips (classic "cold sore")
  - Typically recurrent due to latent herpes simplex virus (HSV) within trigeminal ganglia
- Herpetic whitlow
  - HSV infection of distal fingers
  - Classically seen in dentists, physicians, or nurses, but autoinoculation in children is common
  - Deep, painful vesicles or pustules on fingertips
- Eczema herpeticum
  - Severe, disseminated HSV infection in patients with atopic dermatitis (eczema) or other chronic skin disease
  - Widespread painful vesicles and red erosions, most pronounced in areas of active eczema (see Fig. 11.1)
- Herpes gladiatorum
  - Widespread primary HSV infection occurring in participants in contact sports, such as wrestling and rugby
  - Most commonly affects head, neck, and arms
  - Severe cases may be accompanied by systemic symptoms including fever, malaise, anorexia, and lymphadenopathy

Varicella

BASIC INFORMATION

- Caused by the varicella-zoster virus, which remains latent in sensory ganglia after infection
  - Reactivation in dermatomal distribution causes herpes zoster (shingles)
- Transmitted via direct contact and respiratory droplet
  - Patients who are not immune may also acquire primary varicella from an individual affected by herpes zoster (shingles)
- Incubation period of 10 to 21 days; patients are contagious 1 to 2 days before the eruption begins and until all lesions are crusted over
- See Chapter 45 for details regarding diagnosis and treatment

CLINICAL PRESENTATION

- Begins with prodrome of fever, coryza, chills, malaise, headache, and myalgia
- Skin lesions appear 1 to 2 days later: vesicles on an erythematous base (dewdrops on a rose petal)
  - Typically begins on head and trunk, then progresses to the extremities
  - New lesions continue to develop as older lesions crust over, leading to the characteristic examination finding of lesions in different stages of healing
    - Contrast with smallpox, in which the vesicles are all in the same stage of healing
- Complications include Reye syndrome (encephalopathy and hepatic dysfunction in patients with varicella who are administered aspirin), Guillain-Barré syndrome, hepatitis, encephalitis, and pneumonia
  - Most common complication: secondary infection with *S. aureus* or group A streptococcus
    - Secondary infection presents as an isolated secondary fever, often with local signs of skin infection

Measles

BASIC INFORMATION

- Caused by rubeola virus, a single-stranded RNA virus in the Paramyxovirus family
- More common in developing world; worse disease associated with vitamin A deficiency
- See Chapter 45 for details regarding diagnosis and treatment

CLINICAL PRESENTATION

- Begins with fever and the "three C's": cough, coryza, conjunctivitis (nonpurulent)
- Koplik spots (gray-white papules on buccal mucosa)
- 2 to 3 days later, exanthem begins on the face, then generalizes to trunk and extremities
  - Disappears in same progression 2 to 3 days later
  - Once the fever has peaked, symptoms typically resolve quickly. If a secondary fever develops, consider secondary bacterial infection
  - Complications: pneumonia, otitis, myocarditis, gastroenteritis, encephalitis

Rubella

BASIC INFORMATION

- Caused by an RNA virus in the Togavirus family
- Transmission via respiratory droplet
- See Chapter 45 for details regarding diagnosis and treatment

CLINICAL PRESENTATION

- Prodrome of fever, occipital lymphadenopathy, pharyngitis, coryza
- 2 to 5 days later, a fine erythematous rash appears on the face, then spreads to trunk and extremities

- Rash resolves within 72 hours
- Arthritis and arthralgias are common, particularly in female patients
- Up to 25% of infected persons are asymptomatic, but they may still transmit the disease

Erythema Infectiosum

BASIC INFORMATION

- Erythema infectiosum, also known as fifth disease, is caused by parvovirus B19
- See Chapter 45 for details regarding diagnosis and treatment

CLINICAL PRESENTATION

- Exanthem typically begins with bright red erythema of the cheeks ("slapped cheek" appearance), then progresses to a generalized lacy erythematous eruption on the extremities
- Eruption fades over 2 to 3 weeks but may intermittently recur
  - Triggers include sun exposure, heat, and physical activity
- Arthralgias are present in 10% of infected children but are much more common in adults (60% of infected adults are female; classic presentation is preschool teacher presenting with arthralgias)
- Petechial eruptions may also be caused by parvovirus B19, including papular-purpuric gloves and socks syndrome (PPGSS)
  - Acute onset of symmetric edema of hands and feet, with petechial or purpuric papules
  - May be associated with fever, arthralgias, and oral petechiae
- Parvovirus B19 can also cause transient anemia via suppression of RBC production (binds to P antigen on erythroid precursors). Anemia can be particularly severe in patients with preexisting disorders of red blood cell (RBC) production (or increased RBC destruction), such as sickle cell disease, spherocytosis, thalassemia, and G6PD deficiency

Roseola

BASIC INFORMATION

- Roseola, also known as sixth disease or exanthem subitum, is caused by human herpesvirus (HHV) 6 or 7
- See Chapter 45 for details regarding diagnosis and treatment

CLINICAL PRESENTATION

- Classic presentation is high fever (39°C or more) for 2 to 3 days
- Defervescence is followed by appearance of the classic exanthem, which begins on the trunk and spreads to the face and extremities
- Oral examination: Nagayama spots (erythematous papules on soft palate/uvula)

Hand-Foot-and-Mouth Disease (HFMD)

BASIC INFORMATION

- Classically caused by Coxsackievirus A16 but may be caused by other strains of Coxsackie A, Coxsackie B, or enterovirus 71
- Coxsackie A6 infection is associated with epidemics and more generalized HFMD
- Fecal-oral transmission, with highest incidence in spring and fall

CLINICAL PRESENTATION

- Begins with prodrome of low-grade fevers, malaise
- 24 hours later, eruption appears
  - Gray-white vesicles on palms and soles
    - Some patients, particularly in epidemics of A6 infection, present with more diffuse vesicular eruption
  - Vesicles and erosions throughout oral mucosa

DIAGNOSIS AND EVALUATION

- Clinical diagnosis

TREATMENT

- Supportive care

Other Viral Exanthems

BASIC INFORMATION

- Several additional viral exanthems are common in pediatric patients, without association with a specific viral agent
- These include nonspecific viral exanthems, Gianotti-Crosti syndrome, and unilateral laterothoracic exanthem

CLINICAL PRESENTATION

- Nonspecific viral exanthems
  - Associated with many viral infections, including respiratory viruses, enteroviruses, influenza, parainfluenza, and respiratory syncytial virus
  - Eruption consists of erythematous macules and papules with a diffuse distribution
  - Clinically difficult to differentiate from drug eruptions
- Gianotti-Crosti syndrome
  - Also known as papular acrodermatitis of childhood
  - In Europe, Gianotti-Crosti syndrome is associated with hepatitis B infection
  - In United States, Epstein-Barr virus (EBV) is the most common cause, although the eruption is also associated with cytomegalovirus (CMV), respiratory virus, and many other viral infections (as well as vaccinations)
  - Patients present with red edematous papules on the face, buttocks, and extremities; the trunk is spared
- Unilateral laterothoracic exanthem

- Eruption begins unilaterally, often on the trunk and axilla (photos often show a child with the arm in the air to display the trunk and axilla, the "Statue of Liberty sign")
- The rash may eventually become bilateral, but the initial area remains the most pronounced
- No consistent association with any one specific virus

DIAGNOSIS AND EVALUATION

- These eruptions are diagnosed clinically

TREATMENT

- Supportive care, because these eruptions resolve spontaneously
- Gianotti-Crosti typically has the most protracted course and resolves over 1 to 3 months
- Unilateral laterothoracic exanthem resolves over 1 to 2 months
- Other viral exanthems typically resolve over 1 to 2 weeks without sequelae

Warts

BASIC INFORMATION

- Common viral skin infection, caused by human papillomavirus (HPV)

CLINICAL PRESENTATION

- Verruca vulgaris (common warts)
- Verruca plana (flat wart)
- Verruca plantaris (plantar wart)
- Condylomata acuminata (genital warts)

DIAGNOSIS AND EVALUATION

- Diagnosis is made clinically
- Condyloma (genital warts) in children should prompt consideration of child abuse
  - Alternative modes of transmission in children include autoinoculation, inoculation from a wart on the hand of a caretaker, and vertical transmission

TREATMENT

- Treatment options include expectant management (50%–65% of warts will resolve spontaneously within 2 years), salicylic acid, cryosurgery, and imiquimod

Molluscum Contagiosum

BASIC INFORMATION

- Common viral infection among school-aged children
- Caused by a pox virus
- Presents with pearly, pink umbilicated papules, most commonly involving trunk (see Fig. 11.2)

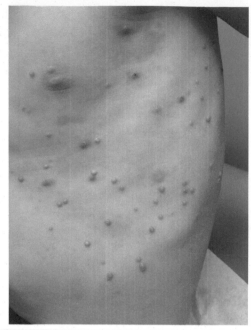

Fig. 11.2. Erythematous to skin-colored, umbilicated papules on the trunk in this patient with molluscum contagiosum.

- Is primarily a clinical diagnosis
- Expectant management if not bothersome, because most have spontaneous resolution over 1 to 2 years; particularly bothersome cases may be treated with Cantharidin or curettage. Imiquimod or tretinoin creams may be helpful in some patients (off-label)

FUNGAL INFECTIONS

Tinea infections

BASIC INFORMATION

- Superficial cutaneous fungal infections (dermatophytoses) are caused by dermatophytes (*Trichophyton tonsurans*, *Trichophyton rubrum*, or *Microsporum canis*)

CLINICAL PRESENTATION

- Tinea infections are categorized by the site involved:
  - Tinea capitis: infection of the scalp, typically seen in children ages 3 to 10 years
    - Characterized by erythema, scale, broken hairs, and alopecia (see Fig. 11.3)
    - Cervical/occipital lymphadenopathy common
    - Kerion is a variant of tinea capitis, in which patients present with a tender, boggy, indurated inflammatory mass, with purulence
    - Patients with tinea capitis may have an associated id reaction ("autoeczematization")
      Id reactions present as monomorphous small skin-colored or erythematous papules on the trunk/extremities
      May present before or after initiation of treatment with antifungals

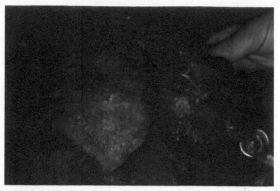

Fig. 11.3. Erythematous, scaly plaques with overlying alopecia in tinea capitis.

  - Although this eruption is self-limited, the rash-associated pruritus typically improves with topical corticosteroids
  - Tinea corporis (also known as "ringworm"): superficial infection of trunk or extremities; clinically characterized by annular erythematous plaques with scaly border and central clearing
  - Tinea pedis (also known as "athlete's foot"): erythematous, pruritic, scaly plaques on plantar and/or dorsal feet, often with involvement of web spaces
  - Tinea manuum: tinea infection of the hand; presents similarly to tinea corporis
  - Tinea faciei: superficial fungal infection of facial skin; often presents with annular scaly plaques, but the scale may be subtle on facial skin, leading to frequent misdiagnosis
  - Tinea cruris (also known as "jock itch"): infection of the groin, inguinal creases, and medial thighs
  - Onychomycosis: fungal infection of the nails (typically toenails); presents as yellow, brown, or white discoloration of the affected nail, with onycholysis (separation from the nail bed) and subungual debris
  - Tinea versicolor: hypopigmented, hyperpigmented, or erythematous patches with fine scale on the chest and upper back
    - Unlike the other superficial fungal infections (which are caused by *Trichophyton* or *Microsporum*), tinea versicolor is caused by *Malassezia furfur* (formerly known as *Pityrosporum ovale* or *orbiculare*)

DIAGNOSIS AND EVALUATION

- Diagnosis is suspected clinically
- Confirm with potassium hydroxide (KOH) preparation of skin scrapings
  - For tinea infections with *Trichophyton* or *Microsporum*, KOH reveals branching hyphae
  - Fungal culture can confirm the presence of *Trichophyton* or *Microsporum*
  - *Microsporum* species fluoresce on Wood's lamp examination, which can aid in clinical diagnosis of tinea capitis (though other causes of tinea capitis, such as *T. tonsurans*, do not fluoresce)
  - In tinea versicolor, KOH preparation shows spores and short hyphae (spaghetti and meatballs)

TREATMENT

- Tinea corporis, pedis, cruris, and manuum are treated with topical antifungals (e.g., ketoconazole cream, terbinafine cream)
- Tinea capitis and faciei are treated with oral antifungal therapy
  - First line for tinea capitis is oral griseofulvin; oral terbinafine or azoles are alternatives
- Topicals are typically ineffective for onychomycosis; if severe or symptomatic, first line is oral terbinafine

Candidiasis

BASIC INFORMATION

- Candida albicans is the most common organism to infect the skin and mucous membranes

CLINICAL PRESENTATION

- Thrush (oral candidiasis) typically affects the tongue, palate, and buccal mucosae. Most commonly seen in infants
- Intertrigo refers to inflammation in the intertriginous areas, such as the neck, groin, intergluteal, and inframammary folds. Not all intertrigo is caused by Candida, but the yeast thrives in this moist, warm environment
- Candidal vulvovaginitis presents as pruritus, erythema, and edema of the labia, and leukorrhea
- Diaper dermatitis is often multifactorial, but Candidiasis should be considered when pustules and satellite lesions are present
- Chronic candidal paronychia presents as chronic nail fold erythema, loss of the cuticle, and often changes in the nail plate

DIAGNOSIS AND EVALUATION

- Diagnosis of candidal infection is clinical but can be confirmed by KOH or fungal culture

TREATMENT

- Thrush: nystatin suspension, massaged into affected mucous membrane
- Intertrigo: topical nystatin
- Vulvovaginitis: intravaginal azole tablets; in adolescents consider a single dose (150 mg) of oral fluconazole
- Diaper dermatitis: topical nystatin or azole antifungals

INFESTATIONS

Scabies

BASIC INFORMATION

- Common skin infestation caused by the mite *Sarcoptes scabiei*, which burrows into the epidermis
- Transmitted by direct contact or by fomites (bedding, clothing)

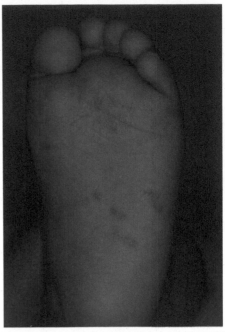

Fig. 11.4. Erythematous papules and linear burrows on the sole in a patient with scabies infestation.

- Infestation typically begins with pruritus, followed by burrows and papules, nodules, or pustules
- Skin lesions are often seen in interdigital web spaces, wrists, umbilicus, groin, palms, and soles (see Fig. 11.4); affected infants often have more widespread involvement, including the trunk, scalp, and extremities
- Diagnosis is confirmed by mineral oil examination of skin scrapings, which reveals mites, eggs, or feces (scybala)
- Treatment of choice is 5% permethrin cream applied from the neck down and rinsed off 8 to 12 hours later, with concurrent treatment of all close contacts. Repeat treatment in 1 week
- Sulfur 6% in petrolatum is an alternative for neonates and pregnant women. Oral ivermectin (off-label) is sometimes considered in immunocompromised patients or severe cases
- Wash all clothing and bedding in hot water to prevent reinfestation

Lice

BASIC INFORMATION

- Three presentations in humans, each caused by a unique species: head lice (*Pediculus humanus capitis*), body lice (*Pediculus humanus corporis*), and pubic lice (*Phthirus pubis*)
- Only the body louse is known to transmit disease in humans (epidemic typhus, relapsing fever, trench fever)
- The head louse and the body louse are similar in appearance: elongated bodies, 1 to 4 mm in size, and six legs; pubic lice are round or crab shaped and also have six legs
- Transmitted by close contact or by fomites such as clothing, hats, or bedding

- Diagnosed clinically by finding live lice or viable nits (0.3–0.8-mm egg sacs) on examination, which are firmly attached to hairs (head and pubic lice) or clothing fibers (body lice) and are difficult to move
- Skin findings include excoriations in the infested areas. "Maculae ceruleae" is an uncommon but characteristic finding in pubic lice, consisting of blue-gray patches on the abdomen and thighs
- First-line treatment for head lice is permethrin 1% cream rinse (though resistance is increasing); additional options include lindane 1% shampoo, malathion 0.5% lotion, ivermectin 0.5% lotion, oral ivermectin, and manual removal of nits
- Treatment for body lice includes improved hygiene, washing of clothing/bedding; can consider addition of permethrin 5% cream or lindane 1% lotion
- Treatment of pubic lice is similar to that of head lice; add topical petrolatum if eyelash involvement is noted

Review Questions

For review QUESTIONS, please go to ExpertConsult.com.

Suggested Readings

1. A Paller and A Mancini. *Hurwitz Clinical Pediatric Dermatology: A Textbook of Skin Disorders of Childhood and Adolescence.* 4th ed.
2. Bernard Cohen. *Pediatric Dermatology.* 4th ed.
3. Marcia Hogeling. *Case-Based Inpatient Pediatric Dermatology.* 2016.

12 Selected Topics in Dermatology

DURI YUN, MD and BRANDI KENNER-BELL, MD

PAPULOSQUAMOUS AND ECZEMATOUS DERMATOSES

Papulosquamous dermatoses refer to rashes that involve papules or plaques with overlying scale and variably associated pruritus. Examples include psoriasis and pityriasis rosea. Eczematous dermatoses refer to rashes where there is significant inflammation with scaly red plaques associated with pruritus and edema within the epidermis. Classic examples include atopic dermatitis and contact dermatitis.

Psoriasis

BASIC INFORMATION

- Accounts for 4% of dermatoses seen in children under 16 years of age; 30% have an immediate family history of psoriasis
- Immune-mediated inflammatory disorder and subsequent expedited proliferation of the epidermis
- Triggers include streptococcal infection, *Staphylococcus aureus*, and Kawasaki disease, and medications such as lithium, beta-blockers, and antimalarials
- See also Nelson Textbook of Pediatrics, Chapter 657, "Diseases of the Epidermis."

CLINICAL PRESENTATION

- Plaque-type psoriasis: symmetric, round, brightly erythematous plaques with overlying silvery white scale most commonly involving the scalp, elbows, knees, and lumbosacral region (Fig. 12.1A)
  - Auspitz sign: removal of scale resulting in punctate bleeding points
  - Woronoff ring: peripheral white ring around psoriatic plaques
  - Koebner phenomenon: isomorphic extension to sites of preceding trauma; this phenomenon is not specific to psoriasis and can occur with other dermatitides (Fig. 12.1B)
- Inverse psoriasis: thin erythematous patches predominantly involving flexural regions: axillae, groin, perineum, central chest, and umbilicus
- Guttate psoriasis: droplike ovoid papules symmetrically distributed on the trunk and extremities; 40% may progress to plaque psoriasis; associated with streptococcal infection of the oropharynx or perianal region or other upper respiratory infection
- Pustular psoriasis: severe variant; collections of numerous pustules overlying an erythematous patch or plaque

- Differential diagnosis: seborrheic dermatitis, tinea capitis/corporis, nummular dermatitis, drug eruption, pityriasis rosea, sarcoidosis

TREATMENT AND MANAGEMENT

- Topical therapy: topical corticosteroid, calcineurin inhibitors (i.e., tacrolimus or pimecrolimus), coal tar, vitamin D_3 analogues (i.e., calcipotriene), retinoids
- Systemic therapy for extensive or refractory cases: methotrexate, cyclosporine, oral retinoids, or biologics including TNF-alpha inhibitors (i.e., adalimumab, etanercept, infliximab)
- Phototherapy (narrowband-ultraviolet B [UVB] therapy)
- Screen for psoriatic arthritis and metabolic syndrome and refer to specialists as needed

Pityriasis Rosea

BASIC INFORMATION

- Self-limited papulosquamous eruption with a possible viral etiology

CLINICAL PRESENTATION

- Herald patch: solitary ovoid peripherally scaly lesion preceding a generalized eruption (Fig. 12.1C)
- Generalized eruption of small papules appearing in crops that follow natural skinfold lines and thus may have a "Christmas tree" orientation on the back. Skin lesions may take 6 weeks to 3 months to clear (Fig. 12.1D)
- Differential diagnosis: tinea corporis, nummular dermatitis, guttate psoriasis, drug eruption, and secondary syphilis in sexually active adolescents

TREATMENT AND MANAGEMENT

- Supportive care for pruritus: antihistamines, topical pramoxine, and mild topical corticosteroids

Atopic Dermatitis

- See Chapter 2 for details

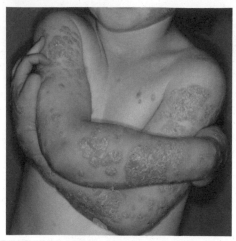

Fig. 12.1A. Plaque psoriasis. Salmon pink erythematous plaques with overlying thick scale. (From Paller AS, Mancini AJ. *Hurwitz Clinical Pediatric Dermatology.* 5th ed. New York: Elsevier; 2016: p. 74, Fig. 4.2.)

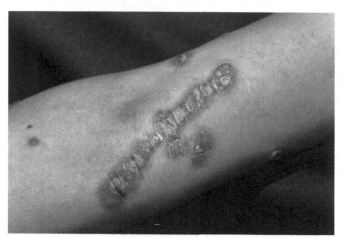

Fig. 12.1B. Koebner phenomenon. Development of linear psoriatic plaque after trauma to the arm. (From Paller AS, Mancini AJ. *Hurwitz Clinical Pediatric Dermatology.* 5th ed. New York: Elsevier; 2016: p. 76, Fig. 4.8.)

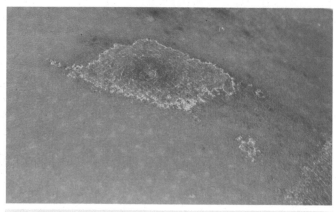

Fig. 12.1C. Herald patch. Ovoid patch with peripheral scale. (From Paller AS, Mancini AJ. *Hurwitz Clinical Pediatric Dermatology.* 5th ed. New York: Elsevier; 2016: p. 89, Fig. 4.38.)

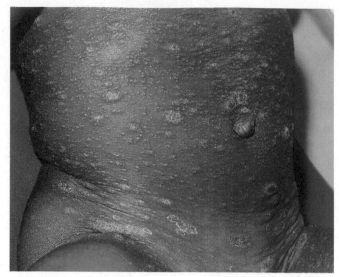

Fig. 12.1D. Pityriasis rosea. Ovoid papules following skinfolds. (From Paller AS, Mancini AJ. *Hurwitz Clinical Pediatric Dermatology.* 5th ed. New York: Elsevier; 2016: p. 90, Fig. 4.42.)

Table 12.1.   Irritant Contact Dermatitis Versus Allergic Contact Dermatitis

	ICD (cytotoxic)	ACD (immune mediated)
Sensitization required	No	Yes
Affect unexposed skin	No	Yes
Dose-related response	Yes	No
Similar response in others with same exposure	Yes	No

ICD, irritant contact dermatitis; *ACD,* allergic contact dermatitis.

CLINICAL PRESENTATION

- Hypopigmented patches involving the face, neck, upper trunk, and proximal extremities, occasionally with fine scale. Symptoms are most apparent after sun exposure
- Differential diagnosis: tinea versicolor, vitiligo, postinflammatory hypopigmentation secondary to atopic dermatitis

TREATMENT AND MANAGEMENT

- Gentle skin care and sun protection to minimize further accentuation of affected skin; mild topical corticosteroids or calcineurin inhibitors may be helpful if scaly

Pityriasis Alba

BASIC INFORMATION

- Common asymptomatic cutaneous disorder representing a nonspecific dermatitis with postinflammatory hypopigmentation

Contact Dermatitis

BASIC INFORMATION

Acute or chronic inflammatory reaction to a substance in contact with the skin, categorized by mode of irritation: cytotoxic versus immune mediated (Table 12.1)

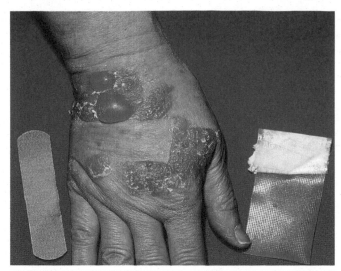

Fig. 12.1E. Acute contact dermatitis from tape. (From Paller AS, Mancini AJ. *Hurwitz Clinical Pediatric Dermatology.* 5th ed. New York: Elsevier; 2016: p. 72, Fig. 3.62.)

- Irritant contact dermatitis (ICD)
  - 80% of contact dermatitis cases
  - Direct cytotoxic effect of chemical on skin cells without distant spread; therefore irritant dose-dependent
  - Common irritants include harsh soaps, bodily fluids such as saliva, stool, and urine
  - Acute ICD presents after limited exposure to irritant, no sensitization (previous exposure) required
  - Chronic ICD presents after repeated exposure to a mild irritant
- Allergic contact dermatitis (ACD)
  - 20% of contact dermatitis cases
  - Type IV immune-mediated hypersensitivity reaction to irritant resulting in delayed onset of symptoms 24 to 96 hours after allergen exposure in sensitized patients
  - Skin previously unexposed to allergen may develop similar dermatitis
  - Nickel and poison ivy are the most common causes of ACD

CLINICAL PRESENTATION

- ICD/ACD
  - Acute: various morphologies, including erythematous patches and plaques that can develop vesicles and bullae with sharp geometric borders corresponding to irritant exposure (Fig. 12.1E)
  - Chronic: lichenified plaques with secondary scaling and fissuring
- Differential diagnosis: atopic dermatitis, psoriasis, lichen simplex chronicus

TREATMENT AND MANAGEMENT

- Avoidance of irritant or allergen and supportive care with topical corticosteroids and emollients
- Systemic steroids with prolonged steroid taper are indicated for severe cases
- Patch test for ACD to identify specific allergens if symptoms persist despite compliant treatment

Acne Vulgaris

BACKGROUND INFORMATION

- Most common skin problem in the United States
- Inflammatory disorder of the pilosebaceous unit with multiple pathogenic factors, including hyperkeratinization, androgen stimulation, bacterial overgrowth, and inflammation

CLINICAL PRESENTATION

- Acne lesions can present initially as microcomedones (subclinical) and progress to open/closed comedones, papules, pustules, nodules, and cysts with adverse sequelae, including dyspigmentation and scarring; there is rarely keloid formation
- Presents as prepubertal acne, ages 7 to 11 years, and adolescent acne after the age of 12 years
- Acne fulminans
  - Rare, severe form of acne vulgaris that presents acutely with painful nodular lesions on the face, chest, shoulders, and back with associated fever, leukocytosis, and musculoskeletal pain

Acne Variants

- Neonatal acne (0–6 weeks)
  - Affects 20% of newborns within the first few weeks of life and spontaneously resolves over 3 to 6 months
  - Differential diagnosis: neonatal cephalic pustulosis, infection, erythema toxicum, eosinophilic folliculitis
- Infantile acne
  - Affects patients between 6 weeks and 12 months of life. Typically presents as comedonal lesions but can also have more inflammatory pustules and papules. Treatment may be indicated to prevent scarring
  - Differential diagnosis: eosinophilic folliculitis, milia
- Mid-childhood acne
  - Onset between 12 months and 7 years of life, and some may be related to underlying endocrine abnormalities. This diagnosis can be considered if there are acneiform lesions and signs of androgen excess in acne patients, including body odor, axillary/pubic hair development, cliteromegaly, or growth acceleration
  - Differential diagnosis: periorificial dermatitis, sarcoidosis

TREATMENT AND MANAGEMENT

- If there is concern for hyperandrogenism, especially in children presenting with acne from 1 to 7 years of age, consider serum testosterone, luteinizing hormone (LH), follicle-stimulating hormone (FSH), dehydroepiandrosterone sulfate (DHEAS), 17-hydroxyprogesterone, prolactin, and radiographic bone age
- Initial management of acne should always include a topical retinoid that is comedolytic and consideration of a topical antibiotic if there is concern for bacterial overgrowth (i.e., benzoyl peroxide ± clindamycin/dapsone)
- For more inflammatory lesions, systemic therapy may be required such as an oral antibiotic, isotretinoin, or oral contraceptives

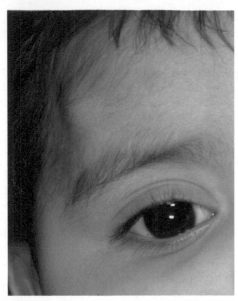

Fig. 12.2A. Dermoid cyst. (From Paller AS, Mancini AJ. *Hurwitz Clinical Pediatric Dermatology*. 5th ed. New York: Elsevier; 2016: p. 27, Fig. 2.37.)

EPIDERMAL, APPENDAGEAL, AND DERMAL TUMORS

Dermoid Cyst

BASIC INFORMATION

- Epithelium-lined cyst formed along embryonic fusion planes presenting as a congenital lesion, classically along the lateral orbital eyebrow along the orbital rim (Fig. 12.2A)
- Approximately 3% can involve the nasal midline (glabella, dorsal nose, columella)
- Differential diagnosis: epidermal cyst, deep hemangioma
- Midline lesions should be evaluated radiographically before invasive diagnostic or therapeutic interventions because there is an increased risk of intracranial communication
- Surgical excision is the recommended treatment

Nevus Sebaceous

BASIC INFORMATION

- Common benign congenital hamartoma of sebaceous elements typically located on the scalp or face

CLINICAL PRESENTATION

- Hairless, yellow-orange plaque, which thickens and develops a pebbly texture during adolescence (Fig. 12.2B)
- After puberty, benign tumors (trichoblastoma, syringocystadenoma papilliferum) and, very rarely, malignant tumors (basal cell carcinoma <1%) can develop within this lesion
- Multiple lesions may be associated with cerebral, ocular, and skeletal abnormalities (Schimmelpenning syndrome)
- Differential diagnosis: epidermal nevus, nevus comedonicus, aplasia cutis congenita

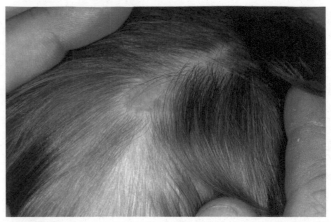

Fig. 12.2B. Nevus sebaceous. (From Paller AS, Mancini AJ. *Hurwitz Clinical Pediatric Dermatology*. 5th ed. New York: Elsevier; 2016: p. 211, Fig. 9.41.)

TREATMENT

- Surgical excision has been recommended due to potential disfigurement and development of secondary neoplasms within this lesion
- Timing of excision depends on size and risks of anesthesia to the patient

Mastocytosis

BASIC INFORMATION

- Spectrum of disorders with mast cell proliferation within the skin and other organs
- See Chapter 4 for details

AUTOIMMUNE DISORDERS

Lichen Sclerosus et Atrophicus

BASIC INFORMATION

- Primarily affects females
- Autoantibodies against extracellular matrix protein-1 and BP180 in the skin
- Associated with risk of squamous cell carcinoma within the affected area, which is decreased by treatment

CLINICAL PRESENTATION

- Anogenital presentation: pruritic hypopigmented atrophic plaques, sometimes with pink inflammatory border or purpura. Perianal/vulvar involvement resembles a figure-of-eight pattern. Associated symptoms include dysuria, constipation, pain, and bleeding (Fig. 12.3A)
  - In males, the dorsum of the glans penis can be involved and is called *balanitis xerotica obliterans*
- Extragenital lesions are typically asymptomatic, slightly raised, flat-topped, white papules or plaques with atrophic "cigarette-paper wrinkling" and often have associated anogenital involvement
- Differential diagnosis: child abuse, vitiligo, irritant or contact dermatitis

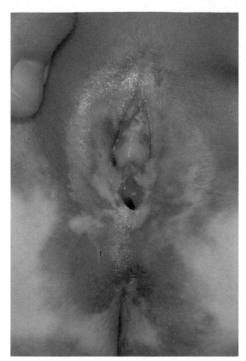

Fig. 12.3A. Lichen sclerosus et atrophicus. (From Paller AS, Mancini AJ. *Hurwitz Clinical Pediatric Dermatology.* 5th ed. New York: Elsevier; 2016: p. 535, Fig. 22.52.)

TREATMENT

- Anogenital
  - High-potency topical steroids for 2 to 3 months for active disease with gradual taper and maintenance treatment with topical calcineurin inhibitors (i.e., tacrolimus ointment or pimecrolimus cream)
  - Plastic surgery for labial fusion or clitoral obliteration and circumcision for male patients presenting with phimosis
  - Stool softeners for patients with associated constipation
- Extragenital
  - Significantly more difficult to treat; topical steroids, retinoids, and UVA1 phototherapy have been reported to be helpful

Vitiligo

BASIC INFORMATION

- Disorder in which melanocytes are targeted by antigen-specific cytotoxic T cells
- Prepubertal onset is associated with a greater likelihood of a family history of vitiligo
- Often associated with other autoimmune disorders, such as hypothyroidism and alopecia areata

CLINICAL PRESENTATION

- Depigmented, smooth patches surrounded by normal pigmented skin; accentuated by Woods lamp evaluation (Fig. 12.3B)
- Favors periorificial regions and bony prominences; exhibits Koebner phenomenon

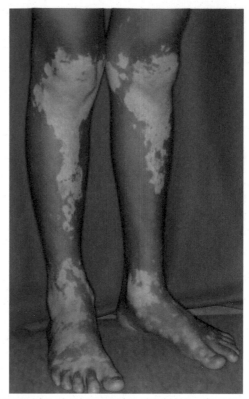

Fig. 12.3B. Vitiligo. (From Paller AS, Mancini AJ. *Hurwitz Clinical Pediatric Dermatology.* 5th ed. New York: Elsevier; 2016: p. 246, Fig. 11.3.)

- Associated with halo nevi (see later)
- Poliosis: patches of white hair in which the melanocytes residing in the hair follicles have been targeted
- Differential diagnosis: pigmentary mosaicism, lichen sclerosus, pityriasis alba

TREATMENT AND MANAGEMENT

- Likelihood of repigmentation depends on the density of hair follicles of the affected skin because they serve as reservoirs of melanocytes. Facial involvement typically recovers more easily than acral areas (i.e., hands and feet)
- Topicals: moderate- to high-potency corticosteroids, calcineurin inhibitors (i.e., tacrolimus ointment or pimecrolimus cream)
- Phototherapy
- Psychosocial support
- Consider screening for thyroid dysfunction and antithyroid antibodies

MELANOCYTIC LESIONS

Congenital Nevus

BASIC INFORMATION

- Subset of melanocytic lesions with an increased risk of malignant transformation to melanoma, particularly in large and giant congenital nevi
- Incidence: 1% of newborns

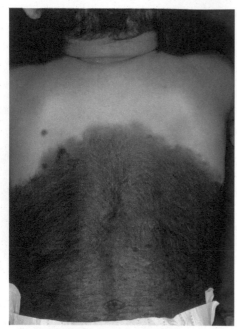

Fig. 12.4A. Giant congenital nevus with satellite lesion. (From Paller AS, Mancini AJ. *Hurwitz Clinical Pediatric Dermatology.* 5th ed. New York: Elsevier; 2016: p. 197, Fig. 9.13.)

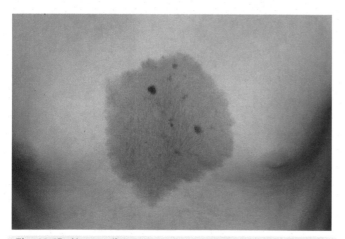

Fig. 12.4B. Nevus spilus. (From Paller AS, Mancini AJ. *Hurwitz Clinical Pediatric Dermatology.* 5th ed. New York: Elsevier; 2016: p. 204, Fig. 9.29.)

CLINICAL PRESENTATION

- Present at birth or within the first year of life
- Categorized by projected diameter size by adulthood: small (<1.5 cm), medium (1.5–20 cm), large (20–40 cm), giant (>40 cm)
- Satellite nevi: smaller disseminated congenital nevi in a patient with a large or giant congenital nevus (Fig. 12.4A)
- Nevus spilus: a combination of dark macules and/or papules within a solitary tan patch (Fig. 12.4B)
- Differential diagnosis: café-au-lait patch, dermal melanocytosis, mastocytoma

TREATMENT AND MANAGEMENT

- Sun protection and regular surveillance
- Observation for smaller lesions; excision for larger lesions and lesions that are difficult to monitor routinely, such as the scalp, back, and groin

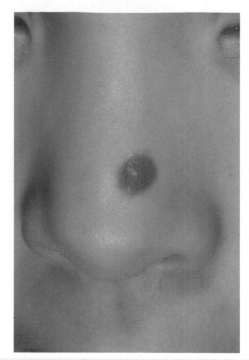

Fig. 12.4C. Spitz nevus. (From Paller AS, Mancini AJ. *Hurwitz Clinical Pediatric Dermatology.* 5th ed. New York: Elsevier; 2016: p. 202, Fig. 9.22.)

- Consider evaluation for neurocutaneous melanosis—leptomeningeal melanocytosis in which nevus cells proliferate within the central nervous system and can present with seizures; magnetic resonance (MR) imaging is recommended in patients with large or congenital nevi with significant number of satellite nevi
- Melanoma screening: congenital nevi with irregular pigment or rapid growth should be biopsied to rule out melanoma; malignant change typically occurs in adulthood. Risk of melanoma in small and medium congenital nevi is very low; the risk is significantly greater in large and giant congenital nevi and can be as high as 3.1%

Spitz Nevus

BASIC INFORMATION

- Subtype of melanocytic nevus that occurs primarily within the first two decades of life
- Smooth dome-shaped pink, red-brown, or black papule (Fig. 12.4C). Some will have surface telangiectasia. Can be congenital or, rarely, agminated (grouped)
- Differential diagnosis: hemangioma, pyogenic granuloma, xanthogranuloma, melanoma
- Biopsy is definitive, and complete excision is recommended because up to 5% of Spitz nevi can recur and are more likely to be misinterpreted as melanoma

Halo Nevus

BASIC INFORMATION

- Due to localized immune response to nevus melanocytes
- Commonly seen in children and adolescents
- Associated with an increased risk of vitiligo

CLINICAL PRESENTATION

- Rim of depigmentation or hypopigmentation around a central nevus
- Typically noted on the trunk
- Differential diagnosis: dysplastic nevus, vitiligo

TREATMENT AND MANAGEMENT

- Observation; halo nevi in adults have been associated with melanoma, but this association has not been found in the pediatric population
- Should the pigmented portion of the halo nevus appear atypical, an excision is warranted
- Perform a complete skin examination to rule out vitiligo elsewhere

VASCULAR DISORDERS

Infantile Hemangioma

BASIC INFORMATION

- Most common benign vascular tumor of childhood
- Risk factors include prematurity, placental complications, and female gender
- Can present as superficial, deep, or combined phenotypes
- Natural history
  - Precursor stage: initially presents at birth as a faint vascular stain, telangiectasia, or even pallor
  - Proliferative stage:
    - Clinically evident by 2 to 3 weeks of life
    - Typically has significant clinical growth for the first year of life with the greatest growth velocity before 6 months of age
  - Involution stage:
    - Color changes from bright red to dull red, purple, or grayish
      Rule of 10s: complete involution by a rate of 10% per year (e.g., 30% by age 3 years, 50% by age 5 years, 90% by age 9 years)

CLINICAL PRESENTATION

- Superficial hemangioma:
  - Bright-red papule or plaque (Fig. 12.5A)
- Deep hemangioma:
  - Subcutaneous, partially compressible with overlying blue hue or prominent venous network (Fig. 12.5B)
- Minimal or arrested growth type
  - Prominent telangiectasis that exhibits very little proliferation during the proliferative stage; prone to ulcerate
- Segmental hemangioma:
  - Involves a broad anatomic region or recognized developmental unit; therefore it often presents unilaterally and sharply demarcated at the midline
  - Higher risk of internal complications
  - PHACE syndrome (*p*osterior fossa anomalies, *h*emangioma, *a*rterial lesions, *c*ardiac abnormalities/aortic coarctation, *e*ye abnormalities)

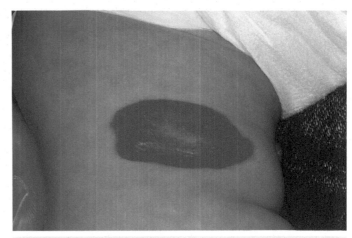

Fig. 12.5A. Superficial hemangioma. (From Paller AS, Mancini AJ. *Hurwitz Clinical Pediatric Dermatology.* 5th ed. New York: Elsevier; 2016: p. 281, Fig. 12.5.)

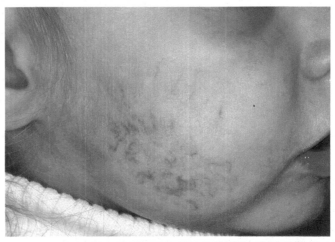

Fig. 12.5B. Deep hemangioma. (From Paller AS, Mancini AJ. *Hurwitz Clinical Pediatric Dermatology.* 5th ed. New York: Elsevier; 2016: p. 281, Fig. 12.8.)

  - LUMBAR syndrome (*l*ower body infantile hemangioma, *u*rogenital anomalies/ulceration, *m*yelopathy, *b*ony deformities, *a*norectal malformations/*a*rterial anomalies, *r*enal anomalies)
- Neonatal hemangiomatosis
  - Multiple cutaneous hemangiomas (>5) with extracutaneous organ involvement
  - Most common extracutaneous organ involved is the liver, which can be asymptomatic or significantly large enough to cause shunting and subsequent high-output cardiac failure, as well as severe hypothyroidism
- Differential diagnosis: port-wine stain, venous malformation, tufted angioma, infantile myofibromatosis, rhabdomyosarcoma

TREATMENT AND MANAGEMENT

- In cases in which the diagnosis is unclear, biopsy is confirmatory with positive glucose transporter 1 (GLUT-1) immunohistochemical staining
- Further workup:

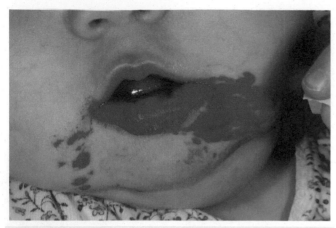

Fig. 12.5C. Hemangioma, beard distribution. (From Paller AS, Mancini AJ. *Hurwitz Clinical Pediatric Dermatology.* 5th ed. New York: Elsevier; 2016: p. 288, Fig. 12.33.)

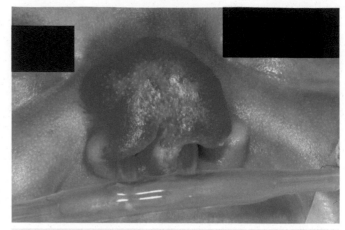

Fig. 12.5D. Hemangioma, nose. Note the destruction of the nasal cartilage and near collapse of the columella from the proliferating hemangioma. (From Paller AS, Mancini AJ. *Hurwitz Clinical Pediatric Dermatology.* 5th ed. New York: Elsevier; 2016: p. 288, Fig. 12.30.)

- Segmental hemangioma of the face or facial hemangioma >5 cm²: PHACE workup should be completed, including an MRI/MRA (MR imaging/angiography) to evaluate for brain and cerebrovascular abnormalities, an echocardiogram for aortic arch abnormalities, and an ocular examination
- Hemangiomas involving the midline lumbosacral region: LUMBAR workup should be completed, including an MRI examination of the spine and a renal ultrasound to rule out spinal and renal abnormalities
- Hemangiomas involving the "beard area" such as the neck, lower lip, chin, preauricular and mandibular area: increased risk of airway involvement; requires otolaryngology evaluation (Fig. 12.5C)
- >5 hemangiomas: complete an ultrasound of the liver and spleen to look for extracutaneous lesions and evaluate for thyroid function
- For small, uncomplicated hemangiomas causing no functional impairment or potential cosmetic disfigurement, observation is the treatment of choice
- Treatment of hemangiomas is indicated when the hemangioma imposes a possible functional impairment such as obstruction of vision, obstruction of hearing, nasal deformity (Fig. 12.5D), parotid involvement, airway involvement, significant liver involvement, or ulceration of the hemangioma
- Treatment, if indicated, is preferably instituted within 6 months of life, and options include topical timolol, topical steroids, systemic propranolol therapy, systemic corticosteroid therapy, and intralesional corticosteroid injections

Table 12.2. Port-Wine Stain–Associated Syndromes

Sturge-Weber syndrome	▪ Segmental port-wine stain (PWS) of the face ▪ Triad of PWS, glaucoma, and leptomeningeal angiomatosis associated with seizures
Klippel-Trenaunay syndrome	▪ Segmental PWS of the extremity ▪ Triad of PWS, gradual venous varicosities, and hyperplasia of the soft tissue and bone
Parkes Weber syndrome	▪ Segmental PWS of the extremity ▪ Triad of PWS, arteriovenous malformation, and hyperplasia of the soft tissue and bone
Macrocephaly-capillary malformation syndrome	▪ Centrofacial capillary malformation ▪ Evaluate for macrocephaly (ventriculomegaly, megalencephaly, and/or cerebellar tonsillar herniation)
Capillary malformation-arteriovenous malformation syndrome	▪ Multiple capillary malformations that develop during childhood instead of at birth ▪ Evaluate for *RASA1* mutation as well as brain/spine imaging due to high risk of AVMs within the brain and spine
Other syndromes associated with PWS	Phakomatosis pigmentovascularis Proteus syndrome Cobb syndrome Bannayan-Riley-Ruvalcaba syndrome Beckwith-Wiedemann syndrome Von Hippel-Lindau disease Rubinstein-Taybi syndrome

Port-Wine Stain

BASIC INFORMATION

- Capillary malformation, typically with congenital onset
- Can be an isolated finding or associated with syndromes (Table 12.2)

CLINICAL PRESENTATION

- Typically presents at birth as a partially blanchable to nonblanchable dark-red to pink patch that is most often noted on the face and typically unilateral
- Grows proportionately with the patient with thickening and darkening over time; can develop vascular blebs on the surface
- Differential diagnosis: nevus simplex (salmon patch), infantile hemangioma

TREATMENT AND MANAGEMENT

- Further evaluation is dependent on the location of the port-wine stain
- Treatment modalities include pulsed dye laser, rapamycin (topical or systemic), and supportive care that includes tinted cosmetics

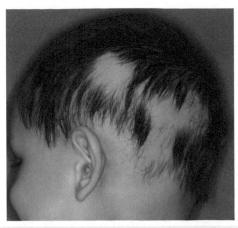

Fig. 12.6A. Alopecia areata. (From Paller AS, Mancini AJ. *Hurwitz Clinical Pediatric Dermatology.* 5th ed. New York: Elsevier; 2016: p. 154, Fig. 7.32.)

HAIR DISORDERS

Alopecia Areata

BASIC INFORMATION

- Most common nonscarring alopecia
- Likely autoimmune-mediated, targeting hair follicles

CLINICAL PRESENTATION

- Acute onset of smooth round or ovoid patches of hair loss (Fig. 12.6A)
- Depigmented or hypopigmented hairs may be seen
- Alopecia totalis
  - Complete loss of scalp hair
- Alopecia universalis
  - Complete hair loss on the scalp, eyebrows, eyelashes, and often body
- Ophiasis pattern
  - Hair loss pattern characterized by involvement of the occipital scalp and extending anteriorly toward the ears
- Characteristic nail changes of fine indentations or "pitting" in a gridlike pattern can be seen
- Differential diagnosis: trichotillomania, tinea capitis, telogen effluvium

TREATMENT AND MANAGEMENT

- Because alopecia areata can be associated with autoimmune thyroid disease, consider evaluating thyroid function and thyroid antibodies for extensive disease or a strong family history of autoimmunity
- Treatment of affected areas does not prevent areas of new involvement, and despite successful treatment, many patients will relapse
- Focal involvement: high-potency topical corticosteroids, excimer laser, topical minoxidil
- Topical immunotherapy with squaric acid or anthralin
- Alopecia totalis/universalis or ophiasis patterns have an unfavorable prognosis
  - Systemic therapies including corticosteroids or methotrexate have been tried with variable results

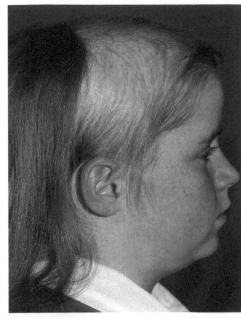

Fig. 12.6B. Trichotillomania. Note the angulated shapes and broken hairs. (From Paller AS, Mancini AJ. *Hurwitz Clinical Pediatric Dermatology.* 5th ed. New York: Elsevier; 2016: p. 160, Fig. 7.45.)

Telogen Effluvium

BASIC INFORMATION

- Non-scarring, diffuse, self-limited alopecia due to an increase in the percentage of hairs in the shedding (telogen) phase of the hair growth cycle.
- Triggers include systemic illness, thyroid deficiency, iron deficiency, dieting changes, rapid weight loss, and occasionally medications
- Characterized by generalized, uniformly decreased scalp hair density.
- Hair pull test should be positive: more than two telogen hairs on a single hair pull
- Evaluate for any dietary or health changes that may have occurred 3 months before onset of symptoms; a dietitian may be helpful if dietary factors play a role
- Reassurance for patients for sentinel events

Trichotillomania

BASIC INFORMATION

- Nonscarring, self-limited traction alopecia due to habitual hair pulling or twisting
- Angulated focal areas of partial hair loss with varying lengths of short, stublike broken hairs (Fig. 12.6B)
  - Can involve the scalp, eyebrows, or eyelashes
- Behavior typically occurs before falling asleep or when the child is preoccupied (i.e., reading, writing, watching television)
- Differential diagnosis: alopecia areata, tinea capitis
- Treatment includes family reassurance and behavior modification

Table 12.3. Epidermolysis Bullosa – Brief Overview

EPIDERMOLYSIS BULLOSA SIMPLEX (EBS)

Cleavage within the epidermis → heals without scarring

EBS	AD	Onset at birth with grouped blisters, particularly in areas prone to friction. Blistering improves with age. Nails may shed and can regrow without dystrophy. Confluent palmoplantar keratoderma. Localized variants have childhood/adolescent onset with blisters prominently on hands/feet (Fig. 12.7a)
EBS with muscular dystrophy	AR	Widespread bullae at birth with muscular dystrophy. Hair/nail/tooth/oral disease

JUNCTIONAL EPIDERMOLYSIS BULLOSA (JEB)

Cleavage at the dermal-epidermal junction → heals with atrophic scarring

JEB	AR	Onset at birth with widespread bullae, and can have mucosal involvement including respiratory and gastrointestinal tract mucosa. Lesions heal with atrophic scarring. Symptoms may improve with time in milder cases. Severe cases have high morbidity and often die by 2 years of age
JEB with pyloric atresia	AR	Severe congenital blistering, hydronephrosis, pyloric atresia, and mucosal erosions

DYSTROPHIC EPIDERMOLYSIS BULLOSA (DEB)

Cleavage below the basement membrane → heals with significant scarring and milia

Recessive dystrophic EB	AR	Onset at birth with widespread blistering, scarring, and milia complicated by mitten deformities and contractures of hands and feet (Fig. 12.7b). Mucous membrane involvement can be complicated by strictures of the gastrointestinal and genitourinary tract. Blister-prone areas are susceptible to cutaneous squamous cell carcinoma and nevi. Patients can have significant dental caries and increased risk of osteoporosis, delayed puberty, cardiomyopathy, and kidney disease. Blisters are prone to secondary infection with *Staphylococcus aureus* and *Pseudomonas aeruginosa*
Dominant dystrophic EB	AD	Less severe than recessive variant. Onset at birth with blistering and milia on trauma-prone areas such as the dorsum of hands, elbows, knees, and lower legs

AD, autosomal dominant; *AR*, autosomal recessive; *EB*, epidermolysis bullosa.

Tinea Capitis

- See Chapter 11

GENODERMATOSES

Ectodermal Dysplasia

BASIC INFORMATION

A group of congenital disorders due to abnormal signaling during development that can affect the hair, teeth, nails, and eccrine (sweat) glands

- Hypohidrotic ectodermal dysplasia (HED): a constellation including hypohidrosis, hypotrichosis, and defective dentition; also has characteristic facies (square forehead with frontal bossing, everted lips, prominent chin, pointed ears, conical incisors, minimal/mild nail changes, and alopecia) and may have immunodeficiency
  - Management goals include prevention of overheating with cool baths and water soaks in hot environments, dental evaluation by 2 years of age (for dental prostheses and implants), and lubricating eye drops
- Hidrotic ectodermal dysplasia: a constellation including normal facies, normal sweating, fine to sparse hair, normal teeth, and prominent nail dystrophy; also includes ocular abnormalities including strabismus, conjunctivitis, and premature cataracts
  - Management goals include monitoring for paronychial infections; minoxidil and tretinoin have been reported to help with hair growth

Incontinentia Pigmenti

BASIC INFORMATION

- X-linked dominant disease due to a NF-kappa-B essential modulator (NEMO) gene mutation, which encodes a subunit of a larger complex that activates NF-KB; lethal in males
- Four cutaneous stages
  - Vesicular stage: vesicles arranged in linear/whorled streaks that resolve by 6 weeks of life
  - Verrucous stage: thickened hyperkeratotic linear plaques that typically resolve by 2 years of age
  - Hyperpigmented: linear/whorled hyperpigmented patches that resolve by adolescence
  - Hypopigmented: hypopigmented linear streaks with decreased hair density
- Other cutaneous symptoms include patchy scarring alopecia and absent or peg-shaped teeth and nail dystrophy
- Requires multidisciplinary approach due to associated abnormalities, including seizures, delayed psychomotor development, and ocular disease

Epidermolysis Bullosa

BASIC INFORMATION

- Group of inherited mechanobullous disorders caused by defects in structural proteins found in the skin that are essential to skin integrity

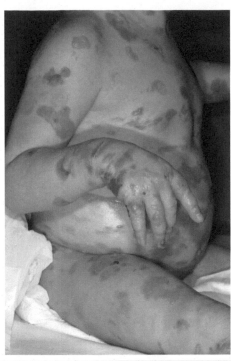

Fig. 12.7A. Epidermolysis bullosa simplex, generalized. (From Paller AS, Mancini AJ. *Hurwitz Clinical Pediatric Dermatology.* 5th ed. New York: Elsevier; 2016: p. 219, Fig. 13.3.)

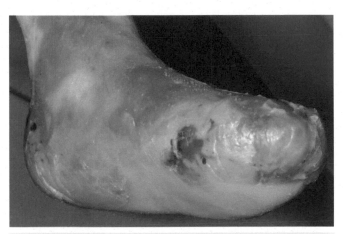

Fig. 12.7B. Recessive dystrophic epidermolysis bullosa. Note the mitten deformity of the foot. (From Paller AS, Mancini AJ. *Hurwitz Clinical Pediatric Dermatology.* 5th ed. New York: Elsevier; 2016: p. 324, Fig. 13.17.)

- Classified by the level of the skin in which the defective structural protein is found and qualified further by disease severity and clinical course
  - Family history is helpful because some are dominantly inherited (Table 12.3)
- Diagnosis is made by skin biopsy samples for immunofluorescence mapping or whole exome sequencing
- Differential diagnosis: bullous mastocytosis, neonatal herpes simplex, bullous impetigo, incontinentia pigmenti
- Supportive care is the mainstay of treatment (protection from friction/overheating, nonstick dressings to open areas, bleach baths and dilute vinegar baths to decrease overgrowth of Pseudomonas and staphylococcal organisms, pain and pruritus management, and nutritional support)

Table 12.4.   Common Forms of Ichthyosis

Ichthyosis vulgaris	Autosomal dominant Presents a few months after birth to early childhood with fine white scales on extensor surfaces, sparing flexures Hyperlinear palms/soles, prone to atopy
X-linked ichthyosis	X-linked recessive, males Mother will have low/absent estrogen in urine/amniotic fluid, resulting in labor that fails to progress Presents within first 6 months of life with large brown scaling involving the entire body with accentuation over the scalp, trunk, and neck with sparing of the palms/soles/face Can be associated with hypogonadism and/or cryptorchidism
Autosomal recessive congenital ichthyoses	Autosomal recessive Group of congenital ichthyoses with AR inheritance, may present with collodion membrane at birth Lamellar ichthyosis: generalized, large, platelike scales causing ectropion and alopecia. Associated with nail dystrophy Congenital ichthyosiform erythroderma: generalized, fine white scaling with erythema
Keratinopathic ichthyoses	Autosomal dominant Group of epidermolytic forms of ichthyosis Presents at birth with blistering or erythroderma which evolve into hyperkeratotic scaling

Hereditary Disorders of Cornification

BASIC INFORMATION

- Group of hereditary disorders characterized by abnormal keratinocyte differentiation and therefore impaired desquamation
- See Table 12.4
- Provide supportive care with emollients and gentle soaps, as well as regular bleach baths, to prevent overcolonization of bacteria

Review Questions

For review questions, please go to ExpertConsult.com.

Suggested Readings

1. Castelo-Soccio L. Diagnosis and management of alopecia in children. *Pediatr Clin North Am.* 2014; 61(2):427–442.
2. Léaute-Labrèze C, Boccara O, Degrugillier-Chopinet C, et al. Safety of oral propranolol for the treatment of infantile hemangioma: a systematic review. *Pediatrics.* 2016;138(4):1–19.
3. Levy R, Lara-Corrales I. Melanocytic nevi in children: a review. *Pediatr Ann.* 2016;45(8):293–298.
4. Paller AS, Mancini AJ. *Hurwitz Clinical Pediatric Dermatology.* 5th ed. New York: Elsevier; 2016.
5. Takeshita J, Grewal S, Langan SM, et al. Psoriasis and comorbid diseases: implications for management. *J Am Acad Dermatol.* 2017;76(3):393–403.

Emergency Medicine and Trauma

13 *Shock*

KATHARINE C. LONG, MD and FRAN BALAMUTH, MD, PhD

Overview of Shock

BASIC INFORMATION

- Shock is characterized as inadequate oxygen delivery and/or extraction of oxygen to meet metabolic demands of vital organs and tissues
- Shock is often categorized based on etiology into the following types (See Table 13.1):
  - Hypovolemic shock
  - Cardiogenic shock
  - Distributive shock
  - Dissociative shock
  - Neurogenic shock
- See also Nelson Textbook of Pediatrics, Chapter 70, "Shock."

COMPENSATED VERSUS UNCOMPENSATED SHOCK

- Majority of pediatric patients present in compensated shock. Features include tachycardia for age, but normal blood pressure, normal mental status and tissue perfusion on exam, and no evidence of end-organ damage on laboratories.
- Uncompensated shock may have variable presentations:
  - some may present with frank hypotension, a hallmark of uncompensated shock
  - others may be normotensive, but suffer significant microvsacular dysfunction. Patients may have altered mental status or poor perfusion on exam. Laboratory data may show evidence of end-organ dysfunction (e.g. elevated liver transaminases, elevated blood urea nitrogen-creatinine ratio [BUN/Cr])

COLD VERSUS WARM SHOCK

- The interplay between cardiac output and systemic vascular resistance in different types of shock yields different clinical examinations
- In certain states (e.g., hypovolemic shock, cardiogenic shock), patients more likely present in cold shock:
  - As a compensatory mechanism, patients have tachycardia, hypotension, increased systemic vascular resistance, and vasoconstraciton. Consequently, they exhibit delayed capillary refill, decreased peripheral pulses, and cold extremities.
  - Cold shock is more common in infants and children due to limited ability to augment stroke volume

- In other states (e.g., distributive shock), patients may present in warm shock:
  - Also called "hyperdynamic" or "vasodilatory" shock because patients have decreased systemic vascular resistance, flash capillary refill, and strong pulses in addition to tachycardia and hypotension.
  - More common in teenagers, adults, and immunosuppressed patients.
- Some states such as septic shock can have a varied picture (i.e. features of warm or cold shock)

Types of Shock

HYPOVOLEMIC SHOCK

Basic Information

- Due to an acute process that decreases circulating blood volume
- Common examples include dehydration or hemorrhage
- Pathophysiology
  - Decreased cardiac output due to decreased preload
  - The body compensates by increasing heart rate (HR) and systemic vascular resistance

Clinical Presentation

- History
  - Gastrointestinal losses from vomiting and/or diarrhea
  - History of blood loss or trauma
  - Plasma losses such as with extensive burns or pancreatitis
  - Extraintestinal water loss such as with heat stroke
- Physical examination
  - Patients usually present with "cold shock" (see previous)
  - May demonstrate signs of dehydration
    - Sunken fontanelle
    - Loss of skin turgor
    - Decreased urine output
    - Altered level of awareness (irritability, somnolence, confusion, anxiety)

TREATMENT

- Restoring intravascular volume is a first priority:
  - 20 mL/kg intravenous (IV) crystalloid fluid bolus up to 60 mL/kg as tolerated
  - Rapid administration of blood products is critical if volume loss is secondary to hemorrhage
- Inotropic/vasoactive agents (e.g. dopamine, epinephrine) may be used, but will have limited effect until intravascular volume is restored.

Table 13.1.   Classification of Shock and Common Underlying Causes

Type	Primary Circulatory Derangement	Common Causes	HR	BP	Capillary Refill
Hypovolemic	Decreased circulating blood volume	Hemorrhage	↑	↓	Delayed
		Diarrhea			
		Diabetes insipidus, diabetes mellitus			
		Burns			
		Adrenogenital syndrome			
		Capillary leak			
Distributive	Vasodilation → venous pooling → decreased preload	Sepsis	↑	Normal or ↓	Flash or delayed
	Maldistribution of regional blood flow	Anaphylaxis			
		Drug intoxication			
Neurogenic	Maldistribution of regional blood flow	CNS/spinal injury	↓	↓	Flash or normal
Cardiogenic	Decreased myocardial contractility	Congenital heart disease	↑	↓	Delayed
		Arrhythmia			
		Hypoxic/ischemic injuries			
		Cardiomyopathy			
		Metabolic derangements			
		Myocarditis			
		Drug intoxication			
		Kawasaki disease			
Obstructive	Mechanical obstruction to ventricular filling or outflow	Cardiac tamponade	↑	↓	Delayed
		Massive pulmonary embolus			
		Tension pneumothorax			
		Cardiac tumor			
Dissociative	Oxygen not appropriately bound or released from hemoglobin	Carbon monoxide poisoning Methemoglobinemia	↑	↓	Normal

BP, Blood pressure; *CNS,* central nervous system; *HR,* heart rate.
Adapted from Marcdante KJ, Kliegman RM. *Nelson Essentials of Pediatrics.* 7th ed. Philadelphia, PA: Elsevier/Saunders; 2015.

CARDIOGENIC SHOCK

Basic Information

- Decreased cardiac output secondary to diminished cardiac contractility
- Common examples include myocarditis, cardiomyopathy, incessant arrhythmias, drug ingestions, and metabolic derangements
- Pathophysiology
  - Decreased myocardial contractility is usually compensated for by increased systemic vascular resistance.

Clinical Presentation

- History
  - Symptoms of heart failure can be vague (e.g. abdominal pain, nausea, dyspnea, altered mental status), so a high index of suspicion is needed to avoid misdiagnosis
  - Previous cardiac disease, syncope, or chest pain
- Physical examination
  - If poor left ventricular function, then may see respiratory distress, rales/crackles as signs of pulmonary overload
  - If poor right ventricular function, then may see jugular vein distention, hepatomegaly, and peripheral edema

- In either case, patients usually present with "cold shock" (see previous)

Diagnosis and Evaluation

- Standard laboratory evaluation outlined previously
- Creatinine kinase, troponin, and/or brain-type natriuretic protein
- Chest radiograph: may find evidence of cardiomegaly and/or pulmonary edema
- ECG

Treatment

- Unlike in other mechanisms of shock (e.g., hypovolemic, septic), fluid resuscitation should be judicious because excessive fluid will not improve cardiac output; rather, it will exacerbate the situation with fluid overload. Boluses of 5 to 10 mL/kg are provided and titrated as tolerated
- Emergent cardiology consultation to attain echocardiogram to evaluate ventricular function with likely transfer to center with pediatric cardiology expertise
- Inotrope infusions are critical for improving systolic performance (dobutamine, epinephrine, milrinone)
- Extracorporeal support for refractory cases

DISTRIBUTIVE SHOCK

Basic Information

- Excessive vasodilation and capillary leak due to a variety of mechanisms (e.g., warm septic shock, drug ingestions, anaphylaxis)
- Pathophysiology
  - Low systemic vascular resistance
  - Capillary leak

Clinical Presentation

- History
  - Risk factors for septic shock: neonatal age, immunodeficiency or suppression, asplenia, central venous line, or bone marrow transplant
  - Risk factors for anaphylaxis: exposure to potential food, medication, or environmental allergens
- Physical examination
  - Classically presents as "warm shock" due to vasodilation; however, it can also present in cold shock in certain scenarios (e.g., with coexisting hypovolemia, progression from warm to cold septic shock)
  - Anaphylaxis: facial or tongue swelling, hypotension, respiratory distress/wheezing/stridor, and urticaria

Treatment

- "Cold" septic shock
  - 20 mL/kg normal saline bolus up to 60 mL/kg as tolerated
  - Vasoactive agents (e.g., epinephrine)
  - Consider hydrocortisone if fluid-refractory catecholamine-resistant shock is suspected
  - Broad-spectrum antibiotics
- "Warm" septic shock
  - 20 mL/kg normal saline bolus up to 60 mL/kg as tolerated
  - Vasoactive agents (e.g., norepinephrine)
  - Consider hydrocortisone if fluid-refractory catecholamine-resistant shock is suspected
  - Broad-spectrum antibiotics
- Anaphylaxis
  - Intramuscular epinephrine 1:10,000 dose of 0.01 mg/kg/dose up to 0.5 mg intramuscular (IM)
  - Consider steroid administration, diphenhydramine, and H2 blocker

NEUROGENIC SHOCK

Basic Information

- Disruption of autonomic pathways of the spinal cord resulting in decreased vascular tone without reflex tachycardia; thus patients may present with hypotension and relative bradycardia
- Common example includes spinal cord injury

Clinical Presentation

- History
  - Traumatic injury from axial load on spinal column
  - Traumatic injury with direct impact to spinal column
- Physical examination
  - Midline spinal column tenderness, pain, step-offs
  - Lack of rectal tone
  - Lack of sensation/tone/strength in upper and/or lower extremities

Treatment

- Spinal immobilization
- Vasoactive agent (e.g. norepinephrine)
- Emergent neurosurgical consultation

OBSTRUCTIVE SHOCK

Basic Information

- Obstruction of blood flow from the heart
- Common examples include tension pneumothorax, cardiac tamponade, or obstructive lesions of the left side of the heart (congenital heart disease)
- Pathophysiology
  - Acute increase in systemic vascular resistance from sudden decrease in cardiac output
  - Functional hypovolemia

Clinical Presentation

- Usually presents with "cold shock," hepatomegaly, and signs/symptoms specific to the underlying etiology:
  - Jugular venous distention, murmur, gallop, diminished heart sounds (cardiac tamponade)
  - Unilateral decreased breath sounds (tension pneumothorax)
  - Poor perfusion, cyanosis (congenital heart disease)

Diagnosis and Evaluation

- Chest radiograph
- Echocardiogram
- Congenital heart disease: four-extremity blood pressure and pre- and postductal saturations

Treatment

- Dependent on etiology
- Ductal-dependent lesions: initiate prostaglandin
- Tension pneumothorax decompression with angiocatheter or chest tube placement
- Cardiac tamponade: pericardiocentesis

DISSOCIATIVE SHOCK

Basic Information

- Impaired oxygen delivery or utilization
- Common examples include severe anemia (see Chapter 36), methemoglobinemia, and carbon monoxide poisoning (details of hemoglobin poisonings provided in Chapter 18)
- Treatment is dependent on etiology (e.g., methylene blue for methemoglobinemia)

Sepsis

BASIC INFORMATION

- SIRS and the sepsis continuum (sepsis, severe sepsis, septic shock) are covered in Chapter 43.
- Given the risk of significant morbidity and mortality with SIRS/sepsis, clinicians must be adept at detecting abnormal vital signs and leukocyte counts for age that comprise the SIRS criteria (see Table 13.2).

Table 13.2.   Age-Specific Vital Signs and Laboratory Values

Age Group	Tachycardia	Bradycardia	Respiratory Rate	Leukocyte Count	Hypotension (SBP)
Birth to 1 week	>180	<100	>50	>34	<59
1 week to 1 month	>180	<100	>40	>19.5 or <5	<79
1 month to 1 year	>180	<90	>34	>17.5 or <5	<75
2 to 5 years	>140	—	>22	>15.5 or <6	<74
6 to 12 years	>130	—	>18	>13.5 or <4.5	<83
13 to <18 years	>110	—	>14	>11 or <4.5	<90

SBP, Systolic blood pressure.
From Prusakowski MK, Chen AP. Pediatric sepsis. *Emerg Med Clin North Am.* 2017;35(1):123–138.

CLINICAL PRESENTATION

- Patients may present in cold or warm shock. Furthermore, patients can also transition from one to the other, classically going from warm shock early in the illness to cold shock if it is allowed to progress
- Fluid-refractory, catecholamine-resistant shock
  - Persistent cardiovascular dysfunction despite 60 mL/kg fluid resuscitation and vasoactive medication (dopamine, epinephrine, or norepinephrine)

DIAGNOSIS AND EVALUATION

Recommended Initial Laboratory Evaluation

- The goal is to isolate the infectious source and to evaluate for organ dysfunction
- Immediate point-of-care blood glucose and arterial or venous blood gas including lactate, electrolytes, and ionized calcium
- Complete blood count with differential
- Complete metabolic panel (including BUN, creatinine, and liver function tests)
- Prothrombin time, partial thromboplastin time, and international normalized ratio (INR) to evaluate for coagulopathy
- Blood culture
- Urinalysis and urine culture
- Inflammatory biomarkers in select cases (e.g., C-reactive protein, procalcitonin)

Imaging

- Consider chest radiography to evaluate for infectious source (e.g. pneumonia) as well as for other non-infectious etiologies of shock (e.g. tension pneumothorax, cardiomegaly, airway obstruction)
- Consider bedside ultrasound for fluid status, cardiac contractility, and/or presence of pericardial effusion

TREATMENT

- 2014 sepsis guidelines state that institutions should have a sepsis protocol in place to standardize therapy with the goal of balancing oxygen delivery with increased oxygen demand
- Most protocols address the following areas:

Cardiovascular Support

- Obtain two points of vascular access, preferably large-bore peripheral IV (PIV; antecubital veins are ideal), intraosseous (IO), or central line
- Fluid resuscitation with 20 mL/kg isotonic crystalloid fluid up to 60 mL/kg as tolerated
  - May need to adjust volume in children with renal or cardiac disease
- Reevaluate patient for signs of fluid overload (rales, hepatomegaly, worsening respiratory status) after each bolus
- If persistently hypotensive despite fluid resuscitation, add vasoactive medication
  - Epinephrine if cold shock
  - Norepinephrine if warm shock
- If in catecholamine-resistant shock, add stress-dose hydrocortisone (e.g. 2 mg/kg/day, 100 mg/m^2/day)

Respiratory Support

- Supplement with FiO$_2$ 100% initially (via nonrebreather mask)
- Endotracheal intubation and mechanical ventilation may be necessary if the patient is unable to maintain the airway (e.g., altered mental status), has respiratory failure (e.g., pneumonia), or demonstrates excessive work of breathing that could be contributing to excessive energy utilization
  - Caution should be employed with intubation because patients may become more hypotensive upon conversion to positive pressure ventilation. Best to optimize hemodynamics if possible before intubation
- The subsequent goal of supplemental oxygen is to maintain oxygen so that pulse oximetry is >90% or PaO$_2$ is between 60 and 80 mm Hg

Infection Control

- Early initiation of broad-spectrum antibiotics to cover Gram-positive and Gram-negative organisms, tailored to the likelihood of drug-resistant bacteria
- Consider local antibiogram when making antibiotic selection for a given institution; some examples include the following:
  - Healthy patient: ceftriaxone *and* vancomycin
  - Immunocompromised/immunosuppressed patients or patients with a central line, chronic medical condition, or recent hospitalization: add pseudomonal coverage (e.g., cefepime and vancomycin)
  - Patients with a suspected intraabdominal source: add anaerobe coverage (e.g., piperacillin/tazobactam and vancomycin)
- Source control is important to combat impermeable collections of bacteria:

- Example: abscess, foreign body, necrotizing soft tissue infections
- Consider surgical consultation

Electrolyte Management

- Hypoglycemia: rapid correction with goal 70 to 150 mg/dL
- Hypocalcemia: correction for goal of ionized calcium ≥1.1 mmol/L

Blood Products

- Packed red blood cell (PRBC) administration
  - Within first 6 hours of acute resuscitation, maintain hemoglobin (Hgb) >10 mg/dL
  - Once tissue hypoperfusion has resolved, goal Hgb >7 mg/dL
- Platelet administration
  - Administer platelets for goal platelet count ≥10/mm^3 if <u>no</u> active bleeding
  - Administer platelets for goal platelet count ≥20/mm^3 if **active** bleeding
- May consider correcting severe coagulopathy with fresh frozen plasma (FFP)

Review Questions

For review questions, please go to ExpertConsult.com.

Suggested Readings

1. Balamuth F, Fitzgerald J, Weiss SL. Shock. In: Shaw KN, Bachur RG, eds. *Fleisher & Ludwig's Textbook of Pediatric Emergency Medicine.* 7th ed. Philadelphia: Wolters Kluwer; 2016.
2. Brierley J, Carcillo JA, Choong K, et al. Clinical practice parameters for hemodynamic support of pediatric and neonatal septic shock: 2007 update from the American College of Critical Care Medicine. *Crit Care Me.* 2009;37:666–688.
3. Cruz AT, Perry AM, Williams EA, et al. Implementation of goal-directed therapy for children with suspected sepsis in the emergency department. *Pediatrics.* 2011;127:e758–e766.
4. Goldstein B, Giroir B, Randolph A. International pediatric sepsis consensus conference: definitions for sepsis and organ dysfunction in pediatrics. *Pediatr Crit Care Med.* 2005;6(1):2–8.
5. Balamuth F, Weiss SL, Neuman MI, et al. Severe sepsis in US Children's Hospitals. *Pediatr Crit Care Med.* 2014;15(9):798–805.

BRUE, SIDS, and Cardiopulmonary Arrest

J. BRYAN COOPER-SOOD, MD and SHRUTI KANT, MD

Brief Resolved Unexplained Event

Infants periodically present to the emergency room or their primary care physician's office after an event in which the infant's color, tone, or behavior suddenly and markedly changes. Historically, this was referred to as an apparent life-threatening event (ALTE), thought to be a precursor of sudden infant death syndrome (SIDS). Over time, studies have suggested otherwise, and in 2016 a consensus statement was released, replacing ALTE with brief resolved unexplained event (BRUE). The statement provides guidelines for the evaluation and management of BRUE. Developing an understanding of BRUE and differentiating low- from high-risk infants can aid the practitioner in providing individualized care and avoiding unnecessary testing and hospitalization.

See also Nelson Textbook of Pediatrics, Chapter 67, "Pediatric Emergencies and Resuscitation."

BASIC INFORMATION

- ALTEs:
  - Historically referred to as "near-miss" SIDS
  - Reasons for transition away from the term ALTE:
    - Despite the apparent "life-threatening" appearance of these events, the majority of patients have low risk of serious medical condition
    - The term placed a psychological burden on the family.
    - The diagnosis rests on the family's perception of the event
    - The idea of a "life-threatening" aspect of these events often prompted further evaluation and hospitalization at cost to the patient, family, and society
- BRUE versus ALTE:
  - Infants who have experienced a BRUE by definition have returned to their baseline and are without a readily identified cause after a history and physical examination
  - New American Academy of Pediatrics (AAP) consensus statement recommends replacing ALTE with BRUE. If the BRUE definition is not applicable, ALTE should be replaced with only a description of the event characteristics
    - For example, a child with a BRUE-like event at home that has not returned to baseline should be defined only by the event characteristics (e.g., apnea, respiratory distress, etc.)
- Epidemiology: studies regarding the prevalence of BRUE are extremely limited

- Cause: the most common causes of BRUE are an area of ongoing investigation

CLINICAL PRESENTATION

- BRUE is sudden, brief (usually less than 1 minute), and unexplained after a thorough history and physical examination, and now a completely resolved episode in which an infant experiences one or more of the following:
  - Central cyanosis or pallor
  - Absent, decreased, or irregular breathing
  - Change in tone
  - A change in the level of responsiveness

DIAGNOSIS AND EVALUATION

- BRUE is a diagnosis of exclusion in which an episode meets the earlier definition criteria; a proper evaluation requires a detailed history with multiple elements (see Table 14.1)

Table 14.1. Areas of Focus for the HPI of a Suspected BRUE Patient

HISTORY OF THE EVENT

What was the child doing at the time of the event (i.e., feeding, sleeping, crying, quietly awake)?

Feeding: Was the BRUE associated with feeding, or did it occur just after feeding? If so, was there spitting up or vomiting before the BRUE? If so, from the nose, mouth, or both? What was the character of the emesis/spit-up (milk-/formula-colored, bloody, etc.)?

Color: Did the child become pale, cyanotic, plethoric, or pallid? What part of the body was affected (in particular, were the changes "central," meaning affecting the whole body and/or the inside of the mouth)?

Respiratory: Was there choking or gagging during the event? Was there irregular, shallow, or absent breathing? Did the child make any stridulous or other abnormal respiratory sounds during the event?

Physical changes: Was the tone increased or decreased? Were there seizure-like jerking movements? Did the child have abnormal eye movements (deviated to one side, rolling in the back of the head, etc.)?

Duration and witnesses: How long did it last? Who saw the event, and are they present or available to provide further history?

INTERVENTIONS (LOWEST TO HIGHEST)

Self-resolved

Gentle stimulation (e.g., blowing air in the child's face; suctioning of the nose or mouth)

Vigorous stimulation (e.g., hard rubbing, yelling at the child or vigorous shaking)

CPR or mouth-to-mouth by a noncertified provider

CPR by a certified provider

Continued

Table 14.1. Areas of Focus for the HPI of a Suspected BRUE Patient—cont'd

PAST HISTORY

Does the child have a history of these events? If so, how many and for how long? Provide a thorough description of each, and who was present?

Past medical history: Particularly prior issues with gastroesophageal reflux disorder, reflux, or respiratory issues

Birth history: Was the child born premature? Was the mother healthy? Were there any issues during the birth or during the stay in the nursery (or in the perinatal period)?

Medications: Does the child take any medications daily, or did the child take any medications on the day of the event or the day before? Are there medications in the home that the child could have accessed?

Family history: Did other infants who were in the home or who were cared for by the parents/caregivers experience such events? Have any died as a result?

Social history: Is there a maternal history of smoking? Is there drug or alcohol abuse in the home? Is there a history of child abuse or involvement of Child Protective Services? What is the parents' capacity to present for care and to see their primary care provider or emergency facilities if needed?

BRUE, Brief resolved unexplained event.

- A review of the event with any witnesses, focusing on the timeline of the event, the severity of the symptoms, and the level of intervention required to aid its resolution
- A past medical history including birth history, growth and developmental history, and the presence or absence of any respiratory or feeding problems
- A family history looking for genetic or metabolic causes or for prior ALTE or SIDS events in the family raising concern for nonaccidental trauma [NAT]
- By definition, the physical examination must be normal, with special attention to:
  - Weight, head circumference, and length
  - Growth pattern of these parameters
  - Age-appropriate vital signs
  - Thorough examination for signs of bruising or other injuries
  - Cardiorespiratory examination to evaluate for signs of lung or cardiac pathology
  - Careful neurologic examination, including baseline tone, strength, and developmentally appropriate reflexes

TREATMENT

- If the history and physical examination are indicative of a causal etiology, the episode is not a BRUE, and management should be tailored to the inciting disorder
- If the history and physical examination are reassuring, patients may be designated as "low risk" or "high risk," which will aid in determining the necessity of certain diagnostic interventions and monitoring
- All of the following must be met to qualify as low risk criteria:
  - Patient must be at least 60 days old
  - Patient was at least 32 weeks at birth and is at least 45 weeks postconceptional age
  - Patient had only one BRUE and no prior history of BRUE
  - The event was brief (less than 1 minute)
  - The patient did not require cardiopulmonary resuscitation (CPR) by a trained medical provider

- Recommendations for these low-risk patients include family education and CPR training, with only a limited diagnostic workup, if necessary (e.g., pertussis testing, electrocardiogram (ECG), brief monitoring with continuous pulse oximetry and serial observation). Further diagnostic workup (e.g., serum studies, urine studies, cerebrospinal fluid [CSF] studies, imaging) and inpatient cardiorespiratory monitoring can be avoided
  - Disposition will depend on reassurance and collaboration with parents (i.e., assessing their level of concern) and ensuring adequate primary care physician follow-up (usually within 12 to 24 hours)
- BRUEs failing to meet low-risk criteria should be managed as clinically indicated, with diagnostic testing targeted at the patient's most likely diagnosis based on history and physical examination:
  - Specific areas to consider for etiologic evaluation:
    - Infectious diseases
      Particularly consider respiratory virus (e.g., respiratory syncytial virus [RSV], influenza) and pertussis infections
      Also consider other serious bacterial infections – community-acquired pneumonia, urinary tract infection (UTI), bacteremia, meningitis, etc.
    - Neurologic disorders
      Consider electroencephalogram (EEG) or the need for head imaging
    - Gastrointestinal (especially reflux)
      Consider fluoroscopic swallow study if recurrent episodes or neurodevelopmental abnormalities present
    - NAT/drug exposure
      Strongly consider if there is any concerning history (e.g., unexplained death in a child in the family, history of previous child abuse or Child Protective Services involvement) or if there are any signs of injury (see Chapter 90 for details)
    - Rare diseases
      Cardiopulmonary anomalies/disease requiring an echocardiogram
      Inborn errors of metabolism requiring further serum testing
- Common (but not universally required) studies for high-risk patients include complete blood cell count (CBC), complete metabolic panel, venous blood gas and lactate, urine toxicology, urinalysis and culture, pertussis testing, respiratory virus testing, blood culture, chest x-ray (CXR), and ECG
- All patients who presented with significant physiologic compromise should be admitted to the hospital for observation and cardiorespiratory monitoring
- Home monitoring after admission for BRUE is not universally recommended but may be an option in certain cases:
  - Premature infants with apnea and bradycardia
  - Airway issues
  - Chronic lung disease
- Prognosis
  - Prognostic data for BRUE, because it has a narrower definition than ALTE, including risk of recurrence and death, is not currently available; the only available prognostic data is from the ALTE literature

- Historic risk of ALTE recurrence: 10% to 25% overall
  - Young and premature infants
  - Multiple events before presentation
  - Viral respiratory infection
- Risk of SIDS after ALTE: approximately 1%
  - ALTE, and therefore BRUE, is likely *not* a precursor to SIDS
  - Most SIDS cases never experience an ALTE before death
  - Difference in peak age ALTE (younger) versus SIDS (older)
  - Difference in time of day ALTE (day) versus SIDS (early a.m.)
  - Interventions to decrease SIDS have not altered incidence of ALTE

Sudden Infant Death Syndrome

SIDS occurs when an infant dies without apparent cause after a thorough forensic and pathologic examination. It continues to be the leading cause of death in infants 1 month to 1 year old; however, studies originating in the 1990s and beyond have led to a better understanding of the pathophysiology and epidemiology of SIDS, including identifying factors that place infants at higher risk for SIDS. This has led to significant preventative efforts resulting in a decline in the number of deaths.

BASIC INFORMATION

- Definition
  - Sudden death of an infant less than 1 year of age
  - Must be unexplained after a forensic case investigation by police, an autopsy, and after a clinical history to exclude other causes
  - In contrast to sudden unexplained infant death (SUID):
    - SUID is a catch-all for all infant deaths
    - Some SUIDs become SIDS after a cause cannot be identified
- Epidemiology
  - Leading cause of death 1 month to 1 year in the United States
  - Highest-risk populations
    - Children at day care centers
    - Boys greater than girls
    - Black and Native American infants
  - Timing of SIDS
    - Median age is 11 weeks
      - 90% between 2 and 4 months
      - May suggest a developmental-/maturation-related cause to SIDS
  - Independent infant risk factors, factors notable for not increasing risk, and factors that mitigate risk of SIDS are included in Table 14.2
  - Independent ante- and postnatal maternal risk factors for SIDS are detailed in Table 14.3
  - 95% of SIDS cases are associated with one of the previous risk factors
  - Notable infant and maternal risk factors:
    - Prematurity

Table 14.2. Independent Infant Risk Factors for and Protective Factors Against SIDS

INFANT RISK FACTORS FOR SIDS

Risk factors in the neonatal period:
  Low birth weight
  Small for gestational age
  Prematurity
Risk factors in the post-neonatal period:
  Prone sleeping position
  Soft sleeping surface
  Loose bedding/accessories in the bed (e.g., plush toys)
  Overheating
  Bed sharing and cosleeping
  Recent gastrointestinal illness
  Decrease in normal activity (i.e., listless or languid)
  Sibling death from SIDS
  Twin death from SIDS
  Use of a car seat or other sitting device for sleep

INFANT FACTORS NOT FOUND TO INCREASE RISK OF SIDS
  Apnea of prematurity
  Recent history of upper respiratory tract infection
  Recent immunization
  History of ALTE

INFANT PROTECTIVE FACTORS
  Breastfeeding
  Supine sleeping
  Use of a fan during sleep (particularly if risk factors are present)
  Immunization (possible)
  Consistent pacifier use

ALTE, Apparent life-threatening event; *SIDS,* sudden infant death syndrome.

Table 14.3. Independent Ante- and Postnatal Maternal Risk Factors for SIDS

POSTNATAL MATERNAL RISK FACTORS FOR SIDS

Smoking in the home
Use of illicit drugs in the home
Inverse relationship with age (i.e., higher risk <20 years old)
Unmarried
Lack of high school education

ANTENATAL RISK FACTORS FOR SIDS

Anemia
Poor gestational weight gain
Urinary tract infection
Sexually transmitted diseases
Brief interval between pregnancies
No or insufficient prenatal care
Perinatal complications of pregnancy (e.g., placenta previa, premature rupture of membranes)

SIDS, Sudden infant death syndrome.

- Peak incidence 4 to 6 weeks earlier than in term infants
- Particularly increased risk in small-for-gestational age (SGA) infants
- Markedly increased risk if not placed in supine position
- Sleep position
  - Odds ratio of SIDS 8.7 in prone and side-lying versus supine position
  - Risk increases as well if normally supine-sleeping infants are placed prone or side-lying
  - Sleep positioners are *not* recommended (linked to infant deaths in late 1990s)
- Sleep environment

Bed sharing, soft and loose bedding, sleeping in car seats or other devices are all associated with increased risk of SIDS

Should not dissuade patients from using car seats for travel, however

Room sharing, however, is recommended—possible SIDS prevention linked with breastfeeding

- Maternal smoking

Apart from nonsupine sleep position, this risk factor is associated with the greatest increased risk of SIDS

Includes smoke and particles in clothing or in other caregivers' clothing (i.e., not just smoking in the home)

- Etiology for SIDS is unclear but is thought to be multifactorial, including:
  - Brainstem immaturity and abnormality
  - Genetic predisposition (whereas multiple polymorphisms have been found in SIDS patients, there is a relatively low rate in siblings and in twins of SIDS victims)
  - Developmental stage (most SIDS occurs between 4 and 6 months of age)
  - Infection
    - Various bacterial and viral pathogens have been suggested
    - Infants with SIDS more likely to have pathogenic bacteria isolated from their autopsies versus healthy infants
  - Prone positioning
    - Possible links with suffocation, obstructive events, increased arousal thresholds, and decreased cerebral oxygenation with prone positioning
  - Cardiac dysfunction (which is controversial because only 10% of those with SIDS had an identified ion-channelopathy)
  - Environmental factors still required (i.e., a multifactorial illness)

CLINICAL PRESENTATION

- Typically present in the early morning when caregivers go to check on infant
- Failed resuscitation efforts by emergency medical services (EMS) and/or emergency department (ED) providers
- No immediate cause is available at the time of presentation

DIAGNOSIS AND EVALUATION

- Thorough evaluation by social work, police, treating physicians, and postmortem evaluation must be performed
  - Death scene investigation: note temperature of room, position, and so forth; can aid in identifying risk factors that may be associated with diagnosis
  - Autopsy: an otherwise well child with frothy-pink fluid from the airway, pulmonary congestion, edema, airway inflammation, and hepatic hematopoiesis
  - Clinical history
    - Identify risk factors associated with SIDS (see previous tables)
    - Collection of applicable information to help complete death investigation

Time last seen

Time found and by whom

Position found

Other details of the room and sleep environment

- Look for family history, particularly for ALTE

May identify NAT as a more likely cause (e.g., Munchausen syndrome by proxy)

Also to identify possible genetic/metabolic disorders in the family

- Differential diagnoses to consider:
  - NAT
    - 1% to 5% of cases designated as NAT are actually fatal child abuse
    - Autopsy should differentiate the two; however, establishing, for example, accidental versus intentional asphyxiation is very difficult
    - Suspect with history of sibling deaths, history of ALTEs in patient or siblings, and in older children.
  - Metabolic disorders
    - Perhaps 1% to 6% of cases of SIDS (before testing was available)
    - Similar family history findings compared with NAT (e.g., sibling death, ALTEs, etc.)
    - Prior episodes of unexplained illness or metabolic abnormalities during illness
  - Cardiac disorders
    - Including channelopathies, arrhythmias
  - Infections
    - Viral and bacterial
  - Genetic disorders
  - Environmental causes
    - Sleep positioning
    - Maternal smoking
    - Other causes

TREATMENT

- Prevention
  - Attempt to address modifiable risk factors. Notable prevention measures to address:
    - Universal back-to-sleep program by all providers who care for infants

Particularly emphasize for SGA and premature infants

    - Prevention of maternal smoking and substance use
    - Optimal sleep environment

Use of a fan

Use of pacifier

Avoid soft bed materials and loose bedding/toys in bed

Avoidance of cosleeping

    - Encourage vaccination and breastfeeding
  - Marked decrease in SIDS deaths as smoking rates have dropped and back-to-sleep programs have been put in place
- Care post-SIDS—on-scene emergency providers
  - Appropriate resuscitative measures if indicated
    - Some infants already in rigor mortis when found
  - Document responses of family, document the environment, and provide emotional support
    - Importance of emotional support by first providers to familial healing after infantile death
  - Appropriate transportation to a pediatric facility preferred

- Care post-SIDS—providers in the ED or other emergency setting
  - Attempt to give structure to family, improving familial outcomes
    - Direct communication, avoiding euphemisms for death, and professional, calm interaction with the family by all staff
    - Consideration of family/other emotional supporters during discussions with family
    - Culturally appropriate discussion, prioritizing contact with infant and associated cultural rituals as applicable
    - Discussion of organ donation
    - Prioritize keepsakes for the family to aid in healing
    - Social support for funeral arrangement, transportation home
    - Referral to SIDS group or individual therapy as appropriate
    - If occurred at a day care, day care must notify other families
  - Debrief for emergency providers
    - Psychological trauma and effects on emergency personnel
    - Time and space to reflect are necessary
    - Goal is to avoid personal and professional negative impacts of stress on providers

Cardiopulmonary Arrest

Cardiopulmonary arrest is a high-stakes, low-frequency presentation in pediatrics, with a variety of causes including, but not limited to, respiratory arrest resulting in cardiac arrest, accidental/NAT, sudden cardiac arrest (SCA), sepsis, and others. Much research has been devoted to prevention and treatment of pediatric cardiopulmonary arrest to avoid its devastating effects. In this chapter we will review the epidemiology, etiology, clinical presentation, prevention, and management of cardiopulmonary arrest.

BASIC INFORMATION

- Epidemiology
  - 0.5 to 20 per 100,000 person-years
  - Bimodal distribution: highest in 0 to 2-year age group, increasing again in the 14- to 25-year age group
    - Survival rate ranges from 27% to 40% for all ages. Highest survival rate is seen in 3 to 13 years old
    - Does not include SIDS deaths
    - Higher incidence in children and adolescents during athletics and post exercise
  - National Center for the Review and Prevention of Child Deaths (NCRPCD)
    - Highest incidence in infants <1 year old
    - Male predominance
    - Highest in Caucasians
- Etiology
  - General trends by age for cardiopulmonary arrest:
    - <1 year old: congenital anomalies followed by maternal complication, SIDS, sepsis, respiratory disorders, and cardiac causes

  - 1 to 4 years old: unintentional injuries followed by congenital anomalies, malignancies, homicides, cardiac and respiratory causes
  - 5 to 11 years old: unintentional injuries followed by suicide, malignancies, homicides, and cardiac causes
  - Of the medically correctable causes, sepsis, respiratory, and cardiac disorders predominate
- SCA
  - A subcategory of cardiopulmonary arrest, particularly important in older children and adolescents
    - In descending order: coronary artery disease, arrhythmias, cardiomyopathies, and congenital heart disease
    - By age:
      Genetic disorders that predispose to SCA
      Ion channelopathies (e.g., Brugada, long QT)
      Cardiomyopathies (hypertrophic, dilated, restrictive)
      Wolff-Parkinson-White syndrome
      <2 years old: congenital heart disease and arrhythmia
      3 to 9 years old: equal distribution of congenital heart disease, hypertrophic cardiomyopathy, long QT, and primary arrhythmia
      10 to 25 years old: equal distribution of primary arrhythmia, congenital heart disease, long QT, and myocarditis
      Genetic causes represent 20% of all etiologies of SCA
- Pathophysiology
  - General cardiopulmonary arrest is usually caused by a mismatch of oxygen demand and supply to tissues. For instance:
    - Respiratory causes: decreased oxygen supply due to primary dysfunction of gas exchange
    - Sepsis: increased oxygen demand due to increased tissue consumption
    - Cardiac causes: inadequate supply of oxygen to the tissues due to circulatory compromise
  - SCA is typically caused by a lethal ventricular tachyarrythmia (e.g. ventricular fibrillation or pulseless ventricular tachycardia) leading to a cessation of oxygen delivery to tissues

CLINICAL PRESENTATION

- Warning signs and symptoms
  - General cardiopulmonary arrest:
    - Patients often demonstrate evidence of end-organ dysfunction before arrest:
      Neurologic: irritability, altered mental status, lethargy
      Cardiovascular: tachycardia, low blood pressure, delayed capillary refill time, poor pulses
      Respiratory: tachypnea, increased work of breathing, hypoxia, hypercapnia
      Gastrointestinal: abdominal distention, abdominal pain, bilious or bloody emesis or stool
      Renal: poor urine output, increase in BUN or creatinine
    - Unexplained tachycardia is always concerning because it is often the first sign of shock and a cardinal sign of end-organ hypoperfusion and dysfunction

Table 14.4. Pediatric Basic Life Support Adapted from the American Heart Association Basic Life Support Program Guidelines (2010)

Age Group	Technique	Compression-to-ventilation Ratio	Depth of Chest Compression	Site of Compression	Rate of Compression
Neonate (0–28 days)	Two thumbs encircling chest or two fingers	3:1	One-third to one-half anterior posterior diameter of chest	Lower third of sternum	120 events/min
Infant (1 month to 1 year)	Two thumbs encircling chest or two fingers	30:2 (15:2 if two rescuers)	One-third to one-half anterior posterior diameter of chest	Lower half of sternum just below nipple line	100 events/min
Child (1 year to signs of puberty)	Heel of one or two hands	30:2 (15:2 if two rescuers)	One-third to one-half anterior posterior diameter of chest	Center of chest at nipple line	100 events/min
Adult (puberty and above)	Heel of two hands	30:2	2 inches	Center of chest at nipple line	100 events/min

- These findings may be present before cardiopulmonary arrest, or a child may simply present to you in cardiopulmonary arrest as the end stage of one of the previous processes
- SCA:
  - Usually presents as an acutely unresponsive child with absent pulses/heart sounds and no breathing
  - 40% to 70% have had subtle warning signs before SCA such as fatigue, light-headedness/syncope, and chest pain (usually during activity)
    40% of families discussed the previous warning signs with their child's clinician before SCA
    25% of child victims of SCA have a family history of SCA before age 50

DIAGNOSIS AND EVALUATION

- In certain cases, cardiopulmonary arrest can be prevented by performing a thorough history, physical examination, appropriate testing, and resuscitative measures
  - For example, close attention to warning signs and symptoms, fluid resuscitation and circulatory support in shock, early antibiotics, etc.
- A diagnosis of cardiopulmonary arrest per the American Heart Association (AHA) Pediatric Advanced Life Support (PALS) program is as follows:
  - Pulseless ventricular tachycardia, pulseless bradycardia, pulseless electrical activity, or the absence of organized cardiac rhythm (e.g., ventricular fibrillation (VF) or asystole)
    - Ventricular tachycardia (VT) or bradycardia with poor perfusion but with a pulse requires immediate intervention but is not technically defined as cardiopulmonary arrest
- Initial labs that may help management in a cardiac arrest include:
  - CBC, metabolic profile, blood gas, and lactate
  - Chest x-ray, ECG, and focused ultrasound assessment

TREATMENT

- The AHA PALS program is the current standard of care for children in peri- or actual cardiopulmonary arrest

- Primary and secondary surveys provide a systematic manner in which to triage organ system assessment because these guide the treatment team in addressing issues with the resuscitation and may provide clues as to the cause of the arrest. See Chapter 15 for the details of the primary and secondary surveys
- CPR is the coordinated delivery of ventilatory breaths with extrathoracic chest compressions, with the goal of providing forward blood flow and maintaining coronary perfusion pressure
  - See Table 14.4 for a summary of CPR guidelines
- Specific algorithms established by the AHA for the treatment of cardiopulmonary arrest in pediatrics are taught in PALS. Although the details of these algorithms are beyond the scope of this review, important concepts are presented here.
  - Pediatric bradycardia with a pulse but poor perfusion:
    - CPR should be initiated if heart rate (HR) <60 beats/min
    - Epinephrine is a first-line therapy after the initiation of CPR; atropine may be considered for cases with increased vagal tone or primary atrioventricular block
    - Transthoracic pacing may be necessary to maintain an adequate HR
  - Pediatric tachycardia with a pulse but poor perfusion:
    - Evaluation of the rhythm for narrow QRS complex (≤0.09 s) or wide QRS complex (>0.09 s) tachycardia is fundamentally important because the former is consistent with sinus tachycardia or supraventricular tachycardia (SVT), whereas the latter is consistent with VT
    - SVT may respond to vagal maneuvers or intravenous (IV) or intra-osseous (IO) adenosine
    - VT may require immediate synchronized cardioversion if a patient is hypotensive or is demonstrating other signs of hemodynamic instability. If clinically stable, cardiology consultation may provide recommendations for antiarrhythmic medications
  - Pediatric cardiac arrest:
    - Characterized by pulselessness; treatment algorithms are generally divided into "shockable" and "nonshockable" rhythms. Regardless, in either case, CPR should be started immediately in the absence of palpable pulses

- Pulseless patients with a "shockable rhythm" (VF or VT) should receive an electrical shock as soon as possible. Persistence of these rhythms will require alternating administrations of epinephrine and further electrical shocks before consideration of antiarrhythmic agents (e.g., amiodarone, lidocaine)
  - Pulseless patients with a "nonshockable rhythm" may have either asystole or any other organized rhythm (e.g., tachycardia, bradycardia, normal rate) called pulseless electrical activity. These patients require intermittent doses of epinephrine
  - Patients with either shockable or nonshockable rhythms require periodic checks of the underlying rhythm because an arrested patient's rhythm may evolve throughout the course of a resuscitation
- Extracorporeal membranous oxygenation (ECMO) with CPR:
  - Large multicenter prospective cohort of 3756 children found that *only* children with cardiac disease who suffered an inpatient cardiac arrest benefited from the addition of ECMO to CPR
    - Intact survival for cardiac patients who received ECMO and CPR in the previous study = 50%
- Management of shock after return of spontaneous circulation (ROSC):
  - In general, the goal is to maintain normothermia, avoid hypo-/hypercapnia and hypo-/hyperoxia, and appropriately manage end-organ hypoperfusion and associated signs of end-organ dysfunction
- Termination of resuscitation
  - Terminating a resuscitation is always a difficult decision
  - Factors to consider:
    - Presence of lividity, such as in SIDS, may lead teams to terminate resuscitation earlier
    - Length of resuscitation >30 min is associated with poor outcomes poor outcomes
    - Administration of >3 doses of epinephrine is usually associated with poor outcome
    - In hospital arrests generally have better outcomes than out of hospital arrests
    - Consider if all reversible causes have been addressed:
      - Presence of shockable rhythm (better outcome)
      - PALS "H's and T's" of potentially reversible causes:
        - Hypoxia, hypovolemia, hypoglycemia, hypothermia, hydrogen ions (acidosis), and hypo-/hyperkalemia
        - Toxins, thrombosis, tamponade, tension pneumothorax, and trauma-related causes
  - In rare instances, intact survival may be seen with prolonged resuscitation (>30 minutes). This is particularly true in the setting of poisonings, primary hypothermic arrest, and patients with cardiac disease resuscitated with ECMO and CPR
- Presence of family during resuscitation:
  - Most parents want to be present
  - Does not appear to negatively impact resuscitation or increase stress experienced by staff
  - In many instances, has been shown to aid in parental adjustment and grieving after death of the child

Table 14.5.   Concerning ECG Findings

Q waves greater than 3 mm in depth in two or more leads—hypertrophic cardiomyopathy

QRS duration more than 120 ms in adults, 100 ms in adolescents <16, and 90 ms in children <4 years old

P-wave amplitude more than 2.5 mm for right atrial abnormality, and P-wave negative component in V1 or V2 of 40 ms and 1-mm amplitude

ST elevation more than 2 mm, depression more than 0.5 mm, or inappropriate age-related T-wave inversion—cardiac ischemia

QT prolongation—long QT syndrome

Delta wave and a short PR interval—Wolff-Parkinson-White syndrome

- Prevention of SCA:
  - Universal screening is controversial
    - Appropriate (correct age and test) yet cost-effective (minimizing false-positives while capturing all patients at risk for SCA) is challenging
    - Randomized controlled trials to determine the ideal age and test (ECG versus echocardiogram) are impractical due to the low prevalence of SCA
    - Studies suggest that ECG screening has a high ratio of cost-effectiveness to health benefit
      - See Table 14.5 for concerning ECG findings for risk of or actual progression to SCA
    - According to the AHA and AAP, the most cost-effective initial screening is *only* a thorough history and physical examination
    - Greater controversy exists in the screening of competitive athletes for risk factors of SCA and is outside the scope of this chapter

Review Questions

For review questions, please go to ExpertConsult.com.

Suggested Readings

BRUE

1. Kahn A. European society for the study and prevention of infant death. Recommended clinical evaluation of infants with an apparent life-threatening event. Consensus document of the European Society for the Study and Prevention of Infant Death. *Eur J Pediatr.* 2004;163(2):108–15.
2. Kiechl-Kohlendorfer U, et al. Epidemiology of apparent life threatening events. *Arch Dis Child.* 2005;90:297–300.
3. McGovern MC, Smith MB. Causes of apparent life threatening events in infants: a systematic review. *Arch Dis Child.* 2004;89:1043–1048.
4. Tieder JS, et al. Management of apparent life-threatening events in infants: a systematic review. *J Pediatr.* 2013;163:94–99.
5. Tieder JS, et al. Brief resolved unexplained events (formerly apparent life-threatening events) and evaluation of lower-risk infants. *Pediatrics.* 2016;5:137:e20160590.

SIDS

6. American Academy of Pediatrics, Hymel KP, Committee on Child Abuse and Neglect, National Association of Medical Examiners. Distinguishing sudden infant death syndrome from child abuse fatalities. *Pediatrics.* 2006;118:421–427.
7. Centers for Disease Control and Prevention (CDC). Sudden infant death syndrome – United States. 1983-1994. *MMWR Morb Mortal Wkly Rep.* 1996;45:859–863.
8. Committee on Pediatric Emergency Medicine. Death of a child in the emergency department. *Pediatrics.* 1994;93:861–862.

9. McClain M. *Sudden Unexpected Infant and Child Death: A Guide for the Emergency Department Personnel*. Boston: Massachusetts Center for the Sudden Infant Death Syndrome; 2008.

10. Task Force on Sudden Infant Death Syndrome. SIDS and other sleep-related infant deaths: expansion of recommendations for a safe infant sleeping environment. *Pediatrics*. 2011;128:1030–1039.

Cardiac Arrest

11. American Heart Association. *Pediatric Advanced Life Support*. Dallas, TX: American Heart Association; 2016.

12. Centers for Disease Control and Prevention (CDC). "Ten Leading Causes of Death and Injury." Injury prevention and control: data and statistics (WISQARS). https://www.cdc.gov/injury/wisqars/leadingcauses.html; 2016.

13. Drezner JA, et al. Warning symptoms and family history in children and young adults with sudden cardiac arrest. *J Am Board Fam Med*. 2012;25:408–415.

14. Mahle WT, et al. Key concepts in the evaluation of screening approaches for heart disease in children and adolescents: a science advisory from the American Heart Association. *Circulation*. 2012;125:2796–2801.

15. Meyer L, et al. Incidence, causes, and survival trends from cardiovascular-related sudden cardiac arrest in children and young adults 0 to 35 years of age: a 30-year review. *Circulation*. 2012;126:1363–1372.

15 Trauma

ANNA WEISS, MD, MSED

Traumatic injury is the most common cause for pediatric emergency department visits and the leading cause of death among children ages 1 to 18 years in the United States. The goal of this chapter is to provide an overview of the evaluation of pediatric trauma patients, starting with elements of the initial examination and resuscitation, followed by details of specific traumatic injuries.

Basic Information

- Although much of the approach to triage and management of traumatic injury in children is derived from the algorithms established by the American College of Surgeons in Advanced Trauma Life Support (ATLS), practitioners caring for injured children must be aware of the ways in which the approach to pediatric trauma is unique:
  - A child is far more likely to suffer multisystem injury than an adult injured by the same mechanism; care should be taken to assess all organ systems carefully—even those that may not initially appear to be injured
  - Unlike adults, children demonstrate hypotension only as a late finding in hemorrhagic shock; practitioners should be wary of tachycardia in injured children and have a high index of suspicion for volume loss as the cause
  - Evaluation of the traumatically injured child must take into account age-determined developmental abilities; standardized scoring systems used for adults (e.g., Glasgow Coma Scale [GCS]) must be altered to take developmental milestones into account
- When determining whether a child should be transferred to definitive care at a dedicated pediatric trauma center, prehospital practitioners and providers practicing in hospitals not designated as trauma centers can use both the GCS and Pediatric Trauma Score (PTS) to determine the disposition of an injured child (Tables 15.1 and 15.2)

Initial Assessment

Practitioners should aim to assess all pediatric trauma victims with a standardized method of evaluation. ATLS outlines recommendations for such an approach, highlighting the primary and secondary surveys as the essential tools for initial assessment.

- Primary survey: assess "ABCDEs"; look for immediately life-threatening injuries
  - A: airway

- Evaluate for airway patency and prepare for endotracheal intubation in patient with poor mental status (GCS <8) and/or concern for impending threat to airway integrity
- B: breathing
  - Assess for spontaneous respirations and adequate air exchange; ensure equal breath sounds in both hemithoraces
  - All trauma patients should receive supplemental oxygen and should be monitored continually with pulse oximetry and (where possible) capnography
- C: circulation
  - Evaluate for adequate cardiovascular function by assessing strength of pulses, capillary refill time, and skin color
  - Control visible bleeding with application of direct pressure and/or a tourniquet where possible
- D: disability
  - Assess neurologic function by measurement of GCS and evaluation of pupillary response
- E: exposure
  - Fully expose patient by removing all clothing to allow for thorough evaluation of all injuries. Use blankets, warmed IV fluids, or radiant warmers as needed to maintain adequate body temperature
- Secondary survey: systematically assess for injury by performing a rapid head-to-toe examination of the injured child

Table 15.1. Modified Glasgow Coma Scale for Children

	Glasgow Coma Scale (GCS)	Infant Coma Scale (ICS)	Score
Eye opening	Spontaneous	Spontaneous	4
	To voice	To voice	3
	To pain	To pain	2
	None	None	1
Verbal response	Oriented	Coos, babbles	5
	Confused	Irritable cry	4
	Inappropriate	Cries to pain	3
	Garbled	Moans to pain	2
	None	None	1
Motor response	Obeys commands	Normal movements	6
	Localizes pain	Withdraws to touch	5
	Withdraws to pain	Withdraws to pain	4
	Flexion	Flexion	3
	Extension	Extension	2
	Flaccid	Flaccid	1

GCS or ICS less than 12 is an indication for transfer to a pediatric trauma center.

Table 15.2. Pediatric Trauma Score

Component	+2	+1	−1
Size	>20 kg	10–20 kg	<10 kg
Airway	Normal	Maintainable	Unmaintainable
Systolic blood pressure	>90 mm Hg	50–90 mm Hg	<50 mm Hg
Central nervous system	Awake	Obtunded/loss of consciousness	Coma/decerebrate
Skeletal finding(s)	None	Closed fracture	Open or multiple fractures
Cutaneous finding(s)	None	Minor	Major/penetrating

PTS less than 8 is an indication for transfer to a pediatric trauma center. Pediatric Trauma Score. From Tepas JJ 3rd et al. The Pediatric Trauma Score as a predictor of injury severity: an objective assessment. *J Trauma,* 1988;28:425–429.

- During the secondary survey, care should be taken to maintain cervical spine immobilization if there is concern for spinal or neck injury. Indications for cervical spine immobilization include the following:
  - Concerning mechanism or anatomic predisposition to C-spine injury
  - GCS <13 or intoxication
  - Neck pain or torticollis
  - Neurologic deficit(s)
- Patients should be log-rolled at least once during the secondary survey to allow for evaluation of often-missed areas of injury, including the back, axillae, and perineum

RADIOLOGY AND LABORATORY STUDIES

- Findings from the primary and secondary surveys will guide imaging choices:
  - Perform computed tomography (CT) of the head for decreased mental status or focal neurologic deficits
  - Perform CT of the abdomen (with IV contrast) for patients with history of blunt abdominal trauma or with evidence of blunt abdominal trauma (e.g., "seat belt sign," hematuria)
  - Focused assessment with sonography for trauma (FAST) examination may be used to look for free fluid in the abdomen and for hemopericardium
    - In children, the role of FAST in trauma is evolving; it does not yet replace CT as a definitive study for detection of intraperitoneal blood, but it may help in prioritizing management goals in the initial postinjury period
  - Screening radiographs help identify immediately life-threatening injuries during the primary survey
    - Cross-table lateral C-spine: identifies 80% of fractures, subluxations, and dislocations; a negative film does not rule out all injuries (e.g., ligamentous)
    - Anteroposterior (AP) chest radiograph: may reveal hemo-/pneumothorax, rib fractures, mediastinal widening, and pulmonary contusions
    - AP pelvis radiograph: if indicated by injury mechanism or findings on examination, may reveal fracture(s) and allow for early pelvic binding to minimize blood loss into the pelvic cavity

LABORATORY STUDIES

- Most trauma patients should receive complete blood count (CBC), urinalysis (for blood), and type and screen
- Additional laboratory testing to consider (depending on mechanism of injury and/or clinical concern): complete metabolic panel (including liver transaminases), amylase, lipase, coagulation studies, blood gas
- For older children, the following may also be appropriate: urine pregnancy test, urine drug screen, serum ethanol level

EARLY RESUSCITATION

- Establish IV access early for administration of fluids and possibly blood products
  - Preferable IV access is two large-bore catheters in bilateral upper extremities. If unable to place two large IV catheters, consider placement of an intraosseous line
  - Avoid extremities in which there is concern for fracture
  - Resuscitation with crystalloid fluids should be started immediately (usually in boluses of 20 mL/kg for hypovolemic shock, and assessment should occur during and after each bolus to evaluate response)
  - Preparations should be made to initiate blood transfusion in patients for whom significant blood loss is a concern
    - Children with no response to 60 mL/kg of crystalloid fluids are likely to need blood products in addition to surgical intervention

SPECIFIC TRAUMA TYPES

Traumatic Injury of the Chest

BASIC INFORMATION

- In children, blunt chest trauma is more common than penetrating trauma to the chest
- Children with thoracic trauma may have injuries to the chest wall and bony thorax as well as to the trachea, bronchi, lung parenchyma, heart and great vessels, esophagus, and diaphragm
- The most common traumatic chest injuries in the pediatric population include lung contusions, hemo-/pneumothorax, and rib fractures

CLINICAL PRESENTATION, EVALUATION, AND INITIAL MANAGEMENT

- When evaluating the chest of a trauma patient, practitioners should take care to thoroughly assess for and take initial steps to stabilize the following potentially life-threatening injuries:
  - Injuries capable of causing respiratory failure:
    - Airway obstruction: such patients should be intubated early and with the assistance of a difficult-airway team when possible

- Injury to the trachea and/or bronchial tree: subcutaneous emphysema, dyspnea, and/or hemoptysis may indicate an injury to the bronchial tree
  - Pulmonary parenchymal injury (secondary to aspiration, contusion, laceration, or hemorrhage): supplemental oxygen and positive-pressure ventilation may assist with both oxygenation and ventilation
  - Chest wall injuries (including rib fractures and flail chest): stabilize the chest wall, and ensure adequate pain management to prevent inadequate respiratory effort
- Injuries causing circulatory failure:
  - Blunt cardiac injury: muffled heart sounds may herald pericardial effusion. Myocardial rupture or injury to great vessels can lead to cardiac tamponade and cardiogenic shock. In cases in which cardiovascular collapse is imminent, pericardiocentesis should be performed, preferably with ultrasound guidance
  - Intrathoracic hemorrhage: laceration of the myocardium and/or great vessels may lead to massive intrathoracic bleeding. Treatment will require IV fluid resuscitation, blood transfusion, and surgical correction as necessary
  - Tension pneumothorax or hemothorax: accumulation of air and/or blood in the pleural cavity will cause a shift of mediastinal structures and a decrease in venous return to the heart. Initial therapy is needle decompression followed by chest tube placement as a definitive stabilizing measure. Note that in children with tension physiology, endotracheal intubation should not be performed until the tension has been relieved

Traumatic Injury of the Abdomen

BASIC INFORMATION

- Weak abdominal musculature and a more pliable skeletal system make children more likely than adults to suffer from intraabdominal injuries due to blunt trauma
- In patients for whom there is significant concern for intraabdominal traumatic injury, practitioners must quickly and carefully determine whether the patient is hemodynamically stable and whether emergent operative control of intraperitoneal bleeding is necessary
- Patients with abdominal trauma often require frequent reassessment because severe intraabdominal injury can evolve over the first minutes to hours after the traumatic event. All children with traumatic injuries to the liver, spleen, pancreas, or hollow viscera should be hospitalized for close observation
- Injuries can be classified as "blunt" or "penetrating," as detailed below
- Penetrating abdominal trauma is less common than blunt (nonpenetrating) abdominal trauma in children; however, it carries extremely high morbidity and mortality secondary to potential for massive hemorrhage and injury to both solid and hollow organs
  - Mainstay of management is treatment of hemorrhagic shock and (in most cases) exploratory laparotomy

Splenic Injuries

BASIC INFORMATION

- The spleen is the intraabdominal organ most commonly injured in traumatic events
- Most serious splenic injuries occur secondary to blunt trauma (e.g., bicycle falls and automobile-pedestrian accidents)
- Given the extreme vascularity of the spleen, the highest risk to the patient from a splenic injury is the risk of life-threatening hemorrhage

CLINICAL PRESENTATION

- May present as either diffuse abdominal pain or local tenderness
- May also present as referred left shoulder pain (Kehr sign)
- Rarely, a patient will have ecchymosis overlying the left upper quadrant
- Often, the only clue to a splenic laceration is hemodynamic instability in the traumatized patient

DIAGNOSIS

- FAST examination may identify free intraperitoneal fluid; however, a negative FAST result does not rule out splenic laceration
- CT of the abdomen with IV contrast is the definitive diagnostic study and will demonstrate the extent of the splenic lesion
- Splenic lacerations are graded based on CT findings; note, however, that the decision about whether to operate is based on the patient's hemodynamic stability and not solely on the radiologic grading of his or her injury

TREATMENT

- Treatment involves volume expansion with crystalloid fluids as well as blood when necessary
- Input from a surgical consultant should also be sought
- Hemodynamically stable patients are managed expectantly with serial abdominal examinations; most life-threatening hemorrhages from splenic injury will occur within the first 24 hours after injury
- Hemodynamically unstable patients may be brought to the operating room for surgical control of bleeding; in some cases, splenectomy is required to achieve definitive hemorrhagic control
- Postsplenectomy, children under 5 years of age will require daily antibiotic prophylaxis, whereas older children may be given antimicrobial prophylaxis for the first 1 to 2 years after the procedure
- Depending upon their age and vaccination status, children who have undergone splenectomy may require repeat inoculation with all or some of the recommended series for *Streptococcus pneumoniae*

Liver Injuries

BASIC INFORMATION

- Blunt liver injury is the most common fatal abdominal traumatic injury in children
- Injury mechanism is generally the same as for blunt splenic injury

CLINICAL PRESENTATION

- As with splenic injuries, traumatic liver injuries may present with diffuse abdominal pain, local right upper quadrant pain, right shoulder tenderness, or right-sided abdominal wall contusion
- They may also present with hemodynamic instability as the only abnormal finding

DIAGNOSIS

- As with splenic injuries, diagnosis and grading of liver injury are via contrast-enhanced CT scan
- FAST examination may demonstrate fluid in the peritoneal cavity; as with splenic injuries, a negative FAST examination does not rule out liver laceration

TREATMENT

- Except for cases of significant hemodynamic instability, nonoperative management of traumatic liver injury with close observation by a trauma surgery service is the standard of care in most pediatric centers

Pancreatic Injuries

BASIC INFORMATION

- Pancreatic injuries usually result from blunt trauma to the epigastrium, most commonly from bike handlebars or from a vehicular lap belt crossing the upper abdomen of an inappropriately restrained child passenger
- Because the pancreas is anatomically well protected within the epigastrium, pancreatic injuries are significantly less common than blunt injuries to other solid organs
- Blunt trauma to the pancreas can lead to the formation of pseudocysts; if extensive, these cysts can disrupt pancreatic ductal flow and lead to enzyme leakage

CLINICAL PRESENTATION

- Diagnosis of traumatic pancreatic injury is difficult because the classic triad of epigastric pain, elevated amylase, and palpable epigastric mass is rarely present
- Pancreatic injuries most commonly present as nonspecific abdominal pain
- In severe cases, leakage of pancreatic enzymes causes peritonitis and the appearance of an acute abdomen

DIAGNOSIS

- Most patients with abdominal trauma will have an amylase drawn as part of their initial workup; although hyperamylasemia is suggestive of pancreatic injury, the absolute numeric value of the result is not indicative of injury severity. Additionally, an amylase level within normal limits does not rule out pancreatic injury
- Most diagnoses of pancreatic trauma are made with contrast-enhanced CT scan, although even CT is imperfect at identifying these elusive injuries

TREATMENT

- The mainstay of therapy for pancreatic injury is nasogastric decompression and bowel rest
- Isolated pseudocysts due to trauma are usually managed nonoperatively because many resolve on their own
- Pseudocysts that persist beyond 6 weeks after injury are generally drained percutaneously

Hollow Viscera Injuries

BASIC INFORMATION

- Injuries to the hollow viscera are most commonly caused by vehicle lap belts, automobile-pedestrian accidents, and nonaccidental trauma
- The mechanism of injury usually entails either compression of the viscera between two hard objects (e.g., lap belt and spine) or shearing force around a point of fixation (e.g., the ligament of Treitz)

CLINICAL PRESENTATION

- Patients with traumatic injury to the hollow viscera generally present with peritonitis and/or fever, which may evolve over several hours after the initial traumatic event
- Certain delayed presentations of hollow viscus injuries may not become clinically apparent until days or weeks after the initial injury
  - Symptoms of duodenal hematoma include bilious emesis, epigastric pain, and distention
  - Although extremely rare, hemobilia usually presents with abdominal pain and signs of upper gastrointestinal bleeding

DIAGNOSIS

- A high index of suspicion is needed to diagnose hollow viscus injuries because plain films demonstrate free air only 50% of the time
- Similarly, CT scans performed in the first few hours after a traumatic injury often miss bowel perforations
- Most hollow viscus injuries are identified in the operating room during laparoscopy or laparotomy in the setting of peritonitis or fever

TREATMENT

- Treatment of hollow viscus injuries is nearly always operative
- The decision to repair or resect the injured bowel depends on the location and extent of the injury

Renal and Urinary Tract Trauma

BASIC INFORMATION

- Renal injuries are nearly always caused by blunt trauma to the abdomen, flanks, or back
- Unlike adults:
  - Children are more likely to suffer traumatic renal injuries due to the relatively larger size of the kidney in children
  - Children do not reliably display hypotension as an indicator of kidney injury
- Luckily, most kidney injuries in children do not require urgent intervention

CLINICAL PRESENTATION

- Renal injuries are usually accompanied by localizing signs, including flank pain, ecchymosis, or mass
- Hematuria is highly specific for kidney injury, but its absence does not rule out trauma to the kidney or its surrounding vasculature
- In cases of high-grade renal fracture, patients may present with significant hemodynamic instability

DIAGNOSIS

- All children with multisystem trauma or with clinical concern for renal trauma should have a urinalysis sent
- FAST examination may detect perinephric fluid in cases of renal trauma, but it is less than 50% sensitive in detecting traumatic kidney injury
- Children with suspected kidney injury should undergo contrast-enhanced CT scan. Renal injuries are graded (I–V) based on CT findings

TREATMENT

- Most patients with renal injuries can be managed expectantly:
  - Grade I injuries can be discharged home and monitored with repeat urinalysis
  - Admission and close observation for at least 24 hours are indicated for Grades II and III injuries. Discharge is dependent on persistent hemodynamic stability and resolution of gross hematuria
  - Grades IV and V injuries are usually managed operatively
- Patients with significant hemodynamic instability may be taken to the operating room for operative management

Traumatic Injury of the Spine

BASIC INFORMATION

- Spinal cord injuries are relatively uncommon in children but may have devastating consequences
- The most common mechanism for spinal cord injuries in children is motor vehicle accidents (either as passenger, pedestrian, or bicyclist)

CLINICAL PRESENTATION, EVALUATION, AND INITIAL MANAGEMENT

- Clinical signs of spinal cord injury:
  - Awake patients: abnormal motor or sensory examination below the level of injury
  - Patients with multiple injuries or altered mental status: paradoxic respirations, priapism, Horner syndrome, abnormal reflexes, decreased perspiration below the level of injury
  - Spinal shock: practitioners should have a low threshold of suspicion in patients with hypotension, relative bradycardia, and a mechanism concerning for spinal cord injury. Other signs include temperature instability and peripheral vasodilation
- Considerations for cervical spine trauma:
  - C-spine should be immediately immobilized in all traumatized children with altered mental status, neurologic deficit(s), neck pain, or history concerning for high-risk mechanism or predisposition to cervical spine injury. Children with suspected spinal cord injuries should be stabilized on a long spine board
  - A cross-table lateral radiograph should be obtained during the secondary survey, followed by AP and odontoid views after initial assessment is complete
  - Children with multisystem injury or altered mental status usually cannot have their c-collar clinically cleared; these children must remain in a stiff collar until definitive imaging (usually magnetic resonance imaging [MRI]) is available (see Fig. 15.1 for cervical spine clinical clearance algorithm)
  - Children can have C-spine dislocations and/or ligamentous injury without evidence of bony abnormality on plain films (spinal cord injury without radiographic abnormality [SCIWORA]); a high index of suspicion should thus be maintained for both ligamentous and cord injuries even in patients with normal-appearing radiographs
- Management goals
  - Aim for normotension to mild hypertension because hypotension will threaten perfusion to the injured spinal cord
  - In spinal shock, initiation and titration of vasopressors is preferable to high-volume fluid resuscitation (unless associated injuries make large volumes of IV fluid necessary)
  - Patients with blunt spinal cord injuries should be treated with 30 mg/kg methylprednisolone within 8 hours of the initial traumatic event

Traumatic Injury of the Head

BASIC INFORMATION

- Traumatic brain injury (TBI) is the leading cause of death and disability among pediatric patients. TBI can be divided into two categories:

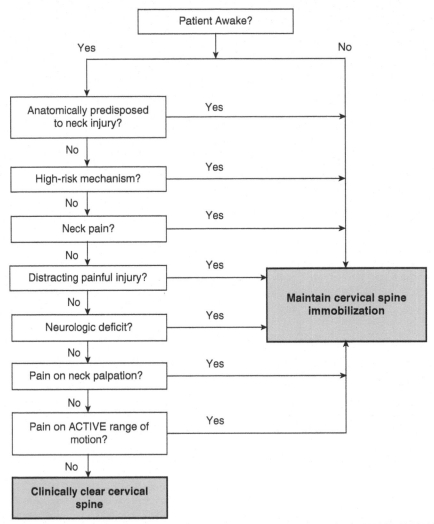

Fig. 15.1. Algorithm for clinically clearing cervical spine. (Data from American College of Surgeons Committee on Trauma. *Advanced Trauma Life Support [ATLS] Student Course Manual.* 9th ed. American College of Surgeons: Chicago, IL; 2012.)

- Primary brain injury: damage to brain parenchyma resulting directly from initial injury (e.g., axonal shearing, laceration by penetrating injury)
- Secondary brain injury: subsequent damage to brain tissue not injured by the initial trauma; most commonly secondary to hypoxia, hypoperfusion, or metabolic derangement
- The mainstays of management for children with TBI are rapid recognition and management of primary brain injury and prevention of secondary brain injury
  - TBI therapies are generally focused on maintaining cerebral perfusion pressure (CPP) to prevent secondary brain injury
  - CPP is the difference between mean arterial pressure (MAP) and intracranial pressure (ICP)
  - Any decrease in MAP or increase in ICP will threaten CPP

INJURIES CAUSING INCREASED ICP

- Epidural hematoma (EDH)
  - Usually the result of a direct localized blow to the head leading to a skull fracture and laceration of epidural vessels

- Classic presentation is initial loss of consciousness (LOC) followed by "lucid interval," although the minority of patients present this way
- Most common presenting symptoms are lethargy, vomiting, and headache
- On noncontrast CT, EDH appears as a high-density, biconvex lesion adjacent to the skull (see Fig. 15.2)
- The mainstay of therapy for EDH is immediate neurosurgical consultation and craniotomy with evacuation of blood contents
- Subdural hematoma (SDH)
  - Usually the result of shearing forces to the brain (e.g., rapid acceleration-deceleration from motor vehicle accident or nonaccidental trauma) leading to tearing of bridging veins in subdural space
  - Most common presenting symptoms are depressed mental status, headache, vomiting, or seizures—with or without initial loss of consciousness at the time of injury
  - On noncontrast CT, SDH will appear as a high-density crescentic lesion in the extraaxial space (see Fig. 15.3)

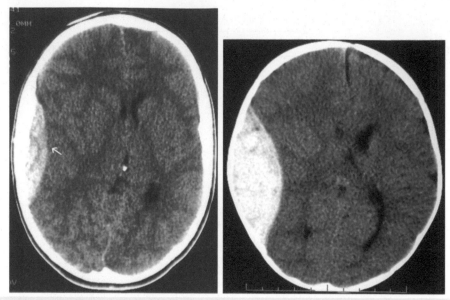

Fig. 15.2. Epidural hematoma. (From Dunoski B, Slovis TL. Update in pediatric imaging. *Advances in Pediatrics,* 2014;61[1]:75–125.)

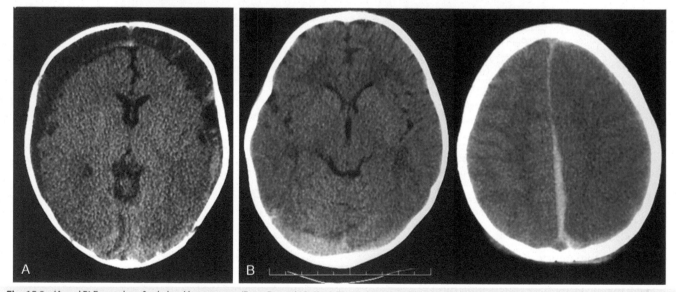

Fig. 15.3. (A and B) Examples of subdural hematoma. (From Dunoski B, Slovis TL. Update in pediatric imaging. *Advances in Pediatrics,* 2014;61[1]:75–125, Fig. 39.)

- Children with nonsevere SDH (no significant mass effect) can usually be managed nonoperatively; severe SDH requires surgical evacuation
- Subarachnoid hemorrhage (SAH)
  - Can result from either a severe direct blow or severe shearing forces that lead to the tearing of small vessels in pia mater
  - SAH alone rarely causes increased ICP; SAH does cause cerebral vasospasm, leading to cerebral hypoxia and diffuse brain swelling (DBS; see Fig. 15.4)
- Diffuse axonal injury (DAI) and DBS
  - DAI is caused by shearing forces similar to those for SDH
  - DBS is caused by DAI and/or by hypoxia/metabolic derangements occurring after initial injury
  - Both DAI and DBS can lead to increased ICP and decreased CPP

MEDICAL MANAGEMENT OF INCREASED ICP

- Whereas some of the aforementioned causes of increased ICP require immediate surgical intervention, others require intensive monitoring and medical management
- Generally, after TBI a delayed brain swelling will occur over 24 to 48 hours, which will further increase ICP; this will threaten CPP and lead to further secondary injury
  - Additionally, hypotension (low MAP) will also yield decreased CPP and therefore should be avoided in TBI patients; it may require aggressive fluid resuscitation and early inotropic/vasopressor support
- Hyperosmolar therapies:
  - Thought to decrease ICP by increasing intravascular osmolarity and "pulling water" from the brain; may also decrease ICP through a rheologic mechanism

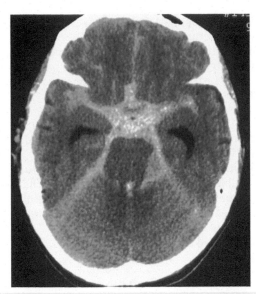

Fig. 15.4. Subarachnoid hemorrhage. (From Hacein-Bey L, Origitano TC, Biller J. Subarachnoid Hemorrhage in Young Adults. *Stroke in Children and Young Adults.* Vol. 2. Saunders Elsevier: Philadelphia; 2009:289–314. Fig. 15.1.)

- May be employed when there is concern for increased ICP and neurosurgical intervention is not indicated or not immediately available:
  - Mannitol: 0.25-1 g/kg/dose as a 20% solution over 10 minutes
  - 3% Hypertonic saline: 5 mL/kg as a one-time IV bolus over 3 to 5 minutes

OTHER HEAD INJURIES

- Concussion
  - Head injury resulting in altered mental status, in which no imaging is performed or in which head CT is normal
  - Most commonly results from falls in young children and from sports in older children
  - Most common presenting symptoms: confusion, headache, nausea and/or vomiting, dizziness, amnesia, difficulty concentrating
  - Patients usually are back to baseline within a week. Patients with persistent symptoms can undergo vestibular therapy as part of a gradual return to school and sports
- Skull fractures
  - Most commonly from falls in infants; also from child abuse and motor vehicle crashes in older children
    - Highest risk group consists of infants under 1 year of age
  - Can occur in any bone of the skull; parietal bone is most common
  - Most commonly present with overlying hematoma; bony abnormalities are difficult to palpate
  - Can be diagnosed with plain film or CT (preferred)
  - Linear skull fractures: more commonly associated with underlying brain injury in older children
    - Isolated linear skull fractures (without underlying brain injury) usually do not require intervention
  - Basilar skull fracture: presents with cerebrospinal fluid rhinorrhea, "raccoon eyes," "battle sign" (bruising over mastoid), hemotympanum

- Depressed skull fractures: usually associated with underlying brain injury and often require surgical intervention
- There is a low threshold for considering child abuse in infants and young children with skull fractures

IMAGING GUIDELINES FOR HEAD INJURIES

- Criteria derived from Pediatric Emergency Care Applied Research Network (PECARN)
  - Children for whom head CT is recommended:
    - Under 2 years with:
      GCS 14 or below
      Any other sign of altered mental status
      Palpable skull fracture
    - 2 years and older with:
      GCS 14 or below
      Any other sign of altered mental status
      Basilar skull fracture
  - Children for whom an observation period may allow avoidance of CT:
    - Under 2 years with none of the following:
      Nonfrontal scalp hematoma
      History of LOC 5 seconds or greater
      Severe mechanism of injury
      Not acting normally per parents
    - 2 years and older with none of the following:
      History of LOC
      History of vomiting
      Severe mechanism of injury
      Severe headache

Dental Trauma

BASIC INFORMATION

- 30% of preschool-aged children suffer injuries to primary teeth; incidence is equal between boys and girls
- Among injuries to permanent teeth, incidence is twice as high among boys
- Serious dental injuries without plausible explanation are concerning for nonaccidental trauma
- High-force dental trauma may be associated with significant head and neck injuries

CLINICAL PRESENTATION, EVALUATION, AND INITIAL MANAGEMENT

- Injuries to primary teeth
  - Avulsion: should not be reimplanted; ensure that entire tooth is accounted for; otherwise consider radiographs of head/neck/chest to rule out intrusion or aspiration
  - Extrusion: removal is necessary if tooth poses aspiration risk; refer to dentist or remove gently
  - Intrusion: will typically re-erupt spontaneously; requires dental evaluation within days to rule out injury to underlying permanent tooth
  - Lateral luxation: no intervention necessary if displacement does not interfere with bite mechanics
  - Concussion or subluxation: soft diet and routine dental follow-up; gray discoloration of concussed tooth suggests pulp necrosis and requires dental evaluation

- Fracture: nonemergent referral to a dentist if concern for root/pulp involvement
- Injuries to permanent teeth
  - Avulsion:
    - Avulsion is a dental emergency requiring immediate intervention because prognosis is inversely proportional to time the tooth is out of place
    - Handle tooth by crown and rinse gently without scrubbing
    - Manually implant in empty socket
    - Keep reimplanted tooth in place either with manual pressure or by having child bite on a piece of rolled gauze
    - Refer for urgent dental evaluation and treatment (usually splinting)
    - If immediate implantation is not possible, store in cold milk or a container of the child's saliva until treatment is available
  - Extrusion, intrusion, and lateral luxation:
    - Require repositioning and splinting by a pediatric dentist
    - Goal is reduction of luxation within 2 hours when possible
  - Concussion and subluxation: nonurgent dental follow-up within days for radiographs to look for root/pulp involvement
  - Fractures:
    - Alveolar ridge fracture: urgent referral to an oral maxillofacial surgeon or dentist
    - Root fracture: prompt (within 48 hours) referral to a dentist for splinting
    - Crown fracture: nonurgent dental follow-up (within days) for bonding as necessary

Extremity Fractures in Children

BASIC INFORMATION

- Details regarding common fractures are covered in Chapter 72.
- Brief overviews of fracture patterns are covered here:
  - Torus "buckle" fractures:
    - Most commonly in distal radius, followed by distal tibia, fibula, and femur
    - Result from axial compression (e.g., fall on outstretched hand)
    - Can be managed with splinting versus cast and nonurgent orthopedic follow-up
  - Plastic deformation "bowing" fractures:
    - Most commonly in the midshaft of ulna, radius, and fibula
    - Longitudinal bowing of plastic long bones in young children
    - If less than 20% of deformity, intervention is rarely needed; otherwise, refer to orthopedics for closed reduction (can be splinted in the interim)
  - Greenstick fractures:
    - Bending of long bone with fracture line that does not extend completely through shaft

- Occur in prepubertal children with pliable bones
- Physeal fractures:
  - Involve the growth plate; therefore can affect growth symmetry if not managed correctly
  - Salter-Harris classification system and management are detailed in Chapter 72.
- Easily missed fracture types:
  - Salter-Harris type I: children with pain over the physis and a normal radiograph should be assumed to have a Salter-Harris type I fracture
  - Toddler's fracture: nondisplaced spiral fracture of the distal tibia; immediately after injury, plain films may be normal; in children with persistent refusal to ambulate, repeat plain films a week after initial injury will usually reveal the diagnosis
  - Nondisplaced supracondylar fracture

Nonaccidental Trauma

BASIC INFORMATION

- Details regarding the approach and diagnosis of nonaccidental trauma (NAT) are covered in Chapter 90
- American Academy of Pediatrics (AAP) imaging recommendations (2015):
  - Skeletal survey: all children under 2 years of age with suspected NAT, especially:
    - Children under 2 years of age with obvious abusive injuries
    - Children under 2 years of age with suspicious injury, including bruising or oral injury in nonambulatory infants
    - Infants and young toddlers with unexplained intracranial injury
    - Infant and toddler siblings of an abused child
  - Head imaging: all patients with suspected abusive head trauma require head CT (in cases of depressed mental status or focal neurologic deficit) and/or MRI (in cases with normal mental status and neurologic examination)

Review Questions

For review questions, please go to ExpertConsult.com.

Suggested Readings

1. American College of Surgeons Committee on Trauma. *Advanced Trauma Life Support (ATLS) Student Course Manual.* 9th ed. Chicago: American College of Surgeons; 2012.
2. Canale ST. Fractures and dislocations in children. In: *Campbell's Operative Orthopedics.* 12th ed. Philadelphia: Mosby; 2012.
3. Lavoie M, Nance ML. Approach to the injured child. In: Shaw KN, Bachur RG, eds. *Fleischer and Ludwig's Textbook of Pediatric Emergency Medicine.* 7th ed. Philadelphia: Lippincott Williams & Wilkins; 2016.
4. Management of shock. In: Chameides L, Samson RA, Schexnayder SM, Hazinski MF, eds. *Pediatric Advanced Life Support Provider Manual.* Dallas: American Heart Association, Subcommittee on Pediatric Resuscitation; 2010;122(18 suppl 3). http://circ.ahajournals.org/content/122/18_suppl_3/S876.long.
5. Stafford PW, Blinman TA, Nance ML. Practical points in evaluation and resuscitation of the injured child. *Surg Clin North Am.* 2002;82:273–300.

16 Bites, Stings, and Wounds

MAMATA V. SENTHIL, MD, MSED

ANIMAL AND INSECT BITES

Dog and Cat Bites

BASIC INFORMATION

- Around 4.5 million dog bites and ~400,000 cat bites in the United States each year, with children being the most commonly injured
- Dog bites account for 80% to 90% of all animal bite injuries
- Most common pathogens include *Pasteurella multocida*, followed by staphylococcus, streptococcus, and anaerobic bacteria

CLINICAL PRESENTATION

- Dog bites often involve the head and neck in younger children and extremities in older children, whereas cat bites more commonly affect the upper extremities
- Puncture wounds are of particular concern given the seemingly innocuous surface injury but the higher risk for deep tissue infection
- Compared with the onset of symptoms from other pathogens, the onset from pasteurella infection is much more rapid and usually occurs within 24 hours, along with significant pain, swelling, and/or drainage at the site of the bite

EVALUATION

- Wound cultures may be obtained for infected-appearing wounds
- Plain radiographs or ultrasonography may be warranted for deep bite wounds near joints or if there is concern for a foreign body

MANAGEMENT

- Thorough irrigation and cleansing of the wound. Avoid high-pressure irrigation of puncture wounds
- Primary closure can be done when the wound is <12 hours old (24 hours if on face) and appears uninfected, and when the cosmetic result is a concern, such as with wounds involving the face. Wounds with higher risk of infection, such as puncture wounds, bites involving hands or feet, or crush injuries, should not be repaired by primary closure
- Administration of tetanus vaccine if the individual has not been adequately vaccinated
- Antimicrobials

- Antibiotic prophylaxis can be given for wounds with higher risk of infection:
  - Puncture wounds
  - Wounds involving hands, genitalia, face, or in close proximity to bone or joints
  - Wounds requiring closure
  - Moderate to severe wound injuries
- Antimicrobial agent should cover *P. multocida* species, which is a common pathogen causing infection after dog bites, cat bites, and cat scratches
  - Amoxicillin-clavulanate is the most appropriate choice for empiric treatment of most human and animal bite wounds. Clindamycin plus trimethoprim-sulfamethoxazole is an alternative regimen for penicillin-allergic patients
- Rabies prophylaxis
  - Postexposure rabies prophylaxis should be given if vaccination status of animal is inadequate or unknown
- Treatment includes the human rabies immune globulin (HRIG) injected around the site of the bites in addition to the four-series rabies vaccine given on days 0, 3, 7, and 14

Human Bites

BASIC INFORMATION

- Human bites are the third most common type of bites seen in the emergency department (ED) after dog and cat bites
- Pathogens from human bites are often mixed aerobic and anaerobic organisms, given the nature of oral flora, and include streptococci, *Staphylococcus aureus*, *Eikenella*, *Fusobacterium*, *Peptostreptococcus*, *Prevotella*, and *Porphyromonas* spp.

CLINICAL PRESENTATION

- Human bites generally appear as semicircular- or oval-appearing areas of erythema or bruising, with or without intact skin
- In young children, bites are often the result of aggression from other children and are most commonly found on the face, upper extremities, or trunk, typically with superficial wounds or intact skin
  - Deep puncture human bites should raise suspicion for child abuse because they are likely caused by an adult
- Bite wounds can also occur in adolescents and older children as a result of closed-fist injuries in which the

patient punches someone in their mouth or teeth. These wounds are at high risk of infection given the proximity of the skin wounds to the joint space of the knuckles

MANAGEMENT

- Prophylactic antibiotics should be administered for bites through the dermis and for wounds involving the hands, given the higher risk of infection
- Antibiotics
  - Should choose an agent with anaerobic coverage and coverage against *Eikenella*. Amoxicillin or amoxicillin-clavulanate are both reasonable options for prophylaxis or treatment of infection

Snake Bites

Pit Vipers (Crotalidae Family) [including Rattlesnakes, Water Moccasins / Cottonmouths, and Copperheads]

BASIC INFORMATION

- Most common venomous snakebite in the United States and typically seen in southern and western states. Rattlesnake envenomations are usually the most clinically severe
- 25% of Crotalidae snakebites are "dry bites" in which no envenomation occurs and only local tissue irritation develops
- Appearance of venomous snakes: triangular-shaped head; elliptical-shaped pupils; large, retractable hollow fangs; heat-sensing pit between eye and nose
- Appearance of nonvenomous snakes: rounded heads, round pupils, no fangs

CLINICAL PRESENTATION

- Local tissue damage with progressive swelling
- Systemic symptoms: tachycardia, hypotension, tachypnea, nausea, vomiting, diarrhea, weakness, light-headedness, diaphoresis, and chills
- Coagulopathy, rhabdomyolysis, increased vascular permeability, neurotoxicity (altered mental status, seizures, paresthesias, fasciculations)

MANAGEMENT

- Constrictive clothing, jewelry, and watches should be removed; avoid tourniquets or pressure dressings
- Keep child warm, at rest, and as calm as possible in a supine position
- Immobilize injured body part to the level of the heart
- Local cleansing and wound care
- Pain control and tetanus vaccine as indicated
- Obtain labs if systemic symptoms are present (complete blood count [CBC], electrolytes, creatinine kinase [CK], coagulants, fibrinogen, D-dimer)

- Indications for pit viper antivenom: consult with medical toxicologist, most effective when given within 6 hours of envenomation
  - Should be given to patients with moderate to severe toxicity or bites to head or neck that may cause airway compromise
  - Patients with mild symptoms can be observed closely for 12 to 24 hours without giving antivenom

Coral Snakes (Elapidae Family)
BASIC INFORMATION

- Coral snakebites are rare. Found predominantly in the southern United States
- Appearance: small, oblong heads; no pit; short, hollow fangs; red and yellow bands adjacent to each other. "Red on yellow, kill a fellow. Red on black, venom lack" helps distinguish from similar-appearing nonvenomous snakes

CLINICAL PRESENTATION

- Little to no tissue damage but can develop neurotoxic effects due to neuromuscular blockade (cranial nerve [CN] palsies: ptosis, dysarthria, dysphagia, respiratory failure)
- Onset of systemic effects can be delayed for hours

MANAGEMENT

- Same initial management as for pit viper bites
- Coral snake antivenom should be administered early given greater risk of neurotoxicity compared with other venomous snakebites

Spider Bites

Black Widow (*Lactrodectus Mactans*)
BASIC INFORMATION

- Typical appearance includes a shiny black body with red hourglass shape on ventral surface of abdomen
- Most common in southeastern region of the United States
- Localized pain usually develops within 5 to 20 minutes of the bite, whereas more widespread symptoms can occur within hours

CLINICAL PRESENTATION

- Local reactions
- Lesions are pale, circular areas with central punctum surrounded by an erythematous ring
- "Lactrodectism": localized muscle pain, rigidity, diaphoresis, weakness, paresthesias, or pain extending to the abdomen or chest
- Systemic reactions
- Younger children more likely to have severe envenomation

- Tachycardia, hypertension, nausea, vomiting, headache, shortness of breath, severe abdominal pain and cramping
- Rarely causes death, but younger children are at higher risk

MANAGEMENT

- Local cleansing and wound care
- Oral analgesics, benzodiazepines for muscle spasms
- Tetanus prophylaxis if needed, antibiotics if signs of superinfection; steroids are not recommended
- Lesions usually *do not* become necrotic; no debridement necessary
- Antivenom is reserved for children <40 kg with confirmed black widow spider bites and moderate to severe envenomation

Brown Recluse (*Loxosceles Reclusa*)

BASIC INFORMATION

- Identified by characteristic violin-shaped marking on portion of the body to which the legs attach; hence a "fiddleback"
- In the United States, predominantly found in midwestern and southeastern states. Most bites occur in the summer months

CLINICAL PRESENTATION

- Local reactions
- Initially painless blister or papule. Symptoms typically occur 2 to 8 hours after bite. Lesions can sometimes become necrotic or ulcerated days to weeks later.
- Localized pain, itching, muscle pain, redness
  - Systemic reactions
  - Fever, nausea, vomiting
  - Rarely causes death, but younger children are at higher risk of severe systemic involvement (e.g., Disseminated Intravascular Coagulation)

MANAGEMENT

- Local cleansing and wound care
- PO (per os) analgesics, antihistamines for itching; tetanus prophylaxis if indicated; antibiotics if signs of superinfection
- Debridement may be necessary for larger necrotic wounds

Prevention of Animal Bites

- Anticipatory guidance should be given to families:
  - Close supervision of small children in the presence of animals
  - Teaching children at an early age safety and respect surrounding household pets
  - Animals with a history of aggression are inappropriate in households with children
  - See also Nelson Textbook of Pediatrics, Chapter 668, "Arthropod Bites and Infestations."

STINGS

Scorpion Stings

BASIC INFORMATION

- *Centruroides sculpturatus,* also known as *C. exilicauda,* is a highly neurotoxic species distinguished by a tubercle at the base of the stinger
- Typically found in southwestern United States and Mexico

CLINICAL PRESENTATION

- Presentation grade varies with degree of envenomation:
  - Grade I: local pain and paresthesias, usually no local inflammation, may not see punctum
  - Grade II: local symptoms that radiate proximally up affected extremity
  - Grade III: either CN *or* somatic skeletal neuromuscular dysfunction
    - CN dysfunction (blurred vision, abnormal eye movement, slurred speech, tongue fasciculations, hypersalivation)
    - Somatic skeletal neuromuscular dysfunction (restlessness, fasciculations, shaking/jerking extremities, opisthotonos)
  - Grade IV: CN *and* somatic skeletal neuromuscular dysfunction
    - Respiratory distress, hyperthermia, pulmonary edema, metabolic acidosis, and multiorgan failure

MANAGEMENT

- Grade I or II: oral analgesics, local wound cleansing and care, tetanus prophylaxis
- Grade III or IV: airway management and intensive care monitoring if needed
- Antivenom: indicated for Grade III or IV Centruroides scorpion stings

Jellyfish Stings

BASIC INFORMATION

- Jellyfish stings most commonly occur in warm and coastal waters around the world

CLINICAL PRESENTATION

- Jellyfish stings occur as a result of envenomation of toxin-producing nematocysts released by jellyfish tentacles
- Patients usually experience immediate pain at the time of the sting, followed by linear, erythematous, urticarial lesions minutes to hours later. These lesions can cause itching, burning, and throbbing, and the pain can radiate
- Lesions are usually localized but intensely pruritic; papular urticarial reactions can recur days later
- Lesions usually resolve within 10 days but can sometimes persist for weeks

MANAGEMENT

- Prompt removal of jellyfish tentacles by brushing off with a plastic object such as a credit card; avoid vigorous rubbing, which can cause further toxin release
- Remedies for jellyfish stings have shown variable effectiveness depending on type of species and geographic area
- In general, studies have shown effectiveness with hot water immersion of the affected limb or application of vinegar (acetic acid) to prevent further envenomation by the nematocysts
- Pain management

Hymenoptera Stings

BASIC INFORMATION

- Hymenoptera species include winged insects (bees, wasps, yellow jackets, and hornets) as well as fire ants

CLINICAL PRESENTATION

- Local reactions: painful, itchy, red swelling at the site of sting. Some people may develop large local reactions (>10 cm) that last for several days
- Systemic allergic reaction: anaphylaxis in venom-allergic

MANAGEMENT

- Stingers should be removed as quickly as possible due to continued venom secretion
- Pseudopustules caused by fire ant stings should not be unroofed
- Local reactions: local wound care, nonsteroidal antiinflammatory drugs (NSAIDs), cold compresses, antihistamines; may consider oral steroids for large local reactions
- Anaphylaxis management if indicated (e.g. intramuscular epinephrine) (see Chapter 3 for details)
- Venom immunotherapy
  - Indicated for any patient, regardless of age, with a systemic reaction and a positive skin test
  - Not usually indicated for children ≤16 years of age with only a cutaneous reaction and no systemic response because their risk for a systemic reaction after a subsequent sting is only ~10%. Indications for venom immunotherapy as outlined by the Task force for the American Academy of Allergy, Asthma and Immunology Practice Parameters. Link to the journal guidelines are here: https://www.jacionline.org/article/S0091-6749(11)00114-X/fulltext#appsecb35

Tick Bites

- Can cause several diseases including Lyme disease, Rocky Mountain spotted fever, ehrlichiosis, babesiosis and tularemia
- Tick removal
  - The longer ticks are attached to skin and the more engorged they are, the higher the likelihood

of transmission of tick-borne diseases. For this reason, removal of a tick as soon as it is noticed is imperative
  - Use tweezers or small forceps to grasp the tick as close to the skin as possible. If no forceps are available, use a paper or cloth between fingers to extract the tick. Pull gently but firmly using steady pressure. Avoid crushing or squeezing the tick
  - After removal, disinfect the skin and wash hands with soap and water
  - Local heat, gasoline, and fingernail polish are ineffective methods for tick removal. Avoid crushing the tick because this can release additional infectious secretions into the wound

Insect Repellants

- Per the American Academy of Pediatrics (AAP) guidelines, insect repellants for children can be used to prevent insect bites, but products for children should contain no more than 30% DEET
- Should be used for outdoors only; once indoors, children should promptly wash off repellant with soap and water and put sprayed clothing in the laundry

WOUNDS

General Wound Care

- Copious irrigation under pressure with tap water or normal saline to remove debris
- Soap and water to cleanse wound
- Intact blisters should be left alone. Broken blisters or necrotic tissue should be debrided

Lacerations

BASIC INFORMATION

- Lacerations in children more commonly occur on the face and scalp as compared with adults. Given the increased vascularity of these locations, wounds are less likely to become infected
- Lacerations over joints are more likely to develop wider scars given increased tension during healing. Horizontal or vertical mattress sutures may be necessary for higher-tension wounds. Deep lacerations often need a two-layer closure with deep dermal absorbable sutures in addition to superficial epidermal sutures
- Staples are an appropriate choice for the scalp, where appearance of scarring is less important; skin adhesives may be ideal for linear, superficial, well-approximated lacerations that are not under tension
- Primary closure should occur within 24 hours
- Antibiotic prophylaxis is usually not indicated, with the exception of animal bites or dirty wounds at risk for infection
- Special case: lip lacerations

Table 16.1. Indications for Tetanus Prophylaxis

History of Tetanus Toxoid Immunization	CLEAN, MINOR WOUNDS		ALL OTHER WOUNDS[1]	
	Tdap or Td[2]	TIG	Tdap or Td[2]	TIG
Uncertain or <3 doses	Yes	No	Yes	Yes
Three or more doses	No[3]	No	No[4]	No

Adapted from the Centers for Disease Control and Prevention (CDC). Prevention of Pertussis, Tetanus, and Diphtheria with Vaccines in the United States: Recommendations of the Advisory Committee on Immunization Practices (ACIP). MMWR Recomm Rep 2018;67(No. RR-2):1–44. https://www.cdc.gov/mmwr/volumes/67/rr/rr6702a1.htm#T6_down.

[1]Includes dirty wounds such as those contaminated with dirt, feces, and saliva; puncture wounds; crush injuries; burns; and avulsions.
[2]For children <7 years, DTaP is the preferred method for tetanus toxoid booster if <3 doses of DTaP have been given. For children >7 years, Tdap is the preferred method, though Td can be given if Tdap booster has already been received previously.
[3]Yes if ≥10 years since last tetanus toxoid–containing vaccine dose.
[4]Yes if >5 years since last tetanus toxoid–containing vaccine dose.

- Most lacerations involving the mucosa of the mouth do not need primary closure, given the high vascularity and rapid healing. However, lacerations involving the lip that cross the vermilion border should be repaired with careful attention paid to realignment of the lip border for optimal cosmetic results. Consultation with plastic surgery may be necessary for more complex lip wounds

Puncture Wounds

MANAGEMENT

- Most puncture wounds through the foot can be managed with thorough irrigation and a tetanus booster if indicated. Cellulitis may develop, with *S. aureus* and *Pseudomonas aeruginosa* being the most common pathogens
- Less common sequelae from puncture wounds include septic arthritis and osteomyelitis
  - A puncture wound through a running shoe or sneaker has a higher risk of pseudomonas infection, and a 10- to 14-day course of antibiotics for *P. aeruginosa* should be considered, such as ciprofloxacin

Tetanus Prophylaxis

- Indications for tetanus prophylaxis in wound management: see Table 16.1 for further details

- A tetanus toxoid booster (Td or Tdap) should be given to the following individuals:
  - All persons with any wound if the tetanus immunization status is unknown or incomplete
  - More than 10 years have passed since last booster in an individual who has minor, clean wounds and has completed the primary immunization series
  - More than 5 years have passed since the last booster in an individual who has more serious wounds and has completed the primary immunization series
- Tetanus immune globulin (TIG) should be given to the following individuals:
  - All persons with more serious wounds and with an unknown or incomplete tetanus immunization status

Review Questions

For review questions, please go to ExpertConsult.com.

Suggested Readings

1. Black KD, Cico SJ, Cagler D. Wound management. *Pediatr Rev.* 2015;36(5):207–216.
2. Garcia VF. Animal bites and *Pasturella* infections. *Pediatr Rev.* 1997;18(4):127–130.
3. Schroeder BJ, Norris RL. Envenomations. In: Kliegman RM, Stanton BM, St. Geme J, Schor NF, eds. *Nelson Textbook of Pediatrics.* 20th ed. Philadelphia: Elsevier; 2016:3452–3459.

17 | *Heat-Related Illnesses and Pediatric Drowning*

COURTNEY E. NELSON, MD and MERCEDES M. BLACKSTONE, MD

Heat-Related Illnesses

Heat-related illnesses include any condition caused by high environmental temperatures and a stressed thermoregulation system. These conditions range from those that are low risk, such as heat rash, to high-risk conditions, such as heat exhaustion and heatstroke.

BASIC INFORMATION

- Heat-related illnesses are caused by excessive external heat exposure, the failure of thermoregulation, or a combination of the two
- Heat-related illnesses can be classified by their severity
  - Heat rash, heat edema, heat syncope, and heat cramps are milder complications of the body's response to excessive heat
  - Heat exhaustion is a moderate complication with significant morbidity, and heatstroke is an absolute emergency that can be fatal
  - Heatstroke is typically divided into nonexertional and exertional heatstroke based on the underlying mechanism
- Heat-related illnesses doubled between 1997 and 2006, and patients <19 years of age represent the majority of cases. There were over 3000 heat-related deaths between 2006 and 2010; of those, patients <1 year of age and patients >65 years of age had the highest rates of death
- Risk factors are shown in Table 17.1
- Pediatric-specific considerations in heat-related illnesses:
  - Children are more vulnerable to ambient heat
    - Greater body surface area to absorb more heat
  - Children have higher endogenous heat production
    - Higher metabolic rate
  - Children are less efficient at heat dissipation
    - Decreased sweating ability
    - Decreased blood volume, limiting heat loss by vasodilation
    - Decreased ability to acclimatize
    - Less likely to rehydrate adequately

PATHOPHYSIOLOGY

- Normal thermoregulation: balance between heat generation and heat loss
  - Thermoregulation occurs in the hypothalamus, and when it is functioning properly, our temperature varies between 36°C and 38°C (96.8°F to 100.4°F)
- Heat is lost in four different ways:

- Evaporation (transfer of heat by converting a liquid to a gas) is our primary means of heat loss and occurs with sweating and panting
- Radiation (transfer of heat through electromagnetic waves) will occur if body temperature is higher than ambient temperature
- Conduction (transfer of heat to adjacent objects) will occur if the body touches colder objects, such as a cooling blanket
- Convection (transfer of heat to air currents) is aided by ambient wind
- Physiology of heat loss: efferent fibers from the hypothalamus direct the autonomic nervous system to facilitate heat loss in the following ways:
  - Tachycardia: increased stroke volume will bring more blood to the periphery and facilitate heat loss by radiation, conduction, and convection
  - Vasodilation: similarly will increase blood flow to the periphery and allow for radiation, conduction, and convection
  - Diaphoresis (sweating): primary means of evaporative heat loss; typically sodium is lost in sweat, as well, ranging from 30 to 65 mmol/L
  - Tachypnea (panting): another means of evaporative heat loss
- Loss of thermoregulation: temperature rises above physiologic set point
  - Evaporation fails at humidity levels >75%
  - Convection, conduction, and radiation fail at ambient temperatures >95°F (35°C)
  - Critical thermal maximum (CTM) is a threshold after which point there is diffuse cell injury through both an inflammatory cascade of cytokines and the denaturing of cellular proteins. Typically this threshold is 42°C for as little as 45 minutes to a maximum of 8 hours, depending on the person

CLINICAL PRESENTATION

- Clinical findings are variable depending on the type of heat-related illness and severity. They can be divided into conditions with a normal core temperature and conditions with an elevated core temperature
- Normal core temperature
  - Heat rash (miliaria rubra): obstruction of sweat glands by either significant sweating or tight clothing, leading to an erythematous, papular (sometimes pustular) rash on the face, trunk, neck, and, although less so, extremities or exposed areas

Table 17.1. Risk Factors for Heat-Related Illnesses

Demographic Risk Factors	Environmental Risk Factors	Medical History Risk Factors
NONEXERTIONAL HEATSTROKE: - Younger age **EXERTIONAL HEATSTROKE:** - High school athletes - Football is the highest risk[1]	- Higher ambient temperatures - Parked cars or closed spaces without air conditioning - Higher humidity - Excess clothing	**ACUTE HISTORICAL RISK FACTORS:** - Inadequate sleep - Alcohol consumption - Poor acclimatization - Dehydration - Recent febrile illness **CHRONIC MEDICAL HISTORY:** - Poor cardiovascular fitness - Obesity - Prior heat-related illness - Sickle cell trait **COMMON MEDICATIONS:** - Psychiatric medications - Anticholinergics - Decongestants - Tricyclic antidepressants - Antihistamines - Benzodiazepines

- Heat edema: mild swelling (nonpitting) in dependent areas (typically only hands and feet) related to vasodilation and poor venous return
- Heat syncope: fainting episode after exertional activity in high ambient temperatures. These episodes typically occur after exercise has ceased; there is vasodilation and poor venous return secondary to muscle relaxation, resulting in poor cerebral perfusion. Patients may present with hypotension and cool, moist extremities
- Heat cramps: severe muscle spasms of the extremities and abdomen after exertional activity in elevated ambient temperatures. Cramping is typically transient but can last a few minutes or longer. The mechanism is related to electrolyte abnormalities, and patients may have hyponatremia, hypokalemia, or hypochloremia on laboratory testing
- Heat exhaustion: multitude of viral illness–like symptoms (fatigue, headache, nausea/vomiting, myalgias) with normal to mildly elevated core temperature (less than 40.6°C). Patients may have hypernatremia due to water depletion or hyponatremia due to electrolyte depletion. Heat exhaustion can be the precursor to heatstroke, and it should be treated aggressively
- Elevated core temperature
  - Heatstroke: distinguished from heat exhaustion by a core temperature >40.6°C and central nervous system (CNS) dysfunction
    - CNS symptoms range from severe headache and irritability to seizure and coma
    - Nonexertional heatstroke tends to be insidious because a patient may not come to medical attention until he or she is obtunded
    - Exertional heatstroke may present in a healthy, young athlete sweating after a strenuous workout, followed by rapid neurologic decline
    - Individuals with heatstroke will be tachycardic and may have significant hypotension related to profound vasodilation. These patients can have significant hyperventilation in an effort to promote more conductive heat loss
    - Muscles spasms and dehydration can lead to rhabdomyolysis or muscle breakdown and subsequent renal disease
    - In the most extreme cases, patients may develop multiorgan dysfunction syndrome (MODS)
    - Laboratory abnormalities may include hyper- or hyponatremia, hypokalemia, hypochloremia, respiratory alkalosis with a metabolic acidosis, transaminitis, coagulopathy, azotemia, and myoglobinuria

DIAGNOSIS AND EVALUATION

- Heat-related illnesses are diagnosed clinically
- Elements of heat rash, heat edema, heat syncope, and heat exhaustion all overlap with heatstroke, but the neurologic dysfunction and temperature of >40°C distinguish heatstroke from the other heat-related illnesses
- One should have a high clinical suspicion for heatstroke given its severe complications; all patients with heat exhaustion should have a core temperature (typically rectal temperature) to evaluate for the risk of heatstroke. All patients with heatstroke need core temperature monitoring
- Laboratory testing is not required in heat rash and heat edema; serum electrolyte levels should be checked in children with heat syncope and heat exhaustion
- Children with heatstroke need comprehensive blood work, including basic electrolyte levels, serum creatinine, hepatic function tests, venous or arterial blood gas measurement, and coagulation studies to evaluate for more significant MODS. In addition, creatinine kinase levels and urine studies are needed to evaluate for muscle breakdown and myoglobinuria
- Consider a urine drug screen if substance abuse is suspected
- Consider an ECG in any patient with significant electrolyte abnormalities
- Consider a chest x-ray in any patient with significant vital sign abnormalities to evaluate for pulmonary edema in the setting of high-output cardiac failure
- Consider a head CT in any patient with persistent neurologic derangement after cooling

TREATMENT

- Environment modification
  - The primary treatment of any heat-related illness is removal from the high temperature environment and removal of all occlusive clothing
  - The National Athletic Trainers Association recommends a motto of "cool first, transfer second" so as not to delay the ultimate treatment of lowering the body temperature
  - Maximize heat loss
    - Fans will promote convective heat loss
    - Cool mist will promote evaporative heat loss
    - Skin exposure and cool blankets or ice packs applied to the axilla or groin will promote conductive heat loss
- Improve venous return
  - Heat syncope is treated by laying the patient supine to improve cerebral blood flow

- Heat edema responds well to extremity elevation
- Hydration with fluid and electrolytes via the oral route or intravascularly will not only improve intravascular volume in the case of syncope but it also will improve electrolyte and extravascular fluid shifts seen with heat edema, heat syncope, heat cramps, and heat exhaustion
- Treatment of heatstroke
  - Heatstroke treatment requires a more aggressive approach because outcomes are directly related to the duration of hyperthermia (goal should be to lower body temperature <104°F or 40°C within 30 minutes)
  - Active evaporative cooling with continuous cool water spraying and fanning
  - Ice water submersion and ice water baths are well described, but the safety of this treatment depends on the patient's mental status
  - Aggressive cooling can be stopped when a goal temperature of 38°C is reached
  - All patients should be placed on oxygen to maximize cerebral oxygen delivery. In severe cases, intubation may be needed if the patient is obtunded and cannot protect his or her airway
  - Intravenous fluids (IVFs) are a mainstay for rehydration in heatstroke for both cardiovascular support and electrolyte repletion
  - In the most critical cases, vasopressors may be needed to maintain adequate perfusion, but they must be used with caution because they will increase the metabolic rate and add to the core temperature
  - In rare cases, hyperthermia can lead to cardiac arrhythmias, which should reverse with temperature lowering; electrical cardioversion is not recommended
  - Benzodiazepines can be used for severe agitation or seizures. They are also believed to help reduce shivering during the cooling process and thus minimize metabolic demand

PREVENTION

- Prevention of heat-related illnesses rests largely on education
- Parents need to be educated on children's vulnerability to heat-related illnesses and on the risks of leaving a child unattended in a parked car or in other locations with high ambient temperatures
- Athletic trainers need to be educated on early signs of heat exhaustion so treatment can be initiated rapidly
- Athletic departments should have a preseason heat acclimatization program
- Athletes should refrain from practice during a febrile illness
- Hydration goals:
  - All athletes should maintain euhydration during practice and games
  - Are weight-based with a goal of less than 3% weight loss from dehydration during practice and games
  - For high school athletes: a goal of 16 oz of water or sports drink 1 hour before exertion, and then 4 to 8 oz of fluid every 15 to 20 minutes during exertion is recommended
  - Rehydration with a sports drink is recommended over water to replace electrolytes lost in sweat

PROGNOSIS

- The majority of heat-related illnesses are not fatal
- Heatstroke has a significant mortality rate
  - Adult nonexertional heatstroke mortality rates are as high as 58%[2]
  - There is limited data on mortality rates of nonexertional heatstroke among children: 231 reported U.S. deaths between 1999 and 2007[3]
  - Exertional heatstroke has a mortality rate of 17% to 70%, depending on the speed with which the patients are treated
  - 100% survival rate reported for those treated immediately[4]

Pediatric Drowning

Drowning is a leading cause of death both in the United States and worldwide. In addition, those who survive a prolonged drowning event can have devastating neurologic impairment. Despite the prevalence and morbidity of drowning, it is largely a preventable cause of death.

BASIC INFORMATION

- Definition:
  - Drowning is defined by the World Health Organization as a "primary respiratory impairment from submersion or immersion in a liquid medium." This includes both fatal and nonfatal submersion injuries
  - "Near drowning," "dry drowning," and "wet drowning" are no longer recommended terminology
- Epidemiology:
  - Second leading cause of accidental death among children <14 years old third leading cause of death worldwide among those 10 to 14 years of age
  - Bimodal distribution: less than 5 years of age or 15 to 25 years of age
  - Non-Caucasian children have higher risk of drowning
- Risk factors:
  - Most drownings occur in previously healthy children
  - Lack of proper adult supervision and overestimation of swimming abilities
  - Comorbid conditions: seizure disorders, cardiac disease, mental disabilities, and psychiatric disease
  - Cardiac arrhythmias such as long QT and channelopathies such as catecholaminergic polymorphic ventricular tachycardia represent up to 30% of drowning cases associated with a primary cardiac arrest
  - Alcohol consumption or substance abuse near open water, particularly in the adolescent population
  - Seasonal: more likely to occur in summer months
  - More likely to occur in afternoon
  - Location: infants are more likely to drown in the bathtub, younger children are more likely to drown in a pool, and older children are more likely to drown in fresh water

Pathophysiology

- Pulmonary complications
  - Primary insult: hypoxia (either due to apnea in an unconscious patient, or to aspiration and laryngospasm in a conscious patient)

- Secondary insult: surfactant disruption caused by fluid shifts across the alveoli after water aspiration, resulting in atelectasis, poor lung compliance, decreased functional residual capacity (FRC), intrapulmonary shunting and, ultimately, acute respiratory distress syndrome (ARDS)
  - Lung compliance is further complicated by particulate aspiration (sand, sewage, vomit, etc.)
- Cardiac injury
  - Hypoxia and metabolic acidosis lead to myocardial injury and to classic progression from tachycardia to bradycardia to pulseless electrical activity (PEA) to asystole
  - Sudden cardiac arrest is less likely and suggests an alternative primary diagnosis leading to drowning, such as long QT or catecholaminergic polymorphic ventricular tachycardia (see Chapter 8)
  - Hypothermia alone can lead to cardiac arrest. Thus in the appropriate clinical setting, resuscitative efforts should be continued in a drowning victim until the core temperature reaches 32°C to 34°C
- Neurologic injury
  - Hypoxic ischemic encephalopathy is the leading cause of death due to drowning
  - The extent of neurologic injury is proportional to the duration of submersion, effective cardiopulmonary resuscitation (CPR), and adequate post-resuscitative care
  - Even in nonfatal drowning cases, up to 20% of patients have permanent neurologic injury
- Multiorgan dysfunction syndrome
  - MODS is seen in up to 18% of pediatric drowning cases with cardiopulmonary arrest
  - Additional injuries may include uremia, transaminitis, thrombocytopenia, and lactic acidosis

CLINICAL PRESENTATION

- Clinical findings on examination: variable depending on the severity
- Neurologic examination: patients have a variety of presentations from alert to comatose. The presenting Glasgow Coma Scale score (GCS) is a prognostic factor
- Lung examination: patients may have a clear lung examination or may have significant rales and work of breathing due to pulmonary edema
- Cardiac examination: patient may progress from tachycardia to bradycardia and asystole. Hypotension is an indicator of poor prognosis
- Musculoskeletal examination: drowning victims are often trauma victims and need a full primary and secondary survey
  - Risk factors for cervical spine (C-spine) injury include shallow water or rocky water drowning, patients found unconscious, and the presence of head or facial trauma

DIAGNOSIS AND EVALUATION

- Diagnosis is seldom in question. Remember to consider child abuse as a possible cause in young children
- Evaluation of the drowning patient is driven by history, symptomatology, and illness severity

- Asymptomatic patients may just need a period of observation; there is no need for routine blood work in the absence of symptoms
- Patients who sustained traumatic injuries as part of their drowning merit laboratory studies and imaging per advanced trauma life support (ATLS) guidelines
- Children with any respiratory symptoms should have a chest radiograph
- Critically ill children and/or those with severe hypothermia need comprehensive laboratory studies to assess for multiorgan system failure
- Consider toxicology screens for adolescent patients where appropriate
- Consider ECG, antiepileptic drug levels, electroencephalogram (EEG) where underlying medical cause such as arrhythmia or seizure is suspected

TREATMENT

- Prehospital:
  - Timely rescue is critical. There is incremental increase in adverse outcomes the longer the submersion time, with short submersions of <5 minutes having the best outcome
  - In a pulseless or apneic patient, CPR should be started immediately because PEA and asystole are common presenting rhythms
    - Bystander CPR is crucial because a short time to quality CPR is a direct predictor of survival
  - C-spine immobilization is not routinely recommended unless a patient had a high-risk mechanism, such as diving, or has signs of head and/or facial trauma.
  - A conscious patient should be placed in the right lateral decubitus position to prevent aspiration because he or she is at a high risk for vomiting
  - Heimlich maneuver is not recommended because it delays resuscitation and could worsen a C-spine injury
  - Rewarming with blankets should begin immediately. More aggressive rewarming measures should wait until arrival at the emergency department (ED)

Airway and Breathing Management

- Conscious patients may need supplemental oxygen or noninvasive positive pressure ventilation to maintain their oxygenation and ventilation
- Unconscious patients, apneic patients, or patients with progressive distress on noninvasive ventilation need endotracheal intubation and mechanical ventilation
- Chest x-ray can be obtained, but findings lag behind injury; serial blood gas measurements may corroborate respiratory failure
- Surfactant replacement is controversial and not recommended
- Although pneumonia is not uncommon after drowning, empiric antibiotic use is not recommended

Circulation Management

- Severe drowning victims are often intravascularly volume depleted and need fluid resuscitation and potentially inotropic or vasoactive support

Hypothermia Management

- Cerebral blood flow decreases by 6% to 7% for every degree drop in core temperature
- Hypothermia management depends on the degree of hypothermia. A low-reading thermometer is necessary for hypothermic patients
  - **Mild hypothermia (32°C to 35°C):** passive external rewarming with external sources of heat such as warm blankets or radiant heat, relies on patient to generate heat
  - **Moderate hypothermia (28°C to 32°C):** active external rewarming with radiant heat, heating pads, warm baths, forced warm air. Beware of core temperature afterdrop, which occurs when extremities are warmed, causing vasodilation and circulation of cold peripheral blood to the core. This can cause hypotension and potentially arrhythmias. Can be avoided by rewarming trunk first
  - **Severe hypothermia (<28°C):** active internal rewarming with warm IVFs, warm humidified oxygen, and potentially lavage of pleural and peritoneal cavities with warm fluids. For most severe cases or when rewarming is inadequate, endovascular warming devices, hemodialysis, or extracorporeal membrane oxygenation (ECMO) should be considered
- Patients should be aggressively rewarmed to a target goal of about 34°C to minimize secondary injuries. There is no established goal rate for rewarming, but one degree per hour is generally accepted. If patient is failing to rewarm at a rate of at least 0.5°C/hr, progress to a more aggressive method
- With rising core temperature, there are increased metabolic demands, and patients can develop secondary injuries. Likewise, arrhythmias are common during the rewarming process
- Disposition:
  - A conscious patient with no signs of respiratory distress should be observed for 6 to 8 hours. If he or she continues to be asymptomatic, he or she may be discharged
  - If any symptoms arise during the observation period, further evaluation and inpatient observation is required
  - Severely ill patients or those requiring resuscitation should be admitted to an intensive care unit
- Long-term care:
  - Once the patient is stabilized and the acute hypoxia is reversed, the goal of inpatient care is to prevent any secondary injuries
    - All electrolyte and acid-base disruptions should be corrected
    - Patients should be kept euglycemic
    - Any seizure activity should be aggressively controlled with antiepileptics
    - Volume status should be closely monitored to maintain adequate cerebral perfusion
- Therapeutic hypothermia:
  - Therapeutic hypothermia compared with normothermia does not significantly affect survival, with a favorable neurologic outcome for drowning victims with out-of-hospital cardiac arrest
  - In addition, there is a trend toward more infectious complications in patients treated with therapeutic hypothermia compared with normothermia

PREVENTION

- Adult supervision is critical to prevention
- Secure fencing and gates around swimming pools have been shown to decrease drowning rates
- Avoiding drugs and alcohol while swimming is also important to drowning prevention, particularly in the adolescent population

PROGNOSIS

- Patients can often survive their pulmonary insult but still have devastating neurologic injury from their cerebral hypoxic insult
- Outcome depends on several factors:
  - Drownings outside the home, witnessed drownings, bystander CPR, the presence of a shockable rhythm, and limited delays between the event and the arrival of emergency medical services (EMS) are all associated with increased survival to hospital admission
  - Patients who are conscious upon arrival to the hospital have an excellent prognosis
  - Submersion time >11 minutes, CPR for >30 minutes, and/or presentation with a body temperature <34°C are associated with worse outcome
- There are many case reports of survival after very prolonged resuscitations in extremely cold water drownings, possibly due to the neuroprotective effects of the mammalian diving reflex

Review Questions

For review questions, please go to ExpertConsult.com.

References

1. Kerr ZY, Casa DJ, Marshall SW, Comstock RD. Epidemiology of exertional heat illness among U.S. high school athletes. *Am J Prev Med.* 2013;44:8–14.
2. Argaud L, Ferry T, Le Q, Marfisi A, Ciorba D, Achache P, et al. Short- and long-term outcomes of heatstroke following the 2003 heat wave in Lyon, France. *Arch Intern Med.* 2007;167:2177–2183.
3. Booth JN, Davis GG, Waterbor J, McGwin G. Hyperthermia deaths among children in parked vehicles and analysis of 231 fatalities in the United States, 1999-2007. *Forensic Sci Med Pathol.* 2010;6:99–105.
4. Demartini JK, Casa DJ, Stearns R, Belval L, Crago A, Davis R, et al. Effectiveness of cold water immersion in the treatment of exertional heat stroke at the Falmouth Road Race. *Med Sci Sports Exerc.* 2015;47:240–245.
5. Quan L, Mack CD, Schiff MA. Association of water temperature and submersion duration and drowning outcome. *Resuscitation.* 2014;85:790–794.

Suggested Readings

1. Howe AS, Boden BP. Heat-related illness in athletes. *Amer J Sports Med.* 2007;35:1384–1395.
2. Kerr ZY, Casa DJ, Marshall SW, Comstock RD. Epidemiology of exertional heat illness among U.S. high school athletes. *Am J Prev Med.* 2013;44:8–14.
3. Causey AL, Tilelli JA, Swanson ME. Predicting discharge in uncomplicated near-drowning. *Am J Emerg Med.* 2000;18(1):9–11.

4. Kieboom JK, Verkade HJ, Burgerhof JG, et al. Outcome after resuscitation beyond 30 minutes in drowned children with cardiac arrest and hypothermia. dutch nationwide retrospective cohort study. *BMJ*. 2015;350:h418.
5. Papa L, Hoelle R, Idris A. Systematic review of definitions for drowning incidents. *Resuscitation*. 2005;65:255.
6. Quan L, Cummings P. Characteristics of drowning by different age groups. *Inj Prev*. 2003;9:163–168.
7. Quan L, Mack CD, Schiff MA. Association of water temperature and submersion duration and drowning outcome. *Resuscitation*. 2014;85:790–794.
8. Watson RS, Cummings P, Quan L, et al. Cervical spine injuries among submersion victims. *J Trauma*. 2001;51:658.

18 Toxicology

DANIELLE CULLEN, MD, MPH and KEVIN C. OSTERHOUDT, MD, MS

Basic Information

- Nearly 3 million calls are made to regional poison control centers in the United States annually (although not all poisonings are reported, with an estimated 4 million people poisoned each year)
- Over half of poisoning exposure cases involve children under 6 years of age
- 80% to 85% of poisonings are unintentional
- More than 90% occur in the home, and most involve a single substance
- Approximately 50% of cases involve nondrug substances: cosmetics, cleaning solutions, plants, and foreign bodies
- Seven basic routes of exposure: envenomation, inhalation, oral, ocular, parenteral, topical, and transplacental
  - Ingestion accounts for >80% of exposures, followed by dermal, inhalation, and ocular routes
- Bimodal distribution of poisoning
  - Exploratory behavior, typically from ages 1 to 5 years
    - More likely to be of male gender, hyperactive-type behavior, and increased finger-mouth activity
  - Drug abuse, depression, experimental risk-taking behaviors in ages 13 to 19 years
- Risks for poisoning:
  - Substance-specific: ease of access, attractiveness, palatability, packaging/child-safety caps, volume contained within single package
  - Environment: acute or chronic stressors, level of supervision
  - See also Nelson Textbook of Pediatrics, Chapter 63, "Poisoning."

Clinical Presentation

- Consider toxic exposure if history is suggestive, or in a child with unexplained symptoms, including metabolic derangements, neurologic symptoms, or hemodynamic effects.
- Important components of history:
  - Amount and concentration of substance ingested
  - Timing
  - Listing of all medications in the home
  - Symptoms noted
- Timing of onset and progression can help generate a list of potential toxicants and predict the severity of the ingestion
- Groupings of physical signs that comprise a particular toxidrome may help suggest the drug class responsible for a poisoning (Tables 18.1 and 18.2)

ALTERED MENTAL STATUS

- Alterations in mental status can range from agitation to coma
- Exclude other causes ("VITAMINS"):
  - Vascular injury (migraine, stroke, etc.)
  - Infection (encephalitis, meningitis, sepsis, etc.)
  - Trauma
  - Asphyxia
  - Metabolic abnormality (hypoglycemia, hyperammonemia, etc.)
  - Intussusception
  - Neoplasm
  - Seizure

DIRECT TISSUE INJURY

- Caustic ingestions may lead to dysphagia, epigastric pain, oral mucosal injury, and low-grade fever.
  - Alkali agents (tasteless) cause liquefactive necrosis
  - Acidic agents (sour) cause coagulation necrosis
- Hydrocarbon ingestions
  - Pulmonary toxicity: chemical pneumonitis by inhalation exposure
  - Ingestion frequently leads directly to emesis, increasing the risk of aspiration pneumonitis

METABOLIC ABNORMALITY

- Alterations in glucose metabolism (hypo- or hyperglycemia)
- Acid-base disturbances
- Osmolal gap
  - Measured osmolality is more than 10 mOsmol/L greater than the calculated osmolality
  - Indicates low-molecular-weight solute other than sodium, glucose, or urea that is at a high enough concentration to raise the osmolality
  - Caused by toxic alcohols: ethanol, methanol, ethylene glycol, propylene glycol, isopropanol

CARDIOVASCULAR COMPROMISE

Hypotension

- May result from volume loss (e.g., vomiting, diarrhea, hemorrhage), alterations in vascular tone (e.g., venodilation, arteriolar dilation), depressed cardiac contractility, and dysrhythmias
- Hypothermia may also contribute to hypotension
- Although most causes of hypotension are associated with compensatory tachycardia, the presentation of hypotension with bradycardia suggests: alpha-II agonists,

Table 18.1. Historical and Physical Findings in Poisoning

ODOR

Bitter almonds	Cyanide
Acetone	Isopropyl alcohol, methanol, paraldehyde, salicylate
Alcohol	Ethanol
Wintergreen	Methyl salicylate
Garlic	Arsenic, thallium, organophosphates, selenium
Violets	Turpentine

OCULAR SIGNS

Miosis	Narcotics (except propoxyphene, meperidine, and pentazocine), organophosphates, muscarinic mushrooms, clonidine, phenothiazines, chloral hydrate, barbiturates (late)
Mydriasis	Atropine, cocaine, amphetamines, antihistamines, cyclic antidepressants, PCP, LSD
Nystagmus	Phenytoin, barbiturates, ethanol, carbamazepine, PCP, ketamine, dextromethorphan
Lacrimation	Organophosphates, irritant gas or vapors
Retinal hyperemia	Methanol
Poor vision	Methanol, botulism, carbon monoxide

CUTANEOUS SIGNS

Needle tracks	Heroin, PCP, amphetamine
Dry, hot skin	Anticholinergic agents, botulism
Diaphoresis	Organophosphates, muscarinic mushrooms, aspirin, cocaine
Alopecia	Thallium, arsenic, lead, mercury
Erythema	Boric acid, mercury, cyanide, anticholinergics

ORAL SIGNS

Salivation	Organophosphates, salicylate, corrosives, strychnine, ketamine
Dry mouth	Amphetamine, anticholinergics, antihistamine
Burns	Corrosives, oxalate-containing plants
Gum lines	Lead, mercury, arsenic
Dysphagia	Corrosives, botulism

INTESTINAL SIGNS

Diarrhea	Antimicrobials, arsenic, iron, boric acid, cholinergics
Constipation	Lead, narcotics, botulism
Hematemesis	Corrosives, iron, salicylates, nonsteroidal antiinflammatory drugs

CARDIAC SIGNS

Tachycardia	Atropine, aspirin, amphetamine, cocaine, cyclic antidepressants, theophylline
Bradycardia	Digitalis, narcotics, clonidine, organophosphates, β-blockers, calcium channel blockers
Hypertension	Amphetamine, LSD, cocaine, PCP
Hypotension	Phenothiazines, barbiturates, cyclic antidepressants, iron, β-blockers, calcium channel blockers, clonidine, narcotics

RESPIRATORY SIGNS

Depressed respiration	Alcohol, narcotics, barbiturates
Increased respiration	Amphetamines, aspirin, ethylene glycol, carbon monoxide, cyanide
Pulmonary edema	Hydrocarbons, organophosphates

CENTRAL NERVOUS SYSTEM SIGNS

Ataxia	Alcohol, barbiturates, anticholinergics, narcotics
Coma	Sedatives, narcotics, barbiturates, salicylate, cyanide, carbon monoxide, cyclic antidepressants, alcohol
Hyperpyrexia	Anticholinergics, salicylates, amphetamine, cocaine
Muscle fasciculation	Organophosphates, theophylline
Muscle rigidity	Cyclic antidepressants, PCP, phenothiazines, haloperidol
Peripheral neuropathy	Lead, arsenic, mercury, organophosphates
Altered behavior	LSD, PCP, amphetamines, cocaine, alcohol, anticholinergics

From Kostic M. Poisoning, Kliegman R, Stanton B, St Geme III J, Schor N. In: Kliegman R. *Nelson Textbook of Pediatrics.* 20th ed. Philadelphia, PA: Elsevier; 2016: Chapter 63, Table 63.2, 447–467.

Table 18.2.   Selected Common Toxidromes

Toxidrome	Vital signs	Mental status	SIGNS					Possible toxins
			Pupils	Skin	Bowel sounds	Other		
Sympathomimetic	Hypertension, tachycardia, hyperthermia	Agitation, psychosis, delirium, violence	Dilated	Diaphoretic	Normal to increased			Amphetamines, cocaine, PCP, bath salts (cathinones), attention deficit/hyperactivity medication
Anticholinergic	Hypertension, tachycardia, hyperthermia	Agitated, delirium, coma, seizures	Dilated	Dry, hot	Diminished	Ileus urinary retention		Antihistamines, tricyclic antidepressants, atropine, jimson weed
Cholinergic	Bradycardia Blood pressure and temperature typically normal	Confusion, coma, fasciculations	Small	Diaphoretic	Hyperactive	Diarrhea, urination, bronchorrhea, bronchospasm, emesis, lacrimation, salivation		Organophosphates (insecticides, nerve agents), carbamates (physostigmine, neostigmine, pyridostigmine), Alzheimer medications, myasthenia treatments
Opioids	Respiratory depression bradycardia, hypotension, hypothermia	Depression, coma, euphoria	Pinpoint	Normal	Normal to decreased			Methadone, buprenorphine, morphine, oxycodone, heroin, etc.
Sedative–hypnotics	Respiratory depression, heart rate normal to decreased, blood pressure normal to decreased, temperature normal to decreased	Somnolence, coma	Small or normal	Normal	Normal			Barbiturates, benzodiazepines, ethanol
Salicylates	Tachypnea, hyperpnea, tachycardia, hyperthermia	Agitation, confusion, coma	Normal	Diaphoretic	Normal	Nausea, vomiting, tinnitus, arterial blood gas with primary respiratory alkalosis and primary metabolic acidosis; tinnitus or difficulty hearing		Aspirin and aspirin-containing products, methyl-salicylate

Modified from Kostic M. Poisoning. In: Kliegman R. *Nelson Textbook of Pediatrics*. 20th ed. Philadelphia, PA: Elsevier; 2016: 447–467.

Table 18.3. Common Dysrhythmias Associated with Toxic Ingestions

Rate	Tachycardia*		Bradycardia
Electrocardiogram finding	Prolonged QT	Widened QRS	Sinus bradycardia
Mechanism	Potassium channel blockade	Sodium channel blockade	
selected agents	■ Amiodarone ■ Antipsychotics (typical and atypical) ■ Arsenic ■ Cisapride ■ Citalopram and other selective serotonin reuptake inhibitors ■ Clarithromycin, erythromycin ■ Disopyramide, dofetilide, ibutilide ■ Fluconazole, ketoconazole, itraconazole ■ Loperamide, methadone ■ Pentamidine ■ Phenothiazines ■ Sotalol	■ Tricyclic antidepressants ■ Diphenhydramine ■ Carbamazepine ■ Cardiac glycosides ■ Chloroquine, hydroxychloroquine ■ Cocaine ■ Lamotrigine ■ Quinidine, quinine, procainamide, disopyramide ■ Phenothiazines ■ Propoxyphene ■ Propranolol ■ Bupropion, venlafaxine (rare)	■ Digoxin ■ Cholinergic agent ■ β-Blocker ■ Calcium channel blocker ■ Clonidine/ guanfacine

*Sinus tachycardia is a common side effect.

sympatholytic agents, membrane-depressant drugs, calcium antagonists, cardiac glycosides, or hypothermia

Hypertension

- Amphetamines cause hypertension and tachycardia through generalized sympathetic stimulation
- Selective alpha-adrenergic agents cause hypertension with reflex (baroreceptor-mediated) bradycardia or even atrioventricular (AV) block
- Anticholinergic agents cause mild hypertension with tachycardia
- Stimulation of nicotinic cholinergic receptors by organophosphates may cause tachycardia and hypertension, followed by bradycardia and hypotension
- Withdrawal with hypertension and tachycardia suggests sedative-hypnotic drugs, ethanol, opioids, or clonidine

Dysrhythmias

- Certain drugs/toxins can predispose patients to rhythm disturbances (Table 18.3).
- Care must be taken to rule out other causes of dysrhythmia that can be caused by toxic exposures:
  - Hypoxemia
  - Hypokalemia
  - Metabolic acidosis
  - Myocardial ischemia or infarction
  - Electrolyte disturbances such as hypocalcemia or hypomagnesemia, or congenital disorders that cause QT prolongation
  - Brugada syndrome

SEIZURES

- Exclude underlying seizure disorder or trauma
- Exposures that can cause seizures can be remembered with the mnemonic PLASTIC (Table 18.4)

Diagnosis and Evaluation

- Every patient with suspected ingestion should be evaluated with a complete history and physical examination

Table 18.4. PLASTIC Mnemonic for Partial Listing of Drugs and Chemicals That May Cause Acute Seizures

"PLASTIC"

P—Phencyclidine, pesticides, phenol, propoxyphene

L—Lead, lithium, lindane, local anesthetics

A—Antidepressants, antipsychotics, anticonvulsants, antihistamines, abstinence syndromes

S—Salicylate, sympathomimetic, strychnine, solvents, shellfish (domoic acid)

T—Theophylline, tricyclic antidepressants, thallium, tobacco (nicotine)

I—Isoniazid, insulin (and other causes of hypoglycemia), insecticides

C—Camphor, cocaine, cyanide/carbon monoxide, chloroquine, cyclonite (C4 plastic explosive), cicutoxin

Data from Osterhoudt KC, Henretig FM. A 16-year-old with recalcitrant seizures. *Pediatr Emerg Care*, 2012;28(3):304–306.

- Primary attention in assessing and stabilizing the airway, breathing, circulation, and mental status
- Key features of the physical examination that can suggest a toxidrome (see Tables 18.3 and 18.4)
  - Vital signs
  - Mental status
  - Pupils (size, reactivity)
  - Nystagmus
  - Skin
  - Bowel sounds
  - Odors
- Additional evaluation may be considered, depending on the agents ingested and the patient's mental status and clinical presentation (Table 18.5)
- Electrocardiogram (ECG)
- Laboratory evaluation:
  - Urine drug screen: drugs of abuse; consider comprehensive urine drug screen
  - Serum drug screen: acetaminophen, salicylates, and alcohol
    Additional serum drug studies of suspected agents can be helpful in determining treatment

Table 18.5. Laboratory and Imaging Clues

ANION GAP METABOLIC ACIDOSIS (MNEMONIC: MUDPILES CAT)

M—methanol, metformin
U—uremia
D—diabetic ketoacidosis
P—propylene glycol
I—isoniazid, iron, massive ibuprofen
L—lactic acidosis
E—ethylene glycol
S—salicylates
C—cellular asphyxiants (cyanide, carbon monoxide, hydrogen sulfide)
A—alcoholic ketoacidosis
T—Tylenol

ELEVATED OSMOLAL GAP

Alcohols: ethanol, isopropyl, methanol, ethylene glycol

HYPOGLYCEMIA (MNEMONIC: HOBBIES)

H—hypoglycemics, oral: sulfonylureas, meglitinides
O—other: quinine, unripe ackee fruit
B—beta blockers
I—insulin
E—ethanol
S—salicylates (late)

HYPERGLYCEMIA

Salicylates (early)
Calcium channel blockers
Caffeine

HYPOCALCEMIA

Ethylene glycol
Fluoride

RHABDOMYOLYSIS

Neuroleptic malignant syndrome, serotonin syndrome
Statins
Mushrooms (*Tricholoma equestre*)
Any toxin causing prolonged immobilization (e.g., opioids, antipsychotics) or excessive muscle activity or seizures (e.g., sympathomimetics)

RADIOPAQUE SUBSTANCE ON ABDOMINAL X-RAY (MNEMONIC: CHIPPED)

C—chloral hydrate, calcium carbonate
H—heavy metals (lead, zinc, barium, arsenic, lithium, bismuth)
I—iron
P—phenothiazines
P—Play-Doh, potassium chloride
E—enteric-coated pills
D—dental amalgam, drug packets

From Kostic M. Poisoning. In: Kliegman R. *Nelson Textbook of Pediatrics.* 20th ed. Philadelphia, PA: Elsevier; 2016: 447–467.

plan: some anticonvulsants, carbon monoxide, digoxin, ethylene glycol, iron, lead, lithium, and methanol
- Urine pregnancy test is indicated for all adolescent female patients
- Basic chemistry panel and blood gas
  Calculate anion gap on any patient with low serum bicarbonate
  Differential is focused by the nature of the anion gap in metabolic acidosis
- If known overdose of acetaminophen, assess liver transaminases and international normalized ratio (INR)

- If prolonged "downtime," measure serum creatine kinase level to evaluate for rhabdomyolysis
- Serum osmolality is helpful as a surrogate marker for a toxic alcohol
- Imaging to consider based on differential diagnosis:
  - Chest x-ray
    - Pneumonitis: hydrocarbon aspiration
    - Noncardiogenic pulmonary edema: salicylate toxicity
    - Foreign body
  - Abdominal x-ray
    - Foreign body: bezoar, radiopaque tablets, drug packets

Treatment

The four main categories of treatment are supportive care, decontamination, enhanced elimination, and specific antidotes.

SUPPORTIVE CARE

- Particular attention to airway, breathing, circulation, and mental status
- If depressed consciousness and suspicion of toxic ingestion:
  - Glucose
  - 100% oxygen supplementation
  - Naloxone

DECONTAMINATION

- Goal of minimizing absorption
- Dermal and ocular decontamination
  - Remove contaminated clothing and particulate
  - Flush with tepid water or normal saline for minimum of 10 to 20 minutes
- Gastrointestinal decontamination
  - Single-dose activated charcoal
    - Most effective within 1 hour of ingestion
    - Ineffective if: caustic/corrosive agent, hydrocarbon, heavy metals, small ions (i.e., lithium), alcohols, water-insoluble compounds
    - Ensure patent or protected airway to minimize risk of aspiration
  - Whole bowel irrigation: polyethylene glycol
    - For slowly absorbed substances (sustained-release or enteric-coated preparations), substances not well absorbed by charcoal, ingested transdermal patches, and drug packets
    - May be combined with use of activated charcoal
    - Ensure patent or protected airway to minimize risk of aspiration
    - Avoid use in cases of bowel obstruction or ileus
  - Syrup of ipecac: risks have been found to outweigh benefits and therefore is no longer recommended
  - Gastric lavage: generally not recommended
    - Place a tube into the stomach to aspirate contents and flush with aliquots of fluid
    - Can cause a vagal response and subsequent bradycardia

Table 18.6. Selected Antidotes

Poison	Antidote	Comments
Acetaminophen	N-Acetylcysteine	Most effective within 16 h of ingestion
Anticholinergic	Physostigmine	May cause bradycardia, heart block, asystole; lowers seizure threshold. Keep atropine nearby Use in TCA poisoning is controversial and should be done only with expert guidance
Benzodiazepine	Flumazenil	Possible seizures, arrhythmias; may precipitate serious withdrawal among habituated
β-Blocking agents	Glucagon	
Carbon monoxide	Oxygen	Half-life of carboxyhemoglobin is 5 hr in room air but 1.5 hr in 100% O_2
Cyclic antidepressants	Sodium bicarbonate	Follow potassium levels and replace as needed
Cyanide	Hydroxocobalamin	Causes red discoloration of body fluids
Digoxin	Digoxin-specific antibodies	Give slowly. Rate- and dose-dependent anaphylactoid reaction can occur
Ethylene glycol or Methanol	Fomepizole	
Sulfonylurea	Octreotide	
Iron	Deferoxamine	Hypotension (worse with rapid infusion rates)
Isoniazid	Pyridoxine	
Lead	Edetate calcium disodium (EDTA)	
	BAL (British anti-Lewisite [dimercaprol])	May cause sterile abscesses. Prepared in peanut oil; do not use in patients with peanut allergy
	Succimer (2,3-dimercaptosuccinic acid ([DMSA])	Few toxic effects; requires lead-free home plus compliant family
Methemoglobinemia	Methylene blue	Coloration may lead to acute apparent decline in pulse oximetry. Take care in G6PD deficiency – methylene blue may contribute to oxidant injury
Opiates	Naloxone	Naloxone causes no respiratory depression.
Organophosphates	Atropine	Physiologic: blocks acetylcholine
	Pralidoxime (2 PAM; Protopam)	Specific: disrupts phosphate-cholinesterase bond

From Kostic M. Poisoning, Kliegman R, Stanton B, St Geme III J, Schor N. In: Kliegman R. *Nelson Textbook of Pediatrics.* 20th ed. Philadelphia, PA: Elsevier; 2016: 447–467.

ENHANCED ELIMINATION

- Urinary alkalinization
  - Enhances elimination of weak acids by forming charged molecules
  - Most useful in salicylate or methotrexate toxicity
  - Continuous infusion of sodium bicarbonate–containing intravenous (IV) fluids, with goal urine pH of 7.5 to 8
  - Closely monitor serum pH and electrolytes for hypokalemia and hypocalcemia
- Hemodialysis
  - For elimination of toxicants with low volume of distribution, low molecular weight, low protein binding, and high water solubility
    - For example, methanol, ethylene glycol, salicylates, theophylline, bromide, lithium, and valproic acid
- Multiple-dose activated charcoal
  - Dosing every 4 to 6 hours for ≤24 hours to enhance elimination
  - Airway and abdominal examination should be assessed before each dose
  - Most commonly considered in the event of significant ingestions of carbamazepine, phenobarbital, quinine, or theophylline
- Lipid emulsion therapy
  - Sequesters fat-soluble drugs and decreases the effect on target organs
    - Verapamil and tricyclic antidepressants

SPECIFIC ANTIDOTES

- Antidotes are available for relatively few toxicants, but when they are given early and appropriately, they are vital in the management of a poisoned patient (Tables 18.6 and 18.7)

Review Questions

For review questions, please go to ExpertConsult.com.

Table 18.7.   Commonly Encountered Toxicologic Exposures

	Clinical Presentation	Diagnosis	Treatment
Acetaminophen	*Early* (within 24 hours): asymptomatic, mild nausea, vomiting, diaphoresis, pallor, lethargy, malaise *Late* (24–96 hours): hepatotoxicity, jaundice, coagulopathy, encephalopathy	▪ Serum acetaminophen level (4 hours after ingestion) ▪ Electrolytes, blood urea nitrogen, creatinine, aminotransferases, coagulation studies	N-acetylcysteine (see Table 18.6)
Alcohol	Ataxia, nystagmus, respiratory depression, disinhibition, somnolence	▪ Ethanol level ▪ Osmolal gap (other toxic alcohols) ▪ Blood gas: metabolic acidosis	▪ Supportive therapy ▪ Hydration ▪ Glucose monitoring/support ▪ Fomepizole, if indicated
Carbon monoxide	Altered mental status: confusion to coma May have "cherry red" lips/skin Severe toxicity: seizures, cardiac ischemia, pulmonary edema	▪ Check carbon monoxide level with co-oximetry ▪ Measure blood cyanide concentration with history of smoke inhalation *Pulse oximetry inaccurate: falsely normal/high	▪ Intubate if soot in mouth/nares ▪ Apply high-flow O_2 regardless of pulse oximetry or pO_2 ▪ Hyperbaric oxygen, as indicated
Iron	Progression in time post ingestion: 30 min to 6 hr: Gastrointestinal (GI) phase: abdominal pain, vomiting, diarrhea, and GI bleeding 6 to 24 hr: Latent (relative stability) phase 6 to 72 hr: Shock and metabolic acidosis 12 to 96 hr: Hepatotoxicity 2 to 8 weeks: Bowel obstruction	▪ Serum iron (4–6 hours after ingestion) ▪ Abdominal x-ray for pills/fragments	▪ Volume resuscitation ▪ Whole bowel irrigation ▪ Deferoxamine, as indicated (see Table 18.6)
Methemoglobinemia	Cyanosis, headache, tachycardia, fatigue, dyspnea, lethargy *Hypoxia does not improve with supplemental oxygen	▪ Direct blood analysis for methemoglobin *Blood gas and pulse oximetry are inaccurate: falsely normal/high PaO_2, pulse oximetry persistently ~85%	Methylene blue (see Table 18.6)
Salicylates	Tachypnea, tinnitus, nausea/vomiting, agitation, confusion, restlessness, pulmonary edema	▪ Plasma salicylate level ▪ Blood gas: primary respiratory alkalosis and primary metabolic acidosis	▪ Avoid intubation if possible ▪ Volume resuscitation ▪ Activated charcoal ▪ Sodium bicarbonate to bind salicylate and enhance excretion
Selective serotonin reuptake inhibitors	Serotonin syndrome, vomiting, tremor, central nervous system (CNS) depression, seizure	▪ ECG: prolonged QTc ▪ If suspect serotonin syndrome: CK, urine myoglobin, creatinine, aminotransferases, coagulation studies, blood gas	▪ Supportive care ▪ Activated charcoal ▪ If seizure: benzodiazepine ▪ If prolonged QRS: bicarbonate ▪ If serotonin syndrome: benzodiazepine ± cyproheptadine
Tricyclic antidepressants	Anticholinergic effects (see Table 18.4), CNS depression, tachycardia	▪ Urine or serum TCA testing ▪ ECG: typically sinus tachycardia, but can develop prolonged QRS and ventricular tachycardia or ventricular fibrillation	▪ Fluid resuscitation ▪ Sodium bicarbonate for cardiac toxicity ▪ Activated charcoal ▪ Benzodiazepines for agitation ▪ If severe instability: lipid emulsion

Suggested Readings

1. Kostic M. Poisoning, Kliegman R, Stanton B, St Geme III J, Schor N. In: Kliegman S, St Geme S, eds. *Nelson Textbook of Pediatrics*. 20th ed. Philadelphia: Elsevier; 2016:447–467.
2. Mowry J, Spyker D, et al. 2014 Annual report of the American Association of Poison Control Centers' National Poison Data System. *Clin Toxicol*. 2015;53:962–1147.
3. O'Donnell K, Osterhoudt K, et al. Toxicologic emergencies. In: Shaw K, Bachur R, eds. *Fleisher and Ludwig's Textbook of Pediatric Emergency Medicine*. 7th ed. Philadelphia: Wolters Kluwer; 2016:1061–1114.
4. Olson K, ed. *Poisoning & Drug Overdose*. 6th ed. New York: McGraw-Hill; 2012.
5. Osterhoudt KC. No sympathy for a boy with obtundation. *Pediatr Emerg Care*. 2004;20(6):403–406.
6. Osterhoudt KC, Henretig FM. A 16-year-old with recalcitrant seizures. *Pediatr Emerg Care*. 2012;28(3):304–306.
7. Wiley J, Osterhoudt K. Poisonings. In: Selbst S, ed. *Pediatric Emergency Medicine Secrets*. 3rd ed. Philadelphia: Saunders; 2015:312–332.

19 Selected Topics in Emergency Medicine

ANNA WEISS, MD, MSc and KATHARINE C. LONG, MD

Thermal Injuries

BASIC INFORMATION

- More than 120,000 children seek care annually in U.S. emergency departments (EDs) for burn-related injuries; despite advances in care, burns are the fourth leading cause of accidental death among children in the United States
- Burns in infants and children under 5 years of age are most frequently from scalding events
- Older children suffer more frequently from flame-related events
- Mortality is directly related to the size of the burn as well as to the accompanying injuries associated with the event (e.g., inhalational injury or blunt trauma)
- See also Nelson Textbook of Pediatrics, Chapter 75, "Burn Injuries."

CLINICAL PRESENTATION

Burn Classification

- Burn severity is classified by both depth and size
- Depth:
  - *Superficial*: epidermis only; painful; red and blanching
  - *Superficial partial-thickness:* epidermis and dermis; painful to temperature and air; blisters; may be weeping, red, and blanching
  - *Deep partial-thickness:* epidermis and dermis; nonpainful; blisters; can be weeping or dry; nonblanching
  - *Full-thickness:* epidermis and full dermis; nonpainful; appearance from waxy and taut to charred; nonblanching
- Size:
  - Expressed as a percentage of total body surface area (TBSA)
  - Most centers use a modified Lund and Browder chart for estimation of TBSA in children (Fig. 19.1)
    - "Rule of nines" for adults: the head, each arm, and each side of each leg are 9% (whereas the anterior and posterior torso are 18% each)
    - Modified rule for infants: "take from the legs" (each side of each leg is 7%) to "double the head" (18%)
  - Superficial burns are *not* included in calculations of % TBSA
- Treatment and prognosis are directly related to a burn's severity classification

HISTORY

- A careful history should be obtained in any patient with a thermal injury, with attention to risk factors that might signal the presence of additional injuries:
  - Children with flame-related burns and/or burns sustained in a closed space may have:
    - Airway compromise
    - Parenchymal lung injury
    - Carbon monoxide (CO) and/or cyanide poisoning
  - Patients who sustained falls in addition to their burns (e.g., during an evacuation attempt) may have blunt traumatic injuries
  - An inconsistent history or patterned thermal injury may indicate nonaccidental burning

DIAGNOSIS AND EVALUATION

Physical Examination

- Should include thorough assessment of the size and depth of the burn itself (see previous) and careful assessment for signs of associated injury:
  - Hypoxemia and/or changes in mental status (concerning for carbon monoxide or cyanide poisoning, head injury, lung injury)
  - Drooling, stridor, or soot in mouth/nares (concerning for airway compromise)
  - Tachypnea, grunting, or retractions (concerning for lung injury)
  - Abdominal pain (concern for blunt trauma)
  - Extremity pain or deformity concern for blunt trauma

DIAGNOSTIC STUDIES

- In children with severe burns, practitioners could consider the following:
  - Serum testing: complete blood count (CBC), BMP, CK, UA, carboxyhemoglobin, serum lactate
  - Chest x-ray (CXR) in children in whom there is concern for inhalation injury

TREATMENT

Minor Burns

- Remove all clothing and jewelry
- Pain control
  - Nonsteroidal antiinflammatory drugs (NSAIDs) usually sufficient; can add opiates as needed

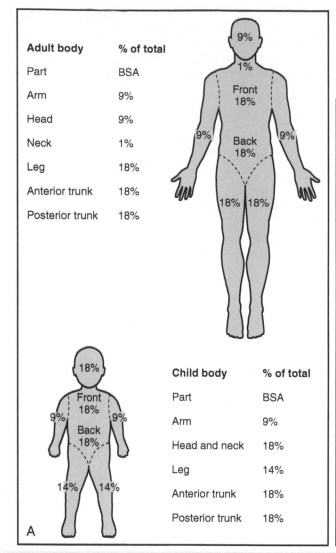

Adult body | % of total

Part	BSA
Arm	9%
Head	9%
Neck	1%
Leg	18%
Anterior trunk	18%
Posterior trunk	18%

Child body | % of total

Part	BSA
Arm	9%
Head and neck	18%
Leg	14%
Anterior trunk	18%
Posterior trunk	18%

Age	0-1	2-4	5-9	10-14	15
A - ½ of head	9½%	8½%	6½%	5½%	4½%
B - ½ of one thigh	9½%	8½%	6½%	5½%	4½%
C - ½ of one leg	9½%	8½%	6½%	5½%	4½%

Fig. 19.1. (A) Estimation of burn size with the "rule of nines." (B) Estimation of burn size with the Lund and Browder method. *BSA*, Body surface area. (From Deutschman CS, Neligan, PJ. *Evidence-Based Practice of Critical Care*. 2nd ed. Philadelphia, PA: Elsevier; 2017, Fig. 76.1.)

- Cooling
  - Cool or room-temperature running water up to 5 minutes
  - Cool or room-temperature soaked gauze up to 30 minutes
  - Never apply ice directly to burned skin
- Cleaning
  - Mild soap and water only; avoid antimicrobial skin cleansers
  - Debride ruptured blisters
- Dressing (for partial-thickness burns; not necessary for superficial burns)
  - Three layers: antimicrobial ointment, nonadherent dressing, dry gauze (n.b. wet dressings may predispose to hypothermia)
  - Antimicrobial ointments to use:
    - Face/head/perineum (or fingers if risk of ingestion): bacitracin
    - Periorbital: bacitracin-polymixin ophthalmic
    - All other burns: silver sulfadiazine (N.B., do not use in patients with sulfa allergy or G6PD)
- Tetanus prophylaxis

Major Burns

- Supplemental oxygen
- Secure airway early if concern for airway compromise
- Establish large-bore intravenous (IV) access
- Treat for cyanide and/or CO poisoning if history or laboratory findings are suggestive of exposure
- Provide adequate pain control
- Consider surgical consultation; in most centers, surgical services manage moderate and severe burns
- Burn care:
  - Debride devitalized skin with sterile saline/water and gauze
  - Partial- and full-thickness burns should be dressed with:
    - Antimicrobial layer
    - Nonadherent dressing
    - Outer layer of dry gauze
    - Consider need for escharotomy in patients with circumferential burns
- Fluid resuscitation:

Table 19.1. Criteria for Referral to a Burn Center

1. Partial-thickness burns covering more than 10% of total body surface area
2. Full-thickness burns (in any amount)
3. Burns that involve the face, hands, feet, genitalia, perineum, or major joints
4. Chemical or electrical burns, including lightning injury
5. Burns with associated inhalation injury
6. Burns in pediatric patients with complex medical history
7. Burns in pediatric patients who require significant social or emotional support
8. Burns in pediatric patients in hospitals without qualified personnel or equipment for the care of children
9. Nonaccidental burns

Data from European Burns Association and American Burn Association.

- Burns are associated with significant fluid shifts and total-body fluid losses
- Use Parkland formula to estimate fluid requirements:
  - 4 mL/kg per percent TBSA burned *plus* 24-hour maintenance fluids
  - One-half of fluids given in first 8 hours; remaining one-half run over next 16 hours
- Use isotonic crystalloids
- If necessary, transfer to a burn center for definitive care (Table 19.1)

Foreign Body Ingestions

BASIC INFORMATION

- In 2014 the American Association of Poison Control Centers reported approximately 128,000 cases of foreign body ingestions with 69% of events occurring in children 5 years of age or younger. 98% of these cases of foreign body ingestion were unintentional
- Over 50% to 90% of foreign bodies pass without incident:
  - 10% to 20% require removal
  - 1% require surgical intervention
- Almost 40% of foreign body ingestions are unwitnessed
- Coins account for 80% of impacted foreign bodies in the esophagus

CLINICAL PRESENTATION

- Majority of patients are asymptomatic
- Concerning clinical presentations:
  - Airway obstruction: stridor, wheezing, or respiratory distress
  - Esophageal obstruction: drooling, gagging, dysphagia, refusal to eat, chest pain
  - Abdominal perforation: abdominal tenderness, rebound tenderness, rigidity

DIAGNOSIS AND EVALUATION

Overview

- Object most commonly impacted in thoracic inlet (~75%)

Table 19.2. Indications for Emergent or Urgent Intervention

- Signs of airway compromise
- Symptoms consistent with esophageal obstruction
- Button battery in the esophagus
- Sharp or long (>5 cm) objects in the esophagus or stomach
- High-powered magnets
- Intestinal obstruction
- Foreign body impacted in the esophagus for more than 24 hours or for an unknown period

Adapted from Wright CC, Closson FT. Updates in pediatric gastrointestinal foreign bodies. *Pediatr Clin North Am*, 2013;60(5):1221–1239, Box 3.

- 10% to 20% in midesophagus and ~20% in distal esophagus
- Almost two-thirds of pediatric ingested foreign bodies are radiopaque

Imaging

- Initial screening with two-view chest radiograph and one- or two-view abdominal films
  - Two-view chest radiograph essential to distinguish coins from button batteries
  - Dedicated airway films as indicated
- Computed tomography (CT) may be indicated if concern remains high
- Consider ultrasound for gastric or vaginal foreign body
- *Not indicated:*
  - Oral contrast studies due to risk of aspiration
  - Laboratory studies are not indicated unless a significant complication is suspected

TREATMENT

- See Table 19.2 for a summary of indications for emergent or urgent endoscopic removal of a foreign body

Coins and Blunt Objects

BASIC INFORMATION

- Account for the majority of impacted foreign body ingestions in children
- 75% of coins in the esophagus pass into the stomach within 6 to 10 hours
- Spontaneous passage rates based on location:
  - 14% in proximal third of esophagus
  - 43% in middle third of esophagus
  - 67% in distal third of esophagus
- Symptoms
  - Upper esophagus: drooling, stridor, respiratory distress
  - Middle or distal esophagus: chest pain, dysphagia, drooling, vomiting

TREATMENT

- Depends on location and symptoms
  - Symptomatic patients warrant urgent endoscopy

- Asymptomatic patients with esophageal coins can be observed for 8 to 16 hours with repeat films at 12 to 24 hours
- Asymptomatic patients with coins in stomach or intestine may be discharged with follow-up and caregiver monitoring of stool
- Follow-up
  - Instruct caregiver to monitor stool for coin passing
  - Repeat films at 2 to 3 weeks and again at 4 to 6 weeks if coin has not passed
  - Elective endoscopy if coin does not pass at 4 to 6 weeks
- Complications
  - Esophageal strictures, fistulas, perforation

Button Batteries

BASIC INFORMATION

- High morbidity if lodged in esophagus due to discharge of electrical current and tissue damage
- Damage to esophagus, including burns and stenosis, occurs within 2 hours of ingestion

DIAGNOSIS AND EVALUATION

- Bilaminar with double ring or halo sign on chest radiograph (Fig. 19.2)
- Visible step-off on lateral view (Fig. 19.3)

TREATMENT

- Make patient NPO and obtain STAT two-view radiograph
- If battery confirmed in esophagus, emergent endoscopy warranted (even if the patient is asymptomatic)
- If battery is in stomach:

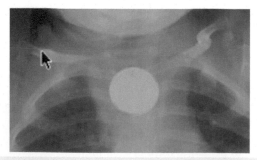

Fig. 19.2. Bilaminar with double ring or halo sign on chest radiograph.

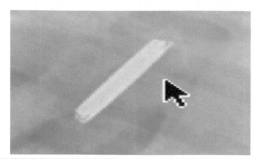

Fig. 19.3. Visible step-off on lateral view.

- If patient is symptomatic, indication for urgent endoscopy removal, regardless of age or battery size
- If a magnet is co-ingested with the battery, endoscopic removal is also warranted, regardless of symptomaticity
- Management of button battery in the stomach (Table 19.3)
- Complications: esophageal perforation, necrosis, fistula, mediastinitis, pneumothorax, pneumoperitoneum

Cylindrical Batteries

BASIC INFORMATION

- Ingested less frequently than button batteries
- Lower risk of caustic injury

TREATMENT

- If battery confirmed in esophagus, emergency endoscopy is warranted
- If battery is in the stomach, consider endoscopy removal if it does not pass in 48 hours
- If battery is in the small intestine, no acute intervention is warranted

Magnets

BASIC INFORMATION

- 50% of magnet ingestions involve ingestion of multiple magnets
- Rare-earth magnets are typically 5 to 10 times stronger than regular magnets and can strongly attract coingested metallic objects in additional to other magnets

DIAGNOSIS AND EVALUATION

- Two-view radiograph of abdomen to evaluate number of magnets ingested
  - Magnets can stack, making multiple radiographic views beneficial

TREATMENT

- Single-magnet ingestion
  - If in stomach or esophagus and coingested metallic object, urgent endoscopy is warranted for removal

Table 19.3. Management of Button Batteries in the Stomach Based on Age of Patient and Size of the Battery

Age	Battery Size	Management
≥5 years	<20 mm	KUB 12–14 days if not passed
	≥20 mm	KUB 24–48 hours if not passed
<5 years	<20 mm	
	≥20 mm	Consider removal in 24–48 hours

KUB, Upright one view abdominal radiograph.

- If no coingestion, consider close monitoring with serial radiographs
- Counsel regarding additional risk if coingested second metallic object
- Multiple-magnet ingestion
  - If in the esophagus or stomach, urgent endoscopic removal
  - If beyond the stomach, keep the patient NPO and admit to monitor in hospital with surgical consult for potential removal
  - Consider use of polyethylene glycol 3350 inpatient if magnets are beyond the stomach and progression through the bowel has slowed
- Complications
  - Intestinal necrosis, ulceration, bowel perforation, and fistula formation
  - Obstruction and volvulus, pneumoperitoneum, peritonitis, sepsis

Additional Categories of Ingestions

SHARP OBJECTS

- If within reach of endoscopy, urgent removal is warranted
- If past the duodenum, follow with serial radiographs for 72 hours; consider surgical consult if object fails to progress
- Monitor for vomiting, worsening abdominal pain, fever, hematemesis, or melena

LONG OBJECTS

- Objects >2 cm in width and/or >5 cm in length are unlikely to pass through pylorus
- Consider nonurgent endoscopic removal

FOOD IMPACTION

- Most commonly occurs with meat
- Increased incidence of underlying esophageal pathology, such as eosinophilic esophagitis or esophageal strictures
- Emergent versus urgent endoscopic removal depending on the child's symptoms/tolerance

Review Questions

For review questions, please go to ExpertConsult.com.

Suggested Readings

1. Bauman B, McEachron K, et al. Emergency management of the ingested magnet: an algorithmic approach. *Pediatr Emerg Care.* 2017. Epub.
2. Carvajal HF, Griffith JA. Burn and inhalation injuries. In: Furhman BP, Zimmerman J, eds. *Pediatric Critical Care.* 3rd ed. Philadelphia: Mosby Elsevier; 2006:1565.
3. D'Souza AL, Nelson NG, McKenzie LB. Pediatric burn injuries treated in U.S. emergency departments between 1990 and 2006. *Pediatrics.* 2009;124:1424–1430.
4. Duke J, Wood F, Semmens J, et al. A study of burn hospitalizations for children younger than 5 years of age 1983-2008. *Pediatrics.* 2011;127e–e971.
5. Gomez R, Candcio LC. Management of burn wounds in the emergency department. *Emerg Me Clin North Am.* 2007;25:135–146.
6. Kramer RE, Lerner DG, et al. Management of ingested foreign bodies in children: a clinical report of the NASPGHAN Endoscopy Committee. *J Pediatr Gastroenterol Nutr.* 2015;60(4):562–574.
7. Kurowski JA, Kay M. Caustic ingestions and foreign body ingestions in pediatric patients. *Pediatr Clin N Am.* 2017;64:507–524.
8. Wright CC, Closson FT. Updates in pediatric gastrointestinal foreign bodies. *Pediatr Clin N Am.* 2013;60(5):1221–1239.

Endocrinology

20 *Hyperglycemia and Hypoglycemia*

BETTY SHUM

DISORDERS OF HYPERGLYCEMIA

Type 1 Diabetes

BASIC INFORMATION

- One of the most common chronic illness in childhood, affecting about 1.93 per 1000 youth age <20 years in the United States
- The prevalence is varied based on gender, age, and ethnicity
  - There is a bimodal distribution with first peak onset in children 4 to 6 years of age and another peak around puberty
  - More commonly affects non-Hispanics whites with equal female to male ratio
- It is an autoimmune disease with destruction of pancreatic insulin-producing beta cells in the islets of Langerhans; this leads to progressive loss of insulin production and results in hyperglycemia, ketoacidosis, and death
- There is a genetic and environmental component to this disease
  - Susceptibility has been associated with allele variation in the human leukocyte antigen (HLA) class II region on chromosome 6
  - Development of type 1 diabetes (T1D) has been strongly associated with HLA DR3-DQ2 and DR4-DQ8 haplotypes in Caucasian patients
  - Monozygotic twins have a concordance rate of 30–65%; dizygotic twins have a concordance rate of 6–10%.
- See also *Nelson Textbook of Pediatrics*, Chapter 589, "Diabetes Mellitus"

CLINICAL PRESENTATION

- Usually presents in three types of settings:
  - Classic new onset
    - Presents to the pediatrician's office with subacute progression of polyuria, polydipsia, polyphagia, and weight loss (over weeks to months)
    - Often found to have hyperglycemia, but no acidosis
  - Diabetic ketoacidosis (DKA; see the following section)
    - Presents with neurologic symptoms (lethargy and confusion), gastrointestinal (GI) symptoms (nausea, vomiting, and abdominal pain), and Kussmaul breathing along with a history of weight loss, polyuria, and polydipsia
    - Found to have hyperglycemia and ketoacidosis
  - Silent presentation

- Patient blood glucose is checked by a parent or grandparent with diabetes and found to have hyperglycemia and be asymptomatic

DIAGNOSIS

- Criteria for diagnosis of diabetes (have one of the following):
  - Hemoglobin (Hgb) A1C ≥ 6.5 *or*
  - Fasting plasma glucose level ≥ 126 mg/dL *or*
  - Two-hour oral glucose tolerance test reading ≥ 200 mg/dL *or*
  - Random plasma glucose level ≥ 200 mg/dL in a patient with classic symptoms of hyperglycemia
- It can be difficult to differentiate T1D from type 2 diabetes (T2D); a few factors favoring T1D include:
  - Elevation of multiple autoantibodies (e.g., glutamic acid decarboxylase antibody, insulinoma-associated protein 2 antibody)
  - Low insulin C-peptide level
  - Family history of autoimmune disease
  - Normal body mass index (BMI)

MANAGEMENT

- Initial management depends on the presentation of symptoms
  - The goal is to restore to euglycemia and to provide patient and parent education
  - Education for patient and parents is very important for management at home, including calculation of insulin doses for carbohydrate coverage, hyperglycemia correction factor, and self-care during sick days
- Types of insulin: there are long acting, intermediate acting, rapid acting, and short acting insulins (see Table 20.1)
  - Basal/bolus insulin regimen: the goal is to provide a more physiological pattern of insulin levels
  - Basal insulin provides steady amount of insulin to cover for time between meals
  - The bolus component (rapid acting insulin) provides insulin for food coverage and to correct hyperglycemia
  - When used, "intermediate" and short-acting forms are often given in combination to minimize the number of injections
  - Delivery methods: insulin can be delivered as subcutaneous injections or delivered through an insulin pump system, which minimizes the number of injections
  - Blood glucose should be checked before meals (three times a day) and before snacks

Table 20.1. Types of Insulin

Insulin Preparation	Onset (h)	Peak (h)	Duration (h)
Rapid acting Lispro, Aspart Glulisine	0.25–0.5	0.5–1	3–4
Short acting Regular	0.5–1	2–3	4–6
Intermediate acting NPH	2–4	6–10	14–16
Long acting Detemir	Slow	6–8	6–24
Glargine	1–2	No peak	20–24

- Sample home routine insulin regimen (*not* in DKA)
  - Total daily dose (TDD) of insulin is calculated as 0.5 unit/kg/day to 1 unit/kg/day; prepubertal children tend to require a lower TDD, and pubertal children will need a higher insulin amount
  - Half of the TDD is given as long-acting insulin and the other half is given as rapid-acting or short-acting insulin to cover for meals
  - Insulin to carbohydrate (I:C) ratio is used to cover the amount of carbohydrate consumed; for example, an I:C ratio of 1:15 means that for every 15 g of carbohydrate consumed 1 unit of insulin will be given
    - To calculate the I:C ratio use the "Rule of 500" by dividing 500 by the TDD
  - Hyperglycemia correction factor is used to provide doses of rapid-acting or short-acting insulin to normalize hyperglycemia for a tight glycemic control; this factor estimates how much 1 unit of insulin would drop the blood glucose concentration
    - To calculate the correction factor, use the "Rule of 1800"
    - Correction factor = 1800 divided by TDD
  - "Sick days": patients with T1DM may develop ketosis when ill (e.g., upper respiratory infection [URI], gastroenteritis); to prevent progression to DKA, patients will need increased insulin requirement reverse the ketosis at home
- "Honeymoon phase"
  - Refers to a period of time after the initial diagnosis of T1D in which patients often require less daily insulin than they will later because they often have some endogenous insulin secretion from remaining beta cells. This period may last several months
- Long-term complications and monitoring
  - Long-term effects of chronic hyperglycemia include risk for microvascular disease (i.e., nephropathy, retinopathy, neuropathy) and macrovascular disease (i.e., coronary artery disease, strokes)
  - Important to have tight hyperglycemia control to prevent these complications
  - Nephropathy:
    - Monitor early disease with microalbuminuria with a urine spot test for albumin to creatinine ratio (positive if ratio is 30–299 mg/g)
    - Start screening at 10 years of age or older and if there has been diabetes for at least 5 years

- Diabetic retinopathy: start screening at 10 years of age and if there has been diabetes for 3 to 5 years; routine ophthalmologic examination annually
- Macrovascular disease: start lipid screen at 10 years of age
- Autoimmune disease:
  - T1D is associated with development of other autoimmune disorders including celiac disease (~10%), autoimmune hypothyroidism, vitiligo, autoimmune adrenalitis, and pernicious anemia
  - Screen for celiac disease every 2 to 3 years and hypothyroidism every 1 to 2 years in follow-up

Diabetic Ketoacidosis

BASIC INFORMATION

- Occurs in about one-quarter of new-onset patients and can present as a critical illness
- Risk factors for presenting in DKA include age < 2 years, ethnic minority, lower socioeconomic status, and lower BMI

CLINICAL PRESENTATION

- Patients may present with sequelae of hyperglycemia and dehydration (e.g., sunken eyes, decreased skin turgor, dry mucous membranes), as well as sequelae of ketoacidosis:
  - Neurologic symptoms (lethargy and confusion)
  - GI symptoms (nausea, emesis, and abdominal pain)
  - Tachypnea, with severe cases developing Kussmaul breathing

DIAGNOSIS

- Initial laboratory tests should include point-of-care (POC) glucose, serum blood glucose, blood gas, comprehensive metabolic panel (CMP), urinalysis (UA) (to check for ketones), and complete blood count (CBC)
- Criteria for DKA include all three of the following:
  - Hyperglycemia: blood glucose > 200 mg/dL
  - Metabolic acidosis: venous pH <7.3 or plasma bicarbonate <15 mEq/L
  - Ketosis: positive in blood or urine
- Severity of DKA is categorized by degree of acidosis

Mild (pH 7.2–7.3), moderate (pH 7.1–7.2), and severe (pH <7.1)

MANAGEMENT

- Fluid resuscitation
  - Patient may present with significant dehydration; isotonic fluids should be given to restore the circulating volume
    - In the pediatric patient, current practice often favors conservative fluid resuscitation to avoid administration of excess volume and possible fluid shifts (e.g., 10 mL/kg 0.9% NaCl per bolus up to 500 mL, with reassessment between each bolus)
  - Following the initial fluid resuscitation, initiate continuous fluids at 1.5 to 2 times the maintenance rate
    - There may be institutional variability in fluid composition, but most use isotonic fluids with a significant amount of supplemental K^+ because patients are often total body K^+ depleted on presentation and will shift potassium intracellularly with the administration of insulin and the correction of acidosis
- Insulin titration:
  - A continuous insulin infusion is usually started immediately to begin correction of the ketosis
    - Start an insulin infusion at a rate of 0.05 to 0.1 unit/kg/h with frequent blood glucose checks
    - An insulin bolus is no longer recommended because some think it could precipitate cerebral edema
  - Dextrose titration with resolution of hyperglycemia:
    - In addition to resolving the ketosis, the insulin infusion will decrease the blood glucose, potentially causing hypoglycemia before the acidosis is corrected
    - In anticipation of this, maintenance fluids with dextrose should be initiated and up-titrated as blood glucose drops below 250 mg/dL
      - For instance, it is common for DKA patients to require D10%-containing fluids (e.g., D10 0.9% NaCl with 40 mEq/L KCl) while on insulin to maintain blood glucose levels > 100 mg/dL
    - Cessation of the insulin infusion may also prevent hypoglycemia; however, doing so will also fail to resolve the ketosis, prolonging the illness
    - On resolution of ketosis and acidosis, patients are usually transitioned to a home insulin regimen (as previously mentioned)

Cerebral Edema

BASIC INFORMATION

- A major complication of DKA (<1%)
  - Classically occurs 4 to 12 hours after starting treatment for DKA
  - Can lead to mortality or permanent neurologic impairments
- Diagnostic criteria exist and are based on clinical findings, not imaging (the head computed tomography [CT] will most likely be normal):
  - Altered mental status change
  - Abnormal response to pain
  - Decorticate or decerebrate posture
  - Cranial nerve palsy

- Persistent bradycardia
- Abnormal neurogenic breathing
- Treatment should proceed as for usual causes of intracranial hypertension (e.g., hyperosmolar therapy with mannitol or 3% hypertonic saline)

Type 2 Diabetes

BASIC INFORMATION

- Increasing prevalence has increased in the United States, representing about 20% of pediatric diabetes; about half of the cases are among adolescents ages 15 to 19 years old
- Caused by an impairment of insulin secretion and insulin resistance leading to hyperglycemia
- Risk factors include genetic disposition, environmental factor, obesity, affects females more than males, and minority group (increased risk in Hispanics, Native Americans, and non-Hispanic blacks)

CLINICAL PRESENTATION

- Physical examination finding: overweight/obese patient, acanthosis nigricans, and hypertension
- Can present in several ways:
  - Asymptomatic
  - Symptomatic (i.e., polydipsia and polyuria)
  - DKA (as previously mentioned)
  - Hyperglycemic hyperosmolar state (see in a later section)

DIAGNOSIS

- Diagnostic criteria of diabetes mellitus (have one of the following):
  - Hb A1C ≥ 6.5 or
  - Fasting plasma glucose level ≥ 126 mg/dL or
  - Two-hour oral glucose tolerance test reading ≥ 200 mg/dL or
  - Random plasma glucose level ≥ 200 mg/dL in a patient with classic symptoms of hyperglycemia
- Unlike type 1 diabetics, type 2 diabetics typically present at the onset of puberty with increased BMI and signs of insulin resistance (acanthosis nigricans, hypertension, dyslipidemia, and polycystic ovary syndrome)
  - A minority of patients with T2D will be antibody positive
- Screening for T2D is indicated in children and adolescents >10 years old or onset of puberty who have a first-degree or second-degree relative with T2D, show signs of insulin resistance, have a mother with gestational diabetes, or are from a high-risk ethnic group (i.e., Hispanics, Native Americans, African American and Asian and Pacific Islanders)

MANAGEMENT

- T2D is managed with both medications and lifestyle changes; lifestyle modification includes weight reduction, which helps increase insulin sensitivity through increased physical activity, and dietary changes

- Metformin is the first-line therapy for medication management of T2D (approved for use in children >10 years of age)
- For a patient with severe hyperglycemia (Hgb A1C ≥ 8.5%), insulin is also used to achieve glucose control
- Other classes of drugs, including sulfonylureas, have not been approved by the US Food and Drug Administration (FDA) for children and adolescents
- Monitor every 3 months with Hgb A1C and screen for other comorbidities including hypertension, dyslipidemia, retinopathy, and nephropathy

Metabolic Syndrome

BASIC INFORMATION

- Refers to a cluster of symptoms that increases the risk for developing T2D and cardiovascular disease
- Criteria for metabolic syndrome as defined by the International Diabetes Federation include abdominal obesity (waist circumference ≥90th percentile for age and sex) and 2 of the following:
  - Hypertension
  - Elevated serum triglycerides (≥150 mg/dL)
  - Low high-density lipoprotein (HDL) cholesterol <40 mg/dL
  - Fasting glucose ≥100 mg/dL
- Screening and diagnosis
  - All pediatric patients should be screened with BMI and blood pressure (BP) at annual physicals
    - By age 9 and 11 years, a non-HDL cholesterol or fasting lipid screening should be performed
    - Children aged 10 years and older who have a family history of T2D and signs of insulin resistance, or at greater risk, should be screened with fasting glucose and Hgb A1C
- Management
  - Lifestyle modification is the main treatment for metabolic syndrome to reduce obesity, insulin resistance, hypertension, and dyslipidemia
    - Behavioral modification includes dietary changes (lower carbohydrate diet) and increasing physical activity
  - Orlistat is the only FDA-approved medication for weight loss in adolescents as young as 12 years old; however, the side effects of steatorrhea and flatulence make it hard to use

Hyperosmolar Hyperglycemic Nonketotic Syndrome

BASIC INFORMATION

- A severe complication of T2D characterized by severe hyperglycemia (>600 mg/dL), hyperosmolarity (serum osmolality >330 mOsm/kg), and dehydration, but no ketonuria or acidosis
- Pathogenesis: the decreased activity of insulin leads to hyperglycemia and increased renal osmotic diuresis with sodium, glucose, and potassium loss; hypernatremia occurs along with dehydration

- However, unlike in DKA, there is adequate suppression of lipolysis, preventing the development of ketoacidosis
- Treatment: fluid resuscitation is very important because these patients have decreased intravascular volume; electrolyte abnormalities are also presented and will need to monitor and correct carefully; may consider starting low-dose insulin infusion after fluid resuscitation has been adequate

DISORDERS OF HYPOGLYCEMIA

BASIC INFORMATION

- The body maintains glucose homeostasis through hormonal feedback, glucose production (gluconeogenesis), and glycogen breakdown (glycogenolysis)
- Hypoglycemia occurs when the appearance of glucose into the plasma is slower than the utilization of glucose
- Glucose is the main source of energy fuel for the brain, which does not synthesize glucose on its own; it is dependent on a constant supply of plasma glucose
  - Low serum glucose can have detrimental neurologic effects including seizures and comas
- The definition of hypoglycemia is having a low serum glucose concentration (<40 mg/dL) and symptoms of hypoglycemia (i.e., lethargy, jitteriness, irritability, even seizures)
  - Patients may have low glucose concentration when fasting but be asymptomatic
  - Given the risk of adverse neurodevelopmental outcome from severe hypoglycemia in neonates, expert consensus has also used a blood glucose concentration of <50mg/dL as the threshold for further evaluation and treatment

PHYSIOLOGY OF FASTING

- The liver is the main source of endogenous glucose via glycogen breakdown and glucose production (gluconeogenesis)
  - Muscle provides a source of glycogen and amino acids for metabolism during fasting
  - The kidneys can also produce smaller amounts of glucose
- During fasting, blood glucose concentration starts to decline, causing the following:
  - First there is a physiologic response to decrease insulin secretion by pancreatic beta cells
  - Counterregulatory hormones glucagon (secreted by pancreatic alpha cells) and epinephrine are secreted to stimulate the liver to undergo glycolysis and breakdown glycogen to glucose
  - By 24 to 48 hours of fasting, gluconeogenesis occurs to make an endogenous glucose supply from amino acids (i.e., alanine and glutamine), lactate, and glycerol (i.e., fat)
  - With prolonged starvation, the body starts breaking down fatty acids to produce ketone bodies to be used by the brain and other tissues for an alternative source of fuel

Table 20.2. Differential Diagnosis for Hypoglycemia

Disorders

Transient neonatal hypoglycemia
- Prematurity
- SGA
- IUGR
- Perinatal stress (sepsis, asphyxia)
- Polycythemia

Transient hyperinsulinism
- Infant of diabetic mother
- Beckwith-Wiedemann syndrome

Persistent hyperinsulinism
- Congenital hyperinsulinism
- Insulinomas (rare in children)

Growth hormone deficiency
- Turner mosaicism
- Hypopituitarism

Cortisol deficiency
- Congenital adrenal hyperplasia
- Adrenal hypoplasia
- Hypopituitarism

Carbohydrate metabolism disorder
- Glycogen storage diseases
- Hereditary fructose intolerance
- Galactosemia

Amino acid disorder
- Maple syrup urine disease

Fatty acid disorder
- Carnitine deficiency
- Fatty acid transport chain defects
- Beta-oxidation enzyme defects

Ketotic hypoglycemia of childhood

Medication exposures
- Insulin and sulfonylureas

IUGR, Intrauterine growth restriction; *SGA*, small for gestational age.

General Approach to Hypoglycemia

- The differential diagnosis for hypoglycemia is dependent on age, family history, and clinical presentation (Table 20.2)
  - Up to 10% of newborns may have hypoglycemia during the first few hours of life
- A "critical sample" of blood is drawn during a hypoglycemic episode to help discern the diagnosis:
  - Serum plasma glucose (to confirm hypoglycemia), insulin, C-peptide, cortisol, growth hormone, free fatty acids, β-hydroxybutyrate, lactate, ammonia, acylcarnitine profile, and urine organic acids
  - The glucagon stimulation test is also helpful in cases of hypoglycemia; the test is performed by giving 1 mg of glucagon intravenously (IV) or intramuscularly (IM); the plasma glucose is checked every 10 minutes up to 30 minutes. One would expect a "normal" response of increase in glucose after glucagon administration

Transient Newborn Hypoglycemia

BASIC INFORMATION

- It is the most common cause of hypoglycemia in neonates and is physiologic in certain instances
- In utero, the fetus receives a constant supply of glucose from maternal circulation via diffusion transport across the placenta; after delivery, the umbilical cord is clamped interrupting the placental supply of glucose, and the newborn undergoes fasting until the first enteral feed
  - During this transition period, a healthy term neonate may have a glucose concentration as low as 30 mg/dL
  - Transient hypoglycemia may result in neonates because of the rapid utilization of the available fuel supply during and after birth, and they also have inadequate hepatic glycogen storage, muscle mass, and fat storage

CLINICAL PRESENTATION

- Presentation may vary:
  - Common nonspecific symptoms include jitteriness, irritability, cyanosis, respiratory distress (apnea or tachypnea), tachycardia, temperature instability, and feeding difficulties
  - Neurologic symptoms include hypotonia, poor suck, and seizures or coma
- These symptoms may also be seen in neonates who have sepsis, hypothermia, inborn errors of metabolism, and neonatal abstinence syndrome
- Risk factors for transient hypoglycemia include the following:
  - Small for gestational age (SGA)
  - Prematurity
  - Intrauterine growth restriction (IUGR)
  - Perinatal stress (birth asphyxia, preeclampsia, and sepsis)
  - Polycythemia
  - Infant of diabetic mother (IDM)
  - Maternal drug exposure (e.g., sulfonylureas, tocolytics)

DIAGNOSIS AND MANAGEMENT

- Obtain a careful perinatal history including risk factors (e.g., perinatal stress, IUGR, prematurity, maternal diabetes) and family history of hypoglycemic disorders
  - In any hypoglycemic neonate, one must also consider sepsis as an etiology
- The American Academy of Pediatrics (AAP) (2011) and the Pediatric Endocrine Society (2015) have slightly different recommendations for the management of neonatal hypoglycemia; presented in the following section is the AAP approach, although various algorithms exist:
  - Screen late preterm and term SGA, IDM/large for gestational age (LGA) infants 30 minutes after the first feed (which is given within the first hour of life)
    - If symptomatic *and* glucose <40 mg/dL, proceed with IV glucose administration
    - If <25 and asymptomatic, feed again and check in 1 hour
      If second postprandial check is also <25, then provide with IV glucose

If second postprandial check is 25 to 40, then continue refeeding and consider IV glucose

If second postprandial check is >40, then discontinue hourly checks

- Continue screening blood glucose prefeed (approximately every 2–3 hours) for the first 24 hours of age

If <35, then feed and check in 1 hour

If second postprandial check is <35, then provide IV glucose

If second postprandial check is 35 to 45, then refeed versus IV glucose

- The need for IV glucose should require evaluation and possible admission to a neonatal intensive care unit
- Persistence of hypoglycemia past 24 to 48 hours may warrant additional investigation for etiology

Hypoglycemic Infant of Diabetic Mother

BASIC INFORMATION

- IDMs are at increased risk for developing neonatal hypoglycemia shortly after birth because of an increase in insulin secretion from the pancreatic islet cells
  - Maternal hyperglycemia leads to fetal hyperglycemia in utero, resulting in hyperplasia of beta islet cells and higher levels of insulin
  - After birth, the neonate is no longer exposed to maternal blood glucose concentration but the insulin level remains high, increasing peripheral glucose utilization and inhibiting glycolysis and lipolysis, resulting in hypoglycemia
- This may persist for 24 to 72 hours

CLINICAL PRESENTATION

- Commonly presented as macrosomia (birth weight >90th percentile) and hypoglycemic with symptoms (i.e., jitteriness, irritability, cyanosis, respiratory distress)
- IDMs are also at risk for polycythemia, which exacerbates hypoglycemia
  - An increase in red blood cells (RBCs) leads to more rapid utilization of plasma glucose
- These infants are also at increased risk of metabolic syndrome and T2D later in life

DIAGNOSIS AND MANAGEMENT

- Diagnosis is clinical based on family history of maternal gestational diabetes, symptoms of hypoglycemia, and response to glucose treatment
- Hypoglycemia will resolve with frequent feeds
- Blood glucose should be screened by 1 hour of life and monitored closely

Hyperinsulinism

BASIC INFORMATION

- Occurs from hypertrophy of beta islet cells resulting in inappropriate secretion of insulin in the presence of hypoglycemia

- Hyperinsulinism may be transient (e.g., IDMs, Beckwith-Wiedemann syndrome, infants with erythroblastosis) or persistent (congenital hyperinsulinism (CHI), see the following section)

Congenital Hyperinsulinism

BASIC INFORMATION

- Most common cause of persistent hypoglycemia in infants; occurs in about 1/50,000 live births
- There are two forms of CHI: transient and persistent
  - The persistent form is caused by genetic mutations involving enzymes and transport channels in the insulin secretion pathway (e.g., *ABCC8*, *KCNJ11*)
  - Usually inherited in an autosomal recessive pattern, but some mutations are autosomal dominant
  - Persistent CHI may present as diffuse involvement of beta islet cells or focal lesions of islet cell hyperplasia

CLINICAL PRESENTATION

- About one-third of neonates are LGA at birth
- It usually presents in a neonate (within the first few hours of life) with persistent symptomatic hypoglycemia, usually requiring higher glucose infusion rates than in transient newborn hypoglycemia
- Some neonates with CHI may present with hypoglycemia later in the first year of life or during childhood

DIAGNOSIS

- Diagnosis is made from clinical presentation of severe hypoglycemia and laboratory testing
- Critical samples would be important to obtain during hypoglycemia, which include:
  - Inappropriately high insulin level and elevated C-peptide level
  - Low ketones (β-hydroxybutyrate) and low free fatty acids
  - Patients will respond to glucagon administration by increasing blood glucose by >30 mg/dL
- Genetic testing may identify mutations, but not all genes are known
- ^{18}F-dihydroxyphenylalanine positron emission tomography (PET) may identify focal lesions amenable to resection (see the following section)

MANAGEMENT

- Medical management
  - The immediate goal is to maintain blood glucose concentrations above 70 mg/dL typically; frequent enteral feeds or IV glucose therapy are used to treat hypoglycemia
  - Diazoxide is used as first-line therapy to suppress insulin secretion; octreotide (somatostatin analog) is a second-line therapy, which works by inhibiting insulin effect and suppression secretion of pancreatic enzyme secretion

- Surgical management: if patients have difficulty controlling hypoglycemia with medical management, they may require near total pancreatectomy (diffuse) or focal resection (for focal disease)

Inborn Errors of Metabolism

- Enzyme defects in carbohydrate, amino acid, and fat metabolism can present with hypoglycemia while fasting in infants and children
- Newborn screening has made a significant impact on diagnosis of inborn errors of metabolism
- For details, see Chapter 49; an overview will be provided here

DISORDERS OF CARBOHYDRATE METABOLISM

- Usually presents with fasting hypoglycemia, mild to moderate ketosis, and may have hepatomegaly; symptoms improve with eating or IV glucose
- Causes include glycogen storage disease, glycogen synthase deficiency, glucose-6-phosphatase deficiency, fructose-1,6-bisphosphatase deficiency, phosphorylase deficiency, and galactosemia

DISORDERS OF AMINO ACID METABOLISM

- Causes include maple syrup urine disease, propionic academia, methylmalonic aciduria, and glutaric aciduria type 1

DISORDERS OF FATTY ACID OXIDATION

- Diagnosis is made with laboratory findings, which include hypoketotic hypoglycemia, elevated free fatty acids and sometimes hyperammonemia
- Causes include carnitine deficiency, branched-chain α-keto acid dehydrogenase complex deficiency, fatty acid transportation defects, and beta-oxidation enzyme defects

Defective counterregulatory hormones

- Deficiency of growth hormone and cortisol can present with hypoglycemia

- Causes include hypopituitarism, adrenal hypoplasia, and congenital adrenal hyperplasia

Ketotic Hypoglycemia of Childhood

BASIC INFORMATION

- The etiology is unclear but may be caused by decreased mobilization of precursors for gluconeogenesis (amino acids and fatty acids) or an imbalance of suppression of glucose utilization by ketone bodies and limited rate of glucose production in the liver
- Typically presents with fasting hypoglycemia (especially during illnesses) at 2 to 5 years of age and usually spontaneously remits before age 10 years
- It is a diagnosis by exclusion
- Laboratory findings include:
  - Elevated growth hormone, cortisol, free fatty acid, and ketones
  - Decreased insulin level and alanine
  - Normal carnitine, lactate, and pyruvate
  - There is no response during the hypoglycemic event when glucagon is given
- Treatment involves preventing hypoglycemia with a high-protein and high-carbohydrate diet, and home monitoring for urinary ketones

Review Questions

For review questions, please go to ExpertConsult.com.

Suggested Readings

1. Kaufman F. Type 1 diabetes mellitus. *Pediatrics in Review.* 2003; 24(9):291–300.
2. Thompson-Branch A, Havranek T. Neonatal hypoglycemia. *Pediatrics in Review.* 2017;38(4):147–157.
3. Wittcopp C, Conroy R. Metabolic syndrome in children and adolescents. *Pediatrics in Review.* 2016;37(5):193–202.

21 Disorders in Sex Differentiation and Pubertal Development

ALYSSA HUANG, MD

Sexual development is a complex process that is influenced by one's chromosomal sex (genetics), gonadal sex (morphology of internal organs and gonads), and phenotypic sex (appearance of external genitalia), which together ultimately influence one's gender identity (one's self-perception of gender). In most children, these features blend and conform; however, in some children the sequence of sexual development does not conform and leads to a disorder of sexual differentiation.

Normal Sexual Development

BASIC INFORMATION

- Both internal and external genitalia form between 6 and 13 weeks of gestation
- During this period of time, both the fetal gonad and external genitalia are bipotential—capable of developing into either normal male or female phenotype
- In the presence of *SRY* gene (*sex-determining region on the Y chromosome*), the fetal gonad differentiates into a testis
    - Testicular Leydig cells secrete testosterone, which stimulates development of wolffian ducts and is also converted by 5α-reductase enzyme into dihydrotestosterone (DHT)
    - DHT leads to external virilization including enlargement and fusion of the labioscrotal folds to form the scrotum, fusion of the penis, and enlargement of the phallus
    - Testicular Sertoli cells secrete müllerian-inhibitory substance (MIS), which leads to regression and disappearance of the müllerian ducts
    - Testosterone promotes wolffian ducts to develop into vas deferens, seminiferous tubules, and prostate
- In the absence of the *SRY* gene, the ovary spontaneously develops from the bipotential gonad
- Research now has shown that female-specific genes are required to develop into a female phenotype
- See also Nelson Textbook of Pediatrics, Chapter 561, "Physiology of Puberty."

NORMAL PUBERTY

- The onset of puberty is marked by pubarche and gonadarche
    - Pubarche: results from adrenal maturation (adrenarche) leading to pubic hair, oiliness of hair and skin, acne, axillary hair, and body odor
    - Gonadarche: maturation of the hypothalamic-pituitary axis leading to increased secretion of gonadal sex steroids
        - For males: testosterone from the testes
        - For females: estradiol and progesterone from the ovaries
        - See Table 21.1 for common physical signs of puberty
- Hypothalamic gonadotropin-releasing hormone (GnRH) is secreted into the pituitary portal system, which stimulates the pituitary gonadotropes to release luteinizing hormone (LH) and follicle-stimulating hormone (FSH) into the circulation
    - GnRH is released in episodic pulses that ensure gonadotropins (FSH and LH) are also released in a pulsatile manner
- In females:
    - FSH stimulates ovarian production of estrogen
- In males:
    - LH stimulates production of testosterone from Leydig cells
    - FSH stimulates the development of the seminiferous tubules
- At the onset of puberty, the amplitude of pulses of gonadotropins and consequent sex steroids increases (first at night and then throughout the day)
- Adrenarche generally occurs several years earlier than gonadarche and is initiated by increase in dehydroepiandrosterone (DHEA) or androstenedione

NORMAL FEMALE PUBERTY

- See Fig. 21.1.
- Thelarche (breast budding) and adrenarche (pubic hair over the mons pubis) are the earliest signs of puberty, which are characteristic of Tanner stage II
    - Onset generally occurs around age 11 years of age (range from 8 to 13 years)
    - Mean age of onset in Caucasian females is 10 years old. Mean age of onset in African-American girls is 9 years
- Completion of puberty ranges from 4 to 5 years
- The peak growth spurt occurs about 1 year after thelarche (around Tanner stages III–IV) and before the onset of menarche
- Females grow about 2 to 5 cm in height before menarche
- Menarche is usually about 2 to 3 years after thelarche and occurs at Tanner stage IV

Table 21.1.   Tanner Staging

	Boys	Pubic Hair	Girls
Tanner I	Prepubertal testes (<2.5 mL); child phallus	Absent	Breasts are preadolescent. There is elevation of the papilla only
Tanner II	Increase in testicular size (>4 mL, length >2.5 cm); the penis does not enlarge. Scrotal skin reddens	Sparse growth of long, slightly pigmented downy hair	Breast bud stage. A small mound is formed by the elevation of both breast and papilla. The areolar diameter enlarges
Tanner III	Testicles enlarge, and phallus also enlarges in length	Hair is darker, coarser, and curled. Spreads sparsely over junction of the pubes	Breast and areola enlargement without any separation of their contours
Tanner IV	Further growth of the testes and scrotum. Increase in size and breadth of the penis	Adult type, but confined to rectangle not on thighs	Formation of mound-on-mound (enlarged areola and papilla form a secondary mound)
Tanner V	Adult (testicles 10–25 mL)	Adult quantity and type with extension to the thighs	Mature female breast as areola has recessed into general contour of the breast

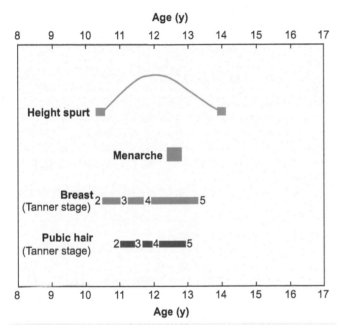

Fig. 21.1. Sequence of pubertal events in average American female.

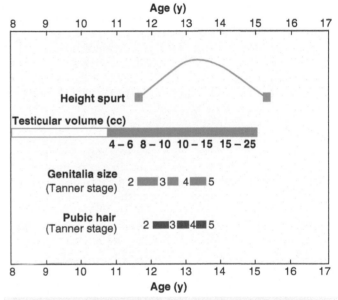

Fig. 21.2. Sequence of pubertal events in average American male.

- Mean ages of menarche are 12.2 and 12.9 years for African-American and Caucasian females, respectively
- Completion of puberty by reaching Tanner stage V occurs at around 13.9 years of age for females

NORMAL MALE PUBERTY

- See Fig. 21.2.
- The first sign of puberty is scrotal thinning followed by testicular enlargement (long diameter >2.5 cm or volume greater than 4 mL)
- This is followed by pubic hair development and axillary hair development (adrenarche)
- Deepening of the voice, facial hair, and acne indicate early stages of puberty
- Sperm development occurs at Tanner stage III. Males are capable of ejaculation and nocturnal emissions
- The growth spurt occurs relatively late in puberty—anywhere from 10.5 to 16 years of age
- Completion of male puberty by reaching Tanner V occurs at around 15.5 years of age for males

Precocious Puberty (PP)

BASIC INFORMATION

- Classically defined as secondary sexual development occurring before age of 9 years in boys or 8 years in girls

CLINICAL PRESENTATION

Premature Thelarche

- Isolated breast development that is usually benign
  - No evidence of linear growth acceleration, rapid breast development, or advanced maturation of bone age
- Most common in toddler girls, but it can present at birth or with older girls
- Associated with higher baseline FSH
- Does not progress and actually regresses over months
- It is not generally associated with PP or early menarche
- However, one should still continue to monitor for any progression of puberty because about 10% of premature thelarche does progress to sexual precocity

Premature Adrenarche/Pubarche

- Caused by elevations in adrenal androgens causing pubic or axillary hair growth
  - Breast development is absent
- Bone age often demonstrates mildly advanced skeletal maturation
- Androgen concentrations are in the early pubertal range
- May present with increased pubertal growth velocity
- Of note, premature adrenarche is associated with normal onset of gonadarche and normal adult final height
- It has been linked to increased cardiometabolic risk factors and risk for polycystic ovarian syndrome

Central Precocious Puberty (CPP)

- Results from gonadarche initiated by premature activation of the hypothalamic-pituitary-gonadal (HPG) axis (i.e. GnRH dependent)
- Follows physiologic pubertal development but occurs too early
- This includes tall stature for age, advanced bone age, increased production of sex steroids, and pulsatile gonadotropin secretion
- Almost any condition that affects the central nervous system (CNS) can precipitate CPP (e.g., hydrocephalus, meningitis, head trauma, epilepsy, irradiation, intracranial tumors)
  - Although CNS masses may cause CPP by disrupting areas that inhibit puberty, others like germinomas may also produce human chorionic gonadotropin (hCG), which can cross-react with the LH receptor leading to PP, which is GnRH independent
- Diagnosis of idiopathic PP occurs about 90% more often in females than in males. Boys have a higher incidence of CNS disorders that initiate PP

Peripheral Precocious Puberty

- Results from gonadarche or adrenarche that does not involve the HPG axis (i.e. GnRH independent)
- McCune-Albright syndrome (MAS): the most common cause of GnRH-independent PP
  - Classic triad:
    - Polyostotic fibrous dysplasia (FD): the most common feature
    - Precocious gonadarche: results from ovarian hyperfunctioning and erratic estrogen secretion
    - Hyperpigmented macules (café-au-lait spots)
  - Occurs more commonly in girls than in boys
  - Results from mutation in the G protein intracellular signaling system and leads to constitutive activation of adenylate cyclase and of cAMP
  - Affected cells in ovary, bone, and skin are commonly affected. Presents with irregular vaginal bleeding and recurrent ovarian cysts
  - Other endocrine organs are also affected, leading to hyperthyroidism and hyperadrenalism (Cushing syndrome); acromegaly or renal phosphate wasting may occur
  - Thus a more clinically relevant definition of MAS = FD + hyperfunctioning endocrinopathy ± café-au-lait spots

- Familial GnRH-independent sexual precocity:
  - Boys may have precocious gonadarche due to constitutive activation of an LH receptor that leads to continuous production and secretion of testosterone
  - Also known as "testotoxicosis"
- The hCG-secreting tumors (from pineal gland or liver) can stimulate LH receptors and lead to increase in testosterone
- Ovarian cysts can also lead to high estrogen levels
- Congenital adrenal hyperplasia (CAH) can cause peripheral PP from excess androgen production by adrenal glands
- Exogenous estrogen or testosterone exposure
  - Estrogen exposures: oral contraceptive pills, estrogen-based creams, phytoestrogens, and endocrine-disrupting chemicals (EDCs)
  - EDCs are exogenous agents that interfere with the synthesis or action of natural hormones: lavender oil, tea tree oil, fennel
- Testosterone exposures: topical testosterone gels

DIAGNOSIS AND EVALUATION

- See Table 21.2 for the differential diagnosis for PP
- Initial evaluation includes thorough history to determine the age of onset, the tempo of pubertal progression, linear growth velocity, and presence of other secondary sex characteristics (acne, body odor, and vaginal bleeding)
- It is key to screen for exogenous exposures and a family history of PP
- Physical examination is key in determining Tanner staging (sexual maturity rating)
  - In females, estrogen leads to breast development, uterine increase, and menarche
  - In males, it is key to note if testes are greater than 2.5 cm (4-mL volume) because this signifies gonadarche
  - If testes are not enlarged but virilization is progressing, the source of androgens may be the adrenal glands or another exogenous source
- Pathology is more likely with rapid progression, higher sexual maturity rating (SMR), accelerated linear growth, advanced bone age, and multiple sex characteristics
- Laboratory work
  - Determine if sex steroid levels are in pubertal range: testosterone, estradiol, DHEA sulfate (DHEAS), or androstenedione
  - Baseline gonadotropins: LH and FSH
    - If these are elevated for the child's age, it is likely that CPP has occurred
    - LH value of more than 0.3 mIU/mL at 8 a.m. is diagnostic for CPP
    - If these are low, it is difficult to interpret because LH and FSH are pulsatile. Thus a GnRH stimulation test is warranted
      - During GnRH stimulation, a child is given a dose of GnRH, and measurements of LH and FSH are obtained
      - FSH is dominant during prepuberty

Table 21.2.   Differential Diagnosis for Precocious Puberty

Central or True Precocious Puberty (Gonadotropin Dependent)	Pseudo or Peripheral Precocious Puberty (Gonadotropin Independent)	Normal-Variant Puberty
▪ Idiopathic ▪ Central nervous system (CNS) tumors (astrocytoma, hypothalamic hamartoma, craniopharyngioma, ependymoma, pineal tumor) ▪ CNS insults: ▪ Cerebral palsy ▪ Hydrocephalus ▪ Irradiation ▪ Trauma ▪ Infection ▪ Granulomatous disease ▪ Subarachnoid cyst ▪ Tuberous sclerosis, Sturge-Weber ▪ Secondary to withdrawal of chronic sex hormone exposure ▪ Gain-of-function mutations of kisspeptin/kisspeptin receptor	▪ Gonadal activation: ▪ McCune-Albright syndrome ▪ Familial testotoxicosis (activating mutation of luteinizing hormone receptor) ▪ Ovarian tumor ▪ Ovarian cyst ▪ Leydig cell tumor ▪ Adrenal: ▪ Estrogen-secreting adrenal tumor ▪ Congenital virilizing adrenal hyperplasia ▪ Adrenal functional adenoma/carcinoma ▪ Human chorionic gonadotropin-producing tumors ▪ CNS chorioepithelioma ▪ CNS Dysgerminoma ▪ CNS Teratoma ▪ Choriocarcinoma ▪ Hepatoma ▪ Teratomas ▪ Other: ▪ Primary hypothyroidism ▪ Exogenous estrogen exposure ▪ Aromatase excess ▪ Exogenous testosterone exposure ▪ Peutz-Jeghers syndrome	▪ Premature thelarche ▪ Premature adrenarche

Data from Long D. Precocious puberty. *Pediatrics in Review*, 36(7)2015.

- ▪ LH is dominant during puberty, and a stimulated level greater than 5 mIU/mL is diagnostic for CPP
- ▪ Thyroid function studies (thyroid-stimulating hormone [TSH] and free T4) should also be obtained because severe primary hypothyroidism can cause incomplete PP
- ▪ 17-hydroxyprogesterone is also recommended to rule out CAH as the cause of sexual precocity
- ▪ Imaging:
  - ▪ Bone age is helpful to determine whether there are any skeletal advancements, including growth plate closure. This would suggest that there is sex hormone exposure
  - ▪ Brain magnetic resonance imaging (MRI) is critical to obtain if there is any suggestion of CNS anomaly or tumor
    - ▪ A diagnosis of CPP mandates that an MRI of the CNS be performed
    - ▪ Compared with girls, boys with PP have higher incidence of CNS disorders leading to PP, and this always warrants brain MRI
  - ▪ Pelvic ultrasound should be considered for girls with isolated vaginal bleeding to evaluate for ovarian cyst or tumor

TREATMENT

- ▪ The major reason for treatment is to preserve adult height and respond to the psychosocial difficulties associated with early puberty and menarche
- ▪ There is a clear benefit in treating children under the age of 6 to preserve adult height (see Table 21.3)
  - ▪ PP can adversely affect a child's self-esteem

Table 21.3.   Treatment Options for Precocious Puberty

Disorder	Treatment	Mechanism
GnRH-dependent central precocious puberty	GnRH agonists	Blocks action of endogenous pulsatile GnRH
GnRH-independent precocious puberty for girls McCune-Albright syndrome Autonomous ovarian cysts	Aromatase inhibitors	Inhibition of ovarian steroidogenesis; regression of cyst and inhibition of follicle-stimulating hormone
GnRH-independent precocious puberty for boys	Testolactone Ketoconazole	Inhibition of P-450 aromatase; blocks estrogen synthesis
Familial testotoxicosis	Spironolactone or flutamide	Antiandrogen inhibition of aromatase→ blocks estrogen synthesis

Modified from Grumbach MM, Kaplan SL. Recent advances in the diagnosis and management of sexual precocity. *Acta Paediatr Jpn.* 1988;30(Suppl):155-175.

- ▪ GnRH-dependent CPP:
  - ▪ Treatment usually with GnRH analogs that maintain a constant serum concentration of GnRH that eliminates the pulsatility of the endogenous GnRH
- ▪ GnRH-independent CPP:
  - ▪ Those with GnRH-independent germ cell tumors or Leydig cell tumors require an inhibitor of testosterone synthesis (i.e., ketoconazole), an antiandrogen (i.e., spironolactone), or aromatase inhibitor (i.e., testolactone or letrozole)
  - ▪ Those with PP due to hormone-secreting tumor require surgical removal
  - ▪ MAS will be unresponsive to GnRH analog; thus it is treated with antiandrogens or antiestrogen

Table 21.4.   Important Causes of Delayed Puberty

Hypogonadotropic hypogonadism

BOTH GENDERS

Congenital
- Isolated gonadotropin deficiency
- Kallmann syndrome and non-X-linked Kallmann syndrome
- Idiopathic
- Multiple pituitary hormone deficiencies
- Septo-optic dysplasia
- Disorders of pituitary organogenesis (e.g., idiopathic hypopituitarism)

- Other inherited syndromes
- Prader-Willi
- Laurence-Moon-Biedl
- Syndromes with midline defects/tumors
- Syndromes with infiltrative disease (e.g., hemochromatosis)

Acquired
- Anorexia nervosa/malnutrition
- Functional gonadotropin deficiency due to chronic illness (e.g., inflammatory bowel disease)
- Central nervous system tumor (e.g., craniopharyngioma, adenoma)

- Central nervous system irradiation
- Central nervous system infiltrative disease (e.g., histiocytosis, sarcoidosis)
- Hyperprolactinemia
- Hypothyroidism

Hypergonadotropic hypogonadism

BOYS

Congenital
- Follicle-stimulating hormone and luteinizing hormone resistance
- Noonan syndrome
- Klinefelter syndrome (small testes but adequate androgen production)

Acquired
- Radiation/chemotherapy
- After surgery for cryptorchidism
- Vanishing testes syndrome
- Infection (e.g., mumps)
- Infarction (e.g., torsion)/trauma

GIRLS

Congenital
- Follicle-stimulating hormone and luteinizing hormone resistance
- Noonan syndrome
- Turner syndrome (gonadal dysgenesis)
- Galactosemia

Acquired
- Radiation/chemotherapy
- Autoimmune ovarian failure

Delayed Puberty

BASIC INFORMATION

- Puberty is delayed when there is no sign of pubertal development by age 13 years in girls (no breast development) and 14 years in boys (no growth of testes or penis)
- In girls, if menarche has not developed by age 15 years, it is considered delayed
- Delayed puberty occurs in about 2.5% of healthy boys
- Table 21.4 lists some common causes of delayed puberty

CLINICAL PRESENTATION

Constitutional delayed puberty

- Some patients with constitutional growth delay can have delayed onset of puberty and significant bone age delay; adult normal height for genetic potential is generally obtained
- A family history of delayed puberty in a parent or sibling is common and reassuring
- Spontaneous puberty usually begins in patients by the time the bone age reaches 12 years in boys and 11 years in girls
- This is a diagnosis of exclusion, and thus other causes must be explored
  - Young women with delayed puberty must be evaluated for primary amenorrhea
- Observation and reassurance are appropriate

- Some boys may be treated with low-dose testosterone to precipitate puberty
- Estrogen has been used in girls with constitutional delay, but there are no clear benefits

Hypogonadotropic hypogonadism

- No spontaneous entry into gonadarche. There may be some degree of adrenarche
- There is normal proportion and growth during childhood; however, during adulthood, eunuchoid proportions develop, which consist of longer-than-normal long bones
- The upper-to-lower segment ratio if lower than the normal of 0.9, and the arm span is often greater than height
  - Isolated gonadotropin deficiency
    - Relatively rare congenital condition caused by complete or partial deficiency of GnRH, leading to decreased or absent secretion of LH and FSH
  - Kallmann syndrome: characterized by isolated gonadotropin deficiency with disorder of olfaction
    - Wide genetic heterogeneity with wide clinical spectrum from those with isolated anosmia, others with abnormal reproduction, and some with both
    - Mutations of the *KAL1* genes on the X chromosome have been implicated
    - This mutation causes GnRH neurons to remain in primitive nasal area and prevent migration to hypothalamus
  - Idiopathic hypopituitarism: congenital absence of various combinations of pituitary hormones
    - May manifest as a male with gonadotropin deficiency, growth hormone deficiency, microphallus, or hypoglycemic seizures
  - Anorexia nervosa
    - Characterized by striking weight loss and psychiatric disorder
    - Decreased gonadotropins occur when excessive dieting, malnutrition, or chronic disease results in weight loss to less than 80% of ideal body weight
    - Results in primary or secondary amenorrhea
    - Pubertal development is absent or minimal
    - Regaining weight to ideal level may not immediately reverse the condition
    - Athletic amenorrhea: due to increased physical activity can lead to decreased gonadotropin and decreased menstrual frequency
  - Chronic or systemic illness:
    - May lead to pubertal delay or amenorrhea secondary to hypothalamic dysfunction
    - Examples include sickle cell disease, inflammatory bowel disease (IBD), cystic fibrosis (CF), celiac disease, chronic renal failure, and rheumatoid arthritis
  - Hypothyroidism inhibits onset of puberty and delays menstrual periods

Hypergonadotropic hypogonadism

- Characterized by elevated gonadotropins and low sex steroid levels due to primary gonadal failure
- Ovarian failure:
  - Diagnosed by elevated gonadotropins
  - In Turner syndrome, gonadal dysgenesis is the common cause of ovarian failure and short stature

Table 21.5. Differential Diagnosis for Delayed Puberty

Causative Condition/ Disorder	Stature	Plasma Gonadotropins	GnRH Test: LH Response	Plasma Gonadal Steroids	Plasma DHEAS	Karyotype	Olfaction
Constitutional delay in growth and adolescence	Short for chronologic age, usually appropriate for bone age	Prepubertal, later pubertal	Prepubertal, later pubertal	Prepubertal, later normal	Low for chronologic age, appropriate for bone age	Normal	Normal
HYPOGONADOTROPIC HYPOGONADISM							
Isolated gonadotropin deficiency	Normal, absent pubertal growth spurt	Low	Prepubertal or no response	Low	Appropriate for chronologic age	Normal	Normal
Kallmann syndrome	Normal, absent pubertal growth spurt	Low	Prepubertal or no response	Low	Appropriate for chronologic age	Normal	Anosmia or hyposmia
Idiopathic multiple pituitary hormone deficiencies	Short stature and poor growth since early childhood	Low	Prepubertal or no response	Low	Usually low	Normal	Normal
Hypothalamic- pituitary tumors	Decrease in growth velocity of late onset	Low	Prepubertal or no response	Low	Normal or low for chronologic age	Normal	Normal
HYPERGONADTROPIC HYPOGONADISM							
Syndrome of gonadal dysgenesis and variants	Short stature since early childhood	High	Hyperresponsive for age	Low	Normal for chronologic age	XO or variant	Normal
Klinefelter syndrome and variants	Normal to tall	High	Hyperresponsive at puberty	Low or normal	Normal for chronologic age	XXY or variant	Normal
Familial XX or XY gonadal dysgenesis	Normal	High	Hyperresponsive for age	Low	Normal for chronologic age	XX or XY	Normal

From Grumbach MM, Styne DM. Puberty. In Wilson JD, Foster DW, eds. *Williams Textbook of Endocrinology.* ed 9, Philadelphia, PA: WB Saunders; 1997. *DHEAS,* Dehydroepiandrosterone sulfate; *GnRH,* gonadotropin-releasing hormone; *LH,* luteinizing hormone.

- Patients with galactosemia, other gonadal dysgenesis, or treated with radiation or chemotherapy are at risk for ovarian failure
- Autoimmune ovarian failure is a less common cause but is more likely if there are other autoimmune conditions such as type 1 diabetes mellitus or autoimmune endocrinopathy syndrome (hypothyroidism, Addison disease, hypoparathyroidism)
- Testicular failure:
  - Klinefelter syndrome: most common cause of testicular failure. It is due to seminiferous tubule dysgenesis
    - Karyotype is 47,XXY, but variants with more X chromosomes are possible
    - Testosterone level may be close to normal because Leydig cell function may be retained; however, seminiferous tubules are lost and lead to infertility
    - LH levels are normal to elevated, and FSH levels are characteristically high

Primary amenorrhea

- Characterized by lack of menarche by 15 years of age
- In the case of normal secondary sexual characteristics development, one must also consider anatomic obstruction by imperforate hymen or vaginal septum
- Mayer-Rokitansky-Küster-Hauser syndrome is characterized by the congenital absence of the uterus
- Additionally, one must consider androgen insensitivity syndrome, in which males do not respond to testosterone. This leads to feminization, absent pubic/axillary hair, and primary amenorrhea. See later for more information

DIAGNOSIS AND EVALUATION

- See Table 21.5 for laboratory results from select causes of delayed puberty
- Laboratory work:
  - Serum gonadotropins to determine if patient has hypo- or hypergonadotropic hypogonadism
  - Key tests include LH, FSH, and either total testosterone or estradiol depending on sex
  - Those with delayed puberty usually have testosterone concentrations less than 40 ng/dL, and anything greater than 50 ng/dL indicates puberty is under way
  - LH greater than 0.3 mIU/mL and estradiol concentration greater than 20 pg/mL in girls suggest puberty onset
  - In both constitutional delay in growth and hypogonadotropic hypogonadism, there are low gonadotropin levels
    - Thus patients may need a GnRH or hCG stimulation test (recall that hCG has LH-like actions on the testes)
  - Those with primary gonadal failure will have strikingly elevated LH and FSH
    - For girls, a karyotype is needed to rule out Turner syndrome
    - For boys with abnormally small testes, a karyotype should be obtained to evaluate for Klinefelter syndrome
- Imaging:
  - Bone age can determine if a patient has skeletal delay, which is commonly seen in constitutional pubertal delay

- Pelvic ultrasound may be helpful in girls with delayed puberty
- It is unnecessary to obtain brain imaging unless there is evidence of hypopituitarism
- For primary care clinicians, it is reasonable to obtain basic testing including LH, FSH, either testosterone or estradiol, and a bone age. Referral to endocrinologist is then advised

TREATMENT

- If the patient has a permanent condition, sex hormone replacement is indicated
- For girls:
  - Transdermal estradiol, low-dose ethinyl estradiol (5–10 µg), or conjugated estrogens in low daily doses and titrated up to mimic puberty
  - Once breakthrough bleeding occurs, cycling with progesterone agent should start to mimic normal increases in gonadal hormones
  - A combined estrogen and progesterone agent (oral contraceptive pill) can be used instead once break-through bleeding has occurred
- For boys:
  - Testosterone can be given intramuscularly every 4 weeks
  - Dose: 50 to 100 mg monthly with gradual increase to 100 to 200 mg monthly
  - Of note, oral agents are not used due to risk of hepato-toxicity
  - For those with constitutional delay in puberty, a 3- to 6-month course of low-dose testosterone can be given to promote spontaneous puberty
- All patients with any form of delayed puberty are at risk for decreased bone mineral density. Thus sufficient calcium intake is essential
- In patients with Turner syndrome, the goal is to promote growth with exogenous growth hormone and induction of secondary sexual characteristics with low-dose cyclic estrogen/progesterone replacement

Disorders of Sexual Differentiation

BASIC INFORMATION

- Atypical genitalia: genitalia that are different from the normal spectrum in males and females but in which the sex can be assigned with a reasonable degree of certainty
- Ambiguous genitalia: minority of babies with atypical genitalia in which the sex of rearing is not apparent
- Both of these categories fall under the disorder of sexual differentiation spectrum
- The prevalence of atypical genitalia is estimated to be 1 in 300 births, whereas ambiguous genitalia may be seen as rarely as 1 in 5000 births
- Sex development
  - Sex determination: depends on the formation of testes or ovary from the bipotential gonad
  - Sex differentiation: development of physical charac-teristics, both internal and external, that are driven by gonadal hormone effects on target tissues

- Defects in either of these processes can lead to atypical genitalia
- Sertoli cells in the testes usually release anti-müllerian hormone (AMH) that leads to regression of müllerian structures
- Disorders of sexual differentiation (DSD) are congenital conditions in which the development of chromosomal, gonadal, or anatomic sex is atypical
- Classified as 46,XX DSD; 46,XY DSD; and sex chromo-somal aberrations

46,XX Disorders of Sexual Development

- Masculinization of external genitalia of genotypic females is generally caused by the presence of excessive androgens during the critical period of development (8–13 weeks of gestation)
- Degree of virilization can range from mild cliteromegaly to the appearance of a male phallus with penile urethra and fused scrotum
- CAH is the most common cause of female ambiguous genitalia
  - See Chapter 25 for details
  - Due to enzyme deficiency that impairs glucocorticoids but does not affect androgen production
  - Impairment in cortisol secretion leads to adrenocorti-cotropic hormone (ACTH) hypersecretion that induces hyperplasia of the adrenal cortex

46,XY Disorders of Sexual Development

- Underdevelopment of male external genitalia occurs due to relative deficiency of testosterone production or action
- The penis is small with various degrees of hypospadias as well as bilateral or unilateral cryptorchidism
- The testes should be located either by palpation or ultra-sound
- Testosterone production can be reduced by the follow-ing:
  1. Disorders of gonadal development
     - If müllerian-inhibiting substance is reduced, a rudimentary uterus or fallopian tubes may be present
  2. Disorders of androgen biosynthesis
  3. Defects in the androgen action
     - Complete androgen insensitivity syndrome (CAIS) is the most dramatic example of resistance to hor-mone due to defect in the androgen receptor. See later for a full description
     - 5-alpha reductase deficiency: presents with predominantly female phenotype or with ambiguous genitalia (particularly perineoscrotal hypospadias)
     - Defect in 5-alpha reductase enzyme leads to in-ability to convert testosterone to potent metabolite DHT, which is critical in the development of male external genitalia

Sex Chromosome and Ovotesticular DSD

- **Turner syndrome** and **Klinefelter syndrome** and mosaic variants are part of this category of DSD

- Mixed gonadal dysgenesis (45,X; 46,XY) can often present with ambiguous genitalia, asymmetric external genitalia, and inguinal hernias

CLINICAL PRESENTATION

- Physical examination and determining normal versus abnormal neonatal genital anatomy is key
- There is a wide spectrum of normal male and female genitalia in terms of phallic size and clitoral and labial appearance
- It is key to note where the urethral opening lies and whether there is fusion of the labioscrotal folds
- For term males
  - Normal stretched penile length in term infants ranges between 2.5 and 4.5 cm
  - In the preterm male infant, penile size varies with gestational age and should be taken into account using penile reference charts
  - Undescended testes are more common in preterm infants
  - The presence of a palpable gonad usually implies the presence of a Y chromosome; however, the gonad could still be an ovary or an ovotestis (where there is both ovarian and testicular tissue in the same gonad)
- For term females:
  - Normal clitoral length ranges from 0.2 to 0.85 cm
  - Note if patient has normal vaginal opening or fusion of labial folds
  - In preterm female infants, the appearance of the labia minora can be prominent
- Excessive exposure to androgens in utero can cause progressive degrees of labioscrotal fusion with phallic enlargement
- The Prader grading system can be used to describe the various degrees of virilization from cliteromegaly to genitalia typically seen in males with urethral opening at the tip of the glans
- See Table 21.6 for key history and physical findings in DSD

DIAGNOSIS AND EVALUATION

- Obtaining a thorough history, particularly family history, may help in the diagnosis
- Most ambiguous genitalia have a genetic cause that can be recessive, X-linked recessive, or in a dominant pattern
- The first step is to determine whether the disorder represents virilization of a genetic female (androgen excess) or underdevelopment of a genetic male (androgen deficiency)
- Karyotype determination is only one of the many factors in deciding gender of rearing
- Statistically, most virilized females have CAH, and about 90% of these have 21-hydroxylase deficiency
- Laboratory work
  - Fluorescence in situ hybridization (FISH) for sex-determining region on the Y chromosome (SRY) and steroid hormone analysis
    - Most babies with SRY will have karyotype of 46,XY, but not all
  - Karyotype

Table 21.6. Key History and Physical Findings in Disorder of Sexual Differentiation (DSD)

MATERNAL HISTORY	GENITAL EXAM
• Prenatal medications • Maternal virilization during pregnancy (voice changes or hirsutism) • Infertility	• Length and size of phallus (stretched length normally 2.5–4.5 cm) • Clitoral length (normally 0.2–0.85 cm) • Presence of gonads in scrotal sac or along line of descent from inguinal canal • Prominence of labia and degree of labial fusion • Position of urethra/urogenital sinus opening • Site of anus
FAMILY HISTORY	**OTHER PHYSICAL EXAMINATION FINDINGS**
• Consanguinity • Ambiguous genitalia • Unexplained neonatal deaths in family • Infertility • Genital surgery	• General appearance (e.g., jitteriness/lethargy due to hypoglycemia or electrolyte abnormality) • Hemodynamic compromise (i.e., shock due to salt-wasting) • Midline defects: cleft palate/lip • Excess pigmentation: areolar pigmentation • Cardiac murmur • Skeletal abnormalities and dysmorphisms

Data from Davies JH, Cheetham T. Recognition and assessment of atypical and ambiguous genitalia in the newborn. *Arch Dis Child.* 2017.

- Blood glucose and electrolytes should be measured because these can be abnormal in the setting of CAH. Hyponatremia, hyperkalemia, and hypoglycemia do not typically manifest until days 4 to 5 of life
- After 48 hours of life, obtain:
  - 17-OH progesterone, which will be elevated several hundredfold in CAH
  - Androstenedione
  - Testosterone
  - AMH: released from Sertoli cells. In males, low levels indicate testicular dysfunction, and high levels can suggest CAIS. In females, AMH is released from the granulosa cells and are a marker for ovarian reserve
- If the defect involves testosterone biosynthesis, an hCG stimulation test may be required
- Genetic testing for specific mutations may be necessary to confirm androgen insensitivity or 5-alpha reductase deficiency
- Imaging
  - Abdominal and pelvic ultrasound provide critical information regarding presence of a uterus, presence of gonads, adrenal anatomy, or renal anatomy

TREATMENT

- Management of ambiguous genitalia involves extensive open discussion with the family regarding the biology of the infant and the likely prognosis
- Treatment is individualized and generally managed by a DSD team including a pediatric endocrinologist, urologist, geneticist, psychologist, and primary care physician
- For those with deficient hormones, the treatment is hormone replacement

- Those with CAH will need replacement of cortisol (hydrocortisone)
- Those with androgen biosynthetic defects may need testosterone replacement
- Surgical restoration of genitalia may be needed
  - The recommendation for reconstructive surgery is controversial; some advocate that surgery be reserved until adolescence so that the child may be involved in decision-making
  - Gonads and internal organs that are not consistent with gender of rearing are often removed
  - Dysgenetic gonads should always be removed due to increased risk of gonadoblastoma or dysgerminoma
- Psychological support of the entire family is also recommended
- The decision to raise a child a specific gender is controversial and the family should be made aware that patients with DSD may change their gender later in life.

Androgen Insensitivity Syndrome

BASIC INFORMATION

- Insensitivity to androgens constitutes the most common cause of disorders of sexual differentiation
- It is reported to be as high as 1 in 20,000
- These are X-linked disorders and are due to defects in the androgen receptor gene

CLINICAL PRESENTATION

- Androgen insensitivity syndrome has a wide clinical spectrum ranging from complete phenotypic females to males with various forms of atypical genitalia to males with normal genitalia but infertility
- All have testes and normal or elevated testosterone levels. The phenotype depends on the degree of androgen insensitivity
- Complete androgen insensitivity: the infant is a complete phenotypic female at birth
  - Both genital and somatic end organs do not respond to androgens in the fetus or at puberty
  - External genitalia are female, and the vagina ends in a blind pouch. There is no uterus
  - Fallopian tubes may or may not be present. Testes are intraabdominal
  - At puberty, aromatization of testosterone brings about feminization of the body, leading to breast development, but menses do not occur, and pubic/axillary hair also does not occur
  - Consider this diagnosis in a phenotypic female with bilateral inguinal hernia and amenorrhea and secondary sexual characteristics
- Partial androgen insensitivity:
  - Due to a gene mutation that encodes for defective but partially functional androgen receptor
  - Variable clinical spectrum: female appearance to those with ambiguous genitalia or predominantly male phenotype

- Can present with micropenis, perineal hypospadias, and cryptorchidism

DIAGNOSIS AND EVALUATION

- As always, a thorough history and physical examination are warranted to look for Tanner staging of the genitals
- Hormone evaluation includes LH, FSH, testosterone, and DHT
  - Testosterone is often elevated
  - DHT is often normal. It is usually decreased in the setting of 5-alpha reductase deficiency
- Genetic testing to look for androgen receptor mutation will confirm the diagnosis

TREATMENT

- Treatment is difficult. In those with complete female phenotypes and characteristics, the testes are usually removed after the condition is discovered
- Seminomas are common by age 50 years old in those with retained testes
- For those with varying phenotypes, the treatment varies and is beyond the scope of the general pediatric boards

Male Gynecomastia

BASIC INFORMATION

- Gynecomastia is the occurrence of mammary tissue in males. It is a fibroglandular mass that measures at least 0.5 cm in diameter
- It is a common condition in adolescence and in newborn males
  - Pubertal gynecomastia is a physiologic phenomenon that occurs in normal boys (~45%–75%). It is a benign, self-limited increase in breast tissue
  - Physiology:
    - Androgens are converted to estrogen by aromatization
    - In early puberty, only modest amounts of androgen are produced, and thus there may be an imbalance with the estrogen produced from aromatization
    - The imbalance in the free androgen to free estrogen ratio allows for greater physiologic estrogen effect on breast tissue
    - Most frequently seen in midpuberty with Tanner stage III–IV pubic hair and testicular volumes of 5 to 10 mL bilaterally
  - Familial gynecomastia occurs in some families, can stimulate Tanner III–V, and will not regress
- Lipomastia ("pseudogynecomastia"): typically seen in obese males. Excess adipose tissue may be mistaken for breast tissue; however, it does not have characteristic firm, rubbery mass
- Pathologic gynecomastia is due to hormonal aberrations, including absolute or relative estrogen excess (including increased peripheral conversion of androgens to estrogen), androgen deficiency, or androgen insensitivity
  - Pathologic gynecomastia can be seen in patients who are genital Tanner stage I to V

- Prepubertal gynecomastia is rare and should always be considered pathologic
  - Characterized by presence of breast tissue without other secondary sexual characteristics

Selected Causes of Pathologic Gynecomastia

ESTROGEN EXCESS

- Neoplasms:
  - Leydig cell tumors secrete estradiol directly
  - hCG-secreting tumors stimulate the testes to preferentially secrete estradiol
  - Adrenocortical tumors also secrete estrogen directly and produce large amounts of DHEA that are converted to estrone in peripheral tissues
- Hyperthyroidism increases aromatization of androgens to estrogens and decreases free testosterone levels by increasing circulating levels of sex hormone binding globulin levels
- Other causes include:
  - CAH
  - Chronic liver or renal disease
  - Obesity (with increased aromatase activity)
  - Medication exposure
    - Those most commonly associated with gynecomastia include ketoconazole, spironolactone, exogenous hormones (androgens, anabolic steroids, estrogens, growth hormone, gonadotropins), soy, marijuana, cimetidine, calcium channel blockers, and first-generation antipsychotics

ANDROGEN INSUFFICIENCY

- Causes of hypogonadism (see previous) may also lead to gynecomastia
  - Primary defect is usually a decreased serum testosterone
  - However, hypergonadotropic hypogonadism also has increased LH, which causes Leydig cells to produce excess estradiol (e.g., Klinefelter syndrome)
    - Klinefelter syndrome is also prone to gynecomastia because patients have excessive aromatase production

ANDROGEN INSENSITIVITY

- X-linked disorder that is caused by mutations in the androgen receptor gene; see previous for further details

CLINICAL PRESENTATION

- Pubertal gynecomastia usually occurs in boys with genital Tanner stage II/III/IV
- Physiologic pubertal gynecomastia can involve one or both breasts, and each breast may develop to a different size
  - Tenderness is common
  - Breast tissue in Tanner stage II most often resolves with time as puberty progresses (often after 2 to 3 years)

- However, if breast tissue is Tanner stage III or above, they have macrogynecomastia, and this likely will not resolve with time

DIAGNOSIS AND EVALUATION

- Appropriate evaluation starts with physical examination with focus on size of breasts, Tanner stage of genitals, size of testicles, abdominal examination for tumors, thyroid examination, and adenopathy
- Only boys with presentations beyond normal pubertal gynecomastia warrant additional workup:
  - This includes atypical Tanner staging (Tanner I or V), atypical age (<10 or >16 years), abnormal pubertal progression, patients requesting surgery, or those with macrogynecomastia (greater than 4 cm in diameter)
- If warranted, initial laboratory evaluation includes:
  - Estradiol, testosterone and LH to rule out LH-secreting tumor; DHEAS to rule out adrenal tumor; and hCG to screen for an hCG-secreting tumor
    - LH stimulates Leydig cells and leads to increased testosterone, which converts to estrogen
  - Screen for thyroid disease (TSH, FT4), renal disease (blood urea nitrogen [BUN], Cr, urinalysis), and liver disease (ALT, AST, bilirubin, albumin, international normalized ratio [INR])
  - If patients have galactorrhea, obtain a prolactin level
  - If there is suspicion for Klinefelter syndrome, a karyotype will confirm the diagnosis
  - If any of the initial screening tests are abnormal, imaging studies are needed to evaluate for tumor

TREATMENT

- As puberty advances, circulating androgen levels rise closer to adult levels
- Within 1 to 3 years, up to 90% of boys have regression of their breast enlargement
  - For physiologic pubertal gynecomastia, the treatment is reassurance
- Treatment of the underlying endocrinopathy or removal of any offending medication or environmental exposure can be sufficient to cause breast tissue regression
- Medical treatment is directed toward blocking effects of estrogen on the breast (tamoxifen), inhibiting its production (testolactone), or administering androgens (danazol) to counterbalance estrogen
  - There are very limited data on treatment of gynecomastia in the pediatric population
  - There is some evidence that early pharmacologic intervention with antiestrogens may diminish persistent pubertal gynecomastia, but treatment with aromatase inhibitors has not been shown to be more effective than placebo
  - Current data are inadequate to recommend medical treatment for idiopathic gynecomastia at this time
- If breast tissue is significant (greater than Tanner III) or causes emotional distress, surgical resection is an option

- However, surgery is not pursued until after puberty is completed because breast tissue can continue to develop as puberty progresses

Anabolic Steroid Use

BASIC INFORMATION

- Performance-enhancing substances are commonly used by children and adolescents to improve athletic performance and appearance
- These substances include over-the-counter dietary supplements and illicit pharmacologic agents, including anabolic steroids
- For most young athletes, the use of these enhancing substances does not produce significant gains over adherence to appropriate nutrition and training program; in fact, the substances may be detrimental to normal growth and development
- Anabolic steroids include a variety of testosterone derivatives that can be taken orally, buccally, by injection, or transdermally
    - Androstenedione is widely promoted as a body-building substance, but it is now classified as a controlled substance
    - DHEA is also available as a nutritional supplement, but it is not androgenic by itself
- The purported mechanism of action is enhancement of protein synthesis by increasing transcription and decreasing catabolism

CLINICAL PRESENTATION

- When to suspect use of anabolic steroids:
    - Patient exhibits changes in behavior—depression, irritability, or increased aggression
    - In males: more rapid increase in muscle strength and mass compared with other athletes, gynecomastia, acne, small testes, low sperm density
    - In females: irregular menstrual cycles, hirsutism, acne, breast atrophy, temporal hair recession, deepening voice, cliteromegaly, increased muscle mass, decreased body fat
    - Can see high hematocrit, low serum LH, and low sex hormone binding globulin
- Long-term side effects:
    - Brain remodeling in adolescents
    - Premature growth plate closure with decreased final adult height

- Acne
- Gynecomastia that is irreversible
- Hair loss/male pattern baldness (irreversible)
- Hypogonadism
- Behavior changes: hypomania, irritability, aggression
- Cardiomyopathy and hypertension
- Increased low-density lipoproteins and decreased high-density lipoproteins
- Cholestatic jaundice and liver tumors

DIAGNOSIS AND EVALUATION

- Screening for substance abuse as part of age-appropriate comprehensive history taking
    - Ask open-ended questions regarding substance use at home, at school, and by peers before progressing to questions about personal use
- The American Academy of Pediatrics (AAP) does not endorse general drug use screening by pediatric health care providers, but there are guidelines for testing when there is clinical suspicion of use
- Detection of anabolic steroids:
    - Androgen use can be detected in urine of such patients

TREATMENT

- Stopping these drugs can be challenging
- Many individuals struggle with body image disorders and depression
- Those who discontinue androgens may become hypogonadal because it may take months for the HPG axis to recover

Review Questions

For review questions, please go to ExpertConsult.com.

Suggested Readings

1. Davies JK, Cheetham T. Recognition and assessment of atypical and ambiguous genitalia in the newborn. *Arch Dis Child.* 2017; 102:968–974.
2. Fuqua JS. Treatment and outcomes of precocious puberty: an update. *J Clin Endocrinol Metab.* 2013;98(6):2198–2207.
3. Kaplowitz P. Delayed puberty. *Pediatr Rev.* 2010;31:189.
4. Long D. Precocious puberty. *Pediatr Rev.* 2015;36(7):319–321.
5. Ma NS, Geffner ME. Gynecomastia in prepubertal and pubertal boys. *Curr Opin Pediatr.* 2008;20:465–470.

22 *Growth Disorders*

ALYSSA HUANG, MD

Growth is a complex process that is influenced by a person's genetic makeup, physical and nutritional status, and psychosocial environment. One of the major goals of pediatrics is to help each child achieve his or her individual potential through monitoring and screening of growth and development. Linear height growth can occur as a continuous process or with periodic bursts of growth and arrest. The process of growth is complex, but despite this, healthy children usually grow linearly in a remarkably predictable manner. Deviation from normal growth patterns is usually one of the first clinical manifestations of chronic, severe disease, or may be the only symptom of parental neglect or abuse. Therefore it is essential for all children to have frequent and accurate assessment of their growth.

See also Nelson Textbook of Pediatrics, Chapter 15, "Assessment of Growth."

Normal Growth

BASIC INFORMATION

- Growth rates differ during intrauterine life, childhood, and adolescence
- Accurate measurement of length/height, weight, and head circumference should be obtained at every health visit and compared with statistical norms on growth charts
- Serial measurements are more useful than a single measurement
- Normal growth patterns have spurts and plateaus, so some shifting on percentile graphs can occur
- Large shifts in percentiles warrant further investigation
- The most common reasons for deviant measurements are technical—faulty equipment or human error. Repeating the measurement is the first step!
- See Table 22.1 for expected growth parameters
- Prepubertal growth
  - Children grow the fastest in the first year of life (about 25 cm/year overall)
  - This rate decreases over time, and children 5 years until puberty will have a growth velocity about 5 cm/year
  - See Table 22.2 for growth rates by age
- Pubertal growth
  - Females: peak velocity of approximately 10 cm/year by sexual maturity rating II to III (age 14–15 years)
    - Growth spurt begins with onset of breast development and reaches peak about 1.5 years before menarche
    - After menarche, only a minimal amount of growth remains
  - Males: peak growth velocity of approximately 12 cm/year by sexual maturity rating IV (age 16–17 years)
- Growth ceases after fusion of the long bone and vertebral epiphyses
- Genetics is a critical determinant of growth; thus it is important to relate patient's height to that of siblings and parents
- Midparental height (MPH):
  - For girls:
    - [(Paternal height inches + Maternal height inches – 5 inches)] / 2
  - For boys:
    - [(Paternal height inches + Maternal height inches + 5 inches)] / 2
- Underlying pathology must be considered if child's growth pattern deviates from parents'

Disorders of Growth

BASIC INFORMATION

- Short stature is defined as subnormal height relative to other children of the same gender and age
  - Common clinical problem that may be a variant of normal growth or may indicate pathology
  - Height < −2 standard deviations (SD; 3%) for age and gender
  - Height more than 2 SD below the MPH target
- The Centers for Disease Control and Prevention growth charts use the 3rd percentile of growth as the demarcation of the lower limit
- Growth failure is slow growth rate regardless of stature and appears as a curve that crosses growth percentile lines downward (see Fig. 22.1C)
- Use the MPH to determine whether the child is growing well in relation to the family genetics
- The presence of height 3.5 SD below the mean, height velocity below the 5th percentile, or height 2 SD below the target MPH requires diagnostic evaluation

Variations of Normal (Table 22.3)

Familial/Genetic Short Stature

- Stature of a child of short parents, who is expected to reach lower than average height and yet is normal for these parents
- Bone age is equivalent to chronologic age

Table 22.1. Rules of Thumb for Growth

WEIGHT

Birth weight is regained by days 10 to 14 of life (approximately 3.5 kg)

Birth weight doubles by 4 months

Birth weight triples by 12 months (approximately 10 kg)

Birth weight quadruples by 24 months

After age 2 years, normal weight gain is about 5 lb/year until adolescence

LENGTH/HEIGHT

Birth length increases by 50% at 1 year

Birth length doubles by 4 years

Birth length triples by 13 years

After age 2 years, average height increase is 2 inches (5 cm)/year until adolescence

HEAD GROWTH

Largest rate of growth is between 0 and 2 months (0.5 cm/week)

Table 22.2. Growth Rates by Age

Age	Growth Rate
Gestation	1.2 to 1.5 cm/week, increasing to 2.5 cm/week
First 2 years of life	15 cm/year
Middle childhood	5 to 6 cm/year
Puberty—peak height velocity	7 to 11 cm/year

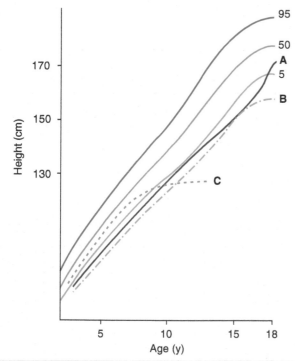

Fig. 22.1. Patterns of linear growth. See text for description of growth patterns indicated by A, B, and C. (From Palma Sisto PA, Heneghan MK. Endocrinology. In: Marcdante KJ, Kliegman RM, eds. *Nelson's Essentials of Pediatrics*. 7th ed. Philadelphia, PA: Elsevier; 2015: 586)

- Normal growth velocity
- See Fig. 22.1B

Constitutional Short Stature

- Caused by reduced tempo of physiologic development
- A child who is preadolescent or adolescent and who starts puberty later than others—"late bloomers"
- Usually a family member had delayed growth or puberty but achieved a normal final height
- Growth deceleration early on, followed by normal growth progression paralleling lower percentile curve, with acceleration late in adolescence
- The bone age is delayed compared with chronologic age
- Normal nutritional status and physical examination
- Observation and reevaluation every 4 to 6 months to ensure progression of growth and puberty
- See Fig. 22.1A

Idiopathic Short Stature

- Height >2 SDs below mean for given age, sex, and population
- No systemic, endocrine, nutritional, or chromosomal abnormality
- Patients have normal birth weight and are growth hormone (GH) sufficient
- Diagnosis of exclusion
- There is FDA approval for GH treatment (Table 22.4)

Short Stature Due to Growth Hormone Deficiency

BASIC INFORMATION

- Occurs in about 1/4000 to 1/10,000 children
- Idiopathic GH deficiency is the most common cause of both congenital and acquired GH deficiency
- GH deficiency can be caused by anatomic defects of the pituitary gland
- GH resistance or insensitivity (**Laron syndrome**) is a rare cause of growth failure and is due to abnormal function or number of GH receptors

CLINICAL MANIFESTATIONS

- Infants with congenital GH deficiency achieve normal or near-normal birth lengths and weight at term
- Growth slows after birth—notably after 2 to 3 years of age
  - Tends to become progressively shorter and elevated weight to height ratio
- "Cherub appearance": chubby, immature appearance
- Other clinical features:
  - Hypoglycemia
  - Prolonged jaundice
  - Microphallus (stretched penile length of <2 cm)
  - Cranial irradiation, head trauma, central nervous system (CNS) infection
  - Family history of GH deficiency
  - Craniofacial midline abnormalities (think of single central incisor)
  - Other pituitary hormone deficiencies
- Generally have normal intellect, unless patient has severe hypoglycemia or severe midline defect of the head and CNS

Table 22.3. Short Stature Summary

	Constitutional "Late Bloomer"	Familial/Genetic Short Stature	Hormone Deficiency: Growth Hormone Deficiency or Hypothyroidism
Growth velocity	Normal (early deceleration followed by later acceleration)	Normal	Decreased
Bone age	Delayed	Normal	Delayed
Family history	Pubertal delay	Short stature	±

Table 22.4. FDA-Approved Indications for Growth Hormone

Growth hormone deficiency
Chronic renal failure with short stature
Turner syndrome
Noonan syndrome
Short stature homeobox-containing gene (SHOX) deficiency
Prader-Willi syndrome
Small for gestational age
Idiopathic short stature

Differential Diagnosis of Short Stature

- Nutrition is the most important factor affecting growth on a worldwide basis
  - Malnutrition is the number one cause of growth failure in the world
  - Failure to thrive may be related to maternal nutritional deprivation or may result from organic illness (malabsorption or hypermetabolic state)
- Psychosocial or deprivation dwarfism in which child develops temporary GH deficiency and shows poor growth as a result of psychological abuse
  - When child is placed in healthier environment, this process reverses and GH physiology normalizes
- See Table 22.5 for a comparison of causes of short stature
- Certain genetic syndromes are associated with short stature:
  - Turner syndrome (see Chapter 35 for details): characterized by karyotype of 45,XO or mosaic karyotype. Presents with short stature, shield chest, wide-spaced nipples, wide carrying angle of upper arms, high-arched palate, gonadal failure, kidney dysplasia, and aortic arch abnormalities
  - Down syndrome (see Chapter 35 for details)
  - Russell-Silver dwarfism
  - Defects in bone development: achondroplasia (see Chapter 35 for details), hypochondroplasia, chondrodystrophies
- Consider genetic syndromes with obesity and decreased height because normal obese children are usually taller than average and have advanced skeletal development and physical maturation:
  - Prader-Willi syndrome (see Chapter 35 for details): fetal and infantile hypotonia, small hands and feet, postnatal acquired obesity, excessive appetite, developmental delay, hypogonadism, almond eyes
  - Laurence-Moon-Bardet-Biedl syndrome: retinitis pigmentosa, hypogonadism, developmental delay, obesity
  - Pseudohypoparathyroidism: short stature, developmental delay with short fourth and fifth digits, resistance to parathyroid hormone and resultant hypocalcemia and hyperphosphatemia

DIAGNOSTIC APPROACH TO SHORT STATURE

- If family or other medical history does not provide a likely diagnosis, consider obtaining screening tests (see Table 22.6)
- GH secreted episodically and mostly during slow-wave sleep
  - Between pulses, GH secretion is usually low. Thus measuring serum GH levels is not useful
  - Indirect measurements of GH (insulin-like growth factor 1 [IGF-1] and insulin-like growth factor-binding protein 3 [IGFBP-3]) are considered better screens for GH deficiency
- If chronic disease or familial short stature are ruled out and routine laboratory work is unremarkable, then GH stimulation testing should be offered, especially to those who are >3.5 SD below the mean, growing poorly, or have height projection that is below target height for family height
  - Additionally, patients with low IGF-1 and IGFBP-3 and clinical concern for short stature would also benefit from GH stimulation testing
- GH stimulation testing
  - Used to determine adequacy of GH secretion
  - Patients are given various substances (intravenous clonidine, arginine, or insulin, which can cause severe hypoglycemia and is not regularly used) to elicit GH secretion, which is measured from the serum every 30 minutes for 2 hours
  - A peak serum GH greater than 7 to 10 ng/mL is considered adequate GH secretion
  - Classic GH deficiency patients do not show an increase in serum GH levels after stimulation
  - There is a high false-positive rate for GH deficiency because about 10% or more of children may not reach normal GH peak after two stimulation tests

TREATMENT

- GH deficiency is treated with recombinant DNA-derived GH (daily injections)
- See Table 22.4 for approved indications for GH treatment

Table 22.5.   Differential Diagnosis

Diagnostic Feature	Hypopituitarism GH Deficiency*	Constitutional Delay	Familial Short Stature	Deprivation Dwarfism	Turner Syndrome	Hypothyroidism	Chronic Disease
Family history positive	Rare	Frequent	Always	No	No	Variable	Variable
Gender	Both	Males more often affected than females	Both	Both	Female	Both	Both
Fades	Immature or with midline defect (e.g., cleft palate or optic hypoplasias)	Immature	Normal	Normal	Turner fades or normal	Coarse (cretin if congenital)	Normal
Sexual development	Delayed	Delayed	Normal	May be delayed	Female prepubertal	Usually delayed, may be precocious if hypothyroidism is severe	Delayed
Bone age	Delayed	Delayed	Normal	Usually delayed; growth arrest lines present	Delayed	Delayed	Delayed
Dentition	Delayed	Normal; delay usual	Normal	Variable	Normal	Delayed	Normal or delayed
Hypoglycemia	Variable	No	No	No	No	No	No
Karyotype	Normal	Normal	Normal	Normal	45,X or partial deletion of X chromosome or mosaic	Normal	Normal
Free T$_4$	Low (with TRH deficiency) or normal	Normal	Normal	Normal or low	Normal: hypothyroidism may be acquired	Low	Normal
Stimulated GH	Low	Normal for bone age	Normal	Possibly low, or high if patient malnourished	Usually normal	Low	Usually normal
Insulin-like growth factor-1	Low	Normal or low for chronologic age	Normal	Low	Normal	Low	Low or normal (depending on nutritional status)
Therapy	Replace deficiencies	Reassurance; sex steroids to initiate secondary sexual development in selected patients	None	Change or improve environment	Sex hormone replacement, GH; oxandrolone may be useful	T$_4$	Treat malnutrition, organ failure (e.g., dialysis, transplant, cardiotonic drugs, insulin)

CRH, Corticotropin-releasing hormone; GH, growth hormone; GnRH, gonadotropin-releasing hormone; TRH, thyrotropin-releasing hormone; T$_4$, thyroxine.
*Possibly with GnRH, CRH, or TRH deficiency.
From Palma Sisto PA, Heneghan MK. Endocrinology. In: Marcdante KJ, Kliegman RM, eds. *Nelson's Essentials of Pediatrics.* 7th ed. Philadelphia, PA: Elsevier; 2015: 587

Table 22.6.   Growth Failure Screening Tests

Test	Purpose
Complete blood count with erythrocyte sedimentation rate/C-reactive protein, liver function tests, albumin	Screening for inflammatory bowel disease or other indicators of chronic disease
Renal function tests: urine, blood urea nitrogen, creatinine	Screening for chronic renal failure with acidosis or renal tubular disease
Serum calcium, phosphate, alkaline phosphatase	Rickets screening
Serum thyroid-stimulating hormone and free thyroxine	Hypothyroidism screening
Insulin-like growth factor 1 and insulin-like growth factor-binding protein 3	Growth hormone deficiency screening
Prolactin	May be elevated or depressed in pituitary disorders
Total IgA and tissue transglutaminase IgA antibody	Celiac disease screening
Karyotype on all females	Determines Turner (XO) or other syndromes
Bone age	Compare with chronologic age and estimate adult predicted height
Brain magnetic resonance imaging	Assesses for congenital midline defects and hypothalamic pituitary tumors (craniopharyngioma, glioma, germinoma)

Table 22.7. Causes of Accelerated Linear Growth

Endocrine-Related Causes	Nonendocrine
Growth hormone excess	Obesity
Thyrotoxicosis	Marfan syndrome
Excess androgen hormones (congenital adrenal hyperplasia or virilizing tumors)	Homocystinuria
	Total lipodystrophy
	Neurofibromatosis
	Chromosomal abnormalities:
Sexual precocity	Klinefelter syndrome, 48,XXYY, 47,XYY

- Side effects of GH therapy
  - Edema, joint pain, local bruising
  - Worsening scoliosis
  - Insulin resistance
  - Rare effects: pseudotumor cerebri, slipped capital femoral epiphysis (SCFE), gynecomastia
- Other concerns with GH therapy
  - Obstructive sleep apnea related to tonsillar hyperplasia in Prader-Willi syndrome
  - Exacerbation of insulin resistance in small for gestational age (SGA), Prader-Willi syndrome
  - Long-term cancer risk
- Contraindications for GH therapy
  - Active malignancy

Tall Stature

BASIC INFORMATION

- Most tall children are normal, and their height is related to their genetics and optimal environment for growth
- Tall stature is concerning only if inappropriate compared with parental height or when linear growth velocity is accelerating too quickly
- There are a number of causes for accelerated growth, both endocrine and nonendocrine (Table 22.7)

CLINICAL PRESENTATION

- Constitutional tall stature
  - Tall children typically have tall parents
  - Body proportions are normal
  - Height has been greater than 97th percentile since childhood
  - Normal height velocity
- Excess of pituitary GH
  - Rare condition among children

- Overgrowth of the mandible, enlargement of hands and feet
  - Thickening of skin
  - Excessive sweating
- Other overgrowth disorders
  - Sotos syndrome: cerebral gigantism. Growth velocity is increased in the first years of life but then decelerates and is parallel to the 97th percentile
    - Large size at birth
    - Macrocrania
    - Large ears
    - Prominent mandible
    - Subnormal intelligence
    - Poor coordination
  - Beckwith-Wiedemann syndrome
    - Macrosomia
    - Macroglossia
    - Omphalocele
    - Hypoglycemia

DIAGNOSTIC APPROACH TO TALL STATURE

- Screen with insulin-like growth factor 1, which will be elevated in those with GH excess (IGFBP-1 may not be elevated in acromegaly)
- Confirm diagnosis with oral glucose load (oral glucose tolerance test), which should suppress GH in normal patient
  - If GH is increased, then an MRI of brain should be obtained to evaluate hypothalamus and pituitary

Review Questions

For review questions, please go to ExpertConsult.com.

Suggested Readings

1. Chianese J. Short stature. *Pediatr Rev.* 2005;26(1):36–37.
2. Chinoy A, Murray PG. Diagnosis of growth hormone deficiency in the pediatric and transitional age. *Clinical Endocrin & Metabolism.* 2016;30(6):737–747.
3. Grimberg A, Divall SA, et al. Guidelines for Growth Hormone and Insulin Like Growth Factor-1 treatment in children and adolescents: growth hormone deficiency, idiopathic short stature, and primary IGF1 deficiency. *Hormone Research Paediatrics.* 2016;86(6):361–397.
4. Reiter EO. Growth and Growth Impairment. In: Rudolph CD, ed. *Rudolph's Pediatrics.* 22nd ed. McGraw Hill Medical; 2011:2014–2024.
5. Rosenfeld RL. Essentials of growth diagnosis. *Endocrinol Metab Clin North Am.* 1996;25:743–758.
6. Zargham S, Crotty JE. Tall stature. *Pediatr Rev.* 2014;35(12):538–539.

23 *Thyroid Disorders*

AYCA ERKIN-CAKMAK, MD, MPH

The hypothalamic-pituitary-thyroid system develops during the first trimester of gestation, and thyrotropin-releasing hormone (TRH) can be detected by 10 to 14 weeks' gestation. The thyroid gland develops from the primitive pharyngeal floor and fourth pharyngobronchial pouch at the base of the tongue, and migrates to the lower neck in front of the laryngeal cartilage. During the first couple of hours after birth, a cold-stimulated TRH/thyroid-stimulating hormone (TSH) surge causes pituitary TSH secretion leading to an abrupt and significant (up to sixfold) increase in circulating T4 and T3 levels. The serum TSH level progressively decreases to a normal level within 3 to 5 days of life, but serum free T4 may remain elevated for weeks.

Congenital Hypothyroidism

BASIC INFORMATION

- Most common endocrinologic disorder
- Incidence is 1/4000 in North America
- Leading *preventable* cause of intellectual disability

ETIOLOGY

- Iodine deficiency: most common cause of congenital hypothyroidism worldwide
- Thyroid gland dysgenesis:
  - Most common cause of congenital hypothyroidism in iodine-sufficient areas
  - Caused by abnormalities during embryologic development, sporadic versus idiopathic
  - Ectopic thyroid gland (two-thirds); aplastic or hypoplastic gland (one-third)
- Dyshormonogenesis (15%)
  - Autosomal recessive mutations in enzymes or ion transporters necessary for production of thyroid hormones
- Iatrogenic
  - Occurs with maternal treatment with radioactive iodine during pregnancy, although it is contraindicated
- Transient hypothyroidism
  - May be caused by multiple causes:
    - Maternal antibodies crossing the placenta (TSH receptor-blocking autoantibodies)
    - Maternal use of antithyroid medication (goitrogenic agents such as methimazole or propylthiouracil [PTU])
    - Relative iodine deficiency during newborn period, in areas of endemic iodine deficiency
    - Maternal consumption of excess iodine during pregnancy (such as SSKI or Lugol solution)

CLINICAL PRESENTATION

- Infants appear clinically normal at birth (in utero growth is not affected by congenital hypothyroidism)
- Initial postnatal symptoms will be nonspecific
  - Large posterior fontanelle (>1 cm in diameter)
  - Macroglossia
  - Goiter
  - Coarse cry
  - Prolonged jaundice
  - Umbilical hernia
  - Abdominal distention
  - Constipation
  - Hypotonia
  - Hypothermia
  - Lethargy
- Late findings:
  - Poor linear growth
  - Developmental delay
  - Delayed tooth development

DIAGNOSIS AND EVALUATION

- Newborn screening collected at 24 to 48 h of life screens for TSH (with or without reflex free T4)
  - Elevated TSH (TSH > 40 mIU/L) is concerning for congenital hypothyroidism
  - Normal TSH with newborn screening will not exclude central hypothyroidism
- In the event of a positive newborn screen:
  - Immediate evaluation of newborn for complete history and physical examination is needed
  - Confirmatory TSH and free T4 (with equilibrium dialysis) is necessary
    - Elevated TSH with low free T4 confirms congenital hypothyroidism
- Maternal and/or baby antibodies should be obtained with known maternal thyroid disease
- Neck ultrasonography can be used to assess presence or absence of thyroid gland, although this is technically difficult in a newborn
- Iodine (I-123) and technetium (TC99m) thyroid scans can be used to determine thyroid gland location and uptake
  - Absent radioactive isotope: thyroid aplasia, maternal thyrotropin-binding inhibitory immunoglobulin (TBI-Ig), thyrotropin beta mutations, TSH-receptor (TSHR) inactivating mutations, and iodide trapping defects
  - Increased uptake consistent with dyshormonogenesis
- X-ray of knee may be useful to assess intrauterine hypothyroidism

TREATMENT

- Levothyroxine treatment should be initiated without any delay
  - Initiation of treatment within 2 weeks of life improves long-term outcomes
  - Initial dose: 10 to 15 µg/kg/day
    - Average term infant (3–4.5 kg) will require ~50 µg levothyroxine daily
  - Goal is to maintain serum FT4 in the upper half of the normal range on therapy
    - Requires monthly monitoring of TSH and free T4 initially; may then space out frequency of checks
- May consider trial off levothyroxine after 3 to 4 years of age if euthyroid status is maintained without any dose increase during early childhood

Central Hypothyroidism

BASIC INFORMATION

- TSH deficiency caused by either congenital or acquired causes
- Congenital TSH deficiency is relatively rare
  - Prevalence of 1/20,000 to 1/30,000 newborns
  - Usually associated with other pituitary hormone deficiencies
    - Can develop because of genetic abnormalities involving the development of hypothalamus (tertiary) or pituitary gland (secondary), and presents as congenital hypothyroidism
  - Isolated TSH deficiency caused by mutational defects of the TSHR or TRH receptor gene
- Can develop as a result of cranial radiation or surgery involving the pituitary gland or hypothalamus

CLINICAL PRESENTATION

- Signs of hypothyroidism
  - Dry skin
  - Dry hair
  - Constipation
  - Cold intolerance
  - Fatigue
  - Difficulty in concentrating
  - Slowed mentation (lethargy and impaired school performance)
  - Delayed puberty
  - Menstrual irregularity
  - Growth delay
  - Bradycardia
  - Weight gain
  - Dyslipidemia
  - Delayed deep tendon reflexes
- Signs of other pituitary hormone deficiencies may be present, including hypoglycemia, polyuria, polydipsia, delayed or precocious puberty, galactorrhea, short stature, and failure to thrive

DIAGNOSIS AND EVALUATION

- Free T4 is low, and TSH is normal/low

- Newborn screening will miss the diagnosis because it will only recognize elevated TSH
- If suspicious about central hypothyroidism, screen for other pituitary deficiencies

TREATMENT

- Levothyroxine replacement therapy (would not be able to trend TSH levels; instead aim for normalization of free T4)
- Monitor thyroid function studies every 3 months for younger children; monitoring can be spaced as growth completed

Hashimoto Thyroiditis (Autoimmune Thyroiditis, Chronic Lymphocytic Thyroiditis)

BASIC INFORMATION

- Most common cause of hypothyroidism in children and adults
- Female predominance 2:1
- Increased prevalence in early to mid-puberty
- Occurs in a genetically predisposed population
  - Family history of autoimmune thyroiditis or other autoimmune diseases present
  - May be part of autoimmune polyglandular syndrome (see Chapter 27)
  - Patients with Down syndrome, Turner syndrome, and type 1 diabetes mellitus (T1DM) should be screened annually

CLINICAL PRESENTATION

- Usually insidious onset, may present only with goiter or firm thyroid gland, often described as having a "rubbery," "pebbly" consistency
  - Goiter present in 70% of children diagnosed with Hashimoto thyroiditis and is often the first manifestation of disease
  - ~80% patients are often otherwise asymptomatic at the time of diagnosis because patients may be euthyroid or have only mild hypothyroidism
- Signs of moderate or severe hypothyroidism may develop:
  - Dry skin
  - Dry hair
  - Constipation
  - Cold intolerance
  - Fatigue
  - Difficulty in concentrating
  - Slowed mentation (lethargy and impaired school performance)
  - Delayed puberty
  - Menstrual irregularity
  - Growth delay
  - Bradycardia
  - Weight gain
  - Dyslipidemia
  - Delayed deep tendon reflexes
- Few may present with thyrotoxicosis (tachycardia, nervousness, etc.)

DIAGNOSIS AND EVALUATION

- In early stages, TSH may be normal with positive antithyroid peroxidase (TPO) antibodies and goiter; later the TSH elevation becomes modest with a normal free T4
- Transient suppression of TSH along with high free T4 may be seen as stored thyroid hormone is released with inflammatory destruction of the gland
- Presence of thyroglobulin (TGL) and/or TPO antibody
  - Sensitivity of anti-TPO antibody > 90%, Anti-TGL antibody > 90%
  - Keep in mind that 10% to 15% of the general population is positive for anti-TPO antibodies
- Characterized by diffuse lymphocytic infiltration with occasional germinal centers
  - Enlarged individual thyroid cells with oxyphilic cytoplasm (the Hurthle cell or Askanazy cell)
- Ultrasound of thyroid gland is recommended for:
  - Palpable thyroid nodule
  - Asymmetric gland
  - Large goiter in which there may be a nodule that is not easy to palpate
  - US finding: enlarged thyroid gland with heterogeneous echogenicity
- I-123 scan: Decreased radioactive iodine uptake

TREATMENT

- Levothyroxine therapy should be initiated with biochemical proof of hypothyroidism
  - Treatment dose depends on age and severity of the symptoms
  - Goal is to keep TSH between 1 and 3 µU/mL
  - Levothyroxine should be taken on an empty stomach in the morning and eating should be delayed 15 to 20 minutes
  - Dairy products and vitamin supplements including calcium and iron interfere with absorption
  - Serum TSH and free T4 should be obtained 4 to 6 weeks after initiation of therapy
- Once biochemically euthyroid, monitor TSH and free T4:
  - Every 4 to 6 months in the growing child
  - Annually once final height is achieved
- Children with goiter or autoantibody positivity without biochemical hypothyroidism should be monitored every 6 months with TSH and free T4

COMPLICATIONS

- Hashitoxicosis
  - Release of stored thyroid hormone from the thyroid gland resulting in a clinical scenario that is difficult to distinguish from Graves disease
    - Unlike Graves disease, hashitoxicosis is a transient, self-limited process and evolves into permanent hypothyroidism
  - Radioactive iodine uptake would be increased
  - Lacks ophthalmologic findings of Graves disease
  - May require beta-blockers to control hyperthyroid symptoms

- Hashimoto encephalopathy (steroid-responsive encephalopathy associated with autoimmune thyroiditis [SREAT])
  - Idiopathic encephalopathy (altered mental status, clonus, seizures) in the presence of positive thyroid autoantibodies
    - Encephalopathy or severity of neurologic symptoms do *not* correlate with thyroid hormone levels or antibody titers
    - The pathogenesis and role of antithyroid antibody remains unclear
  - It is a diagnosis of exclusion
  - The estimated prevalence is 2.1 per 100,000; relatively rare in the pediatric population
  - Responds to corticosteroid therapy

Sick Euthyroid Syndrome

BASIC INFORMATION

- Acute or chronic illnesses among individuals without history of thyroid disease can result in abnormal thyroid hormone profile
- Secondary to changes in iodothyronine deiodinase activity, TSH secretion, thyroid hormone binding to plasma proteins, transport of thyroid hormone into peripheral tissues, nuclear thyroid hormone receptor activity, and TRH secretion
- Dopamine, dobutamine, high-dose steroids, and severe illnesses can result in a transient decrease in TSH secretion

DIAGNOSIS AND EVALUATION

- Low triiodothyronine (T3) levels, normal TSH levels, and increased reverse triiodothyronine (rT3) levels

TREATMENT

- Clinical significance has not been clear, with conflicting results in the literature
- Trials of treatment with T4 or T3 have not shown concrete benefit of replacement, and therefore remain controversial

Iatrogenic Hypothyroidism

BASIC INFORMATION

- Secondary to neck radiation or surgery for medical therapy-resistant Graves disease
- Secondary to medications
  - Thionamides: methimazole, carbimazole (prodrug for methimazole in Europe), and PTU to control hyperthyroidism
  - Lithium
  - Amiodarone
    - Inhibits organification in the thyroid gland
    - Decrease in the formation and release of T4 and T3 (Wolff-Chaikoff effect)
    - Decreases conversion of T4 to T3 resulting in elevated TSH

Thyroid-Binding Globulin Deficiency

BASIC INFORMATION

- X-linked condition affecting 1/4000 to 1/10,000 males
- Low levels of T4 and T3; normal TSH; clinically euthyroid
- Normal FT4 and FT3 and/or low thyroid-binding globulin (TBG) levels

Resistance to Thyroid Hormone

BASIC INFORMATION

- Prevalence is not clear; more than 1000 cases are reported in the literature
- Autosomal dominant in familial cases; 15% to 20 % of cases are sporadic
- Decreased activity of thyroid hormones on their receptors yielding:
  - Generalized resistance to thyroid hormone
  - Pituitary resistance to thyroid hormone
  - Peripheral resistance to thyroid hormone

CLINICAL PRESENTATION

- Clinical presentation depends on the location of the thyroid hormone resistance
- May vary from euthyroid to hyperthyroidism or hypothyroidism
- Deafness is observed in 20%; attention-deficit hyperactivity disorder (ADHD) reported in 50%

DIAGNOSIS AND EVALUATION

- Increased circulating levels of T4 and T3 with a normal or increased serum TSH

TREATMENT

- Important to detect infants with generalized thyroid hormone resistance as early as possible to address relative hypothyroidism and to minimize brain dysfunction, including ADHD
- Indications for treatment
  - An elevated TSH level in the absence of clinical evidence for thyrotoxicosis
  - Failure to thrive
  - Delayed developmental milestones
  - Delayed bone maturation
- Requires three to six times the usual levothyroxine replacement dose

Subclinical Hypothyroidism

BASIC INFORMATION

- TSH elevation with normal levels of circulating thyroid hormones, both T4 and T3
- Mostly asymptomatic

- Thyroid hormone levels should be monitored
- TPO antibody positivity, presence of goiter, increasing TSH levels increase the likelihood of developing hypothyroidism
- Treatment: levothyroxine replacement is not recommended if TSH < 10 *and* no goiter *and* negative antithyroid antibodies, but should be considered in the setting of signs/symptoms of hypothyroidism with increasing TSH (>10) and positive antithyroid antibodies

HYPERTHYROIDISM

Graves Disease

BASIC INFORMATION

- Most common cause of hyperthyroidism in the pediatric population
- Prevalence 1/10,000 in the United States
- Adolescent girls are more likely to be affected than boys
- IgG antibody against TSHR mimics the action of TSH

CLINICAL PRESENTATION

- Goiter
- Tachycardia, palpitations
- Increased pulse pressure
- Weight loss
- Diarrhea
- Polyuria
- Sleep disturbances
- Anxiety
- Heat intolerance
- Restlessness
- Tremor
- Headache
- Difficulty in focusing
- Growth acceleration
- Bone maturation advancement
- Proximal muscle weakness
- Ophthalmopathy: lid lag

DIAGNOSIS AND EVALUATION

- Suppressed TSH along with high free T4
- Thyroid receptor antibody positivity
  - Thyrotropin receptor binding inhibitor immunoglobulins (TRAbs)
  - Thyroid-stimulating immunoglobulin (TSI)
- Radioactive iodine uptake is increased

TREATMENT

- American Thyroid Association guidelines recommend an initial trial with antithyroid drugs and then permanent therapy via radioactive iodine ablation (RAI) or surgical thyroidectomy if remission is not achieved on medical therapy in 2 years or relapse occurs
- 40% to 60% of children and adolescents relapse with medication withdrawal
- Medical therapy

- Methimazole
  - Inhibits thyroid hormone biosynthesis by decreasing oxidation of iodide and iodination of tyrosine
  - Side effects: drug-induced rash, granulocytopenia (affects <1%, typically within the first 3 months of therapy), cholestasis
  - Surveillance: complete blood count (CBC), and liver function studies should be obtained and repeated 8 weeks after initiation of therapy or dose increase
  - Important to counsel patients to seek medical attention if they develop unexplained fever higher than 101.8°F, sore throat, mouth sores, jaundice, or arthritis
- PTU
  - Inhibitor of type 1 deiodinase (T4 to T3 conversion)
  - Potential side effect of irreversible hepatotoxicity prohibits use in children
  - Might be used short term to bridge the RAI or surgery in select cases with severe side effects on methimazole
- Beta-blockers to alleviate cardiovascular symptoms until euthyroid status achieved
- RAI with I-131
  - Beta emission induces an initial radiation thyroiditis, which results in thyroid follicular cell destruction and subsequent hypothyroidism
  - Directed at the hyperthyroid gland, not the underlying autoimmune cause
  - Extrathyroidal manifestations of disease may appear or worsen because of ongoing immunologic process
  - Contraindicated in pregnancy, and pregnancy should be avoided for 6 months following ablation
  - Need to stop antithyroid medication 3 to 5 days before treatment and start low-iodine diet to increase efficiency of the treatment
  - May take up to 2 to 6 months to achieve either a biochemically euthyroid or hypothyroid state; will require levothyroxine replacement after ablation once hypothyroidism develops
- Subtotal or total thyroidectomy
  - Indications:
    - Large thyroid glands (>80 g)
    - Patients who have failed treatment with antithyroid drugs
    - Patients who have low uptake of RAI
    - Severe eye disease
    - Patient's personal preference
  - Patient should be treated with an antithyroid drug, a beta-blocker and inorganic iodine to decrease the vascularity of the gland and control hyperthyroidism transiently
  - Most common complications are scar, transient hypoparathyroidism, and recurrent laryngeal nerve palsy
  - Levothyroxine replacement should be started immediately after surgery

Subacute Thyroiditis (de Quervain Syndrome)

BASIC INFORMATION

- Self-limited inflammation of the thyroid that usually follows an upper respiratory tract infection
- Relatively rare in the pediatric population
- Presents with fever and pain referred to the jaw; thyroid gland may be tender to palpation
  - Signs/symptoms of hyperthyroidism will be present
- Diagnosis: suppressed TSH along with high T4 and T3; decreased radioactive iodine uptake
- Treatment: a self-limited disease, thus antiinflammatory medications to control pain; patients may develop transient hypothyroidism

Neonatal Thyrotoxicosis

BASIC INFORMATION

- Results from transplacental delivery of TSI antibodies from a mother with Graves disease

CLINICAL PRESENTATION

- Symptoms may be masked because of transplacental delivery of maternal antithyroid medications
- Irritability
- Tachycardia (often with signs of cardiac failure simulating cardiomyopathy), including supraventricular tachycardia
- Polycythemia
- Craniosynostosis
- Bone age advancement
- Poor feeding
- Failure to thrive

DIAGNOSIS AND EVALAUTION

- Important to check maternal TSI levels during third trimester, ideally at the time of delivery
- Suppressed TSH along with high free T4

TREATMENT

- Self-limited disease
- Maternal antibodies will degrade over time, and may take up to 6 months
  - May need methimazole and beta-blockers to control transient hyperthyroidism and cardiovascular symptoms
  - Observation without treatment in patients who are minimally affected

THYROID-RELATED NECK MASSES

Thyroid Nodules

BASIC INFORMATION

- 2% of children develop solitary thyroid nodules
- 70% to 80% of nodules are cystic in nature and benign:
  - Follicular adenoma
  - Colloid cysts
  - Thyroglossal duct cysts
  - Chronic thyroiditis

- See Chapter 71 for more information regarding pediatric neck masses.
- Carcinoma of the thyroid is rare in children, but should be suspected in the following "classic" scenarios:
  - A history of therapeutic head or neck irradiation or radiation exposure from nuclear accidents predisposes a child to thyroid cancer
  - A "solid" nodule on ultrasound
  - A "cold" nodule on radioiodine scanning
  - There is a solitary thyroid mass with a consistency differing from that of the rest of the thyroid gland
  - Nodule with rapid growth, hoarseness (recurrent laryngeal nerve involvement)
  - Nodule with metastasis to local lymph nodes or lung
- Papillary and follicular carcinomas represent 90% of childhood thyroid cancers
- Diagnostic workup
  - Thyroid function tests
  - Neck ultrasound
  - In some patients with low TSH, may consider thyroid scan to consider diagnosis of benign hyperfunctioning nodule
  - Fine-needle aspiration (FNA) is most common diagnostic step; however, excisional biopsy may also be necessary

Medullary Thyroid Cancer

BASIC INFORMATION

- Seen with multiple endocrine neoplasia (MEN) 2a or 2b, possibly in a familial pattern (See Chapter 27 for details)
- Arises from parafollicular C cells
- The presence of mutations of the RET protooncogene is predictive of the development of medullary carcinoma of the thyroid
- Genetic screening of other members of the family is indicated after a proband is recognized
- Prophylactic thyroidectomy is indicated for the family members with the same allele

DIAGNOSIS:

- Elevated calcitonin levels, basal or stimulated (pentagastrin stimulation)
  - Histologic

TREATMENT

- Resection of nodule versus subtotal or total thyroidectomy with/without lymph node dissection
  - RAI
  - TGL level could be used for surveillance following total thyroidectomy

Review Questions

For review questions, please go to ExpertConsult.com.

Suggested Readings

1. Brent GA, Weetman AP. Hypothyroidism and thyroiditis. In: Kronenberg H, Larsen PR, Melmed S, Polonsky KS, eds. *Williams Textbook of Endocrinology*. 13th ed. Philadelphia: Elsevier; 2016:416–448.
2. Davies TF, Laurberg P, Bahn RS. Hyperthyroid disorders. In: Kronenberg H, Larsen PR, Melmed S, Polonsky KS, eds. *Williams Textbook of Endocrinology*. 13th ed. Philadelphia: Elsevier; 2016:369–415.
3. Fisher DA, Grueters A. Disorders of the thyroid in the newborn and infant. In: Sperling M, ed. *Pediatric Endocrinology*. 3rd ed. Philadelphia: Saunders Elsevier; 2008:198–226.
4. Fisher DA, Grueters A. Thyroid disorders in childhood and adolescence. In: Sperling M, ed. *Pediatric Endocrinology*. 3rd ed. Philadelphia: Saunders Elsevier; 2008:227–253.
5. Francis GL, et al. Management guidelines for children with thyroid nodules and differentiated thyroid cancer. The American Thyroid Association Guidelines Taskforce on pediatric thyroid cancer. *Thyroid*. 2015;25(7):716–759.
6. Jonklaas B, et al. Guidelines for the treatment of hypothyroidism: prepared by the American Thyroid Association Taskforce on thyroid hormone replacement. *Thyroid*. 2014;24(12):1670–1751.
7. Okawa, et al. Pediatric Graves' disease: decisions regarding therapy. *Curr Opin Pediatr*. 2015;27:442–447.
8. Ross B, et al. 2016 American Thyroid Association guidelines for diagnosis and management of hyperthyroidism and other causes of thyrotoxicosis. *Thyroid*. 2016;26(10):1343–1421.
9. Salvatore D, Davies TF, Schlumberg MJ, Hay ID, Larsen PR. Thyroid physiology and diagnostic evaluation of patients with thyroid disorders. In: Kronenberg H, Larsen PR, Melmed S, Polonsky KS, eds. *Williams Textbook of Endocrinology*. 13th ed. Philadelphia: Elsevier; 2016:334–368.
10. Schlumberg MJ, Sebastiano F, Alexander EK, Hay ID. Nontoxic diffuse goiter, nodular thyroid disorders, and thyroid malignancies In: Kronenberg H, Larsen PR, Melmed S, Polonsky KS, eds. *Williams Textbook of Endocrinology*. 13th ed. Philadelphia: Elsevier; 2016:449–489.

24 Disorders of Calcium Homeostasis

JANET Y. LEE, MD, MPH

Disorders of calcium homeostasis involve the complex interplay among the parathyroid hormone (PTH), calcium, fibroblast growth factor 23 (FGF23), phosphate, $1,25(OH)_2$ vitamin D (calcitriol), and their respective receptors. Understanding the various feedback loops will facilitate interpretation of the laboratory studies because the clinical presentations of hypercalcemia, hypocalcemia, and rickets of all etiologies often overlap. Fig. 24.1 illustrates the key relationships essential in the regulation of calcium, phosphate, and vitamin D.

Hypocalcemia

BASIC INFORMATION

- Hypocalcemia may result from a number of disorders, which may present at various ages depending on the cause of the calcium deficiency (Table 24.1)
  - It is a common occurrence in neonates in the first 3 days of life because of a multitude of factors
- We will provide an overview of the effects and workup for hypocalcemia, as well as a survey of the most commonly encountered disorders

CLINICAL PRESENTATION

- Symptoms may range in severity depending on the cause and severity of hypocalcemia
- Increased neuromuscular excitability
  - Patients may experience significant muscle contractions (tetany) as well as jitteriness, tremulousness, and facial spasms
  - Sustained contractions in the hands and feet, may progress to numbness, stiffness, and tingling; rarely, laryngospasm can lead to apnea, stridor, or cyanosis
  - Chvostek's sign is a muscle twitch at the ipsilateral corner of mouth in response to a light tap over the facial nerve below the maxilla
  - Trousseau's sign is a carpal spasm in the hand caused by inflation of the blood pressure cuff around the ipsilateral arm approximately 15 mm Hg above systolic blood pressure
- Additional neurologic signs/symptoms:
  - Perioral numbness and tingling
  - Irritability and feeding problems
  - Hyperacusis
  - Seizures resistant to anticonvulsants (e.g., hypocalcemic convulsions in hypoparathyroidism can be mistaken for epilepsy)

- Cardiac toxicity:
  - Severe hypocalcemia may lead to hypotension and cardiac failure
  - Electrocardiogram (ECG) may show reduced PR interval, narrowing of the QRS complex, prolonged ST and ST depression, T-wave flattening and inversion, prolonged QTc interval, and prominent U-wave
- Long-term effects:
  - Delayed tooth eruption and soft, irregular enamel formation
  - Cataracts, and other ocular manifestations
  - Dry scaly skin, angular cheilitis, and horizontal lines on the nails may also develop
  - Failure to treat could result in permanent physical and neurocognitive damage

DIAGNOSIS AND EVALUATION

- Interpretation of the serum calcium level should be adjusted for albumin levels because the total serum calcium level declines by 0.8 mg/dL for every 1 g/dL decline in the serum concentration of albumin below 4 g/dL
  - In addition to albumin, blood pH also inversely affects the fraction of ionized calcium (i.e., alkalosis precipitates hypocalcemia)
  - Measurement of ionized calcium may provide a more accurate assessment of hypocalcemia
  - Normal range of calcium varies somewhat by age; look at age-specific reference ranges when available
    - Hypocalcemia is defined as serum calcium <7.5 to 8 mg/dL in newborns with birth weights >1500 g or <7.0 mg/dL in those with birth weights <1500 g
- Additional studies:
  - Serum electrolytes, magnesium, and phosphate
  - Liver function tests (including alkaline phosphatase and albumin)
  - PTH:
    - If not elevated in the setting of hypocalcemia and adequate magnesium levels, then hypoparathyroidism (see the following section) is present
  - 25-OH vitamin D level and $1,25(OH)_2$ vitamin D level
- 24-hour urine calcium/creatinine; if not possible, urine calcium/creatinine ratio may be helpful; normal ranges are age dependent

GENERAL TREATMENT APPROACH

- Acute severe cases require monitoring in an intensive care setting with telemetry

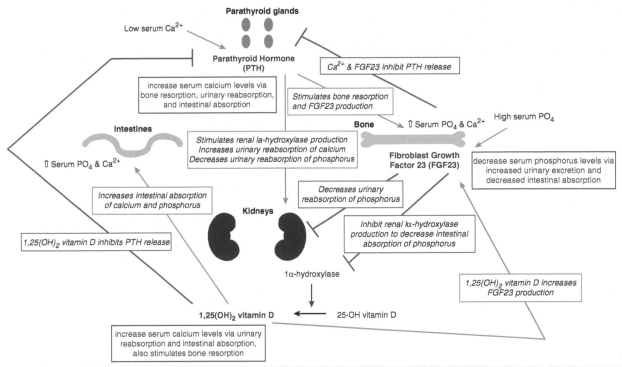

Fig. 24.1. Calcium, phosphate, and vitamin D homeostasis.

Table 24.1. Causes of Hypocalcemia

Neonatal Disorders	Maternal Disorders	Hypoparathyroidism	Other Disorders of Calcium Metabolism	Organ Dysfunction	Medications
Sepsis or perinatal stress/asphyxia	Gestational diabetes	Congenital hypoparathyroidism	Inadequate Ca intake	Renal failure	Furosemide
Low birthweight, prematurity, IUGR	Maternal vitamin D deficiency	DiGeorge syndrome	Vitamin D deficiency	Liver disease	Bisphosphonates
Hyperbilirubinemia	Maternal use of anticonvulsants	Acquired hypoparathyroidism	Hypomagnesemia	Pancreatitis	Calcitonin
Transient neonatal hypocalcemia	Maternal use of magnesium sulfate or alkali		Hyperphosphatemia		Chemotherapies
Late neonatal hypocalcemia			Hypoalbuminemia or hypoproteinemia		Ketoconazole
IDM					Antiepileptic drugs
					Packed red blood cells (i.e., citrate)

IDM, Infant of diabetic mother; *IUGR,* intrauterine growth restriction

- Replete hypomagnesemia if present
- Intravenous (IV) calcium (e.g., calcium gluconate) should be provided if severe hypocalcemia or symptomatic
- Enteral calcium is the most durable method of repletion
- Low phosphorus formula to achieve 4:1 Ca:Phos ratio of supplementation
- Depending on the underlying mechanism of calcium deficiency, forms of vitamin D (cholecalciferol, ergocalciferol, or calcitriol) and/or recombinant human PTH (for hypoparathyroidism, see later section) may be needed
- Long-term monitoring is needed to avoid hypercalcemia, which may have negative consequences (e.g., nephrocalcinosis, pancreatitis)

Selected Causes of Hypocalcemia

Transient (Early-Onset) Neonatal Hypocalcemia

- Occurs within the first 12 to 72 hours of life
- Exaggeration of normal decline in serum calcium levels in the first 1 to 2 days of life
- Maternal hyperparathyroidism, hypercalcemia, or blood transfusion with citrated blood can suppress infant PTH secretion

Late Neonatal Hypocalcemia

- Occurs 5 to 10 days after birth
- Transient hypoparathyroidism caused by immature parathyroid glands

Hyperphosphatemia

- Elevated phosphate levels may reduce serum ionized calcium by a number of mechanisms (precipitating calcium, suppressing vitamin D production, disrupting PTH-mediated bone resorption)
- May be caused by renal failure, excess intake (e.g., laxatives, sodium phosphate enemas, dietary intake), and/or excess cellular release (e.g., tumor lysis syndrome, rhabdomyolysis)

Hypomagnesemia (or Less Commonly, Hypermagnesemia)

- Interferes with PTH release and responsiveness
- Most often caused by malabsorption, aminoglycosides (increase urinary loss of magnesium)

Renal Failure

- Leads to decreased 1-alpha-hydroxylase, essential for conversion of 25-OH vitamin D to $1,25(OH)_2$ vitamin D, which assists with intestinal calcium absorption
- Can ultimately result in secondary and tertiary hyperparathyroidism

Liver Disease

- Leads to impaired 25-hydroxylation of vitamin D

Hypoparathyroidism

BASIC INFORMATION

- A deficiency in PTH can lead to hypocalcemia
- Causes can be divided into the following categories:
  - Congenital hypoparathyroidism
    - Several familial forms exist with autosomal recessive, autosomal dominant, or X-linked recessive inheritances
    - Hypercalciuric hypocalcemia is an autosomal dominant gain-of-function mutation in the calcium-sensing receptor (CASR) that results in depression of PTH secretion despite hypocalcemia, leading to calciuria
    - Other inherited syndromes: Barakat syndrome (hypoparathyroidism-deafness-renal dysplasia [HDR]), Sanjad-Sakati syndrome (hypoparathyroidism-mental retardation-dysmorphism [HRD]), Kenny-Caffey syndrome type 1 (KCS1)
    - Certain mitochondrial disorders (e.g., Kearns-Sayre syndrome, mitochondrial encephalopathy, lactic acidosis, and strokelike episodes [MELAS]) are associated with hypoparathyroidism
  - Iatrogenic
    - Usually secondary to anterior neck surgery such as thyroidectomy (look for neck scar)
  - Acquired
    - Autoimmune forms often exist as part of autoimmune polyendocrinopathy syndrome type 1 (Chapter 27)
    - Infiltrative conditions such as hemochromatosis, iron overload, Wilson disease
  - Idiopathic hypoparathyroidism: diagnosis of exclusion

Table 24.2. Important Physiologic Changes in Bone and Mineral Diseases

Condition	Calcium	Phosphate	Parathyroid Hormone	25(OH)D
Primary hypoparathyroidism	↓	↑	↓	NI
Pseudo hypoparathyroidism	↓	↑	↑	NI
Vitamin D deficiency	NI(↓)	↓	↑	↓
Familial hypophosphatemic rickets	NI	↓	NI (sl↑)	NI
Hyperparathyroidism	↑	↓	↑	NI
Immobilization	↑	↑	↓	NI

25(OH)D, 25-Hydroxyvitamin D; *NI*, normal; *sl*, slight; *↑*, high; *↓*, low.

DIAGNOSIS

- Laboratory evaluation reveals hypocalcemia and elevated phosphorus and a low PTH level (Table 24.2)
  - If hypocalcemia occurs in the setting of adrenal insufficiency, then the hypocalcemia may only be recognized after treatment of the adrenal insufficiency
- Alkaline phosphatase may be normal or low, and $1,25\text{-}(OH)_2D_3$ is usually low
- Hypoparathyroidism should not cause rickets (see the following section)

TREATMENT

- If severely hypocalcemic or symptomatic, provide with IV calcium gluconate and calcitriol
- Patients typically require long-term enteral calcium supplementation dosed multiple times per day, restriction of dietary phosphorus, and vitamin D supplementation (both cholecalciferol/ergocalciferol and calcitriol)
  - Patients with hypercalciuric hypocalcemia should not be provided with vitamin D supplementation because this leads to nephrocalcinosis
- Long-term treatment options include recombinant human PTH analogs

Pseudohypoparathyroidism

BASIC INFORMATION

- Most commonly caused by an autosomal dominant loss-of-function mutation of the stimulatory alpha subunit in G-protein signaling, leading to PTH resistance
  - Patients demonstrate laboratory findings consistent with hypoparathyroidism (i.e., hypocalcemia, hyperphosphatemia) but with an elevated PTH
- Although may present in isolation, there are multiple types of pseudohypoparathyroidism with distinct constellations of findings in addition to endocrinologic abnormalities, of which type 1a is the most common:

- Type 1a causes *Albright's hereditary osteodystrophy*, which includes resistance to thyroid-stimulating hormone, gonadotropins, and growth hormone-releasing hormone and is associated with short stature, cognitive impairment, skeletal abnormalities, and dysmorphia
  - Other type 1a dysmorphic features include:
    - Brachydactyly of the third, fourth, and fifth metacarpals
    - Round face with low nasal bridge
    - Heterotopic intramembranous subcutaneous calcifications
- An entity known as *"pseudopseudohypoparathyroidism"* also exists:
  - May have usual phenotype but with normal serum calcium and phosphate with slightly elevated PTH levels, which eventually can progress to hypocalcemia with age

Rickets and Osteomalacia

BASIC INFORMATION

- A constellation of findings that can be associated with hypocalcemia and/or hypophosphatemia
- If a similar syndrome evolves in a patient with closed growth plates, the result is osteomalacia, demineralized "soft" bone, rather than rickets (i.e., diagnosis of rickets requires open growth plates)
- Rickets and osteomalacia can both be present in children with open growth plates
- The causes of rickets can be broadly grouped into three categories (Table 24.3)

CLINICAL PRESENTATION

- Classically presents with short stature, poor growth, deformities, bone pain, pseudofractures, and fractures
- Bone-related abnormalities:
  - Delayed fontanelle closure, parietal and frontal bossing, craniotabes
  - "Rachitic rosary" is the enlargement of the costochondral junction, which appears as beading along the anterolateral chest
  - Leg bowing with varus or valgus deformities with weight bearing (especially with hypophosphatemic rickets)
  - Dental abscesses or delayed tooth rupture (especially with hypophosphatemic rickets)
  - Widening of joints such as wrists and ankles
- Enthesopathy (disorders of muscle or ligament attachment) caused by calcification of tendons or ligaments
- Harrison's grooves at the lower margin of the thorax as muscle pull diaphragmatic attachments to lower ribs
- Infantile seizures (in hypophosphatasia, these are pyridoxine responsive)

DIAGNOSIS AND EVALUATION

- Laboratory studies:
  - Electrolytes, calcium, phosphate, magnesium, alkaline phosphatase, and albumin
  - Serum PTH
  - 25-OH vitamin D level, 1,25-$(OH)_2$ vitamin D level, C-terminal FGF23
  - Urine evaluation of calcium, phosphate, and creatinine
- Radiographic studies: plain film radiographs particularly of wrists, ankles, and standing films of the legs; show generalized demineralization, bowing deformities, widening of the physes with metaphyseal fraying, cupping, and irregularity
- Genetic studies, if indicated

Vitamin D Deficiency Rickets

BASIC INFORMATION

- A decrease in vitamin D bioavailability yields a decrease in calcium and phosphorus; as a compensatory mechanism, PTH is increased, which incompletely compensates for hypocalcemia (so may be normocalcemic or hypocalcemic) and exacerbates hypophosphatemia
- In addition to the causes listed in Table 24.3, vitamin D deficiency is also associated with obesity and respiratory infections

Table 24.3. Causes of Rickets and Hypophosphatasia

Vitamin D Deficiency Rickets	Vitamin D-Dependent Rickets	Hypophosphatemic Rickets	Hypophosphatasia
Inadequate vitamin D intake (e.g., breastfeeding without supplementation)	Mutations affecting 25-hydroxylase, 1-alpha-hydroxylase, vitamin D receptor	Inadequate intake	*ALPL* gene mutation
Inadequate UV exposure (e.g., dark skin pigmentation, avoidance of sunlight)		Malabsorption, or ingestion of phosphate binders (e.g., aluminum-containing, calcium-containing, or magnesium-containing antacids)	
Malabsorption (e.g., pancreatic dysfunction)		Mutations affecting FGF23 signaling	
Nephrotic syndrome		Fanconi syndrome	
Renal or liver dysfunction			
Phenytoin/phenobarbital use			

UV, Ultraviolet.

- Diagnosis:
  - Low 25-OH vitamin D (but 1,25-[OH]$_2$ vitamin D may still be normal)
  - PTH will be elevated;
  - alkaline phosphatase will be elevated because of increased bone turnover
- Treatment:
  - Calcium supplementation and high doses of vitamin D3 (cholecalciferol) or vitamin D2 (ergocalciferol) are the most common treatment

Vitamin D-"Dependent" Rickets

BASIC INFORMATION

- Unlike in vitamin D deficiency rickets, these disorders are caused by inherited defects in vitamin D processing or downstream signaling
  - The clinical presentation resembles vitamin D deficiency rickets, with timing in the neonatal/infantile period
- Types:
  - 1-alpha-hydroxylase deficiency
    - Formerly known as "pseudovitamin D deficiency rickets" or vitamin D-dependent rickets type 1:
    - Inherited autosomal recessive disorder of 1-alpha-hydroxylase deficiency, yielding impaired conversion of 25-OH vitamin D into 1,25-(OH)$_2$ vitamin D
    - Presents in the first year of life with skeletal disease and severe hypocalcemia and secondary hyperparathyroidism with moderate hypophosphatemia
    - Diagnosis: elevated 25-OH vitamin D and low 1,25-(OH)$_2$ vitamin D levels
    - Treatment: daily administration of high-dose 1,25-(OH)$_2$ vitamin D (calcitriol) and calcium supplementation; may require IV administration depending on severity of disease
  - 25-hydroxylase deficiency
    - Caused by mutations in the gene encoding the enzyme responsible for 25-hydroxylation of vitamin D
    - Treatment: in heterozygotes, calcium supplementation is more effective than vitamin D supplementation; homozygotes respond to high-dose vitamin D supplementation or calcium
  - Hereditary resistance to vitamin D
    - Formerly known as vitamin D-dependent rickets type II
    - Very rare inherited autosomal recessive disorder, usually caused by mutations in the gene encoding the vitamin D receptor, leading to end-organ resistance to vitamin D
    - Normal at birth, develops rickets within first 2 years of life
    - Associated with alopecia in two-thirds of cases, which is caused by lack of vitamin D receptor activity within keratinocytes; this is a marker of disease severity
    - Diagnosis: elevated 25-OH vitamin D and 1,25-(OH)$_2$ vitamin D levels

- Treatment: high-dose calcitriol and calcium supplementation; depending on severity, may not respond to oral treatment and could require IV calcium infusions

Hypophosphatemic Rickets

BASIC INFORMATION

- Vitamin D-resistant rickets was originally used to describe hypophosphatemic rickets that did not respond to vitamin D treatment
- Although acquired phosphate deficiency (e.g., inadequate intake, malabsorption) may cause rickets, there are also inherited forms of hypophosphatemic rickets
- FGF23 is the major phosphate regulator that stimulates phosphaturia (renal phosphate wasting), therefore these can be classified as FGF23 dependent (i.e., high or inappropriately normal FGF23 levels) or FGF23 independent (Table 24.4)
- X-linked hypophosphatemic rickets (XLH)
  - The most common cause of inherited rickets, XLH is caused by mutations in the phosphate regulating endopeptidase on the X chromosome (PHEX) gene, which leads to elevated levels of FGF23 and hypophosphatemia Fig. 24.1
    - FGF23 inhibits 1-alpha-hydroxylase, which decreases conversion of 25-OH vitamin D to 1,25(OH)$_2$ vitamin D which leads to a net decrease in intestinal phosphate absorption
    - FGF23 decreases renal phosphate absorption, leading to renal phosphate wasting
    - The key biochemical finding is low phosphate level and evidence of renal phosphate wasting; serum calcium levels are usually normal
    - PTH levels are usually normal or only slightly elevated
  - Clinical presentation is similar to vitamin D deficiency rickets, with a propensity toward dental abscesses, craniosynostosis, and enthesopathy
    - Bone pain is also characteristic
    - Family history or rickets is typical, although some cases are caused by sporadic PHEX mutations
  - Treatment typically involves phosphate and 1,25-(OH)$_2$ vitamin D (calcitriol) supplementation, which heal rickets and may be able to restore linear growth; after growth plates are fused, some patients no longer require treatment unless bone pain persists

Table 24.4. Causes of Hypophosphatemic Rickets

FGF23-Dependent Hypophosphatemic Rickets	FGF23-Independent Hypophosphatemic Rickets
X-linked hypophosphatemic rickets (*PHEX* mutation)	Fanconi syndrome/rental tubular acidosis
Autosomal dominant hypophosphatemic rickets (*FGF23* mutation)	Hereditary hypophosphatemic rickets with hypercalciuria
Autosomal recessive hypophosphatemic rickets (*DMP1* and *ENPP1* mutations)	—
Ectopic FGF23 production (e.g., McCune-Albright syndrome, tumor-induced osteomalacia)	—

- Traditional treatment modalities are imperfect and place patients at risk of nephrolithiasis, hypercalcemia, and secondary hyperparathyroidism; chronic pain may persist despite treatment
- Burosumab, human monoclonal antibody against FGF23, has been approved for treatment of XLH for individuals 1 year of age or older and have been shown in children to result in improved outcomes in terms of phosphorus levels, pain, rickets healing, and stature with similar or better side effect profile to phosphate and calcitriol

Hypophosphatasia

BASIC INFORMATION

- *ALPL* gene mutations result in decreased alkaline phosphatase activity with varying severity
- Six clinical phenotypes ranging from severe to mild, with pyridoxine (vitamin B_6)-responsive seizures in the severely affected infants
- Treatment is available with asfotase alfa, bone-targeted infusion of alkaline phosphatase replacement therapy

Hypercalcemia

BASIC INFORMATION

- As with hypocalcemia, there are multiple potential causes of hypercalcemia (Table 24.5); total calcium measurements should be adjusted for albumin levels if ionized calcium levels are unavailable

CLINICAL PRESENTATION

- Neonatal period: irritability, anorexia/failure to thrive, lethargy, constipation, fractures caused by osteoporosis
- Short-term additional symptoms:
  - Muscle weakness, fatigue, and headache
  - Abdominal pain, nausea, vomiting, and weight loss
  - Polydipsia/polyuria (nephrogenic diabetes insipidus)

- Fever
- Acute pancreatitis
- Coma or stupor
- Long-term sequelae:
  - Renal failure, nephrolithiasis, or nephrocalcinosis
  - Soft tissue calcifications, brain microcalcifications, skeletal abnormalities, and fractures
  - Emotional lability, depression, or psychosis
  - Eventual cognitive impairment, convulsions, and blindness can develop if untreated
- Hypercalcemic crises (with oliguria, azotemia, and coma) can also occur in severe cases

DIAGNOSIS AND EVALUATION

- Laboratory evaluation:
  - Serum total calcium measurements should be adjusted for albumin levels if ionized calcium levels are unavailable
  - Additional laboratory tests:
    - Serum electrolytes, liver function tests, alkaline phosphatase, magnesium, phosphate, PTH, 25-OH vitamin D level, and 1,25-$(OH)_2$ vitamin D level
  - 24-hour urine calcium/creatinine is preferred; if not possible, urine calcium/creatinine ratio may be helpful
- Renal ultrasound for potential nephrolithiasis
- X-ray: resorption of subperiosteal bone, best seen in phalanges of hands
- ECG: if severe, can show disappearance of P-waves and tall peaking T-waves
- Additional workup is dictated by clinical suspicion for etiology (e.g., evaluation of parathyroid glands in primary hyperparathyroidism)

TREATMENT

- Telemetry monitoring
- Low-calcium formula
- Fluid administration: this is the mainstay of treatment because hypercalcemic individuals are volume depleted because of polyuria
- Furosemide as needed to continue fluid administration

Table 24.5. Causes of Hypercalcemia

Neonate/Infant	Hyperparathyroidism	Excessive Calcium or Vitamin D	Other Causes
Excessive vitamin D ingestion (maternal, neonatal)	Parathyroid hyperplasia, adenoma, carcinoma	Milk-alkali syndrome	Immobilization
Maternal hypoparathyroidism or pseudohypoparathyroidism	MEN 1 and 2a	Exogenous administration of calcium or vitamin D	Drugs (vitamin A, thiazides, lithium)
Subcutaneous fat necrosis of the newborn	McCune-Albright	Granulomatous diseases (e.g., sarcoidosis, TB, cat-scratch fever)	TPN
Williams-Beuren syndrome	Postrenal transplantation		Hypophosphatemia
Various congenital disorders (e.g., *CASR* mutation, hyperthyroidism-jaw tumor syndrome, Jansen-type metaphyseal chondrodysplasia)	Malignancy (i.e., ectopic PTHrP or bone destruction)		Other endocrinologic disorders (hyperthyroidism/thyrotoxicosis, primary adrenal insufficiency, severe congenital hypothyroidism)
	Acute kidney injury and chronic kidney disease caused by secondary and tertiary hyperparathyroidism		

CASR, Calcium-sensing receptor; *MEN*, multiple endocrine neoplasia; *PTHrP*, parathyroid hormone-related protein; *TB*, tuberculosis; *TPN*, total parental nutrition.

- Calcitonin
  - Increases renal clearance of both calcium and phosphate
  - Reduces calcium release from bone by suppressing osteoclasts
  - Tachyphylaxis prevents its use as a long-term solution, so is mainly used for temporizing measures
- Bisphosphonates
  - Acts at the level of osteoclasts as potent inhibitors of bone resorption
  - Reserved for management of chronic hypercalcemia (can cause hypocalcemia if used to treat acute, readily reversible causes of hypercalcemia), typically for malignancy-related hypercalcemia

Selected Causes of Hypercalcemia

PRIMARY HYPERPARATHYROIDISM

- Uncommon in childhood, typically caused by single benign parathyroid adenomas usually apparent after 10 years of age
- Autosomal dominant inheritance patterns have been described in primary hyperparathyroidism
- Also a feature in multiple endocrine neoplasia (MEN) syndromes types 1 and 2a (see Chapter 27)

DIAGNOSIS

- Hypercalcemia in the presence of elevated or inappropriately normal range PTH;
- Rule out familial hypocalciuric hypercalcemia (FHH, below) and consider genetic testing;
- If adenoma is suspected, then imaging to determine location of the adenoma (ultrasound and Tc-99m sestamibi scintigraphy with or without single-photon emission computed tomography [SPECT] are favored over computed tomography [CT] or magnetic resonance imaging [MRI]) or in rare cases, parathyroid venous sampling by interventional radiology if unable to locate with imaging

TREATMENT

- Surgical removal of adenoma(s) if present; recalcitrant or recurrent cases such as parathyroid hyperplasia may require near total or total parathyroidectomy (beware of inappropriate surgery in FHH);
- Some cases may be treated with bisphosphonates and calcimimetics such as cinacalcet if surgery is contraindicated

SUBCUTANEOUS FAT NECROSIS (SCFN) OF THE NEWBORN

- Uncommon, transient benign panniculitis that occurs in first few weeks of life
- Usually full-term infants who have experienced perinatal distress
- Firm subcutaneous nodules on cheeks, buttocks, back, arms, and thighs; histology with fat necrosis, abundant histiocytes, and multinucleated giant cells with granuloma formation

- Thought to be mediated by granulomatous production of 1,25 (OH)2 vitamin D
- Typically resolves over a period of weeks to months but may require treatment

WILLIAMS-BEUREN/WILLIAMS SYNDROME

- Autosomal dominant disorder, deletion in 7q11.23
- Infantile hypercalcemia occurs in approximately 15% of cases, usually in the first years of life with resolution by 4 years of age and possible recurrence in puberty
- Cause of hypercalcemia is unknown, and course is typically mild and transient, but some cases can be severe and life-threatening

HYPERPARATHYROIDISM-JAW TUMOR SYNDROME

- Autosomal dominant disorder characterized by parathyroid adenomas and jaw tumors; other manifestations include polycystic kidneys, renal hamartomas, and Wilms tumor

TRANSIENT NEONATAL HYPERPARATHYROIDISM

- Associated with inadequately treated or untreated maternal hypoparathyroidism or pseudohypoparathyroidism, which leads to hyperplasia of fetal parathyroid glands

NEONATAL SEVERE HYPERPARATHYROIDISM

- Rare disorder with symptoms manifesting shortly after birth
- Caused by CASR inactivating mutation and is biallelic

FHH

- Caused by loss-of-function mutations in CASR; monoallelic mutation results in this familial benign hypercalcemia phenotype
- Often mistaken for primary hyperparathyroidism, which leads to unnecessary multiple parathyroidectomy surgeries

Review Questions

For review questions, please go to ExpertConsult.com.

Suggested Readings

1. Greer FR. Calcium and phosphorus and the preterm infant. *NeoReviews.* 2016;17(4):e195–202.
2. Markowitz M, Underland L, Gensure R. Parathyroid disorders. *Pediatr Rev.* 2016;37(12):524–535.
3. Munns CF, et al. Global consensus recommendations on prevention and management of nutritional rickets. *JCEM.* 2016;101(2):394–415.
4. Razali NN, Hwu TT, Thilakavathy K. Phosphate homeostasis and genetic mutations of familial hypophosphatemic rickets. *J Pediatr Endocrinol Metab.* 2015;28(9-10):1009–1017.

25 *Adrenal Disorders*

TERRY DEAN JR, MD, PhD and LIAT PERL, MD

Adrenal Physiology

BASIC INFORMATION

- Anatomy of adrenal hormone biosynthesis
  - Zona glomerulosa: area of cortex responsible for mineralocorticoid production (e.g., aldosterone)
  - Zona fasciculata: area of cortex responsible for cortisol production
  - Zona reticularis: area of cortex responsible for sex steroid production
  - Adrenal medulla: synthesizes catecholamines
  - Cholesterol from circulating plasma lipoproteins provides the majority of substrate required for steroid biosynthesis
- Hypothalamic-pituitary-adrenal (HPA) axis:
  - Hypothalamus secretes corticotropin-releasing hormone (CRH), which stimulates pituitary release of adrenocorticotropic hormone (ACTH; i.e., corticotropin)
  - ACTH induces the release of cortisol and adrenal androgens. Glucocorticoids feed back to inhibit ACTH and CRH secretion
  - ACTH has little effect on aldosterone production except in excess; otherwise aldosterone is regulated by the renin-angiotensin system and potassium concentration
  - The diurnal rhythm of ACTH and cortisol yields higher levels of both early in the morning and nadirs at night (may take months to years to develop regular rhythmicity)
  - See also Nelson Textbook of Pediatrics, Chapter 574, "Physiology of the Adrenal Gland."

Primary Adrenal Insufficiency

BASIC INFORMATION

- Disorders characterized by insufficient production of cortisol and often aldosterone
- Includes acquired causes (Addison disease) and inherited causes
- In pediatrics, the most common cause is congenital adrenal hyperplasia (CAH) (in ~60%, see below)
- Other causes include autoimmune disease, APECED (autoimmune polyendocrinopathy-candidiasis-ectodermal dystrophy), adrenoleukodystrophy, and isolated glucocorticoid deficiency

CLINICAL PRESENTATION

- Clinical manifestations are a consequence of the underlying hormone deficiencies or excesses

- Glucocorticoid deficiency
  - General constitutional symptoms
    - Anorexia, nausea, vomiting, weight loss
    - Lethargy
    - Weakness, myalgia
  - Hypoglycemia (classically with ketosis)
  - Decreased cardiac output and vascular tone, resulting in hypotension (ranging from orthostasis to shock)
- Aldosterone deficiency
  - May result in salt-wasting and electrolyte abnormalities:
    - Hypovolemia (exacerbates glucocorticoid deficiency effects on the cardiovascular system)
    - Hyponatremia (due to aldosterone deficiency and attempt at blood pressure compensation with arginine vasopressin)
    - Hyperkalemia
    - May also cause hyperchloremic metabolic acidosis
- Age dependence of presentation:
  - It is more usual for infants to present after only a few days of constitutional symptoms with severe illness (e.g., shock), whereas adolescents are more likely to develop subacute/chronic symptoms over days to weeks
- Additional symptoms:
  - Primary adrenal insufficiency is usually accompanied by oversecretion of ACTH, which is associated with hyperpigmentation:
    - Fair-skinned individuals may demonstrate "bronzing"; gingival and buccal mucosa hyperpigmentation may be more sensitive signs on physical examination
  - Overproduction or underproduction of androgens may also occur in some enzyme deficiencies, leading to primary adrenal insufficiency (see Congenital Adrenal Hyperplasia, below)

APPROACH TO ACUTE ADRENAL INSUFFICIENCY

- Rapid recognition and treatment of adrenal insufficiency require vigilance because symptoms may be nonspecific, and there is risk of circulatory collapse
- If there is concern in the acute setting, screening laboratories for electrolytes, glucose, and acid-base status will guide resuscitation
  - ACTH, cortisol, aldosterone, and plasma renin activity at the time of presentation will provide baseline values
  - Clinical presentation may direct additional workup for underlying causes of adrenal insufficiency (see entries later)

Table 25.1. Equipotence Among Steroids Relative to Hydrocortisone

Hydrocortisone	1	1
Prednisolone	4	0.8
Prednisone	5	0.8
Methylprednisolone	7.5	0.5
Fludrocortisone	15	200
Dexamethasone	40	0

- Laboratory tests should not delay administration of stress-dose steroids if clinically indicated
- Administration of stress-dose water-soluble hydrocortisone (e.g., IV hydrocortisone sodium succinate 50–100 mg/m²) should be provided as quickly as possible
  - If height cannot be acquired, one may provide 10 mg for infants, 25 mg for toddlers, 50 mg for children, and 100 mg for adolescents
  - Initial stress dose is followed by an equivalent daily dose divided into 4- to 6-hour dosing
  - Clinical course and consultation with a pediatric endocrinologist will help determine steroid taper and testing for adrenal sufficiency

CHRONIC SUPPLEMENTATION FOR ADRENAL INSUFFICIENCY

- Most causes of primary adrenal insufficiency require chronic steroid replacement therapy for cortisol and aldosterone
  - Patients typically require 10 to 15 mg/m²/day of oral hydrocortisone (or equivalent; see Table 25.1)
  - Patients with aldosterone deficiency generally require fludrocortisone, usually at 0.05 to 0.2 mg daily
  - Replacement of dehydroepiandrosterone (DHEA) may be considered for certain patients.

Addison Disease

BASIC INFORMATION

- Most commonly caused by autoimmune destruction of the adrenals
- May also occur as part of autoimmune polyendocrinopathy syndromes (see Chapter 27)

DIAGNOSIS

- Morning cortisol (best screening test)
- High-dose corticotropin (ACTH) stimulation test to identify adrenal steroidogenic defects
- Low-dose ACTH stimulation test may provide assessment of pituitary-adrenal reserve
- Consider imaging to quantify adrenal gland size (e.g., ultrasound [US], computed tomography [CT], magnetic resonance imaging [MRI])
- Screen for associated autoimmune disorders:
  - Hypoparathyroidism
  - Diabetes
  - Hypothyroidism
  - Premature ovarian failure

Adrenoleukodystrophy

BASIC INFORMATION

- An inherited disorder (most commonly X-linked) that results in impaired β-oxidation of very long chain fatty acids in peroxisomes and subsequent accumulation in body tissues and fluids
- The result is an adrenocortical deficiency and central nervous system (CNS) demyelination and neurodegeneration
- Classic presentation is late-childhood onset of subtle neurologic symptoms and progressive deterioration (i.e., dementia, vision/hearing loss) associated with adrenal insufficiency (which may develop before, coincident with, or after the neurologic symptoms)

Congenital Adrenal Hypoplasia

BASIC INFORMATION

- Disorder of adrenal development resulting in primary adrenal insufficiency, often associated with variable inheritance patterns and syndromes. For instance:
  - X-linked congenital adrenal hypoplasia: the most common form, found in males, and presents with salt-wasting, glucocorticoid insufficiency, and hypogonadotropic hypogonadism
  - IMAGe syndrome: intrauterine growth retardation, metaphyseal dysplasia, adrenal hypoplasia, genitourinary anomalies

Other Acquired Causes of Primary Adrenal Insufficiency

- Infections (e.g., tuberculosis [TB], meningococcemia [i.e., Waterhouse-Friderichsen])
- Drugs:
  - Ketoconazole (direct steroidogenesis inhibition)
  - Etomidate (direct steroidogenesis inhibition)
  - Rifampin (increased liver metabolism of steroids)
  - Phenytoin/phenobarbital (increased liver metabolism of steroids)

Congenital Adrenal Hyperplasia (CAH)

BASIC INFORMATION

- CAH, the most common cause of primary adrenal insufficiency, is a family of autosomal recessive disorders of adrenal steroidogenesis
- The clinical presentation is variable for CAH:
  - The breadth and severity of possible symptoms is determined by the affected enzyme (e.g., 21-hydroxylase deficiency, 11-hydroxylase deficiency; see Table 25.2)

Table 25.2. Diagnosis and Treatment of Congenital Adrenal Hyperplasia

Disorder	Affected Gene and Chromosome	Signs and Symptoms	Laboratory Findings	Therapeutic Measures
21-Hydroxylase deficiency, classic form	CYP21 6p21.3	Glucocorticoid deficiency	↓ Cortisol, ↑ ACTH ↑↑ Baseline and ACTH-stimulated 17-hydroxy-progesterone	Glucocorticoid (hydrocortisone) replacement
		Mineralocorticoid deficiency (salt-wasting crisis)	Hyponatremia, hyperkalemia ↑ Plasma renin	Mineralocorticoid (fludrocortisone) replacement; sodium chloride supplementation
		Ambiguous genitalia in females; postnatal virilization in males and females	↑ Serum androgens	Vaginoplasty and clitoral recession suppression with glucocorticoids
21-Hydroxylase deficiency, nonclassic form	CYP21 6p21.3	May be asymptomatic; precocious adrenarche, hirsutism, acne, menstrual irregularity, infertility	↑ Baseline and ACTH-stimulated 17-hydroxyprogesterone ↑ Serum androgens	Suppression with glucocorticoids
11β-Hydroxylase deficiency	CYP11B1 8q24.3	Glucocorticoid deficiency	↓ Cortisol, ↑ ACTH ↑↑ Baseline and ACTH-stimulated 11-deoxycortisol and deoxycorticosterone	Glucocorticoid (hydrocortisone) replacement
		Ambiguous genitalia in females; postnatal virilization in males and females	↑ Serum androgens	Vaginoplasty and clitoral recession; suppression with glucocorticoids
		Hypertension	↓ Plasma renin, hypokalemia	Suppression with glucocorticoids
3β-Hydroxysteroid dehydrogenase deficiency, classic form	HSD3B2 1p13.1	Glucocorticoid deficiency	↓ Cortisol, ↑ ACTH ↑↑ Baseline and ACTH-stimulated Δ5 steroids (pregnenolone, 17-hydroxy-pregnenolone, DHEA)	Glucocorticoid (hydrocortisone) replacement
		Mineralocorticoid deficiency (salt-wasting crisis)	Hyponatremia, hyperkalemia ↑ Plasma renin	Mineralocorticoid (fludrocortisone) replacement; sodium chloride supplementation
		Ambiguous genitalia in females and males; Precocious adrenarche, disordered puberty	↑ DHEA, ↓ androstenedione, testosterone, and estradiol	Surgical correction of genitals and sex hormone replacement as necessary, consonant with sex of rearing; Suppression with glucocorticoids

↓, Decreased; ↑, increased; ↑↑, markedly increased; *ACTH*, adrenocorticotropic hormone; *DHEA*, dehydroepiandrosterone; *FSH*, follicle-stimulating hormone; *hCG*, human chorionic gonadotropin; *LH*, luteinizing hormone.

- With each enzyme deficiency, there is a spectrum of presentation depending on degree of quantitative enzyme deficit and relative enzyme function

- Affects 1/12,000 to 1/20,000 children; more common in Caucasian than in African-American children
  - Later-onset forms affect 1/1000, with higher frequency among Ashkenazi Jews and Hispanics

21-Hydroxylase Deficiency

BASIC INFORMATION

- Results from mutation in *CYP21A2*, leading to variable quantities or functionality of resultant protein necessary for production of cortisol and aldosterone
  - Similar to causes of acquired primary adrenal insufficiency (e.g., Addison disease), ACTH and CRH are elevated
  - Unlike causes of acquired primary adrenal insufficiency, there is:
    - Hyperplasia of adrenal cortex
    - Increased levels of precursor steroids (e.g., progesterone, 17-OH progesterone)
    - A potential for shunting of 17-OH progesterone to increase androgen biosynthesis

CLINICAL PRESENTATION

- Impaired 21-hydroxylase function represents a continuum of disease, including:
  - "Classic" forms (salt-wasting and simple virilizing) present as neonate or very young child
  - "Nonclassic" forms present later in childhood/adolescence
- The effects of prenatal androgen exposure on genital appearance is variable depending on whether the patient is a genetic male or female:
  - If genetic male (XY):
    - No ambiguous genitalia at birth
    - May have "excessive scrotal pigmentation"
    - Patients are more likely to go undiagnosed until adrenal insufficiency develops

- If genetic female (XX):
  - More likely to have ambiguous genitalia at birth (clitoral hypertrophy that can sometimes even be mistaken for penis with hypospadias, "rugated labia")
    - Salt-losing form has most severe virilization
  - Internal genital organs (ovaries) are normal because affected females have normal ovaries; no testes are present
  - The long-term effect of prenatal exposure of the brain to high levels of androgens is controversial and a subject of much research
- "Salt-wasting classic" CAH
  - Comprises ~70% to 75% of "classic" presentations
  - Presentation is a consequence of insufficient glucocorticoids and aldosterone (hyponatremia, hyperkalemia, nongap metabolic acidosis, dehydration, shock)
  - Classically presents with salt-losing crisis within the first 2 weeks of life
- "Simple virilizing (classic)" CAH
  - ~25% to 30% of individuals with "classic CAH" are able to produce adequate mineralocorticoid (therefore no salt-wasting) but are unable to synthesize glucocorticoids and still have androgen excess
  - May not be diagnosed until 3 to 7 years of age
  - Presentation includes:
    - Accelerated linear growth but may have ultimately stunted growth due to advanced skeletal maturation
    - Premature pubarche
    - Clitoral enlargement (in girls) versus phallic enlargement in the setting of prepubertal testes (in boys)
    - Females may have delayed breast development and amenorrhea unless androgens are suppressed
- "Nonclassic" CAH:
  - Least severe form because cortisol and aldosterone levels are normal
  - Affected females usually have normal genitals at birth
  - Males and females may present with precocious puberty and early pubarche
  - Some may develop hirsutism, acne, and menstrual disorders, but many may be asymptomatic

DIAGNOSIS

- Morning 17-OH progesterone is increased
  - Because milder onsets may have normal or mildly elevated 17-OH progesterone levels, it is common to pursue an ACTH-stimulated 17-OH progesterone level, which is very elevated
    - Confirmatory genotyping is available
- Newborn screening involves measuring 17-OH progesterone
- Electrolyte abnormalities consistent with cortisol and aldosterone deficiency (see previous)
- Other hormonal changes:
  - ACTH is increased
  - Plasma renin activity is increased
  - Aldosterone is decreased
  - Serum androgens are increased
- Prenatal screening can be done from amniotic fluid and chorionic villus sampling (CVS; see later)

TREATMENT

- Treat adrenal crisis (see previous)
- Provide chronic mineralocorticoid (if salt-wasting) and corticosteroid via hydrocortisone (HC)
  - Androgens will normalize because glucocorticoid treatment suppresses excessive production
- May consider surgical management of ambiguous genitals

PRENATAL DIAGNOSIS AND TREATMENT

- Early prenatal diagnosis (e.g., amniocentesis, CVS) can assist in treatment decisions by providing definitive diagnosis of CAH
- Providing the mother with dexamethasone will suppress secretion of steroids by fetal adrenal glands, including adrenal androgens, which ameliorates virilization of female fetuses
- Male fetuses do not require dexamethasone

11β-Hydroxylase Deficiency

BASIC INFORMATION

- Deficiency caused by mutation in the *CYP11B1* gene, leading to the second most common cause of CAH
- Leads to decreased cortisol and high levels of corticotropin, so it may present with symptoms of glucocorticoid insufficiency
  - However, patients may have normal or increased mineralocorticoid hormones (get hypertension, hypernatremia, hypokalemia)
    - Increased androgen production due to shunting of precursors, so patients may have virilizing symptoms described previously
    - Demonstrates elevated levels of 11-deoxycortisol, 11-deoxycorticosterone (DOC), and dehydroepiandrosterone (DHEA) before and after ACTH stimulation test

3β-Hydroxysteroid Dehydrogenase Deficiency

BASIC INFORMATION

- Deficiency of 3β-hydroxysteroid dehydrogenase, resulting in decreased cortisol, aldosterone, and androstenedione, but in increased DHEA
  - Can result in salt-wasting crises
  - Androstenedione and testosterone are not synthesized so:
    - If XX: will appear slightly masculine due to elevated DHEA (weak androgen) and may later have symptoms of androgen excess
    - If XY: no testosterone, will appear so incompletely virilized (small phallus) and may later have symptoms of hypogonadism
- Demonstrates marked elevation of the 17-OH pregnenolone and DHEA
  - May also have 17-OH progesterone elevation; however, at an increased ratio of 17:OH pregnenolone:progesterone (versus decreased ratio in 21-OHase deficiency)

Secondary Adrenal Insufficiency

BASIC INFORMATION

- Most often due to insufficient pituitary release of ACTH
  - Classically due to suppression of the HPA axis by chronic administration of high-dose glucocorticoids (e.g., >10 days) with no or inadequate taper
  - Other causes:
    - Pituitary lesions (e.g., craniopharyngioma)
    - Congenital midline lesions (e.g., septo-optic dysplasia, anencephaly)
    - Midline brain surgery
    - Traumatic brain injury
    - Autoimmune hypophysitis
    - Other congenital diseases (e.g., Prader-Willi syndrome)

CLINICAL PRESENTATION

- More likely to present with symptoms of glucocorticoid insufficiency (see previous)
- Unlike in primary causes, secondary adrenal insufficiency is always characterized by:
  - Low ACTH (no hyperpigmentation)
  - Adequate aldosterone because the renin-angiotensin system is intact (no hyperkalemia, no hyponatremia, no salt-wasting)
- Secondary adrenal insufficiency differs from tertiary adrenal insufficiency, in which there is failure of hypothalamic release of CRH (leading to low ACTH concentrations)
- In presentations including an affected pituitary gland, additional deficiencies may be present (e.g., thyroid hormone deficiency)

DIAGNOSIS AND EVALUATION

- CRH stimulation testing and/or low-dose ACTH stimulation testing remain the most commonly used assays

Cushing Syndrome

BASIC INFORMATION

- Describes a syndrome characterized by an excess of glucocorticoid effects
- Incidence is 2 to 5 per 1 million per year (of which only 10% are in pediatrics)

CLINICAL PRESENTATION

- Common symptoms include:
  - Weight gain with linear growth failure is the most common presentation
  - Hirsutism, acne, amenorrhea, and delayed puberty
  - Generalized centripetal obesity (buffalo hump, moon facies)
  - Violaceous striae (may also have hyperpigmentation if ACTH is elevated)
  - Hypertension
- Uncommon symptoms (<50%) include:
  - Headache
  - Easy bruising
  - Osteopenia
  - Compulsive behaviors and emotional lability
  - Muscle weakness

COMMON CAUSES

- See Table 25.3 for common causes of Cushing syndrome
- Cushing disease
  - Most commonly pituitary microadenomas, detectable with pituitary MRI
- Adrenal tumor
  - Adrenal tumors (adenoma, carcinoma) are more likely to cause Cushing syndrome in young children
- Ectopic ACTH syndrome
  - Most likely caused by tumors such as neuroblastoma, pheochromocytoma, pancreatic tumors, or neuroendocrine thymus tumors
  - Typically results in ACTH levels far higher than those in Cushing disease

DIAGNOSIS AND EVALUATION

- Confirm elevated cortisol:
  - 24-hour urine collection
  - Midnight salivary cortisol sample (usually cortisol is low, so an elevated value should raise suspicion for Cushing syndrome)
- Additional initial testing:
  - Midnight ACTH level
    - In causes with excessive cortisol production (e.g., cortisol-secreting tumors), ACTH is expected to be low
    - In causes with excessive ACTH production (e.g., ACTH-secreting tumors), ACTH is expected to be high; however, ACTH can be normal in some pituitary adenomas
  - Single-dose dexamethasone suppression test:
    - Administration of a single dose of dexamethasone around midnight should suppress 8 a.m. cortisol level (i.e., <5 µg/dL)
    - In Cushing syndrome, 8 a.m. cortisol will be elevated
- Consultation with an endocrinologist will provide guidance regarding the utility and interpretation of the following tests:

Table 25.3. Common Causes of Cushing Syndrome

ACTH-Dependent Cushing	ACTH-Independent Cushing
Cushing disease (ACTH-secreting pituitary adenoma, second most common cause in children >5 years old)	Exogenous corticosteroid use (the most common cause)
Exogenous ACTH use	Adrenocortical tumor (second most common cause in infants)
Ectopic ACTH syndrome (ACTH-secreting disease from nonpituitary site)	Bilateral primary adrenocortical hyperplasia
CRH hypersecretion (rare in pediatrics)	PNAD or Carney complex
	Massive macronodular hyperplasia
	McCune-Albright syndrome

ACTH, Adrenocorticotropic hormone; CRH, corticotropin-releasing hormone; PNAD, primary pigmented nodular adrenocortical disease.

- CRH stimulation testing
  - After a bolus of CRH, ACTH-dependent Cushing syndrome will increase ACTH and cortisol response
  - Conversely, adrenal tumors show an increase in ACTH and cortisol
  - Two-step dexamethasone suppression test may also assist in diagnosis
- Imaging:
  - Depending on the presentation and age of the patient, one may consider abdominal or head imaging (e.g., MRI) to confirm a cause for corticosteroid excess

TREATMENT

- After treatment of the cause of Cushing syndrome (e.g., tumor removal), it is common to continue the patient on supraphysiologic doses of glucocorticoid therapy (i.e., "stress dose") that will be weaned before provided an ACTH-stimulation test to ensure integrity of HPA axis

Pheochromocytoma

BASIC INFORMATION

- Catecholamine-secreting tumors usually arising from chromaffin cells of adrenal medulla (but may develop anywhere along the sympathetic chain)
- Compared with adults, children are more likely to have bilateral disease, extrarenal disease, or multiple tumors
- Can be associated with genetic syndromes (e.g., VHL, MEN, NF1, TS)

SYMPTOMS

- Patients most often present with hypertension (usually sustained)
  - Children rarely present with the classic triad: tachycardia, headache, diaphoresis

- Vague symptoms are common: back pain, abdominal pain, abdominal distention
- Although rare, the presentation may mimic that of type 1 diabetes, with weight loss, polyphagia/polydipsia, and hyperglycemia with impaired glucose tolerance

DIAGNOSIS AND EVALUATION

- 24-hour urinary catecholamines or metanephrines are diagnostic
  - Urinary vanillylmandelic acid (VMA) is no longer used due to false-positive results
- Plasma measurements of free catecholamines and metanephrines may also be used for diagnosis
- Tumor localization is usually obtained via MRI
  - Small tumors may be visualized via ^{123}I-MIBG scanning
- Care should be taken to rule out other causes of excess catecholamines, whether exogenous (e.g., drug abuse) or endogenous (e.g., neuroblastoma, panic attacks)

TREATMENT

- Preoperative management requires careful blood pressure control with alpha- and beta-blocker medications
- Surgical removal is required

Review Questions

For review questions, please go to ExpertConsult.com.

26 Endocrine Dysnatremias

ERIC M. BOMBERG, MD, MAS

Diabetes Insipidus (DI)

BASIC INFORMATION

- Normal physiology:
  - Body water and osmotic homeostasis are balanced by arginine vasopressin (AVP) (also known as antidiuretic hormone [ADH]) signaling and depend on serum osmolality and arterial blood volume
  - AVP (produced in the hypothalamus and stored in the posterior pituitary) activates the renal vasopressin-2 receptor (V2R) at the basolateral membrane of principal cells in the distal convoluted tubule (DCT) and collecting duct. This increases tubular fluid permeability via insertion of water channel aquaporin-2 (AQP2) into the apical membrane. Reabsorption of water via increase in AQP2 channels subsequently allows for the concentration of urine, limiting free water loss
  - AVP also binds V1 receptors (V1R) in vascular smooth muscles, platelets, and hepatocytes, but these effects do not affect the sodium/water balance
- Central DI:
  - Basic defect: deficient production and secretion of AVP
  - Causes:
    - Neurosurgery
    - Brain trauma (e.g. deceleration injury)
    - Brain tumors (e.g. craniopharyngioma, pituitary macroadenoma, germinoma, metastases)
    - Granulomatous (histiocytosis, sarcoidosis)
    - Infectious (meningitis, encephalitis)
    - Autoimmune hypophysitis
    - Genetic (Wolfram syndrome)
    - Developmental (septo-optic dysplasia)
    - Sheehan syndrome
    - Idiopathic
- Nephrogenic DI:
  - Basic defect: renal insensitivity to antidiuretic effect of AVP
  - Causes:
    - Lithium
    - Other medications (e.g. demeclocycline, cidofovir, foscarnet, didanosine, amphotericin B, ifosfamide, etc.)
    - Electrolyte imbalances (hypercalcemia, hypokalemia)
    - Obstructive uropathy
    - Infiltrating lesions e.g. sarcoidosis, amyloidosis, multiple myeloma
    - Sickle cell disease (but more likely to have isosthenuria than true DI)

- Acute tubular necrosis
- Genetic: X-linked recessive (AVP receptor-2 gene) is the most commonly inherited form, but autosomal recessive (AQP2 gene) and autosomal dominant (AQP2 gene) forms exist
- Idiopathic
- See also Nelson Textbook of Pediatrics, Chapter 558, "Diabetes Insipidus."

CLINICAL PRESENTATION

- Excretion of abnormally large volumes of dilute urine (polyuria), often with associated polydipsia
  - Results in urinary frequency, incontinence, nocturia, and enuresis
- May present with either:
  - Hypovolemia and hypernatremia (if patient does not have an intact thirst mechanism or access to free water)
  - Euvolemia and normonatremia (if patient has an intact thirst mechanism and access to free water → polyuria increases thirst, which increases fluid intake to compensate for polyuria)
- In neurosurgery cases, central DI may develop postoperatively!
- In infants: frequent heavy and wet diapers, irritability, increased thirst, hypernatremia
- Associated pituitary endocrinopathies more suggestive of central DI than nephrogenic DI

DIAGNOSIS AND EVALUATION

- Steps to confirming the diagnosis:
  - First, confirm true polyuria; must distinguish from urinary frequency without excess urine volume
  - Exclude other causes of polyuria such as drugs (diuretics) and metabolic causes (hyperglycemia, hypercalcemia, hypokalemia)
  - In adults or children >2 years:
    - Combination of urine volume >40 mL/kg/day, urine osmolarity <300 mOsm/L, and negative glucosuria are diagnostic of DI
  - If diagnosis equivocal, could do water deprivation test
  - With administration of desmopressin (DDAVP):
    - Central DI: urine osmolality (and an equivalent fall in urine output) will rise more than 100% in complete central DI and 15% to 50% in partial central DI
    - Nephrogenic DI: urine osmolality will not rise or will rise only minimally

TREATMENT

- Monitor fluid balance in all cases:
  - Intake (intravenous + oral) = Output (urine output + insensible losses + free water deficit if one is present)
- Nephrogenic DI:
  - May or may not respond to removal of offending agent (i.e., lithium)
  - Low solute diet: decreasing salt intake decreases urine output (urine output dependent upon salt intake)
  - Thiazide diuretics: induce mild hypovolemia → increased reabsorption of sodium and water in the proximal tubules → less water reaches distal tubules that are affected by AVP → decreased urine volume
  - Amiloride (useful in lithium toxicity): blocks epithelial sodium channel (ENaC) in the collecting ducts
  - With or without indomethacin: not often used due to effects on renal function
- Central DI:
  - Treat underlying cause if able
  - DDAVP given intranasally, orally, or by injection
  - Thiazide diuretics (hydrochlorothiazide, chlorthalidone) in combination with a low renal solute formula may be used in infancy
  - For patients without an intact thirst mechanism (adipsia), consider fixed water intake in addition to DDAVP

Syndrome of Inappropriate Antidiuretic Hormone Secretion (SIADH)

BASIC INFORMATION

- Pathophysiology: excess ADH secreted from posterior pituitary or ectopic source → increase in aquaporin channels in the DCT and collecting duct → water retention and excretion of concentrated urine
- Etiology:
  - Central nervous system disorders: hemorrhage, infections, inflammatory disorders, mass lesions, multiple sclerosis
  - Drugs: antipsychotic medications, desmopressin, MDMA (Ecstasy), nonsteroidal antiinflammatory drugs (NSAIDs), opiates, selective serotonin reuptake inhibitors, serotonin norepinephrine reuptake inhibitors, vasopressin, vincristine, carbamazepine, cyclophosphamide, ifosfamide etc.
  - Infections: HIV, Rocky Mountain Spotted Fever
  - Postoperative: nausea, pain, anesthesia
  - Pulmonary disorders: infections, respiratory failure, inflammatory disorders, positive pressure mechanical ventilation
  - Tumors: gastrointestinal, genitourinary, lymphomas, sarcomas, lung cancers

CLINICAL PRESENTATION

- Hyponatremia
  - Acute hyponatremia (onset <24 hours): rare in SIADH

- Neurologic: lethargy, somnolence, weakness, seizures, coma, respiratory arrest, death
- Chronic hyponatremia (onset >72 hours):
  - Often asymptomatic; detected incidentally on laboratory findings
  - May present with anorexia, nausea, vomiting, fatigue, headache, falls

DIAGNOSIS AND EVALUATION

- Diagnosis of exclusion: must rule out other causes of hyponatremia including medications (i.e., diuretics), medical conditions (congestive heart failure, cirrhosis, nephrosis, hypothyroidism, adrenal insufficiency), or other (diarrhea, low solute intake, etc.)
- Findings supporting the diagnosis:
  - Hyponatremia with inappropriately concentrated urine
    - Hyponatremia, hypoosmolality, and urine osmolality >100 mOsm/kg
    - Urinary sodium >40 mmol/L with normal dietary salt intake
  - Clinical euvolemia: no signs of volume depletion (i.e., orthostasis, tachycardia, dry mucous membranes) and usually without volume excess (i.e., edema)
  - Low serum uric acid level
  - Low blood urea nitrogen (BUN) and creatinine

TREATMENT

- Correct the underlying cause!
- Asymptomatic patients (should be corrected slowly):
  - Water restriction (key treatment) ± increased solute intake (salt tabs)
  - Demeclocycline: inhibit effects of ADH in the kidney
  - Urea: increases free water excretion
- Symptomatic patients:
  - Water restriction
  - Hypertonic saline for severe cases with neurologic manifestations
    - Goal is not to correct sodium faster than 6 to 10 mEq per day
    - If sodium corrected too quickly → may cause central pontine myelinolysis (osmotic demyelination syndrome)
  - Loop diuretics: disrupt the medullary concentration gradient, allowing excretion of more dilute urine (of note, thiazide diuretics can worsen hyponatremia)
- Vasopressin receptor antagonists (vaptans) considered for severe, refractory cases

Cerebral Salt Wasting

BASIC INFORMATION

- A controversial diagnosis most often discussed in an intensive care unit setting in which patients present with brisk urine output and hyponatremia, usually associated with brain pathology or postneurosurgical intervention
- Given the controversy of this diagnosis, the details are beyond the scope of this review

Review Questions

For review questions, please go to ExpertConsult.com.

Suggested Readings

1. Ellison DH, Berl H. The syndrome of inappropriate antidiuresis. *N Engl J Med.* 2007;356:2064–2072.

2. Fenske W, Allolio B. Current state and future perspectives in the diagnosis of diabetes insipidus: a clinical review. *J Clin Endocrinol Metab.* 2012;97(10):3426–3437.

3. Robertson GL. Diabetes insipidus: differential diagnosis and management. *Best Pract Res Clin Endocrinol Metab.* 2016;30(2):205–218.

Selected Topics in Endocrinology

TERRY DEAN JR., MD, PhD

Hypopituitarism

BASIC INFORMATION

- The anterior pituitary produces growth hormone (GH), prolactin, thyroid-stimulating hormone (TSH), proopiomelanocortin (precursor of adrenocorticotropic hormone [ACTH]), luteinizing hormone (LH), and follicle stimulating hormone (FSH)
- The posterior pituitary, part of the neurohypophysis, is comprised of projections from the hypothalamus and responsible for secretion of arginine vasopressin (antidiuretic hormone [ADH]) and oxytocin
- For "hypopituitarism," there is most commonly an insufficiency of GH, either alone (GH deficiency; see Chapter 22) or accompanied by deficiencies in other hormones (i.e., "panhypopituitarism")
- Congenital multiple pituitary hormone deficiency
  - Various mutations (e.g., *PROP1*, *POU1F1*, *HESX1*, *LHX3/LHX4*) are responsible for differing constellations of deficiencies, including which hormones are deficient, age of onset, abnormality in pituitary anatomy, and whether there are coexisting anomalies
  - Can be associated with anatomic abnormalities (e.g., congenital absence of pituitary, septooptic dysplasia, anencephaly, holoprosencephaly, midface anomalies such as cleft lip/palate) or other inherited syndromes (e.g., Kallmann, Prader-Willi)
- Acquired pituitary hormone deficiency
  - May be caused by multiple causes:
    - Cranial irradiation
    - Postsurgical (e.g., stalk compromise, vascular compromise)
    - Mass effect (e.g., craniopharyngioma)
    - Trauma (e.g., nonaccidental trauma, motor vehicle accident, birth trauma)
    - Inflammation/autoimmunity (e.g., sarcoidosis, hypophysitis, histiocytosis)
    - Infection (e.g., tuberculosis [TB], toxoplasmosis, meningitis)
    - Idiopathic
  - Acquired causes tend to yield multiple hormone deficiencies
- See also *Nelson Textbook of Pediatrics*, Chapter 107, "The Endocrine System"

CLINICAL PRESENTATION

- Presentation varies, depending on which hormones are deficient and age of onset:

- Neonatal onset (e.g., congenital forms): micropenis, hypoglycemia, excessive urine output, hypothyroid symptoms
- Pediatric onset: short stature with weight gain disproportionate to the slowed linear growth, delayed puberty, delayed tooth development, increased urination, hypothyroid symptoms

EVALUATION AND DIAGNOSIS

- In addition to evaluation for individual hormone deficiencies (e.g., GH, insulin-like growth factor [IGF]-1, IGF-1BP, GH stimulation test, bone age; see Chapters 21–26), imaging is often attained of the pituitary gland (i.e., brain magnetic resonance imaging [MRI]
- Consider genetic testing

TREATMENT

- In the event of a reversible acquired cause of hypopituitarism (e.g., tumor, infection, autoinflammatory disease), the treatment course may be curative
- Hormone replacement therapy should be considered with respect to deficient hormones

Autoimmune Polyendocrine Syndrome

BASIC INFORMATION

- A single patient may have multiple endocrine deficiencies caused by an autoimmune etiology; these disorders have had multiple names, including "autoimmune polyglandular disease" and "polyendocrine deficiency syndromes"
- Autoimmune polyendocrine syndrome (APS) type 1
  - Also known as APECED
    - Autoimmune polyendocrinopathy (especially Addison disease, hypoparathyroidism)
    - Candidiasis (chronic mucocutaneous, almost always precedes the other disorders)
    - Ectodermal dystrophy
    - Patients may have other autoimmune diseases (e.g., alopecia totalis, pernicious anemia, vitiligo, type 1 diabetes mellitus [T1DM])
  - Autosomal recessive inheritance
  - Presents in childhood
  - Affected siblings can have the same or different constellations of symptoms

- APS type II
  - Most common of the immunoendocrinopathy syndromes
  - Features
    - Required:
      - Addison disease ± Hashimoto thyroiditis ± T1DM
    - Also observed:
      - Primary hypogonadism
      - Myasthenia gravis
      - Celiac disease
    - Different combinations of individual disorders have been called different disorders in the past (e.g., Schmidt syndrome = Addison disease + Hashimoto thyroiditis)
  - Typically presents in early adulthood (20–30s)
- APS type III
  - Unlike types 1 and 2, it does not involve the adrenal cortex, but does involve autoimmune thyroiditis
  - Additional coexisting autoimmune disorders include:
    - Organ-specific diseases (e.g., T1DM, pernicious anemia, vitiligo/alopecia, celiac disease, hypogonadism, myasthenia gravis)
    - Systemic autoimmune diseases (e.g., sarcoidosis, rheumatoid arthritis, Sjogren syndrome)
- Immunodysregulation polyendocrinopathy enteropathy X-linked (IPEX)
  - Although not a traditional autoimmune polyglandular disease, it does feature multiple endocrinopathies as part of a general immune dysregulation syndrome
  - Caused by a mutation in *FOXP3*, resulting in loss of regulatory T cells; IPEX-like syndromes caused by mutations in other genes (e.g., *CD25*, *STAT5B*) also exist
  - Features:
    - Autoimmune enteropathy (causes watery diarrhea at <1 month of age)
    - Eczematous rash (in infancy)
    - Early-onset T1DM (in infancy)
    - Hyperthyroidism/hypothyroidism

  - Severe allergies
  - Variable lymphadenopathy/splenomegaly
  - Autoimmune cytopenias, eosinophilia
- Patients are immunocompromised
- Treatment: immune modulation therapy with the goal of T-cell inhibition (cyclosporine, tacrolimus, sirolimus, and steroids); bone marrow transplantation is the only cure (untreated patients often die by 2 years of age)

Multiple Endocrine Neoplasia

BASIC INFORMATION

- These inherited disorders cause benign and/or malignant tumors in at least two endocrine glands (Table 27.1); tumors can also develop in nonendocrine tissues, therefore follow-up often centers on screening for cancers in multiple organs over time
- Multiple endocrine neoplasia (MEN) type 1
  - Disorder caused by mutation in *MEN1* tumor suppressor gene and likely "2-hit hypothesis" for tumor development
  - Results in the development of hyperplasia/neoplasia in multiple endocrine organs
- MEN type 2
  - Two distinct disorders characterized by different mutations in *RET* protooncogene
  - In addition to effects on endocrine organs, MEN type 2b also causes characteristic facies, marfanoid body habitus, and generalized ganglioneuromatosis (see Fig. 27.1)
  - Medullary thyroid carcinoma is a prominent feature in both forms of MEN type 2 and may require prophylactic thyroidectomy; screening for other cancers (e.g., pheochromocytoma) and hormone status (e.g., hyperparathyroidism) may also be necessary

Table 27.1. Multiple Endocrine Neoplasia Syndromes

	MEN Type 1	MEN Type 2a	MEN Type 2b
Distinguishing features	Hyperplasia/neoplasia of: - Pancreas (may secrete gastrin, insulin, VIP, glucagon, pancreatic polypeptide) - Anterior pituitary (may secrete prolactin, GH) - Parathyroid (most common presenting symptom)	Medullary thyroid carcinoma (near 100% penetrance) Pheochromocytoma (in up to 50%, often bilateral or multiple) Parathyroid hyperplasia (in up to 20%, late manifestation)	Medullary thyroid carcinoma Pheochromocytomas Mucosal neuroma (tongue, buccal mucosa, lips, and conjunctivae)
Other	Other MEN1-associated tumors: - Carcinoid tumors - Lipomas - Adrenal tumors - Thyroid adenomas - Thymic neuroendocrine tumor	—	Marfan-like facies, may have peripheral neurofibromas or gangliomas (especially in GI tract) and café au lait patches, "inability to cry tears"
Inheritance	Autosomal dominant	Autosomal dominant	Autosomal dominant
Affected gene	*MEN1*	*RET* (exon 10 or exon 11)	*RET* (exon 16)

GH, Growth hormone; *GI*, gastrointestinal; *VIP*, vasoactive intestinal peptide.

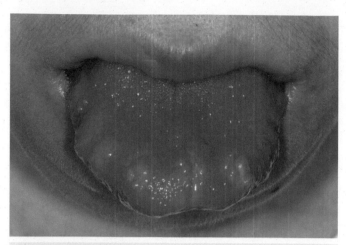

Fig. 27.1. Oral mucosal neuroma in multiple endocrine neoplasia (MEN) type 2b. (From Kliegman, R. M., Stanton, B. F., St Geme, J. W., & Schor, N. F. (Eds.). *Nelson's textbook of pediatrics* (20th ed.), Figure 506-1.)

Review Questions

For review questions, please go to ExpertConsult.com.

Suggested Readings

1. Husebye ES, Anderson MS, Kampe O. Autoimmune polyendocrine syndromes. *NEJM.* 2018;378:1132–1141.
2. Lewis CD, Yeh MW. Inherited endocrinopathies: an update. *Mol Genet Metab.* 2008;94(3):271–282.

Gastroenterology

28 Clinical Approach to Emesis and Diarrhea

NINA N. SAINATH, MD

Diarrhea and emesis both have a long list of etiologies. A careful history and physical examination can help narrow the differential and minimize diagnostic testing.

Emesis

BASIC INFORMATION

- Definition of vomiting: the forceful expulsion of gastric contents
- Vomiting is often preceded by a prodrome, which can include nausea, tachycardia, diaphoresis, pallor, flushing, and retching

CLINICAL PRESENTATION

- Differentiate between vomiting and regurgitation
  - Regurgitation represents expulsion of gastric contents without any of the previous accompanying symptoms
- Age is important
  - Reflux, systemic infections, and anatomic abnormalities are common causes of emesis in infancy
  - Inborn errors of metabolism that present with emesis are usually diagnosed in infancy, but partial enzyme deficiencies can present later
- Establish the pattern of vomiting
  - Acute—an episode of intense vomiting
    - More commonly due to an infectious etiology, obstruction, or a medication/toxin
  - Chronic
  - Cyclical—the patient is healthy between intense episodes of vomiting
    - Consider malrotation with volvulus, metabolic causes, ureteropelvic junction obstruction, and cyclic vomiting syndrome
- Key associated symptoms may help narrow the differential
  - Fevers and diarrhea—suggest an infectious etiology
  - Bilious emesis—strongly consider a partial or complete obstruction
  - Morning emesis—consider etiologies of increased intracranial pressure, although sinusitis and postnasal drip can also cause this
  - Weight loss, poor weight gain, or poor linear growth—consider malabsorptive processes
  - Hematemesis—consider esophagitis, Mallory-Weiss tear, milk protein allergy in an infant, or a bleeding disorder
  - Dysphagia—may indicate esophagitis, achalasia, esophageal stricture, or esophageal dysmotility

- Constipation—may indicate altered bowel motility or anatomic abnormality
  - Consider ileus or pseudoobstruction
  - Consider Hirschsprung disease
- Presence versus absence of abdominal pain
  - A lack of abdominal pain may suggest an extraintestinal etiology of emesis
- Emesis triggered by fasting, illness, or a high-protein meal may be due to an underlying metabolic disorder
- Abnormal gait, abnormal eye movements, personality changes, or developmental delay requires consideration of neurologic or metabolic causes of emesis
- Prior surgical history may increase risk for adhesions or stricture at bowel anastomosis site
- In a neonate with emesis, maternal history of polyhydramnios may suggest congenital obstruction within the gastrointestinal (GI) tract
- Family history or patient history of migraines may occur in patients with cyclic vomiting syndrome
- Key physical examination components
  - Acute dehydration or lethargy may be consistent with infection, toxic ingestion, or cyclic vomiting syndrome
  - Location of abdominal tenderness
  - Bowel sounds
    - May be hypoactive in pseudoobstruction or ileus
    - Can be hyperactive in mechanical obstruction
  - Abnormal neurologic or ophthalmologic examination—consider intracranial mass or bleed

DIAGNOSIS AND EVALUATION

- The differential diagnosis for emesis is broad (Table 28.1). Similarly, the range of possible diagnostic testing and imaging is expansive. The history and physical examination are critical to dictate which are required for a proper evaluation, including whether certain abdominal imaging must be performed emergently to assess for indications for immediate surgery (e.g., appendicitis) or other interventions (e.g., intussusception)
- General laboratories
  - Serum electrolytes
    - Gastric outlet obstruction with repeated emesis is classically associated with hypochloremic hypokalemic alkalosis
    - Blood gas with lactate may evaluate for acid-base disturbances that may also present with emesis (e.g., diabetic ketoacidosis [DKA], ischemic bowel)
  - Complete blood cell count
  - Liver function tests

Table 28.1. Differential Diagnoses of Emesis

INFECTIOUS

- Gastroenteritis
- Extraintestinal infections—otitis media, sinusitis, pneumonia, pharyngitis, meningitis

GASTROINTESTINAL

- Anatomic
  - Bowel obstruction—atresia, pyloric stenosis, distal intestinal obstruction syndrome, stricture from Crohn disease
  - Tracheoesophageal fistula
  - Malrotation with volvulus
  - Intussusception
  - Superior mesenteric artery syndrome
  - Duodenal hematoma
  - Surgical adhesions
- Gastroesophageal reflux disease
- Eosinophilic esophagitis
- Celiac disease
- Milk protein allergy
- *Helicobacter* pylori gastritis
- Appendicitis
- Cholecystitis
- Cholelithiasis
- Pancreatitis
- Hepatitis
- Appendicitis
- Peptic ulcer disease
- Inflammatory bowel disease
- Ménétrier disease
- Motility disorders:
  - Achalasia
  - Gastroparesis
  - Ileus
  - Pseudoobstruction

NEUROLOGIC

- Migraine
- Intracranial mass
- Intracranial hemorrhage
- Hydrocephalus
- Arnold-Chiari malformation
- Pseudotumor cerebri
- Concussion

GENITOURINARY

- Pyelonephritis
- Nephrolithiasis
- Renal tubular acidosis
- Chronic kidney disease with uremia
- Ureteropelvic junction obstruction

ENDOCRINE/METABOLIC

- Diabetic ketoacidosis
- Adrenal insufficiency
- Pheochromocytoma
- Gastrinoma
- Carcinoid syndrome
- Fatty acid oxidation disorders
- Medium-chain acyl-CoA dehydrogenase (MCAD) deficiency
- Partial ornithine transcarbamylase (OTC) deficiency

OTHER

- Medication induced—including chemotherapy
- Toxic ingestion
- Bulimia
- Pregnancy
- Rumination
- Cyclic vomiting syndrome
- Anxiety or depression
- Acute intermittent porphyria
- Stress

- Amylase and lipase
- Serum or urine pregnancy test in a menstruating female
- Urinalysis
  - Low urinary pH in certain types of renal tubular acidosis
  - Presence of blood may indicate nephrolithiasis
  - Presence of white blood cells to screen for a urinary tract infection
- Additional laboratories if history and/or physical are consistent
  - Inflammatory markers
  - Celiac disease screening
  - Infectious stool studies for acute emesis with diarrhea
  - Metabolic labs as evaluation for cyclic vomiting
    - Ammonia, lactate, pyruvate, serum amino acids, urine organic acids, plasma carnitine, and acylcarnitine
  - Urinary δ-aminolevulinic acid and porphobilinogen to evaluate for acute intermittent porphyria
- Radiology
  - Abdominal x-ray—two-view if evaluating for obstruction
  - Abdominal computed tomography (CT)
  - Fluoroscopic studies: esophagram, upper GI with or without small bowel follow-through
    - Order to identify an anatomic abnormality such as esophageal stricture, malrotation, or partial obstruction due to adhesions

- Abdominal ultrasound—especially if evaluating for hepatobiliary or pancreatic pathology, intussusception, or pyloric stenosis
  - Magnetic resonance enterography (MRE)
  - Magnetic resonance imaging (MRI) or CT of the brain
  - Gastric emptying study
- Endoscopy and colonoscopy with biopsies

TREATMENT

- Treatment is ultimately directed at the underlying cause of emesis
- Intravenous hydration may be required if dehydrated
- Correction of electrolyte abnormalities may be necessary
- A number of different antiemetics may be trialed (Table 28.2)

Diarrhea

BASIC INFORMATION

- Definition of diarrhea: either decreased stool consistency and/or increased stool frequency compared with baseline
- See also Nelson Textbook of Pediatrics, Chapter 102, "Digestive System Disorders."

CLINICAL PRESENTATION

- Acute versus chronic

Table 28.2. Commonly Used Antiemetic Medications

Drug class	Drugs	Adverse effects
5-HT$_3$ receptor antagonist	Ondansetron Granisetron	Headache, QT$_c$ prolongation
Anticholinergic	Scopolamine	Sedation, blurry vision, dry mouth, urinary retention
D2 receptor antagonist	Prochlorperazine Chlorpromazine Promethazine	Extrapyramidal side effects
Antihistamine	Promethazine Diphenhydramine Meclizine	Sedation, blurry vision, dry mouth, urinary retention
Benzodiazepines	Lorazepam Diazepam	Sedation, respiratory depression
Corticosteroids	Dexamethasone	Increased appetite, mood swings, adrenal suppression
Cannabinoids	Dronabinol	Sedation, mood changes

5-HT, Serotonin; *D*, dopamine.

- Acute diarrhea lasts less than 2 weeks
- Chronic diarrhea lasts greater than 2 weeks
- Osmotic versus secretory diarrhea
  - Osmotic diarrhea stops when the patient is fasting
  - Secretory diarrhea persists when the patient is fasting
- Key associated symptoms may help narrow the differential:
  - Fevers or presence of blood suggests an infectious or inflammatory etiology
    - *Salmonella*, *Shigella*, *Clostridium difficile*, *Campylobacter*, and certain strains of *Escherichia coli* can have bloody diarrhea
  - The presence of weight loss, poor weight gain, or poor linear growth suggests malabsorption
  - Identify the presence of bulky, greasy, malodorous, or floating stools to suggest steatorrhea (fat malabsorption)
  - Increased flatus or gaseous bowel distention can be consistent with carbohydrate malabsorption
  - Fecal incontinence may indicate fecal impaction with overflow incontinence
- History may provide insight to diagnosis:
  - Assess dietary history: high intake of sugar-sweetened foods and beverages, excess milk intake, or artificial sweeteners may contribute to diarrhea
  - Onset early in life or congenital diarrhea is rare but alters the diagnostic approach (may consider withholding feeds to determine whether the diarrhea is osmotic or secretory)
  - Review medications, including recent antibiotic use
  - Elements of history may suggest an infectious etiology (see Chapter 44 for more details)
    - Recent antibiotic exposure: *C. difficile*
    - Traveler's diarrhea: *E. coli*
    - Common causes of food poisoning: *Staphylococcus aureus*, *Bacillus cereus* (reheated rice)
    - Similar presentation to appendicitis: *Yersinia enterocolitica*
    - Contaminated poultry: *Campylobacter*
    - Seizures: *Shigella*
    - Reptiles, animals, livestock, picnic: *Salmonella*
    - Bloody diarrhea: *Salmonella*, *Shigella*, *Campylobacter*, *C. difficile*, enterohemorrhagic *E. coli* (EHEC), *Y. enterocolitica*

- Communicable diarrhea despite exposure to treated water: *Cryptococcus* (chlorine-resistant)
- Immunocompromised host: *Cytomegalovirus* (CMV), herpes simplex virus (HSV), BK (acute), cryptosporidium, *Mycobacterium avium* complex (MAC)
- Physical examination components:
  - Assess hydration status
  - Location of abdominal tenderness
  - Features of inflammatory bowel disease (IBD): oral ulcers, arthritis, perianal disease, uveitis
  - Skin: disease-specific rashes (IBD and erythema nodosum or pyoderma gangrenosum, celiac disease and dermatitis herpetiformis)
  - Rectal examination to assess for fecal impaction and likelihood of overflow incontinence

DIAGNOSIS AND EVALUATION

- As for emesis, the differential diagnosis of diarrhea is quite broad. The diagnostic approach should be dictated by the clinical scenario
- General laboratories
  - Complete blood cell count
    - Leukocytosis can occur with an infectious or inflammatory process
    - Anemia may be due to blood loss from the GI tract and/or nutritional deficiencies
    - Thrombocytosis may occur with an infectious or inflammatory process.
  - Serum electrolytes
  - Liver function tests
  - Serum albumin, which may be low due to protein losses in the stool and/or malnutrition
- Additional laboratories if history and/or physical are consistent
  - Inflammatory markers
  - Celiac disease screening
  - Plasma peptides: gastrin, vasoactive intestinal peptide
  - Urine—5-hydroxyindoleacetic acid, metanephrines, histamine
- Common stool testing
  - Infectious stool studies
  - Stool hemoccult—measure of microscopic blood in the stool
  - Measures of GI tract inflammation
    - Stool calprotectin
    - Stool white blood cell count
  - Stool osmotic gap: $290 - 2 \times ([Na] + [K])$
    - Secretory diarrhea: osmotic gap <50 mOsm/L Stool Na >90 mmol/L more consistent with secretory diarrhea
    - Osmotic diarrhea: osmotic gap >100 mOsm/L Multiple etiologies Occurs due to the presence of an osmotically active substance that was ingested or is present due to malabsorption/maldigestion
- Targeted testing for malabsorption
  - Xylose testing
    - Rarely used today, it is a diagnostic test for malabsorption due to damaged small intestine mucosa
    - D-xylose is administered enterally, and serum or urine levels are measured several hours later; lower-than-expected levels are seen when the intestinal

barrier is compromised (e.g., IBD, celiac disease, bacterial overgrowth)

■ Fat malabsorption
  ■ Fecal elastase—consistent with pancreatic insufficiency if <200 µg/g stool
  ■ 72-hour fecal fat or coefficient of fat absorption
    Gold standard for measuring fat malabsorption
    Requires a diet of 100 g of fat or more per day
    Fecal fat >7 g/24 hours or a coefficient of fat absorption <93% indicates fat malabsorption
    Generally not clinically practical
  ■ Fat-soluble vitamin deficiency (vitamins A, D, E, and K)
  ■ Triene:tetraene ratio as a measure of essential fatty acid deficiency
■ Carbohydrate malabsorption
  ■ Stool-reducing substances positive (n.b. test does not recognize sucrose and other nonreducing carbohydrates)
  ■ Stool pH <5.5
  ■ Hydrogen breath testing
    Not always clinically available and can be challenging to perform in young or delayed children
    Consider empiric elimination of certain carbohydrates from diet
■ Protein malabsorption
  ■ Hypoalbuminemia—make sure there is no protein loss from the urine

  ■ May have an elevated stool alpha-1 antitrypsin
■ Radiology
  ■ MRE or abdominal CT can help identify bowel inflammation
  ■ Abdominal ultrasound
    ■ Can identify bowel or pancreatic inflammation
■ Upper endoscopy and colonoscopy
  ■ Electron microscopy may be helpful, especially in cases of congenital diarrhea

DIFFERENTIAL DIAGNOSIS

■ Acute diarrhea
  ■ Infectious—viral, bacterial, parasitic
  ■ Medication related—commonly antibiotics
  ■ Toxin induced
  ■ Food allergies
■ Chronic diarrhea (Table 28.3)
  ■ Can be osmotic or secretory
    ■ Causes of secretory diarrhea include:
      Certain forms of congenital diarrhea
      Specific infections—*Vibrio cholerae, E. coli* toxin
      Neuroendocrine tumors

TREATMENT

■ Treatment is disease specific

Table 28.3.   Differential Diagnoses of Chronic Diarrhea

MALABSORPTION/MALDIGESTION

■ Fat malabsorption
  ■ Cholestasis
    ■ Cystic fibrosis
    ■ Biliary atresia
    ■ Primary sclerosing cholangitis
    ■ Progressive familial intrahepatic cholestasis
  ■ Bile acid diarrhea
    ■ Ileal resection due to any etiology
    ■ Cholecystectomy
  ■ Pancreatic insufficiency
    ■ Cystic fibrosis
    ■ Shwachman-Diamond syndrome
    ■ Johanson-Blizzard syndrome
    ■ Chronic pancreatitis
■ Carbohydrate malabsorption
  ■ Lactose intolerance
  ■ Post infectious enteropathy
  ■ Toddler's diarrhea—due to malabsorption of excess fructose intake
  ■ High dietary intake of artificial sweeteners
    ■ Short bowel syndrome
    ■ Small intestinal bacterial overgrowth

INFLAMMATORY DISEASES

■ Celiac disease
■ Inflammatory bowel disease
■ Eosinophilic gastroenteritis
■ Food protein induced enterocolitis
■ Milk protein enterocolitis
■ Collagenous colitis
■ Ischemic colitis
■ Radiation colitis

INFECTIOUS

■ Bacterial gastroenteritis
■ Parasitic gastroenteritis—giardia

NEUROENDOCRINE/ENDOCRINE

■ VIPoma
■ Gastrinoma
■ Carcinoid syndrome
■ Glucagonoma
■ Pheochromocytoma
■ Hyperthyroidism
■ Adrenal insufficiency

CONGENITAL DIARRHEA

■ Malabsorption/maldigestion
  ■ Glucose galactose malabsorption
  ■ Sucrose isomaltase deficiency
  ■ Congenital chloride diarrhea
  ■ Abetalipoproteinemia
  ■ Acrodermatitis enteropathica
  ■ Congenital sodium diarrhea
  ■ Enterokinase deficiency
■ Abnormal enterocyte structure
  ■ Microvillous inclusion disease
  ■ Tufting enteropathy
  ■ Trichohepatoenteric syndrome
■ Abnormal enteroendocrine cells
  ■ Enteric anendocrinosis
  ■ Proprotein convertase 1/3 deficiency
■ Dysregulation of the immune system
  ■ Autoimmune enteropathy
  ■ Very early onset inflammatory bowel disease
  ■ IPEX syndrome

OTHER

■ Fecal impaction and overflow incontinence
■ Irritable bowel syndrome
■ Vagotomy after surgery—dumping syndrome
■ Systemic mastocytosis
■ Micronutrient deficiencies: niacin or zinc deficiency

- Intravenous hydration if dehydrated
- Correction of electrolyte abnormalities if present

Review Questions

For review questions, please go to ExpertConsult.com.

Suggested Readings

1. Canani RB, Castaldo G, Bacchetta R, Martín MG, Goulet O. Congenital diarrhoeal disorders: advances in this evolving web of inherited enteropathies. *Nat Rev Gastroenterol Hepatol.* 2015;12:293–302.
2. Gupta R. Diarrhea. In: Wyllie R, Hyams JS, Kay M, eds. *Pediatric Gastrointestinal and Liver Disease.* 5th ed. Philadelphia: Elsevier Saunders; 2016:104–114.
3. Li BUK, Kovacic K. Vomiting and nausea. In: Wyllie R, Hyams JS, Kay M, eds. *Pediatric Gastrointestinal and Liver Disease.* 5th ed. Philadelphia: Elsevier Saunders; 2016:84–103.
4. Li BUK, Lefevre F, et al. North American Society for Pediatric Gastroenterology, Hepatology, and Nutrition consensus statement on the diagnosis and management of cyclic vomiting syndrome. *JPGN.* 2008;47:379–393.
5. Raman M. Testing for chronic diarrhea. *Adv Clin Chem.* 2017;79:199–244.

Clinical Approach to Gastrointestinal Bleed

LISA FAHEY, MD

Basic Information

- Gastrointestinal (GI) bleeding may present in various manners:
  - Hematochezia: passage of fresh (bright red) blood per rectum, typically mixed in with or on top of stools
  - Melena: very dark or black stool containing partially digested blood
  - Hematemesis: bloody vomit
- There are various causes of GI bleeding, which are classically divided into upper and lower sources of blood (Tables 29.1 and 29.2)
  - Upper GI bleeds occur proximal to the ligament of Treitz
  - Lower GI bleeds occur distal to the ligament of Treitz
- The goal of this chapter is to provide some tools for assessing patients presenting with GI bleeds
- See also Nelson Textbook of Pediatrics, Chapter 306, "Major Symptoms and Signs of Digestive Tract Disorders."

UPPER GI BLEED

- Classically presents with hematemesis and/or melena; however, brisk upper bleeds are also capable of causing hematochezia
- Acute upper GI bleed is a medical emergency because the bleeding can be brisk and result in hemorrhagic shock, compromising the upper airway if there is hematemesis
  - See Table 29.1 for a differential diagnosis for acute upper GI bleeds

LOWER GI BLEED

- Lower GI bleeds classically present with hematochezia
- See Table 29.2 for a differential diagnosis of lower GI bleeds

Clinical Presentation

- The speed of GI bleed as well as whether there is abdominal pain may lend insight into the cause of the bleed (Table 29.3)
- Possible symptoms
  - Related to anemia:
    - Weakness
    - Light-headedness
  - Related to cause of GI bleed:
    - Weight loss
    - Fevers
    - Change in bowel habits
- Physical examination findings

- Assess vital signs. Red flags include:
  - Hypotension
  - Tachycardia
  - Prolonged capillary refill
  - Mental status changes
- Pallor
- Jaundice, ascites, hepatosplenomegaly, and abdominal distention suggest chronic liver disease
- Perianal diseases suggest Crohn disease
- Vascular skin lesions such as hemangiomas and telangiectasias suggest possible GI vascular malformation
- Blood in hypopharynx may indicate a nasopharyngeal etiology of bleeding
- Severe presentation of a GI hemorrhage may lead to shock

Diagnosis and Evaluation

- The history consistent with upper or lower GI bleed may help direct the diagnostic workup
  - Of note, one of the initial determinations for upper GI bleeds is establishing the likelihood of whether the

Table 29.1. Differential Diagnosis of Acute Upper GI Bleeding

Neonates/Infants	Children and Adolescents
Swallowed maternal blood in breastfeeding infants	Peptic ulcer
Peptic ulcer	Esophagitis
Esophagitis	Gastritis
Gastritis	Arteriovenous malformation*
Vascular malformation*	Duodenitis
Duodenitis	Gastric or intestinal duplication
Coagulopathy*	Mallory-Weiss tear
Gastric or intestinal duplication	Mucosal erosions
Mallory-Weiss tear	Dieulafoy lesion (large, tortuous arteriole in wall of GI tract that erodes and bleeds)*
	Esophageal varices (can be due to portal hypertension secondary to liver cirrhosis)*
	Gastric varices
	Use of nonsteroidal antiinflammatory drugs (NSAIDs) or aspirin
	Malignancy*
	Toxic ingestion*
	Foreign body*

*Denotes life-threatening causes that must be ruled out immediately.

Table 29.2. Differential Diagnosis of Lower GI Bleeding

Neonates/Infants	Children and Adolescents
Swallowed maternal blood in breastfeeding infants	Anal fissure
Anal fissure	Meckel diverticulum
Allergic proctocolitis	Volvulus*
Necrotizing enterocolitis*	Intestinal duplication
Meckel diverticulum	Hirschsprung colitis* (if not diagnosed in infancy)
Volvulus*	Intussusception*
Coagulopathy*	Infectious colitis
Intestinal duplication	Vascular malformation*
Hirschsprung colitis*	Juvenile polyps
Intussusception*	Inflammatory bowel disease
Infectious colitis	Small bowel obstruction*
Vascular malformation*	Pseudomembranous colitis
	Ischemic colitis*
	Hemorrhoids

*Denotes life-threatening causes that must be ruled out immediately.

Table 29.3. Associations with GI Bleeding

Causes of Brisk GI Bleed	Causes of *Painful* GI Bleed	Causes of *Painless* GI Bleed
Meckel diverticulum	Intussusception (abdominal pain + "red currant jelly") stools	Meckel diverticulum
Arteriovenous malformation	Volvulus	Juvenile polyps
Esophageal or gastric varices	Small bowel obstruction	
	Inflammatory bowel disease	
	Ischemic colitis	
	Pseudomembranous colitis	

bleeding is nonvariceal or variceal because this dictates management (see later)

- Laboratory tests
  - Complete blood count
    - Hemoglobin/hematocrit to assess degree of anemia
    - Microcytosis may suggest a chronic etiology
  - Blood type and cross
  - Complete metabolic panel, including hepatic function panel, electrolytes, and blood urea nitrogen level
  - Prothrombin time/partial thromboplastin time/international normalized ratio
  - Hemoccult
    - False positive may be due to ingestion of red meat, certain medications including NSAIDs, excessive alcohol, certain vegetables including broccoli, cauliflower, and radishes
  - Gastroccult
  - Apt test in infants to distinguish maternal swallowed blood from infant blood
- Consider nasogastric (NG) lavage with room-temperature normal saline to see whether bright-red blood clears rapidly
  - Bright-red blood return or coffee-ground gastric contents support upper GI bleed

- Consider Meckel scan or radiolabeled red blood cell scan if appropriate
- Stool *Clostridium difficile* toxin testing and stool culture if hematochezia is present

Treatment

- Resuscitation
  - Initial management step: assess airway, breathing, and circulation
    - Securing an airway is of utmost importance, especially in severe upper GI bleeding due to potential for impending altered mental status, blood-filled oropharynx, and hypovolemic, hemorrhagic shock
    - Some scenarios may require this to be done emergently, *before* placing NG tube
  - Aggressively rehydrate with crystalloid or colloid solution
  - For an acute loss, transfuse with packed red blood cells (PRBC) if anemic (e.g., Hb ≤7 g/dL) or impending anemia
    - Note that anemia may not be evident on testing until after reequilibration of fluid between intravascular and extravascular compartments
    - Resuscitation with large quantities of PRBC will necessitate coadministration of platelets and coagulation factors to prevent coagulopathy
  - Correct coagulopathy if applicable
  - Consider NG placement for suspected upper GI bleed for NG lavage
- Initiate IV proton pump inhibitor therapy
- Consider upper endoscopy or colonoscopy to identify cause of the upper or lower GI bleed, respectively, once the patient is stabilized
  - Polypectomy if polyps present
- Consider capsule endoscopy if no bleeding source is identified with endoscopy
  - Consider patency capsule to rule out bowel obstruction
- Consider air- or water-soluble contrast enema if high suspicion for intussusception
- Specific management recommendations for acute varices:
  - Admit patients with suspected acute variceal bleed
  - Rehydrate and transfuse with PRBCs to provide intravascular volume support
  - Initiate pharmacologic therapy as soon as bleed is suspected
    - Somatostatin
    - Somatostatin analog (i.e., octreotide)
  - Endoscopic intervention for active bleeding or varices that have recently bled, including sclerotherapy (i.e., sodium tetradecyl injection) and/or banding
  - Consider balloon tamponade as a temporary measure if bleeding is uncontrollable (e.g., Sengstaken–Blakemore tube placement), until a more definitive therapy can be achieved (i.e., transjugular intrahepatic portosystemic shunt [TIPS] or endoscopic intervention)
  - Consider TIPS if bleeding cannot be controlled or if there is recurrent esophageal variceal bleeding
- Endoscopic interventions for nonvariceal GI hemorrhage:
  - Injection of sclerosing agent (i.e., ethanolamine oleate)

- Injection of epinephrine
- Thermocoagulation with heater probe, monopolar probe, or bipolar probe
- Argon plasma coagulation
- Clips to facilitate hemostasis

Review Questions

For review questions, please go to ExpertConsult.com.

Suggested Readings

1. Hwang JH, Fisher DA, Ben-Menachem T, et al. The role of endoscopy in the management of acute non-variceal upper GI bleeding. *Gastrointest Endosc.* 2012;75:1132–1138.
2. Neidich GA, Cole SR. Gastrointestinal bleeding. *Pediatr Rev.* 2014;35: 243–253.
3. Zawahir S, Blanchard S. GI bleeding. In: Huratado C, Li B, eds. *The NASP-GHAN Fellows Concise Review of Pediatric Gastroenterology, Hepatology and Nutrition.* 2nd ed. Ambler, PA: NASPGHAN; 2017:49–58.

30 Esophageal and Gastric Disorders

BRIDGET C. GODWIN, MD and JENNIFER WEBSTER, DO

ESOPHAGEAL DISORDERS

Gastroesophageal Reflux (GER)

BASIC INFORMATION

- Causes and etiology
  - Description: movement of gastric contents into the esophagus
  - Physiologic reflux: in infants it is caused by open lower esophageal sphincter (LES). Present in all infants at birth, prevalence decreases with age, with peak between 4 and 6 months of age, and 99% of infants having no physiologic reflux at 18 months of age
  - Gastroesophageal reflux disease (GERD) is reflux accompanied by clinical symptoms such as pain, poor feeding, failure to thrive, apnea, or aspiration
  - GERD is the most common esophageal disorder in children

CLINICAL PRESENTATION

- History
  - In infants, GER presents with vomiting, weight loss, arching of the back, irritability, or feeding refusal
  - In older children, GER may present with abdominal pain, chest pain, or chest burning
- Physical signs
  - Weight loss
  - Dental erosions
  - Cobblestoning of the posterior pharynx
- Natural history
  - Long-term risk of dysplasia/Barrett esophagus (uncommon in pediatrics)

DIAGNOSIS AND EVALUATION

- Diagnosis made by history and physical
- Upper gastrointestinal (GI) study is indicated if there is persistent vomiting to rule out malrotation or other structural abnormalities
- pH/impedance probe to determine height and acidity of reflux
- Esophageal manometry to rule out achalasia or rumination
- Endoscopy to evaluate for extent of esophagitis (visual and histologic) and to rule out other causes of symptoms such as eosinophilic esophagitis
- Scintigraphy: milk scan versus solid gastric emptying scan. Not sensitive or specific for reflux, but can evaluate for aspiration (milk scan) and gastroparesis (gastric emptying scan)

TREATMENT

- Reflux precautions: decrease volume of feeds in infants, avoid dietary triggers in older patients, keep upright for 30 minutes after feeds
- Thicken feeds: does not decrease presence of reflux, but decreases height of reflux
- Acid suppression:
  - H2 receptor antagonists (H2RA)—may develop tolerance
  - Proton pump inhibitor (PPI)
    - Superior to H2RAs for treating erosive esophagitis or GERD
    - No controlled studies to support using them empirically in irritable infants
    - May increase risk of community-acquired pneumonia, gastroenteritis, fractures, hypomagnesemia, *Clostridium difficile* infection
- Prokinetic agents such as erythromycin and metoclopramide: not enough evidence to support use of these in GERD
- Surgery/fundoplication: indicated if medical therapy has failed, children have severe GERD dependent on medication, neurologic impairment, or recurrent esophageal bleeding or aspiration. Risks include need for further surgery, retching, bloating, and dysphagia

Eosinophilic Esophagitis

BASIC INFORMATION

- Causes and etiology: chronic antigen-mediated immune disorder
- See also Nelson Textbook of Pediatrics, Chapter 324, "Eosinophilic Esophagitis and Non–Gastroesophageal Reflux Disease Esophagitis."

CLINICAL PRESENTATION

- History
  - Mean age of presentation 8 years old
  - More common in boys than girls
  - Often associated with eczema, asthma, food allergies, allergic rhinitis, and urticaria
  - Symptoms include feeding refusal, vomiting, abdominal pain, dysphagia, food impaction, and chest pain
- Physical signs: failure to thrive, poor weight gain
- Natural history: natural history studies suggest that prolonged active disease most likely leads to stricture formation (Fig. 30.1)

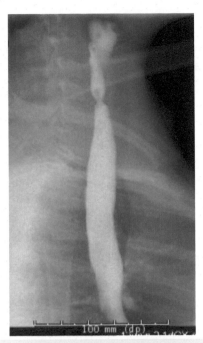

Fig. 30.1. Esophageal stricture.

DIAGNOSIS AND EVALUATION

- Esophagram is needed to evaluate for stricture if symptoms of food impaction or dysphagia (Fig. 30.1)
- Endoscopy: appearance of devascularization, trachealization, esophageal narrowing, microabscesses, and rings
- Eosinophilia of greater than or equal to 15 eosinophils per high powered field on esophageal biopsy with patient on therapy with a PPI

TREATMENT

- Acid suppression with PPI (if eosinophilia resolves, most likely acid reflux versus PPI-responsive esophageal eosinophilia, a separate entity)
- Swallowed corticosteroids: most commonly fluticasone or budesonide
- Multiple options including: food elimination based on allergy testing; food elimination based on patient's diet and most likely cause of allergy; six-food elimination diet versus elemental diet

Pill Esophagitis

BASIC INFORMATION

- Causes and etiology: pill lodged in the esophagus. Most common with tetracycline and ferrous sulfate. Often due to insufficient water intake with pill versus esophageal pathology such as stricture or dysmotility

CLINICAL PRESENTATION

- History: dysphagia and chest pain after taking a pill
- Physical signs: none
- Natural history: may cause ulceration and scarring of the esophagus

DIAGNOSIS AND EVALUATION

- If suspected on history, stop medication or change to a liquid form and observe for improvement

TREATMENT

- Stop medication as described previously
- Antacid therapy
- Sucralfate may help with symptoms

Infectious Esophagitis

BASIC INFORMATION

- Causes and etiology
  - Fungal—95% are candidal. Other causes include Cryptococcus, histoplasmosis, blastomycosis, and aspergillosis
    - More common in immunosuppressed patients
    - May occur in setting of stasis (i.e., from achalasia)
  - Viral—herpes simplex virus (HSV) is the most common
    - May occur in immunocompetent or immunocompromised patients; more common after injury
  - Bacterial—*Mycobacterium tuberculosis* may occur as part of more systemic infection
  - Parasitic—*Trypanosoma cruzi* may lead to megaesophagus

CLINICAL PRESENTATION

- History:
  - Candidal esophagitis: presents with dysphagia, chest pain, vomiting
  - Herpes esophagitis: presents with fever, malaise, dehydration, dysphagia, chest pain
  - Cytomegalovirus (CMV) esophagitis more common in immunocompromised patients
- Physical signs: candidal esophagitis may present with oral thrush

DIAGNOSIS AND EVALUATION

- Endoscopy:
  - Candidal esophagitis: adherent white plaques on esophageal wall in fungal esophagitis. Send biopsies as well as brushings for culture
  - Herpes esophagitis: herpetic vesicles, volcano ulcers with nuclear inclusions, and multinucleate giant cells. Can send viral culture
  - CMV esophagitis: linear ulcerations

TREATMENT

- Fungal esophagitis may be self-limited in healthy individuals or may require therapy with antifungals in healthy or immunosuppressed patients
- Herpes esophagitis may be self-limited versus requiring therapy with acyclovir or foscarnet
- CMV esophagitis: foscarnet or ganciclovir

Table 30.1. Congenital Anomalies of the Esophagus: Basic Information

	Esophageal Atresia/TEF	Esophageal Duplication	Esophageal Stenosis	Esophageal Web	Esophageal Ring
Description	Esophageal atresia: Proximal and distal portions do not communicate TEF: Abnormal communication between trachea and esophagus	Cysts, diverticula, or tubular malformations	Intrinsic esophageal stenosis caused by congenital malformation	Mucosal membrane occluding esophageal lumen. Usually found in proximal esophagus.	Found in distal esophagus. Presents as dysphagia.
Diagnosis	Inability to pass nasogastric tube/x-ray showing coiling in the esophagus	Upper gastrointestinal Chest computed tomography	Esophagram Endoscopy	Endoscopy	Esophagram Endoscopy
Treatment	Surgical repair	Surgical repair	Excision with end-to-end anastomosis	Endoscopy may rupture web. May require dilation.	Dilation Surgical resection

Achalasia

BASIC INFORMATION

- Causes and etiology: a rare esophageal motility disorder in which there is impaired movement of the esophagus as well as inability of the LES to relax

CLINICAL PRESENTATION

- History: chest pain, vomiting, decreased appetite
- Physical signs: weight loss
- Natural history: leads to malnutrition, occasionally dehydration

DIAGNOSIS AND EVALUATION

- Esophagram will show a dilated esophagus and a class "bird's peak" appearance of tapering at the LES
- Esophageal manometry will confirm diagnosis
- Endoscopy may be normal with scope easily passed through LES

TREATMENT

- Endoscopic dilation of the LES
- Surgery: a Heller myotomy to surgically open the LES

Esophageal Varices

BASIC INFORMATION

- A complication most commonly caused by liver disease and portal hypertension; can lead to chronic bleeding (and iron deficiency) as well as acute, life-threatening bleeds
- See Chapter 32 for details.

Congenital Anomalies of the Esophagus

BASIC INFORMATION

- Causes and etiology: occur in ~1 for every 3000 to 5000 live births. Tracheoesophageal fistula and esophageal atresia are the most common

- Types (See Table 30.1):
  - Tracheoesophageal fistula
  - Esophageal atresia
  - Esophageal web
  - Esophageal duplication
  - Esophageal stenosis
  - Esophageal rings

CLINICAL PRESENTATION

- History: consider in infants with persistent vomiting, cough, and/or dysphagia
- Physical signs: failure to thrive, respiratory distress, recurrent aspiration pneumonia

DIAGNOSIS AND EVALUATION

- Diagnose by esophagram or endoscopy

TREATMENT

- Surgical repair or endoscopic dilation

GASTRIC DISEASES

Pyloric Stenosis

BASIC INFORMATION

- The most common surgical disorder of the stomach in infants
- 1 to 3.5 per 1000 live births
- Differential diagnosis includes: antral web, annular pancreas, duodenal stenosis, allergic gastroenteropathy, GERD, intestinal obstruction
- Increased with maternal smoking (2×), bottle-feeding (4×), family history, macrolide antibiotic use under 2 weeks of age (odds ratio 8−13), male (5:1)

CLINICAL PRESENTATION

- Nonbilious projectile vomiting, often described as "wanting to eat" despite the inability to keep milk down
- Persistent emesis results in dehydration, weight loss, failure to thrive
- Laboratory testing: hypercarbia, hypochloremia, alkalosis

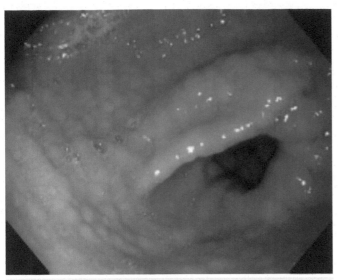

Fig. 30.2. *Helicobacter pylori* gastritis.

DIAGNOSIS AND EVALUATION

- Ultrasound is test of choice: pyloric length >19 mm and thickness >4 mm confirms diagnosis
- Upper GI reveals elongated pyloric channel or "string sign"

TREATMENT

- Laparoscopic pyloromyotomy after correction of electrolytes and acid-base disturbance and restoration of volume status

H. pylori Gastritis

BASIC INFORMATION

- Most common cause of gastritis worldwide; affects ~50% of the world's population
- Selectively colonizes the stomach and produces a potent T-cell response
- Increased risk in developing countries, crowded living conditions, lack of running water, and low socioeconomic status (SES)
- Bacteria releases urease, leading to epithelial damage and inflammation

CLINICAL PRESENTATION

- Ulcer disease
- Iron deficiency anemia
- Reflux

DIAGNOSIS AND EVALUATION

- Gold standard: endoscopy with biopsy
  - Nodularity in the stomach; "cobblestone appearance" (Fig. 30.2)
- Urea breath test
- Stool antigen

TREATMENT

- Triple therapy: amoxicillin + clarithromycin + PPI for 14 days

Other Infectious Causes of Gastritis

- Viral
  - CMV most common (also hepatitis C virus [HCV], Epstein-Barr virus [EBV], HHV7, measles, varicella, influenza, HSV)
  - Most common in immunocompromised patients
  - Diagnosis: CMV inclusions or viral culture on biopsy
  - Treatment: spontaneous recovery in 1 to 2 months or ganciclovir
  - Diagnosis: CMV inclusions or viral culture on biopsy
- Parasitic
  - Anisakis, Eustrongylides, Giardia
- Fungal
  - Candida most common (also cryptosporidiosis and aspergillus)
  - Most common in immunocompromised patients

Reactive Gastritis

BASIC INFORMATION

- Stress gastropathy: secondary to hypoperfusion, typically within 24 hours of a stress event
- Neonatal gastropathy: sick infants in the neonatal intensive care unit (NICU), prostaglandin infusion for PDA
- Traumatic gastropathy: secondary to vomiting

Medication-Induced Gastritis

BASIC INFORMATION

- Most commonly caused by nonsteroidal antiinflammatory drugs (NSAIDs)
- Also caused by valproic acid, dexamethasone, chemotherapy, KCl, iron, long-term fluoride ingestion
- Treatment usually involves PPI or misoprostol for NSAIDs

Peptic Ulcer Disease

BASIC INFORMATION

- Often secondary to medications in children <10 years of age (steroids, NSAIDs)
- Approximately half of cases or idiopathic in nature

CLINICAL PRESENTATION

- Vomiting, epigastric pain several hours after eating
- Perforation possible in young children

DIAGNOSIS AND EVALUATION

- Stool *Helicobacter pylori* antigen
- Seen on endoscopy

TREATMENT

- PPIs

Zollinger-Ellison Syndrome (ZES)

BACKGROUND

- Secretion of gastrin by duodenal or pancreatic neuroendocrine tumors
- Most patients are 20 to 50 years old

CLINICAL PRESENTATION

- Chronic diarrhea caused by high gastric acid output
- Heartburn
- Esophagogastroduodenoscopy (EGD) with multiple peptic ulcers, typically in the first part of the duodenum

DIAGNOSIS AND EVALUATION

- Fasting serum gastrin: >10 times the upper limit is diagnostic of ZES

TREATMENT

- Medical management: PPIs
  - Octreotide if metastatic disease
- Surgical: resection of sporadic gastrinoma (eradicates disease)

EOSINOPHILIC GASTRITIS

BACKGROUND

- 50% of adults have peripheral eosinophilia
- Most often occurs as part of eosinophilic gastroenteritis

CLINICAL PRESENTATION

- Vomiting, abdominal pain, blood loss
- Gastric outlet obstruction

DIAGNOSIS AND EVALUATION

- Endoscopy: friability, erosions, erythema, pseudopolyps
- Histology: eosinophilia

TREATMENT

- Elimination of specific allergens: most commonly milk/soy, egg, and wheat
- Steroids

Ménétrier Disease

BASIC INFORMATION

- Typically presents around 4 years of age
- Associated with CMV infection
- Differential: lymphoma, *H. pylori*, CMV

CLINICAL PRESENTATION

- Vomiting, edema

DIAGNOSIS AND EVALUATION

- upper GI fluoroscopy: giant gastric folds

TREATMENT

- Typically self-limiting in children

Toxic Ingestions

BASIC INFORMATION

- Causes and etiology
  - Alkali agents (dishwasher detergents, drain cleaners) cause liquefaction necrosis with fast-onset transmural inflammation and edema with risk of perforation
  - Acidic agents (toilet bowl cleaners, battery liquids) cause coagulation necrosis and damage to the superficial mucosa
  - Injury depends on concentration of agent
  - Risk of perforation is present for 3 weeks after ingestion while scar is forming

CLINICAL PRESENTATION

- History
  - May be asymptomatic versus present with dysphagia, drooling, chest pain, respiratory distress, or hematemesis
- Physical signs
  - May not be any sign of mucosal injury to the mouth or face
- Natural history
  - May lead to perforation and/or stricture formation
  - 2% with severe caustic esophageal injury may develop esophageal squamous cell carcinoma

DIAGNOSIS AND EVALUATION

- Endoscopy within 24 hours. Recommended to wait >6 hours to observe the full extent of injury

TREATMENT

- Immediately use water to wash face and oral cavity and emergently present to medical care
- Do not induce vomiting

- Patients may undergo placement of nasogastric tube to ensure patency of the esophagus through the postingestion inflammatory process
- Role of antibiotics and steroids is unclear
- Esophageal dilation if needed for stricture formation

Esophageal Injuries

BASIC INFORMATION

- Causes and etiology
  - Mallory-Weiss tear—linear laceration at gastroesophageal (GE) junction due to vomiting
  - Boerhaave syndrome—spontaneous rupture of the esophagus due to vomiting

CLINICAL PRESENTATION

- History
  - Mallory-Weiss: history of vomiting followed by hematemesis or melena
  - Boerhaave syndrome: history of vomiting leading to chest pain
- Physical signs
  - Boerhaave syndrome: subcutaneous emphysema

DIAGNOSIS AND EVALUATION

- Mallory-Weiss: history versus endoscopy within 24 hours because may be healed if scope is delayed
- Boerhaave syndrome: chest x-ray showing unilateral effusion, mediastinal and free peritoneal air. Esophagram will show extravasation of contrast into pleural cavity. CT scan can be used if cannot tolerate contrast

TREATMENT

- Mallory-Weiss: observation, usually self-limited. Interventional endoscopy for bleeding in severe cases
- Boerhaave syndrome: intravenous (IV) fluids, antibiotics, surgery

Foreign Bodies

BASIC INFORMATION

- Ingestions of foreign bodies are a relatively common occurrence in pediatrics. Additional details of ingestions and clinical management are provided in Chapter 19
- Causes and etiology
  - Toys, screws, marbles
  - Magnets
  - Sharp objects
  - Button batteries
  - Pills (see Pill Esophagitis)
  - Food

CLINICAL PRESENTATION

- History
  - Most common between ages 6 months and 3 years
  - May present with chest pain, drooling, fussiness, vomiting, stridor, fever, dysphagia, wheezing, or feeding refusal. May also be asymptomatic
- Physical signs
  - May be no physical signs
  - Drooling, respiratory distress if impacted
  - Crepitus if has led to esophageal perforation
- Natural history
  - Weight loss, decreased oral intake
  - Recurrent aspiration pneumonia
  - Esophageal stricture
  - Tracheoesophageal fistula

DIAGNOSIS AND EVALUATION

- Initial evaluation is x-ray of neck/chest/abdomen—may miss nonradiopaque objects
- Fluoroscopic upper GI study to evaluate for filling defects
- CT scan

TREATMENT

- Urgent endoscopy for removal if:
  - Object is sharp
  - Object is >5 cm long
  - Object is a lithium or button battery (high risk of perforation and injury from electrical cause, leading to life-threatening complications such as tracheoesophageal fistula, esophageal perforation, aortoenteric fistula)
  - Food impaction (consider eosinophilic esophagitis and obtain biopsies at time of removal of food bolus)
  - Signs of respiratory distress
  - Inability to swallow secretions
- Observe for object to pass if none of the previous apply. If it does not pass for >24 hours, remove endoscopically

Bezoars

BASIC INFOMRATION

- Bezoars may complicate certain foreign body ingestions
- Definition: tightly packed collection of partially digested or undigested material
  - Trichobezoar: hair bezoar
  - Lactobezoar: milk based
- Common in patients with delayed gastric motility

Congenital Anomalies of the Stomach

- Table 30.2 reviews congenital anomalies of the stomach

Table 30.2.   Congenital Anomalies of the Stomach

	Gastric Pancreatic Heterotopia	Congenital Gastric Outlet Obstruction	Gastric Duplication	Gastric Volvulus	Congenital Microgastria
Clinical Presentation	Most common in the antrum	1. Pyloric atresia 2. Antral webs	Within the wall of the stomach along greater curvature Presents with palpable cyst, bleeding, obstruction, volvulus, perforation	Presentation triad: 1. Sudden severe epigastric pain 2. Intractable emesis 3. Inability to pass a tube into the stomach	Small, incompletely rotated stomach
Diagnosis And Evaluation	On EGD	X-ray: large dilated stomach EGD: for antral web	Upper GI series Computed tomography or ultrasound: outlines the cyst	Upper GI series CT scan	Upper GI series
Treatment	Incidental finding; no treatment	Surgical repair	Excision or partial gastrectomy	Emergency surgery	• Conservative: small feedings, NJ tube, prokinetic agents • Surgical

EGD, Esophagogastroduodenoscopy; *GI,* gastrointestinal.

Review Questions

For review questions, please go to ExpertConsult.com.

Suggested Readings

1. Blecker U, Gold BD. Gastritis and peptic ulcer disease in childhood. *Eur J Pediatr.* 1999;158:541–546.
2. Bruch SW, Coran AG. Congenital malformation of the esophagus. In: Wyllie R, Hyams JS, Kay M, eds. *Pediatric Gastrointestinal and Liver Disease.* 4th ed. Philadelphia: Elsevier Saunders; 2011:222–231.
3. Dellon ES, Gonsalves N, Hirano I, et al. ACG clinical guideline: evidence based approach to the diagnosis and management of esophageal eosinophilia and eosinophilic esophagitis (EoE). *Am J Gastroenterol.* 2013;108:679–692.
4. Feldman M, Friedman LS, Brandt LJ. Anatomy, histology, embryology, and developmental anomalies of the stomach and duodenum. In: Feldman M, Friedman LS, Brandt LJ., eds. *Sleisenger and Fordtran's Gastrointestinal and Liver Disease.* 9th ed. Philadelphia: Elsevier Health Sciences; 2010.
5. Koletzko S, Jones NL, Goodman KJ, et al. Evidence-based guidelines from ESPGHAN and NASPGHAN for Helicobacter pylori infection in children. *J Pediatr Gastroenterol Nutr.* 2011;53:230–243.
6. Kramer RE, Lerner DG, Lin T, et al. Management of ingested foreign bodies in children: a clinical report of the NASGPHAN Endoscopy Committee. *J Pediatr Gastroenterol Nutr.* 2015;60:562–574.
7. Sah B, Mamula P, Ford CA. Review of foreign body ingestion and esophageal food impaction management in adolescents. *J Adolesc Health.* 2014;55:260–266.
8. Teitelbaum JE. Mouth and esophagus. In: Kleinman RE, Sanderson IR, Goulet O, et al., eds. *Walker's Pediatric Gastrointestinal Disease.* 5th ed. Hamilton, Ontario: BC Decker; 2008:7–17.
9. Vandeplas Y, Rudolph CD, Di Lorenzo C, et al. Pediatric gastroesophageal reflux clinical practice guidelines; joint recommendations of the North American Society for Pediatric Gastroenterology, Hepatology and Nutrition (NASPGHAN) and the European Society for Pediatric Gastroenterology, Hepatology, and Nutrition (ESPGHAN). *J Pediatr Gastroenterol Nutr.* 2009;49:489–547.

31 Intestinal Disorders

MAIRE CONRAD, MD, MS and ELIZABETH CLABBY MAXWELL, MD

ABDOMINAL EMERGENCIES

Appendicitis

BASIC INFORMATION

- One of the most common surgical conditions affecting children and adults
- Requires diagnostic consideration, evaluation, and prompt surgery referral
- Results from obstruction of appendix lumen (typically by fecal matter) and development of ischemic breakdown of the mucosa from impaired blood flow
- Complicated by proliferation of gastrointestinal (GI) bacterial organisms that cause infection, gangrene, and perforation
- See also Nelson Textbook of Pediatrics, Chapter 343, "Acute Appendicitis"

CLINICAL PRESENTATION

- Classic: periumbilical pain that migrates to the right lower quadrant (RLQ)
- Anorexia, nausea, vomiting
- Fever
- Atypical: persistent periumbilical pain or hip pain (retroperitoneal position of appendix)
- Pain may temporarily improve after a perforation
- Differential diagnoses: see Table 31.1

DIAGNOSIS AND EVALUATION

- High degree of clinical suspicion if symptoms/signs present
- Laboratory studies (may be normal, and none are specific to appendicitis)
  - White blood cells (WBC) >10,000 cells/mL
  - Neutrophils >7000 cells/mL
  - Sterile pyuria
  - Elevated C-reactive protein (CRP)
  - Imaging
- Plain films—may detect:
  - Fecalith
  - Distended loop of bowel in RLQ ("sentinel loop")
  - Free air after perforation
- Ultrasound
  - Can detect noncompressible appendix, para-appendiceal fluid, abscess
  - Operator dependent
- Computed tomography (CT) scan
  - Most extensively used with high sensitivity and specificity
  - Intravenous (IV) and PO (per os) contrast ideal
  - Exposes child to ionizing radiation

TREATMENT

- Prompt referral for surgical evaluation and open versus laparoscopic appendectomy
- IV fluids
- Broad-spectrum IV antibiotics to cover gram negative and anaerobic bacteria (e.g., ceftriaxone plus metronidazole)
- Perforation/abscess: may defer appendectomy to follow a period of IV antibiotics ± percutaneous drainage

Intussusception

BASIC INFORMATION

- Anatomic condition of invagination of one segment of bowel into the lumen of an adjacent segment and distal propagation within the bowel lumen, commonly referred to as a "telescoping" motion
- Believed to be caused by unbalanced forces during a peristaltic wave that encounters a focal abnormality in the bowel wall
  - Focal abnormality may be a pathologic "lead point" but is often thought to be lymphoid hyperplasia in the bowel wall in "idiopathic" cases
- Terminology
  - Intussusceptum: advancing tube of proximal intestine
  - Intussusceptions: distal recipient intestine
- Telescoping bowel leads to compression of vascular supply and compromised venous drainage
- Most common cause of intestinal obstruction from 3 months to 6 years
  - 80% of cases in childhood are ileocolic but can occur in any location
  - 60% occur in first year of life; peak incidence between 6 and 12 months
  - Idiopathic cases more common in children under 2 years
- Cases of pathologic lead point are more common in children older than 2 years: juvenile polyp, lymphoid hyperplasia, hypertrophied Peyer's patches, lymphoma, Meckel's diverticulum, Henoch-Schönlein purpura (HSP)

CLINICAL PRESENTATION

- Symptoms of intestinal obstruction
  - Colicky abdominal pain
  - Emesis, which can be bilious
- Symptom-free periods between bouts of colic, although patients may be described as incredibly tired-appearing or lethargic between paroxysms of pain
- Classically described as a "sausage-shaped palpable abdominal mass"
- Diarrhea in 10%

Table 31.1. Differential Diagnosis for Appendicitis

Infection (Including Yersinia, Campylobacter, viral gastroenteritis)
Constipation
Volvulus
Meckel's diverticulum
Intussusception
Henoch-Schönlein purpura
Urinary tract infection
Crohn disease
Pelvic inflammatory disease
Pregnancy/Ectopic pregnancy
Ovarian cyst/torsion
Testicular torsion
Right lower lobe pneumonia
Mesenteric adenitis
Nephrolithiasis
Pyelonephritis
Neutropenic typhlitis
Lymphoma

- Hypovolemia, pallor, diaphoresis; late sign: passage of blood/mucus per rectum
- Classic triad occurs in less than one-third of patients: colicky abdominal pain, vomiting, passage of "currant jelly" stools

DIAGNOSIS AND EVALUATION

- Plain abdominal film
  - To exclude perforation
  - Although it can be normal, a paucity of gas in right abdomen or soft tissue mass indenting the colon may be seen
- Ultrasound
  - "Doughnut" or "target" sign in cross-sectional view
  - "Pseudokidney sign" in longitudinal view
- CT can diagnose but is rarely used

TREATMENT

- Nonoperative reduction
  - Air enema with fluoroscopic guidance is the preferred nonoperative strategy in most pediatric institutions
  - Hydrostatic reduction with saline or barium enema may also be used
  - Pneumatic reduction during endoscopy
  - Possible complications: perforation (especially if prolonged symptoms for >3 days), tension pneumoperitoneum
  - Enema reduction contraindicated in shock or peritonitis
- Operative reduction
  - Indications: unsuccessful nonoperative reduction, suspicion for pathologic lead point, perforation during reduction (risk of 0.5% to 1%)
  - Necrotic tissue is removed
  - Pathologic lead point resected if discovered

Malrotation of the Bowel and Volvulus

BASIC INFORMATION

- Rotational and fixation abnormalities of the intestine
- During normal development, midgut herniates out of abdominal cavity, then rotates 270 degrees counterclockwise around axis of superior mesenteric artery (SMA). Midgut reenters abdomen at 10 to 12 weeks' gestation and is fixated with the duodenal-jejunal junction fixed to posterior abdominal wall to left of the spine at the ligament of Treitz, and the cecum is fixed to the RLQ
- Absence of fixation predisposes to intestinal torsion around vascular supply and midgut volvulus
- One-third of cases are associated with congenital anomalies including intestinal atresia, web, Meckel's diverticulum, Hirschsprung disease, mesenteric cyst, extrahepatic biliary anomalies
- Congenital diaphragmatic hernia, gastroschisis, and omphalocele all have malrotation

CLINICAL PRESENTATION

- Malrotation: can be asymptomatic and incidentally found on imaging. True incidence is unknown
- Volvulus: may be acute (e.g., bilious emesis with complete obstruction) or chronic (e.g., gastroesophageal reflux, recurrent abdominal pain, vomiting, poor weight gain)
- Majority detected in first month of life but can present at any age (up to 40% detected in adulthood)

DIAGNOSIS AND EVALUATION

- Radiology testing: upper GI series is gold standard for diagnosis
- Evolving evidence on role of ultrasound but operator dependent
- Barium enema helpful in equivocal cases to look for cecum positioning
- Typically see normal bowel gas pattern on plain film
- If malrotation with volvulus, upper GI may have corkscrew appearance as contrast passes from duodenum to jejunum, or bird beak appearance at obstruction from the luminal narrowing

TREATMENT

- Correct electrolytes and volume status because acute presentation may require resuscitation
- Surgery: Ladd's procedure, even if asymptomatic, due to risk for catastrophic volvulus

Meckel's Diverticulum

BASIC INFORMATION

- Most common congenital anomaly of GI tract
- Rule of twos:
  - Occurs in 2% of population
  - ~2 feet from ileocecal valve

- 2 inches long
- Present in patients younger than 2 years old 50% of the time
  - "2 types of tissue" (usually with ectopic mucosa)
- Occurs in one to four males to every one female
- Due to incomplete obliteration of omphalomesenteric duct, resulting in outpouching of ileum on antimesenteric side at 40 to 100 cm proximal to ileocecal valve
- True diverticulum: contains all three layers of bowel wall (mucosa, muscularis, serosa)
- May contain ectopic mucosa—most commonly gastric, which can ulcerate and bleed

CLINICAL PRESENTATION

- Majority are asymptomatic
- May cause acute or chronic painless rectal bleeding due to peptic ulceration of ectopic gastric mucosa
- Alternatively, it may cause small bowel obstruction due to:
  - Lead point for intussusception
  - Prolapsed diverticulum through persistent omphalomesenteric defect
  - Volvulus of ileum around a persistent fibrous band from tip of Meckel's to umbilicus
  - Loop of intestine involved with internal hernia produced by aberrant right vitelline artery or fibrous band arising from associated mesentery
  - Incarcerated Meckel's diverticulum within inguinal hernia (Littre hernia)
- May lead to perforation and peritonitis and mimicking acute appendicitis
  - Trisomy 18 with increased risk of this

DIAGNOSIS AND EVALUATION

- Meckel's scan: technetium-99 m pertechnetate scintigraphy
  - Gastric parietal cells take up intravenously administered technetium-99, revealing gastric mucosa in RLQ
  - Give H2 receptor antagonist before study to help increase uptake and retention of tracer
  - 85% to 95% sensitivity and specificity in children; lower in adults
- Video capsule endoscopy
- Double-balloon enteroscopy
- Arteriography
- Diagnostic laparoscopy for negative workup and high clinical suspicion

TREATMENT

- Laparoscopic removal to prevent further bleeding episodes
- For incidental findings of Meckel's, removal is controversial
  - Conservative management if found incidentally by radiologic study
  - Surgical removal if found incidentally during operation for another medical issue

Necrotizing Enterocolitis

BASIC INFORMATION

- Inflammatory disease of the intestine with poorly understood pathophysiology

- Up to 10% of preterm infants <1500 g can be affected
- Has high rate of mortality

CLINICAL PRESENTATION

- Risk for necrotizing enterocolitis (NEC) high in preterm babies until 36 weeks postconception
- Up to 25% of cases can occur in term or near-term infants
- Enteral nutrition may predispose to NEC because unfed babies rarely develop it
- Highly variable presentation leads to difficult definitive diagnosis
  - Feeding intolerance
  - Abdominal distention
  - Bloody stools
  - Gastric residuals
  - Bacteremia in up to one-third of cases
  - Shock, death

DIAGNOSIS AND EVALUATION

- WBC with left shift, thrombocytopenia, disseminated intravascular coagulation (DIC)
- Electrolyte abnormalities, metabolic acidosis
- AXR: fixed dilated loop of bowel, pneumatosis intestinalis
- In certain centers, ultrasound of the bowel may provide additional diagnostic information about the presence of NEC

TREATMENT

- NPO
- IV antibiotics to prevent sepsis and peritonitis
- Gastric decompression
- Half of cases require surgical management
  - Absolute indication for surgery is pneumoperitoneum
  - Also indicated if clinical worsening in setting of maximized medical therapy
  - Repair of perforation
  - Resection of necrotic bowel

CONGENITAL INTESTINAL MALFORMATIONS

Interruption in normal embryonic development can lead to congenital intestinal malformations, commonly resulting in obstruction.

Duodenal Atresia

BASIC INFORMATION

- Incidence: 1 in 5000 to 10,000 live births
- Result of failed recanalization of duodenum after week 7 of gestation, possibly due to ischemic event or genetic factors
- Duodenal atresia is more common than jejunal and ileal atresias (see later)
- Four different types that describe the nature of atresia and whether bowel is continuous
- Commonly associated with other congenital anomalies, such as Trisomy 21, vertebral, anal atresia, trachea-esophageal,

and renal defects (VATER), malrotation, annular pancreas, biliary tract anomalies, and cardiac and mandibulofacial anomalies

CLINICAL PRESENTATION

- Prenatal polyhydramnios secondary to inability to swallow and absorb amniotic fluid
- Obstructive symptoms within first 2 days of life
  - Feeding difficulties
  - Bilious emesis
  - Abdominal distention

DIAGNOSIS AND EVALUATION

- Prenatal ultrasound
- Plain film with "double bubble": dilated proximal duodenum and stomach
- Administration of barium for upper GI study could lead to aspiration
- Could consider barium enema to look for disuse microcolon to differentiate from malrotation
- Confirmed diagnoses often require additional imaging for associated defects, including echocardiogram, renal ultrasound, and vertebral radiography

TREATMENT

- Place nasogastric or orogastric tube to decompress stomach and minimize aspiration
- Supportive management with IV fluids
- Surgery when clinically stable: side-to-side or end-to-side duodenoduodenostomy or duodenojejunostomy

Jejunal and Ileal Atresia

BASIC INFORMATION

- Occurs due to ischemic insult due to intussusception, perforation, volvulus, hernia strangulation, thromboembolism during pregnancy
- Associated with maternal smoking and cocaine use during pregnancy
- Incidence is 1 to 3 in every 10,000 live births
- Less common to be associated with other congenital anomalies
- Hereditary multiple intestinal atresia caused by autosomal recessive TTC7A mutation, which is important for intestinal epithelium and thymus development so can lead to very early onset inflammatory bowel disease and combined immunodeficiency

CLINICAL PRESENTATION

Signs and Symptoms

- Bilious emesis in first 2 days of life
- History of maternal polyhydramnios
- Abdominal distention
- Feeding difficulties
- Hyperbilirubinemia
- Distal lesions can present with failure to pass meconium

DIAGNOSIS AND EVALUATION

- Prenatal ultrasound detection of dilated, echogenic bowel and excess maternal amniotic fluid
- Abdominal x-ray (AXR): multiple dilated loops of intestine, air fluid levels
  - "Triple bubble": dilated stomach, duodenum, and proximal jejunum
  - Peritoneal calcifications suggest meconium peritonitis due to perforation
  - Raises question of meconium ileus, cystic fibrosis (CF)
- Barium enema to distinguish atresia from other obstructive disorders
  - Jejunoileal atresia typically associated with microcolon

TREATMENT

- Gastric decompression and supportive care until surgical management can be provided
- Complications:
  - Stenosis at anastomosis, short gut syndrome
  - Long-term complications may be related to prematurity, associated anomalies, infection, short gut syndrome, oral feeding intolerance
- 90% survival

Omphalocele

BASIC INFORMATION

- Midline abdominal wall defect through umbilicus involving umbilical cord
- Herniation of viscera covered by thin three-part membrane that develops at 5 to 10 weeks' gestation
- Failure of lateral abdominal wall folds
- Occurs in 1/4000 to 1/6000 live births
- Risks of dried-out viscera, hypothermia, dehydration, and infection

CLINICAL PRESENTATION

- 4- to 12-cm wall defect
- Shiny translucent membrane covering small intestine and possibly other abdominal organs
- Up to 70% have additional congenital anomalies
  - Bowel atresia
  - Chromosomal abnormalities (Trisomy 13, 18, 21)
  - Beckwith-Wiedemann syndrome
  - Cardiac anomalies
  - Renal anomalies
- Almost all will have malrotation
- Commonly have long-term intestinal dysmotility and gastroesophageal reflux

DIAGNOSIS AND EVALUATION

- Diagnosed by prenatal ultrasound—abdominal contents outside abdomen
- Should plan for delivery at tertiary care center

TREATMENT

- Immediately cover exposed viscera with sterile, moist, nonadherent dressing to maintain sterility and prevent evaporation
- Start IV fluids and antibiotics on day of life (DOL) 0
- Two management strategies of giant omphalocele
  - Staged surgical closure after multiple operations
    - Silo (Silastic funnel protecting bowel from injury, minimizing evaporation losses, visualize perfusion) used to expand abdominal capacity
  - Nonoperative delayed closure by epithelialization of the sac
    - Apply topical medication such as silver sulfadiazine, povidone-iodine, or silver nitrate to membrane to promote eschar formation, then granulation and neoepithelialization
    - Followed by repair of remaining ventral hernia neoepithelialization
- Total parenteral nutrition may be necessary if enteral feeds cannot be tolerated or if there are issues with motility
- Small omphalocele infant mortality rate: 13% to 25%
  - Higher mortality rate with giant omphalocele
    - Larger defect
    - Increased visceroabdominal disproportion
    - Higher frequency of associated anomalies
  - Other negative prognostic factors
    - Rupture of sac
    - Perinatal respiratory distress
    - Younger gestation age

Gastroschisis

BASIC INFORMATION

- Full-thickness abdominal wall defect to the right of umbilicus
- No sac or membrane covering herniated intestine
- Prevalence: 1/20,000 to 1/30,000 pregnancies

CLINICAL PRESENTATION

- ≤5-cm wall defect
- Typically only small bowel herniates, but can have other abdominal organs
- Covered by thin inflammatory peel; has abnormal, matted appearance
- 10% to 20% will also have associated intestinal anomalies such as atresia
- Almost all will have malrotation
- Commonly have intestinal dysmotility and gastroesophageal reflux

DIAGNOSIS AND EVALUATION

- Diagnosed by prenatal ultrasound—abdominal contents outside abdomen
- Thickened intestines due to chronic amniotic fluid exposure
- Elevated maternal serum alpha fetoprotein

TREATMENT

- Silo (Silastic funnel protecting bowel from injury, minimizing evaporation losses, visualize perfusion) used to expand abdominal capacity
- Surgical repair of abdominal wall defect
- Total parenteral nutrition may be necessary if cannot tolerate enteral feeds or if issues with motility
- 5% to 10% risk of adhesions
- 90% to 95% survival

Hirschsprung Disease

BASIC INFORMATION

- Disorder of distal intestinal motility
- Congenital absence of ganglion cells in the myenteric plexuses of rectum and distal colon caused by failure of normal migration of neural crest cells during fetal development (weeks 5–12)
- Extent of aganglionic segment is variable
- Abnormal innervation results in absence of relaxation of affected bowel segment, impaired propagation of peristalsis, lack of rectoanal inhibitory reflex (RAIR) upon distention of rectum
- Incidence is 1/5000 live births
- 70% of cases are isolated, and 30% have associated anomalies (e.g., neurologic, cardiovascular, urologic, other GI anomalies)

CLINICAL PRESENTATION

- Constipation and distal pseudoobstruction characterized by enlargement of proximal colon where ganglion cells are present
- Delayed passage of meconium in the neonatal period—95% of healthy infants pass meconium on day 1 of life
- 80% to 90% diagnosed in newborn period
- Symptoms/signs
  - Constipation with abdominal distention
  - Bilious emesis
  - Lack of encopresis in a constipated child
  - Normal or thin-caliber stools
- Rectal exam
  - Tight anus
  - Empty/collapsed rectal vault
- Enterocolitis
  - Foul-smelling, explosive diarrhea
  - Fever
  - Abdominal distention
  - Can progress to potentially fatal toxic megacolon/shock
    - Still at risk for this complication even after surgical correction

DIAGNOSIS AND EVALUATION

- Consider diagnosis in patients with particular presentations:
  - Delayed passage of meconium (beyond 24 to 48 hours after birth)
  - Any infant with difficulty stooling

- Constipation that develops before toilet training
- Suspected functional constipation in an older child that fails to respond to conventional therapies
- Diagnostic Testing
  - Unprepped contrast enema: caliber change between small or normal distal aganglionic segment and dilated proximal segment (transition zone)
  - Anorectal manometry demonstrating absence of RAIR
  - Rectal suction biopsy: can be done in infants without sedation – several biopsies between 2 and 4 cm above anal margin
  - Full-thickness rectal biopsy: gold standard for diagnosis but requires general anesthesia
- Pathology of rectal biopsy to confirm diagnosis
  - Absence of ganglion cells
  - Positive staining for acetylcholinesterase
  - Hypertrophic nerve fibers

TREATMENT

- Surgical resection of the aganglionic segment of bowel and reconstruction with normal proximal bowel
- Postsurgical issues
  - Constipation
  - Encopresis
  - Enuresis
  - Rarely: obstruction, fistula
- Prompt recognition and supportive management of enterocolitis

Meconium Ileus

BASIC INFORMATION

- Impacted thick meconium in distal small bowel leads to obstruction
- Associated with ileal atresia, ileal perforation, meconium peritonitis, and volvulus
- Can be the presenting feature of CF in up to 20% of cases
- Presents as abdominal distention, bilious vomiting, and no passage of meconium in newborn period
- Associated complications include malrotation, intestinal atresia, or perforation
- Treat with contrast enema and N-acetylcysteine, which may relieve obstruction if no other complication is detected
- If complicated or if enema does not relieve obstruction, proceed with surgical creation of ileostomy with N-acetylcysteine lavage

Small Left Colon Syndrome

BASIC INFORMATION

- Presents in newborn as distal intestinal obstruction similar to anatomic (imperforate anus) or functional obstruction (Hirschsprung disease)
- Barium enema demonstrates abrupt intestinal caliber transition near or at splenic flexure
- Consider diagnosis only after excluding Hirschsprung disease
- Rare finding, but half of reported cases present with maternal history of gestational diabetes mellitus

Intestinal Duplication Cyst

BASIC INFORMATION

- Cystic or tubular structures attached to intestine that share common blood supply, with lining resembling that of the GI tract (intestinal, gastric, or pancreatic tissue typically)
- Occurs in 1 in 4500 to 10,000 births
- Most commonly in jejunum and ileum, followed by colon, stomach, duodenum, and esophagus
- Can be asymptomatic or cause obstruction, chronic pain, volvulus, or abdominal mass
- If present, ectopic gastric tissue can lead to bleeding, ulceration, and perforation
- Usually diagnosed with prenatal ultrasound or on CT/MRI
- Treatment is surgical, even if the finding is incidental

Anal Atresia

BASIC INFORMATION

- Also known as imperforate anus
- Can result in:
  - Narrow anal opening
  - Anal opening in wrong location
  - Membrane covering anal opening
  - Intestine not connected to anus
  - Fistula connecting anal pouch to perineum, urethra in males or to vagina, fourchette, or bladder in females
- Incidence is 1 in 5000 live births; more common in males and with Trisomy 21 or other congenital disorders
- Frequently associated with other congenital anomalies such as VACTERL syndrome (vertebral anomalies, anal atresia, cardiac malformations, tracheoesophageal fistula, esophageal atresia, renal anomalies, limb anomalies)

CLINICAL PRESENTATION

- Anus not patent or abnormally located on physical examination of newborn
- No stool within 24 to 48 hours of birth
- Stool excreted through vagina, penis, scrotum, or urethra
- If fed or diagnosis is missed, neonate will show obstructive signs and symptoms, including vomiting and distended abdomen
- Mild anal atresia may not be apparent until age 3 years, when fecal continence is expected, because there can be abnormalities to anal sphincters

DIAGNOSIS AND EVALUATION

- Prenatal ultrasound
- Physical examination
- Requires complete evaluation for other congenital anomalies before any surgical intervention (especially anomalies associated with VACTERL)

TREATMENT

- Surgery to correct specific defect: often requires diversion colostomy and anoplasty before reconnection

INTESTINAL COMPLICATIONS

Short Bowel Syndrome

BASIC INFORMATION

- Most common cause of intestinal failure because it is often the result or a complication of congenital intestinal malformation that requires intestinal resection (e.g., NEC, volvulus)
- Reduction of functional intestinal surface area leading to nutrient, fluid, and/or electrolyte malabsorption
- Severity of complications related to short bowel syndrome varies with:
  - Length of remaining bowel
  - Presence of ileocecal valve
  - Dependence on long-term parenteral nutrition
  - Prematurity and associated comorbidities
- Management of short bowel focuses on:
  - Feeding tolerance, malnutrition, weight loss
  - Dehydration, electrolyte disturbances
  - Complications related to parenteral nutrition dependence (e.g., total parenteral nutrition cholestasis) and central line (e.g., central line infection)
- Function of remaining bowel gradually improves, typically over 5 years after loss of bowel

TREATMENT

- IV fluids, total parenteral nutrition, tube feeding
- Enteral feeding is best stimulus for intestinal adaptation
- Reduce GI secretions with acid blockade (proton pump inhibitors, H2 receptor antagonists).
- Bowel-lengthening surgical procedures and small bowel transplantation may provide palliation of disease.

Chronic Intestinal Pseudoobstruction

BASIC INFORMATION

- Severe impairment of GI propulsion resulting in symptoms suggestive of partial or complete intestinal obstruction in the absence of any lesion restricting or occluding the intestinal lumen
- Can occur in any segment of GI tract, most typically small or large intestine
- Most severe form of GI dysmotility, potentially lethal consequences
- Often delayed diagnosis
- Rare, but unknown incidence/prevalence due to frequency of misdiagnoses
- Primary or secondary causes (Table 31.2)

Table 31.2. Causes of Chronic Intestinal Pseudoobstruction

GENETIC CAUSES

- Autosomal dominant: *SOX10*
- Autosomal recessive: *RAD21, SGOL1, TYMP, POLG*
- X-linked: *FLNA, L1CAM*

SECONDARY CAUSES

- Neurologic disorders
- Metabolic, including mitochondrial disease
- Paraneoplastic syndrome
- Neurotropic viruses
- Autoimmune disorder
- Celiac disease
- Neuromuscular disorders
- Radiation enteritis
- Endocrine disorders
- Medications/drugs

CLINICAL PRESENTATION

- Can vary depending on segment of GI tract involved
- Abdominal pain and distention that worsen in severity during acute episodes of pseudoobstruction
- Nausea, vomiting, constipation, diarrhea, early satiety, anorexia
- Often presents with malnutrition due to limited oral intake to lessen symptoms and malabsorption related to altered intestinal transit due to dilated bowel loops
- Intestinal stasis can lead to small-intestinal bacterial overgrowth
- Higher risk for volvulus due to dysmotility, dilatation, adhesions, or malrotation
- Urologic involvement is often seen in pediatric cases as well

DIAGNOSIS AND EVALUATION

- Mainly clinical diagnosis after ruling out mechanical cause of obstruction
- Typically requires AXR or possible CT scan
- Evaluate for underlying diseases or drug exposures
- Endoscopy to look for luminal obstruction, celiac disease, or eosinophilic GI disorder
- GI manometry to differentiate mechanical from functional forms of subocclusion of intestine

TREATMENT

- Nutritional support
- Medications
- Intestinal transplantation

Small Intestinal Bacterial Overgrowth (SIBO)

BASIC INFORMATION

- In healthy humans, biliary and pancreatic secretions, antegrade peristalsis, and the intestinal mucus layer limit the growth and overproduction of bacteria in the small intestine, and the ileocecal valve inhibits retrograde translocation of bacteria from colon to ileum

- In states with intestinal wall injury (e.g., inflammation, radiation), dysmotility, or short bowel syndrome, patients may develop bacterial overgrowth
- May present with malabsorptive weight loss, steatorrhea (bile acid deficiency), or vitamin and mineral deficiencies (e.g., fat-soluble vitamins, Fe, B_{12})
- Diagnosis: small-intestinal aspiration and culture (demonstrates $>10^5$ colony-forming units per milliliter of bacteria)
- Glucose or lactulose breath tests to measure an increase (peak) in breath hydrogen resulting from small-intestinal bacterial fermentation before the prolonged peak from normal colonic fermentation
- Treatment strategies focused on modifying GI microbiota through the use of probiotics, ciprofloxacin, metronidazole, amoxicillin-clavulanic acid, cefoxitin

MALABSORPTIVE DISORDERS

Celiac Disease

BASIC INFORMATION

- T-cell immune-mediated systemic disorder caused by ingestion of wheat gliadin and related prolamins in barley and rye
- Genetic predisposition in individuals with human leukocyte antigen (HLA) DQ2 and/or DQ8 positivity; high concordance in twins and HLA-identical siblings
- Antitissue transglutaminase (TTG) antibodies are characteristic
- Prevalence of symptomatic celiac disease is 1/1000

CLINICAL PRESENTATION

- Intestinal symptoms/signs (variable and age-dependent):
  - Failure to thrive, chronic diarrhea, vomiting, abdominal distention, anorexia
- Extraintestinal symptoms/signs:
  - Muscle wasting, irritability, anemia, short stature, dermatitis herpetiformis (chronic, pruritic, blistering eruption over extensor surfaces around elbows, knees, and buttocks), aphthous stomatitis, enamel hypoplasia, infertility, neurologic (seizures, ataxy, polyneuropathy), idiopathic pulmonary hemosiderosis (Lane-Hamilton syndrome)
- Associated diseases:
  - Type 1 diabetes mellitus, autoimmune endocrinopathies, IgA deficiency, connective tissue disorders, Down syndrome, Turner syndrome

DIAGNOSIS AND EVALUATION

- Diagnosis is made by duodenal biopsy/histologic findings plus full remission on gluten-free diet
- Positive serologic panel that normalizes after gluten-free diet adds weight to the diagnosis

- Laboratory evaluation
  - Serologic tests
    - Anti-TTG antibodies have strong sensitivity and specificity for celiac disease
    - Endomysial antibody testing can be used if IgA TTG test is equivocal
    - Must check for IgA deficiency
    - Deamidated gliadin antibodies (IgG and IgA) added in patients <5 years old
  - HLA
    - Strong negative predictive value if DQ2 and DQ8 absent
    - Up to one-third of healthy population has at least one celiac HLA type
- Diagnostic pathology of duodenum
  - Villous atrophy, elongated crypts, increased intraepithelial lymphocytes
  - Marsh criteria developed and validated to characterize severity of histologic abnormalities
  - Histologic changes alone are not pathognomonic for celiac disease and can be seen in other enteropathies

TREATMENT

- Gluten-free diet is the cornerstone of management
- Diet must exclude wheat, rye, barley; serologic tests should normalize by ~1 year after treatment initiation
- Treat dermatitis herpetiformis with dapsone
- Symptomatic and asymptomatic patients should follow the gluten-free diet because it protects against development of malignancy (small bowel adenocarcinoma, enteropathy-associated T-cell lymphoma)

Protein-Losing Enteropathy (PLE)

BASIC INFORMATION

- Abnormal protein loss from the GI tract
- Manifestation of several GI and non-GI tract diseases
- Causes: abnormal protein leakage across the gut (mucosal erosion/inflammation), decreased protein uptake by lymphatic system, lymphatic obstruction (intestinal lymphangiectasia), metabolic (congenital disorders of glycosylation)

CLINICAL PRESENTATION

- Diarrhea: fat and/or carbohydrate malabsorption
- Edema: dependent, extremity, facial
- Pleural or pericardial effusion

DIAGNOSIS AND EVALUATION

- Clinical signs: highly variable, and determined by degree of protein loss and underlying disease process/cause
- Laboratory findings
  - Decreased serum proteins: albumin, α1-antitrypsin, ceruloplasmin, hormone-binding proteins, transferrin
  - Malabsorption of fat-soluble vitamins
  - Hypogammaglobulinemia (IgA, IgG, IgM)
  - Lymphocytopenia

- Diagnosis established noninvasively with elevation of stool a1-antitrypsin or fecal calprotectin
- Exclude urinary protein loss and liver disease as the source of low serum proteins
- Small bowel contrast study shows "stacked coins"—thickened or edematous folds
- Endoscopy: may see white specks on mucosa or mucosal inflammation

TREATMENT

- Treatment of underlying process
- Congenital disorder of glycosylation 1b is treatable with mannose
- Intestinal lymphangiectasia: treated with high-protein, low-fat diet, medium-chain fatty acid supplementation
- Fontan procedure related PLE: treatment goal to reduce systemic venous pressure medically and/or surgically

Disaccharidase Deficiencies

BASIC INFORMATION

- Disaccharidases are glycoproteins in the apical portion of the microvillus membrane of enterocytes
- Disaccharidases break down a-glycosidic linkages between monosaccharides so they can be transported across the brush border
- Four types:
  - Sucrase-isomaltase – sucrose → fructose + glucose
  - Lactase-phlorizin hydrolase – lactose → glucose + galactose
  - Maltase-glucoamylase – glucose + glucose oligosaccharides
  - Trehalase – glucose
- Etiology may be primary or secondary
  - Primary/congenital
    - Sucrase deficiency most common
    - Congenital lactase deficiency is rare
    - Intestinal biopsy often normal
  - Secondary: results from intestinal mucosal damage from insult—infection, inflammation, toxicity, radiation, celiac disease, malnutrition
    - Intestinal biopsy can be useful to find an underlying cause
    - Multiple deficiencies are common
    - Prevalence of secondary lactase deficiency
    - Increases with age (75% of adult population with adult-type hypolactasia)
    - Preterm infants with relative lactase deficiency that resolves

CLINICAL PRESENTATION

- Symptoms coincide with ingestion of the implicated disaccharide and are absent when that disaccharide is avoided
  - Nausea and vomiting
  - Abdominal pain
  - Diarrhea
  - Abdominal distention, flatulence

DIAGNOSIS AND EVALUATION

- Sucrase-isomaltase
  - Sucrose hydrogen breath test
    - 2 g/kg sucrose bolus given orally
    - Increase in breath hydrogen >20 ppm in 2 hours postingestion
    - Can have false negative if on antibiotics, abnormal motility
- Duodenal biopsies with absent sucrase activity
- Lactase (enzyme is complexed with phlorizin hydrolase)
  - Diagnosis
    - Clinical diagnosis: lack of symptoms on lactose-free diet—typically sufficient
    - Breath hydrogen test after lactose ingestion
    - Duodenal biopsies with decreased/absent lactase activity

TREATMENT

- General: avoidance of offending disaccharide; treatment of underlying cause
- Sucrase-isomaltase: low-sucrose/low-starch diet; supplemental sucrase enzyme (lyophilized *Saccharomyces cerevisiae*, liquid yeast sucrase)
- Lactase: yeast-derived lactase supplements taken with milk products

Toddler's Diarrhea

BASIC INFORMATION

- Chronic nonspecific diarrhea of childhood
- Age 6 months to 5 years
- Up to 10 loose stools, typically during the day, can occur immediately after eating
- Growth and weight gain are typically appropriate and normal
- Abdominal pain is atypical
- Lack of infection, blood in the stool
- Treatment: limit fruit juice and excessive fluid intake; increase dietary fiber

INFLAMMATORY DISORDERS

Inflammatory Bowel Disease (IBD)

BASIC INFORMATION

- Comprised of Crohn disease (CD) and ulcerative colitis (UC)
- Chronic disorder resulting in inflammation of the GI tract
- Pathogenesis: environmental exposures and a maladaptive response to GI flora generating a dysregulated inflammatory cascade in genetically susceptible individuals
- Natural history of IBD for an individual patient cannot yet be predicted

Table 31.3. Crohn Disease Versus Ulcerative Colitis

	Crohn Disease	Ulcerative Colitis
Clinical	Abdominal pain Diarrhea Perianal disease Weight loss, growth failure	Rectal bleeding Bloody diarrhea Abdominal pain No perianal disease Risk for toxic megacolon
Endoscopic	Involves any part of gastro-intestinal tract (mouth to anus) Discontinuous ("skip lesions") Rectal sparing Fistulae, abscess, stricture Linear ulcers	Colon only Continuous No rectal sparing ± Backwash ileitis No fistulae, abscess, stricture
Pathology	Transmural involvement Granulomas Crypt abscesses	Inflammation limited to mucosa No granulomas Crypt abscesses

Table 31.4. Extraintestinal Manifestations of Inflammatory Bowel Disease

Dermatologic	Pyoderma gangrenosum (UC > CD) Erythema nodosum (CD > UC) Alopecia Bowel-associated dermatosis-arthritis syndrome Oral ulcers (CD > UC)
Rheumatologic	Arthritis—peripheral, nonerosive Enthesitis Sacroiliitis Ankylosing spondylitis (UC > CD)
Ophthalmologic (CD > UC)	Uveitis Episcleritis Iritis
Hepatic/pancreas/biliary	Primary sclerosing cholangitis (UC > CD) Autoimmune hepatitis (UC > CD) Pancreatitis Cholelithiasis
Musculoskeletal	Osteopenia Osteoporosis
Hematologic	Anemia—iron deficiency or chronic disease Venous thrombosis (UC > CD)
Urologic	Nephrolithiasis
Oncologic	Increased risk of cancer

CD, Crohn disease; *UC,* ulcerative colitis.

- Crohn disease behavior often evolves after diagnosis, with increasing risk of progression from an inflammatory phenotype to stricturing and/or fistulizing disease over time

CLINICAL PRESENTATION

- Key clinical, endoscopic, and histologic features of CD and UC are highlighted in Table 31.3.
- Extraintestinal manifestations: see Table 31.4
  - Correlating with bowel disease activity: peripheral arthritis, Erythema nodosum, anemia
  - *Not* correlating with bowel disease activity: primary sclerosing cholangitis (PSC), sacroiliitis, ankylosing spondylitis

DIAGNOSIS AND EVALUATION

- Review growth chart: growth failure can be an important early sign; often precedes GI symptoms
- Laboratory evaluation
  - Typical biochemical abnormalities: leukocytosis, anemia, thrombocytosis, hypoalbuminemia
  - Serum inflammatory markers: erythrocyte sedimentation rate (ESR) and CRP often elevated
  - Laboratory analysis may be normal
  - Rule out enteric infections, including *Clostridium difficile*, before endoscopy
- Endoscopy (esophagogastroduodenoscopy and colonoscopy) with confirmatory biopsies demonstrating chronic inflammatory changes is diagnostic gold standard
- Fecal calprotectin
  - Cytosolic protein released by activated neutrophils
  - Elevated concentrations in the stool if GI inflammation is ongoing
  - Cutoff of >200 to 300 μg/g has been suggested as optimal combination of sensitivity and specificity
  - Fecal calprotectin cannot distinguish between inflammation from IBD versus infection, malignancy, or nonsteroidal antiinflammatory drug (NSAID) use; cannot determine the location of disease in the bowel; and has been found to be elevated in healthy infants and toddlers
  - Valuable as a noninvasive marker of disease activity after diagnosis
- IBD serology: several serum autoantibodies have been described in IBD
  - Atypical perinuclear antineutrophil cytoplasmic antibodies (pANCA) in UC and anti-*Saccharomyces cerevisiae* antibodies (ASCA) in CD
  - No sufficient data to support IBD serologic testing for screening evaluation of suspected IBD
- Imaging to evaluate the small bowel at diagnosis to assess for extent of disease—see Table 31.5
  - Choice depends on availability, ability of patient to cooperate with the test, radiation exposure, and cost
  - Barium enemas are generally discouraged in this population

TREATMENT

- Goals: resolution of symptoms, optimal growth, mucosal healing
- Medical treatment options: see Table 31.6
- Approach to treatment is based on disease severity
- Systemic corticosteroids are increasingly being avoided due to negative systemic side effects but may still have a role in acute management of flare (particularly in UC) once infection is excluded
- Pediatric gastroenterologists employ differing strategies for achieving and maintaining remission, with recent evidence supporting early use of biologic therapy in moderate to severe disease to spare steroids and promote mucosal healing
- Patients who present with a milder disease course do not require biologic therapy at diagnosis to induce remission

Table 31.5.   Small Bowel Imaging Options in Inflammatory Bowel Disease

	Identifies	Advantages	Disadvantages
SBFT	• Small bowel only • Bowel wall thickening • Luminal narrowing • Fistulae	• Widely available • Technically easy to perform • No sedation • Lower cost	• Low sensitivity • Low specificity • Ionizing radiation
CT/CTE	• Small and large bowel • Abscess, fistula, obstruction	• Rapid scan time • High resolution to detect subtle abnormalities • No sedation needed • Extraluminal information	• Ionizing radiation
MRI/MRE	• MRE: Small and large bowel • Pelvic MRI: perianal disease	• No radiation • Dynamic assessment of active versus chronic inflammatory changes • Extraluminal information	• Longer test • Requires patient lay still • Cannot sedate safely after enteral contrast • Expensive
US/CE-US	• Small and large bowel • Bowel wall thickening • Luminal narrowing • Intra-abdominal fluid collection/abscess	• No radiation • No sedation • Low cost • Does not require contrast • Visualize lesions out of reach of standard endoscopy;	• Operator dependent • Not widely available
VCE	Small bowel mucosal lesions including ulcers, erosions, fissures, strictures	• Older children may swallow without need for endoscopic placement/anesthesia	• No ability to biopsy • Incomplete study due to slow transit or obscured views • Risk of obstruction requiring surgical removal

CT, Computed tomography; *CE-US,* contrast-enhanced ultrasound; *CTE,* CT enterography; *MRE,* magnetic resonance enterography; *MRI,* magnetic resonance imaging; *SBFT,* upper GI with small bowel follow-through; *US,* ultrasound; *VCE,* video capsule endoscopy.

Table 31.6.   Medical Therapies in Pediatric Inflammatory Bowel Disease

Medications	Indications/Advantages	Disadvantages, Side Effects, and Risks
5-aminosalicylates • Mesalamine • Balsalazide • Sulfasalazine	Locally decreased bowel inflammation Often first-line therapy in UC Well tolerated	Headache Allergy: worsening GI symptoms (3%–5% of patients) Less efficacy data for CD
Corticosteroids	Decrease active inflammation in acute flare (particularly in UC) Immediate relief Budesonide: Enteral release/locally acting with high first pass metabolism decreasing systemic side effects	No mucosal healing Patients may develop tolerance Negative effects: growth, bone mineral density Adrenal suppression Cosmetic: hirsutism, acne, moon facies Disrupt mood, sleep Increase risk of infection
Antibiotics • Metronidazole • Ciprofloxacin	Decrease inflammation by decreasing pro-inflammatory bacteria in the GI tract Perianal disease, abscess, postoperative prophylaxis	Worsening diarrhea *Clostridium difficile* infection Antibacterial resistance
Immunomodulators • Azathioprine • 6-mercaptopurine • Methotrexate	Effective maintenance agents in UC and CD May be effective for perianal disease	Slow onset of action Risk of hepatotoxicity, leukopenia Methotrexate: highly teratogenic; nausea Risk of malignancy Live vaccines should be avoided
Biologics • Infliximab (Ifx) • Adalimumab	Blocks pro-inflammatory cytokine TNFα Mucosal healing in CD and UC Treats perianal disease Improves growth Rapid onset of action (Ifx > adalimumab)	May form antibodies: increases risk of allergic reaction and decreases efficacy Increased risk of infections Risk of malignancy Live vaccines must be avoided Risk of autoimmune symptoms/diseases: psoriasis, lupus
• Vedolizumab	Inhibit T-lymphocyte migration into tissues Gut specific—less risk of progressive multifocal leukoencephalopathy	Slower onset of effect versus biologics Very limited pediatric data
Enteral nutritional therapy	Induces remission in CD Nonimmunosuppressive	Less clear benefit in UC Sustainability/compliance in long-term use

CD, Crohn disease; *GI,* gastrointestinal; *UC,* ulcerative colitis.

Henoch-Schönlein Purpura (HSP)

BASIC INFORMATION

- Acute leukocytoclastic vasculitis with significant GI manifestations (as well skin, kidney, and joint involvement)
- See Chapter 83 for details beyond the GI-relevant information here
- GI manifestations include:
  - Colicky abdominal pain from edema and hemorrhage of the bowel wall
  - Pain worse after eating
  - Nausea, vomiting, GI bleeding (occult versus overt bleed)
  - Ileoileal intussusception
  - Perforation
  - Pancreatitis
  - Rare gallbladder involvement
- GI imaging
  - Ultrasound: bowel wall thickening, intussusception, hepatomegaly, gall bladder (GB) wall thickening
  - Barium study: thickened mucosal folds, small barium flecks (ulcers), mucosal scalloping
  - CT: bowel wall thickening, engorged mesenteric vessels
- Endoscopy
  - Grossly: erythema, edema, petechiae, erosions, ulcerations, purpura
  - Histologically: gastritis, duodenitis
  - Treatment
    - Supportive care
    - Avoid NSAIDs if renal involvement or with GI bleeding
    - Steroids have controversial role in treating GI symptoms
    - Interventions may be required for intussusception

Microscopic Colitis

BASIC INFORMATION

- Umbrella term for lymphocytic colitis and collagenous colitis
- Uncommon in children (occurs most often in middle-aged women)
- Can occur in patients with celiac disease
- Unclear etiology: medications (NSAIDs) and autoimmune conditions have implicated associations

CLINICAL PRESENTATION

- Copious watery, nonbloody diarrhea
- Cramping abdominal pain

DIAGNOSIS AND EVALUATION

- Celiac disease should be excluded (though colitis does not improve on gluten-free diet)
- Biopsies required throughout the colon (even visually normal areas)

- Histologic abnormalities: may have varied severity, ranging from absent histology to frank lymphocytic infiltration of crypts and surface epithelium

TREATMENT

- It is unclear which treatments are able to provide definitive improvement
- Possible causal medications should be stopped
- 5-ASA or budesonide may be effective therapy

OTHER INTESTINAL DISORDERS

Rectal Prolapse

BASIC INFORMATION

- Mucosal or full-thickness protrusion of rectum through the anus
- Males > females
- Etiology (underlying cause is often not identified)
  - Most common is constipation
  - Acute diarrhea
  - CF
  - Parasitic infection
  - Juvenile polyps
  - Malnutrition
  - Pelvic floor weakness
- Clinical presentation: concentric rings of rectal mucosa protruding through anal verge
- Often presents during period of toilet training
- If recurrent or pronounced, test for parasitic infection and screen for CF
- Treatment: often self-resolves but can be manually reduced
- Treat underlying/primary factor if identified
- If persistent, there are surgical options available

Hemorrhoid

BASIC INFORMATION

- Much more common in adulthood than childhood (peak incidence between 45 and 65 years)
- Arise from a plexus of dilated veins from superior and inferior hemorrhoidal veins
- Located in submucosal layer of lower rectum
- Classified by anatomic origin within the anal canal and by degree of prolapse
- Clinical presentation: often incidentally found on examination of asymptomatic child
- Symptomatic hemorrhoids uncommon in childhood, but symptoms include bleeding, prolapse, pain/discomfort, fecal soiling, and pruritus
- Common clinical settings
  - Straining from chronic constipation
  - Crohn disease
  - Anal infection that has spread to veins
  - Portal hypertension

Table 31.7. Familial Polyposis Syndromes

	Familial Adenomatous Polyposis	Juvenile Polyposis Syndrome	Peutz-Jeghers Syndrome
Genetics	▪ Prevalence 1/10,000 births ▪ Autosomal dominant ▪ *APC* gene ▪ 20%–30% spontaneous mutation	▪ Prevalence 1/100,000 ▪ Fully penetrant ▪ Several identified genes ▪ 40% spontaneous mutation	▪ Prevalence 1/50,000 to 1/200,000 live births ▪ Autosomal dominant ▪ *STK11* gene
Clinical features	▪ 100s of colorectal adenomas in childhood ▪ Almost all develop colorectal cancer without colectomy by fifth decade of life ▪ Other related malignancies: gastric fundic gland polyps in antrum and small bowel, duodenal adenomas, hepatoblastoma Extracolonic manifestations: ▪ bone: osteomas, exostosis, sclerosis ▪ teeth: impacted, unerupted, supernumerary ▪ connective tissue: desmoid tumors, intraabdominal adhesions, fibroma, subcutaneous cysts ▪ eyes: congenital hypertrophy of retinal pigment epithelium ▪ CNS: glioblastomas	*Infantile:* anemia, rectal bleeding, diarrhea, protein-losing enteropathy *Juvenile:* ▪ 50–200 colon polyps over the life span *Diagnosis:* ▪ ≥5 juvenile polyps in the colon ▪ juvenile polyps in other parts of the GI tract ▪ any juvenile polyp in a patient with positive family history of polyps Present with GI bleeding, anemia, prolapsed rectal polyps, pain, diarrhea *Extracolonic manifestations:* ▪ digital clubbing ▪ macrocephaly ▪ alopecia ▪ cleft lip/palate ▪ congenital heart disease ▪ GU abnormalities ▪ mental retardation	Mucocutaneous pigmentation/ freckling: ▪ mouth ▪ nose ▪ perianal area ▪ hands/feet Hamartomatous polyps throughout GI tract—primarily in small bowel Often present with intussusception, bleeding, anemia
Management and cancer screening	Annual colonoscopy until colectomy Colectomy eliminates risk of inevitable colorectal cancer Timing of colectomy: ▪ second to third decade of life ▪ when patient has large numbers of adenomas ▪ high-grade dysplasia	Premalignant condition with risk of cancer increasing with age Genetic workup of index cases to determine causative gene for testing of family members Surveillance colonoscopy every 2 years in affected children Colectomy for patients with cancer, dysplasia, high polyp burden	Polypectomy to prevent obstruction and intussusception Routine endoscopic surveillance by 8 years of age (earlier if symptomatic) Video capsule endoscopy preferred for small bowel evaluation At risk for other malignancies: pancreas, lung, testes, breast, uterus, ovaries, cervix

CNS, Central nervous system; *GI*, gastrointestinal; *GU*, genitourinary.

▪ Diagnosis based on history and physical examination, although anoscopy or proctosigmoidoscopy may be indicated for further assessment
▪ Goal of treatment is to address symptoms
▪ Conservative management
  ▪ Sitz baths, proper anal hygiene
  ▪ High-fiber diet, hydration, stool softeners
  ▪ Analgesics (systemic, topical)
  ▪ Short course of topical steroid
▪ Nonoperative management (ligation, sclerotherapy, ablation) or surgical treatments in refractory cases

Polyposis Syndromes

BASIC INFORMATION

▪ Two primary polyp types in pediatrics
  ▪ Adenomatous polyps: familial adenomatous polyposis
  ▪ Hamartomatous polyps
    ▪ Solitary juvenile polyp (benign)
    ▪ Juvenile polyposis syndrome
    ▪ Hamartomatous polyp syndromes
    ▪ Peutz-Jeghers syndrome

CLINICAL PRESENTATION

▪ GI symptoms

▪ Painless rectal bleeding: most common manifestation of colonic polyp
  ▪ Abdominal pain
  ▪ Altered bowel habits
  ▪ Prolapse of polyp/rectum
▪ May be asymptomatic
▪ May be part of a syndrome with other clinical features (Table 31.7)
▪ Juvenile polyp
  ▪ Solitary juvenile polyps present at a mean age of 4 years
  ▪ Up to 40% of patients will have an additional polyp, necessitating a full colonoscopic examination at the time of presentation of the first polyp
  ▪ If there is only a solitary polyp with no family history of polyps, no further screening is indicated unless there are clinical signs of a subsequent polyp

DIAGNOSIS AND EVALUATION

▪ Full colonoscopy and polypectomy to remove symptomatic polyp
▪ Careful and complete family history to identify features of polyposis syndromes, especially specifics of any cancers in the family
▪ May require genetic and/or familial cancer clinic to fully evaluate families
▪ Treatment outlined in Table 31.7

Superior Mesenteric Artery (SMA) Syndrome

BASIC INFORMATION

- Extrinsic compression of duodenum by superior mesenteric artery anteriorly and aorta posteriorly
- Thought to arise due to loss of protective fat pad after rapid weight loss

CLINICAL PRESENTATION

- Symptoms
  - Obstructive symptoms: abdominal pain, vomiting (bilious)
  - Early satiety
  - Nausea
- Clinical associations
  - Rapid weight loss
  - Orthopedic/spinal or abdominal surgery
  - Anorexia, prolonged bed rest

DIAGNOSIS AND EVALUATION

- Upper GI contrast series demonstrating cutoff of the duodenum just to the right of midline
- Duodenal obstruction may be accompanied by dilatation of proximal duodenum/stomach

TREATMENT

- Relief of obstruction
- Improved nutrition: often via nasojejunal (NJ) tube feedings
- Positioning in left lateral or prone position may relieve symptoms
- Prokinetic agents
- May require total parenteral nutrition and/or surgical management in severe cases

Review Questions

For review questions, please go to ExpertConsult.com.

Suggested Readings

1. Bauman, et al. Management of giant omphaloceles: a systematic review of methods of staged surgical vs nonoperative delayed closure. *J Pediatr Surg*. 2016;51(10):1725–1730.
2. Gangopadhyay A, Pandey V. Anorectal malformations. *J Indian Assoc Pediatr Surg*. 2015;20(1):10–15.
3. Gourlay DM. Colorectal considerations in pediatric patients. *Surg Clin North Am*. 2013;93(1):251–272.
4. Graziano K, et al. Asymptomatic malrotation: diagnosis and surgical management. An American Pediatric Surgical Association outcomes and evidence based practice committee systematic review. *J Pediatr Surg*. 2015;50(10):1783–1790.
5. Kay MA, Eng KB, Wyllie RA. Colonic polyps and polyposis syndromes in pediatric patients. *Current Opinion in Pediatrics*. 2015;27(5):634–641.
6. Morris G, Kennedy Jr A, Cochran W. Small bowel congenital anomalies: a review and update. *Curr Gastroenterol Rep*. 2016;18(4):16.
7. Rosen MJ, Dhawan A, Saeed SA. Inflammatory bowel disease in children and adolescents. *JAMA Pediatr*. 2015;169(11):1053–1060.

32 *Hepatobiliary Disorders and Liver Failure*

NICOLE A. HAMES, MD, FAAP, MICHAL ROZENFELD BAR LEV, MD and ORITH WAISBOURD-ZINMAN, MD

Approach to Elevated Liver Enzymes

- Laboratory testing of liver enzymes is used to identify liver injury and type of injury, assess liver function, and monitor for disease progression
- Causes of liver injury include infections, autoimmune processes, damage or obstruction to the biliary system, toxins, various genetic disorders, and tumors
- Laboratory data should be used along with appropriate history and physical examination
- Tests that detect liver injury:
  - Alanine aminotransferase (ALT): released from damaged hepatocytes; more specific than AST (~24 hours)
  - Aspartate aminotransferase (AST): released from damaged hepatocytes. Also found in muscle, kidney, brain, pancreas, lung, leukocytes, and red blood cells
  - Lactic acid dehydrogenase (LDH): least specific to liver injury
- Tests that detect impaired bile flow or cholestasis:
  - Alkaline phosphatase (ALK): found in liver, kidney, bone, placenta, intestine, and white blood cells (WBCs). In pediatrics, must consider linear growth
  - Gamma-glutamyl transpeptidase (GGT): found in biliary epithelia and hepatocytes, as well as kidney, brain, pancreas, spleen, and small intestine. Can be low or normal in certain pediatric cholestatic diseases (e.g., PFIC1, PFIC2, bile acid synthesis defects). Levels vary by age and are highest in neonates
  - Direct bilirubin (equals conjugated bilirubin plus delta bilirubin bound to albumin). Indicates biliary obstruction or hepatocyte dysfunction
- Tests of liver synthetic capacity:
  - Albumin: synthesized in the liver. Decreased level can be seen in starvation, gastrointestinal (GI) or kidney losses, or liver dysfunction. Half-life of 20 days
  - Prothrombin time (PT): elevated PT after administration of parenteral vitamin K indicates liver dysfunction
- Tests of hepatic metabolic function:
  - Ammonia: multiple metabolic abnormalities caused by specific inherited deficiencies of enzymes that reside almost exclusively in the liver, such as the urea cycle defects, can have a primary or secondary effect on the liver
  - See also Nelson Textbook of Pediatrics, Chapter 355, "Manifestations of Liver Disease."

Approach to Hepatomegaly

- Hepatomegaly can be transient during acute infection (e.g., Epstein-Barr virus [EBV]); however, persistent hepatomegaly requires investigation
  - Hepatomegaly can be caused by inflammation, storage (fat, various storage diseases), infiltration (tumors), or congestion
  - Liver span increases linearly with age. Hepatomegaly is defined as liver span above the normal limit for age
  - Simply noting the degree that the liver edge is below the rib margin may be misleading because of the lung hyperinflation
- If hepatomegaly is confirmed, consideration should be given to the firmness of the liver. Left lobe hypertrophy and a firm consistency are seen in advanced fibrosis/cirrhosis. Of note, in advanced cirrhosis the liver can also be small
- Look for signs of chronic liver disease on physical examination (e.g., spider angioma, palmar erythema)
- Spleen size is part of the physical examination of any liver disease. Long-standing liver disease with cirrhosis is accompanied by portal hypertension (PHTN) and, as a result, splenomegaly from congestion
  - Splenomegaly can also be seen in various storage diseases not related to cirrhosis and PHTN

Bilirubin Metabolism and Jaundice

- Bilirubin metabolism
  - Unconjugated bilirubin is end product of heme breakdown
  - Bilirubin is imported into liver, conjugated, and excreted into bile (Fig. 32.1)
  - Once excreted into small intestine, some bile acids are reabsorbed and transported back to the liver, a process called *enterohepatic circulation*
- Unconjugated hyperbilirubinemia
  - Caused by bilirubin overproduction (i.e., excessive heme breakdown; see Chapter 36), impaired hepatic uptake, or impaired conjugation of bilirubin (see Fig. 32.2)
  - Unconjugated bilirubin is not water soluble and will not appear in urine. After conjugation, excretion in the bile, and enterohepatic circulation, it will appear in the urine as urobilinogen
- Conjugated hyperbilirubinemia
  - Conjugated bilirubin >1 mg/dL if total bilirubin <5 mg/dL or conjugated bilirubin >20% of total if serum bilirubin >5 mg/dL

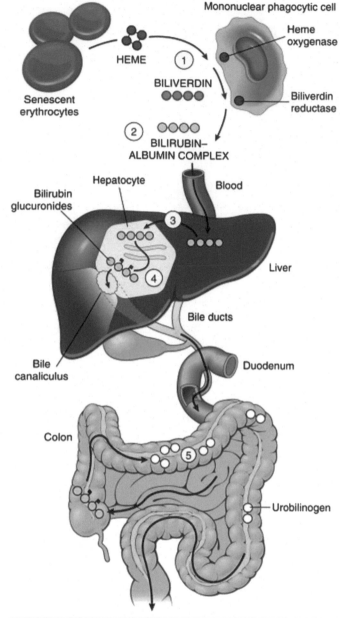

Fig. 32.1. Bilirubin metabolism and elimination. (From Kumar V, Abbas AK, Aster JC. *Robbins basic pathology*, 9th ed. Philadelphia, PA: Elsevier; 2013, p. 605, Fig. 15-1.)

- Conjugated hyperbilirubinemia is never normal
- Results from impaired excretion of conjugated bilirubin into biliary system or from mechanical obstruction of bile flow
- Conjugated bilirubin is water soluble and will be excreted in the urine and thus cause dark urine. When there also is an obstruction of bile flow, the stool is acholic (see Table 32.1)
- Differential diagnosis is broad (see Fig. 32.3)

Neonatal Jaundice

BASIC INFORMATION

- Majority of infants have elevated serum bilirubin concentrations in the first week of life
- Physiologic jaundice

Table 32.1. Features of Prehepatic, Hepatic, and Posthepatic Jaundice

Type of Jaundice	Prehepatic Jaundice	Hepatic Jaundice	Posthepatic Jaundice
Unconjugated bilirubin	Elevated	Elevated	Normal
Conjugated bilirubin	Normal	Elevated	Elevated
Urine Color	Normal	Dark	Dark
Stool Color	Normal	Normal	Pale/Acholic

- Term used to describe a large number of otherwise healthy infants with jaundice
- Etiology is multifactorial, including increased bilirubin production (polycythemia, shorter half-life of fetal red blood cells) and decreased conjugation (decreased glucuronyl transferase activity) and excretion of bilirubin (decreased stooling)
- Pathologic jaundice
  - Jaundice is considered pathologic if any of the following is true:
    - Jaundice develops before 24 hours of life
    - Jaundice persists beyond 10 days of life
    - Serum bilirubin exceeds 12 mg/dL
    - Conjugated bilirubin is equal to or greater than 20% of total serum bilirubin
- Differential for neonatal jaundice is often organized by pathophysiologic categories (see Figs. 32.2 and 32.3) or by postnatal age (Table 32.2) because several diagnoses have distinct time courses of presentation

CLINICAL PRESENTATION

- Jaundice can become clinically apparent when bilirubin concentrations are greater than 2 mg/dL
- Jaundice is often apparent first in head and neck and progresses in a cephalopedal direction; however, visual assessment has not been shown to be a reliable method for detecting significant hyperbilirubinemia in infants
- At higher bilirubin levels, infants can present with poor feeding and lethargy
- Kernicterus or bilirubin encephalopathy describes the acute (poor feeding, high-pitched cry, hypotonia), subacute (seizures, hypertonia, irritability), and chronic (extrapyramidal disorders, hearing loss, paralysis of upward gaze) neurotoxic effects of hyperbilirubinemia (unconjugated) in infants

DIAGNOSIS AND EVALUATION

- Bilirubin level (serum or transcutaneous) should be monitored in all newborns
- Risk factors: any jaundice in the first day of life, jaundice in a sibling, ABO or Rh incompatibility, gestational age <38 weeks, cephalohematoma, exclusive breastfeeding, Asian/Indian ethnicity, G6PD deficiency
- Pregnant women should have blood type, Rh status, and direct Coombs
- If mother is not tested or baby has pathologic jaundice, the baby should have blood type, Rh status, and direct Coombs testing; can be done from cord blood when available

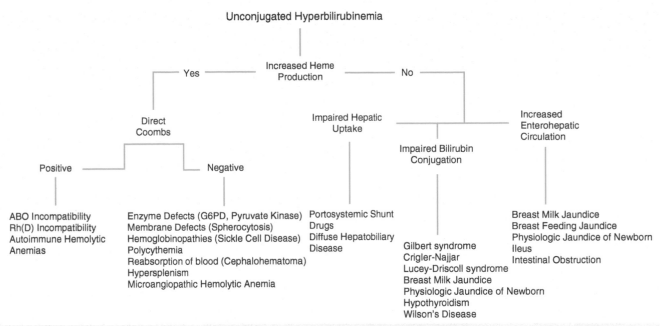

Fig. 32.2. Causes of unconjugated hyperbilirubinemia.

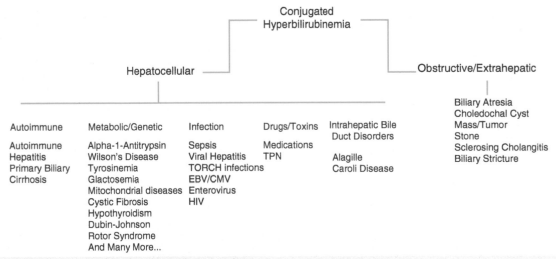

Fig. 32.3. Causes of conjugated hyperbilirubinemia.

- Initial laboratory testing includes fractionated bilirubin (conjugated and unconjugated), complete blood count (CBC), reticulocyte count, blood type and Coombs, blood smear, and electrolytes if there is concern about dehydration
- Consider G6PD testing in boys
- Check newborn screen
- Less common laboratory evaluation to consider depending on history and initial response to treatment includes hemoglobin electrophoresis, thyroid function tests, liver enzymes, PT/PTT (partial thromboplastin time), blood culture and urine culture, urine for reducing substances, urine organic acids, and serum amino acids
- Liver ultrasound (US) or other hepatobiliary imaging are often reserved for conjugated hyperbilirubinemia (see Neonatal Cholestasis section) or severe/refractory cases

TREATMENT

- Identify and treat the underlying cause of jaundice
- Treatment for unconjugated hyperbilirubinemia includes phototherapy and exchange transfusion
- Phototherapy
  - Blue-green light causes photoisomers and oxidation products, which are excreted more readily in the urine
  - Safest and most effective way to decrease serum bilirubin levels and risk of kernicterus
  - Use American Academy of Pediatrics (AAP) guidelines published phototherapy nomogram for infants >35 weeks of age to determine when phototherapy is indicated
  - Phototherapy is initiated much earlier for infants less than 35 weeks of age or with birth weight less than 2000 g

Table 32.2.   Causes of Neonatal Jaundice and Age of Onset

Age	Less Than 24 Hours of Life	2 Days to 2 Weeks of Life	Greater Than 2 Weeks of Life
Causes of Jaundice	ABO Incompatibility Rh Incompatibility G6PD deficiency Pyruvate kinase deficiency Hereditary spherocytosis Congenital TORCH infections	Physiologic jaundice of newborn Breastfeeding jaundice Breast milk jaundice Polycythemia Cephalohematoma Infection (UTI, sepsis) Crigler-Najjar Type I and Type II Lucey-Driscoll syndrome Gilbert syndrome	Breast milk jaundice Infection (UTI, sepsis) Hypothyroidism Pyloric stenosis Neonatal hepatitis Cholestasis syndromes

- Side effects of phototherapy include diarrhea, rash, fluid losses, temperature instability, and bronze baby syndrome
- Bronze baby syndrome: rare, reversible complication of phototherapy; gray-brown discoloration of skin, serum, and urine, as well as hepatic dysfunction
- Exchange transfusion: if serum bilirubin remains above the exchange transfusion threshold despite initiation of intensive phototherapy (refer to AAP guidelines published nomogram for exchange transfusion)
- Other treatment options that can be utilized in specific conditions and that are discussed in appropriate sections below

Breastfeeding Jaundice

BASIC INFORMATION

- Decreased milk intake in a breastfeeding infant results in decreased stool output, decreased excretion of bilirubin in the stool, and increased enterohepatic circulation
- Presents between days 2 and 7 of life, usually in exclusively breastfed infants
- Associated with decreased stools and can have decreased wet diapers and excessive weight loss from birth weight
- Encourage breastfeeding at least 8 to 12 times per day for first week of life
- Consider intravenous (IV) fluids or formula supplementation if there is dehydration and limited breast milk supply
- Phototherapy as indicated based on risk factors, age, and bilirubin level

Breast Milk Jaundice

BASIC INFORMATION

- Biochemical cause of breast milk jaundice remains incompletely understood
- Increased enterohepatic circulation and decreased activity of glucuronyl transferase enzyme are suspected mechanisms
- Onset around day 5 to 10 of life, peaks at 1 to 2 weeks of life, and can last up to 3 to 12 weeks of life
- Often does not reach bilirubin levels that require treatment unless other risk factors are present

- Temporary interruption of breastfeeding for 48 hours is rarely needed but may be tried for higher bilirubin levels
- Phototherapy as indicated based on risk factors, age, and bilirubin level

Gilbert Syndrome

BASIC INFORMATION

- Mutation in promoter region of gene encoding UGT1A1 enzyme responsible for glucuronidation, resulting in <50% normal enzyme activity
- Autosomal recessive inheritance
- 8% of the general population has Gilbert syndrome

CLINICAL PRESENTATION

- Episodic jaundice during fasting, illness, physical stress
- Physical examination, other than jaundice, is normal

DIAGNOSIS AND EVALUATION

- Mild unconjugated hyperbilirubinemia (typically <5 mg/dL); otherwise normal liver enzymes
- Biopsy not needed for diagnosis but will show normal liver with decreased UGT enzyme staining
- Most cases will be diagnosed clinically. Genetic sequencing of *UGT1A1* gene available for atypical cases

TREATMENT

- Benign course; no treatment necessary

Crigler-Najjar

BASIC INFORMATION

- Mutation in gene encoding UGT1A1 bilirubin-conjugating enzyme (in Gilbert syndrome the mutation is in the promotor of the same gene), resulting in completely absent (type I) or <10% activity (type II)
- Autosomal recessive inheritance

CLINICAL PRESENTATION AND DIAGNOSTIC EVALUATION

- Type I: severe unconjugated hyperbilirubinemia (total bilirubin 15–45 mg/dL), progressive jaundice from birth, high risk of kernicterus
- Type II: moderate unconjugated hyperbilirubinemia (total bilirubin 8–25 mg/dL), slightly lower incidence of kernicterus
- Liver function testing otherwise normal; liver biopsy is seldom necessary but would show a normal liver with decreased UGT staining
- Sequencing UGT1A gene can confirm diagnosis

TREATMENT

- Type I
  - Lifelong phototherapy
  - May need exchange transfusion
  - Definitive therapy is liver transplant
- Type II
  - Phototherapy
  - Phenobarbital to induce remaining enzyme activity
  - Oral binding agents (e.g., cholestyramine)

Rotor Syndrome

BASIC INFORMATION

- Defective transporter for hepatocyte reuptake of conjugated bilirubin circulating in liver sinusoids
- Autosomal recessive inheritance
- Presents with episodic jaundice, or icterus; otherwise a normal examination
- Increased with pregnancy and steroid hormones
- Initial laboratory evaluation: conjugated hyperbilirubinemia; otherwise normal liver enzymes
- Follow-up evaluation reveals increased total urine coproporphyrin levels; biopsy usually not required (would show normal liver with absent staining for defective enzyme); genetic sequencing rarely performed
- Benign course; no treatment

Dubin-Johnson Syndrome

BASIC INFORMATION

- Defective transporter resulting in impaired excretion of conjugated bilirubin into bile
- Autosomal recessive inheritance
- Presents with chronic mild jaundice/icterus; may have mild hepatomegaly
- Increased with pregnancy and steroid hormones
- Initial laboratory evaluation: mixed hyperbilirubinemia
- Follow-up evaluation: total urinary coproporphyrin excretion is normal, but predominance of coproporphyrin I; biopsy not needed (grossly liver is black; histology is normal except for dense pigmentation); can sequence gene for transporter
- Benign course; no treatment

Table 32.3. Risk Factors for Cholelithiasis in Children
RISK FACTORS
Age: rises through adolescence
Gender: 3:1 female to male ratio
Obesity
Hemolytic disease: sickle cell disease, thalassemias, and any other cause of chronic hemolysis
Genetics: Hispanic and Native American ethnicity have increased risk, other genetic diseases
Biliary stasis: lack of gallbladder stimulation such as in long-term total parenteral nutrition
Ileal disease/resection: causes malabsorption of bile salts and limits bile salt pool
Medications: oral contraceptives, ceftriaxone, furosemide, cyclosporine, and others
Pregnancy
Hypertriglyceridemia
Cystic fibrosis

OBSTRUCTIVE BILIARY DISEASES

Cholelithiasis

BASIC INFORMATION

- Overall incidence is rising
- See Table 32.3 for risk factors
- Types of stones:
  - Cholesterol stones:
    - Increased cholesterol secretion or decreased bile secretion
    - Stones >50% cholesterol by weight
    - Yellow-white in color
    - Radiolucent
  - Bilirubin stones:
    - Increased unconjugated bilirubin and calcium
    - Black or brown in color
    - Mostly radiopaque
  - Mixed stones:
    - Mixed pathophysiology with increased bile pigment as well as cholesterol
    - Often seen with biliary tract infection
    - Brown to orange in color

CLINICAL PRESENTATION

- Often asymptomatic: asymptomatic stones detected in up to 50% of children
- Symptomatic cholelithiasis: also known as biliary colic; right upper quadrant (RUQ) or epigastric pain with nausea and vomiting; worse with fatty foods
- Choledocholithiasis: consider when increased direct/conjugated bilirubin and/or dilation of the common bile duct
- Can also cause biliary pancreatitis

DIANGOSIS AND EVALUATION

- US to look for stones or dilatation of biliary tree
- X-ray is insensitive because many stones are radiolucent

- MRCP (magnetic resonance cholangiopancreatography) is more sensitive if common bile duct stones are suspected
- Laboratory results may suggest complications described previously: elevated bilirubin, or elevated pancreatic enzymes if biliary pancreatitis, and so forth

TREATMENT

- Cholecystectomy:
  - Laparoscopic when possible
  - Evaluate risk of common bile duct stone because this may change the approach (i.e., preoperative endoscopic retrograde cholangiopancreatography [ERCP] or intraoperative common bile duct [CBD] exploration)
- ERCP: for common bile duct stones; may extract stone and sphincterotomy or dilation of papilla
- Medical:
  - Ursodiol: decrease cholesterol saturation, typically improve symptoms, may dissolve the stones themselves
  - Other less commonly used options: antibiotics, extracorporeal shock wave lithotripsy

Cholecystitis

BASIC INFORMATION

- Etiology: gallbladder stasis is common to all causes
  - Gallstones are primary cause in most cases
  - Acalculous cholecystitis is associated with severe illness or underlying condition; represents higher proportion of cholecystitis in pediatric patients
  - External compression of biliary tree
  - Structural abnormalities
  - Trauma

CLINICAL PRESENTATION

- Fever, RUQ pain, and leukocytosis
- Murphy sign: pain and inspiratory arrest when palpating in area of gallbladder during inspiration
- Elevated direct and total bilirubin, although marked elevation of bilirubin, GGT, and ALK should raise suspicion of choledocholithiasis
- Transaminases are normal or slightly elevated

DIAGNOSIS AND EVALUATION

- US to look for gallstones, gallbladder wall thickening, pericholecystic fluid, and sonographic Murphy sign
- Hepatobiliary iminodiacetic acid (HIDA) scan: sensitive but occasional false positive results

TREATMENT

- NPO, IV fluids, analgesia
- Antibiotics often used but of questionable benefit
- Acalculous cholecystitis can often be managed nonoperatively
- Cholecystectomy
  - Laparoscopic is preferred

- Timing is controversial; if symptoms improve with medical treatment, often done in the first 1 to 2 weeks after presenting

CHOLESTATIC LIVER DISEASES

Neonatal Cholestasis

BASIC INFORMATION

- Cholestasis is defined as reduced bile flow resulting in retention of biliary substances within the liver normally excreted into bile and intestinal lumen
- Cholestasis is always pathologic, and prompt differentiation is mandatory. Some causes are treatable when addressed in a timely manner
  - Any formula-fed icteric infant at 2 weeks of age should be evaluated for cholestasis with total serum bilirubin and direct bilirubin level
  - Breastfed otherwise healthy infants can be followed clinically for mild jaundice until 3 weeks of age, at which time they should undergo laboratory evaluation if they appear icteric
  - Preterm infants are at high risk for cholestasis due to prolonged parenteral nutrition. However, they should have full evaluation for cholestasis as do term infants
- It affects 1:2500 term infants
- The most common causes are biliary atresia (BA) (25%–40%) and an array of uncommon genetic disorders (25%)
- Treatable causes that can present with cholestasis and should be diagnosed early include BA, bacterial sepsis, galactosemia, tyrosinemia, panhypopituitarism, bile acid synthetic defects, and obstructive gallstones

CLINICAL PRESENTATION

- Elements of the history and physical examination may be able to provide clues as to the underlying etiology for neonatal cholestasis (see Table 32.4)

APPROACH TO EVALUATION

- May be divided into intrahepatic disease, such as injury to hepatocytes or bile ducts (infectious, metabolic, "idiopathic," paucity of intrahepatic bile ducts), and extrahepatic disease, such as extrahepatic bile duct injuries or obstruction (e.g., BA; see Table 32.5 for differential diagnosis)
- Initial evaluation should include:
  - Characteristics and severity of liver disease:
    - Glucose, ALT, AST, GGT, total direct serum bilirubin, and total protein, as well as liver synthetic function (albumin, PT/INR [international normalized ratio])
  - Bacterial cultures: as dictated by clinical assessment
  - Evaluate treatable causes: tyrosinemia, galactosemia, thyroid-stimulating hormone (TSH), FT4, cortisol (review local newborn screen)
  - Fasting abdominal US with Doppler evaluates for structural abnormalities (e.g., choledochal cyst, BA)

Table 32.4. Clues to Diagnosis of Neonatal Cholestasis

FAMILY HISTORY

Consanguinity	Autosomal recessive disorders
Cholestasis in parents or siblings	CF, A1AT deficiency, PFIC, Alagille, other genetic conditions
Repeat fetal loss/early demise	Gestational alloimmune liver disease
Spherocytosis/other hemolysis	Aggravate conjugated hyperbilirubinemia

PRENATAL HISTORY

Ultrasound findings	Choledochal cyst, absent gallbladder
Cholestasis of pregnancy	PFIC, mitochondrial disorders
Acute fatty liver of pregnancy	Neonatal LCHAD deficiency
Maternal infection	TORCH

INFANT HISTORY

Prematurity	Risk of neonatal hepatitis
Small for gestational age	Risk of cholestasis, TORCH
Alloimmune hemolysis, G6PD deficiency, hydrops fetalis	Increased risk for cholestasis
Infection	UTI, CMV, HIV, sepsis, TORCH
Newborn screen	Tyrosinemia, galactosemia (United States)
Nutrition	Galactosemia, inherited fructose intolerance, parenteral nutrition associated
Growth	Genetic/metabolic disease
Vision	Septo-optic dysplasia
Hearing	PFIC1, TJP2
Vomiting	Metabolic diseases, bowel obstruction, pyloric stenosis
Stooling	Delayed: CF, panhypopituitarism; Diarrhea: infection, metabolic Acholic: obstructive
Urine	Dark: cholestasis; metabolic disease
Excessive bleeding	coagulopathy, vitamin K deficiency
Irritability, lethargy	metabolic disease, sepsis, panhypopituitarism
Abdominal surgery	Necrotizing enterocolitis, intestinal atresia

PHYSICAL SIGNS

Ill-appearing	Sepsis, metabolic disease
Situs inversus, dextrocardia	Biliary atresia
Congenital heart defects	Allagile
Dysmorphism	Allagile
Large anterior fontanelle	Hypothyroidism
Hepatosplenomegaly	Hypothyroidism
Splenomegaly	Storage, hematologic diseases
Absent red reflexes (congenital cataract)	Galactosemia
Direct visualization of stool pigment	Acholic: obstructive

CF, Cystic fibrosis; CMV, cytomegalovirus; PFIC, familial intrahepatic cholestasis.

- Targeted evaluation is based on the index of suspicion as supported by the history and physical examination
  - Metabolic: ammonia, lactate, cholesterol, urine for organic acids, urine for bile salts
- ID: polymerase chain reaction (PCR) for cytomegalovirus (CMV), herpes simplex virus (HSV), listeria
- Genetic: whole exome sequencing, sweat test, *CFTR* testing
- Imaging: spinal x-ray (vertebrae), echocardiogram, cholangiogram
- Liver biopsy
- Consultations: ophthalmology, cardiology, metabolic/genetic, surgery, nutrition

TREATMENT

- Nutrition is paramount
  - Medium chain triglycerides (MCT) do not require bile salts for intestinal absorption and should be supplemented (MCT-based formula or supplementation)
  - Fat-soluble vitamin deficiencies are common and should be evaluated and replaced early
- Pruritus is common secondary to elevated circulatory bile acids
  - Ursodeoxycholic acid may help improve bile flow
  - Antipruritic drugs may improve symptoms
    - Cholestyramine, rifampin, phenobarbital, naltrexone
  - Partial external biliary diversion is a surgical conduit that drains the gallbladder out to the skin
- Treatment of complications (e.g., PHTN, ascites, variceal hemorrhage, hypersplenism)
- Liver transplantation when indicated

Biliary Atresia (BA)

BASIC INFORMATION

- The most common identifiable cause of jaundice in the first 3 months of life. 1:6000 in Taiwan, 1:12,000 in the United States, 1:19,000 in Canada, and 1:18,000 in Europe
- Three groups:
  - 84% nonsyndromic
  - 6% syndromic with at least one malformation but no laterality defect (e.g., situs inversus)
  - 10% syndromic with laterality defect—common splenic anomalies
- Most cases (85%) comprise an obliteration of the entire extrahepatic biliary tree
- Etiology unknown. Theories include an intrauterine insult due to genetic, viral, toxin, or autoimmune-mediated process
- Screening infants after birth is not universal. In high-risk locations (Taiwan), stool color cards that help detect acholic stools are used

CLINICAL PRESENTATION

- Usually appear otherwise healthy at birth and initially grow normally, which may deceive the parents or physician into believing that the jaundice is physiologic or due to breast milk
- Acholic stools

Table 32.5.   Differential Diagnosis of Neonatal Cholestasis

Disease	Presentation	Gene(s)
MULTISYSTEM DISEASE		
Alagille syndrome	GGT, cholesterol increased; eye, cardiac, vertebral anomalies Liver biopsy: paucity of bile duct (may be normal in first months)	*JAG1; NOTCH2*
ARC (arthrogryposis - renal dysfunction - cholestasis) syndrome	Lax skin, limb contracture, renal tubular acidosis, normal GGT	*VPS33B; VIPAR*
CDG (congenital disorder of glycosylation)	Multisystemic	Numerous genes
Cystic fibrosis	Elevated sweat chloride; liver biopsy: possible ductular proliferation	*CFTR*, chloride channel
Mitochondrial disorders	Multisystemic	Nuclear and mitochondrial genes
Neonatal ichthyosis sclerosing cholangitis syndrome	Hypotrichosis, alopecia, cholestasis	*Claudin-1* CLDN1
Hypothyroidism	Treatment with Eltroxin	
Panhypopituitarism	Low pituitary hormones, adrenal insufficiency, septo-optic dysplasia, liver biopsy: paucity of bile ducts MRI: microadenoma or absent sella	
Trisomy 21	Typical stigmata	Unknown
EXTRAHEPATIC BILE DUCT ABNORMALITIES		
Biliary Atresia	Acholic stools; liver biopsy: proliferation of bile ducts, bile plugs; US: possible absence of gallbladder; 5%–10% other malformations/situs inversus	Unknown
Choledochal cyst	Abdominal mass; US: cyst	
Choledocholithiasis	Acholic stools; US: stones	*ABCB4/MDR3*
Perforation of common bile duct	Ascites without liver disease	
Neonatal sclerosing cholangitis	Rare. Increased GGT; liver biopsy: small duct destruction; cholangiography: pruning of small bile ducts May progress to biliary cirrhosis	Autosomal recessive. Gene unknown
HEPATOCELLULAR DISEASE		
Alpha-1 antitrypsin deficiency	Accumulation of A1AT in ER of hepatocytes. Increased GGT, low serum A1AT, ZZ or SZ variants	Autosomal recessive; SERPINA1 antiprotease
Bile acid synthetic defects/ Conjugation defect	Normal GGT, cirrhosis, fat-soluble vitamins deficiency, Dx: analysis of urinary bile acids Tx: oral bile acid supplementation	*CYP7B1; AKRID1 (SRD5B1)*, HSD3B7, BAAT, BAL
PFIC1	Normal GGT; diarrhea, failure to thrive; liver biopsy/EM helpful	*ATP8B1*: canalicular and intestinal floppase
PFIC2	Normal GGT; liver biopsy/EM helpful	*ABCB11*, defect in bile salt export pump (BSEP)
PFIC3	Increased GGT May present later in life	*ABCB4, MDR3* deficiency affecting phosphatidyl-choline extraction into bile
Tight junction protein 2 mutation	Severe cholestasis	*TJP2*
Aagenaes syndrome	Familial cholestasis with lymphedema of lower limbs. >50% normal life span	Chromosome 15q
Transient neonatal cholestasis (neonatal hepatitis)	GGT, ALK 200–400; ALT AST 80–200 IU/L; liver biopsy negative for obstruction	*PFIC* polymorphism
INBORN ERRORS OF METABOLISM		
Urea cycle defects		
Citrin deficiency	Normal liver enzymes	*SLC25A13*
OTC deficiency	Hyperammonemia	*OTC*
Carbohydrate metabolism		
Galactosemia	Cholestasis and liver dysfunction Congenital cataract *E. coli* sepsis	GALT, galactose-1 phosphate uridyltransferase
Amino acid metabolism		
Tyrosinemia type 1	May present with liver failure, Fanconi-related nephropathy, or seizures Urine: elevated succinylacetone Treatment: NTBC	FAH, fumaryl acetoacetate hydrolase
Lipid metabolism		

Table 32.5.   Differential Diagnosis of Neonatal Cholestasis—cont'd

Disease	Presentation	Gene(s)
Niemann-Pick type C	Splenomegaly	*NPC1*, acid sphingomyelinase
Lysosomal acid lipase deficiency (Wolman)	Hepatomegaly, hepatic steatosis, liver failure; US: hyperechoic liver	*LIPA*
INFECTIONS		
TORCHES	Toxoplasma, rubella, CMV, herpes simplex virus, syphilis, hepatitis ABC	
Bacteremia, sepsis		
Urinary tract infection		
Others		
Idiopathic neonatal cholestasis	Familial or sporadic	Unknown
Zellweger syndrome	Progressive degeneration of liver and kidney, marked hypotonia	Peroxisomal disorder; autosomal recessive
Gestational Alloimmune Liver Disease	Iron deposition in liver, heart, and endocrine glands leading to multiorgan failure and death. Tx: IVIG in next pregnancies	Maternal Ab directed against fetal liver

CMV, Cytomegalovirus; *GGT,* gamma-glutamyl transpeptidase; *IVIG,* intravenous immunoglobulin; *MRI,* magnetic resonance imaging; *US,* ultrasound.

DIAGNOSIS AND EVALUATION

- Abdominal US is useful in excluding choledochal cyst or gallstone disease causing extrahepatic bile duct obstruction. It may demonstrate an absent or abnormal gallbladder or other features suggestive, but not diagnostic, of BA
  - "Triangular cord sign" may be seen representing a cone-shaped fibrotic mass cranial to the bifurcation of the portal vein
- Limited specificity precludes the use of hepatobiliary scintigraphy as a stand-alone test. Definitively demonstrable bile flow decreases likelihood of BA
- Limited specificity of MRCP, ERCP, Percutaneous transhepatic cholecysto-cholangiography (PTCC) provides a limited role in diagnosis of BA
- Liver biopsy demonstrates histopathologic findings of bile duct proliferation, bile plugs, and fibrosis; is the most supportive test in the evaluation of BA
- Intraoperative cholangiography and histologic examination of the duct remnant are the gold standard to diagnose BA

TREATMENT

- Treatment of BA is surgical reestablishment of bile flow with Kasai hepatoportoenterostomy (HPE)
  - Timely diagnosis is important to optimize the response to the HPE; if performed within the first 60 days of life, 70% will establish bile flow; after 90 days of life, less than 25% will have bile flow
  - Survival rates with native liver decrease as the age at surgery increases from less than 45 days to 90 days

Alagille Syndrome (ALGS)

BASIC INFORMATION

- An autosomal dominant multisystem disorder
- The most common form of familial intrahepatic cholestasis (1:30,000)

- Mutations *JAG1* and *NOTCH2* are found in 95% and 5% of patients with ALGS, respectively

CLINICAL PRESENTATION

- Clinical criteria for the diagnosis include:
  - Cholestatic jaundice with paucity of bile ducts on liver biopsy
    - Jaundice may improve with age
  - Alagille facies (broad forehead; small, pointy chin)
  - Posterior embryotoxon on eye examination
  - Butterfly vertebrae
  - Renal disease
  - Cardiac defects (most commonly peripheral pulmonic stenosis or tetralogy of Fallot)

DIAGNOSIS AND EVALUATION

- Evaluate for associated abnormalities
- Laboratory workup
  - GGT extremely elevated (×20 upper limits of normal [ULN])
  - Elevated ALT and serum bile acids
- Liver biopsy: paucity of bile ducts
  - May be normal until 6 months of age

Choledochal cyst

BASIC INFORMATION

- Five subtypes of saccular dilatation in the intrahepatic and/or extrahepatic biliary tree
- Presentation: jaundice, acholic stools, and palpable abdominal mass
  - May present with cholangitis
- Diagnosis: abdominal US, MRCP
- A diagnosis of choledochal cyst in a cholestatic neonate should always prompt careful evaluation for BA
- Increases risk for cholangiocarcinoma
- Treatment: surgical resection

Cholestasis Beyond Infancy

BASIC INFORMATION

- The most common causes for cholestasis in the older child are acute viral hepatitis and exposure to hepato-toxic drugs or herbs
  - Causes for neonatal cholestasis described earlier should also be excluded
- Other causes that are more specific in the older child include:
  - Biliary obstruction: cholelithiasis; biliary cyst with complications (e.g., cholangitis, stricture, cholangio-carcinoma)
  - Genetic-metabolic:
    - Wilson disease
      - 40% to 60% will present with symptoms during the second decade
    - Alpha-1 antitrypsin deficiency
    - PFIC
  - Autoimmune:
    - Autoimmune hepatitis/sclerosing cholangitis
    - Inflammatory bowel disease—associated

Autoimmune Liver Disease (AILD)

BASIC INFORMATION

- Chronic hepatic inflammation; immune mediated; manifested by elevated serum aminotransferase levels, liver-associated autoantibodies, and hypergammaglobulinemia
- Signs of chronicity
  - Duration of liver disease more than 3 to 6 months
  - Evidence of chronic decompensation (low albumin and platelet count)
  - Physical stigmata of chronic liver disease (clubbing, spider telangiectasia, splenomegaly, ascites)
- Three types of AILD:
  - Autoimmune hepatitis (AIH): hepatocyte specific
  - Autoimmune sclerosing cholangitis (AISC): cholangio-pathy, intra- and extrahepatic
    - May overlap with AIH
  - De novo hepatitis: in liver transplant recipients whose initial disease was not autoimmune
- Etiology: activation of immune system by a triggering factor in genetically susceptible individuals
  - Risk factors: HLA DR3 DR4 DR7; AIRE mutation (autoimmune polyendocrinopathy candidiasis ectodermal dystrophy)

CLINICAL PRESENTATION

- Wide spectrum: asymptomatic, fulminant hepatic failure, subtle complaints (fatigue, malaise, behavioral changes, anorexia, amenorrhea), cirrhosis with stigmata of chronic liver disease (ascites, bleeding varices, encephalopathy)
- Extrahepatic manifestations: arthritis, vasculitis, nephritis, thyroiditis, Coombs-positive anemia, rash

Table 32.6. Clinical and Laboratory Features of Autoimmune Hepatitis

	AIH type 1	AIH type 2
Auto-Abs	ANA Anti-smooth muscle Anti-soluble liver Ag Atypical pANCA	Anti-LKM1 Anti-liver cytosol 1 Anti-LKM3
Age	Any age	Children and young adults
Gender	Female 75%	Female 95%
Other autoimmunity	Common	APECED (Autoimmune Polyendocrinopathy Candidiasis Ectodermal Dystrophy)
Severity	Variable	Severe
Histopathology at presentation	Mild to cirrhosis	Advanced
Tx failure	Not frequent	Frequent
Relapse post drug withdrawal	Variable	Common
Need for long-term tx	Variable	100%

AIH, Autoimmune hepatitis.

DIAGNOSIS AND EVALUATION

- Table 32.6 provides an overview of the clinical and laboratory features of autoimmune hepatitis
- Laboratory workup includes:
  - Elevated ALT, AST
  - Bilirubin that is normal or mildly elevated
  - ALK and GGT that are normal to slightly elevated in AIH but increased in AISC
  - Impaired liver synthetic function
    - Low albumin
    - Prolonged PT: due to vitamin K deficiency as well as impaired synthesis of coagulation factors
  - Low WBC, Hb, and platelets when hypersplenism ensues
  - Elevated IgG level observed in most patients
  - Characteristic pattern of autoantibodies defines distinct subgroups
    - Up to 20% may be seronegative at presentation
    - Antisoluble liver antigen signifies worse prognosis
- Liver biopsy: inflammatory infiltrate consisting of lymphocytes and plasma cells that expand portal areas and penetrate the lobules (interface hepatitis); variable necrosis and fibrosis spanning neighboring portal triads or between a portal triad and a central vein (bridging fibrosis)
- Imaging studies
  - Abdominal Doppler ultrasonography: rules out structural or vascular etiology of liver disease
  - Magnetic resonance (MR) cholangiography: screening for evidence for sclerosing cholangitis

TREATMENT

- Treatment should be started promptly upon diagnosis after ruling out infectious, or other, diagnoses:

Table 32.7. Hepatitis B Serology

Serologic Marker	Acute Hepatitis	Immune: Past Infection	Immune: Past Vaccination	Chronic Hepatitis	Inactive Carrier
HBsAg	+	–	–	+ >6 months	+
Anti-HBs	–	+	+	–	–
Anti-HBc	+	+	–	+	+
HBeAg	+	–	–	± Presence indicates high infectivity	–
Anti-HBe	–	+	–	–	+

- Prednisone 1 to 2 mg/kg/day (max. 40–60 mg/day)
- Slow tapering down according to decreased aminotransferase levels over 4 to 8 weeks
- Maintenance prednisone dose: 0.1 to 0.3 mg/kg/day
- Add azathioprine to maintenance treatment regimen
  - Follow for hepatotoxicity and use drug metabolite levels for monitoring
- Optional drugs for treatment failure: mycophenolate mofetil, tacrolimus, sirolimus, cyclosporin
- Ursodeoxycholic acid for AISC or overlap syndrome
- Liver transplantation for end-stage liver disease or fulminant hepatic failure

PROGNOSIS

- 80% remission rate with initial treatment
- Criteria for treatment withdrawal:
  - 3 years of sustained remission
  - Normal transaminases and IgG
  - Negative/low autoantibody titer
  - Repeat liver biopsy with no inflammation
- 25% to 40% meet criteria for treatment withdrawal; however, 50% of them relapse.
  - AIH type 2 patients usually cannot withdraw treatment
- Steroid-resistant hepatitis:
  - Nonadherence to medications most common
  - Reevaluate for AISC and Wilson disease
- Recurrence rate in liver allograft: 15% to 40% of AIH transplanted patients

INFECTIOUS HEPATITIS

Hepatitis A

BASIC INFORMATION

- See Chapter 45 for details.
- Presents with acute onset of nausea, anorexia, vomiting, fever, fatigue, abdominal pain, and jaundice
- Young children can be asymptomatic or have mild symptoms; there is no chronic form of hepatitis A
- Laboratory evaluation: marked elevation of serum aminotransferases; serum anti-HAV IgM detects acute illness, whereas anti-HAV IgG positive with past infection or vaccination
- No specific treatments or supportive care
- Prevention efforts include vaccination and hand hygiene

- Postexposure prophylaxis: recommended for previously unvaccinated persons within 2 weeks of hepatitis A exposure; hepatitis A vaccine for healthy children 12 months and older; immune globulin for infants under 12 months of age, patients with chronic liver disease, or patients who are immunocompromised

Hepatitis B (HBV)

BASIC INFORMATION

- See Chapter 45 for details
- Vertical, parenteral, percutaneous, or sexual transmission
- Typically presents with anorexia, malaise, fever, and jaundice during acute infection; patients may progress to chronic infection
- Many genotypes with varying prevalence and clinical course
- Risk of developing chronic disease varies with age of acquisition; higher in infants and younger children
- Diagnosed by serologic testing and interpretation detailed in Table 32.7
- Liver biopsy shows ground glass pattern of hepatocytes
- Treatment with interferon and nucleoside analogs is considered if ALT >1.5× normal and serology suggests active infection; generally treatment is reserved for chronic HBV. Trending HBV DNA (via PCR) and HBeAg assess for treatment response. Chronic HBV requires periodic screening for hepatocellular carcinoma with alpha-fetoprotein and US
- Liver transplant is associated with a high rate of recurrence
- Prevention:
  - Universal vaccination of infants and high-risk adult contacts, universal precautions, and appropriate postexposure prophylaxis
  - Infants born to HBsAg-positive mothers need HBV immune globulin and HBV vaccine within 12 hours of birth
  - HBV immune globulin for postexposure prophylaxis *if* previously unvaccinated

Hepatitis C (HCV)

BASIC INFORMATION

- See Chapter 45 for details
- Perinatal transmission of HCV (the most common cause of HCV in pediatrics) is 1% to 7% and is two- to threefold higher with concomitant HIV infection

- Risk factors for transmission: high maternal viral load (>600,000 IU/mL), internal monitoring of the fetus, prolonged rupture of membranes, and fetal anoxia around the time of delivery
- Often symptomatic, may have jaundice; chronic infection develops in majority (60% to 85% of cases)
- Risk factors for severe disease: HBV or HIV coinfection, immunosuppression
- Associated with autoimmune hepatitis, cryoglobulinemia, and glomerulonephritis
- Infection acquired in infancy can result in spontaneous resolution or chronic HCV
- Diagnosis: HCV antibody for screening if over 18 months of age; HCV RNA for screening in children younger than 18 months; positive serology testing requires HCV RNA testing for confirmation of active infection
- Liver biopsy may be helpful for grading severity of disease and ruling out other causes
  - Biopsy shows portal lymphoid aggregates, with sinusoidal lymphocytes with fibrosis being a later finding
- Close follow-up without treatment is often the initial plan because most children have mild inflammation with very slow progression of fibrosis. Treat children with persistent elevation of liver enzymes or progressive disease (treatment may vary by genotype)
  - In children under the age of 12 years, pegylated interferon and ribavirin are still the only FDA-approved treatment; however, new medications, including nucleotide analog (sofosbuvir) and combination of sofosbuvir and ledipasvir (inhibitor of NS5A), are currently approved for chronic hepatitis C in adults and children above 12 years of age
  - Monitor HCV RNA to assess response to therapy
- Liver transplant results in infection of the graft in >95% of cases without proper treatment

Hepatitis D

BASIC INFORMATION

- Vertical, parenteral, or sexual transmission
- Replication requires coinfection with hepatitis B; coinfection with hepatitis B accelerates hepatitis B–associated liver injury
- Presents with nausea, anorexia, vomiting, fatigue, abdominal pain, and jaundice
- Diagnosis: anti–hepatitis D antibody
- Treatment: generally supportive therapy

Hepatitis E

BASIC INFORMATION

- Fecal-oral transmission
- Geographic variation of genotypes
- Presents with self-limited illness with features of nausea, anorexia, vomiting, fatigue, diarrhea, and jaundice; severe disease more likely in pregnant women or those with underlying liver disease or immunosuppression

Table 32.8. Nonalcoholic Fatty Liver Disease Subtypes

Phenotype	Definitions
NAFLD	Inclusive term, full spectrum of disease
	Fatty infiltration of the liver in the absence of alcohol, genetic disease, or medications
	Fat >5% of liver by imaging, direct quantification, or histology
NAFL	Steatosis without specific changes
NASH	Steatosis with inflammation, with or without hepatocyte injury/fibrosis
	Type 1 balloon degeneration of hepatocytes
	Type 2 portal inflammation
NAFLD with fibrosis	NAFL or NASH with fibrosis (periportal, portal or sinusoidal, or bridging)
NAFLD with cirrhosis	Cirrhosis in the setting of NAFLD

NAFL, Nonalcoholic fatty liver disease; *NAFLD,* nonalcoholic fatty liver; *NASH,* nonalcoholic steatohepatitis.

- Diagnosis: anti–hepatitis E virus antibody; serum or stool PCR is available
- Treatment: generally supportive therapy

Nonalcoholic Fatty Liver Disease (NAFLD)

BASIC INFORMATION

- NAFLD is a chronic liver disease resulting from excessive fat accumulating in the liver
- NAFLD is the most common liver disease in children in the United States due to its association with obesity; it has become the leading indication for liver transplantation in adults
- NAFLD can result in progressive fibrosis and lead to end-stage liver disease
- Risk factors in pediatric cohorts: obesity, male gender, white or Hispanic race, hypertriglyceridemia, insulin resistance, obstructive sleep apnea, panhypopituitarism
- The different subtypes are summarized in Table 32.8

CLINICAL PRESENTATION

- In most cases, there are no symptoms from the liver disease in patients with NAFLD until the stage of cirrhosis

DIAGNOSIS AND EVALUATION

- NAFLD is a diagnosis of exclusion
- Differential diagnosis of hepatic steatosis is listed in Table 32.9
  - Other diseases and medications can cause fatty infiltration of the liver (e.g., hepatitis C, Wilson disease, amiodarone, corticosteroids, lysosomal acid lipase deficiency)
- Consider liver biopsy when there is increased risk for nonalcoholic steatohepatitis (NASH) (ALT >80 U/L, splenomegaly, AST/ALT >1, type 2 diabetes, panhypopituitarism)
  - Liver US or CT scan is not recommended for quantification of steatosis

Table 32.9. Differential Diagnosis of Hepatic Steatosis

Genetic–Metabolic	Medications	Dietary Causes	Infections
NAFLD (nonalcoholic fatty liver disease)	Amiodarone	Protein-energy malnutrition	Hepatitis C genotype 3
Fatty acid oxidation and mitochondrial disorders	Corticosteroids	Alcohol abuse	
Citrin deficiency	Methotrexate	Rapid surgical weight loss	
Wilson disease	Antipsychotics	Parenteral nutrition	
Uncontrolled diabetes			
Lipodystrophies			
Lysosomal acid lipase deficiency			
Familial combined hyperlipidemia			
Abeta/hypobetalipoproteinemia			

NAFLD, Nonalcoholic fatty liver.

- Screening indications
  - Patients 9 to 11 years of age:
    - Obese children (BMI >95th percentile)
    - Overweight patients (BMI 85%–94%) with additional risk factors
  - Screen sooner in cases of severe obesity, family history of NAFLD/NASH, or hypopituitarism
  - Siblings and parents of children with NAFLD/NASH with risk factors
- Screening method
  - ALT: persistently elevated (>3 months) more than two times
  - If normal, repeat every 2 to 3 years or sooner if indicated

TREATMENT

- First-line treatment for all children with NAFLD is lifestyle modifications to improve diet and increase physical activity
- No currently available medications or supplementations are recommended
  - Metformin, vitamin E, vitamin C, and vitamin D did not prove better than placebo in the treatment of NAFLD/NASH
- Bariatric surgery is not recommended as a specific therapy for NAFLD given lack of outcome data
- There is an increased risk for early atherosclerosis and cardiovascular disease with NAFLD, as well as increased risk for hypertension. It is recommended to screen for dyslipidemia and monitor blood pressure in patients with NAFLD
- It is also recommended to annually screen the patient for diabetes using either fasting glucose level or hemoglobin A1C

METABOLIC LIVER DISEASES

Wilson Disease

BASIC INFORMATION

- Autosomal recessive inheritance
- Mutation in gene encoding a transmembrane copper transporting protein—AT7B
- Inability to export copper from hepatocytes into bile and decreased synthesis of ceruloplasmin
- Copper accumulates in liver first, then in other tissues (basal ganglia, cornea, kidney)
- Epidemiology
  - Prevalence is 1:30,000
  - Often presents in childhood, but typically in the second decade of life; rarely presents before 3 years of age

CLINICAL PRESENTATION

- Liver disease often precedes neurologic symptoms, especially in the first decade of life; often presents as acute hepatitis
- Central nervous system (CNS) symptoms (usually occur in second or third decade of life)
  - Basal ganglia involvement
    - Dystonia
    - Fine motor problems
    - Gait disturbances
  - Psychiatric symptoms: can present with depressive, impulsive, or psychotic features
  - Kayser-Fleischer ring on an eye examination often presents when there are neurologic symptoms
- Coombs negative hemolytic anemia, proximal tubular deficit, cardiac problems, osteopenia

DIAGNOSIS AND EVALUATION

- Elevated liver enzymes (classically AST > ALT and bilirubin > ALK)
- Serum ceruloplasmin is low (<20 mg/dL)
- 24 h urine copper is high (>100 µg/24 h)
- Liver biopsy including quantitative copper content (>250 µg dry weight)
- Genetic testing is available when diagnosis is questionable and for screening siblings

TREATMENT

- Initial treatment is copper chelating agent: penicillamine or trientine dihydrochloride
- Zinc supplementation interferes with copper absorption; can be monotherapy after chelation or in asymptomatic individuals
- Avoid foods with high copper content

- Transplant for those with fulminant liver failure or severe liver disease who are failing medical therapy

Alpha-1 Antitrypsin Deficiency

BASIC INFORMATION

- A1AT enzyme inhibits neutrophil proteases and elastases
- Autosomal codominant inheritance
- Multiple phenotypes
  - MM is the normal phenotype
  - MS, SS, and MZ are associated with mild to moderate deficiency
  - ZZ and SZ are associated with severe deficiency
- Mutations leads to A1AT protein misfolding and accumulation in liver cells
- Epidemiology
  - Most common genetic cause of liver disease in children; 1 in 12,000 live births
  - More common with European ancestry
  - Consider in all infants with cholestasis and children with chronic hepatitis

CLINICAL PRESENTATION

- Liver and pulmonary disease
- Direct hyperbilirubinemia in newborns
- 10% to 15% of those with ZZ phenotype present with liver disease in the first few years of life
- Severity of liver disease varies widely
- Emphysema typically presents in the fourth and fifth decades of life
- Increased risk of antineutrophil cytoplasmic antibodies (ANCA)–positive vasculitis, panniculitis, glomerulonephritis, and chronic pancreatitis

DIAGNOSIS AND EVALUATION

- Increased ALT/AST, alkaline phosphatase, and GGT
- Decreased levels of serum A1AT less reliable than phenotype because it is acute phase reactant
- Liver biopsy with periodic acid Schiff (PAS)–positive diastase-resistant globules from accumulation of A1AT protein

TREATMENT

- No specific therapies
- Fat-soluble vitamin supplements, MCT oil, and ursodeoxycholic acid when cholestasis
- Liver transplant for end-stage liver disease (also eliminates emphysema progression)
- Screen all family members

Hepatorenal Tyrosinemia

BASIC INFORMATION

- See Chapter 49 for additional details
- Autosomal recessive inheritance
- Most severe disorder of tyrosine metabolism
- Defect in fumarylacetoacetate hydrolase in tyrosine catabolism
- Unmetabolized fumarylacetoacetate causes oxidative injury in liver and kidney

CLINICAL PRESENTATION

- Hepatomegaly and failure to thrive in infancy
- Can present as acute or chronic liver disease
- Hepatosplenomegaly, ascites, edema, and elevated liver enzymes
- Hepatic synthetic dysfunction with hypoglycemia, hypoalbuminemia, and coagulopathy
- Increased risk of hepatocellular carcinoma
- Other organ involvement
  - Renal tubular dysfunction, rickets
  - Neurologic symptoms (pain, paresthesias, paralysis)
  - Hemolytic anemia
  - Cardiomyopathy

DIAGNOSIS AND EVALUATION

- Newborn screen detects excess of succinyl acetone
- Tyrosine levels can be false positive due to transient tyrosinemia of newborn
- Elevated urine succinyl acetone is most diagnostic

TREATMENT

- Dietary restriction of tyrosine and phenylalanine
- Nitisinone inhibits step in tyrosine degradation and reduces accumulation of toxic metabolites
- Hepatocellular carcinoma screening with alpha-fetoprotein
- May need liver ± kidney transplant if not responsive to medical therapy

Drug- and Toxin-Induced Liver Injury

BASIC INFORMATION

- Liver is the main site for drug and toxin metabolism and is particularly susceptible to injury
- Most common in children: acetaminophen, antimicrobial and CNS agents
- Drug metabolism in the liver:
  - Phase 1: enzymatic activation (e.g., cytochrome P450 system = CYP) of the substrate to reactive intermediates
    - Pathologic induction of the enzymes can lead to hepatotoxicity
      - Intercurrent infection, starvation, drug interactions
  - Phase 2: enzymatic conjugation of reactive intermediates (e.g., glutathione)
  - Phase 3: energy-dependent excretion of drug metabolites and conjugates
- CYP3A4 is the primary hepatic CYP that metabolizes many drugs and toxins. Poorly expressed in fetus. By 1 month, 30% of adult value. By 6 to 12 months, 50% of adult value

Table 32.10. Clinical Presentation and Histopathology of Specific Causes of Drug-Induced Liver Injury

Disease	Drug
Centrilobular necrosis	Acetaminophen Halothane
Steatosis Microvesicular Macrovesicular	Valproic acid Tetracycline Ethanol
Acute hepatitis	Isoniazide
Chronic hepatitis	Nitrofurantoin Methyldopa
General hypersensitivity	Sulfonamides Phenytoin
Fibrosis	Methotrexate
Cholestasis	Chlorpromazine Erythromycin Estrogens
Sinusoidal obstruction syndrome	Irradiation plus busulfan Cyclophosphamide
Portal and Hepatic vein thrombosis	Estrogens Androgens
Biliary sludge	Ceftriaxone
Hepatic adenoma or hepatocellular carcinoma	Oral contraceptives Anabolic steroids
Hepatitis and Hepatic failure	Mushroom (*Amanita phalloides*) Chinese herbs Other herbal and dietary supplements

- Induced by: phenytoin, phenobarbital, rifampicin →nontherapeutic drug levels
- Inhibited by: erythromycin, cimetidine →toxic drug levels
- Genetic polymorphism of phase 1, 2, or 3 enzymes may increase risk of drug toxicity
- Inherited mitochondrial disorder is associated with sodium valproate hepatotoxicity
- Chemical hepatotoxicity:
  - Dose-dependent
    - Direct damage to hepatocyte by peroxidation of membrane lipids or denaturation of proteins (e.g., carbon tetrachloride, trichloroethylene)
    - Indirect injury by interfering metabolic pathways or distorting cellular constituents (e.g., acetaminophen, 6-mercaptopurine)
  - Idiosyncratic—independent of dose and may depend on other factors, including genetic polymorphisms and immune-mediated hypersensitivities

CLINICAL PRESENTATION

- Certain drugs/toxins are associated with specific clinical presentations or histopathology (see Table 32.10)

DIAGNOSIS AND EVALUATION

- Detailed history is key
- Clinical signs and symptoms: nonspecific. Needs high index of suspicion
- Laboratory features: variable
  - ALT, AST, bilirubin, GGT, ammonia, pH, INR, albumin

- Slight elevation of ALT and AST (×2−3) can occur during therapy and often resolves with continued treatment
- Toxicology serum and urinary screen
- Liver biopsy: may be necessary

TREATMENT

- Mainly supportive therapy; however, specific treatments are available for certain causes:
  - Corticosteroids—in immune-mediated reactions
  - N-acetyl cysteine stimulates glutathione synthesis. May prevent or attenuate acetaminophen hepatotoxicity when administered within 16 hours after acute overdose. May improve survival of patients with severe liver injury up to 36 hours after ingestion
  - IV L-carnitine—for valproic acid hepatotoxicity
- Orthotopic liver transplantation may be required for hepatic failure

Portal Hypertension (PHTN)

BASIC INFORMATION

- Definition: elevation of portal pressure >10 to 12 mm Hg (normal = 7)
- Etiology: obstruction to portal blood flow along the course of portal venous system; prehepatic, intrahepatic, posthepatic (see Table 32.11)
- Obstruction of portal flow leads to the development of collateral circulation (varices in esophagus, stomach, peristomal, duodenum, colon, and rectum) that can rupture and bleed
  - Congestive gastropathy refers to vascular ectasia in the stomach

CLINICAL MANIFESTATIONS

- GI bleeding
  - Bleeding from esophageal varices—most common presentation
    - May be life-threatening
  - Precipitated by minor febrile illness, cough, nonsteroidal antiinflammatory drugs (NSAIDs)
- Signs of chronic liver disease: jaundice, palmar erythema, vascular telangiectasia
- Growth retardation
- Ascites: with intrahepatic causes of PHTN
- Caput medusa: dilated vessels carrying blood from portal to systemic circulation around umbilicus
- Portal hypertensive biliopathy: cholestasis and liver dysfunction due to external compression of biliary tree by cavernous transformation of portal vein
- Splenomegaly with or without hypersplenism
- Encephalopathy
- Classic clinical presentations of portal hypertension
  - Portal vein obstruction: normal physical examination and lab
  - Congenital hepatic fibrosis: enlarged hard liver with minimal disturbance of function
  - Hepatopulmonary syndrome: respiratory failure that develops in >10% of patients with PHTN due to microvascular dilatation and intrapulmonary right-to-left shunting of blood

Table 32.11. Etiologies of Portal Hypertension

Prehepatic	Intrahepatic	Posthepatic

▪ Infection:
  ▪ neonate: omphalitis
  ▪ child: appendicitis, peritonitis
▪ Portal vein thrombosis:
  ▪ Neonate: dehydration, sepsis
  ▪ Child: IBD-associated hypercoagulable state, biliary tract infection, primary sclerosing cholangitis, Factor V Leiden
▪ Portal vein malformations: agenesis, atresia, stenosis, cavernous transformation
▪ AV fistula with increased portal flow: congenital or acquired
	▪ Acute and chronic hepatitis
	▪ Congenital hepatic fibrosis
	▪ Cirrhosis – predominant causes include:
	▪ Biliary atresia
	▪ Autoimmune hepatitis
	▪ Primary sclerosing cholangitis
	▪ Chronic viral hepatitis
	▪ Genetic-metabolic liver diseases: Wilson, Alpha 1 anti-trypsin deficiency, Allagile syndrome, glycogen storage disease type IV, hereditary fructose intolerance, cystic fibrosis
	▪ Malignancy
		▪ Budd-Chiari syndrome – obstruction of flow between efferent hepatic veins, inferior vena cava, and right atrium. Causes include:
		  ▪ Hypercoagulable states
		  ▪ Malignancy
		  ▪ Collagen vascular diseases, Behçet's disease, IBD
		  ▪ Infection – aspergillosis
		  ▪ Trauma
		▪ Sinusoidal obstruction syndrome (venoocclusive disease): occlusion of the central venules. Usually after irradiation, chemotherapy, or ingestion of certain herbal remedies.

IBD, Inflammatory bowel disease.

DIAGNOSIS AND EVALUATION

- Doppler ultrasonography: patency of portal vein and direction of flow. Hepatofugal (reverse) flow associated with variceal bleeding
- Selective arteriography of celiac axis, superior mesenteric artery, and splenic vein may assist in surgical planning for decompression
- Best noninvasive predictors of PHTN in children:
  - Platelet count
  - Spleen length measured by US
  - Serum albumin
- If hypoxia is present, then one must evaluate for hepatopulmonary syndrome
  - Contrast-enhanced echocardiography may show, in the left heart, delayed appearance of microbubbles from a saline bolus injected into a peripheral vein
- Endoscopy for detecting varices
  - Increased risk for bleeding: large size, red spots

TREATMENT

- Treatment for PHTN consists of emergency therapy for life-threatening hemorrhage and prevention of initial or subsequent bleeding
- There is a lack of strong studies in children to establish optimal treatment strategy
- Emergency treatment:
  - Fluid resuscitation: crystalloid and rapid packed red blood cell (PRBC) transfusion
  - Correct coagulopathy: vitamin K, platelets, fresh frozen plasma (FFP)
  - NPO + nasogastric tube
  - IV H2-blockers or proton pump inhibitors (PPI) (reduce risk of bleeding from gastric erosions)
  - Medications that decrease splanchnic blood flow:
    - Vasopressin or an analog
      - Side Effects: vasoconstriction, hypoperfusion of vital organs
    - Nitroglycerin patch
    - Somatostatin analog (octreotide)
  - Endoscopic sclerotherapy or banding of varices
    - Complications: more with sclerotherapy versus banding—bleeding, bacteremia, ulceration, and stricture formation
  - Sengstaken-Blakemore tube: mechanical compression
    - Risk for pulmonary aspiration and rebleeding

- Surgical intervention to decrease portal blood flow
  - Nonselective portacaval shunt
    - Risk for hepatic encephalopathy (HE)
  - Selective shunting: mesocaval shunt, distal splenorenal shunt, rex shunt (superior mesenteric vein to left portal vein bypass, for portal vein thrombosis)
  - Transjugular intrathoracic portosystemic shunt (TIPS)
    - Bridge to liver transplantation
    - Stent placed radiologically between right hepatic vein and portal vein branch
  - Orthotopic liver transplantation
- Primary prophylaxis of bleeding is controversial in children
- Secondary prophylaxis of bleeding with beta-blockers (propranolol) in adults decreased variceal hemorrhage and improved long-term survival. There is limited published data in pediatric patients

PROGNOSIS

- PHTN secondary to intrahepatic disease has poor prognosis
- Indications for liver transplantation:
  - Hepatopulmonary syndrome—the only effective therapy
  - Progressive liver disease and variceal bleeding
  - PHTN secondary to hepatic vein obstruction and sinusoidal obstruction syndrome
- Portal vein obstruction—bleeding episodes improve with age due to collateral circulation
  - Neurocognitive defects may signify encephalopathy due to natural portosystemic shunts
  - Portal biliopathy due to compression of bile duct from dilated collaterals
  - These complications may be treated or prevented with Rex shunt

Ascites

BASIC INFORMATION

- Definition: accumulation of fluid within the abdominal cavity
- Causes:
  - Portal hypertensive
  - Non−portal hypertensive

Renal, cardiac, infectious, GI, neoplastic, gynecologic, pancreatic, systemic lupus erythematosus (SLE), ventriculoperitoneal shunt, hypothyroidism, eosinophilic, chylous accumulation

CLINICAL PRESENTATION

- Mild: abdominal distention
- Moderate: early satiety, dyspnea
- Severe: physical signs—bulging flanks, shifting dullness, fluid wave, "puddle" sign
- Tense: umbilical herniation

DIAGNOSIS AND EVALUATION

- Abdominal paracentesis
  - Serum-ascites albumin gradient (SAAG)
    - >1.1 g/dL: PHTN
    - <1.1 g/dL: other causes

TREATMENT

- Treat etiology
- Sodium restriction
- Diuresis (e.g., furosemide, spironolactone)
- Supplemental albumin may aid
- Large-volume paracentesis or TIPS in refractory cases
- Risk for primary bacterial peritonitis

Acute Liver Failure

BASIC INFORMATION

- Acute liver failure (ALF) is a rapidly progressive clinical syndrome that is the final common pathway for many separate liver diseases

CLINICAL PRESENTATION

- Hepatic dysfunction with hypoglycemia, coagulopathy, and encephalopathy, with jaundice as a late feature
- Typically, a healthy patient presents with flu-like prodrome, with malaise, myalgia, nausea, vomiting, and jaundice
- Current encephalopathy scores were developed for adults with cirrhosis and portal hypertension and not ALF
- The interval between the apparent onset of jaundice HE is used to characterize subtypes of pediatric ALF: hyperacute, acute, and subacute
- Laboratory tests: increased transaminases, hyperbilirubinemia, coagulopathy. Rapidly falling enzymes with worsening coagulopathy suggest exhaustion of hepatocyte mass

DIAGNOSIS AND EVALUATION

- Adult definition: onset of HE and coagulopathy within 8 weeks of onset of liver disease in absence of preexisting liver disease

- Pediatric definition: biochemical evidence of liver injury with coagulopathy not responding to vitamin K, in the absence of preexisting liver disease. INR >1.5 if the patient has HE or >2 without
- Evaluate for potential etiology
  - A specific etiology cannot be found in about 50% of pediatric patients
  - Toxins and medications: acetaminophen, anticonvulsants, mushrooms, isoniazid, etc.

TREATMENT

- Supportive care
  - Manage intracranial pressure (ICP) and multiorgan failure while awaiting recovery of liver function or liver transplant
  - IV fluids with glucose to avoid hypoglycemia
  - Encephalopathy: medical therapy with lactulose. Consider mannitol, hyperventilation, hypothermia, or barbiturate coma for cerebral edema
  - Coagulopathy: correct PT/INR with FFP or recombinant factor VII only in the setting of active bleeding or in anticipation of an invasive procedure
- Specific Therapies
  - Acetaminophen →N-acetylcysteine
  - Drug-induced →remove offending drug
  - Galactosemia →remove dietary lactose
  - Tyrosinemia →NTBC
  - FAO defects →IV glucose and avoid fasting
  - Wilson disease →liver transplantation
  - AIH →corticosteroids
  - Herpes →acyclovir
  - Neonatal hemochromatosis →IV immunoglobulin (IVIG), plasmapheresis; IVIG in future pregnancies
- Liver transplantation if liver does not recover

Review Questions

For review questions, please go to ExpertConsult.com.

Suggested Readings

1. Fawaz R, Baumann U, Ekong U, Fischler B, Hadzic N, Mack CL, et al. Guidelines for the evaluation of cholestatic jaundice in infants: joint recommendations of the North American society for pediatric gastroenterology, hepatology and nutrition and the european society for pediatric gastroenterology, hepatology and nutrition. *J Pediatr Gastroenterol Nutr.* 2017;64:154–168.
2. Kerkar N, Mack CL. Autoimmune hepatitis. In: Suchy FJ, Sokol RJ, Ballistreri WF, eds. *Liver Diseases In Children.* 4th ed. New York, NY: Cambridge University Press; 2014:311–321.
3. Khalaf R, Phen C, Karjoo S, Wilsey M. Cholestasis beyond the neonatal and infancy periods. *Pediatr Gastroenterol Hepatol Nutr.* 2016;19(1): 1–11.
4. Liberal R, Vergani D, Mieli-Vergani G. Paediatric autoimmune liver disease. *Dig Dis.* 2015;33(suppl 2):36–46.
5. Manns mp, Lohse AW, Vergani D. Autoimmune hepatitis – Update 2015. *J Hepatol.* 2015;62:S100–S111.
6. Suchy FJ, Sokol RJ, Ballistreri WF, eds. *Liver Diseases In Children.* 4th ed. New York, NY: Cambridge University Press; 2014:311–321.
7. Vos MB, Abrams SH, Barlow SE, Caprio S, Daniels SR, Kohli R, et al. NASPGHAN clinical practice guidelines for the diagnosis and treatment of nonalcoholic fatty liver disease in children. *J Pediatr Gastroenterol Nutr.* 2017;64:319–334.

33 *Pancreatic Disorders*

J. NAYLOR BROWNELL, MD

Exocrine Pancreatic Insufficiency (EPI)

BASIC INFORMATION

- Definition
  - Alteration in pancreatic function, usually via a decrease in exocrine secretion, leading to maldigestion
- Causes and etiology
  - Inherited
    - Cystic fibrosis (CF) is the most common inherited cause of EPI (see Chapter 77 for details about CF)
      ΔF508 mutation accounts for 66% of known mutations; sweat chloride test is the gold standard for confirmation of diagnosis
      50% of children have EPI at birth; 85% have EPI by 1 year of age
    - Shwachman-Diamond syndrome (SDS) is the second most common cause of EPI (see Chapter 38 and below)
      Presentation is variable, usually before 3 years of age
      Triad of EPI (diarrhea/steatorrhea and failure to thrive), bone marrow dysfunction (cytopenias), and skeletal abnormalities
    - Johanson-Blizzard syndrome is a rare cause
      Presentation is variable; always includes EPI and nasal cartilage hypoplasia, leading to characteristic "bird beak" appearance of the nose
      Patients may also have failure to thrive, microcephaly, hearing loss, and hypothyroidism
    - Certain metabolic disorders, including some fatty acid (FA) oxidation defects, organic acidemias, and mitochondrial respiratory chain disorders
  - Acquired
    - Chronic pancreatitis may lead to EPI through gradual fibrous replacement of the pancreas
    - Surgical resection (Whipple, total pancreatectomy with islet cell autotransplantation)

CLINICAL PRESENTATION

- Physical signs
  - Failure to thrive and significant weight loss
  - Steatorrhea and diarrhea
  - Metabolic bone disease
- Natural history
  - Malabsorption of macro- and micronutrients results in malnutrition manifested by growth failure, organ dysfunction, and eventually cardiovascular events

DIAGNOSIS AND EVALUATION

- Serum laboratory abnormalities
  - Prealbumin is more likely than albumin to be low in EPI

- Serum trypsinogen
  - Most abundant zymogen in pancreatic secretions
  - Elevated in infants with CF and EPI due to impaired release of pancreatic enzymes—used in newborn screening for CF
    - Level drops as the CF infant ages, and patients usually have below-normal values by age 5 years, reflecting exocrine insufficiency
  - In most other cases of exocrine insufficiency, trypsinogen is low
- Fat-soluble vitamin deficiencies (i.e. Vitamins A, D, E, K)
  - Includes prolonged prothrombin time (PT) due to vitamin K deficiency
- Electrolyte abnormalities due to diarrhea
  - Hypokalemia
  - Hypocalcemia
  - Hypomagnesemia
- Measurement of exocrine pancreatic function typically through indirect methods
  - 72-hour fecal fat collection is the gold standard for diagnosing EPI
    - Shows decrease in coefficient of fat absorption
    - More sensitive in mild EPI
    - Technically difficult, and child must be on a full-fat diet before testing
  - Fecal elastase-1
    - Values will be lower in patients with EPI
    - Less sensitive in mild EPI
    - Falsely lowered values in loose stool (e.g., diarrhea due to another cause)

TREATMENT

- Cornerstone of therapy is pancreatic enzyme replacement therapy (PERT)
  - Based on body weight and dietary fat intake
  - Administered before all meals and snacks
  - Monitoring response to therapy
    - Weight gain
    - Decreased stool frequency and improved consistency
    - Improvement in fecal elastase-1 (not affected by enzyme supplementation)
- Fat-soluble vitamin supplementation

Shwachman-Diamond Syndrome (SDS)

BASIC INFORMATION

- Etiology
  - 90% to 95% of cases are due to an autosomal recessive mutation in *SBDS* gene on chromosome 7q11

- Destruction of pancreatic acini with fatty replacement is etiology of EPI; however, ducts and islet cells remain intact
- See also Nelson Textbook of Pediatrics, Chapter 349, "Disorders of the Exocrine Pancreas."

CLINICAL PRESENTATION

- Physical signs
  - Pancreatic insufficiency (steatorrhea, failure to thrive)
    - EPI is transient and may actually improve over time
  - Cytopenias
    - Primarily neutropenia
  - Skeletal abnormalities
    - Due to metaphyseal dysostosis
- Natural history
  - Short stature and poor weight gain continue throughout life, and recurrent pyogenic infections may lead to sepsis and mortality
  - Increased risk of myelodysplastic syndrome and acute myeloid leukemia

DIAGNOSIS AND EVALUATION

- Laboratory abnormalities
  - Cytopenias: neutropenia, thrombocytopenia, anemia
  - Consistent with EPI, as described earlier; fat-soluble vitamin and electrolyte abnormalities in serum, as well as abnormalities in fecal fat and elastase and a low serum trypsinogen
  - Normal sweat test (differentiates SDS from CF)
  - Mutations in *SBDS* gene on chromosome 7
- Radiologic abnormalities
  - X-rays: widened, irregular metaphyses, thickened and irregular growth plates
  - Abdominal imaging: hypodense appearance of the pancreas due to fatty replacement

TREATMENT

- EPI is treated with PERT, but therapy may not improve growth
  - Improvement in EPI naturally occurs in adolescence, reducing the need for PERT in 50% of patients
- Fat-soluble vitamin supplementation may be needed
- Monitor cytopenias and for leukemic transformation with serial complete blood counts (CBCs), and perform bone marrow biopsies
- Early dental evaluation and follow-up is recommended for surveillance of enamel defects

Acute Pancreatitis (AP)

BASIC INFORMATION

- Definitions
  - Acute pancreatitis is a reversible process characterized by acinar cell injury leading to a local inflammatory response accompanied by edema with or without hemorrhage or necrosis

- Acute recurrent pancreatitis is diagnosed if a patient has had two or more discrete episodes with an intervening return to baseline
- Causes and etiologies
  - See Table 33.1
  - 15% to 30% of cases will have no identifiable cause
- Natural history
  - Most cases resolve in 7 to 10 days without complications
  - 6% to 25% may develop SIRS response and require advanced support
  - 15% may develop pseudocysts; most resolve without intervention
  - Mortality ranges from 2% to 10%, usually associated with systemic illness

CLINICAL PRESENTATION

- Physical signs
  - Acute epigastric abdominal pain with or without radiation to the back is the most common symptom:
    - Can be vague or nonspecific, such as irritability in infants
  - Nausea/vomiting also common
  - Turner sign—bluish discoloration of flanks
  - Cullen sign—bluish discoloration around umbilicus
    - Both Turner and Cullen signs are late findings

DIAGNOSIS AND EVALUATION

- Diagnosis of AP requires ≥2 of three criteria:
  - Abdominal pain
  - Increased serum amylase and/or lipase ≥3× the upper limit of normal
    - Lipase is more sensitive for pancreatitis than amylase
  - Radiographic evidence of pancreatic inflammation
    - Abdominal ultrasound is the modality of choice
      Will demonstrate enlarged and hypoechoic pancreas with peripancreatic fluid and inflammation
    - Computed tomography (CT) may be useful if ultrasound is nonspecific or late in course to identify etiologies
- Laboratory results otherwise may be abnormal related to etiology

TREATMENT

- Fluid management
  - Early aggressive administration of intravenous fluids (IVF) demonstrates decreased morbidity and mortality in adult studies
    - 1.5× to 2× maintenance fluid requirements
  - pH-buffering solution such as lactated Ringer's has improved outcomes in adults versus normal saline
  - Monitor for electrolyte abnormalities, including hypocalcemia and coagulopathy
  - Monitor fluid status because it is common to have intravascular hypovolemia but total body fluid overload
- Pain control

Table 33.1.   Etiologies of Acute Pancreatitis in Children

TRAUMA

Fall on bike handlebars

Seat belt injury in motor vehicle collision

Child abuse

MEDICATIONS

Valproic acid

Thiopurines
Azathioprine
6-mercaptopurine

Antineoplastic agents
L-asparaginase
Cytarabine

Antibiotics
Metronidazole
Tetracyclines

Furosemide

Mesalamine

Acetaminophen overdose

TOXINS

Organophosphate poisoning

Alcohol

Scorpion venom

Heroin

Amphetamines

CONGENITAL ANATOMIC ABNORMALITIES

Pancreas divisum

Annular pancreas

OBSTRUCTION

Duodenal ulcers/Crohn disease

Tumors in the head of the pancreas or papilla

Biliary disease
Sludge
Cholelithiasis
Choledochal cyst

METABOLIC ABNORMALITIES

Diabetic ketoacidosis

Hypercalcemia

Hypertriglyceridemia

Malnutrition

INFECTION

Bacterial
Mycoplasma
Salmonella

Viral
Adenovirus
Enterovirus (Coxsackie virus)
Paramyxoviruses (mumps, measles)
Herpesviruses (herpes simplex, varicella, cytomegalovirus)
HIV
Hepatitis A, B, and E

Fungal
Aspergillus

SYSTEMIC ILLNESS

Hemolytic-uremic syndrome

Henoch-Schönlein purpura

Systemic lupus erythematosus

Juvenile idiopathic arthritis

Crohn disease

Pancreatic-sufficient cystic fibrosis

Sickle cell disease

Kawasaki disease

Sepsis

Shock

AUTOIMMUNE PANCREATITIS

GENETIC MUTATIONS

PRSS1 (cationic trypsinogen deficiency)

CFTR (cystic fibrosis transmembrane conductance regulator)

SPINK1 (serine protease inhibitor)

CTRC (chymotrypsin C)

- Parenteral narcotic analgesia is preferred
- No evidence that opioids exacerbate pancreatitis or prolong recovery through sphincter of Oddi spasm
- Nutrition
  - No evidence for gut rest; it is contraindicated in severe disease
  - Early feeding PO or enterally via nasogastric/nasojejunal (NG/NJ) is recommended
    - Full oral feeds may resume when symptoms improve in mild disease
    - Enteral nutrition via NG or NJ in the first 48 hours of disease improves outcomes
  - No evidence to support clear-liquid or low-fat diet when feeds are initiated
  - No evidence to support low-fat diet in preventing recurrence
  - In the event of recurrence of pain, consider pausing feeds and resuming again in 24 hours; an increase in pancreatic enzymes without symptoms is not an indication to stop feeding
- Antibiotics
  - No evidence for antibiotics in uncomplicated pancreatitis
  - Indicated for infected necrotic pancreatitis—a rare complication
- Endoscopy
  - Endoscopic retrograde cholangiopancreatography (ERCP) is indicated in rare cases of obstruction
- Surveillance
  - No indication for repeating laboratory testing or imaging unless course worsens or etiology is unclear
- Local complications
  - Should be suspected if abdominal pain worsens or the patient develops leukocytosis, fever, or signs of sepsis
  - Fluid collections may develop in up to 15% of patients; most resolve without intervention
    - Acute peripancreatic fluid collections have no encapsulation and may be monitored; usually resolve in <2 weeks
    - Pseudocysts are a rare late complication (>4 weeks after onset) and are encapsulated
    - Acute necrotic collections have necrotic components and are not encapsulated
      - Some may become infected, requiring antibiotics or drainage

- Walled-off necrosis is a rare late complication (>4 weeks after onset) and contains necrotic tissue within a well-defined wall
  - Typically require antibiotics and drainage

Chronic Pancreatitis (CP)

BASIC INFORMATION

- Definition
  - Progressive inflammatory process with irreversible fibrotic replacement of the pancreatic parenchyma, leading to permanent loss of both exocrine and endocrine function
- Causes and etiology
  - Any cause of AP, if recurrent, may lead to CP after multiple episodes
  - Genetic disorders are the most common cause in pediatrics
    - Cationic trypsinogen mutation (*PRSS1* gene)
    - Chymotrypsin C mutation (*CTRC* gene)
    - Serine protease inhibitor mutation (*SPINK1*)
    - Cystic fibrosis (*CFTR* gene)
      - 10% to 20% of patients with pancreatic-sufficient CF will eventually have CP
  - Obstructive causes
    - Congenital anomalies
      - Pancreas divisum is present in 20% of patients with CP
      - Annular pancreas
      - Choledochal cysts are frequently seen with pancreaticobiliary ductal malformations
    - Acquired strictures
      - Trauma—ductal scarring and malformation after initial insult can lead to recurrent and CP
      - Previous episodes of pancreatitis
      - Postoperative from biliary surgery
  - Autoimmune
    - Autoimmune pancreatitis
      - Associated with elevated serum IgG4
    - As a complication of recurrent pancreatitis in other autoimmune disorders

CLINICAL PRESENTATION

- Repeated episodes of AP
- Physical signs
  - Acute epigastric abdominal pain is the most common symptom
  - Nausea/vomiting with or without anorexia
  - Symptoms of EPI
    - Failure to thrive
    - Steatorrhea/diarrhea
- Natural history

- 40% to 70% of patients with CP will develop diabetes mellitus
- Increased risk of pancreatic adenocarcinoma in patients with CP
- Opioid dependence in up to 40% of patients with CP

DIAGNOSIS AND EVALUATION

- Diagnosis of CP requires typical imaging findings plus one or more of three criteria:
  - Abdominal pain
  - Exocrine pancreatic insufficiency
    - Typically diagnosed via fecal elastase or 72-hour fecal fat
  - Endocrine pancreatic insufficiency
    - Typically diagnosed via oral glucose tolerance test
- Imaging findings
  - Irregular contours of pancreatic duct represent strictures and fibrosis
  - Heterogenous echotexture represents fibrous parenchymal changes
  - Ultrasound, magnetic resonance cholangiopancreatography (MRCP), or CT appropriate to visualize changes
- Laboratory markers
  - Amylase and lipase may be only mildly elevated due to blunted response from EPI

TREATMENT

- Treat acute episodes as AP (see earlier)
- Pain control
  - Short- and long-acting narcotics may be used conservatively in the acute setting
  - Chronic analgesia with tricyclic antidepressants and gabapentin somewhat effective in adults
- Nutrition
  - PERT for EPI
  - Fat-soluble vitamin supplementation if necessary
- Surgical management
  - Resection should be considered for chronic pain or otherwise poor quality of life

Review Questions

For review questions, please go to ExpertConsult.com.

Suggested Readings

1. Pohl JF, Easley DJ. Pancreatic insufficiency in children. *Pract Gastro.* 2003;27:38–48.
2. Pohl JF, Uc A. Pediatric pancreatitis. *Curr Opin Gastroenterol.* 2015;31: 380–386.
3. Suzuki M, Sai JK, Shimizu T. Acute pancreatitis in children and adolescents. *World J Gastrointest Pathophysiol.* 2014;5:416–426.
4. Uc A, Fishman DS. Pancreatic disorders. *Pediatr Clin North Am.* 2017;64(3):685–706.

34 *Functional Gastrointestinal Disorders*

NOAH HOFFMAN, MD, MSHP

Functional gastrointestinal disorders in children are a group of challenging clinical problems. The Rome criteria are a group of symptom-based diagnostic criteria that are used to diagnose and classify functional disorders in gastroenterology. In the 2016 Rome IV diagnostic criteria, disorders are defined by their characteristic symptoms not attributable to another medical condition. Of note, the criteria do not require particular diagnostic testing to rule out other conditions. This allows the clinician to make the diagnosis of a functional disorder in a positive fashion based on a specific constellation of symptoms rather than by making a diagnosis of exclusion.

Cyclic Vomiting Syndrome

BASIC INFORMATION

- Median onset between 3 and 7 years of age, but can occur from infancy through adulthood
- Prevalence is reported to be between 3% and 6% in younger children
- A personal or family history of migraine is often observed in children with cyclic vomiting syndrome (CVS)

CLINICAL PRESENTATION

- Characterized by periods of unremitting nausea and vomiting lasting hours to days
  - The primary symptom is vomiting rather than abdominal pain
  - Symptoms and episodes are stereotypical in each patient
  - Episodes are separated by weeks to months with a return to baseline health in between
- Rome criteria require two or more such episodes within a 6-month period

DIAGNOSIS AND EVALUATION

- Positive diagnosis based on the previous criteria, which cannot be attributed to another condition after an appropriate evaluation
- The differential diagnosis includes anatomic, inflammatory, neurologic, and metabolic disease, especially in those children who present early
- Cannabis use should be considered in the differential diagnosis of adolescents presenting with symptoms like those described previously.
  - Chronic use of cannabis will predate the onset of CVS-like symptoms.
  - Cannabis use should be strongly suspected if adolescent patients report symptomatic relief related to showering or bathing.

- Testing for metabolic conditions should be considered at the onset of symptoms before the administration of IV fluid, especially in younger children

TREATMENT

- Abortive medical therapies for episodes include aggressive IV hydration and antiemetics drugs
- Prophylactic therapies:
  - First-line prophylactic medical therapies include cyproheptadine for children under age 5 years and amitriptyline for children over age 5 years
  - Propranolol is a second-line option
- Cognitive behavioral therapy may be helpful
- Coenzyme Q10, L-carnitine, and other mitochondrial cofactors have also been used

Abdominal Migraine

BASIC INFORMATION

- Epidemiology is similar to that of CVS. Family history of migraine headache is important
- In contrast to cyclic vomiting, pain is the predominant symptom in the case of abdominal migraine

CLINICAL PRESENTATION

- Includes all of the following, occurring at least twice:
  - Paroxysmal episodes of intense abdominal pain lasting 1 hour or more. Abdominal pain is always the most distressing symptom
  - Episodes are separated in time by weeks to months
  - Pain interferes with regular activities
  - Pattern and symptoms are stereotypical in each individual patient
  - Pain is associated with at least two of the following: anorexia, nausea, vomiting, headache, photophobia, and pallor
- Likely share a common physiology with CVS and migraine headache. Both abdominal migraine and CVS can evolve into migraine headaches later in life
- Episodes are often triggered by stress and/or fatigue

DIAGNOSIS AND EVALUATION

- Diagnosis can be made in a positive fashion based on the previous criteria
- A thorough history and physical examination should be used to determine the need to evaluate for other causes of recurrent abdominal pain, including pancreatitis,

intermittent bowel obstruction, renal stones, cholelithiasis, and other obstructive processes, and for metabolic disorders

TREATMENT

Frequency and severity of the episodes determine the need for prophylactic treatment.
Tricyclic antidepressants such as amitriptyline, propranolol, and cyproheptadine can be considered.

Rumination Syndrome

BASIC INFORMATION

- Rumination syndrome is defined by the repeated regurgitation and rechewing or expulsion of food that usually begins after ingestion of a meal. Rumination can occur at any age, but adolescent females seem to be at higher risk
- There is often a triggering event such as a gastrointestinal infection, traumatic psychosocial experience, or psychiatric disturbances before the onset of rumination
- See also Nelson Textbook of Pediatrics, Chapter 23, Rumination and Pica."

CLINICAL PRESENTATION

- Rumination occurs when intragastric pressure increases due to contraction of lower abdominal muscles. This contraction of lower abdominal muscles is voluntary in rumination
- Importantly, it is not preceded by or associated with retching and is often described as "effortless"
- Although not associated with retching, rumination can be associated with abdominal pain, heartburn, nausea, and other gastrointestinal symptoms

DIAGNOSIS AND EVALUATION

- The diagnosis is made based on regurgitation of food not preceded by retching and not occurring in sleep and that is not explained by another medical condition after an appropriate evaluation
  - Importantly, an eating disorder must be ruled out
  - The differential diagnosis including gastroesophageal reflux disease (GERD), gastroparesis, achalasia, and eating disorders should be considered before making the diagnosis
  - In some cases, the presence of R-waves on esophageal manometry can help confirm the diagnosis

TREATMENT

- Successfully overcoming rumination requires that the patient and family understand the condition as a learned (if not voluntary) behavior
- Treatment may consist of behavioral therapy, including diaphragmatic breathing and reswallowing, as well as other psychologic therapies

- Medical management of associated symptoms such as nausea and heartburn may be helpful

Functional Dyspepsia

BASIC INFORMATION

- Functional dyspepsia can present at any age in childhood
- It can be described as a form of irritable bowel syndrome (IBS) that is defined by symptoms in the upper gastrointestinal tract
- Functional dyspepsia should be considered in the differential diagnosis of GERD, gastroparesis, and peptic ulcer disease

CLINICAL PRESENTATION

- Rome IV criteria for functional dyspepsia include symptoms of postprandial fullness, early satiety, and/or epigastric pain or burning that is not associated with defecation. Symptoms must be present for at least 4 days per month
- The symptoms are not explained by another medical condition after an appropriate evaluation

DIAGNOSIS AND EVALUATION

- Diagnosis is made clinically based on the previously described criteria
- Because the differential diagnosis includes various inflammatory conditions of the upper gastrointestinal tract, upper endoscopy should be considered to evaluate for the differential diagnosis. However, according to Rome IV criteria, upper endoscopy is not necessary

TREATMENT

- For pain-predominant symptoms, acid suppression therapy can be helpful. Proton pump inhibitors appear to be superior to H2 blockers
- For early satiety, prokinetic medications such as erythromycin may be helpful
- Tricyclic antidepressants and cyproheptadine can also be considered

Irritable Bowel Syndrome

BASIC INFORMATION

- IBS in children refers to abdominal pain that is associated with changes in defecation
- Prevalence in school-age children is between 2% and 5%
- The diagnostic criteria described previously reflect the most common clinical presentations, which can occur at ages throughout childhood
- IBS is divided into subtypes reflecting the predominant stool pattern:
  - IBS with diarrhea
  - IBS with constipation
  - IBS with constipation and diarrhea
  - Unspecified IBS

CLINICAL PRESENTATION

- Diagnostic criteria are abdominal pain at least 4 days per month that does not resolve with treatment of constipation and is associated with one or more:
- Defecation
- Change in stool frequency
- Change in form or appearance of stool
- Although IBS is common, the evaluation must include a careful examination for the presence of alarm features that might suggest an alternative diagnosis
- Alarm features in the evaluation of chronic abdominal pain include persistent right upper or right lower quadrant pain, dysphagia or odynophagia, persistent vomiting, gastrointestinal blood loss, nocturnal diarrhea, perirectal disease, and extraintestinal manifestations including arthritis, involuntary weight loss, deceleration of linear growth, delayed puberty, or otherwise unexplained fevers

DIAGNOSIS AND EVALUATION

- The diagnosis is made clinically in the proper clinical context, as noted previously
- A thorough history and physical examination should be used to determine the need to evaluate for infection, celiac disease, carbohydrate malabsorption, and inflammatory bowel disease, among others, before making the clinical diagnosis
- Specifically, fecal calprotectin is a useful noninvasive screen for intestinal mucosal inflammation

TREATMENT

- Pharmacologic therapies include those used to target the symptom of chronic pain, including tricyclic antidepressants and cyproheptadine. Antispasmodic drugs also have a role
- Behavioral treatments such as cognitive behavioral therapy focusing on coping mechanisms play an important role
- Dietary therapies including optimization of dietary fiber intake and the low-FODMAP diet (i.e. low intake of short-chain carbohydrates) can also be recommended

Functional Abdominal Pain—Not Otherwise Specified

BASIC INFORMATION

- Functional abdominal pain—not otherwise specified (FAP-NOS) describes a syndrome of functional abdominal pain that does not meet criteria to be classified as functional dyspepsia, IBS, abdominal migraine, or others
- FAP-NOS is found at a prevalence of 1.2% among children in the United States

Clinical Presentation

- Episodic or continuous abdominal pain that does not occur solely during physiologic events such as eating, menses, or defecation
- A careful history and physical examination should be performed to exclude the alarm features noted previously in the section about IBS

DIAGNOSIS AND EVALUATION

- A diagnostic evaluation should be considered to reassure the family, although by definition, associated signs and symptoms to guide such an evaluation are limited

TREATMENT

- Amitriptyline, selective serotonin reuptake inhibitors (SSRIs), hypnotherapy, and cognitive behavioral therapy can all be considered

Review Questions

For review questions, please go to ExpertConsult.com

Suggested Readings

1. Hyams JS, Di Lorenzo C, et al. Childhood functional gastrointestinal disorders: child/adolescent. *Gastroenterology.* 2016;150:1456–1468.
2. Koppen I, Nurko S, et al. The Pediatric Rome IV criteria: what's new? *Expert Rev Gastroenterol Hepatol.* 2017;24:1–4.
3. Korterink J, Rutten J, et al. Pharmacologic treatment in pediatric functional abdominal pain disorders: a systematic review. *J Pediatr.* 2015;166:424–431.
4. Levy R, Langer S, et al. Cognitive-behavioral therapy for children with functional abdominal pain and their parents decreases pain and other symptoms. *Am J Gastroenterol.* 2010;105:946–956.
5. Li BU, Lefevre F, Chelimsky GG, et al. North American Society for Pediatric Gastroenterology, Hepatology, and Nutrition consensus statement on the diagnosis and management of cyclic vomiting syndrome. *J Pediatr Gastroenterol Nutr.* 2008;47:379–393.

Genetics and Dysmorphology

35 Selected Topics in Genetics and Dysmorphology

LEAH K. DOWSETT

Modes of Inheritance

BASIC INFORMATION

- Autosomal dominant (AD)
  - One copy of a change to a gene results in disease (heterozygous)
  - Condition appears in every generation, with males and females equally affected (see Fig. 35.1)
  - Associated with advanced paternal age
  - See Table 35.1 for examples of conditions following an AD pattern of inheritance.
- Autosomal recessive (AR)
  - Both copies of a change to the gene must be present for the disease to result (homozygous)
  - Disease usually involves genes that code for enzymes (e.g., inborn errors of metabolism)

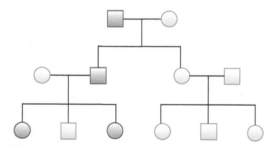

Fig. 35.1. Autosomal dominant inheritance pedigree. Affected individuals are represented by pink. Males are squares; females are circles. Male-to-male transmission with no skipped generations. (From Carey JC, Bamshad, MJ. Clinical genetics and dysmorphology. In: Rudolph CD, et al. *Rudolph's Pediatrics*, 22nd ed. McGraw-Hill; 2011: Fig. 170.1.)

- Condition appears in siblings, but not in parents or children of the affected individual (see Fig. 35.2)
- Risk is 25% for each pregnancy to couples who are both carriers of the same disease
- See Table 35.1 for examples of conditions that follow an AR pattern of inheritance
- X-linked
  - Due to changes in the gene on the X chromosome
  - Males are more likely to manifest given they have only one copy of the X chromosome; females are often carriers (or show mild expression in females with skewed X inactivation)
    - Incidence is often higher in males than females
    - Affected males will pass the mutation to all of their daughters (carriers) but *never* to their sons (see Fig. 35.3)
  - One-third of cases of lethal X-linked diseases are due to de novo mutations
  - Although most X-linked conditions are recessive (XLR), some are X-linked dominant (XLD; see Table 35.1)
- Mitochondrial inheritance
  - Mitochondrial DNA (mtDNA) replicates independently of nuclear DNA
  - All mitochondria are supplied by the oocyte, so mtDNA of any individual is maternally derived
    - A female with a mutation in her mtDNA passes it on to *all* her children (see Fig. 35.4)
  - Heteroplasmy occurs when there is more than one population of mitochondria in the oocyte
  - Conditions that follow a mitochondrial pattern of inheritance include MELAS (mitochondrial

Table 35.1. Modes of Inheritance for Common Genetic Conditions

Autosomal Dominant	Autosomal Recessive	X-Linked Recessive
Achondroplasia	Congenital adrenal hyperplasia	Duchenne muscular Dystrophy
Crouzon syndrome	Cystic fibrosis	Hemophilia A/B
CHARGE	Phenylketonuria	Lesch-Nyhan syndrome
Ehlers-Danlos	Sickle cell disease	
Familial adenomatosis Polyposis	Tay-Sachs disease	
Hereditary breast/ovarian cancer	Congenital myasthenia syndrome	**X-LINKED DOMINANT**
Li-Fraumeni syndrome	Jeune asphyxiating thoracic dystrophy	Incontinentia pigmenti
Marfan syndrome	Alpers-Huttenlocher syndrome	Rett syndrome
Neurofibromatosis 1	Leigh syndrome*	Fragile X syndrome
Neurofibromatosis 2		
Noonan syndrome		
Osteogenesis imperfecta		
Treacher Collins syndrome		
Tuberous sclerosis complex		
Huntington disease		
Denys-Drash syndrome		

*Can also follow a mitochondrial pattern of inheritance.

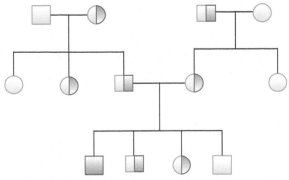

Fig. 35.2. Autosomal recessive inheritance pedigree. Affected individuals are pink; heterozygotes are partially shaded pink. (From Carey JC, Bamshad, MJ. Clinical genetics and dysmorphology. In: Rudolph CD, et al. *Rudolph's Pediatrics*, 22nd ed. China: McGraw-Hill; 2011: Fig. 170.2.)

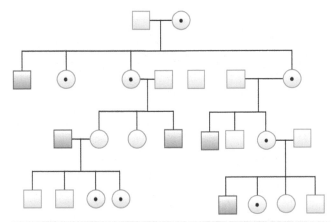

Fig. 35.3. X-linked recessive inheritance pedigree. Affected individuals are shaded pink; heterozygous carries are dotted. Only females transmit the disorder to their sons. Affected fathers transmit the trait to all their daughters. (From Carey JC, Bamshad, MJ. Clinical genetics and dysmorphology. In: Rudolph CD, et al. *Rudolph's Pediatrics*, 22nd ed. China: McGraw-Hill; 2011: Fig. 170.3.)

encephalomyopathy, lactic acidosis, and stroke-like episodes) and Leigh syndrome (both mitochondrial and AR inheritance)

- Uniparental disomy (UPD)
  - In UPD, the patient inherits two copies from one parent's chromosome (instead of one from each parent), leading to identical chromosomal markers on both
  - Conditions that follow a UPD pattern of inheritance include Prader-Willi syndrome, Angelman syndrome, and Beckwith-Wiedemann syndrome
- Trinucleotide repeat expansion
  - DNA appears as repeat sequences of three bases that will cause disease when the number of copies exceeds a certain threshold
  - Conditions caused by trinucleotide repeat expansions include fragile X syndrome, Friedreich Ataxia, and Huntington disease
- Multifactorial
  - Several conditions are attributed to interactions between the genes and environment
  - Do not follow a Mendelian pattern of inheritance

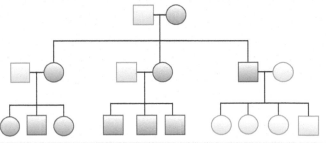

Fig. 35.4. Mitochondrial inheritance pedigree. Affected mothers pass condition to all their children.

- Conditions such as cleft lip and palate, neural tube defects, and hypertrophic pyloric stenosis are attributed to multifactorial inheritance

Teratogens

BASIC INFORMATION

- Certain in utero exposures are associated with a constellation of effects, depending on the timing and degree of the insult. Classic examples are provided in Table 35.2

ANEUPLOIDY SYNDROMES

Trisomy 21 (Down syndrome)

BASIC INFORMATION

- Down syndrome is due to the presence of a third chromosome 21 in each cell, causing disruption of normal development
- Not inherited (although Robertsonian translocations have a high risk of recurrence)
- Risk increases with advanced maternal age
- Occurs in 1/800 newborns
- The majority of cases are due to nondisjunction in the maternal gamete; aside from nondisjunction, translocations and mosaicism are other etiologies of this condition
  - If there is a history of trisomy 21 due to nondisjunction, there is an added 1% risk in addition to usual age-related risk for recurrence
  - For unbalanced translocations (3%–4% of cases):
    - Recurrence risk for paternal 21:21 translocation is 100%
    - Recurrence risk in 21:14 translocation is 16% if maternal and 5% if paternal

CLINICAL PRESENTATION

- Face
  - Epicanthal folds with up-slanting palpebral fissures
  - Brushfield spots of the iris
  - Flat nasal bridge
- Neurologic
  - Hypotonia
- Cardiovascular (CV)

Table 35.2. Teratogenic Exposures

Critical Period	INFECTIOUS DISEASES Agent	Key Clinical Features	DRUGS/CHEMICALS Agent	Key Clinical Features
Early pregnancy (0–20 weeks gestational age [GA])	Rubella	Deafness Cataracts Heart defects Intellectual disability	Methotrexate	Craniosynostosis Craniofacial anomalies Underossified skull Limb defects
	Varicella zoster	Skin scarring Chorioretinitis Limb reduction defects		
	Herpes	Central nervous system effects Vertical transmission Miscarriage		
Late pregnancy (20–40 weeks GA)	Syphilis	Abnormal teeth/bones Intellectual disability	Angiotensin receptor blockers (ARBs)	Renal dysgenesis Skull ossification defects Oligohydramnios
	Toxoplasmosis	Blindness Hydrocephalus Intellectual disability		
Entire pregnancy	Parvovirus	Hydrops Miscarriage Stillbirth	Lead	Miscarriage Stillbirth
	Cytomegalovirus	Microcephaly Hearing loss Low birth weight Intellectual disability	Valproic acid	Spina bifida Craniofacial anomalies Preaxial defects Hypospadias
			Tobacco	Premature delivery Miscarriage Stillbirth
			Warfarin	Nasal hypoplasia Stippled epiphyses Developmental delay
			Thalidomide	Limb reduction Limb hypoplasia Ear anomalies
			Isotretinoin	Central nervous system defects Missing thymus Conotruncal defects Intellectual disability Miscarriage
			Alcohol	Fetal alcohol syndrome Heart defects Intrauterine growth restriction Intellectual disability Miscarriage

Data from Rudolph CD, et al. *Rudolph's Pediatrics*, 22nd ed. McGraw-Hill; 2011.

- Congenital heart disease (conotruncal defects including complete atrioventricular canal [CAVC] defect are most common)
- Gastrointestinal (GI)
  - GI malformations (duodenal atresia, tracheoesophageal fistula [TEF], Hirschsprung, imperforate anus)
  - Celiac disease
- Extremities
  - Fifth finger clinodactyly
  - Single transverse palmar crease
  - Sandal gap toes
- Heme
  - Transient myeloproliferative disorder affects up to 10% of infants with Down syndrome
  - Lifetime risk of leukemia is 1%
- Other
  - Obstructive sleep apnea in >50%
  - Obesity
  - Hearing loss occurs in 75% by adulthood

- See Fig. 35.5

DIAGNOSIS AND EVALUATION

- Laboratory testing
  - Confirmatory karyotype
  - CBC and thyroid function tests (TFTs) at birth, then annually
- Imaging
  - Echocardiography
  - X-ray cervical spine only if symptomatic (neck pain, head tilt, gait instability, clumsiness, spasticity/weakness/hyperreflexia)
  - Abdominal imaging (e.g., kidney, ureter, and bladder [KUB], abdominal ultrasound [US], or upper GI/small bowel follow-through [UGI/SBFT]) if concerned for duodenal atresia
- Polysomnography by 4 years to evaluate for obstructive sleep apnea (OSA)

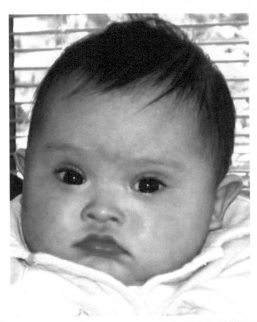

Fig. 35.5. Trisomy 21. (Courtesy Dr. Lynne M. Bird, Children's Hospital, San Diego. From Jones et al. *Smith's Recognizable Patterns of Human Malformation*, 7th ed. Philadelphia, PA: Elsevier Saunders; 2013.)

TREATMENT AND MANAGEMENT

- Early intervention and continued supportive services throughout adulthood
- Routine ophthalmology and ENT (ear, nose, throat)
- Primary care providers must be wary of autoimmune disorders and the lifelong increased risk of leukemia
- Overall life expectancy is reduced

Trisomy 18 (Edwards syndrome)

BASIC INFORMATION

- Edwards syndrome is due to a third copy of chromosome 18 in every cell, causing disruption in normal development
- Not inherited
- Risk increases with advanced maternal age
- Occurs in 1/5000 newborns (F > M)
- Aside from nondisjunction, translocations (partial trisomy 18) and mosaicism (mosaic trisomy 18) are other etiologies of this condition
- See Fig. 35.6 and Table 35.3 for clinical presentation and details

Trisomy 13 (Patau syndrome)

BASIC INFORMATION

- Patau syndrome is due to a third copy of chromosome 13 in every cell, causing disruption in normal development
- Not inherited
- Risk increases with advanced maternal age
- Occurs in 1/16,000 newborns
- Aside from nondisjunction, translocations (partial trisomy 13) and mosaicism (mosaic trisomy 13) are other etiologies of this condition

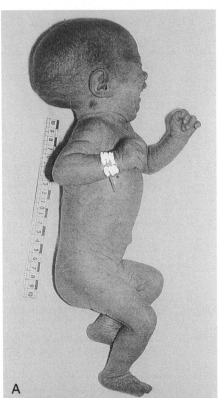

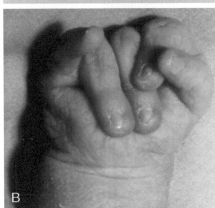

Fig. 35.6. Trisomy 18. (A) Profile of an infant with prominent occiput and low-set, malformed ears. (B) Clenched hand with overlapping digits and hypoplastic nails. (A, From Turnpenny PD, Ellard S. *Emery's Elements of Medical Genetics*, 14th ed. Philadelphia, PA: Elsevier; 2012: Fig. 18-6. B, From Peter T et al: *Emery's Elements of Medical Genetics*. 14th ed. Philadelphia: Elsevier Saunders; 2012)

- See Fig. 35.7 and Table 35.3 for clinical presentation and details

SYNDROMES WITH CRANIOSYNOSTOSIS

Crouzon Syndrome

BASIC INFORMATION

- Premature fusion of the skull bones (craniosynostosis) due to a mutation in *FGFR2*, causing increased signaling of the protein
- AD inheritance

Table 35. 3.   Distinguishing Features Between Trisomy 18 and 13

	Trisomy 18	Trisomy 13
Genetics	Nondisjunction is the most common etiology for this condition, although translocations and mosaicism can also occur.	Nondisjunction is the most common etiology for this condition, although translocations and mosaicism can also occur.

Examination findings	Face:
	    Micrognathia
	    Low-set ears
	Neurologic:
	    Microcephaly
	    Hypertonia
	    Severe intellectual disability
	    Myelomeningocele
	Cardiovascular:
	    Congenital heart disease (ventricular septal defect, atrial septal defect, patent ductus arteriosus)
	Genitourinary:
	    Cryptorchidism
	Extremities:
	    Clenched fists (overlapping digits 2/3 and 5/4)
	    Rocker-bottom feet
	Other:
	    Intrauterine growth restriction
	    Renal anomalies (horseshoe, polycystic, hydronephrosis)
		Face:
		    Microphthalmia
		    Midline defects (e.g., cleft lip/palate)
		    Dysplastic ears
		Neurologic:
		    Microcephaly
		    Hypotonia
		    Severe intellectual disability
		    Seizures
		    Hearing loss
		    Cutis aplasia/holoprosencephaly
		Cardiovascular:
		    Congenital heart disease
		Gastrointestinal:
		    Omphalocele
		Extremities:
		    Clenched fists
		    Polydactyly
		Other:
		    Renal anomalies

Dx/evaluation	Laboratory testing: confirmatory karyotype Imaging: echocardiogram, abdominal ultrasound	Laboratory testing: confirmatory karyotype Imaging: echocardiogram, renal bladder ultrasound, brain MRI, EEG, audiology evaluation
Natural history	50% die within the first week, 90% by the first year	50% die within the first month, 70% by the first year
Tx/management	Supportive care	Supportive care

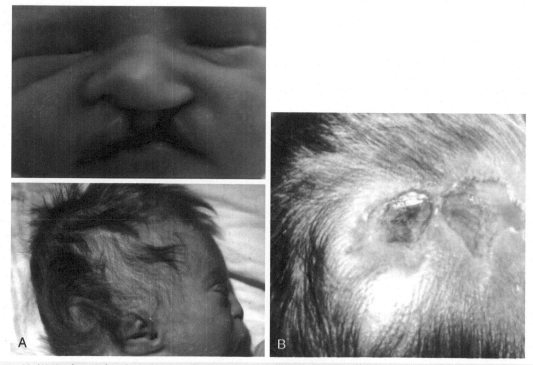

Fig. 35.7. Trisomy 13. **(A) Newborn infant frontal and profile views. (B) Cutis aplasia.** (A, Courtesy of David A. Clark MD, Albany, NY. From Darius J Adams, David A Clark: Common Genetic and Epigenetic Syndromes, Pediatric Clinics of North America 2015, 62(2): 411-426. B, From Jones et al. *Smith's Recognizable Patterns of Human Malformation*, 7th ed. Philadelphia, PA: Elsevier Saunders; 2013: p. 21.)

- Occurs in 1/16 million newborns
- Most common craniosynostosis syndrome
- Differential diagnosis
  - Pfeiffer syndrome (features include craniosynostosis, hearing loss, and pollux/hallux varus ± syndactyly)
  - Apert syndrome (features include craniosynostosis, hearing loss, and prominent syndactyly)

CLINICAL PRESENTATION

- Face
  - Prominent forehead
  - Hypertelorism
  - Proptosis
  - Midface hypoplasia
  - Cleft lip/palate
  - Beaked nose
  - Prognathism
- Neurologic
  - Normal intelligence
- Extremities
  - Normal extremities

DIAGNOSIS AND EVALUATION

- Laboratory testing
- *FGFR2* molecular genetic testing
- Imaging
  - Spinal x-rays to evaluate for vertebral anomalies
  - Computed tomography/magnetic resonance imaging (CT/MRI) as needed for surgical correction and to monitor for progressive hydrocephalus over time

TREATMENT

- Multidisciplinary team required for corrective surgery (craniotomy, frontoorbital advancement) within the first 6 months of life
- Multiple surgeries required over a lifetime
- Progressive hydrocephalus surveillance
  Common problems include dental issues, hearing loss, and progressive hydrocephalus

SYNDROMES WITH PUBERTAL PHENOTYPES

Turner Syndrome

BASIC INFORMATION

- Turner syndrome occurs when the second copy of the X chromosome in females is altered or missing, causing abnormal development
- Not inherited
- Occurs in 1/2500 newborn females; not associated with advanced maternal age
- Aside from monosomy X, some patients do have a mosaic form of Turner syndrome
- See Fig. 35.8 and Table 35.4 for details.

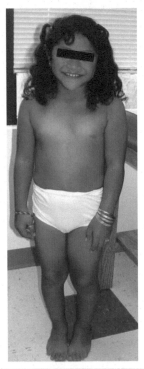

Fig. 35.8. Turner syndrome. (Courtesy Dr. Lynne M. Bird, Children's Hospital, San Diego. From Jones et al. *Smith's Recognizable Patterns of Human Malformation.* 7th ed. Philadelphia, PA: Elsevier Saunders; 2013.)

Noonan Syndrome

BASIC INFORMATION

- Noonan syndrome is due to a mutation in multiple genes (*PTPN11*, *SOS1*, *RAF1*, and *RIT1*), causing constitutive activation of the RAS/MAPK cell signaling pathway, which disrupts cell growth and division
- AD inheritance
- Occurs in 1/1000 to 1/2500 people
- Characterized by facial dysmorphology, congenital heart defects, short stature, and variable developmental delays
- See Fig. 35.9
- Differential diagnosis
  - Turner syndrome
  - Cardiofaciocutaneous syndrome
  - Costello syndrome

Klinefelter Syndrome

BASIC INFORMATION

- Klinefelter syndrome occurs when males have an extra copy of the X chromosome (47,XXY) due to meiotic nondisjunction, causing reduced testosterone production and abnormal sexual development
- Not inherited
- Occurs in 1/500 to 1/1000 newborn males

Table 35. 4.   Distinguishing Features Between Turner and Noonan Syndrome

	Turner	Noonan
Genetics	Chromosome aneuploidy and mosaicism	Gene mutations in the *RAS/MAPK* pathway

Examination findings	Face:
	    Webbed neck, redundant nuchal skin
	    Low posterior hairline
	Cardiovascular:
	    Shield chest with wide-spaced nipples
	    Congenital heart defects (**left**-sided: bicuspid aortic valve is the most common; also aortic coarctation)
	Extremities:
	    Congenital lymphedema (hands and feet)
	    Dysplastic nails
	    Skeletal abnormalities (short fourth and fifth metacarpals, cubitus valgus, scoliosis, congenital hip dislocation)
	Other:
	    Short stature
	    Renal abnormalities (horseshoe kidney, duplex collecting system)
		Face:
		    Webbed neck
		    Low-set, posteriorly rotated ears
		    Hypertelorism
		    Down-slanting palpebral fissures
		    Epicanthal folds
		    Ptosis
		    Ocular anomalies
		Cardiovascular:
		    Pectus carinatum or excavatum
		    Wide-spaced nipples
		    Congenital heart defects (**right**-sided: Pulmonary vein stenosis, atrial septal defect, hypertrophic cardiomyopathy)
		Genitourinary:
		    Cryptorchidism
		    Heme
		    Coagulopathy
		Extremities:
		    Lymphatic dysplasia
		    Other
		    Short stature

Dx/evaluation	Laboratory testing Confirmatory karyotype (FISH or array in cases of mosaicism) Elevated serum FSH/LH, estradiol is low Thyroid function tests Imaging Echocardiogram Renal bladder ultrasound Ophthalmology evaluation for nonsyndromic hearing loss Audiology (strabismus and hyperopia)	Laboratory testing Multigene panel (e.g., *PTPN11, SOS1, RAF1, RIT1*) CBC with diff, PT/PTT Urinalysis Imaging Echocardiogram and ECG Renal bladder ultrasound X-ray chest/spine MRI if symptomatic Ophthalmologic evaluation (strabismus, refractive errors, amblyopia, nystagmus) Audiology
Natural history	Normal intelligence, may have visuospatial learning differences Most individuals have delayed puberty (amenorrhea, breast development limited to breast buds, minimal pubic hair) and infertility due to streaked ovaries with premature ovarian failure; also has significant growth retardation due to estrogen insufficiency	Normal parameters at birth, but develop postnatal growth failure by 1 year of age Facial features variable from infancy to adulthood
Tx/management	Growth hormone therapy Estrogen therapy by 13 if no spontaneous puberty Increased risk for diabetes Surveillance due to higher risk for autoimmune disorders (e.g., hypothyroidism, celiac disease, inflammatory bowel disease)	Growth hormone therapy Orchiopexy when indicated Routine CV management Treatment of coagulopathies (avoid aspirin) Referral to early intervention

CLINICAL PRESENTATION

- Neurologic
- Developmental delay
    - Genitourinary (GU)
    - Microorchidism
    - Micropenis
    - Hypospadias
- Other
    - Tall stature (easily confused for Marfan syndrome)
    - Gynecomastia

DIAGNOSIS AND EVALUATION

- Laboratory testing
    - Confirmatory karyotype

TREATMENT AND MANAGEMENT

- Infants appear normal at birth
- Delayed puberty and infertility occur
- Testosterone replacement therapy in adolescence if no spontaneous puberty
- Consider testicular biopsy to retrieve sperm for future fertility through intracytoplasmic sperm injection (ICSI)
- There is increased risk for testicular and breast cancer
- Other sex aneuploidy syndromes
    - 47,XXY syndrome: males are taller than average and have normal sexual development; variable learning disabilities, delayed speech development, and autism spectrum disorders are common

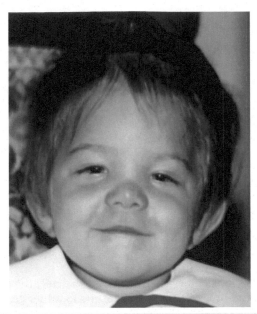

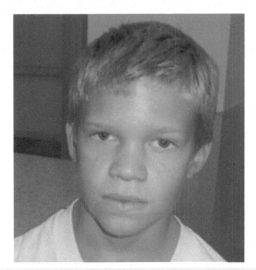

Fig. 35.10. Fragile X syndrome. (From Tsai A et al. Chromosomal disorders and fragile X syndrome. In Carey WB et al. [eds]. *Developmental-Behavioral Pediatrics*, 4th ed. Philadelphia, PA: Elsevier; 2009.)

Fig. 35.9. Noonan syndrome. (Courtesy Dr. Jacqueline Noonan, University of Kentucky, Lexington. From Jones et al: *Smith's Recognizable Patterns of Human Malformation*. 7th ed. Philadelphia: Elsevier Saunders; 2013.)

- 47,XXX syndrome: females are taller than average and have normal sexual development; variable learning disabilities, delayed speech, and behavioral differences are common. Seizures and kidney anomalies occur in 10%

Fragile X Syndrome (FRX)

BASIC INFORMATION

- Cognitive impairment condition due to a trinucleotide CGG repeat expansion in *FMR1*, causing deficiency of the FRMP protein that leads to abnormal synapse development
- XLD inheritance
- Occurs in 1/4000 males

CLINICAL PRESENTATION

- Face (see Fig. 35.10)
  - Long, narrow face
  - Large ears
  - Prominent jaw
  - Tall forehead
- Neurologic
  - Intellectual disability (the most common cause of *inherited* intellectual disability, although the second most common cause of *genetic* intellectual disability because trisomy 21 is more common)
  - Speech delay
  - Behavioral issues (impulsivity, hyperactivity, anxiety)
- GU
  - Macroorchidism
  - Extremities
  - Pes planus
- See Fig. 35.10

DIAGNOSIS AND EVALUATION

- Laboratory testing
  - *FMR1* molecular genetic testing and CGG allele repeat sizes
    - Normal: 5 to 44 repeats
    - Intermediate: 45 to 54 repeats
    - Premutation: 55 to 200 repeats
    - Full mutation: 200+ repeats

TREATMENT AND MANAGEMENT

- Mild to moderate intellectual disability with developmental delay apparent by 2 years
- Early intervention and routine management as issues arise (strabismus, reflux, seizures, mitral valve prolapse, hypertension)
- Fragile X–associated tremor ataxia syndrome (FXTAS) is characterized by late-onset progressive cerebellar ataxia in premutation-range males; a parkinsonian condition
- Female carriers can be symptomatic and often have premature ovarian failure
- Anticipation (transmission to subsequent generations leads to expansion due to unstable *FMR1* alleles)

Prader-Willi Syndrome (PWS)

BASIC INFORMATION

- PWS is due to maternal UPD (inheriting two copies of chromosome 15 from their mother), causing loss of function to several genes in this region
- UPD inheritance
- Occurs in 1/10,000 to 1/30,000 people
- Other mechanisms such as chromosome 15 deletion and imprinting are rare etiologies of PWS

CLINICAL PRESENTATION

- Face
  - Bitemporal narrowing
  - Triangular mouth
- Neurologic
  - Hypotonia
  - Global developmental delay
  - Mild to moderate intellectual disability
  - Behavior problems (compulsiveness, stubbornness, manipulative)
- GI
  - Feeding difficulties
  - Hyperphagia in childhood
- GU
  - Hypoplastic genitalia
  - Endocrine
    - Delayed puberty
    - Short stature
    - Osteoporosis
- Extremities
  - Small hands/feet
- Other
  - Short stature
  - Poor growth in early childhood, obesity in late childhood/adolescence

DIAGNOSIS AND EVALUATION

- Laboratory testing
  - Methylation testing of the Prader-Willi critical region on chromosome 15
  - Annual TFTs

TREATMENT AND MANAGEMENT

- Treatment is mostly supportive
- Growth hormone therapy to help normalize height and maintain lower body mass index (BMI)
- Sex hormone replacement at puberty
- Bisphosphonates for osteoporosis
- Most individuals are infertile

SYNDROMES WITH DERMATOLOGIC FINDINGS

Neurofibromatosis Type 1 (NF1)

BASIC INFORMATION

- Pigmentary changes and nerve sheath tumors due to a mutation in NF1 (tumor suppressor), causing a nonfunctional version of neurofibromin (found in oligodendrocytes and Schwann cells) that cannot regulate cell growth and division, leading to neurofibroma formation
- AD inheritance (50% are inherited from a parent, and 50% are de novo)
- Occurs in 1/3000 to 1/4000 individuals

CLINICAL PRESENTATION

- Diagnostic criteria (2+ of the following):
  - 6 hyperpigmented café-au-lait macules (5 mm in children, 15 mm postpuberty)
  - 2+ neurofibromas or 1 plexiform neurofibroma
  - Axillary or inguinal freckling (often appears in late childhood)
  - Optic glioma (<10 years of age)
  - 2+ Lisch nodules (iris hamartomas, <20 years of age)
  - Tibial pseudoarthrosis or sphenoid dysplasia
  - First-degree relative with NF1 (although a significant percentage are de novo mutations)

DIAGNOSIS AND EVALUATION

- Laboratory testing
  - NF1 molecular genetic testing will detect the most common cause; however, testing for other genes may be necessary if the clinical presentation is consistent with NF but the NF1 testing is normal
- Imaging
  - MRI for detection and monitoring of internal neurofibromas over time, including monitoring for signs of cerebrovascular disease
  - Unidentified bright objects (UBOs) visualized in 50% of children with NF1

TREATMENT AND MANAGEMENT

- Annual physical examination with routine blood pressure and scoliosis monitoring
- Annual ophthalmologic examination in children (optic glioma should be diagnosed quickly)
- Most children meet criteria by 8 years of age because features increase with age
- Normal intelligence, though most affected individuals have learning differences
- Seizures are more common than in the general population, can occur at any age
- NF1-associated tumors that occur in the absence of other findings include pheochromocytomas, gliomas, juvenile myelomonocytic leukemia, and breast cancer
- Consider MRI if clinically suspecting internal tumors
- Routine tumor surveillance and management
- Prenatal preimplantation genetic diagnosis can be considered

Neurofibromatosis Type 2 (NF2)

BASIC INFORMATION

- Benign schwannomas and nerve tumors due to a mutation in NF2 (tumor suppressor gene), causing a complete loss of function of merlin protein, causing uncontrolled cell division
- AD inheritance, but requires a second hit to trigger tumor formation
- Occurs in 1/33,000 people

CLINICAL PRESENTATION

- Clinical diagnosis is made by fulfilling one of the following sets of criteria:
  - Bilateral vestibular schwannomas
  - First-degree relative with NF2 and a unilateral schwannoma or any two of the following: meningioma, schwannoma, glioma, neurofibroma, posterior subcapsular lenticular opacities
  - Unilateral schwannoma and any two of those listed previously
  - Multiple meningiomas and unilateral schwannoma or any two of the following: schwannoma, glioma, neurofibroma, cataract
- Other features include hearing loss, tinnitus, balance difficulties, mononeuropathy, and café-au-lait macules

DIAGNOSIS AND EVALUATION

- Laboratory testing
  - *NF2* molecular genetic testing
- Imaging
  - MRI/CT head if symptomatic
- Audiology evaluation
- Ophthalmology evaluation

TREATMENT AND MANAGEMENT

- Symptoms typically appear during adolescence or early 20s
- Annual MRI head >10 years of age
- Surgical treatment of vestibular schwannomas (avoid radiation therapy)

Tuberous Sclerosis Complex (TSC)

BASIC INFORMATION

- Benign tumor growth due to a mutation in *TSC1* or *TSC2*, causing abnormal hamartin and tuberin production (tumor suppressors), which leads to uncontrolled cell growth and division
  - Mutations in *TSC2* may also be associated with mutations in *PKD1*, so patients may also have polycystic kidney disease
- AD inheritance
- Occurs in 1/6000 people

CLINICAL PRESENTATION

- Physical examination signs (presence of 2+)
  - >3 Hypopigmented macules (Ash leaf spots—seen best with ultraviolet [UV] light)
  - Shagreen patch (50%)
  - Facial angiofibromas ~4 years old (75%)
  - Ungual fibromas (20%)
  - Cortical tubers (80%)
  - Subependymal giant cell astrocytomas (SEGAs, 10%)
  - Lymphangioleiomyomatosis (LAM, 80% of females by age 40 years)
  - Renal angiomyolipomas (70%)
  - Cardiac rhabdomyomas (50%)
  - Retinal hamartomas (40%)

- Natural history
  - Neuropsychiatric features include autism, attention deficit/hyperactivity disorder (ADHD), cognitive impairment, disruptive behaviors, anxiety, and depression
  - Epilepsy is a common complication

DIAGNOSIS AND EVALUATION

- Laboratory testing
  - *TSC1* and *TSC2* molecular genetic testing
- Imaging
  - Brain MRI: surveillance of cortical tubers, radial glial bands, and subependymal nodules (the latter of which can develop into SEGA and cause obstructive hydrocephalus)
  - Electroencephalography (EEG)
  - Echocardiography
  - Renal bladder US (RBUS)
- Ophthalmologic evaluation

TREATMENT AND MANAGEMENT

- mTOR inhibitor therapy for progressing SEGAs; may require neurosurgery
- Infantile spasms and seizures are common; obtain EEG if suspected
- Vigabatrin for seizures (requires visual field surveillance)
- Brain MRI every 3 years for patients <25 years of age if asymptomatic to monitor for SEGAs
- CT every 5 to 10 years in asymptomatic females >18 years of age to monitor for LAM

Incontinentia Pigmenti

BASIC INFORMATION

- XLD inheritance due to mutation in *IKBKG*; males usually fetal lethal
- Classic skin findings along the lines of Blaschko include a blistering rash in infancy, swirling macular hyperpigmentation in childhood, and linear hypopigmentation in adulthood
- Diagnosis by molecular sequencing of *IKBKG*
- Surveillance for seizures and retinal detachment
- Management includes a multidisciplinary team approach with early intervention, dental, ophthalmology, and neurology

SYNDROMES WITH UNIQUE BEHAVIORAL PHENOTYPES

Angelman Syndrome (AS)

BASIC INFORMATION

- AS is due to deletion of the maternal segment of chromosome 15 or paternal UPD (inheriting two copies of chromosome 15 from their father), causing loss of function of *UBE3A*

- PWS is due to maternal UPD (inheriting two copies of chromosome 15 from their mother), causing loss of function to several genes in this region
- Chromosome 15 deletion or UPD inheritance
- Occurs in 1/12,000 to 1/20,000 people

CLINICAL PRESENTATION

- Neurologic
  - Microcephaly (by age 2 years)
  - Seizures (by age 3 years)
  - Sleep disturbance
  - Cognitive impairment:
    - Developmental delay/intellectual disability
    - Severe speech impairment (often nonverbal)
  - Movement disorder:
    - Ataxia
    - Hypermotoric movements (arm tremors, jerky movements, clumsiness)
  - Personality traits:
    - Happy demeanor, with inappropriate laughter
    - Excitable, with hand-flapping movements

DIAGNOSIS AND EVALUATION

- Laboratory testing
  - *UBE3A* molecular genetic testing
  - Methylation testing of the 15q11.2-q13 region on chromosome 15
- Imaging
  - EEG

TREATMENT AND MANAGEMENT

- Developmental delay becomes apparent between 6 and 12 months of age
- Treatment is mostly supportive with early intervention and behavioral support
- Avoid carbamazepine, vigabatrin, and tiagabine for seizure management

Lesch-Nyhan Syndrome (LNS)

BASIC INFORMATION

- LNS is due to mutations in *HPRT1*, causing hyperuricemia due to decreased hypoxanthine-guanine phosphoribosyltransferase activity; X-linked recessive inheritance
- Classic findings include developmental delay, hypotonia, both extrapyramidal and pyramidal involvement, and self-injurious behavior
- Diagnosis by molecular sequencing is confirmatory. Clinical diagnosis is suspected in males with developmental delay with characteristic neurologic, cognitive, and behavioral disturbances. Suggestive laboratory results include hyperuricemia and low HRPT enzyme activity
- Management is directed at controlling overproduction of uric acid with allopurinol, baclofen for spasticity, and other modalities to reduce complications from self-injurious behaviors

Rett Syndrome

BASIC INFORMATION

- Brain disorder (de novo) due to a mutation in *MECP2*, leading to production of MeCP2 protein, which is critical for normal brain function
- XLD inheritance
- Occurs in 1/8500 females
- Differential diagnosis
  - Angelman syndrome
  - Cerebral palsy
  - Autism

CLINICAL PRESENTATION

- Neurologic
  - Microcephaly
  - Seizures
  - Stereotypies (hand-wringing)
  - Gait ataxia
  - Bruxism
  - Sleep disturbance
  - Neuropsychiatric disturbance (agitation)
  - Developmentally normal until regression occurs ~18 months of age
- GI
  - Constipation
  - Extremities
  - Small hands/feet
- Other
  - Failure to thrive (FTT)
  - Scoliosis

DIAGNOSIS AND EVALUATION

- Laboratory testing
  - *MECP2* molecular genetic testing
- Imaging
  - ECG to rule out prolonged QTc
  - EEG

TREATMENT AND MANAGEMENT

- Treatment focuses on symptoms with a multidisciplinary approach (i.e., antiepileptic drugs [AEDs] for seizures, melatonin for sleep disturbance, selective serotonin reuptake inhibitors [SSRIs] for agitation, fiber for constipation)

Williams Syndrome

BASIC INFORMATION

- Causes and etiology
  - Williams syndrome due to a deletion of chromosome 7 (including ~30 genes, including ELN), causing abnormal elastin production, leading to CV and connective tissue problems
  - Although not typically inherited, transmission is AD
  - Occurs in 1/7500 to 1/10,000 people

CLINICAL PRESENTATION

- Face
  - "Elfin facies"
    - Broad forehead with bitemporal narrowing
    - Periorbital fullness
    - Malar hypoplasia
    - Long philtrum
    - Full lips with side mouth
  - Prominent earlobes
- Neurologic
  - Stellate iris
  - Friendly—"cocktail party personality"
  - Intellectual disability
- CV
  - Supravalvular aortic stenosis with or without coarctation
  - Other vascular abnormalities include pulmonary artery stenosis and renal artery stenosis
- GI
  - Hernias (umbilical, inguinal)
  - Rectal prolapse
- Endocrine
  - Hypothyroidism
  - Hypercalcemia
- Other
  - FTT
  - See Fig. 35.11

DIAGNOSIS AND EVALUATION

- Laboratory testing
  - Chromosomal microarray (fluorescence in situ hybridization [FISH], multiplex ligation-dependent probe amplification [MLPA])
  - *ELN* molecular genetic testing

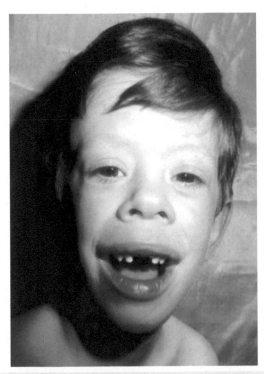

Fig. 35.11. Williams syndrome. (From Jones KL, Smith DW. The Williams elfin facies syndrome: a new perspective. *J Pediatr.* 1975;86:718, with permission.)

- Serum/urine calcium
- TFTs
- Imaging
  - Echocardiography
  - RBUS
- Audiology evaluation
- Ophthalmology evaluation

TREATMENT AND MANAGEMENT

- Supportive care and early intervention
- Monitor for hypercalciuria
- Aggressive management of constipation given risk of rectal prolapse

Huntington Disease (HD)

BASIC INFORMATION

- Progressive brain disease due to a mutation in *HTT*, causing a CAG trinucleotide repeat expansion that leads to the production of an elongated huntingtin protein, which then gets cut into smaller, toxic fragments that accumulate in neurons and disrupt their normal function
- AD inheritance with anticipation (repeat increases in size, causing earlier onset of signs and symptoms in progressive generations)
- Occurs in 3/100,000 to 7/100,000 people of European ancestry
- Mean age of onset is 35 to 44 years, with a survival of 15 to 18 years after onset
  - The juvenile form begins in childhood or adolescence. Affected individuals live 10 to 15 years from onset because this form is more progressive
- Symptoms are primarily motor and psychiatric
  - Early symptoms include clumsiness and psychiatric symptoms (irritability, anxiety, depression)
  - This progresses to involuntary movements, dystonia, and chorea, with the development of speech difficulties and general weakness
  - Late symptoms include rigidity, bradykinesia, and inability to walk/speak
  - Treatment involves neuroleptic, antiparkinsonian, and psychiatric agents, with long-term follow-up by neurology and psychiatry
- Diagnosis provided by *HTT* molecular genetic testing
- Differential diagnosis
  - Early-onset familial Alzheimer disease
  - Hereditary cerebellar ataxia
  - Creutzfeldt-Jakob disease

SYNDROMES WITH DISORDERED GROWTH

Achondroplasia

BASIC INFORMATION

- Dwarfism due to a de novo single-base pair mutation in *FGFR3*, causing increased activation of the growth factor receptor; 99% of individuals have Gly380Arg

- AD inheritance (>80% are de novo mutations)
- Occurs in 1/15,000 to 1/40,000 newborns

CLINICAL PRESENTATION

- Face
  - Macrocephaly with frontal bossing
  - Midface hypoplasia
- Neurologic
  - Normal intelligence
- Extremities
  - Short arms and legs (especially proximally, known as "rhizomelic shortening")
  - Bowed legs (genu varum)
  - Lumbar lordosis
  - Trident fingers
- Other
  - Short stature, dwarfism
  - Sleep apnea

DIAGNOSIS AND EVALUATION

- Laboratory testing
  - *FGFR3* molecular genetic testing
  - Polysomnography in infancy
- Imaging
  - Skeletal survey
  - Consider baseline head CT to evaluate foramen magnum for stenosis

TREATMENT AND MANAGEMENT

- Common health problems include sleep apnea, obesity, recurrent otitis media, lordosis, kyphoscoliosis, and hydrocephalus
- Normal life span
- Growth hormone supplementation is *ineffective*
- Avoid contact sports, diving, gymnastics, and exercise caution with intubation given atlantoaxial instability; most common cause of early death is respiratory insufficiency from a small thorax and neurologic deficit from cervicomedullary junction compression
- Consider ventriculoperitoneal (VP) shunt for hydrocephalus
- Monitor for hearing loss and middle ear problems
- Orthopedist referral if necessary
- Monitor for spinal stenosis in adults with neurologic examination
- Routine management of sleep apnea because it is a common complication

Arthrogryposis Multiplex Congenita (AMC)

BASIC INFORMATION

- AMC refers to the multiple joint contractures that occur in neonates with congenital myasthenic syndromes (CMS) due to lack of in utero fetal movement
- There are several genes that fall into various CMS subtypes, most commonly *RAPSN* mutations, and diagnosis is based on molecular genetic studies; AR inheritance

- Features include joint contractures, neonatal hypotonia, ptosis, high arched palate, poor feeding, and respiratory insufficiency (pulmonary hypoplasia, small thorax)

Jeune Asphyxiating Thoracic Dystrophy (JATD)

BASIC INFORMATION

- JATD is a skeletal dysplasia characterized by disordered bone growth due to mutations in several genes (including *IFT80*, *TTC21B*, and *DYNC2H1*); AR inheritance
- Classic features include a narrow "bell-shaped" chest, short ribs, shortened limbs, and polydactyly
- Clinical diagnosis is confirmed with molecular genetic studies
  Also:
  Beckwith-Wiedemann Syndrome (BWS). Please see section on Wilms tumor risk later

SYNDROMES WITH CONNECTIVE TISSUE PHENOTYPES

Marfan Syndrome (MS)

BASIC INFORMATION

- Connective tissue disorder due to a mutation in *FBN1*, causing reduced amounts of fibrillin-1 (forms microfibrils that provide strength and flexibility to connective tissue) and excess growth factor release leading to tissue instability and overgrowth
- AD inheritance
- Occurs in 1/5000 people
- Differential diagnosis
  - Homocystinuria
  - Loeys-Dietz syndrome

CLINICAL PRESENTATION

See Table 35.5

DIAGNOSIS AND EVALUATION

- Laboratory testing
  - *FBN1* molecular genetic testing
- Imaging
  - Annual echocardiography
  - Intermittent surveillance of aorta with CT or magnetic resonance angiography (MRA) beginning in adolescence

TREATMENT AND MANAGEMENT

- Features of MS become apparent anytime from infancy to adulthood
- Majority of individuals survive into mid- to late adulthood
- Use of beta-blockers and angiotensin receptor blockers is recommended to reduce hemodynamic stress
- Avoid contact sports due to risk of aortic dilation/dissection

Table 35.5.   Clinical Presentation in Marfan Syndrome vs Ehlers-Danlos Syndrome

	Marfan Syndrome	Classic Ehlers-Danlos Syndrome
Face	Long, narrow face Enophthalmos Down-slanting palpebral fissures Malar hypoplasia Micro/retrognathia High-arched palate with dental crowding	n/a
Neurologic	Normal intelligence Ectopia lentis Myopia	Normal intelligence Hypotonia Delayed motor development
Cardiovascular	Pectus excavatum or carinatum Aortic dilation or dissection Mitral valve prolapse	Mitral valve prolapse Aortic root dilation (nonhypermobile type)
Gastrointestinal	n/a	Hernias Rectal prolapse
Dermatologic	Striae	Skin hyperextensibility Widened atrophic scars Smooth skin Molluscoid pseudotumors Subcutaneous spheroids Easy bruising
Extremities	Arachnodactyly Reduced elbow extension Positive wrist/thumb sign	Joint hypermobility Easy dislocations/subluxations Cramping
Other	Tall stature Pneumothorax Scoliosis	Fatigue Chronic pain

- Pneumothorax can occur; avoid positive pressure when possible (playing wind instrument, scuba diving)
- Multidisciplinary cares including ophthalmology, cardiology, orthopedics, and cardiothoracic surgery
- Pregnancy in women with this condition requires high-risk management

Ehlers-Danlos Syndrome (EDS)

BASIC INFORMATION

- Connective tissue defects due to a mutation in *COL5A1* or *COL5A2* (for the classic type, just a few of over a dozen genes implicated with EDS) causing disruption in collagen production, interaction, or processing
- AD inheritance for the classic form; AR inheritance in a few other forms of EDS
- Occurs in 1/5000 people (combined prevalence)
- Aside from the classic type (I and II, described here), there are several other forms, including:
  - Hypermobile type III
  - Vascular type IV
  - Kyphoscoliotic type VI

CLINICAL PRESENTATION

- See Table 35.5

DIAGNOSIS AND EVALUATION

- Laboratory testing
  - *COL5A1* and *COL5A2* molecular genetic testing
- Imaging

- Annual echocardiography with aortic dilation or mitral valve prolapse

TREATMENT AND MANAGEMENT

- Physiotherapy and early intervention in children with the classic type
- Non-weight-bearing exercises promotes strength, but avoid those that strain joints
- Pregnancy in affected women should be monitored closely
- The vascular type (IV) is associated with life-threatening complications due to unpredictable blood vessel rupture (internal bleeding, stroke, peritoneal perforation, organ rupture, and shock)

Osteogenesis Imperfecta (OI)

BASIC INFORMATION

- Group of disorders affecting bone malformation due to mutations in *COL1A1* and *COL1A2*, causing abnormal type I collagen production leading to bone brittleness
- AD inheritance primarily (AR forms do exist)
- Occurs in 6/100,000 to 7/100,000 people
- Although there are several forms of OI, 90% are due to mutations in *COL1A1* and *COL1A2*
- Radiographic findings, including fractures of varying ages, can be suggestive of OI

CLINICAL PRESENTATION

- Face
  - Triangular-shaped face
  - Large skull

- Neurologic
  - Normal intelligence
  - Hearing loss
- Other
  - Easy bruising

DIAGNOSIS AND EVALUATION

- Types of OI
  - OI type I: classic nondeforming OI with blue sclerae
  - OI type II: perinatally lethal OI
  - OI type III: progressively deforming OI
  - OI type IV: common variable OI with normal sclerae
- Laboratory testing
- *COL1A1* and *COL1A2* molecular genetic testing
- Imaging
- Skeletal survey (fractures, wormian bones, "codfish" vertebrae, osteopenia)

TREATMENT AND MANAGEMENT

- Bisphosphonate infusion to decrease bone resorption
- Growth hormone (GH) to increase linear growth
- Multidisciplinary cares including involvementfrom orthopedics, rehabilitation, dentistry, and ENT

SYNDROMES WITH DIFFICULT AIRWAYS

Treacher Collins Syndrome (TCS)

BASIC INFORMATION

- TCS is due to zygomatic and mandibular bone hypoplasia caused by mutations in *TCOF1*, causing abnormal treacle protein, which plays a critical role in facial bone development in early embryogenesis; AD inheritance
- Classic features include eyelid colobomas, sparse eyelashes, microretrognathia, choanal atresia, and microtia
- Diagnosis through molecular sequencing of *TCOF1* is confirmatory in up to 90% of cases; *POLR1D* and *POLR1C* mutations account for ~8%
- Airway difficulties are common in the neonatal period. Surveillance for hearing loss, ophthalmologic defects, and feeding difficulties is routine. Craniofacial reconstruction is also a consideration
- See Fig. 35.12

Pierre-Robin Sequence (PRS)

BASIC INFORMATION

- PRS is a set of abnormalities consisting of micrognathia, glossoptosis, and airway obstruction
- Additional features include cleft palate. If the patient has these findings in conjunction with myopia and skeletal abnormalities, consider a diagnosis of Stickler syndrome

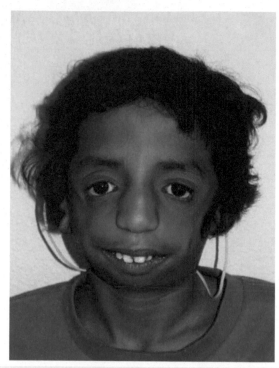

Fig. 35.12. Treacher-Collins syndrome. (Courtesy Dr. Lynne M. Bird, Children's Hospital, San Diego. From Jones et al. *Smith's Recognizable Patterns of Human Malformation*, 7th ed. Philadelphia, PA: Elsevier Saunders; 2013.)

- Mutations in *SOX9* are most often found in patients with isolated PRS. Though most mutations are de novo, the inheritance pattern follows the condition with which it is associated

Goldenhar Syndrome

BASIC INFORMATION

- Goldenhar syndrome belongs to a spectrum of malformations referred to as craniofacial microsomia (CFM), primarily involving structures derived from the first and second branchial arches
- Characteristic findings include facial asymmetry, microtia, preauricular tags, microphthalmia, and cleft lip/palate. Epibulbar dermoid is associated with the Goldenhar phenotype
- Diagnosis is based on clinical findings. Gene involvement is unknown. No specific inheritance pattern
- Multidisciplinary cares with a craniofacial team is recommended

Russell-Silver Syndrome (RSS)

BASIC INFORMATION

- RSS is due to abnormal methylation of the 11p15.5 (35%–50%) and maternal UPD of chromosome 7 (10%)
- Classic features include postnatal growth restriction (normal head circumference), FTT, feeding difficulties, triangular facies with a prominent forehead and pointed chin, and clinodactyly. Males can have cryptorchidism and micropenis

- Diagnosis is made clinically based on physical findings (postnatal growth restriction with normal head circumference and typical features) and confirmed with methylation analysis, deletion/duplication studies, and array for UPD7
- Surveillance of growth, hypoglycemia, and speech are routine
- Multidisciplinary cares (including referral to urology and endocrinology and GI when appropriate)

SYNDROMES WITH WILMS TUMOR RISK

Beckwith-Wiedemann Syndrome (BWS)

BASIC INFORMATION

- BWS is an overgrowth syndrome due methylation defects on chromosome 11 imprinting centers within the BWS critical region, causing disruption in the regulation of genes in this area and overgrowth
- Chromosome 11 methylation defects, UPD inheritance, AD pattern of inheritance
- Occurs in 1/13,500 people

CLINICAL PRESENTATION

- Face
  - Macroglossia
  - Nevus flammeus
  - Infraorbital creases
  - Earlobe creases
- GI
  - Omphalocele, umbilical hernia
  - Visceromegaly
- Endocrine
  - Hypoglycemia
  - Hyperinsulinism
- Other
  - Macrosomia
  - Hemihypertrophy
  - Renal anomalies (medullary dysplasia, nephrocalcinosis)
  - Embryonal tumors (Wilms, hepatoblastoma, neuroblastoma, rhabdomyosarcoma)

DIAGNOSIS AND EVALUATION

- Laboratory testing
  - DNA methylation studies of BWS critical region
  - Chromosomal microarray (to confirm microdeletions/duplications, or paternal UPD)
  - Karyotype (to confirm inversions or translocations)
  - Alpha-feto protein level
- Imaging
  - RBUS
  - Abdominal US

TREATMENT AND MANAGEMENT

- Not all affected individuals have features present at birth, but in utero findings that are suggestive of this diagnosis include placental mesenchymal dysplasia
- Growth rate slows after 8 years of age
- Tumor surveillance
  - Abdominal US every 3 months until 8 years
  - AFP levels every 3 months until 4 years
  - Annual RBUS from 8 years to adolescence

Denys-Drash Syndrome (DDS)

BASIC INFORMATION

- DDS is characterized by diffuse mesangial sclerosis (leads to end-stage renal disease [ESRD] in adolescence) and gonadal dysgenesis due to mutations in *WT1*; AD inheritance
- Diagnosis made through molecular sequencing of *WT1*
- Surveillance for Wilms tumor necessary because this affects up to 90% of individuals. Renal transplant is routine for management to avoid renal failure and potential tumor development
- Males with DDS are infertile

WAGR Syndrome

BASIC INFORMATION

- WAGR syndrome is due to deletion of the short arm (p) of chromosome 11 that includes several genes (*PAX6*, *WT1*), causing Wilms tumor, aniridia (or cataracts, glaucoma, nystagmus), GU anomalies (hypospadias, cryptorchidism, streak ovaries, bicornuate uterus), and mental retardation (with behavioral issues such as ADHD, anxiety, obsessive compulsive disorder [OCD], autism spectrum disorder)
- Not inherited; occurs in 1/500,000 people
- Diagnostic laboratory testing includes: chromosomal microarray, FISH, alpha-feto protein (AFP)
- Supportive cares and early intervention are recommended; ophthalmologic evaluation every 6 months <8 years
- Routine US surveillance for Wilms tumor until 9 years of age

Isolated Hemihyperplasia (IH)

BASIC INFORMATION

- IH, characterized by asymmetric overgrowth of the body, is caused by abnormal methylation or paternal UPD of 11p15
- Typical areas of asymmetric overgrowth include the chest, kidneys, limbs, and soft tissues
- Diagnosis is made through methylation studies and chromosomal microarray
- It is associated with increased risk of embryonal cancers in childhood. Risk for Wilms tumor is 20%

SYNDROMES WITH HEREDITARY CANCERS

Li-Fraumeni Syndrome (LFS)

BASIC INFORMATION

- Increase in risk of cancers due to mutations in *CHEK2* and *TP53*, causing abnormal DNA repair
- AD inheritance
- Cancers most associated include soft tissue sarcomas, osteosarcoma, premenopausal breast cancer, brain tumors, leukemias, and adrenocortical carcinoma, but can occur anywhere
- Clinical criteria
  - Proband with sarcoma <45 years
  - First-degree relative with any cancer <45 years
  - First- or second-degree relative with any cancer at any age
- Diagnostic laboratory testing: *TP53* and *CHEK2* molecular genetic testing
- Surveillance guidelines
  - Breast cancer monitoring with annual breast MRI and biannual clinical breast examination for patients >20 years of age
  - Annual pelvic examination and mammography is recommended for women >40 years of age
  - Prophylactic mastectomy is an option for patients with germline *TP53* mutations
  - Surveillance with routine colonoscopy every 2 to 3 years for patients >25 years of age
  - Avoid radiation and carcinogen (sun, tobacco, alcohol) exposure

Hereditary Breast/Ovarian Cancer (HBOC)

BASIC INFORMATION

- Caused by a mutation in *BRCA1* or *BRCA2* (tumor suppressor genes), causing damage to the DNA repair system
- AD inheritance
- Clinical signs
  - Breast cancer, <50 years at time of diagnosis
  - Ovarian cancer
  - Multiple primary breast cancers in one or both breasts
  - Male breast cancer
  - Family history of multiple breast cancers
- Diagnostic laboratory testing: *BRCA1* and *BRCA2* molecular genetic testing
- Surveillance
  - Monthly self-breast examination, with clinical examinations annually for patients >25 years of age
  - Annual breast MRI for patients >25 years of age
  - Annual mammogram for patients >30 years of age
  - Annual transvaginal US and CA-125 concentration for patients >35 years of age
  - Men are also at risk
    - Monthly self-breast examination, with annual clinical examinations, for men >35 years of age
    - Annual prostate cancer screening for patients >45 years of age
- Treatment of manifestations per National Comprehensive Cancer Network (NCCN) guidelines (may consider prophylactic mastectomy/oophorectomy; oral contraceptives may reduce ovarian cancer risk)

SYNDROMES WITH MITOCHONDRIAL PHENOTYPES

Alpers-Huttenlocher Syndrome (AHS)

BASIC INFORMATION

- AHS is due to mutations in *POLG*, causing abnormal production of the alpha subunit of polymerase gamma, leading to reduced ability to replicate DNA; AR inheritance
- Classic triad: intractable epilepsy, psychomotor regression, liver disease
- Diagnosis includes mitochondrial genome molecular genetic testing, *POLG* molecular genetic testing, and liver function tests
- Surveillance includes EEG (epilepsia partialis continua), MRI if indicated, baseline pulmonary function tests, avoidance of valproic acid and sodium divalproate for seizure management, and dose reductions of hepatically metabolized medications to avoid toxicity
- Supportive cares through multidisciplinary team management are encouraged

Leigh Syndrome

BASIC INFORMATION

- Leigh syndrome is due to a mutation of one of 75+ different genes within the mitochondrial genome, causing abnormal oxidative phosphorylation within the respiratory chain; AR inheritance
- Classic examination findings include lactic acidosis, FTT, hypotonia, peripheral neuropathy, and hypertrophic cardiomyopathy
- Diagnosis through mitochondrial genome molecular genetic testing, blood + cerebrospinal fluid (CSF) lactate levels, muscle biopsy, and respiratory chain enzyme studies. MRI shows bilateral symmetric hypodensities in the basal ganglia
- Surveillance includes supportive management and routine surveillance of new symptoms, sodium bicarbonate to treat acidosis, and antiepileptic drugs to treat seizures (avoiding valproic acid)
- Supportive cares through multidisciplinary team management are encouraged

Mitochondrial Encephalomyopathy, Lactic Acidosis, and Stroke-Like Episodes (MELAS)

BASIC INFORMATION

- MELAS is due to a mutation in one of several mitochondrial genes (*MT-TL1* and others), leading to inability of the mitochondria to produce energy, use oxygen, or make proteins; mitochondrial inheritance
- Classic examination findings include *m*itochondrial *e*ncephalomyopathy, *l*actic *a*cidosis, and *s*troke-like episodes. Other symptoms include muscle weakness, headaches, vomiting, vision impairment, hearing loss, and diabetes mellitus
- Diagnosis includes mtDNA molecular genetic testing, including *MT-TL1*, lactic acidosis in blood + CSF, elevated CSF protein, muscle biopsy, and respiratory chain studies. Muscle biopsy reveals ragged red fibers
- Development is initially normal; symptoms typically begin in childhood with stroke-like episodes presenting in patients <40 years of age (arginine for acute treatment, MRI when indicated). Surveillance includes routine ECG, echocardiography, TFTs, and ophthalmologic evaluation. Avoidance of medications with mitochondrial toxicity
- Supportive cares through multidisciplinary team management are encouraged

HIGH-YIELD SYNDROMES

22q11.2 Deletion Syndrome

BASIC INFORMATION

- Causes and etiology
  - 22q11.2 deletion syndrome due to a common 3 Mb deletion (containing 30–40 genes) that occurs on chromosome 22, causing abnormal development of the pharyngeal arches
  - AD inheritance
  - Occurs in 1/4000 people

CLINICAL PRESENTATION

- Face
  - Hooded eyelids, ptosis
  - Abnormal auricles
  - Bulbous nose with anteverted nares
  - Palate abnormalities
  - Asymmetric crying facies
- Neurologic
  - Developmental delay
  - Psychiatric disorders (ADHD, anxiety, autism spectrum disorder, schizophrenia)
- CV
  - Congenital heart disease (tetralogy of Fallot [ToF], conotruncal defects, interrupted aortic arch)
- GI
  - Feeding difficulties
- Endocrine
  - Hypocalcemia
- Extremities
  - Arachnodactyly
- Other
  - Renal anomalies
  - Immune dysfunction
- See Fig. 35.13

DIAGNOSIS AND EVALUATION

- Laboratory testing
  - 22q11.2 deletion molecular genetic testing (array or MLPA or FISH)
  - Serum calcium
  - Parathyroid hormone (PTH)
  - IgG levels
- Imaging
  - RBUS
  - Video laryngoscopy

TREATMENT AND MANAGEMENT

- Multidisciplinary team approach
- Standard treatment for congenital heart disease
- Calcium replacement as needed
- If immunodeficient, no *live* vaccines
- Postvaccine Ab titers

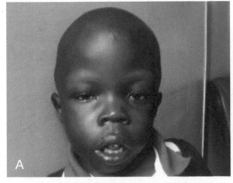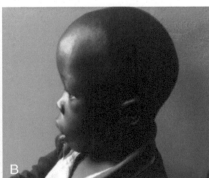

Fig. 35.13. 22q11.2 Deletion syndrome. (A) Frontal view. (B) Profile view. (From Wonkam, Ambroise; Toko, Ricardo; Chelo, David : The 22q11.2 deletion syndrome in congenital heart defects: prevalence of microdeletion syndrome in cameroon, *Global Heart* 12 (2) : 115-120.)

Cri-du-Chat (5p Minus Syndrome)

BASIC INFORMATION

- Cri-du-chat is due to a deletion of the short arm (p) of chromosome 5, causing the loss of *CTNND2*, which is associated with severe intellectual disability; not inherited
- Classic physical examination findings include a high-pitched cry, hypertelorism, low-set ears, microcephaly, micrognathia, congenital heart defects, cleft palate, and hypotonia
- Diagnosis via SNP chromosomal microarray. Echocardiography if there is concern for congenital heart disease (CHD)
- Management includes supportive cares and early intervention

CHARGE Syndrome

BASIC INFORMATION

- Multiple anomalies due to a mutation in *CHD7*, causing insufficiency of the chromatin helicase DNA binding protein 7, thought to play key roles in embryonic development by affecting chromatin structure and gene expression
- AD inheritance
- Occurs in 1/8500 to 1/10,000 people
- Differential diagnosis
  - 22q11.2 deletion syndrome
  - Kallmann syndrome
  - VACTERL association (see later)

CLINICAL PRESENTATION

- Physical examination signs
  - C: eye coloboma (with or without microphthalmia)
  - H: heart anomalies (conotruncal defects, arch abnormalities)
  - A: choanal atresia
  - R: growth retardation
  - G: GU (microphallus) and GI malformations
  - E: ear anomalies (helix malformation, deafness) and extremities (clubfoot, absent tibia)
  - Other:
    - Tracheoesophageal fistula or esophageal atresia
    - Dysphagia
    - Facial palsy
    - Orofacial clefts
    - Hand anomalies (square palm, short fingers, finger-like thumb, hockey-stick palmar crease)

DIAGNOSIS AND EVALUATION

- Laboratory testing
  - *CHD7* molecular genetic testing
- Imaging
  - Echocardiography
  - Temporal bone CT
  - RBUS
- Airway evaluation and associated anesthesia risk
- Audiology evaluation
- Feeding evaluation

TREATMENT AND MANAGEMENT

- 20% to 25% mortality in patients <1 year of age
- Patients are expected to have variable degrees of intellectual disability
- Deaf-blind service referral for those who qualify
- Testing for hypogonadotropic hypogonadism if puberty is delayed in patients >14 years of age
- Multidisciplinary cares based on systemic involvement
- Attention to psychiatric issues such as obsessive-compulsive disorder, pervasive developmental disorder, and ADHD

VACTERL Association

BASIC INFORMATION

- Individuals diagnosed with VACTERL association have at least three of the following characteristic features:
  - Vertebral defects
  - Anal atresia
  - Cardiac defects
  - Tracheo-Esophageal fistula
  - Renal anomalies
  - Limb abnormalities
- Unclear genetic etiology; occurs sporadically; diagnosis is clinical
- Management is mostly symptomatic

Wolf-Hirschhorn Syndrome (WHS)

BASIC INFORMATION

- WHS is due to a deletion of the Wolf-Hirschhorn syndrome critical region short arm (p) of chromosome 4 (includes *NSD2*, *LETM1*, and *MSX1*), causing physical abnormalities and intellectual disability; not inherited
- Classic physical examination findings include a "Greek warrior helmet" appearance (hypertelorism, high forehead with prominent glabella, and a broad/flat nasal bridge), microcephaly, cleft lip/palate, CHD, GU malformations, hypotonia, and structural brain anomalies
- Diagnosis by SNP chromosomal microarray
- Surveillance with plasma IgA levels, CBC, and renal function tests. Imaging should include echocardiography, MRI, and EEG when indicated. Consider routine liver US to screen for hepatic adenomas
- Supportive cares through multidisciplinary team management are encouraged

Cat eye syndrome (CES)

BASIC INFORMATION

- CES is due to a duplication of a critical region on chromosome 22 (22pter > q11), causing trisomy or tetrasomy that leads to its characteristic features; not inherited

- Classic physical examination findings include down-slanting palpebral fissures, iris colobomas, cleft palate, cardiac defects, renal anomalies, anal atresia, short stature, and skeletal anomalies
- Diagnosis via SNP chromosomal microarray
- Supportive cares and expectant management are encouraged because clinical presentation can be extremely variable. Most patients have a normal life expectancy and are mild to borderline normal in terms of intellectual abilities

Review Questions

For review questions, please go to ExpertConsult.com.

Suggested Readings

1. Carey JC, Bamshad MJ. Clinical genetics and dysmorphology. In: Rudolph CD, et al., ed. *Rudolph's Pediatrics.* 22nd ed. China: McGraw-Hill; 2011:677–747.
2. Hunter A. Medical genetics: the diagnostic approach to the child with dysmorphic signs. *CMAJ.* 2002;167(2):367–372.
3. Jones KL, Jones MC, Del Campo M. *Smith's Recognizable Patterns of Human Malformation.* 7th ed. Philadelphia: Elsevier Saunders; 2013.
4. Levy PA, Marion RW. Human genetics and dysmorphology. In: Marcdante KJ, ed. *Nelson Essentials of Pediatrics.* 6th ed. Philadelphia: Saunders Elsevier; 2011:167–186.
5. GeneReviews [Internet]. University of Washington, Seattle; 1993-2017 [cited 2017 Feb 05]. Available from: http://www.genereviews.org/.
6. National Library of Medicine (US). Genetics Home Reference [Internet]. *Bethesda (MD): The library.* 2013. [cited 2017 Feb 05]. Available from: https://ghr.nlm.nih.gov/.
7. Reardon W, Donnai D. Dysmorphology demystified. *Arch Dis Child Fetal Neonatal Ed.* 2007;92:225–229.

Hematology

36 Anemia and Erythrocyte Disorders

ARUN GURUNATHAN, MD

Anemia Overview

BASIC INFORMATION

- In clinical practice, anemia is usually defined as a reduction in blood hemoglobin (Hgb) concentration and/or hematocrit
  - Generally below the 2.5th percentile
  - Normal ranges vary based on age, race, and sex (Table 36.1)
    - African Americans have slightly lower Hgb
- Characterization of anemias
  - Morphology: red blood cell (RBC) size as noted by mean corpuscular volume (MCV): microcytic, normocytic, or macrocytic
    - MCV changes with age; it is above adult range as a newborn, then drops below adult range later on in infancy, and then gradually rises (Table 36.1)
  - Morphology: changes in RBC shape/appearance (e.g., hypochromia, sickle cells, spherocytes)
  - Physiology: decreased production or increased destruction/loss
    - Often assessed via corrected reticulocyte count (CRC)
      Normal reticulocyte count is generally around 0.5% to 1.5%
      CRC = Reticulocyte Count × (Patient Hematocrit/ Normal Hematocrit)
      CRC <1.0 represents inadequate production response to anemia
      CRC >2.0 suggests an appropriately increased bone marrow production response to ongoing RBC destruction (hemolysis), sequestration, or loss (bleeding)

- Physiologic anemia of infancy
  - After birth, a baby receives oxygen directly from the atmosphere as opposed to from maternal circulation, and this increase in availability of oxygen causes a sharp drop in erythropoiesis
    - In term infants, Hgb nadir of 9 to 11 g/dL at 8 to 12 weeks of age
    - Preterm infants nadir lower (7 to 9 g/dL Hgb) and earlier (4 to 6 weeks of age) due to lower levels of Hgb at birth, decreased RBC lifespan and suboptimal erythropoietin response.
    - No treatment needed in cases of otherwise healthy infants.
    - See also Nelson Textbook of Pediatrics, Chapter 447, "The Anemias."

CLINICAL PRESENTATION

- Important historical facts
  - Features that suggest different normal range for Hgb/hematocrit: age, sex, race, and ethnicity
  - External factors: poor diet, medications, toxic and infectious exposures
  - Chronic diseases
  - General symptoms of anemia: weakness, fatigue, decreased exercise tolerance
  - Features that may suggest hemolytic anemia: darkening of urine, family history of jaundice or of needing splenectomy, or early-onset gallstones
- Physical examination
  - Pallor (assess at sites where capillary beds are visible, such as conjunctiva, nail beds, or palms)
  - Cardiac: tachycardia, flow murmur. If prolonged and severe, can see signs of heart failure
  - Features that may suggest hemolytic anemia: scleral icterus, jaundiced skin, splenomegaly

EVALUATION

- Initial testing should include a complete blood count (CBC) to confirm anemia and assess for pancytopenia.
  - If not pancytopenic, assess MCV and CRC, with further testing to be done based on these results and the information on history and physical (Fig. 36.1)
- Other laboratory findings in hemolysis: indirect hyperbilirubinemia, decreased haptoglobin, increased lactate dehydrogenase (LDH), and aspartate transaminase (AST)

Table 36.1. Hemoglobin and MCV Values

Age (years)	Hemoglobin (g/dL)		MCV (µm³)	
	Mean	Lower Limit	Mean	Lower Limit
0.5–1.9	12.5	11	77	70
2–4	12.5	11	79	73
5–7	13	11.5	81	75
8–11	13.5	12	83	76
12–14 female	13.5	12	85	78
12–14 male	14	12.5	84	77
15–17 female	14	12	87	79
15–17 male	15	13	86	78

MCV, Mean corpuscular volume.
Modified from Brugnara C, Oski FJ, Nathan DG. *Nathan and Oski's Hematology of Infancy and Childhood,* ed 7, Philadelphia, PA: Saunders; 2009: 456.

INITIAL MANAGEMENT OF SEVERE ANEMIA

- Patients with chronic profound anemia are at risk for cardiorespiratory compromise with excessive fluid
  - Only give crystalloid fluid boluses if necessary for hemodynamic stability and when there is not enough time to administer packed RBCs (PRBCs), and use smaller volumes and reassess patient after each bolus
    - Risk of worsening anemia and compromising oxygen-carrying capacity with excessive crystalloid fluids
  - If needing to give PRBCs a general rule of thumb is to provide aliquots equal in size to the Hgb concentration, run over 4 hours
    - For example, give 4 mL/kg PRBCs to a child with an Hgb of 4 g/dL (run over 4 hours, and reassess before deciding whether to give more PRBCs)
    - Transfusion goal is to resolve significant symptoms, not normalization of Hbg concentration

MICROCYTIC ANEMIA WITH LOW/ INADEQUATE RETICULOCYTES

Iron Deficiency Anemia (IDA)

BASIC INFORMATION

- Most common nutritional deficiency; most often seen in toddlers aged 1 to 3 years and adolescent females, but can be seen in any age group if diet very low in iron
- Worldwide, a common cause of IDA is gastrointestinal (GI) blood loss from hookworms or schistosomiasis, but this is much less common in the United States
- Etiology in toddlers
  - Iron stores built up in neonatal period (as Hgb concentration falls and iron is reclaimed and stored) are depleted by 9 months of age if poor iron intake
  - Switch from breast milk or formula to whole bovine milk (low iron content, blood loss from milk protein colitis)
    - Especially at risk if >24 oz/day
- Etiology in adolescent females
  - Combination of adolescent growth spurt and menstrual blood loss
  - Highest risk in teenagers who are or have been pregnant
- Time line of hematologic abnormalities: red cell distribution width (RDW) rise → MCV drop → Hgb drop
- Nonhematologic effects of IDA
  - Impaired psychomotor function
  - Impaired intellectual function
    - Changes may not be fully reversible even after iron treatment

CLINICAL PRESENTATION

- Specific features that may suggest IDA
  - Drinking >24 oz/day cow's milk
  - Pica
    - Can result in ingestion of lead-containing substances leading to lead poisoning
  - Menorrhagia
  - Koilonychia (spoon-shaped fingernails)

DIAGNOSIS AND EVALUATION

- CBC: microcytic anemia
  - RDW should be elevated
  - Mentzer index = MCV/RBC
    - >13 suggestive of IDA, <13 suggestive of thalassemia (see below)
  - Screening
    - Generally screen toddlers at least once
    - Recommendations for checking CBC in adolescents vary, but at the very least recommended to check CBC if diet low in iron-rich foods or if excessive menstrual bleeding
- If history, examination, and CBC are all consistent with IDA in a toddler or adolescent female, no other laboratory work is needed
  - For other children, recommend also doing reticulocyte count, lead level if concern on history, review of blood smear (should see hypochromic, microcytic erythrocytes), and screen stools for occult blood

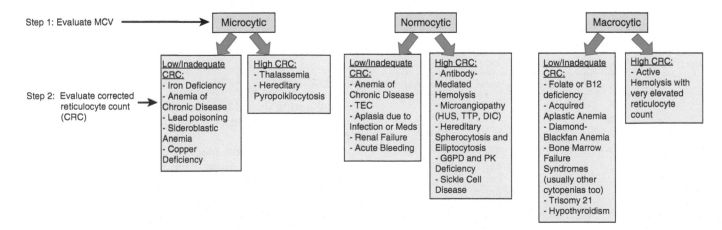

Fig. 36.1. Evaluation of anemia. (Modified from Brunetti M, Cohen J: *The Harriest Lane Handbook*, ed 17, Philadelphia, PA: Elsevier Mosby; 2005: 338.)

Table 36.2. Laboratory Studies in Microcytic Anemias

Test	Iron Deficiency Anemia	Thalassemia	Anemia of Chronic Disease
Hemoglobin	Decreased	Decreased	Decreased
MCV	Decreased	Decreased	Normal to decreased
RDW	Increased	Normal	Normal to increased
RBC	Decreased	Normal to increased	Normal to decreased
Serum ferritin	Decreased	Normal	Increased
Total iron binding capacity	Increased	Normal	Decreased
Transferrin saturation	Decreased	Normal	Decreased

Modified from Kliegman RM, Stanton BF, St. Geme JW, et al, editors: *Nelson Textbook of Pediatrics,* 19th ed. Philadelphia, PA: Elsevier; 2011: 1656.

- If not clearly consistent with isolated IDA and/or anemia does not respond to iron therapy, check iron studies (ferritin, total iron binding capacity, transferrin saturation) and Hgb electrophoresis (Table 36.2)
  - Serum iron can be normal in IDA!

PREVENTION

- Infants
  - For full-term and premature formula-fed infants, the formula should supply the required iron (1 mg/kg/day elemental iron for full-term infants, 2–4 mg/kg/day for premature infants)
  - For breastfed full-term infants, iron supplementation (1 mg/kg/day elemental iron, max. 15 mg) should start at 4 months of age
  - Breastfed premature infants should start an iron supplement after 2 weeks of age (2–4 mg/kg/day elemental iron, max. 15 mg)
- Older children: ensure proper diet
  - Iron-rich foods
    - Meats (red meat, pork, poultry, seafood)
    - Green leafy vegetables (especially spinach)
    - Dried Fruit (e.g., raisins, apricots, dates)
    - Iron-fortified pastas/cereals
    - Beans
  - Also encourage foods rich in vitamin C (increases absorption of iron)
  - No more than 16 oz/day of cow's milk

TREATMENT

- Elemental iron therapy (3 mg/kg/day if Hgb >9, 4–6 mg/kg/day if Hgb <9)
  - Ideally give on an empty stomach; do not take with milk (decreases absorption); giving with orange juice can help (vitamin C increases absorption)
  - Side effects
    - GI symptoms: dark stools, constipation, stomach cramping
    - Darkened urine

- Gray staining of teeth and gums (prevent this by brushing teeth and/or rinsing with water after administration)
- Enteral iron is first-line, but intravenous (IV) iron can be considered when patient is intolerant of or refractory to enteral formulations
- Monitor response
  - Check Hgb no later than 1 month into therapy (Hgb should rise at least 1 g/dL)
    - If needing to assess response quickly, can assess reticulocyte count (should start to increase in 2 to 3 days)
  - If CBC is improving but not normalized, continue supplementation and recheck CBC at least every 2 to 3 months
  - Once normalized, continue iron supplementation for about 2 months to replace iron storage pools

Lead Poisoning

BASIC INFORMATION

- Major sources of lead exposure include paint (especially in houses built before 1978 or in imported toys), imported cosmetics, soil near sources of lead, water from lead-soldered plumbing, and food or beverages stored in lead-containing vessels
- In the United States lead has been removed from gasoline and paint and is no longer used in toys/vessels/pottery; however, that is not necessarily the case in other parts of the world
- Iron deficiency can increase susceptibility to lead poisoning due to increased lead absorption

CLINICAL PRESENTATION

- Neurologic effects
  - In children, the most serious symptoms affect the central nervous system, with subtle changes (such as decreased IQ and changes in behavior) occurring at lower levels and severe effects (such as seizures and encephalopathy) occurring at higher levels (often >100 mcg/dL)
  - Blood lead levels (BLLs) >10 mcg/dL have been shown to affect cognitive and behavioral development, although neurocognitive effects are thought to be possible at even lower BLLs
- Renal effects
  - Can see subtle abnormalities in renal tubular dysfunction associated with aminoaciduria and glycosuria, with progression to chronic interstitial nephritis with prolonged high-level lead exposure
- GI effects
  - Intermittent abdominal pain and emesis, constipation

DIAGNOSIS AND EVALUATION

- Elevated venous BLL
  - Capillary blood sampling is simpler to perform but can have false positives, so all patients with elevated BLLs on capillary samples should have confirmatory venous blood testing

- No amount of lead in the blood is considered "normal." Specific interventions for lead poisoning start at BLLs ≥5 mcg/dL

TREATMENT

- Lead levels between 5 and 44 mcg/dL
  - Retest BLL (within 1 to 3 months if <15 mcg/dL; otherwise within 1 to 4 weeks)
  - Identify and remove potential sources of environmental exposure
  - Nutritional counseling with regard to calcium (competes with lead for binding sites in the body) and iron/vitamin C (correction of iron deficiency decreases lead absorption)
- Lead levels >44 mcg/dL
  - Chelation therapy (oral succimer is generally first-line if asymptomatic; dimercaprol and CaNa2-EDTA if symptomatic)
  - Patients are often admitted for chelation therapy, especially if BLL ≥70 mcg/dL

MICROCYTIC ANEMIA AND HIGH RETICULOCYTES

Thalassemia

BASIC INFORMATION

- Defects in alpha- or beta-globin gene production
  - Four genes produce alpha-globin; two genes produce beta-globin
  - Normal hemoglobin (HgbA) = 2 alpha-globin chains + 2 beta-globin chains = "$\alpha_2\beta_2$"
  - Hemoglobin A$_2$ (HgbA$_2$) = 2 alpha-globin chains + 2 delta-globin chains = "$\alpha_2\delta_2$." Normally makes up 1-3% of all hemoglobin
- Thalassemia is considered a chronic hemolytic anemia
- Epidemiology
  - Alpha and beta thalassemia are most commonly seen in persons of African and Southeast Asian descent (also persons of Mediterranean descent in the case of beta thalassemia)
- Alpha thalassemia
  - Carrier: one-gene deletion ($\alpha-/\alpha\alpha$): not anemic, normocytic
  - Trait: two-gene deletion ($\alpha-/\alpha-$) or ($\alpha\alpha/--$): mild anemia, generally asymptomatic (can be incorrectly diagnosed as iron deficiency anemia)
  - Hemoglobin H (HgbH) disease: three-gene deletion ($\alpha-/--$): moderate to severe anemia characterized by the presence of beta-globin tetramers (β_4) known as Hemoglobin H (HgbH)
  - Hgb Barts/hydrops fetalis: no alpha-globin genes, fatal
- Beta thalassemia
  - "β" = normal beta-globin gene; "β^+" = somewhat defective gene with reduced beta-globin synthesis; "β^0" = severely defective gene with absent beta-globin synthesis
  - Thalassemia trait/minor: (β/β^+) or (β/β^0): mild anemia, generally asymptomatic

Table 36.3. Findings in Alpha Thalassemia

Disorder	Genotype	Anemia Severity	Hemoglobin Electrophoresis
Carrier	$\alpha\,\alpha/\alpha-$	None (mean corpuscular volume normal)	Normal (<3% Hgb Barts at birth)
Trait	$\alpha\alpha/--$ or $\alpha-/\alpha-$	Mild	Normal (3%–8% Hgb Barts at birth)
HgbH disease	$\alpha-/--$	Moderate	5%–30% HgbH (20%–40% Hgb Barts at birth)
Hydrops fetalis	$--/--$	Fatal	No HgbA, HgbF, or HgbA$_2$

Hgb, Hemoglobin; *HgbA,* normal hemoglobin; *HgbF,* fetal hemoglobin; *HgbH,* beta-globin tetramers (β_4); *HgbA$_2$,* $\alpha_2\delta_2$.

Table 36.4. Findings in Beta Thalassemia

Disorder	Genotype	Anemia Severity	Hemoglobin Electrophoresis
Minor/trait	β/β^0 or β/β^+	Mild	HgbA$_2$ and/or HgbF increased
Intermedia	Most commonly β^+/β^+	Moderate	HgbA$_2$ and/or HgbF increased
Major	β^0/β^0	Severe	No HgbA, only HgbA$_2$ and HgbF

HgbA, Normal hemoglobin; *HgbF,* fetal hemoglobin; *HgbA$_2$,* $\alpha_2\delta_2$.

- Thalassemia intermedia: (β^+/β^+): present with anemia around 2 years of life; may need chronic hypertransfusion therapy starting in the second/third decade of life
- Thalassemia major: (β^0/β^0) or (β^+/β^0): presence of anemia

CLINICAL PRESENTATION

- Specific features that may suggest thalassemia
  - Skeletal abnormalities, especially in beta-thalassemia major (e.g., frontal bossing, "hair-on-end" radiographic appearance of the skull, short limbs)
  - Hepatosplenomegaly

DIAGNOSIS AND EVALUATION

- See Tables 36.3 and 36.4
- Microcytosis is generally more pronounced than in iron deficiency
  - Mentzer index (MCV/RBC) <13 is suggestive of thalassemia
- Newborn screening (NBS)
  - Normal NBS Hgb evaluation reveals the presence of fetal hemoglobin (HgbF) and HgbA; thus the NBS result is "FA"
  - An NBS result of only "F" suggests an absence of HgbA (or a premature infant), which may be consistent with beta thalassemia major. Beta thalassemia trait would not be detected
  - Presence of Hgb Barts (tetramers of fetally expressed γ-chains) on newborn screen (e.g., "FA Barts") indicates loss of at least one alpha-globin gene, consistent with alpha thalassemia carrier, trait, or HgbH disease

- Hemoglobin electropheresis
  - Alpha thalassemia
    - Usually normal in carrier and trait
    - HgbH (β_4) may be seen in HgbH disease, but absence does not rule it out
    - Alpha-globin gene analysis available if needing to confirm diagnosis
  - Beta thalassemia
    - Trait/minor and intermedia: HgbA decreased, HgbA$_2$ ($\alpha_2\delta_2$) and HgbF ($\alpha_2\gamma_2$) often increased
    - Major: HgbA absent, only HgbA$_2$ and HgbF present

TREATMENT

- Generally no treatment is required for alpha thalassemia trait and carrier or for beta thalassemia minor
- Chronic transfusion therapy in beta thalassemia major and most cases of beta thalassemia intermedia and HgbH disease
  - Monitor for iron overload because iron chelation therapy is often required
- Hematopoietic stem cell transplantation is a potential curative option in beta thalassemia major

NORMOCYTIC ANEMIA WITH LOW/INADEQUATE RETICULOCYTES

Transient Erythroblastopenia of Childhood (TEC)

BASIC INFORMATION

- Most common acquired red cell aplasia in children
- Occurs in children between 6 months and 3 years of age (most children older than 12 months)
- Temporary suppression of hematopoiesis
  - Often follows a viral illness, although no specific virus has been found to be a consistent etiologic factor

CLINICAL PRESENTATION

- Anemia develops gradually
- Can be symptomatic if anemia is severe

DIAGNOSIS AND EVALUATION

- Other cell lines may be affected
  - Neutropenia can occur in up to 20% of cases
  - Platelets normal or elevated
- Distinguishing TEC from Diamond Blackfan anemia
  - Look at differences in age, MCV, HgbF, and erythrocyte adenosine deaminase (Table 36.5)
- Distinguishing TEC from RBC aplasia from parvovirus B19 infection in a patient with chronic hemolysis or immunocompromise
  - Look for features to suggest hemolysis or immune compromise and signs of parvovirus ("slapped cheek" appearance, adults with arthralgias)

Table 36.5. Comparing Diamond Blackfan Anemia and Transient Erythroblastopenia of Childhood

	Diamond Blackfan Anemia	Transient Erythroblastopenia of Childhood
Median age of onset	3 months	24 months
Antecedent illness	None	Viral illness
Abnormal physical examination	25%	0%
Adenosine deaminase	Increased	Normal
High mean corpuscular volume at diagnosis	80%	5%
High HbF at diagnosis	100%	20%

HgbF, fetal hemoglobin.
Modified from Nathan DG, Orkin SH, Ginsburg D, et al, editors: *Nathan and Oski's Hematology of Infancy and Childhood*, ed 6, vol 1. Philadelphia, PA: WB Saunders; 2003: 329.

TREATMENT

- Often no treatment needed, and children recover within 1 to 2 months
- RBC transfusion may be necessary for severe anemia
- Reevaluate for other diagnosis if requiring >1 transfusion or no signs of recovery by 2 months postdiagnosis

NORMOCYTIC ANEMIA WITH HIGH RETICULOCYTES

Membranopathies

BASIC INFORMATION

- Hereditary spherocytosis
  - Most common inherited abnormality of the RBC membrane
  - Usually autosomal dominant, less commonly autosomal recessive
  - Most common molecular defects are abnormalities in ankyrin or spectrin
  - Most common among persons of Northern European origin
- Hereditary elliptocytosis
  - Autosomal dominant, except for hereditary pyropoikilocytosis, which is autosomal recessive
  - More common among West Africans

CLINICAL PRESENTATION

- Variable severity of symptoms
  - Some patients are asymptomatic into adulthood, but other children develop severe hemolytic anemia with pallor, jaundice, fatigue, and exercise intolerance
- In hereditary spherocytosis and severe hereditary elliptocytosis, the spleen is generally enlarged after infancy
- About half of unsplenectomized hereditary spherocytosis patients ultimately develop bilirubin gallstones
- Susceptible to hypoplastic/aplastic crises from infection (especially parvovirus B19)

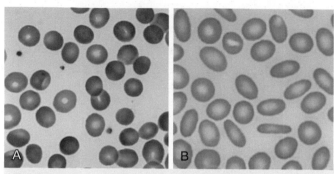

Fig. 36.2. (A) Hereditary spherocytosis. (B) Hereditary elliptocytosis. (From Kliegman RM, Stanton BF, St. Geme JW, et al, eds. *Nelson Textbook of Pediatrics*, 19th ed. Philadelphia, PA: Elsevier Mosby; 2011: 1161 [Fig. 452.4].)

DIAGNOSIS AND EVALUATION

- Other laboratory findings: increased mean corpuscular Hgb concentration (MCHC), findings of hemolysis (see "Evaluation" section of Anemia Overview)
  - Spherocytes (decreased or absent central pallor) or elliptocytes (oval or pencil-shaped) on smear (Fig. 36.2)
  - Some patients are asymptomatic into adulthood, but other children develop severe hemolytic anemia with pallor, jaundice, fatigue, and exercise intolerance
- Osmotic fragility traditionally is used in diagnosis of hereditary spherocytosis and hereditary elliptocytosis, but results may be positive in immune and other hemolytic anemias, and up to 20% of patients can have normal results
  - Ektacytometry is a more sensitive test

TREATMENT

- Supplement with folic acid to prevent deficiency and subsequent decrease in hematopoiesis
- Splenectomy (spherocytes and elliptocytes almost exclusively destroyed in spleen) can eliminate most of the hemolysis, although this is generally done only in severe cases
  - Ideally wait until after 5 years of age to avoid heightened risk of postsplenectomy sepsis in younger children
  - Give vaccines against encapsulated organisms (*Streptococcus pneumoniae*, *Neisseria meningitidis*, and *Haemophilus influenzae* B) before splenectomy
  - Penicillin prophylaxis after splenectomy

G6PD Deficiency

BASIC INFORMATION

- G6PD catalyzes a reaction that produces NADPH, which protects RBCs from oxidant threats that would otherwise cause precipitation of Hgb (Heinz bodies) or damage RBC membrane
- This is an X-linked disorder, so it is much more common in males (rare occurrence in heterozygous females if exaggerated inactivation in normal X chromosome during lyonization)

Table 36.6. Agents That Can Precipitate Hemolysis in G6PD Deficiency

ANTIMICROBIALS
Sulfonamides
Dapsone
Nitrofurantoin
Primaquine and chloroquine

OTHER MEDICATIONS
Methylene blue
Probenecid
Aspirin

CHEMICALS
Benzene
Naphthalene

ILLNESS
Diabetic ketoacidosis
Hepatitis
Sepsis

Modified from Rakel R, editor: *Conn's Current Therapy*, Philadelphia, PA: WB Saunders; 1994: 341.

- G6PD defect in Americans of African descent (G6PD A−) is less severe than G6PD defect in Americans of Mediterranean descent (G6PD B−)

CLINICAL PRESENTATION

- Most patients have no clinical manifestations of illness unless hemolysis is precipitated by infection, medication, or fava beans that increase oxidant stress on RBCs (Table 36.6). Symptoms begin within hours to a few days after exposure to the offending agent
- Chronic hemolytic anemia can be seen in certain enzyme variants that have profound deficiency of G6PD
- G6PD deficiency can produce hemolysis in the neonatal period without a precipitating agent
- If a pregnant woman ingests oxidant drugs and the fetus is G6PD-deficient, hemolytic anemia may be apparent at birth

DIAGNOSIS AND EVALUATION

- Other lab findings: Heinz bodies and bite cells in smear, findings of hemolysis (see "Evaluation" section of Anemia Overview)
- G6PD activity
  - Test a few weeks after a hemolytic episode. Testing during or immediately after a hemolytic episode may produce a misleading normal result because the RBCs that remain are the ones that have higher enzyme activity

TREATMENT

- Screening males of ethnic groups with significant G6PD deficiency (Mediterranean, African, certain Asian groups), and patients who test positive should avoid oxidant drugs and foods
- Discontinue any oxidant agent once found to have G6PD deficiency. If severe hemolysis occurs, may require RBC transfusions to provide support until recovery occurs after the oxidant agent is discontinued

Sickle Cell Disease (SCD)

BASIC INFORMATION

- Hemoglobin S (HgbS) is the result of a single base-pair change in the beta-globin gene which converts a glutamic acid to valine.
- SCD-SS is the most common form, occurring when both beta-globin genes have the sickle cell mutation
- There are many compound heterozygotes in which one beta-globin gene has the sickle mutation and the second beta-globin has a different mutation; SCD-SC and SCD-Sβ-thal (either SCD-Sβ$^+$ or SCD-Sβ^0) are the most common examples
  - Hemoglobin C (HgbC) is the result of a beta-globin base-pair change that converts the glutamic acid to lysine.
- With advancements in care and support, life expectancy of patients with SCD-SS currently in their 50s
- Sickle cell trait: one normal beta-globin (HgbA) and one beta-globin with sickle cell mutation

CLINICAL PRESENTATION

SCD-SS and SCD-Sβ^0

- Generally asymptomatic in the first few months of life due to HgbF
- Immune/infectious complications
  - Functional asplenia can occur as early as 6 months of age and generally occurs by 5 years of age
  - Increased risk of infection and death from bacterial infection, especially encapsulated organisms (*S. pneumoniae*, *N. meningitidis*, and *H. influenzae* B)
  - Increased risk of osteomyelitis (most common organism is still *Staphylococcus aureus*, but much higher incidence of Salmonella osteomyelitis compared with the general population)
  - Infection is the best known etiology of acute chest syndrome (see Management of Acute Chest Syndrome below for more details)
  - Risk of severe red cell aplasia leading to significantly worse anemia (which can precipitate other complications such as acute chest syndrome or stroke) with reticulocytopenia with parvovirus B19 infection
    - Occurs due to temporary cessation of erythropoiesis in the setting of decreased RBC life span in SCD
- Pain complications
  - Dactylitis (also known as hand-foot syndrome)
    - Often the first manifestation of pain in children, generally occurring within the first 2 years of life
    - Manifests with symmetric or unilateral swelling of hands and/or feet
  - Vasoocclusive crisis (pain crisis)
    - Thought to occur when blood flow is disrupted in the microvasculature by sickle cells, causing tissue ischemia
    - Precipitating causes of pain crises include physical stress, infection, dehydration, hypoxia, acidosis, cold
    - Abdominal pain crises can have presenting symptoms mimicking acute abdominal complaints such as appendicitis, cholecystitis, and pancreatitis
  - Priapism
    - Involuntary painful penile erection lasting longer than 30 minutes
    - Refractory priapism is defined as prolonged priapism beyond several hours
  - Avascular necrosis
    - Painful osteonecrosis of bone (most often femoral or humeral head) due to interruptions in blood supply
- Lung disease
  - Acute chest syndrome
    - Defined as radiographic evidence of new consolidation *plus* at least one of the following: fever, hypoxia, tachypnea, increased work of breathing, chest pain, wheezing, new cough
  - Risk of developing pulmonary hypertension (a major risk factor for death in adults with SCD)
- Neurologic complications
  - Without intervention, about 20% of patients will have a silent stroke, and 10% of patients will have an overt stroke before adulthood
  - Other neurologic complications include headache, seizures, cerebral venous thrombosis, and posterior reversible encephalopathy syndrome
- Risk of splenic sequestration
  - Presents as acutely enlarged spleen and Hgb below patient's baseline; may also have thrombocytopenia
- Risk of iron overload if needing regular blood transfusions
- Patients at risk of developing cardiomyopathy (diastolic dysfunction with chamber dilation)
  - At risk for cardiorespiratory compromise from fluid overload if large amounts of IV fluids/blood products are given too quickly

Sickle Cell Disease SC (SCD-SC)

- Children can have the same complications as those with SCD-SS, but frequency generally is less
- SCD-SC patients also have increased incidence of retinopathy, chronic hypersplenism, splenic sequestration, and renal medullary carcinoma

Sickle Cell Trait

- Typically normal life span
- Complications can include splenic infarcts and/or pain crises at high altitudes, hyposthenuria (inability to concentrate urine), hematuria, bacteriuria, and increased risk of renal medullary carcinoma

DIAGNOSIS AND EVALUATION

- In the United States this is most often diagnosed via newborn screen
  - "FS" result = Most likely SCD-SS or SCD-Sβ^0
  - "FAS" = Most likely sickle cell trait
  - "FSC" = Most likely SCD-SC
- Hgb electrophoresis
  - HgbA > HgbS = Sickle cell trait
  - HgbS >> HgbF, no HgbA = SCD-SS or SCD-Sβ^0
  - HgbS >> HgbA and HgbF = Most likely SCD-Sβ$^+$
  - HgbS and HgbC: SCD-SC

PROPHYLAXIS

- Infectious prophylaxis
  - Vaccines as per standard schedule. Additionally, 23-valent pneumococcal vaccine at 2 and 5 years of age, meningococcal ACWY vaccine starting at 2 years of age, and meningococcal B vaccine starting at 10 years of age
  - Penicillin prophylaxis until at least 5 years of age (longer if prior history of pneumococcal infection)
- Stroke prophylaxis
  - Transcranial doppler (TCD)
    - Generally done every 12 to 18 months from 2 to 16 years of age
    - Blood flow velocity >200 cm/s increases risk of stroke
  - If abnormal TCD results despite hydroxyurea, then generally do periodic RBC transfusions versus erythrocytapheresis to keep HgbS concentration <30%
- Prophylaxis against other complications
  - Hydroxyurea
    - Increases HgbF concentration
    - Found to decrease rate of vasoocclusive pain crises, rate of acute chest syndrome, and need for blood transfusions by about 50%
    - Also lowers the risk of stroke
    - Primary toxicity from hydroxyurea is myelosuppression
  - Studies are ongoing regarding the possible role of selectin inhibitors as prophylaxis against vasoocclusive pain crises
  - L-glutamine is an emerging therapeutic to reduce SCD-related complications (including pain crises)
  - Regular incentive spirometer use when admitted for a pain crisis reduces frequency of subsequent acute chest syndrome (do not limit opioids solely to prevent acute chest syndrome)

TREATMENT/MANAGEMENT

- Management of vasoocclusive pain crisis
  - Generally starts with acetaminophen or nonsteroidal antiinflammatory drug (NSAID) and supportive care (hydration, heat packs); if not controlled, then escalation to a short- and/or long-acting oral opioid
  - Some patients require admission for IV opioid and IV NSAID
- Management of priapism
  - Generally start with supportive therapy, such as sitz bath or analgesic medications
  - If lasting >4 hours, urology should aspirate blood from the corpora cavernosa followed by irrigation with dilute epinephrine
- Management of fever
  - Considered a medical emergency requiring prompt medical evaluation
  - Blood culture is drawn, and patients generally receive an intramuscular (IM) or IV third-generation cephalosporin or penicillin derivative to complete at least a 24-hour rule-out
  - Outpatient management should be considered only for those with the lowest risk of bacteremia in which there are no concerns for ability to come back to medical attention if clinically worsening or positive blood culture
- Management of acute chest syndrome
  - Infection is the best known etiology
    - Obtain CBC and blood culture
    - Antimicrobial therapy with a macrolide and third-generation cephalosporin or penicillin derivative
    - Consider RBC transfusion if Hgb is below baseline (especially if hypoxemic)
- Management of stroke
  - Immediate management of patient with acute focal neurologic deficit: prompt neurologic evaluation; keeping O_2 sat >95%; neuroimaging; laboratory testing (CBC/retic, type and screen, coagulation studies, basic metabolic panel [BMP]); simple RBC transfusion, if needed, to get Hgb up to approximately 10 mg/dL; IV fluids
  - Exchange transfusion to reduce HgbS percentage to <30%
- Management of aplastic crisis
  - Test for parvovirus B19 (those who are pregnant should avoid exposure to the patient until testing results are negative)
  - Consider RBC transfusion (generally no more than 10 mL/kg at a time to prevent acute fluid overload)
- Management of splenic sequestration
  - small (5-10 mL/kg) normal saline boluses as needed if severe intravascular hypovolemia
  - RBC transfusion if symptomatic from anemia (usually start with 5 mL/kg)
    - Smaller volumes are used because these fluid/blood product infusions can cause an "autotransfusion" phenomenon whereby the patient's RBCs exit the spleen after a fluid/RBC infusion. If a large RBC transfusion is given and there is also autotransfusion, the rise in Hgb may be large enough to result in a hyperviscosity syndrome

Neonatal Hemolytic Anemia

CLINICAL PRESENTATION AND MANAGEMENT

- Neonatal ABO incompatibility
  - Most common cause of hemolysis in the newborn
  - Occurs when mother produces antibodies against the infant's blood type (most often when mother is type O and infant is type A or B)
  - Incompatibility occurs in 20% to 25% of pregnancies, although hemolytic disease develops in only about 10% of such pregnancies (possibly related to low antigenicity of ABO factors in the fetus)
  - Most cases are mild, with jaundice usually the only clinical manifestation (may need phototherapy if indirect hyperbilirubinemia is high enough). Transfusions are rarely needed
- Erythroblastosis fetalis (hemolytic disease of the newborn)
  - Transplacental transfer of Rh-positive antibodies (from a previously sensitized Rh-negative mother) to an Rh-positive fetus
  - If anemia is severe enough, it leads to compensatory hyperplasia of erythropoietic tissue, leading to massive hepatosplenomegaly; once the compensatory system is exceeded, this can lead to cardiac decompensation, anasarca, and circulatory collapse
  - Injection of anti-D gamma globulin (RhoGAM) into the mother immediately after delivery of each Rh-positive infant helps prevent sensitization and risk of disease in future pregnancies

Non-Neonatal Autoimmune Hemolytic Anemia (AIHA)

BASIC INFORMATION

- A number of agents and disorders can lead to immune-mediated destruction of RBCs (Tables 36.7 and 36.8)
  - May be idiopathic or relate to infections, immunologic diseases, immunodeficiency diseases, neoplasms, and medications

CLINICAL PRESENTATION

- General clinical findings: pallor, jaundice, fatigue, hemoglobinuria
- AIHA associated with "warm" (IgG) autoantibodies
  - In addition to general clinical features, may have splenomegaly (spleen is the primary site of destruction of IgG-coated RBCs and extravascular hemolysis)
  - Ages 2 to 12 years: usually transient, preceded by an infection, resolves after 3 to 6 months, and responds well to treatment
    - Unlikely to have underlying systemic disorder, very low mortality rate
  - Children >12 years: prolonged and chronic course, variable response to treatment
    - More likely to be associated with underlying systemic disease

Table 36.7. Causes of Autoimmune Hemolytic Anemia

Warm Reactive Autoantibodies	Cold Reactive Autoantibodies
Idiopathic	Idiopathic
Lymphoproliferative disorders	Lymphoproliferative disorders
Nonlymphoid neoplasms (e.g., ovarian tumors)	Infections (*Mycoplasma pneumoniae*, Epstein-Barr virus)
Connective tissue disorders (e.g., lupus)	Congenital or tertiary syphilis
Chronic inflammatory diseases (e.g., ulcerative colitis)	Paroxysmal cold hemoglobinuria

Modified from Rakel R, editor: *Conn's Current Therapy*, Philadelphia, PA: WB Saunders; 1995: 305.

Table 36.8. Selected Drugs That Can Cause Immune-Mediated Hemolysis

Quinidine
Sulfonamides
Rifampin
Insulin
Isoniazid INH)
Penicillins
Acetaminophen
Alpha-methyldopa
Ibuprofen

Modified from Hoffman R, Benz EJ, Shattil SJ, Furie B, Cohen HJ, Silberstein LE, et al, In: *Hematology: Basic Principles and Practice*. 3rd ed. Philadelphia, PA: Churchill Livingstone; 2000:624.

- AIHA associated with "cold" (IgM) autoantibodies
  - Less common in children than in adults, and more frequently results in an acute, self-limited episode of hemolysis
    - Most commonly due to viral syndromes, especially mycoplasma and Epstein-Barr virus
  - Exposure to cold can heighten IgM-mediated intravascular hemolysis
- Paroxysmal cold hemoglobinuria
  - IgG cold-reactive antibody that causes intravascular hemolysis at cold temperatures
  - Most reported cases are self-limited and usually associated with nonspecific viral infections

DIAGNOSIS AND EVALUATION

- Positive direct antiglobulin test (direct Coombs) demonstrates antibodies bound to RBCs
- Positive indirect Coombs test demonstrates unbound antibody in the serum
- Distinguishing type of AIHA
  - Reaction is positive with IgG and negative with C3: warm–hemolytic anemia, idiopathic, or drug-associated
  - Reaction is positive with IgG and C3: warm–hemolytic anemia, idiopathic, or associated with lupus
  - Reaction is negative with IgG and positive with C3: cold–hemolytic anemia (occasionally also paroxysmal nocturnal hemoglobinuria if testing is done at 37°C)
    - Other findings in cold–hemolytic anemia: clumped RBCs on smear, high titer cold agglutinins
- Once AIHA is confirmed, assess whether it is idiopathic or whether there is a clear infectious, medication, or systemic disease etiology

TREATMENT

- Patients with mild anemia (>9 g/dL) and no evidence of cardiac compromise may not require treatment
- If hemolysis is severe enough to cause significant anemia or symptoms, first-line treatment is glucocorticoids
  - IV immunoglobulin (IVIG), plasmapheresis, and rituximab are second-line options
- Transfusions may be necessary in immediately life-threatening situations but provide only transient benefit until the effect of other treatments is realized
- Treatment may involve removal of the offending drug or management of underlying disease condition

Microangiopathic Hemolytic Anemias (HUS, TTP)

BASIC INFORMATION

- Microangiopathic hemolytic anemia (MAHA): non-immune hemolysis resulting from intravascular RBC fragmentation, often involving abnormalities in the microvasculature
- Hemolytic uremic syndrome (HUS): most commonly due to Shiga toxins from *Escherichia coli* O157:H7 and O104:H4 causing direct damage to renal epithelial/mesangial cells and vascular endothelial cells

- Other causes of HUS include HIV, *S. Pneumoniae*, medications (some examples include quinine, some chemotherapy, and cyclosporine)
  - Atypical HUS can occur and may not be associated with diarrhea; often relates to genetic abnormalities of the complement regulatory proteins; tends to have a worse prognosis
- Thrombotic thrombocytopenic purpura (TTP)
  - Severe deficiency of ADAMTS13 metalloprotease (cleaves von Willebrand factor); generally a hereditary deficiency or acquired deficiency due to autoantibody
  - High mortality rate if not promptly treated

CLINICAL PRESENTATION

- HUS triad: MAHA, thrombocytopenia, renal failure
  - In Shiga toxin–associated HUS, there is often a history of exposure to farm animals, undercooked meat, or contaminated water
- TTP pentad: MAHA, thrombocytopenia, renal failure, neurologic symptoms, and fever
  - In some cases of TTP, not all features are present

DIAGNOSIS AND EVALUATION

- Thrombocytopenia; lab findings consistent with hemolytic anemia (See "Evaluation" section of Anemia Overview)
- Presence of schistocytes (fragmented RBCs) on blood smear
- Stool culture and Shiga toxin assay if there is concern for HUS
- Measurement of ADAMTS13 activity if there is concern for TTP (may take several days to get result)

TREATMENT

- Shiga toxin HUS ("typical HUS"): supportive care with IV fluids and transfusions if there is significantly symptomatic anemia; if there are severe renal issues, temporary dialysis may be required
  - Generally avoid treatment with antibiotics because destruction of bacteria can lead to more toxin in the blood and therefore worse HUS symptoms
- Atypical HUS: anticomplement therapy with eculizumab (antibody against terminal complement)
- TTP: plasmapheresis is often needed (mortality as high as 90% before use of plasmapheresis)
  - If TTP is strongly suspected, do not wait for results of ADAMTS13 activity testing before initiating plasmapheresis

MACROCYTIC ANEMIA WITH LOW/INADEQUATE RETICULOCYTES

Vitamin B$_{12}$ and Folate Deficiency (Megaloblastic Anemia)

BASIC INFORMATION

- Megaloblastic anemia is a macrocytic anemia characterized by ineffective erythropoiesis

- Often has associated thrombocytopenia and leukopenia
- Blood smear generally shows large (often oval) RBCs, with characteristic hypersegmented (more than five lobes) neutrophils
- Almost all cases of childhood megaloblastic anemia are due to folate or B$_{12}$ deficiency but in rare cases are caused by inborn error of metabolism
- Pernicious anemia: vitamin B$_{12}$ deficiency due to the stomach not making intrinsic factor, which is necessary for the intestines to absorb vitamin B$_{12}$

CLINICAL PRESENTATION

- Vitamin B$_{12}$ deficiency
  - Dietary sources include meats and dairy (vegans are at higher risk of deficiency)
  - Because there are large body stores of vitamin B$_{12}$, it generally takes years of inadequate intake to develop symptoms
    - Starts with paresthesias, ataxia, and vibration/proprioception deficits. Can progress to severe weakness, spasticity, paraplegia, and bowel/bladder incontinence
- Folate deficiency
  - Dietary sources include green vegetables, fruits, nuts, beans, eggs, meats, and cow's milk
  - Because body stores of folate are limited, anemia will occur after 2 to 3 months on a folate-poor diet
    - Classic scenario is folate deficiency in infant drinking goat's milk (has much less folate than cow's milk)
  - Unlike vitamin B$_{12}$ deficiency, generally do not see neurologic symptoms

DIAGNOSIS AND EVALUATION

- Check vitamin B$_{12}$ and folate levels
  - Serum folate is a less expensive test but only reflects short-term folate balance; RBC folate provides a longer-term look at folate status
    - Perform RBC folate if serum folate is equivocal
  - If megaloblastic anemia is present but vitamin B$_{12}$ and folate levels are borderline, check methylmalonic acid and homocysteine (vitamin B$_{12}$ is needed for them to be metabolized, so their levels would be high in vitamin B$_{12}$ deficiency)
- Schilling test is more cumbersome and not readily available; not commonly used anymore
- Pernicious anemia: check for antiintrinsic factor antibodies

TREATMENT

- Folic acid and/or vitamin B$_{12}$ medications (depending on which is deficient), along with dietary modifications
  - Rule out vitamin B$_{12}$ deficiency before treating a patient with megaloblastic anemia with folate: folic acid can partially reverse some of the hematologic abnormalities of B$_{12}$ deficiency, but the neurologic symptoms will still progress
- Parenteral B$_{12}$ for pernicious anemia

Diamond Blackfan Anemia

BASIC INFORMATION

- Defect in erythroid progenitor cell, leading to increased apoptosis
  - In about 25% of cases, mutations are seen in the *RPS19* gene
- About half of cases are familial, generally with an autosomal dominant inheritance pattern

CLINICAL PRESENTATION

- Pallor with profound anemia usually becomes evident by 2 to 6 months of age; 90% of cases are recognized in the first year of life
- Growth retardation occurs in about one-third of children
- Congenital malformations are detected in about 35% to 45% of children
- Most commonly, craniofacial abnormalities such as hypertelorism and thumb abnormalities are present

DIAGNOSIS AND EVALUATION

- Macrocytic anemia with reticulocytopenia, but no hypersegmented neutrophils or other characteristics of megaloblastic anemia
- Elevated HgbF, "i" antigen (red blood cell membrane antigen that is strongly expressed in the fetal/neonatal period but afterwards is typically only weakly expressed), and erythrocyte adenosine deaminase activity

TREATMENT

- Corticosteroids are mainstay of therapy, with 80% of patients responding initially
  - Once effectiveness established, gradually wean down to lowest effective dose
- In patients who never respond to or become refractory to steroids, perform RBC transfusions at 1- to 2-month intervals
  - Chelation therapy is needed as excess iron accumulates
- Bone marrow transplant can be curative, though generally considered only if HLA-matched sibling donor is available (survival much lower with alternative donor transplants)

Hemoglobin Poisonings

- Conditions such as methemoglobinemia and carbon monoxide poisoning are not anemias but do affect the ability of Hgb to carry oxygen and deliver it to tissues. These conditions are covered in more depth in Chapter 18

Review Questions

For review questions, please go to ExpertConsult.com

Suggested Readings

1. Gajjar R, Jalazo E. Hematology. In: Engorn B, Flerlage J, editors. *The Harriet Lane Handbook*: 12th ed. Philadelphia, PA: Elsevier. 305–333
2. Lerner NB, Segel GB, DeBaun MR, Frei-Jones M, Vichinsky E. Diseases of the Blood. In: Kliegman RM, Stanton BF, St. Geme JW, Schor NF. *Nelson Textbook of Pediatrics*. 20th ed. Philadelphia: Elsevier; 2016:2304–2359.
3. Orkin SH, Nathan DG, Ginsburg D, Look AT, Fisher DE, Lux S. In: *Nathan and Oski's Hematology and Oncology of Infancy and Childhood*. 8th ed. Philadelphia, PA: Elsevier; 2015.

37 Platelet Disorders and Coagulopathies

TIFFANY F. LIN, MD

Normal hemostasis of your blood is a balance of the appropriate initiation of clotting and the process of fibrinolysis. This balance allows you to stop bleeding when needed while preventing the spontaneous formation of obstructive clots in one's circulatory system. The key players in clotting to prevent excessive bleeding are functional amounts of the following in appropriate quantities: platelets, von Willebrand factor, and clotting factors. Variations in the amounts of those products or their ability to function appropriately can cause excessive bleeding and/or clotting; these disorders will be the focus of this chapter.

See also Nelson Textbook of Pediatrics, Chapter 484, "Platelet and Blood Vessel Disorders."

Overview of Bleeding Diatheses

BASIC INFORMATION

- Bleeding is due to a problem in one of the following steps of normal coagulation (see Table 37.1)
  - Vascular damage or trauma
    - Examples include repetitive nose picking causing bleeding, bruising with venipuncture, a surgical procedure causing bleeding, or a collagen vascular disease causing easy bruising
    - Bleeding appears at the site of vessel injury
  - Platelet adhesion and aggregation
    - Examples include decrease in platelet number, platelet function (congenital dysfunction or medication-acquired platelet dysfunction), von Willebrand amount or function (von Willebrand is important in platelet adhesion), or consumption of platelets (hemolytic uremic syndrome [HUS], thrombotic thrombocytopenic purpura [TTP], Kasabach-Merritt phenomenon)
    - Typical bleeding due to these causes includes petechiae, purpura, and mucosal bleeding such as epistaxis and menorrhagia
  - Formation of the fibrin clot
    - Examples include decrease in clotting factors such as hemophilia A and B, lack of vitamin K causing decreased clotting factors (liver failure, hemorrhagic disease of the newborn), or consumption of the clotting factors (DIC)
    - Typical bleeding due to these causes includes spontaneous bleeding including intracranial bleeds and, more often, hemarthroses. Purpura and bruising can still occur
- Laboratory findings of various causes of bleeding (Table 37.2)
  - Complete blood count (CBC) gives platelet number

- Abnormal mean platelet volume (MPV) and platelet morphology are clues consistent with a congenital platelet abnormality
- Prothrombin time/international normalized ratio (PT/INR) measures the extrinsic coagulation pathway and is sensitive to deficiencies of the vitamin K–dependent factors 2, 5, 7, and 9
- Partial thromboplastin time (PTT) measures the intrinsic coagulation pathway and is sensitive to deficiencies of factors 8, 9, and 11

Thrombocytopenias

BASIC INFORMATION

- The causes of thrombocytopenia can generally be categorized as caused by increased destruction, decreased production, or sequestration
- Thrombocytopenias with increased platelet destruction:
  - Immune thrombocytopenia (ITP)
  - Neonatal alloimmune thrombocytopenia (NAIT)
  - Kasabach-Merritt phenomenon
- Thrombocytopenias with decreased platelet production:
  - Thrombocytopenia-absent radius (TAR)
  - Wiskott-Aldrich syndrome (WAS)
  - Other congenital syndromes that can exhibit thrombocytopenia include Trisomies 21, 18, and 13 and Noonan syndrome
- Splenomegaly leads to thrombocytopenia by sequestration of a large volume of blood when the spleen is enlarged (for which splenectomy or treatment of underlying cause of splenomegaly can recover the platelet count)

CLINICAL PRESENTATION

- Physical signs of bleeding usually are not present unless the platelet count is consistently below 50,000 (often not until under 30,000 in neonates). Presentation may include the following:
  - Cephalohematoma with or without association to the birth extraction technique
  - Muscular hematoma after medication or immunization injection
  - Intracranial hemorrhage
  - Excessive bleeding with procedures

DIAGNOSIS AND EVALUATION

- CBC with differential and platelet count should be performed

- Morphology can be helpful because the platelet count is not only decreased in WAS but also small in size with an MPV of less than 5 fL (microthrombocytopenia).
  - In neonates, head ultrasound may monitor for evidence of intracranial hemorrhage
- Physical examination may give clues as to congenital platelet deficiencies (e.g., TAR)

TREATMENT

- In general, supportive care is recommended for most causes of thrombocytopenias. For some etiologies detailed later, platelet transfusions can be instituted for persistently low platelet count. Otherwise, routine first aid to achieve hemostasis is still important, such as pressure and topical agents

Table 37.1.   Causes of Bleeding

	BLEEDING	
Vascular Trauma	**Platelet Adhesion/ Aggregation Problem**	**Fibrin Clot Problem**
Repetitive nose picking	Decreased platelets number (immune thrombocytopenia, neonatal alloimmune thrombocytopenia)	Hemophilia A
Surgical procedure	Congenital platelet problem	Hemophilia B
Collagen vascular disease	Wiskott-Aldrich syndrome	Liver failure
	Glanzmann thrombasthenia	Hemorrhagic disease of newborn
	Thrombocytopenia-absent radius	
	von Willebrand disease	Disseminated intravascular coagulation

Immune Thrombocytopenia

BASIC INFORMATION

- Formerly known as idiopathic thrombocytopenia, or immune thrombocytopenic purpura; now known as immune thrombocytopenia (ITP)
- Mechanism is thought to be an autoimmune disease; it can be first presentation of other systemic autoimmune diseases (e.g., lupus)

CLINICAL PRESENTATION

- Peak incidence between ages 2 and 5 years with a slight male predominance, commonly preceded with a nonspecific viral illness (or rarely associated with preceding measles, mumps, and rubella [MMR] vaccination)
- Platelet count can be as low as <10,000 or slightly decreased below normal
- Most often presents with petechiae and bruising
- Mucosal bleeding at diagnosis ("wet" purpura, hematuria, epistaxis, or gastrointestinal or vaginal bleeding) portends a higher rate of serious hemorrhage

DIAGNOSIS AND EVALUATION

- CBC and smear
  - Evaluate for platelet clumping because this can falsely lower platelet count
  - Typical platelets present on blood smear are enlarged, which suggests early platelet formation by the bone marrow precursors
- Bone marrow evaluation is indicated only in patients without a typical presentation (i.e., other cell lines down or symptoms concerning for malignancy) or if there is an inadequate response to front-line treatment

Table 37.2.   Laboratory Findings in Bleeding Disorders

Disorder	PT	PTT	Platelet Count	Other
Hemophilia	nl	↑	nl	- Hemophilia A has low factor 8 - Hemophilia B has low factor 9
vWD	nl	Slightly increased due to decrease in half-life of factor VIII secondary to vWF dysfunction	nl (usually)	vWD Type 2B is associated with low platelet count
Vitamin K deficiency or liver dysfunction	↑	Increased in late dysfunction, slightly increased in early deficiency/dysfunction	nl	Warfarin is a vitamin K antagonist so causes elevated PT/INR as well and is used for anticoagulation
Thrombocytopenia (immune thrombocytopenia, thrombocytopenia-absent radius, Kasabach-Merritt)	nl	nl	↓	
Platelet function defect (Glanzmann, Bernard-Soulier, aspirin exposure, nonsteroidal antiinflammatory drug exposure)	nl	nl	nl or ↓	Depending on the type of platelet function defect, they can be decreased in number or abnormal in morphology or normal but nonfunctioning

INR, International normalized ratio; *nl*, normal limits; *PT*, prothrombin time; *PTT*, partial thromboplastin time; *vWD*, von Willebrand disease.

- Antiplatelet antibody testing is available but lacks sensitivity, so it is not performed routinely
- Full history and physical examination for any type of bleeding is important to guide management decisions
- Classification of ITP
  - Newly diagnosed ITP
    - Within the first 3 months of diagnosis
  - Persistent ITP
    - Ongoing ITP from 3 months to 1 year after diagnosis
  - Chronic ITP
    - ITP present for longer than 1 year

TREATMENT

- Natural history
  - In pediatrics, often spontaneously remits within the first 3 months. Approximately 80% of pediatric patients achieve remission in the first year
  - Treatment is related to the prevention of bleeding complications
- Supportive care
  - Restrict high-risk physical activities (contact sports)
  - Avoid antiplatelet medications (i.e., nonsteroidal anti-inflammatory drug [NSAIDs], aspirin)
- Treatment is not necessarily indicated if there is no significant bleeding or mucosal bleeding regardless of platelet count
  - Presence of mucosal bleeding or other bleeding is an indication for therapy
  - Options for treatment include:
    - Intravenous immune globulin infusion (IVIG)
    - Anti-D immune globulin for Rh-positive patients
    - Glucocorticoids (contraindicated if patient has any concern for possible hematologic malignancy)
    - Immunosuppressants and splenectomy are considered for chronic ITP patients
    - Platelet transfusions are ineffective when provided alone
  - Life-threatening bleeding
    - Intracranial bleeding should be treated immediately with a combination of large-volume platelet transfusions, IVIG, and high-dose glucocorticoids
- Monitoring
  - Monitor weekly platelet count in the ambulatory setting until resolved or stable
  - Monitor clinically for evidence of bleeding
  - Retreatment may be necessary in about one-third of patients initially diagnosed

Neonatal Alloimmune Thrombocytopenia (NAIT)

BASIC INFORMATION

- Occurs due to the development of antibodies created by the mother against the neonate's platelets; for instance, the mother develops an antibody against fetal platelet antigen inherited from the father or from platelet antigens from prior pregnancies/exposures. Consequently, the mother will have normal platelet counts, whereas the baby will be thrombocytopenic

- Differential diagnosis includes neonatal infection or other complications of pregnancy or neonatal autoimmune thrombocytopenia (associated with maternal ITP causing maternal and neonatal thrombocytopenia)

CLINICAL PRESENTATION

- Generally presents in the first 72 hours of life
- Often can be monitored because nadir of thrombocytopenia occurs in the first few days of life and improves as maternal antibodies are cleared by age 6 months

TREATMENT

- In neonates, recommend platelets >30,000, if possible, to prevent intracranial hemorrhage
- Consider maternal platelet transfusion in NAIT if the mother has a normal platelet count
- Parental platelet phenotype testing can be useful for future pregnancy management

Kasabach-Merritt Phenomenon

BASIC INFORMATION

- Platelet consumption within a vascular malformation (e.g., large hemangioma) that can cause severe thrombocytopenia
- Treatment of the vascular malformation or use of anticoagulation decreases platelet consumption in patients with Kasabach-Merritt phenomenon

Thrombocytopenia with Absent Radii Syndrome (TAR)

BASIC INFORMATION

- Autosomal recessive or autosomal dominant inheritance
- Clinical syndrome of thrombocytopenia is associated with congenital absence of radius (but does not have thumb abnormalities); may have cardiac and renal disease as well
- Can present with variable levels of thrombocytopenia throughout life
- Treatment may be required in the setting of planned surgical procedures

Wiskott-Aldrich Syndrome (WAS)

BASIC INFORMATION

- X-linked disorder with a mutation in the WAS protein

CLINICAL PRESENTATION

- Classic triad consists of immune deficiency, eczema, and microthrombocytopenia

DIAGNOSIS AND EVALUATION

- Morphology can be helpful because platelets in WAS are small in size with an MPV of less than 5 fL (microthrombocytopenia)

TREATMENT

- Thrombocytopenia can be variable and may require supportive treatment for any life-threatening bleeding
- Primary management is related to immune deficiency because the patient is deficient in T- and B-cell immunity, which predisposes the patient to common infections (e.g., recurrent acute otitis media (AOM), skin abscesses), severe bacterial infections, and fungal/viral infections
- WAS patients are also predisposed to autoimmunity of other organs and cell lines, as well as at risk for developing hematologic malignancy
- Treatment for WAS often can include bone marrow transplant with indication based on severity of phenotype, patient's immunologic risk factors, and availability of donor

Platelet Function Defects

- Congenital platelet function defects
  - Glanzmann thrombasthenia: congenital abnormality in platelet aggregation receptor
  - Bernard-Soulier syndrome: congenital abnormality in platelet adhesion receptor
- Medication-induced platelet function defects
  - Aspirin causes platelet function defects for the life span of the platelets (5–7 days)
  - NSAIDs cause platelet function defects for the half-life of the drug
  - Selective serotonin reuptake inhibitors and antiepileptics cause variable abnormalities in platelet function
- Renal disease–associated defects
  - Uremia can cause platelet function defects

von Willebrand Disease (vWD)

BASIC INFORMATION

- von Willebrand factor functions to bind platelets to collagen, facilitate the platelet plug formation, and protect factor VIII from degradation (extends its half-life)
- Three types of vWD: types 1, 2, and 3
  - Type 1 vWD is the most common type and has a clinical incidence of close to 1 in 1000

CLINICAL PRESENTATION

- Variable clinical presentation based on different types
- Most often diagnosed in older children or young adults (with the exception of type 3)

Table 37.3. von Willebrand Disease Types and Subtypes

	von Willebrand antigen (vWF:Ag)	Ristocetin cofactor (VWF:RCo)	Factor VIII level	von Willebrand multimer analysis
	Laboratory Results			
1	↓	↓ (proportional to vWF:Ag level)	↓ (mild)	↓ (global decrease in the amount of multimers)
2A	normal or ↓	↓↓	normal or ↓	↓ (complete loss of high-molecular-weight multimers)
2B	normal or ↓	↓↓	normal or ↓	↓ (with thrombocytopenia)
2M	↓	↓↓	normal or ↓	↓ (without loss of high-molecular-weight multimers)
2N	normal	normal	↓↓	normal
3	↓ (none detectable)	↓ (none detectable)	↓↓	↓ (none detectable)

- Characterized by mucosal bleeding (epistaxis, uterine bleeding, bleeding with dental procedures)
- Seldom is associated with intracranial hemorrhage or hemarthrosis

DIAGNOSIS AND EVALUATION

- Clinical suspicion should lead to sending a panel of tests: von Willebrand antigen, ristocetin cofactor levels, factor VIII level, and consideration of multimer analysis testing (see Table 37.3)
- Type 1
  - Most common type of bleeding disorder; commonly via autosomal dominant inheritance
  - 1% of population will test positive, but only 1% of that proportion has clinical symptoms, so start with a clinical history
  - Blood type O patients have a lower level of von Willebrand antigen than the general population
  - Characterized by a low von Willebrand antigen level with a correspondingly low ristocetin cofactor activity
- Type 2
  - Functional defect in von Willebrand factor (rather than a quantitative deficiency in type 1 or 3)
  - Subtype of type 2 is dependent on mutation and its effect on the molecule: can affect platelet binding abilities, production of high-molecular-weight multimers, or the ability to protect factor VIII from degradation
- Type 3
  - Autosomal recessive; diagnosis is based on undetectable levels
  - No von Willebrand antigen is detected or made
  - Severe bleeding manifestations

TREATMENT

- Treatment is largely supportive care
- DDAVP can transiently increase endogenous von Willebrand factor release from the storage pools in the Weibel-Palade bodies of the endothelium
  - It is contraindicated in certain types of type 2 von Willebrand disease because it will release dysfunctional von Willebrand factor and potentially worsen the ongoing bleeding
  - It is not useful in type 3 von Willebrand
  - DDAVP is also used for treatment of diabetes insipidus and can cause water retention leading to hyponatremia, so fluid status must be monitored closely
- Antifibrinolytic therapies (e.g., aminocaproic acid) help promote clot stability and can be used as an adjunct therapy, especially with mucosal bleeding
- A few plasma-derived factor VIII products contain a therapeutic amount of functional von Willebrand factor and can be administered before surgery or for severe bleeding

Hemophilia

BASIC INFORMATION

- Coagulation factors are required to create a thrombin clot that stabilizes the initial platelet plug formed by von Willebrand antigen and platelets
- Types
  - Hemophilia A is a condition with a low or missing amount of factor VIII (eight)
  - Hemophilia B is a condition with a low or missing amount of factor IX (nine)
  - Hemophilia A and B are X-linked recessive gene defects
  - There are other rare congenital bleeding disorders caused by deficiencies of factor II (prothrombin), factor V, factor X, factor XI (hemophilia C), and factor XIII

CLINICAL PRESENTATION

- Bleeding
  - Most common type of bleeding with hemophilia is hemarthrosis
  - Other bleeding that can occur includes muscle hematomas and intracranial bleeding
  - Patients also have bleeding with surgery or other provocation
- Natural history and complications
  - Severity and frequency of bleeding depend on endogenous factor levels (Table 37.4)
  - The majority of patients with hemophilia A have the severe phenotype, and half of the patients with hemophilia B have the severe phenotype
  - 30% of patients do not have a known family history
  - Pooled plasma-donated product was used before the availability of recombinant factor products, leading to infectious complications when this therapy was first introduced decades ago, including HIV and hepatitis C

Table 37.4. Hemophilia Classification and Severity

Amount of factor	<1%	1% to 5%	>5% to 30%
Classification	Severe	Moderate	Mild
Signs	Spontaneous bleeding possible, hemarthrosis, muscle hematoma	Spontaneous bleeding rare, hemarthrosis, muscle hematoma	Infrequent bleeding usually secondary to trauma

- Complications occur based on decreased mobility from repeated joint bleeds and subsequent arthropathy

DIAGNOSIS AND EVALUATION

- Classic history for hemophilias includes bleeding with circumcision, muscle hematoma after immunizations, unexplained intracranial hemorrhage, severe bleeding in a male, or known family history of hemophilia should prompt testing
- PTT is prolonged with low levels of factor VIII and IX and often with normal PT levels
- Factor VIII and factor IX levels can be measured directly
- Genetic testing can confirm the diagnosis
  - The most common mutation is inversion 22 for hemophilia A
- Daughters of patients with hemophilia are obligate carriers

TREATMENT

- For patients with severe disease, prophylaxis is recommended to start at a young age before a target joint or a significant bleed occurs
- Treatment and prophylaxis involve home IV infusions
- Factor VIII product is dosed by international units (IU). Every IU per kg of body weight of factor VIII should raise your factor VIII level by 2%
  - Half-life of factor VIII is around 12 hours, so prophylaxis dosing is given three times a week or every other day
- Factor IX product is dosed by IU. Every IU per kg of body weight of factor IX should raise your factor XI level by 1%
  - Half-life of factor XI is around 20 to 24 hours, so prophylaxis dosing is given twice a week
- DDAVP can be used to transiently increase the secretion of von Willebrand antigen and prolong the half-life of factor VIII in patients with mild hemophilia A
- Treatment of an acute bleed is aimed at keeping factor product levels close to normal to help the body achieve adequate hemostasis
  - Brain bleeds require levels at 100%
  - Muscle bleeds or joint bleeds require levels at 50%
  - Repeated joint bleeds can lead to long-term joint arthropathy, which is the rationale behind use of prophylactic factor replacement to prevent joint bleeds
- 20% to 30% of patients will unfortunately develop an inhibitor to factor products and will require immune tolerance therapy and bypassing agents

Other Causes of Inadequate Fibrin Clot Formation

- Vitamin K deficiency causes lack of factor products, preventing proper fibrin clot formation
  - Vitamin K is a fat-soluble vitamin that is required for formation of factors 2, 7, 9, and 10
  - Hemorrhagic disease of the newborn is due to vitamin K deficiency at birth and can be prevented by administration of vitamin K at birth
  - Warfarin is used as an anticoagulant, and it functions by being a vitamin K antagonist
  - Severe liver failure causes lack of factor product production, specifically the vitamin K–specific factors
- Disseminated intravascular coagulation (DIC)
  - DIC is an inflammatory complication of infections, specifically sepsis, causing unregulated consumption of factor products
  - This deficiency (secondary to consumption) of factor products causes clinical bleeding

Causes of Thrombosis

BASIC INFORMATION

- Thrombosis is the opposite of bleeding and is caused by an imbalance in Virchow's triad
  - Virchow's triad describes three items that are associated with thrombosis or clot formation: endothelial injury that signals need for a clot to form, stasis of blood flow, and hypercoagulability
- Congenital causes of hypercoagulability are found more often in pediatric patients who present with a clot

- Congenital causes of hypercoagulability
  - Factor V Leiden mutation
  - Prothrombin 20210 mutation
  - Protein C deficiency
  - Protein S deficiency
  - Antithrombin deficiency
  - Hyperhomocysteinemia
  - Elevated factor VIII levels
- Acquired hypercoagulable states can be present in pediatric patients who present with a clot
  - Acquired causes of abnormal Virchow's triad
    - Indwelling central line
    - Cancer
    - Recent trauma or surgery
    - Obesity
    - Pregnancy or supplemental estrogen use
    - Prolonged immobility
    - Antiphospholipid antibody syndrome
    - Inflammatory bowel syndrome
    - Nephrotic syndrome

Review Questions

For review questions, please go to ExpertConsult.com.

Suggested Readings

1. Neunert C, Lim W, Crowther M, et al. The American Society of Hematology 2011 evidence-based practice guideline for immune thrombocytopenia. *Blood.* 2011;117:4190–4207.
2. Nichols WL, Hultin MB, James AH, et al. von Willebrand disease (VWD): evidence-based diagnosis and management guidelines, the National Heart, Lung, and Blood Institute (NHLBI) Expert Panel report (USA). *Haemophilia.* 2008;14:171–232.
3. Srivastava A, Brewer AK, Mauser-Bunschoten EP, et al. Guidelines for the management of hemophilia. *Haemophilia.* 2013;19:e1–e47.

38 *Selected Topics in Hematology*

JESSICA FOSTER, MD

Neutropenia

Neutropenia is a common finding in pediatric patients. Most often this is transient and related to a viral infection or another transient cause. Rarely, it can be associated with congenital neutropenia syndromes. The major associated complications include bacterial and fungal infections, which usually arise only when the neutropenia is severe and prolonged.

BASIC INFORMATION

- Defined as absolute neutrophil count (ANC) less than 1500
  - 1000 to 1500: mild
  - 500 to 1000: moderate
  - Less than 500: severe
  - Less than 200: very severe
- Infectious risks discussed further in Chapter 40
- Divided into congenital and acquired causes (see Table 38.1)
  - Congenital isolated neutropenias
    - Severe congenital neutropenia (SCN), including Kostmann syndrome
      Majority caused by mutations in *ELANE* gene
      Presents with persistent severe neutropenia with associated mouth ulcers and infections
      Although the majority are treatable with granulocyte colony-stimulating factor (G-CSF), up to 20% are at risk of myelodysplastic syndrome (MDS) and acute myeloid leukemia (AML)
    - Cyclic neutropenia
      Caused by mutations in *ELANE* gene, usually autosomal dominant inheritance
      Neutrophil count nadirs occur regularly every 3 to 6 weeks; neutropenia accompanied by fevers, oral ulcers, and sometimes infections
      After confirmation of regular cycles of neutropenia and molecular genetics, treatment with G-CSF may be considered
    - Benign ethnic neutropenia
      Primarily affects patients of African, Middle Eastern, and Jewish descent
  - Common acquired causes
    - Viral infection
      Usually resolves within 1 to 2 weeks
    - Autoimmune neutropenia
      Previously called "benign chronic neutropenia" or "primary autoimmune neutropenia"

Primarily occurs in infants <2 years old—median age 7 to 9 months
Neutrophil-specific antibodies cause a *noncyclic* neutropenia with little increase in risk of pyogenic infections
May detect antineutrophil antibodies (ANA) in serum, but may require repeated testing
90% resolve within 2 years
- Alloimmune neutropenia:
  Prenatal sensitization of mother results in maternal IgG Ab to fetal neutrophil antigens
  Neutropenia present at birth
  May lead to increased risk of neonatal infections depending on severity of neutropenia
  Neutrophil count usually recovers by 7 weeks, but can take months
- Medication-induced neutropenia
  Common causes include anticonvulsants, penicillin, Bactrim, and chemotherapeutic drugs
  If neutropenia is severe, recommend changing agents
  If neutropenia is mild, OK to watch and wait

CLINICAL PRESENTATION

- Infections
  - Acute onset of severe neutropenias has a higher risk of infection than chronic neutropenias; similarly, neutropenias associated with other affected cell lines (e.g., monocytopenia, lymphocytopenia) are worse
  - Bacterial: skin infections (e.g., cellulitis, furunculosis), diarrhea
  - Fungal
- Stomatitis and oral ulcers are very common in neutropenia

DIAGNOSIS AND EVALUATION

- Complete blood count (CBC) with differential
  - If otherwise asymptomatic or if there is concern for viral infection, repeat CBC in 3 to 4 weeks
  - If persistently low, then proceed with workup for infections, autoimmune causes (e.g., ANA), or other immune disorders (e.g., quantitative IgG, lymphocyte subsets)
  - History may suggest testing for exocrine pancreas dysfunction (i.e., Shwachman-Diamond), vitamin deficiencies (e.g., folate, B_{12}), or skeletal studies (for metaphyseal chondrodysplasia)

Table 38.1. Causes of Neutropenia

	Congenital Causes	Acquired Causes
Isolated neutropenias	Severe congenital neutropenia	Autoimmune neutropenia (autoantibodies)
	Cyclic neutropenia	Alloimmune neutropenia (maternally passed on to baby)
	Benign ethnic neutropenia	Infections: childhood viral infections, sepsis, HIV
		Drugs: anticonvulsants, penicillin, Bactrim, chemotherapy
Neutropenias usually coexisting with other cytopenias	Metabolic disorders: glycogen storage disease, Pearson syndrome, methylmalonic acidemia, Gaucher disease	Systemic lupus erythematosus
	Immune disorders: common variable immune deficiency, severe combined immunodeficiency, Hyper-IgM	Hypersplenism (also associated with thrombocytopenia)
		Bone marrow infiltration (e.g., malignancy)
		Myelodysplastic syndromes
		Vitamin deficiencies (e.g., B_{12}, folate)

- Bone marrow biopsy if persistent neutropenia or pancytopenia
- Genetic testing of *ELANE* genes if there is clinical concern for congenital neutropenia syndrome

TREATMENT

- G-CSF may be used to increase neutrophil counts
- Infection precautions
  - Antibiotics and antifungals are often used to treat infections
  - Prophylactic antifungals are often provided for very severe neutropenia
  - Rectal temperatures are generally avoided if ANC <1000
- Bone marrow transplant sometimes necessary for SCN

Pancytopenia

The approach to pancytopenia in a pediatric patient varies based on the age, physical examination findings, and additional laboratory findings. After ruling out an oncologic process, the next evaluation is whether there is decreased production or increased destruction of cells. Also important to consider in the pediatric population are the congenital bone marrow failure syndromes, each with unique characteristics and genetic abnormalities.

BASIC INFORMATION

- Definition: decreased quantity of cells in at least two cell lines (anemia, thrombocytopenia, and/or leukopenia)
- Causes and etiology
  - Congenital causes (see Table 38.2)
    - Fanconi anemia (FA)
      Also called "congenital aplastic anemia"
      Inherited disorder leading to defective DNA repair
      Autosomal recessive inheritance
        More than 15 genes have been identified, all involving the FA pathway that responds to DNA damage
        80% to 90% of patients have mutation in *FANCA, FANCC,* or *FANC*

Typically patients develop bone marrow failure by age 5 to 10 years
- Shwachman-Diamond syndrome (SDS) (for details, see Chapter 33)
  Inherited disorder leading to exocrine pancreatic insufficiency, bone marrow failure, and skeletal abnormalities
- Dyskeratosis congenita (DC)
  Inherited disorder due to mutation in telomere maintenance genes
  Results in dystrophy of hair and nails and bone marrow failure
- Pearson syndrome (see Chapter 49)
  Mitochondrial disorder resulting in bone marrow failure, exocrine pancreatic insufficiency, and developmental and growth delays; unlike in SDS, Pearson syndrome patients have significant neurologic/muscle impairment
- Congenital amegakaryocytic thrombocytopenia (CAMT)
  Autosomal recessive disorder in the thrombopoietin receptor, *MPL*
  Presents with severe thrombocytopenia at birth and eventually progresses to pancytopenia
- Acquired causes of pancytopenia (see Table 38.3)
  Divided into increased destruction/pooling and decreased production

CLINICAL PRESENTATION

- Symptoms related to the cell lines affected
  - Anemia: fatigue, headache, pallor
  - Thrombocytopenia: bleeding, bruising, petechiae
    - Symptoms usually present only when platelets less than 20,000
  - Leukopenia: frequent infections, fevers
- Physical findings and symptoms associated with specific congenital causes (see Tables 38.2 and 38.4)
  - FA: short stature, abnormal thumbs/radii, microcephaly, renal abnormalities, cardiac defects
  - Shwachman-Diamond syndrome: growth delay, loose stools, problems with bone formation and density/skeletal changes, hepatomegaly
  - DC: abnormal skin, hair, nails, and teeth; pulmonary fibrosis

Table 38.2.   Congenital Causes of Pancytopenia

	Fanconi Anemia	Shwachman-Diamond Syndrome	Dyskeratosis Congenita	Pearson Syndrome	Congenital Amegakaryocytic Thrombocytopenia
Clinical findings	Short stature, abnormal thumbs/radii, microcephaly, café au lait spots, renal abnormalities, cardiac defects	Steatorrhea, failure to thrive, skeletal abnormalities, hepatomegaly	Dystrophic hair and nails, reticular skin pigmentation, oral leukoplakia, pulmonary fibrosis	Steatorrhea, failure to thrive, developmental delay, metabolic acidosis, neurologic/ muscle impairment	normal
Complete blood count findings	Pancytopenia (macrocytic anemia)	Neutropenia > anemia > pancytopenia	Pancytopenia	Macrocytic anemia evolving into pancytopenia	Severe thrombocytopenia at birth, eventually pancytopenia
Diagnostic test	Chromosomal breakage study	Pancreatic enzyme concentrations, genetic testing	Telomere length study	Bone marrow shows vacuoles in precursor cells and ringed sideroblasts	Bone marrow shows absence of megakaryocytes
Gene involved/ inheritance	*FANC* family/autosomal recessive	*SBDS*/autosomal recessive	Numerous, Involved in telomere maintenance/varies	Mitochondrial DNA deletion/ maternal (mitochondrial) inheritance	*MPL*/autosomal recessive
Treatment	Bone marrow transplant, androgen therapy	Pancreatic enzyme supplementation, bone marrow transplant	Bone marrow transplant, androgen therapy	Supportive care, usually fatal in infancy	Bone marrow transplant
Increased cancer risk?	Yes: leukemia, myelodysplastic syndrome, squamous cell carcinomas, head and neck cancers	Yes: leukemia	Yes: leukemia, squamous cell carcinomas, head and neck cancers	No	Yes: leukemia

Table 38.3.   Acquired Causes of Pancytopenia

Increased Destruction	Decreased Production
Disseminated intravascular coagulopathy	Drugs: ■ Sulfonamides ■ Antiepileptics ■ Chloramphenicol
Hypersplenism	Infections: ■ Sepsis ■ Epstein-Barr virus ■ Cytomegalovirus ■ HIV
Autoimmune/Evans syndrome	Nutritional deficiency: ■ Severe B_{12} deficiency ■ Severe folate deficiency ■ Copper deficiency
	Chemical/radiation exposure
	Paroxysmal nocturnal hemoglobinuria
	Idiopathic aplastic anemia

Table 38.4.   Comparing Clinical Manifestations of Inherited Marrow Failure Syndromes

	Fanconi Anemia	Shwachman-Diamond Syndrome	Diamond Blackfan Anemia	Thrombocytopenia-Absent Radius
Age of presentation	School age	Infancy to School age	Infancy	Infancy
CLINICAL ABNORMALITIES:				
Distinctive facial features			X	X
Upper extremity	X		X	X
Thumb	X		X	
Renal	X		X	X
HEMATOLOGIC FINDINGS:				
Anemia	X	X	X	
Thrombocytopenia	X	X		X
Neutropenia	X	X		

DIAGNOSIS AND EVALUATION

- Screening laboratory evaluation
  - CBC with differential
    - Congenital bone marrow failure syndromes often have macrocytic anemia
  - Reticulocyte count: low in production problems
  - Hemoglobin electrophoresis: congenital bone marrow failure syndromes often have elevated fetal hemoglobin
  - Lactate dehydrogenase (LDH) and uric acid: elevated in leukemia
  - Chromosomal breakage: positive in FA
  - Pancreatic enzyme concentrations: low in SDS
  - Telomere length testing: shortened in DC
- Bone marrow biopsy
  - Decreased production (genetic or acquired) shows marrow replaced by fat
  - Increased destruction shows normal to high number of hematopoietic precursor cells
- Other diagnostics
  - For SDS, one may consider abdominal imaging to confirm pancreatic involvement (e.g., ultrasound, magnetic resonance imaging [MRI], computed tomography [CT])

TREATMENT

- Supportive care
  - Transfusions as needed for anemia or thrombocytopenia.
  - G-CSF for neutropenia or antibiotics for infections or prophylaxis may be necessary
- Treat underlying cause
  - Congenital causes
    - Bone marrow transplant needed for most
    - Androgen therapy can be helpful for anemia and thrombocytopenia but is less helpful for white blood cells
    - Monitor for secondary cancers
    - Follow up with additional specialists: gastrointestinal (GI), pulmonary, dental, and so forth
    - For SDS, patients often require pancreatic enzymes in youth (but some may not need lifelong supplementation)
  - Acquired causes
    - Remove/treat inciting agent
    - Immunosuppressive therapy may be necessary for some disorders

Erythrocytosis (Polycythemia)

BASIC INFORMATION

- Definition: hematocrit (Hct) >60% from free-flowing *venous* sample
  - Capillary samples have 5% to 25% higher Hct values, depending upon perfusion to the area
- Etiology
  - Primary polycythemia
    - Due to intrinsic factors, without elevated erythropoietin (EPO) production
    - Congenital
      Inherited defects in EPO receptor

- Acquired
  Polycythemia vera
  Myeloproliferative neoplasm
  Extremely rare in pediatrics
- Secondary polycythemia
  - Due to increased EPO production
  - Congenital
    Rare hemoglobin variants and other genetic changes that alter oxygen delivery or sensing
  - Acquired
    Secondary to hypoxia
    Cyanotic congenital heart disease
    Chronic pulmonary disease
    High altitude
    Abnormal production of EPO
    Benign and malignant tumors
    Excess hormones: corticosteroids, growth hormone, androgens
    Kidney disease
- Neonatal polycythemia
  - Defined as Hct >65%
  - Occurs in 1% to 5% of healthy term newborns
  - Increased fetal hematopoiesis
    Infants of diabetic mothers
    Placental insufficiency/intrauterine growth restriction (IUGR)
    Chromosomal abnormalities—in particular, trisomies
    Maternal-fetal hemorrhage
  - Increased passive transfusion
    Twin-twin transfusion
    Delayed cord clamping

CLINICAL PRESENTATION

- Symptoms:
  - Ruddy facial complexion
  - If Hct is >65, patient can develop:
    - Headache
    - Joint pain
    - Thrombosis, including stroke and pulmonary embolus (PE)
    - End-organ damage, including heart failure, altered mental status, renal insufficiency, and disseminated intravascular coagulopathy (DIC)
- Complications specific to neonatal polycythemia
  - Necrotizing enterocolitis
  - Hypoglycemia
  - Hypocalcemia

DIAGNOSIS AND EVALUATION

- CBC
- Basic metabolic panel (including calcium); frequent glucose monitoring
- Thorough history and physical examination to evaluate for secondary causes
- In neonates: evaluation for maternal hemorrhage, in utero causes of hypoxia, increased transfusion of blood to baby (twin or delayed cord clamp)
  - Consider chromosomal analysis if other physical signs are suggestive

TREATMENT

- Asymptomatic with Hct between 60% and 70%: hydrate aggressively
- Symptomatic: exchange transfusion with saline

Transfusion Reactions

BASIC INFORMATION

- Transfusion reactions can be divided based on timing, with "early onset" reactions occurring within 4 to 24 hours of completion of a transfusion and "delayed" reactions occurring days to weeks after transfusion. Additionally, transfusion reactions can be divided into those causing hemolytic and nonhemolytic reactions.

Early, Nonhemolytic Reactions

- Febrile nonhemolytic transfusion reactions (FNHTR)
  - Increase in patient temperature 1°C that is unexplained by other patient factors
  - Most common reaction: estimated incidence of 1% for packed red blood cells (PRBC) and 10% for platelets
  - Secondary to either:
  - Accumulation of cytokines in the transfusion product
  - Antileukocyte antibodies
- Allergic reaction
  - Most cases idiopathic, secondary to unknown protein in donor plasma or storage media
  - Rarely also reported secondary to IgA in infused product that is given to IgA-deficient patient
- Transfusion-associated circulatory overload (TACO)
  - Caused by increased transudative pressure in the lungs when blood volume expansion occurs too quickly
  - Most likely to occur in patients with cardiopulmonary compromise at baseline
- Transfusion-related acute lung injury (TRALI)
  - Leading cause of transfusion-related death
  - Two-hit mechanism mediated by neutrophils
    - Patient has underlying condition that sequesters neutrophils in lungs
    - Infused product contains anti-HLA or anti-HNA antibodies that activate the neutrophils and form leukoagglutinins
- Acute bacterial infections
  - Most likely to occur with platelets because they are stored at room temperature
  - Can cause sepsis immediately during or after infusion

Delayed, Nonhemolytic Reactions

- Infections
  - Viral: hepatitis B, hepatitis C, HIV, cytomegalovirus (CMV), West Nile
  - Parasites: babesia, malaria, Chagas disease, leishmaniasis
- Acute hemolytic transfusion reactions
  - Classically occurs when given ABO-mismatched blood
  - Preexisting IgM antibodies immediately bind to infused RBCs. IgM activates complement pathway, producing massive intravascular hemolysis

- True emergency; can be fatal with as little as 30 mL transfused
- Delayed hemolytic transfusion reaction (DHTR)
  - Caused by one of the minor RBC antigens (e.g., Kell) to which a patient becomes sensitized from prior blood exposure
  - Upon reexposure, IgG antibodies lead to extravascular hemolysis via macrophages in the spleen, liver, and bone marrow
  - Typically occurs 3 to 14 days after transfusion and rarely >2 weeks after a transfusion
  - Generally less severe than acute hemolytic reactions

CLINICAL PRESENTATION

- Acute transfusion reactions can be difficult to distinguish between different causes because clinical presentations overlap
- Frequent common symptoms include fever, chills, tachycardia, and difficulty breathing
  - Allergic reactions: range from mild urticarial to full anaphylaxis
  - TACO: dyspnea, tachycardia, jugular vein distention (JVD), headache
  - TRALI: range from mild dyspnea to severe pulmonary edema
    - Not cardiogenic in nature; can be distinguished from TACO by normal cardiac pressures
  - Acute hemolytic transfusion reactions: fever, rigors, flank pain, shortness of breath, chest pain, anxiety, warmth/pain at site of infusion, shock, renal failure, DIC
    - Hemoglobinemia can lead to red palms
    - Hemoglobinuria can lead to bright red/dark urine
  - Delayed hemolytic transfusion reactions: more indolent presentation, including fever, worsening anemia, jaundice

DIAGNOSIS AND EVALUATION

- CBC, reticulocyte count
- Blood culture
- Laboratory testing for hemolysis: bilirubin, LDH, haptoglobin, urinalysis
- Antibody screen/cross-matching
- Chest x-ray (CXR), B-type natriuretic peptide (BNP), troponin for suspected TACO and TRALI
  - CXR looks similar for both TACO and TRALI with bilateral diffuse infiltrates

TREATMENT

- Any acute reaction: stop transfusion
  - Always stop the transfusion first because acute hemolytic reactions can be quickly fatal!
- Supportive care: acetaminophen, diphenhydramine, vasopressors, and so forth, as needed
- Acute hemolytic reaction: aggressive hydration. May require steroids, intravenous immunoglobulin (IVIG), or plasma/red blood cell exchange
- Delayed hemolytic reaction: expectant management, occasionally requires additional transfusion
- Prevention of reactions

- Febrile nonhemolytic
  - Leukocyte-reduced blood can reduce risk but does not completely eliminate risk
  - Acetaminophen premedication does *not* prevent febrile reactions
- Allergic reactions
  - Washed products to prevent transmission of plasma proteins
  - Use IgA-deficient donors for patients with IgA deficiency
  - Benadryl premedication is often used, but there are limited data to support its use
- TACO
  - Slow infusion and limit additional fluids going in at the same time
- TRALI
  - If TRALI is suspected, inform the blood bank that will do testing of antibodies on the donor. If antibodies are found, that donor will be deferred from future donations to prevent potential future TRALI reactions

Review Questions

For review questions, please go to ExpertConsult.com.

Suggested Readings

1. Remon JI, Raghavan A, Maheshwari A. Polycythemia in the newborn. *NeoReviews*. 2011;12(1):e20–e28.
2. Savage W. Transfusion reactions. *Hematol Oncol Clin North Am*. 2016;30(3):619–634.
3. Segel GB, Halterman JS. Neutropenia in pediatric practice. *Pediatr Rev*. 2008;29(1).
4. Sharma R, Nalepa G. Evaluation and management of chronic pancytopenia. *Pediatr Rev*. 2016;37(3):101–111.

Immunology

39 Clinical Approach to Suspected Immune Deficiency

ALICE CHAN, MD, PhD

Children frequently visit their pediatricians for infections because the immune system is developing. It is important to recognize when a child's history of infections should raise concern for an underlying immunodeficiency. This section focuses on general characteristics of patients with immunodeficiency and the basic evaluation and treatment for these patients.

Basic Information

Aspects from a patient's clinical history can be suggestive of a primary immunodeficiency. Whereas certain patterns of infections can be indicative of deficiencies in particular aspects of the innate (e.g., macrophages, neutrophils, natural killer [NK] cells) or adaptive (e.g., B cells, T cells) immune systems, the following provide some general "red flags" for clinicians upon which to consider further immunologic evaluation:

- Frequency of infection
  - Four or more new ear infections per year
  - Two or more serious sinus infections
  - Two or more pneumonias per year
  - Two or more systemic bacterial infections per year
- Severity of infection
  - Need for prolonged intravenous (IV) antibiotics or hospitalizations to clear infections
  - Deep skin or organ abscesses
  - Two or more months of antibiotics without improvement
- Nature of organism
  - Recurrent infection with the same organism
  - Need for surgical intervention for clearance of the infection (myringotomy tubes, drainage, lobectomy)
  - Infection with opportunistic pathogens (e.g., persistent thrush in the mouth, *Pneumocystis jirovecii*, cytomegalovirus [CMV] viremia)
  - Infection from attenuated vaccine strains (e.g., rotavirus, bacillus Calmette-Guerin [BCG], varicella, measles)
- Presence of comorbidities
  - Failure to thrive, weight loss, growth retardation
  - Chronic diarrhea
  - Nonhealing wounds
  - Autoimmunity or chronic inflammation
  - Lymphoproliferative disorder
- Family history

- Recurrent or severe infections
- Consanguinity
- Gender predisposition (i.e., only males affected)
- Family history of a primary immunodeficiency

Clinical Presentation

Patient presentation may vary depending on the component of the immune system that is deficient. More details of specific disorders are provided in Chapters 40 to 42.

- Combined immunodeficiency
  - Bacterial, viral, and fungal infections, as well as opportunistic infections
  - Failure to thrive
  - Chronic diarrhea
- Humoral deficiency
  - Onset of infections usually after 4 to 6 months, when maternal antibodies wane
  - Recurrent, severe upper and lower respiratory tract infections (otitis media, sinusitis, and pneumonia)
  - Failure to thrive
  - Chronic diarrhea
  - Hepatomegaly, splenomegaly
  - Abnormal lung examination (rales, rhonchi)
  - Digital clubbing
- Phagocytic disorders
  - Soft tissue infections requiring surgical debridement
  - Several dental infections leading to premature tooth loss
  - Recurrent anorectal infections
- Complement disorders
  - Recurrent or severe bacterial infections
  - Autoimmune manifestations such as lupus
- Additional clinical findings suggestive of specific immunodeficiency
  - Ataxia telangiectasia: ataxia, telangiectasia, loss of developmental milestones
  - DiGeorge syndrome: congenital cardiac disease, hypocalcemia, dysmorphic facies
  - Hyper IgE syndrome: coarse facial features, chronic-infected eczema, cold abscesses
  - Wiskott-Aldrich syndrome: petechiae, easy bleeding, eczema

Diagnosis and Evaluation

- General screening laboratory evaluation for immune deficiency
  - Complete blood count (CBC) with differential (to evaluate for quantitative deficiency, e.g., lymphopenia)
  - Lymphocyte subsets: CD3 T cells, CD4 T cells, CD8 T cells, B cells, and NK cells
  - Immunoglobulin levels: IgG, IgA, IgM, IgE
  - Vaccination response if vaccinated: tetanus, diphtheria, pneumococcal
  - CH50 to screen for complement disorders
- Obtain cultures or other testing to determine infecting organism
- Imaging for assessment of infection or organ involvement
- Referral to an immunologist

Treatment

- Prompt initiation of empiric antibiotic therapy while awaiting culture results
- Certain immune deficiencies may require therapies to aid and/or replace the immune defect:
  - Immunoglobulin replacement therapy may be indicated for some humoral deficiencies
  - Hematopoietic stem cell transplant or gene therapy may be necessary to reconstitute an immune system

- Prophylactic measures may also be required for certain immunodeficiencies
  - Long-term prophylactic antibiotics/antifungals may be indicated
  - In general, patients are recommended to avoid live-virus vaccines (an immunologist may help determine whether there are exceptions)
  - Postexposure infectious prophylaxis (e.g., antibiotics, immune globulin administration)
  - Patients are recommended to receive irradiated, leukocyte-reduced, CMV-negative blood products

Review Questions

For review questions, please go to ExpertConsult.com.

Suggested Readings

1. Ballow M. Approach to the patient with recurrent infections. *Clin Rev Allergy Immunol.* 2008;34(2):129–140.
2. Buckley RH. *Diagnostic and Clinical Care Guidelines for Primary Immunodeficiency Diseases.* 3rd ed. Towson, MD: Immune Deficiency Foundation; 2015.
3. Costa-Carvalho BT, Grumach AS, Franco JL, Espinosa-Rosales FJ, Leiva LE, King A, et al. Attending to warning signs of primary immunodeficiency diseases across the range of clinical practice. *J Clin Immunol.* January 2014;34(1):10–22.
4. Locke BA, Dasu T, Verbsky JW. Laboratory diagnosis of primary immunodeficiencies. *Clin Rev Allergy Immunol.* 2014;46(2):154–168.

40 *Phagocyte Disorders*

ALICE CHAN, MD, PhD

Phagocytic disorders can be divided into two groups: primary and secondary causes. Primary causes result from a defect in the development, migration, or microbicidal activity of the phagocytes. Secondary causes can result from reduced circulating phagocytes, such as from autoantibodies or bone marrow suppression. The following section focuses on primary causes of phagocytic disorders, which include chronic granulomatous disease, leukocyte adhesion deficiency, myeloperoxidase (MPO) deficiency, and Chediak-Higashi syndrome. Neutropenias are covered in Chapter 38.

See also Nelson Textbook of Pediatrics, Chapter 130, "Disorders of Phagocyte Function."

Chronic Granulomatous Disease (CGD)

BASIC INFORMATION

- Affects function of neutrophils and monocytes
- Phagocytic cells are unable to kill catalase-positive organisms because they are unable to generate reactive oxygen species by the nicotinamide adenine dinucleotide phosphate (NADPH) oxidase
- Inheritance: X-linked or autosomal recessive
  - Female carriers of the X-linked CGD can have a mixed population of functional neutrophils due to random X inactivation. However, female carriers usually do not have increased infections
  - Four gene defects: $gp91^{phox}$ (X-linked, most common cause), $p22^{phox}$, $p47^{phox}$, $p67^{phox}$
  - Five gene defects: CYBB (gp91phox, X-linked), CYBA (p22phox), NCF1 (p47phox), NCF2 (p67phox), and NCF4 (p40phox)
  - Severe glucose-6-phosphate dehydrogenase (G6PD) deficiency may also present with chronic granulomatous disease

CLINICAL PRESENTATION

- Onset from infancy to young adulthood
- Catalase-positive bacterial and fungal infections, which include *Staphylococcus aureus*, Serratia species, Nocardia species, Aspergillus species, and Burkholderia species
  - Recurrent lymphadenitis
  - Bacterial abscesses affecting lung, perianal area, liver, spleen
  - Recurrent osteomyelitis at multiple sites in the small bones of the hands and feet
  - Inflammatory bowel disease Crohn-like with granulomas
  - Can have wound healing complications such as fistula formulation

- Family history of recurrent infection or unusual catalase-positive organism

DIAGNOSIS AND EVALUATION

- Assessing NADPH oxidase function
  - Nitroblue tetrazolium dye (NBT): patients fail to reduce yellow water-soluble tetrazolium dye to insoluble blue formazan pigment
  - Dihydrorhodamine (DHR) test: flow cytometry–based assay to detect conversion of DHR to rhodamine when neutrophils are activated
- Complete blood count (CBC) can indicate normal or low neutrophil count, so not helpful for diagnosis
- Obtain cultures to determine infective organism; imaging for evaluation of infection and to monitor for resolution of the infection

TREATMENT

- Prophylactic antimicrobial agents (bacterial and fungal)
- Abscess drainage
- Interferon gamma to lower frequency of infections
- Glucocorticoids for treatment of autoinflammatory manifestations
- Hematopoietic stem cell transplant or gene therapy may provide definitive treatment

Leukocyte Adhesion Disorder (LAD)

BASIC INFORMATION

- Defect in the ability of neutrophils to leave circulation and migrate to the site of infection
- Inheritance: autosomal recessive
- Two main types
  - Type 1
    - Defect in CD18 (encoded by *ITGB2*), which is important for leukocyte migration
  - Type 2
    - Defect in glycosylation of CD15s because of abnormal fucose metabolism due to mutations in the guanosine diphosphate–fucose transporter gene (encoded by *SLC35C1*)

CLINICAL PRESENTATION

- Recurrent skin bacterial infection with impaired pus formation
  - Perirectal infections
  - Omphalitis
  - Poor wound healing

273

- Periodontitis usually associated with tooth loss
- Classically associated with delayed umbilical cord separation at greater than 4 weeks (although less common with improved umbilical cord care with alcohol wipes)
- LAD type 1 unique features
  - Phenotypic variability that correlates with the level of CD18 expression
- LAD type 2 unique features
  - Infections tend to be less severe than in type 1
  - Associated abnormalities: short stature, abnormal facies, cognitive impairment

DIAGNOSIS AND EVALUATION

- Leukocytosis, usually a white blood cell count (WBC) >15 (and far higher when infected)
- LAD type 1: absent or reduced CD18 expression by flow cytometry
- LAD type 2: lack of sialyl-Lewis X on neutrophils
  - Associated with the Bombay Hh blood group
- Obtain cultures to identify organism
- Imaging for evaluation of infection and to monitor for resolution of infection

TREATMENT

- Prophylactic antibiotics
- Hematopoietic stem cell transplant for certain types
- Dietary oral fucose may be beneficial in type 2

Myeloperoxidase (MPO Deficiency)

BASIC INFORMATION

- Most common inherited neutrophil function disorder
- Autosomal recessive
- MPO is found in neutrophil azurophil granules
- Catalyzes conversion of hydrogen peroxide and chloride ions to hypochlorous acid

CLINICAL PRESENTATION

- Tends to be clinically benign or asymptomatic
- Rarely disseminated candida in patients with diabetes

DIAGNOSIS AND EVALUATION

- Flow cytometry for neutrophil MPO

TREATMENT

- No treatment is usually indicated

Chediak-Higashi Syndrome (CHS)

BASIC INFORMATION

- Abnormal fusion of intracellular granules in vesicle trafficking due to autosomal recessive defect in *LYST* gene

CLINICAL PRESENTATION

- Recurrent bacterial infections, usually in skin and respiratory tract (classically with staphylococcus and streptococcus)
- Oculocutaneous albinism, partial (also with "silvery streaks of hair")
- Tooth loss
- Progressive neurologic abnormalities such as peripheral neuropathy
- Mild coagulation defects with platelet dysfunction
- Aggressive lymphoproliferative disorder, with an Hemophagocytic Lymphohistiocytosis (HLH)-like syndrome

DIAGNOSIS AND EVALUATION

- Blood smear showing giant neutrophil granules
- Hair shaft shows abnormal melanin clumping

TREATMENT

- Prophylactic antibiotic
- Hematopoietic stem cell transplant
- See Table 40.1 for a summary of phagocyte disorders

Review Questions

For review questions, please go to ExpertConsult.com.

Table 40.1. Phagocyte Disorders

	Chronic Granulomatous Disease	Leukocyte Adhesion Disorder	Myeloperoxidase Deficiency	Chediak-Higashi Syndrome
Onset	Young	Variable	Variable	Young
Inheritance	X-linked recessive, autosomal recessive	Autosomal recessive	Autosomal recessive	Autosomal recessive
Characteristic infection	Catalase positive organisms	Bacterial		Bacterial
Pathognomonic signs				Silvery hair streaks
Complete blood count		High white blood cell count		
Diagnostic test	Nitroblue tetrazolium dye, dihydrorhodamine	Flow cytometry for CD18 or CD15	Flow cytometry for neutrophil myeloperoxidase	Neutrophil granules on blood smear

Suggested Readings

1. Hanna S, Etzioni A. Leukocyte adhesion deficiencies. *Ann N Y Acad Sci.* 2012;1250:50–55.
2. Holland SM. Chronic granulomatous disease. *Clin Rev Allergy Immunol.* 2010;38(1):3–10.
3. Segal BH, Holland SM. Primary phagocytic disorders of childhood. *Pediatr Clin North Am.* 2000;47(6):1311–1338.

41 Humoral and Combined Immunodeficiencies

ALICE CHAN, MD, PhD

Adaptive immunity is composed of humoral and cellular immunity. Humoral immunity is mediated by antibodies made by B cells, whereas cellular immunity is mediated by T cells. Defects in humoral immunity include agammaglobulinemia, common variable immunodeficiency (CVID), IgA deficiency, and transient hypogammaglobulinemia of infancy (THI). Cellular immunodeficiency includes severe combined immunodeficiency (SCID), Wiskott-Aldrich syndrome (WAS), and hyper IgM syndrome (HIMS).

Agammaglobulinemia

BASIC INFORMATION

- X-linked
  - Loss of function mutation in Bruton tyrosine kinase (BTK) results in failure in B-cell development
- Autosomal recessive
  - Multiple gene causes
  - Defects in B-cell maturation and function

CLINICAL PRESENTATION

- Usually presents around 4 to 6 months, when the maternal antibodies wane
- Recurrent bacterial infection of the respiratory tract, usually encapsulated bacteria
  - Most common: otitis media, pneumonia, sinusitis
  - Less common: sepsis, osteomyelitis, arthritis, meningitis
- Viral infections
  - Enteroviruses, echovirus
  - Meningoencephalitis (can be particularly severe), chronic hepatitis
- Bronchiectasis can develop in the setting of recurrent and chronic respiratory infections
- Patients may demonstrate failure to thrive if they have a history of multiple infections; they may also have abnormally small/absent tonsillar tissue and lymph nodes

DIAGNOSIS AND EVALUATION

- Absent B cells (CD19+ or CD20+; T cells [CD3+] are intact)
- Absent or low IgG (called *hypogammaglobulinemia*)
- Monitoring of pulmonary disease
- May consider genetic testing for BTK in males

TREATMENT

- Immunoglobulin replacement therapy
- Prompt initiation of antibiotics for infection
- Inactivated vaccinations to provide T-cell immunity
- Prophylactic antibiotic in certain cases

Common Variable Immunodeficiency (CVID)

BASIC INFORMATION

- Defect in humoral deficiency due to multiple genetic causes

CLINICAL PRESENTATION

- Recurrent sinopulmonary infections with variable onset (>2 years old)
- Gastrointestinal (GI) symptoms: diarrhea, malabsorption, steatorrhea, protein-losing enteropathy
  - Giardia infection
  - Bacterial overgrowth
- Also at increased risk of autoimmune disorders (e.g., rheumatoid arthritis)
- Some may present with malignancies (e.g., lymphoma) without having frequent infections

DIAGNOSIS AND EVALUATION

- Low IgG and either low IgA or low IgM
- Normal lymphocyte subsets
- Poor responses to vaccines (e.g., low antipneumococcal titers, low antitetanus/diphtheria titers)

TREATMENT

- Immunoglobulin replacement therapy
- Immunosuppressive medications if autoimmune manifestations are present

IgA Deficiency

BASIC INFORMATION

- Low to absent IgA production

CLINICAL PRESENTATION

- Most patients are asymptomatic, but some may have recurrent sinopulmonary and GI infections
- Atopy
- Autoimmune diseases, usually celiac disease

DIAGNOSIS AND EVALUATION

- Low to absent IgA with normal IgG, IgM, and IgE

TREATMENT

- No specific therapy

Transient Hypogammaglobulinemia of Infancy (THI)

BASIC INFORMATION

- Prolonged physiologic hypogammaglobulinemia of infancy

CLINICAL PRESENTATION

- Recurrent respiratory infections
- Onset is around 4 to 6 months, when maternal antibodies wane
- Self-resolves by 6 years of age

DIAGNOSIS AND EVALUATION

- Low IgG, two standard deviations below mean of age-matched controls
- Normal vaccine responses
- Normal lymphocyte subsets including B cells

TREATMENT

- Usually no immunoglobulin replacement needed

Severe Combined Immunodeficiency (SCID)

BASIC INFORMATION

- Gene defects
  - X-linked: *IL2RG*
  - Autosomal recessive: *ADA, JAK3, IL7RA, RAG1, RAG2*
- Defect in cellular immunity with absent T cells and impaired B-cell function

CLINICAL PRESENTATION

- Onset usually before 3 months of age with severe/recurrent infections
- Types of infections

- Bacterial
- Viral: cytomegalovirus (CMV), Epstein-Barr virus (EBV), herpes simplex virus (HSV), respiratory syncytial virus (RSV), adenovirus
- Fungal: candida, aspergillus
- Opportunistic organisms: *Pneumocystis jirovecii*, cryptosporidium
- Attenuated vaccines: rotavirus, varicella, bacillus Calmette–Guérin (BCG)
- Associated symptoms: deficient immune tissues (absent lymph nodes, tonsils, thymus), failure to thrive, chronic diarrhea
- Omenn syndrome: subset of patients can have this presentation
  - Lymphadenopathy
  - Hepatosplenomegaly
  - Diffuse erythroderma
- Graft versus host–like manifestations due to maternal T cells—such as rash

DIAGNOSIS AND EVALUATION

- Complete blood count (CBC) with differential with low absolute lymphocyte count (i.e., lymphopenia)
- Absent to low T-cell receptor circles (TRECS; part of newborn screen in most states)
- Lymphocyte subset findings may be indicative of different gene diagnoses:
  - T minus, B+, NK+
  - T minus, B+, NK minus
  - T minus, B minus, NK+
  - T minus, B minus, NK minus
- Low to absent immunoglobulin levels
- Low to absent lymphocyte proliferation
- Absent thymus on imaging
- Monitoring for viral infections (CMV, EBV, adenovirus)

TREATMENT

- Prophylactic antimicrobials against bacterial, viral, and fungal infections
- Immunoglobulin replacement therapy
- Vaccines will not provide immunologic protection; live vaccines may be harmful
- Transfusions of blood should be irradiated, leukocyte reduced, and CMV negative
- Hematopoietic stem cell transplant or gene therapy because complete SCID is often fatal by 2 years old (some "leaky SCID" may have delayed/variable course)
- Enzyme replacement is indicated for adenosine deaminase (ADA) deficiency

Wiskott-Aldrich Syndrome (WAS)

BASIC INFORMATION

- X-linked inheritance of mutation in WASP (WAS protein)
- Combined T-cell and B-cell immunodeficiency

CLINICAL PRESENTATION

- Classic triad of eczema, petechiae (a distinguishing feature for WAS), and immunodeficiency
- Recurrent infections
  - Sinopulmonary infections
  - Severe viral infections such as varicella
- Risk for malignancy

DIAGNOSIS AND EVALUATION

- Low platelets and small in size (called "microthrombocytopenia"; see Chapter 37 for additional information)
- Eosinophilia
- Elevated IgE
- Poor vaccine responses

TREATMENT

- Immunoglobulin replacement
- Hematopoietic stem cell therapy or gene therapy
- Splenectomy for low platelets but increases infection risk

Hyper IgM Syndrome (HIMS)

BASIC INFORMATION

- Defect in class switch recombination (i.e., the ability of B cells to switch from IgM to IgG, IgA, and IgE)
- X-linked: *CD40L* mutation
- Autosomal recessive: multiple gene causes

CLINICAL PRESENTATION

- Pulmonary infections
- GI infections
- Infections
  - Encapsulated bacteria
  - Enterovirus infections
  - *Pneumocystis jirovecii*
  - Cryptosporidium

DIAGNOSIS AND EVALUATION

- Normal to elevated IgM, but with low IgG, IgA, and IgE

TREATMENT

- Immunoglobulin replacement
- Prophylactic antibiotic
- Hematopoietic stem cell transplant or gene therapy

Review Questions

For review questions, please go to ExpertConsult.com.

Suggested Readings

1. Ballow M. Primary immunodeficiency disorders: antibody deficiency. *J Allergy Clin Immunol.* 2002;109(4):581–591.
2. Chinn IK, Shearer WT. Severe combined immunodeficiency disorders. *Immunol Allergy Clin North Am.* 2015;35(4):671–694.

42 Selected Topics in Immunology

ALICE CHAN, MD, PhD

Complement Disorders

BASIC INFORMATION

- Part of the innate immune system comprised of plasma and membrane proteins used to kill or opsonize pathogens, modulate inflammation, and clear dying cells (i.e. apoptotic bodies)
- Three pathways: classical, alternative, lectin
- See also Nelson Textbook of Pediatrics, Chapter 134, "Disorders of the Complement System."

CLINICAL PRESENTATION

- Recurrent infections
  - Classical complement deficits: increased risk for encapsulated infections
  - Terminal complement deficits: recurrent systemic infections to *Neisseria gonorrhoeae* or *N. meningitides*
- Autoimmune manifestations such as lupus (with glomerulonephritis) and atypical hemolytic uremia syndrome
- Angioedema, specifically for C1-esterase inhibitor deficiency (see Chapter 4 for details)

DIAGNOSIS AND EVALUATION

- see Table 42.1
- CH50: assesses classical complement pathway
- AH50: assesses alternative complement pathway
- Absence of specific complement proteins can be tested
  - C1 esterase inhibitor defect (especially if angioedema)

TREATMENT

- Early antibiotic treatment of suspected infections
- Vaccination
- Prophylactic antibiotic
- Treatment of autoimmune manifestations with immunosuppression

Table 42.1. Complement Testing

Defect	CH50	AH50
Early classical complement defect (C1, C2, C4)	Absent to low	Normal
Early alternative complement defect	Normal	Absent to low
Terminal complement defect (C5, C6, C7, C8, C9)	Absent to low	Absent to low

- Replacement of missing complement component may be helpful (e.g., recombinant C1 esterase, fresh frozen plasma)
- Hematopoietic stem cell transplant if deficient protein produced in the hematopoietic compartment

Syndromes Associated With Immunodeficiency

BASIC INFORMATION

- DiGeorge syndrome (see Chapter 35 for details)
  - Defect in the development of the third and fourth pharyngeal pouches, which results in abnormal thymic development, cardiac defects, and parathyroid developmental abnormalities
  - 22q11.2 deletion or *TBX1* mutation
  - Variable immunodeficiency from partial to complete T-cell deficiency
- Ataxia telangiectasia (see Chapter 58 for details)
  - Defect in the *ATM* gene that encodes a protein involved in monitoring DNA repair and synthesis
- CHARGE syndrome (see Chapter 35 for details)
  - Can be due to mutation in *CHD7*
  - Associated immune deficits
    - Decreased T-cell numbers and function
    - Impaired antibody production
- Hyper IgE syndrome (HIES)
  - Also known as Job syndrome
  - Mutations in *STAT3*
  - Autosomal dominant or sporadic

CLINICAL PRESENTATION

- Syndromes can have variable degrees of immunodeficiency
- DiGeorge syndrome
  - Dysmorphic facies: low-set ears, hypertelorism, micrognathia, bulbous nose, short philtrum with small mouth, high-arched palate
  - Hypocalcemia
  - Congenital cardia defects
  - Feeding difficulties
  - Renal abnormalities
  - Psychiatric disorders
- Ataxia telangiectasia
  - Loss of motor milestones
  - Ataxia due to cerebellar involvement
  - Telangiectasia

- Recurrent sinopulmonary infections
- Increased risk of malignancy
- Radiation sensitivity
- Progressive respiratory decline
- Endocrine abnormalities: diabetes, gonadal dysgenesis
- CHARGE syndrome
  - **C**oloboma of the eye
  - **H**eart defects
  - **A**tresia of the choanae
  - **R**etardation of growth
  - **G**enital or urinary defects
  - **E**ar anomalies
- HIES
  - Eczema
  - Cold abscesses (i.e., not warm or red)
    - Usually from *Staphylococcus aureus*
  - Recurrent pneumonias with pneumatoceles
    - Usually from *Staphylococcus aureus*
    - Can get superinfected with pseudomonas and aspergillus
  - Mucocutaneous candidiasis
  - Craniofacial dysmorphisms: coarse facies, wide nose, deep-set eyes
  - Skeletal abnormalities: short stature, retained teeth, frequent bone fractures

DIAGNOSIS AND EVALUATION

- Complete blood count (CBC) with differential
- Lymphocyte subsets for evaluation of T cells
- Immunoglobulin levels
- Lymphocyte proliferation
- Vaccine titers
- Testing specific for DiGeorge
  - Karyotype, fluorescence in situ hybridization (FISH) to assess 22q11.2 deletion, ot TBX1 gene sequencing
  - Low calcium levels
- Testing specific for ataxia telangiectasia
  - Elevated alpha fetoprotein
  - Monitor pulmonary status
  - Limit radiation exposure
- Labs seen in HIES
  - Elevated IgE

- Eosinophilia
- *STAT3* sequencing

TREATMENT

- Potential immune therapies pending degree of immunodeficiency
  - Prophylactic antibiotics
  - Immunoglobulin replacement therapy
- DiGeorge-specific therapies
  - Calcium and vitamin D supplementation if hypocalcemia
  - Thymic transplant
  - Cardiac repair if congenital heart disease
- Ataxia telangiectasia–specific therapies
  - Chest physiotherapy
  - Limit radiation exposure
- HIES
  - Prophylactic antibiotics
  - Skin emollients
  - Immunoglobulin replacement in some cases
  - Surgical intervention for drainage

Review Questions

For review questions, please go to ExpertConsult.com.

Suggested Readings

1. Mahmoudi M, Mollnes TE, Kuijpers TW, Roos D. Complement deficiencies. In: Rezaei N, Aghamohammadi A, Notarangelo LD, eds. *Primary immunodeficiency diseases: definition, diagnosis, and management.* Verlag Berlin-Heidelberg: Springer; 2008:235–249.
2. McDonald-McGinn DM, Sullivan KE, Marino B, Philip N, Swillen A, Vorstman JA, et al. 22q11.2 deletion syndrome. *Nat Rev Dis Primers.* 2015;1:15071.
3. Rothblum-Oviatt C, Wright J, Lefton-Greif MA, McGrath-Morrow SA, Crawford TO, Lederman HM. Ataxia telangiectasia: a review. *Orphanet J Rare Dis.* 2016;11(1):159.
4. Yeganeh M, Gambineri E, Abolmaali K, Tamizifar B, Espanol T. Other well-defined immunodeficiencies. In: Rezaei N, Aghamohammadi A, Notarangelo LD, eds. *Primary immunodeficiency diseases: definition, diagnosis, and management.* Verlag Berlin-Heidelberg: Springer; 2008: 251–290.

Infectious Diseases

Definition of Sepsis

SYSTEMIC INFLAMMATORY RESPONSE SYNDROME (SIRS)

- Two out of four of the following criteria:
  - Core temperature: >38.5°C or <36°C
  - Heart rate:
    - Tachycardia: mean heart rate >2 standard deviations (SD) above normal range for age *or* persistent elevation over 0.5 to 4 hours
    - Bradycardia: in children <1 yr of age—heart rate <10th percentile for age for 0.5 hours
    - Absence of other causes: pain, medications that could cause tachycardia or bradycardia, any other external stimuli
  - Respiratory rate:
    - >2 SD above mean for age *or*
    - Acute need for mechanical ventilation not related to anesthesia or neuromuscular disease
  - Leukocyte count elevated or depressed for age, or >10% immature neutrophils

SEPSIS

- SIRS with suspected or proven infection, or clinical syndrome associated with high probability of an infection

SEPTIC SHOCK

- Sepsis with cardiovascular dysfunction, defined as:
  - Any of the following signs, despite 40 mL/kg of isotonic fluid resuscitation in 1 hour
    - Hypotension: systolic blood pressure <2 SD for age, or <5th percentile for age
    - Two of the following signs:
      Capillary refill >5 seconds
      Urine output <0.5 mL/kg/h
      Unexplained metabolic acidosis: base deficit >5 mEq/L
      Increased arterial lactate more than two times the upper limit of normal
      Core to peripheral temperature gap of >3°C
  - Need for vasoactive drug to maintain blood presure
- Severe sepsis:
  - Sepsis with any one (or more) of the following
    - Cardiovascular dysfunction (defined earlier)
    - Acute respiratory distress syndrome

- Two or more organ system dysfunctions: respiratory, renal, neurologic, hematologic, hepatic
  - See also Nelson Textbook of Pediatrics, Chapter 70, "Shock."
- The terms "sepsis" and "septic shock" have been revised since these classic definitions, with current consensus favoring focus on evidence of end-organ dysfunction and cellular/metabolic abnormalities that arise when sepsis results in inadequate oxygen delivery (e.g. rise in lactate).

Approach to Neonatal Infections and Sepsis

BASIC INFORMATION

- Early versus late onset:
  - Early onset:
    - Diagnosed within 7 days of birth
    - Acquired before or during delivery due to vertical maternal transmission
  - Late onset:
    - Diagnosed between 7 and 90 days after birth
    - Usually due to organisms acquired in the hospital or community after delivery
- Risk factors for neonatal sepsis (see Table 43.1)

CLINICAL PRESENTATION

Must have high index for suspicion because symptoms can be nonspecific and eventually become fulminant

- Clinical signs and symptoms
  - General: temperature instability—fever or hypothermia, poor feeding, decreased urine output
  - Neurologic: irritability or lethargy, full or bulging fontanel, abnormal tone, seizure-like activity
  - Cardiovascular: pallor, poor perfusion, tachycardia or bradycardia without clear explanation
  - Respiratory: apnea or signs of respiratory distress, cyanosis
  - Gastrointestinal (GI): abdominal distention, vomiting, hepatosplenomegaly
  - Heme: jaundice, petechiae, purpura or bleeding

DIAGNOSIS AND EVALUATION

- Obtain cultures from the following sites: blood, urine, cerebrospinal fluid (CSF)

Table 43.1. Risk Factors for Neonatal Sepsis

Maternal infections during gestation or labor

Maternal chorioamnionitis—defined as maternal fever during delivery with or without the following:
- Maternal leukocytosis
- Maternal or fetal tachycardia
- Uterine tenderness
- Purulent or malodorous vaginal discharge or amniotic fluid

Maternal colonization with group B streptococcus, herpes simplex virus, or *Neisseria gonorrhoeae*

Prolonged rupture of membranes (≥18 hours)

Prematurity

Infant with cardiac, respiratory, metabolic disease, or congenital abnormality that could increase susceptibility to infection

- Need at least 1 mL of fluid for cultures because yield can be low in early neonatal sepsis
- Attempt to obtain all cultures before antibiotics if able
- CSF culture indicated as part of sepsis evaluation in all infants under 28 days of age
- May avoid CSF culture in older, well-appearing infants with fever in the setting of reassuring laboratory results, no other signs concerning for sepsis, or clear viral etiology
- At the time of this writing, the American Academy of Pediatrics (AAP) is developing guidelines for indications for lumbar puncture in evaluating febrile young infants
- Complete blood count (CBC):
  - Leukocytosis or increased immature neutrophils: immature—total neutrophil ratio ≥0.2
  - Neutropenia also can be associated with fulminant infection
  - Thrombocytosis or thrombocytopenia
    - Thrombocytopenia can be seen in neonatal fungal infections
- Urinalysis: leukocytosis with leukocyte esterase or nitrites can point to urinary tract infection (UTI)
- CSF studies:
  - CSF WBC count: >10 to 20 mm^3 is suggestive of infection; normal value varies based on age
  - CSF chemistry: elevated protein, low glucose
    - Low glucose is specific for bacterial meningitis
  - CSF Gram stain: WBC or bacteria
- Acute-phase reactants: CRP and procalcitonin can be elevated within 12-24 hours of onset of infection
- Chest x-ray (CXR): evidence of pneumonia
- No clear criteria or "sepsis scores" have been established

TREATMENT

- Organisms causing neonatal sepsis or meningitis:
  - Bacteria:
    - Typically organisms inhibiting maternal genitourinary or lower gastrointestinal (GI) tract
    - Most common are *Escherichia coli* and group B streptococcus (GBS)
      Note: intrapartum GBS prophylaxis reduces risk for early-onset disease (0–7 days) but does *not* decrease risk for late-onset disease in the infant (>7 days)

- Other: non–*E. coli* Gram-negative bacilli (*Pseudomonas aeruginosa* hospital-acquired infection), *Staphylococcus aureus*, *Streptococcus pneumoniae*, group A streptococcus, enterococcus
  - *Listeria monocytogenes*: rare cause of sepsis in neonates <28 days of age, but currently appropriate coverage is still recommended
- Viruses:
  - Herpes simplex virus (HSV): highest risk in 0 to 21 days of life when transmitted during delivery; has high morbidity and mortality
  - Enterovirus: can present with meningitis-like symptoms, usually benign course
  - Respiratory viruses: influenza, RSV, etc.
    Of note, even with infants with a respiratory viral infection, there is still a risk of UTI; thus urine studies may still be warranted for febrile young infants even if viral testing is positive!
  - Cytomegalovirus (CMV) can present with neonatal sepsis
- Empiric antimicrobial therapy
  - Infants within first month of life
    - Aminoglycoside or third-generation cephalosporin
    - Ampicillin (to cover listeria and enterococcus)
    - Acyclovir if risk factors for HSV (<21 days of age, maternal genital HSV lesions during delivery, relatives with cold sores)
  - Infants 30 to 60 days of life:
    - Third-generation cephalosporin
  - Other considerations:
    - Ceftriaxone has been reported to displace bilirubin from albumin binding sites. Use alternative third-generation cephalosporins such as cefotaxime in:
      Neonates (<28 days of age) who are receiving IV calcium-containing products
      Neonates (<28 days of age) with hyperbilirubinemia
      Premature infants
    - If there is concern for meningitis, cephalosporins have better CNS penetration than aminoglycosides
    - Add vancomycin if patient appears ill or there is risk for methicillin-resistant *S. aureus* (MRSA) or resistant *S. pneumoniae*
    - Premature infants who remain hospitalized since birth are at risk for pseudomonal infections
      Consider fourth-generation cephalosporin, piperacillin-tazobactam, or carbapenem
    - Consider amphotericin in ill-appearing, extremely low birthweight infants at risk for disseminated fungal infections, who are not responding to antibacterial therapy

Infections in Immunocompromised Hosts

MALIGNANCY

- Increased risk of opportunistic infections due to neutropenia, chemotherapeutic agents, and malignancy itself
  - Viral infections: increased risk for Epstein-Barr virus (EBV), CMV, HSV, and varicella, in addition to viruses that are pathogenic in healthy hosts

- Bacterial infections:
  - *P. aeruginosa, E. coli, Enterobacter* spp., and *Klebsiella* spp. can lead to septic shock with high risk of mortality if not promptly treated
  - *S. aureus* and *S. pneumoniae* can cause more fulminant disease
  - Viridans streptococci can cause systemic disease in patients with mucositis
- Opportunistic fungal infections:
  - Candida, aspergillus are the most common
  - Other fungal infections include: mucor, fusarium
- Fever and neutropenia
  - Definition
    - Fever: temperature ≥38.3°C
    - Neutropenia: absolute neutrophil count <500 cells/mm^3
      - There is some increased risk for infection if absolute neutrophil count is <1000 cells/mm^3
  - Evaluation
    - Lack of neutrophils results in absence of inflammatory response, so localizing a source of infection can be challenging
    - Examine the oropharynx, lungs, skin, nail beds, intravascular catheter sites, perineum, and anus for any signs of inflammation
  - Empiric therapy
    - Pseudomonas is an important cause of mortality in neutropenic patients, so this must be covered in empiric therapy in addition to broad Gram-positive and Gram-negative coverage
    - Monotherapy can be considered in well-appearing patients without evidence of shock
      - Examples: cefepime, piperacillin-tazobactam, or carbapenem
    - Addition of second agent is common for "double Gram-negative coverage" (e.g., aminoglycoside), especially if a patient is clinically unstable or has history of resistant organisms
    - Indications for the addition of vancomycin:
      - Severe mucositis
      - Risk of catheter-related infection
      - Hypotension/shock
      - History of colonization or prior infection with MRSA
    - Considerations for the addition of antifungal agents:
      - Persistent fever >96 hours
      - Patients with relapsed acute lymphoblastic leukemia, acute myeloblastic leukemia, or post–bone marrow transplant are at higher risk
      - Consider echinocandins (caspofungin, micafungin) or amphotericin as first line

ASPLENIA

- Includes anatomic (e.g., congenital asplenia, postsplenectomy) or functional asplenia (e.g., polysplenia, splenic dysfunction caused by sickle cell disease)
- Patients are at increased risk for infections due to:
  - Encapsulated bacteria: *S. pneumoniae, Haemophilus influenzae, Neisseria meningitidis*
  - Can cause sepsis, pneumonia, meningitis, and osteomyelitis

- Due to absence of splenic macrophages, which are key in phagocytosis of the opsonized encapsulated bacteria
- *Salmonella* spp, *S. aureus*
- Protozoal illnesses: malaria and babesiosis
- Prevention and prophylaxis
  - Delay elective splenectomy if possible: risk of infection is lower in patients who have spleen removed later in life
  - Additional immunizations
    - All vaccines, including live virus vaccines, are safe in this population
    - In patients undergoing planned splenectomy, immunizations should be completed as recommended at least 2 weeks before surgery
    - Pneumococcal conjugate vaccine: PCV 13
      - Standard series of vaccines is recommended for asplenic patients
      - For incompletely vaccinated children of ages 2 to 5 years:
        - One additional PCV 13 dose if child has received three prior doses
        - Two additional PCV 13 doses given 8 weeks apart if child is unimmunized or has received less than three prior doses
      - For incompletely vaccinated children older than 5 years of age:
        - Administer one dose of PCV 13 only if it has never been previously administered
    - Pneumococcal polysaccharide vaccine: PPSV 23
      - All doses of PCV 13 should be completed before PPSV 23 vaccine
      - Give first dose of PPSV 23 at ≥24 months of age and second dose 5 years later
      - Give PPSV 23 a minimum of 8 weeks after most recent PCV 13 dose
    - Meningococcal quadrivalent conjugate vaccines (ACWY)
      - Includes MenHibrix, MenVeo, and Menactra
      - Administer to all asplenic children aged 2 months or older
      - Minimum age and dosage schedule varies by vaccine
      - Menactra (MCV4-D) should not be given within 4 weeks of PCV 13 because it can interfere with antibody response
    - *H. influenzae* type b conjugate vaccine
      - All asplenic patients <5 years of age should receive a routine series or appropriate catch-up dosages
      - Unimmunized patients with asplenia >5 years of age should receive one dose of Hib vaccine. This is not routinely recommended for healthy unimmunized patients
  - Prophylaxis: penicillin V or amoxicillin daily
    - Strongly recommended for all patients with asplenia until at least 5 years of age, and for at least 1 year after surgical splenectomy (although some centers may opt to continue prophylaxis into adulthood)
    - Duration of prophylaxis is not clearly established. Many centers continue prophylaxis until 18 years of age or into adulthood for asplenic patients, especially if they have other comorbidities that increase risk for pneumococcal disease

BURN INJURY

- Increased risk of infection due to damaged skin barrier and alterations in systemic immune response due to neutropenia and/or impaired complement and phagocyte function
- Common infections in burn patients:
  - Gram-positive organisms: seen in early post-burn period
    - Most common: *S. aureus*, coagulase-negative staph
    - Other: enterococcus, streptococcus, listeria, corynebacterium
  - Gram-negative organisms:
    - Thought to be secondary to translocation from GI tract
    - Most common: *P. aeruginosa*
    - Other: *E. coli*, enterobacter, klebsiella, serratia, acinetobacter
  - Fungi
    - Most common: *Candida*
      - Can cause local disease; 3% to 5% have disseminated candidemia
    - Other fungi: due to exposure to spores in ground or water at the time of injury
    - Aspergillus, Mucor, Fuzarium
  - Viruses:
    - Increased risk for CMV, HSV, and varicella-zoster virus

CONSIDERATIONS IN OTHER SPECIAL POPULATIONS

- HIV/AIDS
  - Active HIV/AIDS infection results in impaired cellular immunity, increasing risk for many opportunistic infections. See Chapter 45 for details.
- Malnutrition
  - Protein-calorie malnutrition is associated with impaired cellular-mediated immune response, with degree of infection risk increasing with severity of malnutrition
  - Increased rates of pneumonia, diarrheal illnesses, and tuberculosis (TB) documented in undernourished children in low- and middle-income nations
  - Increased rates of viral infections such as measles, varicella, HSV, and hepatitis in this population
  - Higher likelihood of sepsis and mortality from common childhood infections
- CNS disease
  - Thermoregulation primarily occurs in preoptic area and anterior hypothalamus
  - Children with CNS disease, specifically with defects in corpus callosum and hypothalamic function, can have poor temperature regulation
    - This can result in hypothermia or an inability to mount fever response to infections
    - This can also lead to "autonomic fevers" triggered by immature thermoregulatory mechanisms in the absence of infection
- Infections associated with intravascular catheters:
  - Types of infection:
    - Bloodstream infection: organisms can form biofilms around catheters
      - Usually no localized symptoms

- Skin and soft tissue infection: exit site or tunnel tract infection
  - Can see erythema, fluctuance, or drainage around catheter insertion site
- Organisms: contamination by skin or GI flora
  - Gram-positive cocci, Gram-negative bacilli, fungal etiologies
  - *S. aureus*, coagulase-negative staphylococci, and pseudomonas are common
  - Also consider mycobacteria and *Candida*
- Treatment:
  - Empiric therapy: vancomycin with an antipseudomonal agent (e.g. cefepime, ceftazidime, piperacillin-tazobactam)
  - Usually proceed with 10 to 14 days of targeted systemic antibiotic therapy after identification of the causative organism
  - Indications for catheter removal:
    - Clinical deterioration despite adequate antibiotic therapy
    - Persistent positive blood cultures >72 hours
    - Certain organisms: *S. aureus*, pseudomonas, candida or other fungus, mycobacteria

Transmission and Prevention of Infectious Diseases

PREVENTION OF VECTOR-BORNE DISEASES (TICKS AND MOSQUITOES)

- General precautions
  - Educate families about illnesses that are spread via ticks and mosquito bites
  - Wear clothing that covers exposed skin (arms, legs, neck) when in high-risk areas
  - Use insect repellents when entering high-risk areas:
    - Recommendations for repellent use
      - Do not apply over cuts, wounds, sunburned skin, or around eyes and mouth
      - Do not spray onto the face—spray on the hands, then apply to the face
      - Do not apply *under* clothing
      - Wash hands after application
      - Do not allow children to handle repellents; do not apply to children's hands
      - When back indoors, wash repellent-treated skin with soap and water
    - Permethrin:
      - Most effective against ticks but also works against mosquitoes and other arthropods
      - Spray onto clothes only (not directly onto skin)
      - Ensure children are not chewing on clothes or other applied surfaces
    - DEET:
      - Concentration <30% is approved by AAP for use in children older than 2 months
      - Most effective against mosquitoes but also works against ticks
      - Effective for 2 to 12 hours and often requires reapplication
    - Others: picaridin, oil of eucalyptus, IR3535

- Prevention of mosquito-borne infections
  - Prevent breeding of mosquitoes by removing sources of standing water (e.g., clogged rain gutters, cans/buckets that could collect rainwater) and routinely cleaning and treating swimming pools
  - Avoid outdoor activity at times of high mosquito activity (dusk, dawn)
    - Note: mosquitoes that transmit West Nile virus and dengue have also been found to bite during the day; mosquitoes that transmit malaria are usually active at night
  - Protect skin from mosquitoes (cover exposed skin and use repellents and mosquito nets/screens)
    - Mosquito traps and electronic bug zappers have not been shown to be effective
- Prevention of tick-borne infections
  - Avoid areas with high risk for tick infestation (e.g., dense woods, humid environments)
  - If living in or near a high-risk area:
    - Examine pets routinely for ticks
    - Keep play equipment in sunny and/or dry areas and dense shrubs; keep leaves raked
    - Dry outdoor clothing on high heat to kill unattached ticks
  - If entering a tick-infested area:
    - Wear clothing that covers exposed skin and apply tick repellents
    - Inspect for ticks daily, ideally within 2 hours of coming indoors
      - Focus on areas of tight clothing, axilla, groin, head, neck, and behind ears
  - Remove any attached ticks as soon as they are discovered because risk of transmission of pathogens increases with duration of tick attachment
    - Risk of pathogen transmission is highest if the tick is engorged or has been attached for 36 hours or more
  - Method for tick removal is as follows:
    - Use forceps or tweezers to grasp the tick close to the skin
    - Gently pull outward without twisting motions
    - Examine closely for remaining tick parts embedded in the skin
    - Wash bite site with soap and water
  - Monitor for symptoms of tick-borne illnesses:
    - Testing of attached ticks for spirochetes is not recommended
    - Chemoprophylaxis for Lyme disease is not typically indicated after a tick is found
      - However, a dose of doxycycline as prophylaxis may be considered within 72 hours of tick removal:
        - In certain endemic areas for children over 8 years of age
        - Only if the tick is engorged or suspected to be attached for more than 36 hours
    - Chemoprophylaxis for other tick-borne illnesses is not indicated

PREVENTION OF RECREATIONAL WATER–ASSOCIATED ILLNESSES

- Recreational water use includes:
  - Swimming pools, water parks, and fountains
  - Oceans, lakes, and rivers
  - Hot tubs

- Pathogens that are commonly transmitted via recreational water use
  - Cryptosporidium: oocysts remain infectious for up to 10 days, even in chlorinated water
  - Giardia: survives for up to 45 minutes in chlorinated water but longer in lakes and streams
- Infection control measures:
  - Do not enter recreational water in the following situations:
    - Open wounds or sores
    - Active emetic/diarrhea illness:
      - If diagnosed with cryptosporidiosis, remain out of the water for at least 2 weeks after resolution of symptoms
      - If shigella or norovirus, remain out of water for 1 week after resolution of symptoms
  - Avoid ingestion of recreational water
  - Shower with soap before entering recreational water as well as after exiting
  - Check children's diapers every 30 to 60 minutes, or if they are toilet-trained, take bathroom breaks every 60 minutes
    - Practice hand hygiene around diaper changes, toilet breaks, and before eating or drinking

INFECTIONS TRANSMITTED VIA BREASTFEEDING

- Contraindications for breastfeeding
  - Maternal HIV: even if appropriately treated with antiretrovirals
  - Maternal HSV with lesions on the breast—can be transmitted via direct contact
    - Can resume breastfeeding once breast lesions resolve
    - Can feed from unaffected breast if affected breast lesions are completely covered
  - Maternal active TB:
    - Can resume breastfeeding once mother has received at least 2 weeks of treatment and sputum is negative
- Other considerations
  - Mastitis:
    - Safe to breastfeed while receiving antibiotic therapy. May need to discontinue temporarily after drainage of abscess
  - Maternal hepatitis B:
    - Safe to breastfeed; risk of transmission is minimal if infant receives vaccine and immune globulin within 12 hours of birth
  - Maternal hepatitis C:
    - Transmission is theoretically possible but has not been documented. Safe to breastfeed, but consider discontinuing if nipples are cracked or bleeding
  - Other conditions that are compatible with breastfeeding: rubella, malaria, toxoplasmosis

TRANSMISSION OF INFECTIONS IN CHILD CARE CENTERS

- Viral infections of the respiratory and GI tracts are most commonly transmitted via contact in child care centers
- Children are often infectious 2 to 3 days before they manifest symptoms of the illness
- Child care providers should receive all routine immunizations and a preemployment tuberculin skin test

Table 43.2. Recommendations for Exclusion from Child Care Settings for Children with Communicable Diseases

Disease	Exclusion Recommendations
SKIN	
Skin lesions	Exclude if lesions are weeping or draining and cannot be covered with a waterproof dressing
Rash with fever	Exclude until medical evaluation determines noncommunicable cause
Impetigo	Exclude until 24 hours after antibiotic initiation
RESPIRATORY	
Oral lesions	Exclude if unable to contain drool
Impetigo	Exclude until 24 hours after antibiotic initiation
Streptococcal pharyngitis	Exclude until 24 hours of treatment complete
GASTROINTESTINAL	
Vomiting	Exclude until symptoms have resolved (or if evaluation reveals noncommunicable cause and patient is able to maintain hydration)
Salmonella nonserotype Typhi	Exclude until diarrhea resolves, but no stool cultures needed
Salmonella Typhi	Exclude until diarrhea resolves and three negative stool cultures
Shiga toxin–producing *Escherichia coli* or shigella	Exclude until diarrhea resolves. Check state regulations for stool cultures: usually need two negative

Table 43.3. Recommendations for Exclusion from Child Care Settings for Children with Vaccine-Preventable Viruses

Vaccine- Preventable Viruses	Exclusion Recommendations	Recommendations for Management of Contacts
Measles	Exclude until 4 days after beginning of rash	Immunize children without evidence of immunity within 72 h. If unimmunized: exclude until 2 weeks after the onset of rash in last child with measles.
Mumps	Exclude until 5 days after onset of parotid gland swelling	Immunize children without evidence of immunity. If unimmunized, exclude for at least 26 days after onset of parotitis in last child with mumps.
Varicella	Exclude until all lesions have dried and crusted (at least 6 days after onset)	Immunize contacts within 3 to 5 days of exposure. Varicella-zoster IgG for neonates, immunocompromised patients, or pregnant contacts who do not have evidence of immunity.

- Pregnant women should be careful about transmission of parvovirus and CMV, which can be harmful for fetal development
- Conditions that do not require exclusion:
  - Common cold
  - Rash without fever or changes in behavior
  - Conjunctivitis without fever, changes in behavior, and no more than one other case of concurrent conjunctivitis
  - HIV, chronic hepatitis B, and colonization with MRSA
  - Mild diarrhea
    - Stool should be contained in the diaper for younger children. Toilet-trained children should remain continent. Stool frequency should be less than two stools above normal for that child
- Precautions for general illnesses and specific communicable diseases are provided in Table 43.2 and Table 43.3

HOSPITAL INFECTION CONTROL

- Contact isolation: use of gloves and gown when in contact with the patient or immediate patient surroundings
  - Use in patients with history of infection or colonization with multidrug-resistant organisms (e.g., vancomycin-resistant enterococci, MRSA, multidrug-resistant Gram-negative bacilli)

- Use in patients with vomiting or diarrhea, abscess, or draining wounds that cannot be covered
  - *Clostridium difficile* and norovirus are transmitted through spores, which may not be reliably destroyed by alcohol-based sanitizing agents. Handwashing is preferred
- Droplet isolation: use of masks and eye guards as well as gown and gloves when within 3 to 6 feet of the patient
  - Use droplet with contact isolation for respiratory infections, meningitis, and fever with a rash
- Airborne isolation: use of masks and negative-pressure air-handling systems within the patient's immediate surroundings
  - Use airborne isolation for measles
  - Use airborne along with contact isolation for patients with suspected or confirmed TB and varicella infection, and for immunocompromised patients with zoster infections

Review Questions

For review questions, please go to ExpertConsult.com.

Suggested Readings

1. Chusid MJ, Rotar MM. Infection prevention and control. In: Kliegman RM, Stanton BF, St. Geme JW, et al., eds. *Nelson Textbook of Pediatrics.* 12th ed. Philadelphia: Elsevier; 2016:1260–1264.

2. Goldstein B, Giroir B, Randolph A. International pediatric sepsis consensus conference: definitions for sepsis and organ dysfunction in pediatrics. *Pediatr Crit Care Med.* 2005;6(1):2–8.

3. Michaels MG, Green M. Infections in immunocompromised persons. In: Kliegman RM, Stanton BF, St. Geme JW, et al., eds. *Nelson Textbook of Pediatrics.* 12th ed. Philadelphia: Elsevier; 2016:1287–1295.

4. Patel JA, Williams-Bouyer N. Infections in burn patients. In: Cherry JD, Harrison GJ, Kaplan SL, et al., eds. *Feigin and Cherry's Textbook of Pediatric Infectious Diseases.* 7th ed. Philadelphia: Elsevier/Saunders; 2014:1047–1062.

5. Prevention of illnesses associated with recreational water use. In: Kimberlin DW, Brady MT, Jackson MA, Long SS, eds. *Red Book®: 2015 Report of the Committee on Infectious Diseases.* American Academy of Pediatrics; 2015:216–218.

6. Prevention of mosquitoborne infections. In: Kimberlin DW, Brady MT, Jackson MA, Long SS, eds. *Red Book®: 2015 Report of the Committee on Infectious Diseases.* American Academy of Pediatrics; 2015:213–215.

7. Prevention of tickborne infections. In: Kimberlin DW, Brady MT, Jackson MA, Long SS, eds. *Red Book®: 2015 Report of the Committee on Infectious Diseases.* American Academy of Pediatrics; 2015:210–213.

8. Shapiro ED, Baltimore RS. Epidemiology and biostatistics of infectious diseases. In: Cherry JD, Harrison GJ, Kaplan SL, et al., eds. *Feigin and Cherry's Textbook of Pediatric Infectious Diseases.* 7th ed. Philadelphia: Elsevier/Saunders; 2014:95–128.

9. Stoll BJ, Shane AL. Infections of the neonatal infant. In: Kliegman RM, Stanton BF, St. Geme JW, et al., eds. *Nelson Textbook of Pediatrics.* 12th ed. Philadelphia: Elsevier; 2016:909–925.

10. Transmission of infectious agents via human milk. In: Kimberlin DW, Brady MT, Jackson MA, Long SS, eds. *Red Book®: 2015 Report of the Committee on Infectious Diseases.* American Academy of Pediatrics; 2015:127–132.

11. Waggoner-Fountain, LA. Childcare and communicable diseases. In: Kliegman RM, Stanton BF, St. Geme JW, et al., eds. *Nelson Textbook of Pediatrics.* 12th ed. Philadelphia: Elsevier; 2016:1264–1268.

12. Wolf J, Flynn P. Infections associated with medical devices. In: Kliegman RM, Stanton BF, St. Geme JW, et al., eds. *Nelson Textbook of Pediatrics.* 12th ed. Philadelphia: Elsevier; 2016:1295–1298.

44 *Bacteria*

SALWA SULIEMAN, DO

Bacterial infections represent an important area of general pediatric knowledge. An exhaustive description of each organism is beyond the scope of this chapter; therefore, key areas of content knowledge will be discussed. The bacteria in this chapter are organized in a way that maximizes retention of information for the board exam. Basic microbiology is shown in Fig. 44.1 to aid your review.

HIGH-YIELD GRAM-POSITIVE COCCI

Streptococcus pyogenes

BASIC INFORMATION

- Also called Group A Streptococcus (GAS)
- Gram-positive cocci in chains
- Leading pathogenic bacteria in children in the United States
- Colonizes upper respiratory tract
- Tissue penetration in the oropharynx leads to transient bacteremia and subsequent invasive disease
- Three mechanisms of human disease
  - Suppuration
  - Toxin production
  - Immune-mediated disease
- See also *Nelson Textbook of Pediatrics*, Chapter 183, "Group A Streptococcus"

CLINICAL PRESENTATION

- Most common disease processes are pharyngitis and impetigo
- See Table 44.1 for various group A *Streptococcus* (GAS) infections
- For details on GAS pharyngitis, see Chapter 71
- For details on scarlet fever, see Chapter 11
- For details on rheumatic fever, see Chapters 7 and 81

DIAGNOSIS AND EVALUATION

- Culture of abscess, blood, cerebrospinal fluid (CSF), pharyngeal swab, pleural fluid, pus, urine
- Rapid antigen test done on pharyngeal swab (~80% sensitive)
- Antistreptolysin O (ASO) and anti-DNAse B are antibodies produced after GAS infection
  - Most useful in assessing for rheumatic fever because elevation of either one is a minor criterion in diagnosis
- *Arcanobacterium haemolyticum* may present similarly to GAS pharyngitis (tonsillar exudates, mild fever, cervical adenopathy, possible scarlatiniform rash), can be isolated on throat culture, and may be treated similarly

TREATMENT

- Uniformly susceptible to penicillins
  - Inpatient: penicillin G, ampicillin, clindamycin
  - Outpatient: penicillin VK, amoxicillin, clindamycin
- Treatment of GAS infections is important to prevent progression to acute rheumatic fever

Staphylococcus aureus

BASIC INFORMATION

- Gram-positive cocci in clusters
- Methicillin-sensitive *S. aureus* (MSSA) versus methicillin-resistant *S. aureus* (MRSA)
- Most common pathogen isolated in children in the United States responsible for:
  - Superficial and invasive infections
  - Most common cause of septic arthritis
  - Frequent cause of pneumonia after influenza infection
  - Major nosocomial pathogen
  - Toxin mediated disease
- Colonizes human skin, nails, pharynx, perineum, vagina
- Risk factors
  - Atopic dermatitis
  - Intravenous (IV) drug abusers
  - Indwelling catheters
  - Health care personnel
- Methicillin resistance increasing in the community (up to 50% colonization)

CLINICAL PRESENTATION

- Table 44.2 shows clinical manifestations of various staphylococcal infections
- Toxic shock syndrome
  - Mediated by toxic shock syndrome toxin-1 (TSST-1)
  - Association with high-absorbency tampons
  - Criteria:
    - Fever >38.9°C
    - Diffuse macular erythroderma
    - Desquamation 1 to 2 weeks after onset of symptoms
    - Hypotension
    - Multisystem involvement: three or more of the following
      1. Gastrointestinal (GI): vomiting or diarrhea at onset of illness
      2. Muscular: myalgias or creatine phosphokinase (CPK) level $\geq 2\times$ upper limit of normal

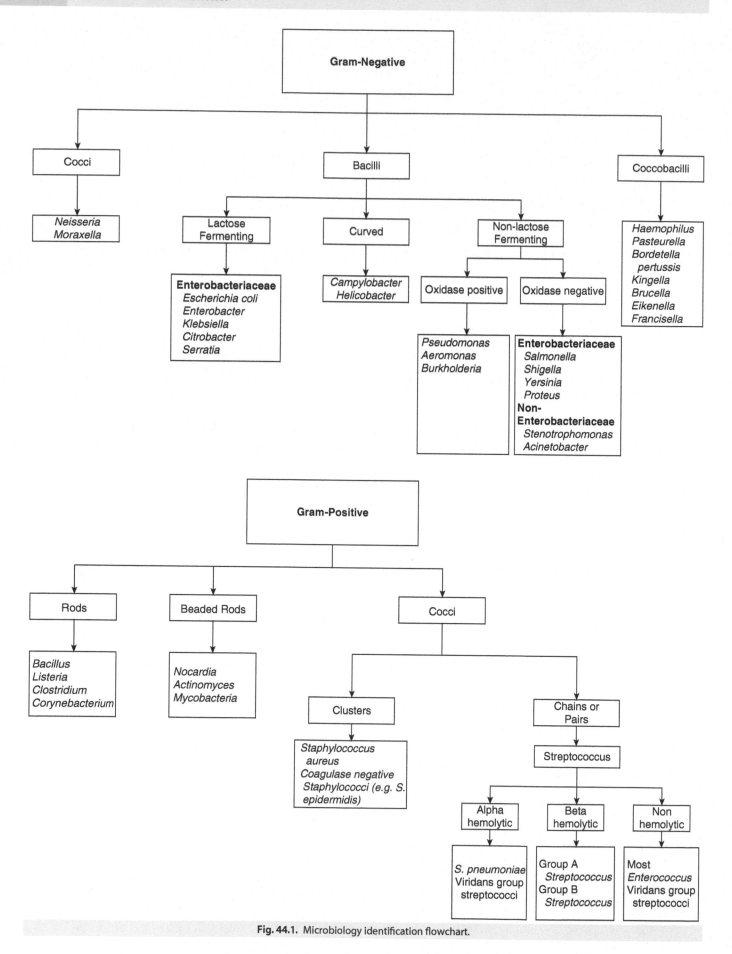

Fig. 44.1. Microbiology identification flowchart.

Table 44.1. Clinical Manifestations of *Streptococcus pyogenes*

Organ System	Clinical Syndrome
Head and neck	▪ Cervical lymphadenitis ▪ Mastoiditis ▪ Otitis media ▪ Peritonsillar/retropharyngeal abscess ▪ Pharyngitis ▪ Sinusitis
Musculoskeletal	▪ Fasciitis ▪ Myositis ▪ Osteomyelitis ▪ Septic arthritis
Pulmonary	▪ Pneumonia ▪ Empyema
Skin and soft tissue	▪ Blistering distal dactylitis ▪ Cellulitis ▪ Erysipelas ▪ Perianal cellulitis ▪ Vaginitis
Systemic	▪ Sepsis ▪ Toxic shock syndrome
Nonsuppurative complications	▪ Acute rheumatic fever ▪ Pediatric autoimmune neuropsychiatric disorder ▪ Sydenham chorea ▪ Post-streptococcal arthritis ▪ Post-streptococcal glomerulonephritis

Table 44.2. Clinical Manifestations of *Staphylococcus aureus*

Skin and soft tissue infection	▪ Abscess, cellulitis, impetigo, mastitis, paronychia, pustulosis, wound infection ▪ Ocular infection ▪ Purulent conjunctivitis, endophthalmitis, orbital/periorbital cellulitis
Musculoskeletal infection	▪ Diskitis, osteomyelitis, pyomyositis, septic arthritis ▪ Major cause of hematogenous osteomyelitis ▪ Diskitis in children <5 years old
Upper respiratory tract infection	▪ Lymphadenitis, nasolacrimal duct abscess, suppurative parotitis, peritonsillar abscess, retropharyngeal abscess, tracheitis
Lower respiratory tract infection	▪ Lung abscess, pneumonia ▪ Increased incidence of pneumonia after influenza infection
Cardiovascular infection	▪ Bacteremia, endocarditis, pericarditis, sepsis, septic thrombophlebitis ▪ Most common cause of infective endocarditis across all age groups
Central nervous system infection	▪ Brain abscess, meningitis ▪ Direct extension of adjacent focus (i.e., sinusitis) ▪ Postsurgical ▪ Seeding of the brain during bacteremia ▪ Spinal abscess
Device-related infection	▪ Central line–associated bloodstream infection ▪ Exit-site catheter infection ▪ CSF shunt infection
Toxin-mediated disease	▪ Staphylococcal scalded skin syndrome ▪ Toxic shock syndrome ▪ Food poisoning

3. Mucous membrane: vaginal, oropharyngeal, conjunctival hyperemia
4. Renal: blood urea nitrogen (BUN) or creatinine ≥2× upper limit of normal, urinary sediment with pyuria without urinary tract infection (UTI)
5. Hepatic: total bilirubin, serum glutamic oxaloacetic transaminase (SGOT), aspartate aminotransferase (AST), or alanine transaminase (ALT) ≥2× upper limit of normal
6. Hematologic: platelets < $100,000/mm^3$
7. Central nervous system (CNS): disorientation or alteration in consciousness without focal signs
▪ Negative results for:
1. Blood, throat, CSF cultures
2. *Rickettsia*, *Leptospira*, or rubeola titers

DIAGNOSIS AND EVALUATION

▪ Culture or polymerase chain reaction (PCR) from affected site
 ▪ Abscess/wound site, blood, bone, CSF, pleural fluid, pus, synovial fluid

TREATMENT

▪ *Staphylococcus aureus* (MSSA or MRSA) is always resistant to penicillin, ampicillin, and amoxicillin
▪ Minor superficial infections
 ▪ Topical 2% mupirocin
▪ Empiric therapy for skin and soft tissue infection
 ▪ Cefazolin, cephalexin, clindamycin, doxycycline, trimethoprim (TMP)/sulfamethoxazole (SMX)
  ▪ Clindamycin resistance is emerging, with about 20% to 25% resistance for both MSSA and MRSA
 ▪ Vancomycin reserved for severe disease or known resistance
▪ Empiric therapy for invasive infections
 ▪ Vancomycin ± oxacillin or nafcillin
▪ Definitive therapy
 ▪ Treatment based on susceptibilities
  ▪ MSSA
   IV: nafcillin or oxacillin, cefazolin
   Oral: cephalexin
  ▪ MRSA
   IV: vancomycin
   Oral: clindamycin, TMP/SMX, doxycycline
 ▪ Other options include linezolid, daptomycin, quinupristin-dalfopristin
 ▪ Aminoglycosides synergistic with beta-lactam antibacterials, but are not sufficient for monotherapy

Coagulase Negative Staphylococcus

BASIC INFORMATION

▪ Gram-positive cocci in clusters
▪ Normal skin flora
▪ Most common species: *S. epidermidis*, *S. hominis*, *S. capitis*, *S. warneri*, *S. saprophyticus*, *S. lugdunensis*

- Common cause of bacteremia in patients in the intensive care unit (ICU) and patients that are immunocompromised because of cancer or transplantation
- Disruption of skin barrier leads to infection
  - Surgery, catheter placement, insertion of a prosthesis
- No toxin production leads to indolent course of infection
- Produces biofilms

CLINICAL PRESENTATION

- Bacteremia and catheter-associated bloodstream infection
  - Most common contaminants in blood cultures so true infection is unlikely in an otherwise healthy host with no risk factors and that is otherwise well-appearing
  - If systemic signs are present, true infection likely
  - If subtle signs, then would get repeated blood cultures; two positive cultures for the same pathogen indicate likely infection
- Neonatal sepsis
  - Most frequent cause of late-onset sepsis in very low birth weight infants
    - Likely caused by central catheter contamination
- Necrotizing enterocolitis and neonatal focal intestinal perforation
- Endocarditis
- CSF shunt infection and meningitis
- Peritonitis associated with a peritoneal dialysis catheter
  - Most common bacterial pathogen (40%)
- UTI
  - Adolescent and young adult females
  - *S. saprophyticus*

DIAGNOSIS AND EVALUATION

- Culture of blood, abscess, CSF, pus, urine

TREATMENT

- Intrinsic resistance to penicillin, methicillin, and gentamicin
- Empiric therapy: vancomycin
- Other options include daptomycin and linezolid
- Treatment based on susceptibilities

Streptococcus agalactiae, GBS

BASIC INFORMATION

- Also called Group B Streptococcus (GBS)
- Gram-positive cocci in pairs and chains
- Colonizes maternal genital and lower GI tract; mothers are rarely symptomatic
- Neonates become colonized vertically
  - Ascending infection in utero or at delivery
- Maternal GBS screening and prophylaxis has significantly decreased early-onset disease, but late-onset disease rates are unchanged
  - Up to 50% of neonates born to GBS(+) mothers, but only ~1% will develop invasive disease

CLINICAL PRESENTATION

- Early-onset disease (<7 days, usually within 24 hours)
  - Apnea, bradycardia, fever, irritability, lethargy, respiratory distress
  - Commonly present with bacteremia, sepsis, and/or pneumonia; meningitis uncommon (~10%)
- Late-onset disease (7–89 days)
  - Fever, irritability, poor feeding
  - Commonly present with bacteremia and meningitis; also may have arthritis and/or osteomyelitis
- Very late onset disease (≥3 months)
  - Bacteremia

DIAGNOSIS AND EVALUATION

- Culture of abscess, blood, CSF, pus, urine
- CSF profile with elevated white blood cells (WBCs), low glucose, and elevated protein
- Antigen testing done rarely in CSF or serum
- Screening testing via nucleic acid amplification test (NAAT)/(PCR)
- Maternal testing
  - Rectal and vaginal swabs at 35 to 37 weeks

TREATMENT

- Therapy
  - Empiric: ampicillin and gentamicin
  - Definitive: penicillin G or ampicillin
- Intrapartum prophylaxis
  - Indications
    - Positive GBS screening culture in late pregnancy
    - GBS bacteriuria at any time during the pregnancy
    - Previous infant with GBS disease
    - Unknown GBS status at onset of labor *plus* one of the following:
      - <37 weeks' gestational age
      - Rupture of membranes ≥18 hours
      - Intrapartum temperature ≥38°C
      - GBS NAAT positive
  - Prophylaxis regimens
    - Must be given four or more hours before delivery
    - Penicillin G or ampicillin IV
    - Penicillin allergic without anaphylaxis: cefazolin
    - Penicillin allergic with anaphylaxis: clindamycin
      - Assuming isolate is clindamycin susceptible

Streptococcus pneumoniae

BASIC INFORMATION

- Gram-positive cocci
- Alpha hemolytic
- Polysaccharide capsule defines serogroup and provides protection from host defenses
- Transmitted by respiratory droplet
- Colonizes nasopharynx in healthy children
- Most children acquire disease in the first 2 years of life with peak at 6 to 12 months

- Leading bacterial cause of community-acquired pneumonia, acute otitis media, sinusitis, and meningitis
- Vaccination
  - Conjugate vaccine (PCV)
    - Immunogenic at 2 months of age, induces memory production, and reduces nasal carriage
    - Initial vaccine with 7 strains, current vaccine with 13 strains
    - US standard is a 4-dose series at 2, 4, 6, and 12 to 15 months
  - Polysaccharide vaccine (PPV)
    - Immunogenic in children >5 years and healthy adults, but minimal efficacy in children <2 years
    - Given to patients at high risk of invasive disease at 2 years of age, and again 5 years later for two lifetime doses:
      - Immunocompromised patients, sickle cell disease, asplenia, cochlear implants, CSF leaks, diabetes mellitus, chronic heart disease, chronic lung disease

CLINICAL PRESENTATION

- Acute otitis media
- Conjunctivitis
- Community-acquired pneumonia
  - Infants and young children
    - Fever, respiratory symptoms, ± cough, vomiting, abdominal distension
    - Scattered consolidations
  - Older children
    - Prodrome of viral upper respiratory infection, then acute-onset fever, chills, chest pain, shortness of breath
    - Lobar consolidation
  - Complications include abscess, effusion, empyema, and necrosis
- Meningitis
  - Classic triad: fever, neck stiffness, altered mental status
  - Infants
    - Bulging fontanelle, irritability, poor feeding, seizures, vomiting
  - Children
    - Focal neurologic deficit, drowsiness, headache, neck stiffness, vomiting
- Musculoskeletal (MSK) infections
  - Pyogenic arthritis
  - Osteomyelitis
- Sinusitis
- Soft tissue infection
  - Buccal and periorbital cellulitis
  - Erysipelas

DIAGNOSIS AND EVALUATION

- Culture of abscess, blood, CSF, pleural fluid, pus, urine
- PCR of blood, CSF, and pleural fluid
- CSF profile with elevated WBC (neutrophil predominance), low glucose, and elevated protein
- Urine antigen tests not useful

TREATMENT

- Acute otitis media and pneumonia
  - Outpatient
    - Drug of choice: high-dose amoxicillin (80–90 mg/kg/day)
    - Alternatives: amoxicillin/clavulanate, cefuroxime, cefdinir, ceftriaxone
    - Penicillin allergy: clindamycin, azithromycin
  - Inpatient
    - Drug of choice: high-dose ampicillin (200 mg/kg/day)
    - Alternatives: ceftriaxone, cefotaxime
    - Penicillin allergy: clindamycin
- Meningitis
  - Empiric therapy: vancomycin + ceftriaxone
  - Definitive therapy guided by susceptibilities
  - Dexamethasone can be given before or with antibiotics for infants and children >6 weeks old with possible pneumococcal meningitis

Enterococcus

BASIC INFORMATION

- Anaerobic gram-positive cocci
- Lives in the GI tract
- Presents as bacteremia, intra-abdominal infection, UTI
- May be found on blood culture, urine culture, wound culture
- Treatment based on susceptibilities of the organism
  - Ampicillin, vancomycin, daptomycin, linezolid are common agents to treat *Enterococcus*
  - *Enterococcus* is intrinsically resistant to cephalosporins (therefore cephalosporins provided for treatment of presumed UTI will not treat enterococcal UTI)

HIGH-YIELD GRAM-NEGATIVE RODS

Pseudomonas aeruginosa

BASIC INFORMATION

- Gram-negative bacilli
- Ubiquitous in nature including soil and water
- Opportunistic pathogen
  - Causes infection in patients with underlying or immunocompromised conditions
  - Also a major cause of health care–associated infections
- Risk factors
  - Immune suppression, neutropenia
  - Cystic fibrosis
  - Burn patients

CLINICAL PRESENTATION

- Community-acquired infections
  - Keratitis: contact lenses
  - Otitis externa: swimmer's ear

- Endocarditis: IV drug abuse
- Osteomyelitis: puncture wound of foot
- Folliculitis: hot tub folliculitis
- Nosocomial infections
  - Central line–associated bloodstream infection
  - Ventilator–associated pneumonia
  - UTI
  - Surgical site infection
- Special populations
  - Immunocompromised/neutropenia
    - Sepsis
    - Central line–associated bloodstream infection
    - Ecthyma gangrenosum: erythematous, tender lesions with central necrosis
  - Burn patients
  - Cystic fibrosis
    - Pneumonia
    - Chronic inflammation

DIAGNOSIS AND EVALUATION

- Culture of any bodily fluid including blood, CSF, wound drainage, abscess, sputum, tissue, urine
- PCR of blood and CSF

TREATMENT

- Treatment guided by susceptibilities
- Increasing resistance rates dictate definitive therapy
- Anti-pseudomonal agents include:
  - Ceftazidime, cefepime, ceftazidime/avibactam, piperacillin/tazobactam, meropenem, imipenem, ciprofloxacin, levofloxacin, gentamicin, amikacin, colistin, polymyxin B
- Empiric therapy: cefepime or piperacillin/tazobactam
- Fever and neutropenia empiric therapy: ceftazidime, cefepime or piperacillin/tazobactam

Escherichia coli

BASIC INFORMATION

- Gram-negative bacilli
- Lives in the GI tract
- Enterohemorrhagic (EHEC): shiga-toxin producing, causative agent of hemolytic-uremic syndrome (HUS)
- Enterotoxigenic (ETEC): traveler's diarrhea
- Enteropathogenic (EPEC): gastroenteritis

CLINICAL PRESENTATION

- Bacteremia, acute gastroenteritis, meningitis, UTIs
- Careful evaluation for development of HUS
  - Bloody diarrhea, thrombocytopenia, anemia, abnormal renal function
  - See Chapter 36 for details

DIAGNOSIS AND EVALUATION

- Culture of blood, CSF, stool, or urine
- PCR testing of CSF and stool

TREATMENT

- GI disease is self-limited and should not be treated, especially if diagnosed with HUS
- Otherwise, treatment of other illnesses is based on susceptibilities
- Empiric therapy with penicillins, cephalosporins, TMP/SMX, quinolones

Haemophilus influenzae

BASIC INFORMATION

- Gram-negative, encapsulated coccobacilli
- Multiple types designated by their capsules, A through F, and nontypeable
- Colonizes the upper respiratory tract
- *H. influenzae* type B (HIB) was previously the leading cause of meningitis until the vaccine was developed
- Transmitted by droplets or contact with respiratory secretions

CLINICAL PRESENTATION

- May present as buccal cellulitis, purulent conjunctivitis, epiglottitis, meningitis, acute otitis media, pneumonia, pyogenic arthritis, sepsis, sinusitis

DIAGNOSIS AND EVALUATION

- Culture or PCR of blood, CSF, respiratory sample, urine

TREATMENT

- Treatment based on susceptibilities
- Empiric therapy with ampicillin/sulbactam, amoxicillin/clavulanate, ceftriaxone, fluoroquinolones; resistant to first-generation cephalosporins
- HIB chemoprophylaxis (i.e., rifampin) should be given to certain contacts:
  - If a household has children <4 years old who are not fully vaccinated or anyone who is immunocompromised, then all household members should receive chemoprophylaxis
  - If there are ≥2 cases of invasive HIB disease within 60 days at a child care facility that also has unimmunized or underimmunized children in attendance, then all attendees and providers should receive chemoprophylaxis, regardless of age or vaccine status

COMMON GASTROINTESTINAL INFECTIONS

Campylobacter Species

BASIC INFORMATION

- Gram-negative curved bacillus
- Common cause of bacterial gastroenteritis and traveler's diarrhea (the most common cause in developed countries)

- Transmitted via contaminated food such as undercooked poultry and meat, unpasteurized dairy such as milk and cheese, and contaminated water

CLINICAL PRESENTATION

- Acute onset within 24 to 48 hours
- Generalized malaise, fever, bloody stools, tenesmus, abdominal cramps
- Extraintestinal manifestations can occur such as bacteremia, meningitis, and septic arthritis
- Immune-mediated complications: Guillain–Barre syndrome, reactive arthritis, erythema nodosum

DIAGNOSIS AND EVALUATION

- Stool culture or PCR testing

TREATMENT

- Supportive care recommended
- Treatment only for those with severe symptoms or immunocompromised
  - Drug of choice: erythromycin or azithromycin

Salmonella Species

BASIC INFORMATION

- Gram-negative bacilli
- Common cause of gastroenteritis, bacteremia, and focal infections including brain abscess, meningitis, and osteomyelitis
  - Most common cause of foodborne outbreaks
- ~100 serotypes that infect humans
- Most common species
  - Nontyphoidal
    - *S. typhimurium*, *S. enteritidis*
    - Main symptom is gastroenteritis
    - One-third of cases in children <4 years of age
    - Worldwide distribution
      Increased incidence in developing countries in which food and water contamination is high
    - Reservoirs: birds, mammals, reptiles
      Animals: chicken, turkey, duck, sheep, cow, pig
      Pets: turtle, snake, lizard, iguana, chick, duckling, hedgehog
    - Foodborne
      Fresh or thawed poultry (beef, pork)
      Raw or undercooked eggs (Caesar salad, eggnog)
    - Incubation period short, 12 to 36 hours
  - Typhoidal
    - *S. typhi*, *S. paratyphi* A/B/C
    - Causes of typhoid and paratyphoid fever
    - 27 million illnesses and 600,000 deaths annually
    - Distribution in Southcentral and Southeast Asia, and southern Africa
    - US cases are mostly in travelers to endemic areas, especially India
    - Humans are reservoirs

- Transmission via ingestion of contaminated food or water from a chronic carrier or acutely infected person
- Incubation period long, 7 to 14 days
- Risk factors
  - Sickle cell anemia
  - Inflammatory bowel disease
  - Chronic granulomatous disease
  - Immunodeficiency including chemotherapy, organ transplantation, and HIV

CLINICAL PRESENTATION

- See Table 44.3

DIAGNOSIS AND EVALUATION

- Fecal WBCs often present
- Culture of blood, bone marrow, CSF, pus, stool, tissue
  - If suspicion for typhoid fever, blood cultures may yield evidence of bacteremia
  - Multidrug resistance common; therefore susceptibilities important
- PCR of blood and stool
- Infants <3 months old with positive stool cultures warrant further evaluation for bacteremia (i.e., blood culture); if blood cultures are positive, consider evaluation for CNS involvement (i.e., lumbar puncture [LP]) or Musculoskeletal (MSK) complications

Table 44.3. Clinical Manifestations of *Salmonella* Infection

Nontyphoidal **Salmonella species** *S. enteritidis* *S. typhimurium*	Gastroenteritis - Nausea, vomiting, crampy abdominal pain - Diarrhea with water, blood, and/or mucus - Fever - Toxic megacolon and systemic toxicity can occur Bacteremia - 1% to 5% of cases, less common compared to typhoidal disease Extraintestinal focal infection - Osteomyelitis and septic arthritis - Meningitis - Rare: empyema, pneumonia, UTI - Occurs at preexisting anatomic abnormalities - Higher incidence in infants <2 months of age Asymptomatic infection - Prolonged shedding in children <5 years old - Median length: 7 weeks - Convalescent (≤1 year) and chronic (>1 year) carriage is caused by asymptomatic biliary tract disease ("typhoid Mary")
Typhoidal **Salmonella species** *S. typhi* *S. paratyphi*	Enteric fever - Increasing fever that becomes unremitting - Anorexia, headache, lethargy, malaise; seizures may be seen - Abdominal pain, hepatosplenomegaly - Intestinal hemorrhage and intestinal perforation are amongst the most feared complications - Dactylitis - Rose spots usually seen on chest and abdomen Asymptomatic infection - See previous section

UTI, Urinary tract infection.

TREATMENT

- Rapid rehydration may be necessary if there are excessive fluid losses
- Therapy not recommended for uncomplicated gastroenteritis
- Therapy is recommended for bacteremia, enteric fever, focal infections, immunocompromised patients (HIV, sickle cell disease, cancer), or infections in infants <3 months of age
- Empiric therapy: third-generation cephalosporin (i.e., ceftriaxone)
- Treatment based on susceptibilities
  - Options include ampicillin/amoxicillin, azithromycin, TMP/SMX; third-generation cephalosporin may be warranted in severe cases in which parental therapy is indicated
  - Fever can persist for 5 to 7 days despite appropriate therapy
  - Antibacterial therapy can prolong shedding
- Length of therapy
  - Bacteremia, enteric fever: 10 to 14 days
  - Meningitis: 28 days
  - Osteomyelitis: 4 to 6 weeks
- Prevention: vaccination
  - Travelers to endemic areas
    - 2 to 5 years old
      Injectable typhoid vaccine
      Immunity for 2 years
    - 6+ years old
      Oral typhoid vaccine
      Immunity for 5 years

Shigella Species

BASIC INFORMATION

- Gram-negative bacilli
- Causes gastroenteritis
- ~50 serotypes that infect humans
- Classified by serogroups
  A: *Shigella dysenteriae*
  B: *S. flexneri* (most common in developing countries)
  C: *S. boydii*
  D: *S. sonnei* (most common in the United States)
- Highly contagious (very few bacteria needed to cause disease)
- Highest incidence in children 12 to 36 months old
- US seasonality in late summer and fall
- Developing countries with tropical climates have infection year-round, worse in summer and rainy seasons
- Transmission mostly person to person, some fecal-oral
  - Child care–associated outbreaks common
  - Very hardy organism, can survive on surfaces and in food for up to 30 days
    - Milk, eggs, oysters, shrimp, flour

CLINICAL PRESENTATION

- Fever
- Diarrhea with water, blood, and/or mucus
- Crampy abdominal pain, tenesmus
- *S. dysenteriae* can cause more severe disease
  - Pseudomembranous colitis, toxic megacolon, intestinal obstruction/perforation, appendicitis, and HUS
- Notable for having relatively frequent neurologic manifestations (10%–45%)
  - Seizures, lethargy, confusion, hallucinations, headache
- Less common: conjunctivitis, neonatal infection, reactive arthritis, UTI, vulvovaginitis

DIAGNOSIS AND EVALUATION

- Fecal WBCs often present
- Culture of stool
- PCR of stool

TREATMENT

- Rapid rehydration
- Empiric antibiotics may be required for severe illness, suspected bacteremia, in the immunocompromised host, or those at high risk of transmission through shedding (e.g., workers in day cares or long-term facilities, food handlers)
- Empiric therapy: third-generation cephalosporin (i.e., ceftriaxone)
- Treatment based on susceptibilities
  - Options include ampicillin/amoxicillin, azithromycin, cefixime, fluoroquinolones, TMP/SMX
  - Azithromycin is generally the preferred first-line therapy

Helicobacter pylori

BASIC INFORMATION

- Gram-negative spiral-shaped bacilli
- Lives in the mouth and stomach
- Person-to-person spread, mostly fecal-oral transmission

CLINICAL PRESENTATION

- Mostly asymptomatic in children
- Rarely see gastritis and duodenal ulcer disease in children

DIAGNOSIS AND EVALUATION

- Endoscopy with biopsies staining for *H. pylori*

TREATMENT

- Protein pump inhibitor (PPI) + amoxicillin + metronidazole
- Length of therapy: 3 weeks

Clostridium difficile

BASIC INFORMATION

- Anaerobic, Gram-positive bacillus
- Forms spores, lives in the environment
- Once ingested, colonizes the GI tract

- When gut microbiota becomes disrupted (antibacterials), gastroenteritis or colitis develops
- Once ingested, colonizes the GI tract
- *C. difficile* spores are very resistant to heat and cleaning products and can survive on surfaces for long periods of time; they are also resistant to alcohol-based hand-sanitizing liquids

CLINICAL PRESENTATION

- Asymptomatic colonization
- Diarrhea, fever, abdominal pain, bloody diarrhea
- Pseudomembranous colitis, toxic megacolon

DIAGNOSIS AND EVALUATION

- Two-step testing: enzyme immunoassay (EIA) followed by toxin testing
- PCR testing
- Endoscopy showing mucosal plaques and/or pseudomembranes

TREATMENT

- Discontinue the precipitating antibacterial agent
- First line: metronidazole enterally for 10 to 14 days
- Second line: vancomycin enterally for 10 to 14 days
- Other options: fidaxomicin, fecal transplant
- For severe disease including toxic megacolon, IV metronidazole is indicated with the consideration of vancomycin given either enterally or as an enema

ATYPICAL RESPIRATORY INFECTIONS

Mycoplasma pneumoniae

BASIC INFORMATION

- Pleomorphic bacteria without a cell wall; therefore not able to perform traditional Gram staining
- Transmitted via aerosolized droplets
- Causes include community-acquired pneumonia in children >5 years of age
  - Primarily a disease of adolescents and young adults

CLINICAL PRESENTATION

- Pulmonary disease
  - Young children
    - Rhinorrhea, pharyngitis, otitis media, croup, bronchiolitis, pneumonia
  - Older children and adolescents
    - Malaise, myalgia, pharyngitis, headache, low-grade fever, sinus pain, ear pain
    - Upper or lower respiratory tract disease "Walking pneumonia"
    - Characteristic course
      - Constitutional symptoms resolve and persistent, intractable nonproductive cough
      - Similar symptoms to pertussis infection
    - Associated with asthma exacerbations
- Extrapulmonary disease
  - Encephalitis/meningoencephalitis
    - Most common extrapulmonary site
  - Arthritis
  - Bell's palsy
  - Erythema multiforme
  - Pericarditis
  - Hemolytic anemia

DIAGNOSIS AND EVALUATION

- Chest radiography may demonstrate variable findings:
  - Bilateral interstitial infiltrates
  - Unilateral, segmental consolidations
  - Pleural effusion
  - Hilar adenopathy
- Organism is difficult to culture
- Serology (IgM and IgG)
  - Acute and convalescent titers showing a fourfold or greater rise in titer indicate recent infection
- PCR is more sensitive/specific and can be sent from CSF, nasal swab, nasopharyngeal swab, throat swab, sputum
- Cold agglutinins are neither sensitive nor specific for mycoplasma

TREATMENT

- Role of antibacterials is uncertain, best given in the first 3 to 4 days of illness
- Cell wall active agents do not work because mycoplasma lacks a cell wall
- Drugs of choice: azithromycin, clarithromycin, erythromycin

Chlamydia/Chlamydophila pneumoniae

BASIC INFORMATION

- Gram-negative obligate intracellular coccobacilli
- Presentation: atypical pneumonia with persistent cough in school-aged children or young adults
  - Unlike usual causes of bacterial pneumonia, associated with laryngitis and loss of voice
  - May also present with extrapulmonary manifestations (e.g., meningoencephalitis, arthritis, myocarditis)
- Diagnosis: serology (IgM and IgG); culture or PCR of respiratory specimen, blood, or tissue
- Treatment: tetracyclines (tetracycline/doxycycline) or macrolides (azithromycin/clarithromycin)

Bordetella pertussis

BASIC INFORMATION

- Gram-negative coccobacilli
- 15 million cases of pertussis annually in the world
- Highest age-related risk are infants <2 months of age
- Transmission by airborne droplets, highly contagious

CLINICAL PRESENTATION

- Three stages
  - Catarrhal
    - Rhinorrhea, sneezing, fever
    - Cough starts
  - Paroxysmal
    - Classic "whooping" cough with paroxysms
    - Apnea, gasping, choking
    - Post-tussive emesis
  - Convalescent
    - Cough persists
    - Malnutrition
- Young infants may present with apnea, general respiratory distress, and/or seizures, but not necessarily paroxysmal coughing

DIAGNOSIS AND EVALUATION

- Marked leukocytosis with lymphocytosis (absolute lymphocyte count [ALC] often higher than 9,400) in serum during late catarrhal and paroxysmal stages
- Culture or PCR of deep nasopharyngeal aspirate, nasal wash, flexible swab in posterior pharynx
  - PCR is method of choice
- Serology (IgG)
- Chest radiography
  - Perihilar infiltrates
  - Consolidation
  - Pneumothorax and pneumomediastinum
- Evaluate for complications
  - Apnea
  - Secondary bacterial infections (pneumonia, otitis media)
  - Respiratory failure (apnea, pneumonia, pulmonary hypertension)
  - Sequelae of forceful coughing (eyelid petechiae, scleral hemorrhage, muscle soreness)

TREATMENT

- All infants <12 months of age should be treated if diagnosed within *6 weeks* of cough
- All children >1 year of age should be treated if diagnosed within *21 days* of cough
- Drugs of choice: azithromycin, clarithromycin, erythromycin
- All household contacts should be given postexposure prophylaxis, regardless of age or immunization status
- Ensure vaccination is up to date
  - Standard five dose series of DTaP in children 6 weeks to 6 years old
  - Single dose of Tdap in children 11 to 12 years old
  - Pregnant women during pregnancy or immediately postpartum

Corynebacterium diphtheriae

BASIC INFORMATION

- Aerobic, Gram-positive bacilli
- Produces the toxin that causes diphtheria

- Ubiquitous in nature
- Spread via droplet or direct contact with secretions
- Cutaneous lesions can also spread disease
- Endemic in certain parts of the world, all US disease is imported
- Vaccination has dramatically decreased overall disease burden

CLINICAL PRESENTATION

- Pharyngeal injection and edema
- Unilateral or bilateral tonsillar membrane formation
  - "Leatherlike" pseudomembrane that firmly adheres to underlying tissue; removal will result in bleeding
  - Severe respiratory involvement may result, with extensive neck swelling and upper airway obstruction
- Cutaneous disease: superficial ulceration with graybrown membrane
- Exotoxin manifestations may cause systemic complications: myocarditis, renal tubular necrosis, peripheral neuropathy

DIAGNOSIS AND EVALUATION

- Culture of ulceration or membrane
- PCR can be done at the Centers for Disease Control and Prevention (CDC)

TREATMENT

- Equine diphtheria antitoxin (dose determined by membrane characteristics and illness course) in addition to erythromycin or penicillin for 14 days
- Exposure prophylaxis:
  - All exposed persons should receive the vaccine, regardless of immune status
  - Close contacts of affected patients should receive chemoprophylaxis (e.g., penicillin G, erythromycin)
  - All exposed persons should have pharyngeal cultures and have close follow-up for development of symptoms
    - Pharyngeal carriers should be treated

SEXUALLY TRANSMITTED INFECTIONS

Chlamydia trachomatis

BASIC INFORMATION

- Gram-negative obligate intracellular coccobacilli
- One of the leading causes of pelvic inflammatory disease (PID) in the United States (the most common reportable sexually transmitted infection [STI] in the United States); see Chapter 92 for additional details for chlamydial STI/PID/lymphogranuloma venereum (LGV)
- One of the leading causes of blindness in the world

CLINICAL PRESENTATION

- Divided into several "serovars" capable of causing distinct infections:
  - Trachoma serovars:
    - Chronic follicular conjunctivitis followed by corneal ulceration and blindness
    - Spreads through contact with secretions from infected eyes or eye-seeking flies
    - Does not cause STI or other oculogenital infections
  - Oculogenital serovars:
    - Adult conjunctivitis or pharyngitis
    - Neonatal conjunctivitis: purulent eye discharge usually within the first 2 weeks after delivery (but should be suspected for all infants <30 days old)
    - Pneumonia in infancy: insidious onset of cough (classically: "staccato," nonproductive) with bilateral interstitial infiltrates and hyperinflation at 3 to 12 weeks of life (but should be considered up to 4 months old); ~50% will have had neonatal conjunctivitis
    - STI: most patients asymptomatic, rarely causes discharge and dysuria; also causes epididymitis/proctitis in men
    - Association with Reiter syndrome
  - LGV serovars:
    - Asymptomatic genital papule or ulcer progressing to unilateral acute lymphadenitis with bubo formation

DIAGNOSIS AND EVALUATION

- Culture
- NAAT
  - Conjunctiva, nasopharynx of infants
  - Cervical swab, urethral swab, urine
    - For urine, generally prefer first 20 to 30 mL, not clean catch

TREATMENT

- Trachoma: azithromycin as a single dose
- Neonatal conjunctivitis: azithromycin for 3 days or erythromycin for 14 days (topical antibiotics are insufficient for treatment, and antibiotic topical prophylaxis at birth will not prevent perinatal transmission)
- Pneumonia in infancy: azithromycin for 3 days or erythromycin for 14 days
- STI: azithromycin as a single dose or doxycycline for 7 days (if >8 years old)
  - Of note, all patients with gonorrhea should also be treated for chlamydia
  - Patients should abstain from sexual intercourse for 1 week
  - Screening guidelines covered in Chapter 92; also pregnant women are screened at their first visit as well as in the third trimester if <25 years old; test of cure is recommended for pregnant women
- LGV: doxycycline or erythromycin for 21 days

Neisseria gonorrhoeae

BASIC INFORMATION

- Gram-negative diplococci
- A leading cause of STI
  - Ocular, pharynx, urethra, cervix, rectum
- See Chapter 92 for additional details

CLINICAL PRESENTATION

- Perinatal infections
  - Scalp abscess
  - Ophthalmia neonatorum: bilateral purulent discharge 2 to 5 days after birth (treatment is required to avoid corneal ulceration and globe rupture; all newborns are provided with ophthalmic antibiotics at birth because silver nitrate is insufficient)
  - Disseminated disease: pyogenic arthritis with pseudoparalysis
- Child and adolescent infections
  - Genital tract infection (e.g., urethritis, cervicitis, PID)
  - Pharyngitis: the majority of patients are asymptomatic, but may present with sore throat, fever, and cervical adenopathy; will not be diagnosed on group A strep culture
  - Disseminated disease:
    - Tenosynovitis-dermatitis: fever chills, rash (painful hemorrhagic or vesiculopapular lesions on palmar and plantar surfaces, which may contain gonococci) and polyarthralgia (especially of the fingers)
    - Suppurative arthritis: monoarticular arthritis
    - Less common manifestations include carditis, meningitis

DIAGNOSIS AND EVALUATION

- Culture
- NAAT

TREATMENT

- Increasing rates of antibiotic resistance (e.g., fluoroquinolones, oral third-generation cephalosporins); cefixime is also declining in efficacy
- Perinatal infections
  - Cefotaxime or ceftriaxone
- STIs
  - Ceftriaxone plus azithromycin/doxycycline (must treat for chlamydia)

Treponema pallidum (Syphilis)

BASIC INFORMATION

- Spiral-shaped bacilli (spirochete)
- Invades host through cutaneous abrasions or mucous membranes
- Transmission
  - Sexual contact (including oral sex)
  - Vertical transmission from mother to child
- See Chapter 92 for additional details

CLINICAL PRESENTATION

- Three classic stages
  - Primary syphilis
    - Incubation period 1 to 4 weeks
    - Occurs in ~30% of patients
    - Development of a chancre: a single, painless papule with red base that erodes to form an ulcer
    - Reactive lymphadenopathy often present
    - Resolves in 3 to 6 weeks without treatment
  - Secondary syphilis
    - Incubation period 6 to 12 weeks
    - Rash
      - Palms, soles, trunk
      - Mucous membranes
        - Condyloma lata, flat wart-like papules in genital area
        - Mucous patches on tongue
    - Painless generalized lymphadenopathy
    - CNS disease can occur
    - Systemic symptoms including fever and malaise
    - Resolves in 3 to 12 weeks without treatment
  - Tertiary syphilis
    - Occurs in 30% of patients that are untreated
    - Neurosyphilis
      - Incubation period 2 months to 30 years
      - Cranial nerve palsies, sensorineural deafness, hydrocephalus, stroke, mental status changes
      - Argyll Robertson pupil (reacts to accommodation and not light)
      - Tabes dorsalis (demyelination of spinal cord)
    - Cardiovascular syphilis
      - Incubation period 10 to 40 years
      - Aneurysms, aortic root dilation, coronary artery disease
    - Late benign syphilis (gummas)
      - Benign lesions in skin and bone that can be destructive and cause scarring
- Congenital syphilis
  - Untreated maternal primary or secondary syphilis results in 60% to 90% transmission rate
  - Transmission transplacental with dissemination to bloodstream
  - Early disease (<2 years old)
    - Stillbirth or premature birth
    - Bone lesions
      - Periostitis and osteitis of long bones
      - Pseudoparalysis of affected extremity
    - Generalized lymphadenopathy
    - Hepatosplenomegaly
    - Nasal discharge "snuffles"
    - Pneumonia
    - Rash
      - Desquamation involving palms and soles
      - Petechiae
  - Late disease (>2 years old)
    - Bone lesions
      - Frontal bossing, saddle nose, saber shins
    - Dental lesions
      - Hutchinson peg-shaped teeth, notched central incisors
    - Skin lesions
      - Rhagades (linear scars at angle of mouth and nose)

DIAGNOSIS AND EVALUATION

- Serology is gold standard: treponemal and nontreponemal
- Traditional algorithm is nontreponemal test followed by confirmation with treponemal, but a reverse method is used in some locations
- Nontreponemal (screening tests)
  - Rapid plasma reagin (RPR), Venereal Diseases Research Laboratory (VDRL) test
  - Detects antibodies against substances released by the bacteria about 4 to 8 weeks after primary infection
  - Monitors disease progress
  - False positives common: autoimmune diseases, rickettsial infection, other treponemal infections
  - Reported out in dilutions
    - Fourfold change is considered significant in either direction
    - Example: 1:4 is fourfold lower than 1:16
- Treponemal (confirmatory tests)
  - Fluorescent treponemal antibody-absorbed test (FTA-ABS), microhemagglutination test for *T. pallidum* (MHA-TP), *T. pallidum particle* agglutination test (TP-PA)
  - Detects antibodies to the bacteria itself
  - Once positive, stays positive for life
  - Cannot use this test for monitoring of infection
- Testing algorithm
  - Congenital syphilis
    - If maternal testing positive for both nontreponemal and treponemal testing, then infant needs evaluation under certain circumstances
    - Please refer to the *Red Book* for testing algorithm under topic heading Syphilis
    - Common evaluation for congenital syphilis includes:
      - Physical examination
      - Serum RPR
      - Blood counts, liver function tests
      - Head ultrasound
      - Radiograph of long bones
      - Hearing screen
      - CSF evaluation including VDRL
  - Acquired syphilis
    - Serum RPR
      - If positive, a treponemal test should be used for confirmation
    - CSF VDRL
      - If concerned about CNS disease

TREATMENT

- Primary, secondary, early latent disease: benzathine penicillin G ×1 dose
- Late latent disease: benzathine penicillin G weekly ×3
- Neurosyphilis: aqueous penicillin G ×10 to 14 days
- Congenital infection: aqueous penicillin G ×10 days
- Penicillin allergy: tetracycline or doxycycline
- Complication of therapy: Jarisch–Herxheimer reaction

MYCOBACTERIA

Mycobacterium tuberculosis

BASIC INFORMATION

- Acid-fast bacilli
- One-third of the world's population infected with *M. tuberculosis* (TB)
  - Endemic in parts of Africa and Asia
  - Decreasing incidence in United States because of better TB testing and control efforts
  - Frequent coinfection with HIV
- Airborne transmission
- Long incubation period of 3 to 12 weeks
- Bacille Calmette–Guerin (BCG) vaccine is used for protection in endemic countries

CLINICAL PRESENTATION

- Thoracic disease
  - Pulmonary
    - Most children do not develop any symptoms
    - May present with mild fever, cough, dyspnea, failure to thrive
  - Pleural
  - Pericarditis
- Extrathoracic disease
  - Disseminated disease (miliary tuberculosis)
    - Lesions in bone marrow, liver, lung, spleen
    - Anorexia, cough, fever, generalized lymphadenopathy, malaise, weight loss
  - Lymphatic disease (scrofula)
    - Supraclavicular, cervical, submandibular lymph nodes most commonly involved
    - Unilateral, fixed, nontender
  - CNS
    - Meningitis
  - MSK disease
    - Spine (Pott disease)
    - Osteoarthritis, osteomyelitis (knee, hip, elbow, ankle)
  - Abdominal/genitourinary tract
    - Enteritis, peritonitis
    - Renal, male and female genital tracts
  - Cutaneous
    - Caused by direct inoculation, hematogenous seeding, lymph node rupture
  - Congenital
    - Very rare (<400 cases in literature), mother with pelvic TB infects infant
- Latent tuberculosis infection (LTBI)
  - Positive tuberculin skin test (TST) or interferon-γ release assay (IGRA) with no evidence of clinical infection or abnormal chest imaging

DIAGNOSIS AND EVALUATION

- Testing methods
  - Prior BCG vaccination is not a contraindication to tuberculin testing
  - TST

Table 44.4. Interpretation of TST Results by Diameter of Induration

Threshold for "Positive" Test Result	Patient population
Induration ≥5 mm	Close contact with an infected person Suspected active TB infection • Abnormal chest radiograph or abnormal clinical exam • Immune suppression (e.g., HIV infection, organ transplant recipients)
Induration ≥10 mm	Children at increased risk of disseminated disease: • Age ≤4 years of age • High-risk medical conditions such as diabetes mellitus, chronic renal failure, malnutrition, lymphoma Children with likelihood of increased exposure to TB: • Born in a TB endemic area • Travel to a TB endemic area • Exposure to high-risk populations such as homeless, illicit drug users, nursing homes, institutionalized, incarcerated
Induration ≥15 mm	Children ≥4 years without risk factors

HIV, Human immunodeficiency virus; *TB,* tuberculosis.

- Positive test based on induration, not erythema
- Table 44.4 shows TST interpretation and indications for TB testing
  - IGRA (QuantiFERON TB-Gold)
    - Blood test assessing for lymphocyte response to specific TB antigens
    - Does not detect atypical mycobacteria or antigens in BCG vaccine, which reduces false-positive testing compared with TST
- Children for whom immediate TST or IGRA is indicated
  - Contacts of people with confirmed or suspected TB
  - Children with radiographic or clinical findings suggesting TB
  - Recent immigration from endemic countries including international adoptees
  - Travel history to countries with endemic infection
- Preferred testing by age
  - Children <2 years of age: TST preferred
  - Children ≥2 years of age: TST or IGRA
  - If a patient has had BCG vaccine, IGRA preferred
- Positive TST or IGRA testing
  - Without symptoms, chest radiograph should be performed
    - If negative imaging, diagnosis of LTBI
    - If positive, assess for active TB disease (see the following section)
  - With symptoms, chest radiograph should be done in addition to assessing for disease (see the following section)
- Assessing for disease
  - Culture or PCR
    - Sputum, gastric aspirate, bronchial washing, pleural fluid, CSF, urine, or tissue
    - Susceptibilities important in guiding therapy because multidrug-resistant TB is increasing
  - Induced sputum in children >5 years

- Three early morning gastric aspirates in children <5 years because induced sputum is difficult to obtain
- LP should be obtained in children <24 months of age to rule out meningitis

TREATMENT

- Latent infection
  - Isoniazid and rifapentine once weekly for 12 weeks
  - Rifampin daily for 4 months
  - Isoniazid daily for 9 months
- Active infection
  - Rifampin, isoniazid, pyrazinamide, ethambutol (RIPE) therapy for 2 months followed by isoniazid and rifampin for 4 months
  - Treatment based on susceptibilities
  - Adjunctive steroids are given in cases of meningitis and pericarditis
  - Directly observed therapy used to ensure control of infection

Nontuberculous Mycobacteria

BASIC INFORMATION

- Acid-fast bacilli
- Common species in children
  - *M. avium* complex (MAC), *M. abscessus*, *M. fortuitum*, *M. marinum*
- Ubiquitous in the environment
  - Soil, fresh and tap water, domestic and wild animals
- Peak incidence in late winter and spring and in ages 1 to 5 years old
- Transmission via inhalation of spores, direct inoculation, ingestion
- Risk factors:
  - Contaminated wounds
  - Cystic fibrosis
  - Immune suppression or organ transplantation
  - Indwelling catheters
  - Tympanostomy tubes
  - Tumor necrosis factor-alpha inhibiting agents (infliximab, etanercept)

CLINICAL PRESENTATION

- Cutaneous infection
  - Skin nodule, nonhealing ulcer, cellulitis, abscess
- Disseminated infection (MAC)
  - Fever, weight loss, night sweats, abdominal complaints
  - HIV patient with CD4 count <100
- Lymphadenitis
  - Most common manifestation in children
  - Unilateral, nontender anterior cervical or submandibular lymph nodes
  - Overlying skin becomes violaceous and sinus tracts can develop
  - Systemically well, no constitutional symptoms
- Pulmonary infection
  - Bronchiectasis, particularly in cystic fibrosis patients

- Fever, weight loss, fatigue, cough
- Enlarged mediastinal and/or hilar lymphadenopathy
- Skeletal infection
  - Tenosynovitis
  - Osteomyelitis including vertebral

DIAGNOSIS AND EVALUATION

- Culture or PCR of blood, tissue, sputum, bronchial washings
- Slow-growing organisms that can take up to 12 weeks to grow
  - Classified into rapid growers (within 7 days) and slow growers (2–12 weeks)

TREATMENT

- General principle: requires multidrug therapy for an extended period of time if not surgically excised
- Cutaneous infection
  - Clarithromycin/azithromycin + rifampin
- Lymphadenitis
  - Surgical excision common
  - Clarithromycin/azithromycin + rifampin
- Pulmonary infection
  - Clarithromycin/azithromycin, ethambutol, rifampin
- Disseminated disease
  - Clarithromycin/azithromycin, ethambutol, ± rifampin

HIGH-YIELD BACTERIA WITH UNIQUE PRESENTATIONS

Kingella kingae

BASIC INFORMATION

- Anaerobic, Gram-negative rod
- Lives in the mouth and pharynx of children typically <5 years of age, but implicated in musculoskeletal diseases more than respiratory tract infections
- Highest incidence in children 6 to 24 months of age
- Spread by person-to-person contact, particularly children in day care
- Outbreaks of infections have been noted in child care facilities

CLINICAL PRESENTATION

- Classically presents after a recent upper respiratory tract infection or stomatitis with MSK disease (i.e., septic arthritis, osteomyelitis, diskitis)
- Systemic disease may occur (e.g., bacteremia, endocarditis, pneumonia, meningitis)

DIAGNOSIS AND EVALUATION

- Culture
  - Difficult to grow on standard media
  - Synovial fluid and/or bone aspirate inoculated into a blood culture bottle
- PCR of synovial fluid, abscess fluid, or tissue

TREATMENT

- Empiric therapy: first-generation, second-generation or third-generation cephalosporin
- Treatment based on susceptibilities
  - Typical definitive therapy cephalexin orally
  - Susceptible to penicillins, cephalosporins, macrolides, TMP/SMX, fluoroquinolones
  - Variable resistance to vancomycin and clindamycin (and may be missed by empiric therapies for osteomyelitis with vancomycin or clindamycin monotherapy)
- Length of therapy depends on site of infection

Neisseria meningitidis

BASIC INFORMATION

- Gram-negative diplococci
- Leading cause of bacterial infections in children causing purulent meningitis and sepsis
- High mortality: 10% to 15%
- Six main disease-causing strains: A, B, C, W135, X, Y
  A: most common in Asia and Africa
  B: common in the United States, associated with college outbreaks
  C: common in the United States
- Normal flora of the nasopharynx
- Asymptomatic carriage maintains spread and herd immunity
- Transmitted via respiratory droplet requiring close, direct contact
- Risk factors:
  - Functional or anatomic asplenia
  - Complement deficiency
  - HIV infection
  - Military recruits
  - First-year college students
- Vaccination has decreased the incidence of disease
  - Types of vaccines
    - Conjugate vaccines (MenACWY)
      Menactra and Menveo protects against serogroups A, C, Y, W135
    - Recombinant protein vaccines (MenB)
      Bexsero and Trumemba: protects against serogroup B
  - Timing of vaccines
    - Healthy children
      MenACWY (two doses) at 11 to 12 years old and 16 years old
      MenB (two-dose or three-dose series) at 16 to 23 years old
    - Children with risk factors
      MenACWY starting at 2 months of age

CLINICAL PRESENTATION

- Asymptomatic carriage is most common form of infection
- Bacteremia, meningitis, sepsis (meningococcemia)
  - Rapid deterioration and death can occur within 12 to 24 hours
- Symptoms
  - Fever
  - Rash (nonblanching, petechiae, purpura), necrotic skin lesions
  - Headache, photophobia
  - Neck stiffness
  - Vomiting
  - Lethargy

DIAGNOSIS AND EVALUATION

- Culture of blood, CSF, tissue, or urine
- PCR of blood, CSF

TREATMENT

- Empiric therapy: third-generation cephalosporin (cefotaxime or ceftriaxone)
- Definitive therapy based on susceptibilities, typically penicillin
- Typical length of therapy: 7 days
- Prophylaxis should be given to close contacts with potential exposure to secretions
  - Household members, day care or school contacts, health care workers
  - Rifampin for four doses, ciprofloxacin for one dose, or ceftriaxone for a single intramuscular (IM) dose

Clostridium botulinum

BASIC INFORMATION

- Anaerobic Gram-positive bacilli
- Forms spores, lives in the environment
- Neurotoxins cause botulism
- Infants at higher risk because GI tract cannot resist spores like children and adults
- Foodborne: improper preparation, preservation, or storage of food (canned goods)
- Wound: contamination with soil

CLINICAL PRESENTATION

- Descending symmetric paralysis
- Weakness, hypotonia
- Constipation

DIAGNOSIS AND EVALUATION

- Detection of toxin in stool

TREATMENT

- Infants: botulism IV immunoglobulin (BabyBIG)
- Children and adults: botulism antitoxin (BAT)
- Supportive care (which may include endotracheal intubation and mechanical ventilation for respiratory failure)
- Antibacterial therapy not recommended unless there is secondary infection

TICKBORNE ZOONOSES

Borrelia burgdorferi (Lyme Disease)

BASIC INFORMATION

- Spirochete
- Transmitted by the brown *Ixodes* tick on feeding and engorgement with blood
- Endemic in New England and mid-Atlantic states
- Seasonal distribution in spring and summer when ticks are active

CLINICAL PRESENTATION

- Early localized disease
  - Characterized by a single erythema migrans lesion (classically referred to as "bulls eye" lesion)
  - Appears 1 to 2 weeks after tick bite, not painful or pruritic, and may be accompanied by vague influenza-like symptoms
  - Rash may not appear in up to 25% of cases
- Early disseminated disease
  - Appears ~1 to 4 months after tick bite, characterized by multiple erythema migrans lesions, fever, myalgias and flulike symptoms
  - May also cause neurologic manifestations (e.g., cranial nerve [CN] VII palsy, meningitis) or carditis (e.g., prolonged PR interval, heart block)
- Late disseminated disease
  - Appears 6 to 12 months after the tick bite
  - Characterized by arthritis (monoarticular or oligoarticular), especially of the large joints (e.g., knees)
  - May be accompanied by chronic CNS disease or acrodermatitis chronica atrophicans on the extensor surfaces
- Southern tick-associated rash illness (STARI) following a bite from the "lone star" tick *Amblyomma americanum* typically in the southeastern United States may present with rashes similar to Lyme disease, however, without neurologic, cardiac, or joint involvement and no evidence of *B. burgdorferi* infection

DIAGNOSIS AND EVALUATION

- Two-step test: serology (IgM and IgG), followed by western blot
  - Positive test = 2 of 3 IgM bands, 5 of 10 IgG bands
  - IgG and IgM antibodies may persist for years despite adequate treatment and clinical cure
  - Specificity of antibody testing is far from 100%, therefore there is a high false-positive rate
  - Sensitivity of antibody testing is also weakest early in disease (i.e., early localized disease)
  - Lyme antibodies may cross-react with *T. pallidum* and Epstein–Barr virus antibody testing
- PCR testing only useful in joint fluid; high rate of false negatives from other fluids

TREATMENT

Early localized disease:
- Doxycycline twice daily for 10 days
- Amoxicillin three times daily for 14 days
- Cefuroxime twice daily for 14 days

Extracutaneous disease:
- Isolated facial palsy: doxycycline twice daily for 14 days
- Arthritis: any oral agent above for 28 days
- Carditis: any oral agent above OR ceftriaxone for 14 to 21 days
- Meningitis: doxycycline orally or ceftriaxone for 14 days
- For third-degree heart block or refractory disease: ceftriaxone can be considered
- Doxycycline can be used regardless of age

PREVENTION

- DEET or permethrin may provide protection
- Tick removal should be accomplished by grasping with fine-tipped tweezers as close to skin as possible
  - Antibiotics are not recommended for routine prophylaxis
  - Risk of transmission is highest in a tick that has been attached for >36 hours

Rickettsial Diseases (Rocky Mountain Spotted Fever, Ehrlichiosis, Anaplasmosis)

BASIC INFORMATION

- *Rickettsia rickettsii*
  - Causes Rocky Mountain spotted fever (RMSF), a potentially fatal disease if unrecognized and untreated
  - Gram-negative bacilli
  - Infects endothelial cells of blood vessels causing primarily small vessel vasculitis
  - Transmitted by black American dog tick bites
  - Two-thirds of cases in five states: Arkansas, Missouri, North Carolina, Oklahoma, and Tennessee
  - Seasonal incidence in warm weather, April through September
- *Ehrlichia* species
  - Causes ehrlichiosis
  - Gram-negative cocci
  - Infected *Amblyomma americanum* tick bites humans and spreads disease
  - Incidence in males > females
  - Endemic in southeastern and south central United States
- *Anaplasma* species
  - Causes anaplasmosis
  - Gram-negative cocci
  - Infected *Ixodes scapularis* tick bites humans and spreads disease
  - Incidence in males > females
  - Endemic in northeastern and northcentral United States

CLINICAL PRESENTATION

- *R. rickettsii*
  - Classic triad of fever, headache, rash
    - Significant neurologic symptoms may accompany the headache, ranging from photophobia to lethargy and altered mental status
    - Rash
      Presents 2 to 5 days after other symptoms
      Starts peripherally on wrists/ankles and spreads centrally to trunk and face
      - Although associated with RMSF, a rash on the palms and soles can be associated with other diagnoses (drug hypersensitivities, infective endocarditis, *T. pallidum*, *N. meningitidis*, enteroviruses)
      Erythematous, blanching maculopapular rash (see http://www.cdc.gov/MMWr/preview/mmwrhtml/figures/r504a1f15.gif) progresses to petechial rash (see www.cdc.gov/MMWr/preview/mmwrhtml/figures/r504a1f16.gif)
  - Other symptoms include nausea, vomiting, myalgias, abdominal pain, periorbital edema
  - Severe disease includes acute respiratory distress syndrome (ARDS), cardiac failure, disseminated intravascular coagulation
  - History of tick bite or tick exposure absent in up to 50% of cases
- *Ehrlichia* and *Anaplasma*
  - Incubation period 5 to 21 days
  - Fever, headache, malaise, myalgia
  - Anorexia, diarrhea, nausea, and vomiting more common in children than adults
  - While frequently referred to as "rashless RMSF," it can present with a variable rash:
    - *Ehrlichia*: 66%
    - *Anaplasma*: 10%
    - Macular, papular, maculopapular, petechial
    - Involves trunk (spares palms and hands)
  - Severe disease including meningitis/encephalitis, ARDS, GI bleeding, disseminated intravascular coagulation (DIC), and renal failure more common with ehrlichiosis

DIAGNOSIS AND EVALUATION

- *R. rickettsii*
  - Routine labs: anemia, thrombocytopenia, hyponatremia, hypoalbuminemia
  - Serology (IgM and IgG) or PCR of blood
    - Initial serum sample frequently negative
    - Repeat serology 3–4 weeks later (convalescent titers) can be obtained to confirm infection
    - Single titer ≥1:64 is probably for infection
  - Immunohistochemical staining of tissue
- *Ehrlichia* and *Anaplasma*
  - Routine laboratory tests: leukopenia (more likely than in RMSF), thrombocytopenia, elevated liver transaminases (more likely than in RMSF), hyponatremia
  - CSF: elevated WBC, elevated protein
  - Serology (IgM and IgG)
    - Initial serum sample frequently negative

- Repeat serology 3–4 weeks later (convalescent titers) can be obtained to confirm infection
  - Fourfold rise in titer
- PCR of blood and CSF
- Intraleukocytic morulae in blood, CSF, or bone marrow
- Immunohistochemical staining of tissue

TREATMENT

- Doxycycline for all age groups
- Empiric therapy should be initiated while awaiting confirmatory tests because disease can be life-threatening
- Consider alternate diagnosis if no improvement within 72 hours of starting antibacterial
- Length of therapy 7 to 10 days or at least 3 days after defervescence

Francisella tularensis (Tularemia)

BASIC INFORMATION

- Gram-negative coccobacilli
- Transmitted by ticks, but also potentially mosquitos and flies
- Reservoirs include rabbits and small animals; therefore can be transmitted through bites, consumption of infected meat, or contact/inhalation from carcass

CLINICAL PRESENTATION

- Ulceroglandular disease
  - Presents a few days after the initial bite with a well-demarcated ulcer with black base, followed by painful lymphadenopathy and constitutional symptoms
- Oculoglandular disease
  - Occurs after direct inoculation of the eye, presents with conjunctivitis followed by ocular ulcer and lymphadenopathy
- Other presentations are variable and include sepsis, GI disease, pulmonary disease

DIAGNOSIS AND EVALUATION

- Serology (IgM and IgG)
- Cultures of wound or blood (laboratory needs to be notified

TREATMENT

- Aminoglycosides, tetracyclines, or fluoroquinolones

Babesia microti (Babesiosis)

BASIC INFORMATION

- Protozoans responsible for malaria-like illness
- Present with fever and hemolytic anemia, with onset ~1 to 4 weeks after a bite
- Immunocompromised or asplenic individuals are especially vulnerable

- Diagnostic testing includes serologies and PCR; "Maltese cross" formations on blood film are pathognomonic (and are not seen in malaria)
- Treatment regimen should be guided by disease severity and with the aid of an Infectious Disease consultant; agents include atovaquone and macrolides

OTHER ZOONOSES

Bartonella henselae (Cat Scratch Disease)

BASIC INFORMATION

- Gram-negative bacillus
- Causative agent of cat scratch disease
  - Cats are a major reservoir and vector for transmission to humans
  - Inhabits the mouth of cats and is transmitted primarily by scratches
- Common cause of unilateral regional lymphadenitis and fever of unknown origin in children
- Highest incidence in southern states
- Seasonal distribution in fall and winter

CLINICAL PRESENTATION

- Localized disease
  - Regional lymphadenopathy
    - Axilla > cervical > submandibular > inguinal
  - Constitutional symptoms
    - Malaise, fatigue, headache, anorexia
  - Fever
- Systemic disease (less common)
  - Fever, rash, weight loss, abdominal pain, hepatosplenomegaly
  - Encephalopathy/encephalitis, endocarditis, meningitis, neuroretinitis, osteomyelitis
- Timing
  - Incubation period 7 to 12 days followed by erythematous papule at inoculation site
  - Papule regresses spontaneously and lymphadenitis develops in 2 to 4 weeks

DIAGNOSIS AND EVALUATION

- Serology (IgM and IgG)
- PCR testing of tissue
- Abdominal ultrasound can show microabscesses in liver and spleen
- Lymph node biopsy shows granulomas

TREATMENT

- Supportive care because most cases are self-limited
- Needle aspiration for relief of painful nodes with marked fluctuance (incision and drainage not warranted)
- Antibacterials for systemic involvement (e.g., hepatitis, encephalitis, endocarditis, osteomyelitis)
  - Azithromycin ± rifampin, TMP/SMX, ciprofloxacin, gentamicin

Chlamydia/Chlamydophila psittaci (Psittacosis)

- "Parrot fever" caused by Gram-negative obligate intracellular coccobacilli transmitted via inhalation of aerosols from the respiratory tract secretions, eye secretions, urine, or feces of infected birds (all domestic and wild birds)
- Presentation: atypical pneumonia, mild influenza-like illness
- Diagnosis: acute and convalescent serology (IgM and IgG)
- Treatment: tetracyclines (tetracycline/doxycycline) *or* macrolides (azithromycin/clarithromycin)

Listeria monocytogenes

BASIC INFORMATION

- Anaerobic Gram-positive bacillus, can resemble cocci
- Ubiquitous in the environment
- Transmission
  - In utero
  - Foodborne
    - Raw foods including fruits, vegetables, milk, fish, poultry, and meat
    - Ready-to-eat meat products at supermarkets and deli counters
    - May be transmitted via raw milk or ice cream

CLINICAL PRESENTATION

- Infection during pregnancy
  - Mild gastroenteritis or influenza-like symptoms
  - Infects placenta
- Neonatal infection
  - One-third of cases result in stillbirth or spontaneous abortion; placenta and neonatal organs classically described as having "white nodules," which are microabscesses
  - Early-onset sepsis
  - Late-onset meningitis
- Bacteremia, gastroenteritis, meningitis, rhombencephalitis

DIAGNOSIS AND EVALUATION

- Culture of blood and CSF
- PCR of CSF

TREATMENT

- Ampicillin

Yersinia enterocolitica

BASIC INFORMATION

- Gram-negative coccobacilli
- Zoonotic GI disease
- Lives in domestic and wild animals
  - Cattle, cats, dogs, goats, pigs, rabbits, rodents, sheep, wild boars
  - Pigs are primary reservoir

- Transmission
  - Eating pork and pork intestine (chitterlings)
  - Contaminated dairy products (e.g., "unpasteurized" or raw milk) or water
  - Infections more common in winter months and in children <5 years old

CLINICAL PRESENTATION

- Enterocolitis
  - Fever
  - Abdominal pain
  - Bloody diarrhea
  - Mesenteric lymphadenitis (pseudoappendicitis) and terminal ileitis in older children
- Extraintestinal
  - Most common: bacteremia
    - Increased incidence in young children and persons with iron overload
  - Less common: liver, kidney, or splenic abscesses, pancreatitis, pharyngitis, osteomyelitis

DIAGNOSIS AND EVALUATION

- Culture of stool, blood, bile, urine, joint fluid, lymph node, throat swab
- PCR testing of stool

TREATMENT

- Supportive care for uncomplicated enterocolitis, especially if immunocompetent
- Immunocompromised patients or those with extraintestinal manifestations warrant antibacterials (e.g., third-generation or fourth-generation cephalosporins, TMP/SMX, fluoroquinolones)
- Definitive therapy guided by susceptibilities

Brucella

BASIC INFORMATION

- "Brucellosis" caused by Gram-negative coccobacilli
- Infectious disease of animals that can be transmitted to humans (zoonosis)
  - Cattle, goats, sheep, swine, dogs, rodents
  - Transmitted by direct contact with infected animals, their carcasses, or their milk
  - Typical scenario is ingestion of raw milk (goat, cow, camel) and/or raw cheeses
- Occurs worldwide, but main distribution is the Mediterranean basin, Arabian Peninsula, Indian subcontinent, Eastern Europe, and parts of Mexico and Central and South America

CLINICAL PRESENTATION

- Fever, malaise, joint pains, hepatosplenomegaly, headaches
- Osteoarticular manifestations prominent
  - Knees, hips, ankles
  - Classic presentation of a child is fever and limp

DIAGNOSIS AND EVALUATION

- Blood, bone marrow, CSF, or tissue for culture or PCR testing
- Serology (IgM and IgG) with antibody titer >1:160

TREATMENT

- Younger than 8 years: TMP/SMX plus rifampin
- Older than 8 years: doxycycline plus streptomycin or gentamicin or rifampin
- Length of therapy: 42 to 45 days, longer in cases of severe disease

Pasteurella multocida

BASIC INFORMATION

- Gram-negative coccobacilli
- Lives in the oropharynx of most dogs, cats, swine, rats, opossums, rabbits, fowl, and possibly humans
- Transmitted via animal bites or scratches, particularly cats

CLINICAL PRESENTATION

- Wound infections develop rapidly after an animal bite/scratch
- Drainage from the site
- Regional lymphadenopathy and fever common
- Less common manifestations
  - Tenosynovitis, osteomyelitis, septic arthritis, meningitis

DIAGNOSIS AND EVALUATION

- Culture of blood, CSF, tissue, urine
- Serology (IgM and IgG)

TREATMENT

- Generally susceptible to penicillin but can have some beta-lactamase production
- Drug of choice: amoxicillin/clavulanate, cefuroxime
- Other options: fluoroquinolones, tetracyclines, TMP/SMX

Leptospira

BASIC INFORMATION

- "Leptospirosis" caused by spirochete transmitted through urine from infected animals (e.g., rodents, cattle, pigs, horses, dogs) or contaminated soil/water
- Classic biphasic illness
  - Up to 4 weeks after exposure, may present with influenza-like symptoms and increasing transaminases (with jaundice), followed by a more severe illness ("Weil disease") with a wide variety of presentations (i.e., icteric liver failure, azotemia, vasculitis, meningitis, shock)
- Diagnosis: serology (IgM and IgG) or DNA PCR
- Treatment: penicillins/cephalosporins, macrolides, or doxycycline depending on clinical scenario

Coxiella burnetii (Q Fever)

BASIC INFORMATION

- Intracellular Gram-negative organism
- Transmitted by breathing aerosolized droplets or coming into contact with infected animal feces, urine, and milk (e.g., sheep, goat, cattle)
- Persons working on farms with exposure to newborn animals and carcasses are at increased risk
- Presentations range from influenza-like illness to more severe disease (e.g., pneumonia, granulomatous hepatitis); chronic disease may result in endocarditis
- Diagnosis: serology (IgM and IgG), acute and convalescent titers needed, PCR during early phase before antibody can be detected
- Treatment:
  - Acute disease: doxycycline for 14 days
    - TMP-SMX could be considered for children <8 years old
  - Chronic disease: requires follow-up with an infectious disease specialist for management of long-term antibiotics (e.g., doxycycline, hydroxychloroquine)

Yersinia pestis (Plague)

BASIC INFORMATION

- Gram-negative coccobacilli
- Maintained in rodents and their fleas (rats, rabbits, prairie dogs, bobcats, coyotes, squirrels, mice)
- Transmitted by flea bites, handling infected tissue or body fluids, or aerosolized droplets from patients with pulmonary manifestations
- Four classic presentations include the bubonic plague (characterized by swollen, tender lymph nodes, often inguinal), septicemic plague, pneumonic plague, and meningitic plague
- Bubonic plague most common in pediatrics (91%)
- Diagnosis:
  - Should be considered in those with travel to plague-endemic areas (Africa, Asia, Americas rarely)
  - Culture from blood, bubo aspirate, sputum, or CSF, laboratory should be notified
- Treatment: cephalosporins, tetracyclines, fluoroquinolones, aminoglycosides

Bacillus anthracis (Anthrax)

BASIC INFORMATION

- Gram-positive bacillus, transmitted by contact with infected animals or animal products; also a potential agent of bioterrorism
- Presentation depends on route of entry
  - Contact: painless ulcer with black eschar
  - Inhalation ("wool sorter's disease"): initially with hemorrhagic mediastinitis, causing respiratory symptoms and fever; followed by a pneumonia stage with respiratory failure and shock
  - Ingestion: enterocolitis with possible bloody stools, followed by bacteremia and sepsis
- Diagnosis: culture of wound or blood, laboratory should be notified, PCR at reference labs
- Treatment: ciprofloxacin or doxycycline; antitoxin is available
- Vaccine is available for those with increased risk (e.g., farmers, livestock handlers); however, it is not licensed for children under 18 years old

Review Questions

For review questions, please go to ExpertConsult.com.

Suggested Readings

Kimberlin DW, Brady MT, Jackson MA, Long SS, eds. *Red Book: 2015 Report of the Committee on Infectious Diseases*. 30th ed. Elk Grove Village, IL: American Academy of Pediatrics; 2015.

Reynolds MG, Holman RC, Curns AT, et al. Epidemiology of cat scratch disease hospitalizations among children in the United States. *Pediatr Infect Dis J*. 2005;24:700–704.

Lewinsohn DM, et al. Official American Thoracic Society/Infectious Diseases Society of America/Centers for Disease Control and Prevention Clinical Practice Guidelines: Diagnosis of Tuberculosis in Adults and Children. *Clin Infect Dis*. 2017;64(2):111–115.

Randis TM, Baker JA, Ratner AJ. Group B streptococcal infections. *Pediatr Rev*. 2017;38(6):254–262.

Long S, Prober C, Fischer M. *Principles and Practice of Pediatric Infectious Diseases*. 5th ed. Philadelphia: Elsevier; 2017.

45 *Viruses*

LORI KESTENBAUM HANDY, MD, MSCE

This is a survey of common pediatric viral infections, with the most typical signs and symptoms listed with each infection. By no means an exhaustive resource (because there exist multiple deviations from classic presentations), this chapter will provide a foundation necessary for board review (and for a career as a pediatrician).

VACCINE-PREVENTABLE VIRAL INFECTIONS

Also includes rotavirus, hepatitis A and B (see Gastrointestinal Viral Infections), poliovirus (see "Other Common Viral Systemic Infections"), and Rabies (see Additional Infections)

Measles Virus

BASIC INFORMATION

- *Paramyxoviridae* family
- Humans are the only host
- Transmission: direct contact with droplets; airborne; *highly* communicable
- Measles vaccine licensed in 1963; now a two-dose series at 1 and 4 years of age
- Sporadic outbreaks due to unvaccinated populations
- Incubation period is 8 to 12 days from exposure; children are infectious 4 days before and 4 days after rash
- See also Nelson Textbook of Pediatrics, Chapter 246, "Measles."

CLINICAL PRESENTATION

- Acute illness with fever, cough, coryza, and conjunctivitis (3 C's)
- Maculopapular rash beginning on face and spreading down (often likened to "dumping a can of paint on someone's head"), begins 3 to 5 days after initial symptoms
- Koplik spots: pathognomonic—small red spots with blue-white centers on oral mucosa
- Complications: otitis media, pneumonia, croup, diarrhea, encephalitis
- Subacute sclerosing panencephalitis (SSPE): degenerative neurologic disease occurring about 10 years after infection; presents with mental deterioration and seizures and is usually fatal

DIAGNOSIS AND EVALUATION

- Serum IgM: detectable for 1 month after rash
- Increase in serum IgG in paired titers; vaccinated patients have positive IgG, necessitating measurement of increase in titers
- RNA polymerase chain reaction (PCR), preferably from throat or nasopharynx
- Report suspected cases to public health agency immediately

TREATMENT

- Vitamin A decreases morbidity, mortality
- Airborne isolation for 4 days after rash
- Postexposure prophylaxis:
  - Exposed, unvaccinated patients who can receive vaccine should be vaccinated within 72 hours of exposure
  - In the event of measles outbreak or travel to endemic areas, children 6 to 11 months of age can receive early vaccination
  - Postexposure intramuscular immunoglobulin or intravenous immunoglobulin (IVIG) (measles-specific products are not available): treat within 6 days of exposure for:
    - Pregnant women without immunity
    - Immunocompromised hosts regardless of vaccination status
    - Severely immunocompromised HIV patients

Mumps Virus

BASIC INFORMATION

- *Paramyxoviridae* family
- Humans are the only host
- Transmission: person-to-person contact
- Mumps vaccine licensed in 1967, with only sporadic outbreaks in the United States
- Incubation ranges from 12 to 25 days after exposure

CLINICAL PRESENTATION

- Swelling of parotid glands; orchitis occurs if after puberty
- Rare complications: arthritis, myocarditis, thrombocytopenia, hearing loss
- Maternal mumps in first trimester may be associated with spontaneous abortion/intrauterine fetal death

DIAGNOSIS AND EVALUATION

- RT-PCR from buccal swabs, throat specimens, spinal fluid, or saliva; change in acute and convalescent titers
- Look for other causes of parotitis (e.g., bacterial infection, autoimmune disease, anatomic obstruction)

TREATMENT

- Supportive care
- Keep children out of school for 5 days from onset of parotitis
- "Immunity to mumps" is considered if there is documentation of vaccine series (one dose for adults not at high risk), lab confirmation of disease, or a date of birth before 1957

Rubella Virus

BASIC INFORMATION

- *Togaviridae* family
- Humans are the only host
- Transmission: Person-to-person contact; droplet contact from nasopharyngeal secretions
- Vaccine licensed in 1969; outbreaks occur in underimmunized populations

CLINICAL PRESENTATION

- Many infections asymptomatic
- Generalized erythematous maculopapular rash with fever and lymphadenopathy, possibly conjunctivitis
- Pregnancy: infection can lead to miscarriage, fetal death, or congenital rubella syndrome (CRS)
  - Anomalies: ophthalmologic, cardiac (patent ductus arteriosus [PDA], peripheral pulmonary artery stenosis [PPAS]), sensorineural hearing loss, behavioral disorders, meningoencephalitis, microcephaly, mental retardation
  - Manifestations at birth: growth restriction, pneumonitis, bone disease, hepatosplenomegaly, thrombocytopenia, dermal erythropoiesis (blueberry muffin lesions)

DIAGNOSIS AND EVALUATION

- IgM positive within 5 days
- Congenital cases IgM positive from birth to 3 months
- Culture, PCR from throat/nasal specimens possible for sporadic cases or outbreaks

TREATMENT

- Supportive care

Varicella-Zoster Virus

BASIC INFORMATION

- Member of the *Herpesviridae* family
- Humans are the only host
- Transmission: contact with upper respiratory mucous membranes or conjunctiva, airborne transmission if patient has open vesicles
- In utero infection: transplacental transmission
- Vaccine introduced in the United States in 1995; now a two-dose series

CLINICAL PRESENTATION

- Primary infection: "chickenpox," a vesicular rash ("dewdrops on a rose petal") with lesions in varying stages of development, accompanied by fever
  - Complications: bacterial superinfection, pneumonia, acute cerebellar ataxia, encephalitis
- Immunocompromised patients: more severe disease with prolonged eruption of lesions, higher fever, and dissemination to organs including liver, lung, and CNS
- Breakthrough disease in vaccinated patients: wild-type varicella-zoster virus (VZV) infection that is milder than disease in unvaccinated patients, with fewer lesions, less fever, atypical rash, and faster recovery
- Zoster: virus becomes latent in sensory ganglia and reactivates in dermatomal distribution as a group of vesicles with pain and itching. Zoster in immunocompromised patients can disseminate like primary infection
- Fetal infection: maternal infection in first or second trimester can lead to limb hypoplasia, CNS damage, scarring of skin, and ophthalmologic abnormalities

DIAGNOSIS AND EVALUATION

- PCR: for skin lesions; can distinguish wild type from vaccine strain
- Direct fluorescent antibody stain (DFA), viral culture, and Tzanck smear all possible from vesicular fluid
- Serology: acute and convalescent titers; limited use for demonstrating immunity from vaccination
- Immunocompromised hosts should be evaluated with chest x-ray (CXR), liver function tests (LFTs), and potentially lumbar puncture if concern for CNS infection

TREATMENT

- For primary infections:
  - Immunocompetent patients: antivirals not indicated for otherwise healthy children; initiate acyclovir for those children with increased risk of severe disease (children over 12, chronic illness, receiving salicylates or steroids)
  - Immunocompromised patients: IV acyclovir; initiate within 24 hours for both primary infection and zoster
  - Do not give salicylates due to concern for Reye syndrome
  - Exclude children from school/day care until lesions are crusted or no new lesions appear within 24 hours (if patient's lesions do not crust)
  - Hospitalized patients require airborne precautions
- Postexposure prophylaxis:
  - Vaccinate those without evidence of immunity, aged 12 months or older
  - VariZIG (varicella immune globulin) should be given to those who cannot receive vaccine and are at risk of severe disease (immunocompromised children, pregnant women, select infants)
- Zoster: lesions must be covered; otherwise exclude from school or day care until lesions have crusted; some may consider antiviral therapy if early in the zoster course

Influenza Virus

BASIC INFORMATION

- Member of the *Orthomyxovirus* family; three types (A, B, C)
- Most disease caused by influenza A or B
- Each season different subtypes circulate, classified by H and N (hemagglutinin and neuraminidase)
- Transmission: person-to-person via respiratory droplets
- Influenza vaccine administered each year developed in anticipation of strains that will be circulating; effectiveness varies each season

CLINICAL PRESENTATION

- Acute febrile illness with headache, fatigue, myalgias, and cough; pharyngitis, rhinorrhea, and potentially abdominal symptoms
- Severe infections can be fatal: viral sepsis, viral pneumonia, encephalitis, myocarditis
- Complications: secondary infection by group A *Streptococcus*, *Staphylococcus aureus*, and *S. pneumoniae*
- Pregnant patients are at high risk of complications

DIAGNOSIS AND EVALUATION

- PCR of nasopharyngeal specimen, rapid molecular assays, other rapid diagnostics
  - Sensitivity/specificity varies by test manufacturer
  - Testing best to be done in first 72 hours of illness via nasopharyngeal wash

TREATMENT

- Two antiviral classes: neuraminidase inhibitors and adamantanes
  - Oseltamivir (neuraminidase inhibitor) first line, often provided early in disease course for best effect; hospitalized pediatric patients with severe illness typically warrant full course of treatment even if beyond the first 48 hours of symptoms
  - Adamantanes are not recommended due to inactivity against influenza B and resistance in influenza A
  - Outpatients: treated based on risk factors and severity of illness
- Postexposure prophylaxis (antiviral medications) available for certain populations

Human Papillomavirus

BASIC INFORMATION

- DNA viruses in the *Papillomavirus* family
- Transmission: person-to-person, skin-to-skin contact, usually sexually transmitted
- Vaccine available covering nine most prevalent serotypes and high-risk serotypes
- Rare transmission: birth canal leading to respiratory papillomatosis in the infant

CLINICAL PRESENTATION

- May be asymptomatic and clear spontaneously
- Skin warts or warts on mucous membranes (genital warts)
- Associated with cervical (99% of cases), anogenital, and oropharyngeal cancers
  - Types 16 and 18 account for 70% of cervical cancer

DIAGNOSIS AND EVALUATION

- Diagnosis of warts is by physical examination
- Respiratory papillomatosis: biopsy lesion via endoscopy
- Pap smears: screen cervical specimens
- Biopsy for lesions suspicious for oncologic process
- Detect virus in lesions via detection of nucleic acid

TREATMENT

- Warts may regress; otherwise remove by physical or chemical methods
- Precancerous lesions managed by excision or location destruction
- Cancerous lesions managed by an oncologist

RESPIRATORY VIRAL INFECTIONS

Rhinovirus

BASIC INFORMATION

- RNA in the *Picornaviridae* family
- ~100 serotypes, with immunity providing little protection from new infection
- Transmission: person-to-person

CLINICAL PRESENTATION

- Common cold; can have pharyngitis, otitis media, bronchiolitis, or pneumonia
- Symptoms may last up to 2 weeks
- Associated with asthma exacerbations

DIAGNOSIS AND EVALUATION

- PCR, nasopharyngeal specimen

TREATMENT

- Supportive care
- Droplet precautions for hospitalized children

Parainfluenza Virus

BASIC INFORMATION

- RNA viruses in the *Paramyxoviridae* family
- Four types cause human infection
- Transmission: person-to-person, respiratory droplets, fomites

CLINICAL PRESENTATION

- Croup (most common cause of croup in children), bronchiolitis or pneumonia, primarily in infants and young children
- Infection does not provide complete immunity
- Immunocompromised hosts: prolonged/severe lower respiratory tract disease

DIAGNOSIS AND EVALUATION

- Culture possible; multiplex PCR, nasopharyngeal specimen, now available

TREATMENT

- Supportive care
- Oxygen for hypoxia
- Croup treatment: racemic epinephrine, corticosteroids

Respiratory Syncytial Virus

BASIC INFORMATION

- RNA virus of the *Paramyxoviridae* family
- Humans are the only host
- Transmission: contact with secretions, large droplets, and fomites

CLINICAL PRESENTATION

- Occurs annually in winter and early spring
- Acute respiratory tract infections
- Most children infected at least once by age 2 years
- 20% to 30% have bronchiolitis or pneumonia with first infection
- High-risk patients: prematurity, congenital heart disease, chronic lung disease (CLD), immunodeficiency

DIAGNOSIS AND EVALUATION

- Rapid diagnostics (immunofluorescent and enzyme immunoassays)
- Culture, multiplex PCR, and nasopharyngeal specimen will detect coinfections

TREATMENT

- Supportive care
- Hydration, suctioning, and oxygen if patient is consistently <90% saturated
- Respiratory support as needed; no definite evidence that steroids, DNAse, or bronchodilators are effective; hypertonic saline is increasingly used for symptomatic relief, with some evidence of reduction of length of hospital stay
- Ribavirin for potentially life-threatening infection
- Infection control policies important to reduce health care–associated infection, including use of contact precautions, cohorting, and visitor screening

- Palivizumab (monoclonal antibody, five doses during respiratory syncytial virus [RSV] season) can be considered to reduce risk of lower respiratory tract infection in children at high risk of severe disease. Practitioners should review the most recent guidelines for indications, but general inclusion criteria include: premature infants, very young infants, those with CLD or congenital heart disease, and those with suppressed immune systems.

Human Metapneumovirus

BASIC INFORMATION

- RNA virus in the *Paramyxoviridae* family
- Humans are the only host
- Transmission: by contact with infected secretions

CLINICAL PRESENTATION

- Respiratory infections occur mainly during winter and early spring
- Bronchiolitis in infants
- Also presents as pneumonia, croup, or upper respiratory infection (URI); may lead to asthma exacerbation or otitis media

DIAGNOSIS AND EVALUATION

- PCR is commercially available for nasopharyngeal specimens

TREATMENT

- Supportive care

GASTROINTESTINAL VIRAL INFECTIONS

Also see Adenovirus, Enteroviruses, Epstein-Barr virus (EBV), and Cytomegalovirus (CMV)

Rotavirus

BASIC INFORMATION

- RNA virus in the *Reoviridae* family
- Common cause of gastroenteritis in young children
- Vaccines are now part of infant vaccine series—significantly reduced incidence
- Virus remains in stool many days before and after infection
- Transmission is fecal-oral

CLINICAL PRESENTATION

- Fever and vomiting followed by watery diarrhea
- Illness lasts 3 to 8 days
- Hospitalization for severe hydration
- Immunocompromised patients: prolonged infection

DIAGNOSIS AND EVALUATION

- Enzyme immunoassay (EIA), immunochromatography, and latex agglutination assays are available
- PCR of stool specimen

TREATMENT

- Supportive care with IV fluids and/or electrolytes
- Children with ongoing diarrhea should remain out of child care settings

Norovirus and Sapovirus

BASIC INFORMATION

- RNA viruses of the *Caliciviridae* family
- Transmission: person-to-person via fecal-oral route, contaminated food, or surface contact

CLINICAL PRESENTATION

- Norovirus: gastroenteritis, either as sporadic cases or as outbreaks
  - Classically causes outbreaks in populated areas such as schools, cruise ships, and health care facilities
  - Is a predominant cause of pediatric gastroenteritis
- Sapovirus: sporadic acute diarrhea; at times may cause outbreaks

DIAGNOSIS AND EVALUATION

- Multiplex PCR of stool specimens available for both viruses

TREATMENT

- Supportive care, with rehydration either with oral solutions or IV, if needed
- Hand hygiene is critical

Hepatitis A Virus

BASIC INFORMATION

- RNA virus in the *Picornaviridae* family
- Transmission: person-to-person via fecal-oral route
- Vaccine licensed in 1995; infection rates in the United States are declining
- Countries without vaccine: most children infected in first decade
- Does not become a chronic infection

CLINICAL PRESENTATION

- Acute illness: fever, fatigue, jaundice, decreased appetite, nausea
- Children <6: 30% will be symptomatic
- Children >6: illness more often symptomatic and prolonged

DIAGNOSIS AND EVALUATION

- Patients can be tested by serology 5 to 10 days after symptoms start
- Serum PCR is available

TREATMENT

- Supportive care
- Postexposure prophylaxis:
  - Unvaccinated patients exposed to hepatitis A virus should receive a dose of vaccine (preferred) or pooled intramuscular immune globulin (IGIM) within 14 days of exposure
  - Exposure includes household or sexual contact, newborn infants to exposed mother, child care staff, health care workers in close contact with infected patient, and infected food handlers

Hepatitis B Virus

BASIC INFORMATION

- DNA virus of the *Hepadnavirus* family
- Transmitted through blood or body fluids (semen, vaginal secretions, cerebrospinal fluid [CSF], amniotic fluids) primarily from individuals with chronic infection
- Percutaneous exposures such as needlesticks, sexual contact, and perinatal exposure are the most common sources of infection
- Vaccine series is initiated at birth in the United States

CLINICAL PRESENTATION

- Acute infection: varies from a mild illness without specific symptoms to clinical hepatitis with jaundice
- Can have extrahepatic manifestations, including papular acrodermatitis (Gianotti-Crosti, also seen with EBV)
- Chronic infection: younger patients are more likely to go on to develop chronic infection and may have growth delay
- Resolved infection: antibody to hepatitis B (HBV) surface antigen with clearance of HBsAg
- Long term: premature death, cirrhosis, hepatocellular carcinoma

DIAGNOSIS AND EVALUATION

- Serology and serum PCR; serology is useful to demonstrate acute infection, chronic infection, or resolved infection (see Figs. 45.1, 45.2)

TREATMENT

- Acute HBV: supportive care
- Chronic HBV:
  - Interferon and antivirals are FDA approved to limit progression to cirrhosis or hepatocellular carcinoma
  - Ensure receipt of hepatitis A vaccine; periodically screen LFTs and alpha-fetoprotein; and perform liver ultrasound

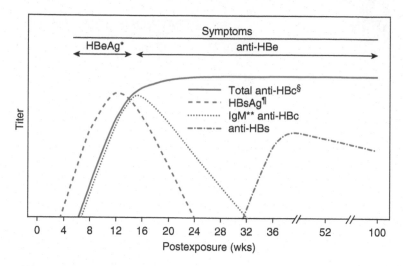

* Hepatitis B e antigen.
↑ Antibody to HBeAg.
§ Antibody to hepatitis B core antigen.
¶ Hepatitis B surface antigen.
** Immunoglobulin M.
↑↑ Antibody to HBsAg.

Fig. 45.1. Typical serologic course of acute hepatitis B infection with recovery. (From Centers for Disease Control and Prevention. Recommendations for identification and public health management of persons with chronic hepatitis B virus infection. *MMWR Recomm Rep*, 2008;57[RR-8]:3.)

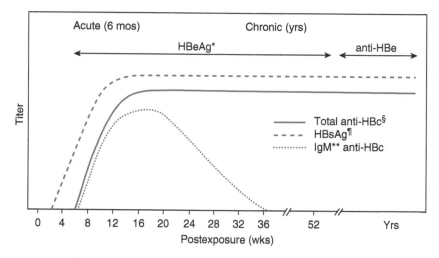

* Hepatitis B e antigen.
↑ Antibody to HBeAg.
§ Antibody to hepatitis B core antigen.
¶ Hepatitis B surface antigen.
** Immunoglobulin M.

Fig. 45.2. Typical serologic course of acute hepatitis B infection with progression to chronic hepatitis B infection. (From Centers for Disease Control and Prevention. Recommendations for identification and public health management of persons with chronic hepatitis B virus infection. *MMWR Recomm Rep*, 2008;57[RR-8]:4.)

- Postexposure prophylaxis:
  - Neonates born to a mother who is HBsAg positive should receive HepB vaccine and hepatitis B immunoglobulin (HBIG), with testing for infection at 9 to 12 months of age; those who receive HBIG and first dose of vaccine can safely breastfeed
  - Unimmunized older children exposed to a known positive source should receive HBIG and HepB vaccine as soon as possible; series must be completed
  - Exposed children who have been immunized should have titers checked; if the child has had an inadequate response to vaccine, that child should receive a single dose of vaccine and HBIG
  - Detailed guidelines are available if source is unknown, pending the child's immunization status

Hepatitis C Virus

BASIC INFORMATION

- RNA virus in the *Flaviviridae* family
- Six hepatitis C (HCV) genotypes
- Spread by blood exposure: injection drug use, sexual partners, receipt of blood products before 1992; maternal-fetal transmission can occur but not at as high a rate as in hepatitis B

CLINICAL PRESENTATION

- Acute infection: asymptomatic, or mild hepatitis and possible jaundice
- Chronic infection: most children with acute infection develop chronic HCV; complications include liver failure leading to death or liver transplant

DIAGNOSIS AND EVALUATION

- Qualitative detection of RNA (nucleic acid amplification test [NAAT])
- Antibody testing (cannot be used in first 18 months of life due to persistence of maternal antibody)

TREATMENT

- Refer to a hepatitis specialist; regimens include peginterferon and ribavirin
- Antiviral agents available for adults may become available for pediatric patients in the future

HERPES FAMILY VIRUSES

Includes varicella (see Vaccine-Preventable Viral Infections)

Cytomegalovirus

BASIC INFORMATION

- Member of the *Herpesviridae* family
- Transmission: person-to-person contact through secretions, blood products
- Can be transmitted intrauterine, intrapartum from cervical secretions, and postpartum from breast milk
- Persists after infection with intermittent shedding

CLINICAL PRESENTATION

- Asymptomatic infections are common
- Congenital (cCMV): 10% of infants are symptomatic
  - Symptoms: intrauterine growth restriction, microcephaly, jaundice, purpuric rash, hepatosplenomegaly, intracerebral calcifications, retinitis with potential for developmental delay, sensorineural hearing loss
- Adolescents/adults: Prolonged fever and mild hepatitis
- Immunocompromised hosts: pneumonia, colitis, retinitis, thrombocytopenia, leukopenia, hepatitis

DIAGNOSIS AND EVALUATION

- Shell vial culture (unique vial supporting CMV growth) and immunofluorescence antibody for early antigen (EA) detection
- Immunoglobulins: paired titers to demonstrate increase over time
- Immunocompromised hosts: viral DNA from serum by PCR

TREATMENT

- Immunocompromised hosts: intravenous ganciclovir (induction and maintenance)
- Valganciclovir: oral prodrug of ganciclovir; only for specific uses in pediatric transplant patients
- Neonates with symptomatic cCMV: oral valganciclovir for 6 months; monitor for bone marrow suppression

Epstein-Barr Virus

BASIC INFORMATION

- Member of the *Herpesviridae* family
- 90% of adults have had an EBV infection
- Transmission: person-to-person contact, blood products
- Persists after infection with intermittent shedding for life

CLINICAL PRESENTATION

- Young children: mild or asymptomatic infections
- Older children: fever, exudative pharyngitis, lymphadenopathy, hepatosplenomegaly with atypical lymphocytes on complete blood count (CBC)
- Rare but severe complications: aseptic meningitis, encephalitis, splenic rupture, hematologic derangements, pneumonia, orchitis, myocarditis
- Associated with lymphoproliferative disorders: fatal infections with EBV in patients with X-linked lymphoproliferative syndrome, posttransplant lymphoproliferative disease, and Burkitt lymphoma

DIAGNOSIS AND EVALUATION

- Heterophile antibody test: diagnose about 85% of infections in children and adolescents >4 years old during second week of infection
- Antibody testing: used to determine timing of infection (see Table 45.1)
  - Viral capsid antigen (VCA) immunoglobulin G and M class
  - EA diffuse staining
  - EBV nuclear antigen: EBNA
- EBV serum PCR: Useful in immunocompromised patients
- In cases of pharyngitis/lymphadenopathy, it is common to see a pronounced atypical lymphocytosis

TREATMENT

- Exposure to amoxicillin/ampicillin leads to a characteristic nonallergic morbilliform rash

Table 45.1. Serologic Testing for Epstein-Barr Virus Infection

Infection Status	VCA IgG	VCA IgM	EA (D)	EBNA
No prior infection	–	–	–	–
Acute	+	+	±	–
Recent	+	±	±	±
Past	+	–	±	+

EA, early antigen; *EBNA*, Epstein-Barr virus nuclear antigen; *VCA*, viral capsid antigen.
Data from Epstein-Barr virus infections. In: Kimberlin DW, Brady MT, Jackson MA, Long SS, eds. *The Red Book*. Committee on Infectious Diseases: American Academy of Pediatrics; 2015:336–340.

- Uncomplicated infections: supportive care; limit collision supports until full recovery to reduce risk of splenic rupture
- Short course of steroids for impending airway obstruction

Herpes Simplex Virus

BASIC INFORMATION

- Member of the *Herpesviridae* family; herpes simplex virus (HSV)-1 and HSV-2 cause clinical infections
- Transmission: person-to-person contact at time of active infection, reactivation, or asymptomatic viral shedding
- Virus remains latent

CLINICAL PRESENTATION

- Neonatal disease (first month of life)
  - Transmitted to newborns during birth through contact in the genitourinary (GU) tract or via ascending infection
  - Highest risk of transmission if mother has primary genital infection at time of delivery
  - Can present as sepsis, fever, rash, lethargy, abnormal liver function, meningitis, or seizures
  - Disseminated disease (liver, lungs, and potentially CNS)
  - CNS disease: localized to the CNS with potential skin involvement
  - Skin-eye-mouth disease: disease localized to these three areas
- Childhood infections: about 25% of school-age children have been infected; some are asymptomatic
  - Gingivostomatitis is the most common
- Adolescents/adults: genital herpes
- Additional manifestations
  - Eczema herpeticum: herpes infection of skin in patients with atopic dermatitis
  - Encephalitis, Bell's palsy, ocular
  - Reactivation of the latent virus occurs as herpes labialis (perioral vesicles) and genital herpes (vesicular lesions in GU region); more severe in immunocompromised hosts

DIAGNOSIS AND EVALUATION

- Neonatal specimens: sample CSF and blood; swab mouth, nasopharynx, conjunctivae, and anus to send for culture and potentially PCR
- Viral culture is the gold standard for surface specimens in evaluation of neonates
- PCR assays in workup of neonate for detection of CNS infection or viremia
- PCR or cell culture: genital lesions or mucocutaneous lesions
- Type-specific antibodies are available

TREATMENT

- Neonatal infections: IV acyclovir followed by oral suppression
- Genital infection: acyclovir or valacyclovir at the time of infection, or for suppression
- Mucocutaneous infection: limited data on benefit of mucocutaneous infection
- Immunocompromised hosts and HSV encephalitis: IV acyclovir

OTHER COMMON SYSTEMIC VIRAL INFECTIONS

Many viral illnesses present with an exanthem and a pattern of associated symptoms. The classic progressions of symptoms are outlined in Tables 45.2 and 45.3.

Human Herpesvirus Type 6 (Roseola)

BASIC INFORMATION

- Member of the *Herpesviridae* family
- Humans are the only host
- Transmission: contact with secretions, particularly from asymptomatic shedding

CLINICAL PRESENTATION

- 80% of children have a nonspecific febrile illness
- 20% have high fever for 3 to 7 days *followed* by erythematous maculopapular rash
- Febrile seizures are common as a complication

DIAGNOSIS AND EVALUATION

- Limited use of tests because results cannot change management
- Serology conversion from negative to positive is helpful in documenting infection
- PCR (serum) of viral DNA is possible; must be interpreted in the clinical scenario

TREATMENT

- Supportive care
- Antiviral use in serious disease in immunocompromised hosts may benefit the patient

Table 45.2.   Viral Exanthems

Virus	Rash	Associated Signs/Symptoms	Population at Risk
Measles	Maculopapular rash beginning on face and spreading down body, begins 3 to 5 days after initial symptoms	Fever, cough, coryza, conjunctivitis; Koplik spots	Previously was common in young children; now seen in unvaccinated children of any age
Rubella	Generalized erythematous maculopapular rash	Fever, lymphadenopathy	All cases in United States are congenitally acquired
Varicella zoster virus	Vesicular pruritic rash with lesions in _varying_ stages of development	Fever	Unvaccinated, immunocompromised patients
Herpes simplex virus	Vesicular lesions or ulcerations on mucocutaneous surfaces	May be associated with pain and fever; superinfection in eczema herpeticum	Neonates: risk of significant morbidity/mortality; otherwise, up to 25% of school-age children infected
Herpesvirus 6	Erythematous maculopapular rash (roseola)	Fever _precedes_ rash by 3 to 7 days; febrile seizure common complication	Children <5 years of age
Parvovirus B19	"Slapped cheeks" rash with circumoral pallor _or_ full-body lacy rash beginning on trunk, moving outward	Mild systemic symptoms (i.e., low-grade fever, upper respiratory symptoms)	Mild illness in most children; patients with hemolytic anemia can have aplastic crisis
Enteroviruses	Variety of presentations, including hand-foot-and-mouth, nonspecific maculopapular rash, petechiae, urticarial eruptions	Nonspecific febrile illness with symptoms including pharyngitis, stomatitis, conjunctivitis; more severe cases of meningoencephalitis, hepatitis, pneumonia	Neonates at risk of more severe disease
Smallpox	Deep-seated, firm, round, and well-circumscribed vesicles or nodules, followed by crusting and leaving depigmentation. Lesions are in _same_ stage of development	Sudden onset of high fever, severe headache, backache, and malaise, followed by oral lesions, _then_ rash	Eradicated worldwide

Table 45.3.   Congenital Viral Infections (see also: Toxoplasmosis)

Rubella	Manifestations at birth: growth restriction, pneumonitis, bone disease, hepatosplenomegaly, thrombocytopenia, dermal erythropoiesis (blueberry muffin lesions) Anomalies: Ophthalmologic, cardiac (patent ductus arteriosus [PDA], peripheral pulmonary artery stenosis [PPAS]), sensorineural hearing loss, behavioral disorders, meningoencephalitis, microcephaly, mental retardation
Cytomegalovirus	Most common intrauterine infection Manifestations at birth: intrauterine growth restriction, microcephaly, jaundice, purpuric rash, hepatosplenomegaly, intracerebral calcifications, retinitis Sequelae: potential developmental delay, sensorineural hearing loss, seizure disorder
Herpes simplex virus	Intrauterine infection: extremely rare. Infants have skin lesions including vesicles, ulcerations, and scarring; chorioretinitis, central nervous system (CNS) disease including microcephaly Infection at time of delivery: can present as sepsis, fever, rash, lethargy, abnormal liver function, meningitis, or seizures 1. Disseminated disease (liver, lungs, and potentially CNS) 2. CNS disease: localized to CNS with potential skin involvement 3. Skin-eye-mouth disease: disease localized to these three areas
Human immunodeficiency virus (HIV)	Infants may appear well at birth; consider infection in infants that are failing to thrive, have opportunistic infections, lymphadenopathy, hepatosplenomegaly
Varicella zoster virus	Congenital varicella syndrome: extremely rare due to maternal infection in first half of pregnancy; manifestations include low birth weight, hypertrophic skin lesions, cataracts, microphthalmia, chorioretinitis, microcephaly, seizures
Parvovirus B19	Fetal loss if infection in mother occurs <20 weeks; maternal infection associated with pleural and pericardial effusions, anemia, and hydrops fetalis; most intrauterine infections do not have long-term sequelae for surviving pregnancies

Parvovirus B19 (Erythema Infectiosum)

BASIC INFORMATION

- Nonenveloped, single-stranded DNA virus in the _Parvoviridae_ family
- Humans are the only host
- Transmission: contact with respiratory secretions, blood products, mother to fetus

CLINICAL PRESENTATION

- Erythema infectiosum or "fifth disease"
- Mild systemic symptoms _followed by_ distinct rash of "slapped cheeks" with circumoral pallor
- Full-body lace-like rash that starts on the trunk and moves outward to the arms, legs, and buttocks
- Patients with hemolytic anemia (sickle cell): aplastic crisis
- Parvovirus in pregnancy: fetal hydrops; highest risk before 20 weeks of gestation

DIAGNOSIS AND EVALUATION

- IgM antibodies indicate infection in prior 2 to 3 months
- IgG antibodies persist lifelong
- PCR (serum) assays are available; detect low levels of virus that may be past infection

TREATMENT

- Supportive care
- Transfusion for aplastic crises

Adenovirus

BASIC INFORMATION

- DNA viruses, *Adenoviridae* family
- >50 serotypes exist, each associated with different types of disease
- Transmission: serotypes causing respiratory tract infections—person-to-person contact, airborne droplets, and fomites
- Transmission: gastrointestinal tract infections—transmitted fecal-oral route

CLINICAL PRESENTATION

- Respiratory tract infections: fever, congestion, cough, tonsillitis, otitis media, conjunctivitis
- Enteric infections: gastroenteritis
- Occur throughout childhood, community outbreaks cause URIs, conjunctivitis, or gastroenteritis

DIAGNOSIS AND EVALUATION

- DFA for rapid identification
- Multiplex PCR (nasopharyngeal or stool) for respiratory and gastrointestinal infections

TREATMENT

- Supportive care
- Control measures require hand and respiratory hygiene; contact precautions for the entire illness with conjunctivitis or gastroenteritis

Enteroviruses (Echo-, Coxsackie-, Numbered Entero-, Poliomyelitis)

BASIC INFORMATION

- Members of the family *Picornaviridae*
- Nonpolio enterovirus: more than 100 serotypes, including coxsackie and echovirus
- Humans are the only known host
- Transmission: fecal-oral, respiratory, and perinatal
- Poliovirus: few regions of the world have wild-type polio virus circulating or vaccine-derived polioviruses
- Poliovirus vaccine available: inactivated or oral
- Last natural case in United States 1979

CLINICAL PRESENTATION

- Nonpolio presentations:
  - Nonspecific febrile illness; can include pharyngitis, stomatitis, hand-foot-mouth disease, and conjunctivitis/ uveitis
  - CNS: aseptic meningitis, encephalitis
  - GI: vomiting, diarrhea, hepatitis
  - Cardiovascular: myopericarditis
  - Neonates: viral sepsis including meningoencephalitis, hepatitis, pneumonia
  - Enterovirus D68: mild to severe respiratory illness
  - Enterovirus (EV) 70 and coxsackievirus A24: associated with hemorrhagic conjunctivitis
- Polio: majority of infections are asymptomatic; 1% of patients have asymmetric acute flaccid paralysis

DIAGNOSIS AND EVALUATION

- PCR nasopharyngeal aspirates, stool, swabs of conjunctiva, rectum, throat
- PCR sterile sites: blood, CSF, urine
- Serotype for epidemiologic purposes only

TREATMENT

- Supportive care
- Immunodeficient patients with chronic EV meningoencephalitis may benefit from IVIG

ADDITIONAL INFECTIONS

Human Immunodeficiency Virus

BASIC INFORMATION

- Cytopathic lentiviruses in *Retroviridae* family
- Humans are the only known host
- Virus remains latent in peripheral mononuclear cells, CNS, bone marrow, and GU tract
- Transmission: blood (percutaneous exposure or transfusion), semen and vaginal secretions (sexual contact), and human milk (breastfeeding)
- Mother-to-child transmission: in utero, at time of delivery, or through breastfeeding

CLINICAL PRESENTATION

- Varied clinical presentation; initial viral infection followed by progressive weakening of immune system leading to acquired immunodeficiency syndrome (AIDS)

- Initial presentation: fever, adenopathy, enlarged liver or spleen, failure to thrive, developmental delay, lymphoid interstitial pneumonia
- May present with opportunistic infection: candidal infection, severe viral illness (VZV, CMV, HSV), invasive bacterial infection, *Pneumocystis jirovecii* (PJP), cryptosporidium, *Toxoplasma gondii*, mycobacterial infections
- IRIS: immune reconstitution inflammatory syndrome—worsening of symptoms after initiation of antiviral medications, usually related to an underlying infection
- Encephalopathy: more common in untreated patients
- Infants with HIV with AIDS-defining illness in first 6 months: worse prognosis

DIAGNOSIS AND EVALUATION

- Infants: infants born to mothers with HIV will have positive antibody tests due to passive acquisition of antibodies. Test with nucleic acid testing (DNA or RNA)
- Children >18 months of age: any licensed HIV test available can be used with referral to HIV specialist for confirmation and management
- CDC recommends diagnostic HIV testing and opt-out screening as part of routine care beginning at age 13 years

TREATMENT

- Pediatric HIV treatment recommendations change over time
- Antiretroviral therapy (ART): regimens should be managed by a clinician trained in care of pediatric patients with HIV; therapy goals include suppression of viremia, maintaining immune system, and minimizing adverse drug effects
  - All children <1 year of age should receive ART
  - Mother-to-child transmission reduced by antepartum, intrapartum, and postnatal antiretroviral prophylaxis
- Condom use reduces HIV transmission; abstinence is the only definitive method to prevent sexual transmission
- Pre- and postexposure prophylaxis are available

Rabies virus

BASIC INFORMATION

- RNA virus in the *Rhabdoviridae* family
- Transmission: bites of infected animals; rarely, transplantation of infected organs or corneas. Worldwide, human infections most often occur from rabid dog bites

CLINICAL PRESENTATION

- Rapidly progressive neurologic disease including hydrophobia, anxiety, pain, pruritus, and dysautonomia
- Almost all infections are fatal

DIAGNOSIS AND EVALUATION

- Diagnose infection in animals by detecting rabies virus antigen in brain tissue
- Antemortem diagnosis for humans by DFA on skin biopsy specimens, isolation of virus from saliva, or antibody in serum or CSF

TREATMENT

- Postexposure prophylaxis is critical to prevent infection
- Bites of dogs, cats, and ferrets: if the animal is healthy, observe for 10 days and give the patient prophylaxis only if signs of rabies develop; if the animal is rabid, suspected of being rabid, or unknown, provide rabies vaccine and rabies immunoglobulin
- Bites of bats, skunks, raccoons, foxes, most carnivores, and woodchucks: consider rabid unless the area is known to be rabies-free and provide vaccination and rabies immunoglobulin
- Experimental treatment protocols exist once patients are symptomatic

Arbovirus (West Nile Virus, Dengue Fever)

BASIC INFORMATION

- RNA viruses transmitted to humans through the bites of infected arthropods
- Common arboviruses: dengue, West Nile virus (WNV), chikungunya, yellow fever
  - WNV: transmitted by mosquitos; humans are dead-end hosts, birds serve as reservoir
  - Dengue fever: four types, transmitted by *Aedes aegypti*; humans are main host
  - Chikungunya: transmitted by the same mosquitos as dengue
- Consider in travelers from Caribbean, Latin America, South Asia

CLINICAL PRESENTATION

- WNV:
  - Most people are asymptomatic; symptoms include an acute febrile illness, headache, myalgia, arthralgia
  - Rare: CNS disease (meningitis, encephalitis, or acute flaccid paralysis)
- Dengue:
  - Most people are asymptomatic; symptoms include acute febrile illness with diffuse pain ("breakbone fever"), rash, leukopenia, petechiae, and minor bleeding; can progress to dengue hemorrhagic fever or shock due to plasma leakage
  - Severe dengue: vomiting, abdominal pain, bleeding ("hemorrhagic fever"), respiratory distress, shock, thrombocytopenia

- Chikungunya:
  - Most infected people will develop symptoms; usually presents with fever and joint pain, but may include headache, myalgia, arthritis, and rash

DIAGNOSIS AND EVALUATION

- WNV: Serum or CSF IgM; if negative at presentation, retest 10 days later
- PCR serum and CSF or tissue specimens at time of illness in immunocompromised hosts
- Dengue: PCR serum or serology (IgM)

TREATMENT

- Supportive care

Review Questions

For review questions, please go to ExpertConsult.com.

Suggested Readings

1. Kimberlin DW, Brady MT, Jackson MA, Long SS, eds. *Red Book: 2015 Report of the Committee on Infectious Diseases*. Elk Grove Village, IL: American Academy of Pediatrics; 2015.
2. Kliegman RM, Stanton BMD, St. Geme J, Schor NF. *Nelson Textbook of Pediatrics*. 20th ed. Philadelphia: Elsevier; 2015.
3. Long SS, Pickering LK, Prober CG, eds. *Principles and Practice of Pediatric Infectious Diseases*. 4th ed. Philadelphia: Saunders; 2012.
4. https://www.cdc.gov/.

46 Fungi, Worms, and Parasites

LESLIE ANNE ENANE, MD

FUNGI

Candida

BASIC INFORMATION

- Candidal disease is caused by several species:
  - Most common and most virulent: Candida albicans
  - Increasingly prevalent: C. parapsilosis
- Illnesses range from those in immunocompetent hosts (thrush, dermatitis, vulvovaginitis) to those affecting primarily immunocompromised patients (esophagitis, chronic mucocutaneous candidiasis, invasive candidiasis)
- Invasive candidiasis includes deep-seated infections, such as candidemia, as well as dissemination to the central nervous system (CNS), eyes, liver, spleen, kidneys, or bone. Considered a disease of "modern medicine," particularly affecting immunocompromised and intensive care unit (ICU) patients;
  - Invasive candidiasis is associated with high mortality

CLINICAL PRESENTATION

- Clinical presentations of local infections are presented in Table 46.1
- Risk factors for invasive candidiasis are presented in Table 46.2
- Candidemia: presentation is nonspecific and similar to bacteremia/bacterial sepsis
  - Infants: temperature instability, feeding intolerance, hypoglycemia, abdominal distention, apnea, respiratory distress, hypotension
  - Immunocompromised children: persistent fever
  - Laboratory findings: thrombocytopenia, leukocytosis, or leukopenia
- Meningoencephalitis: commonly presents with candidemia
  - Lumbar puncture (LP) to rule out meningoencephalitis associated with candidemia
  - CNS disease may present without apparent abnormalities on cerebrospinal fluid (CSF) studies
  - Consider head imaging to evaluate for complications
- Other sites of focal organ involvement may result from invasive candidiasis
- Chronic disseminated candidiasis: seen primarily in patients with leukemia, often identified after immune recovery. Associated with nausea, vomiting, abdominal pain, and hepatosplenomegaly. Candidal lesions in liver and spleen

DIAGNOSIS AND EVALUATION

- Local infections: diagnosed clinically. Confirmation with Gram stain or potassium hydroxide preparation of scraping: demonstrates budding yeast, pseudohyphae
  - Esophagitis: can be diagnosed clinically; if no response to treatment, should perform endoscopy and biopsy; consider other opportunistic infections
- Candidemia:
  - Sensitivity of blood cultures to detect *Candida* is relatively low, particularly in neonates (because lower volumes of culture are obtained)
  - Organ involvement may be seen in the absence of positive blood cultures
  - Evaluate for dissemination and involvement of other sites: CNS, eyes, liver, spleen, kidneys, heart (endocarditis)
  - Neonates: obtain ultrasound of head and abdomen, LP, eye examination, echocardiogram

TREATMENT

- Treatment for local infections is discussed in Table 46.1.
  - Invasive candidiasis:
  - Candidemia should prompt removal of central venous catheters (CVC) as soon as possible and within 24 hours. Delayed removal is associated with increased mortality and morbidity, including worse neurodevelopmental outcomes in infants
  - Neonates: amphotericin B should be used for initial treatment and for severe disease. Treatment duration: 3 weeks from clearance of blood cultures
  - Pediatric patients: an echinocandin (e.g., caspofungin, micafungin) should be used for initial therapy. If echinocandin-resistant infection is suspected, initiate treatment with amphotericin B
  - Once susceptibilities are known, and if the patient is stable with repeat blood cultures negative, he or she may be transitioned to fluconazole (if isolate susceptible). Treatment duration: 2 weeks from clearance of blood cultures
- Meningoencephalitis: consider addition of flucytosine (5-FC) to antifungal treatment
- Antifungal resistance among non-*albicans* species:
  - C. glabrata and C. krusei: resistance to fluconazole; some strains with resistance to amphotericin B
  - C. lusitaniae: resistance to amphotericin B

Table 46.1.   Localized *Candida* infections

Localized Disease	Clinical Presentation	Risk Factors	Treatment
Dermatitis	Well-demarcated, erythematous rash with "satellite lesions." Involves wet, macerated skin (e.g., in the diaper area and neck folds for infants).	Infants, immunocompromised patients, diabetes, pregnancy, overweight, any moist or sweaty conditions (e.g., wearing binding clothing).	Topical nystatin. Area should be kept dry.
Oropharyngeal candidiasis (thrush)	Thick, white plaques on the tongue, buccal mucosae, or oropharynx.	Infants, immunocompromised patients, use of steroid inhaler.	Oral nystatin. Systemic fluconazole for refractory disease or for immunocompromised patients.
Vulvovaginitis	White vaginal discharge, pruritus, dysuria.	Adolescent and adult women, antibiotic therapy, pregnancy, diabetes, HIV.	Topical therapy, or one dose of 150-mg oral fluconazole.
Esophagitis	Pain or difficulty swallowing.	Immunocompromised patients, particularly with HIV/AIDS.	Systemic antifungal therapy. HIV-infected patients should be initiated on antiretroviral therapy.
Chronic mucocutaneous candidiasis	Persistent *Candida* infections of the skin, nails, and mucosal surfaces.	Defects in T-cell immunity.	Fluconazole.
Isolated candiduria	Candida isolated on urine culture from Foley catheter.	Immunocompetent patients with Foley urinary catheter.	Removal of Foley catheter. Antifungal treatment is not recommended unless patient is at high risk for dissemination (i.e., neutropenic, or premature neonate, or will undergo urologic manipulation).

Table 46.2.   Risk Factors for Invasive Candidiasis

- Prematurity
- Extremely low birth weight
- Broad-spectrum antibiotics
- Central venous catheter
- Endotracheal tube
- Parenteral nutrition
- Gastrointestinal surgery
- Necrotizing pancreatitis
- Hyperglycemia
- Corticosteroids
- H2 blocker or proton pump inhibitor (PPI)
- Immunocompromising conditions: hematologic malignancy, chemotherapy, organ transplantation, primary immunodeficiency

Aspergillus

BASIC INFORMATION

- Disease is caused primarily by *Aspergillus fumigatus* (most common), *A. flavus*, *A. niger*, *A. terreus*, and *A. nidulans*
- Host defenses against *Aspergillus* involve both neutrophil and macrophage activity
- Invasive aspergillosis is seen in immunocompromised children: chemotherapy patients (particularly with prolonged neutropenia, as in treatment of acute myelogenous leukemia), bone marrow transplant patients (particularly with mismatched or unrelated donor), patients on immunosuppression for graft-versus-host disease, transplant patients on antirejection therapies, and patients with chronic granulomatous disease (CGD). Also occurs in diabetes mellitus and chronic steroid therapy
- Allergic bronchopulmonary aspergillosis (ABPA) is seen most commonly in patients with cystic fibrosis (CF) or asthma

CLINICAL PRESENTATION

- Invasive aspergillosis: pulmonary disease, invasive sinusitis, CNS disease, skin infection, and disseminated disease
  - Extremely high mortality, particularly with persistent immunocompromised state
  - Presentation is nonspecific, particularly in severely immunocompromised patients. *Most common presentation in this population is persistent fever*
  - Pulmonary: fever, cough, chest pain, shortness of breath, hemoptysis, pneumothorax.
    - Classic chest x-ray (CXR) findings (more typical of adults): "halo sign" in neutropenic patients and "air crescent sign" on neutrophil recovery
    - CGD patients: chronic pulmonary infection may spread to involve pleura, vertebrae, and chest wall, and may disseminate
  - Invasive sinusitis: fever, nasal congestion, epistaxis, pain or swelling involving the face or eye, headache, vision changes
    - Rhinoscopic examination: areas of decreased sensitivity or blood flow, ulcerated or blackened necrotic lesions
    - Invasive sinusitis rapidly extends into the orbits and CNS
  - CNS disease: either from hematogenous dissemination (e.g., from lung) or direct extension from sinus disease. May present with headache, nausea, vomiting, altered mental status, seizures, or focal neurologic signs.
    - Potential for mycotic aneurysm, thrombosis, ischemic or hemorrhagic infarction, and abscess/empyema
  - Pulmonary aspergilloma: noninvasive "fungus ball" that forms in preexisting lung cavity, typically apical location. May present without symptoms or with cough, hemoptysis, and weight loss

- ABPA: hypersensitivity to *A. fumigatus* allergens in the setting of *A. fumigatus* colonization of bronchi. Results in bronchial inflammation, obstruction, wheezing (e.g., "the asthma that just isn't getting better"), pulmonary infiltrates, bronchiectasis, and ultimately fibrosis

DIAGNOSIS AND EVALUATION

- Identification of *Aspergillus* on culture or evidence on tissue biopsy is the gold standard
- Invasive aspergillosis:
  - Pulmonary aspergillosis: bronchoalveolar lavage (BAL) should be performed where feasible but has relatively low sensitivity
  - Sinusitis: rhinoscopic examination and biopsies
  - Positive serum galactomannan suggests invasive aspergillosis.
    - False-positive results may be seen (e.g., with therapy with piperacillin-tazobactam)
    - False-negative results may be seen (e.g., in CGD patients)
- Pulmonary aspergilloma:
  - Compatible imaging
  - *Aspergillus* identified on sputum culture
  - Positive *Aspergillus* antibodies
- ABPA:
  - Compatible clinical presentation in a patient with CF or asthma
  - Diagnosis requires elevated IgE antibody to *A. fumigatus*. Supporting criteria include elevated total IgE level, IgG antibody to *A. fumigatus*, peripheral eosinophilia, and skin reactivity to *A. fumigatus* antigens

TREATMENT

- Invasive aspergillosis: voriconazole; surgical debridement for localized invasive disease
- *A. terreus* is resistant to amphotericin B
- Pulmonary aspergilloma: typically treated with surgical resection
- ABPA: corticosteroids to control inflammation. Itraconazole to reduce the burden of infection

Endemic Mycoses

BASIC INFORMATION

- Endemic mycoses are differentiated on the basis of exposure to endemic areas (Table 46.3), and clinical features of each

- Travel history is key to diagnosing endemic mycoses in patients who have traveled to or moved from an endemic area
- Increased risk of exposure with activities causing inhalation of aerosolized spores (Table 46.3)

CLINICAL PRESENTATION

- All can be asymptomatic or subclinical. Typically self-limited, but can progress to chronic, severe, or fatal forms of disease
- Histoplasmosis: flu-like illness with fever, cough, chest pain, headache, myalgias/arthralgias, fatigue, and weight loss
  - May present as "a pneumonia that just isn't getting better"
  - Erythema multiforme and erythema nodosum may be seen
  - Progressive disseminated infection: increased risk for infants and for immunocompromised patients (e.g., on chemotherapy on immunosuppressive agents, including tumor necrosis factor alpha [TNF-α] inhibitors)
    - Fever, cough, weight loss, diarrhea, hepatosplenomegaly, lymphadenopathy, cytopenias; more likely to look like sepsis with disseminated intravascular coagulation (DIC) and acute respiratory distress syndrome (ARDS)
    - HIV: fever, rash, weight loss, immune reconstitution syndrome
- Coccidiomycosis: pulmonary infection: fever, cough, chest pain, malaise, weight loss, headache
  - "Classic" presentation includes erythema multiforme or erythema nodosum at presentation
  - Dissemination to bone/joints, skin, or meninges can occur—for example, in neonates, pregnant women, and immunocompromised patients, notably those on TNF-α inhibitors
- Blastomycosis: fever, cough, chest pain. Symptoms may be persistent and progress to weight loss, night sweats, or hemoptysis. May be associated with erythema nodosum
  - Includes subacute-to-chronic development of characteristic skin lesions that are well circumscribed; often painless papules/nodules/plaques that become violaceous and verrucous with microabscess in the center; usually heal with scar
  - May progress to disseminated disease, including infection of skin, bones/joints, or CNS

Table 46.3. Regions and Risk Factors for Endemic Mycoses

Disease	Causative Organism	Geographic Regions	Risks for Exposure
Histoplasmosis	*Histoplasma capsulatum* var. *capsulatum*	Midwestern and southeastern United States: Ohio and Mississippi River valleys; Central and South America	Living near or working at a construction or excavation site, cleaning basement or attic, gardening, caving, exposure to barns *Note:* Strongly associated with presence of bird or bat guano
Coccidiomycosis	*Coccidioides immitis* and *C. posadasii*	Southwestern U.S. states; Central and South America	Construction sites, archaeologic sites, military training, dust clouds from earthquake
Blastomycosis	*Blastomyces dermatitidis*	Basins of the Mississippi, Ohio, Missouri, and St. Lawrence Rivers; Great Lakes region; eastern Ontario, Canada	Exposure to endemic waterways, beaver dams, hunting, logging, spoiled/rotten wood (e.g., hunters) *Note:* Symptoms or diagnosis of blastomycosis in pet dog may be a clue

DIAGNOSIS AND EVALUATION

- Histoplasmosis:
  - CXR: mediastinal adenopathy and patchy pulmonary infiltrates
  - May become calcified, but less likely to become cavitary (e.g., blastomycosis)
  - Pathology: necrotizing granulomas, yeasts
  - *Histoplasma* immunodiffusion and complement fixation assays; *Histoplasma* antigen in urine, blood, BAL, or CSF
- Coccidiomycosis:
  - CXR: pulmonary infiltrates, hilar adenopathy, cavities, and/or effusion
  - Spherules may be seen on samples from tissue or body fluid
  - May be isolated on culture; laboratory staff should be alerted if coccidiomycosis is suspected given biohazard risk
  - Urine antigen test, serologies, immunodiffusion and complement fixation tests
- Blastomycosis:
  - CXR: pulmonary infiltrate with possible cavitation/ nodules/effusion
    - Unlike other mycoses, unlikely have hilar/mediastinal lymphadenopathy
  - Organism may be seen on examination of BAL or sputum ("broad-based budding yeast")
  - May be isolated on culture of specimens
  - *Histoplasma* urine antigen test may be positive due to cross-reactivity

TREATMENT

- Histoplasmosis: treatment for severe illness, prolonged disease, or immunocompromised patients
  - Pulmonary disease: itraconazole
  - Disseminated infection: amphotericin B for initial therapy; itraconazole for consolidation therapy
  - HIV: long-term suppressive therapy with itraconazole; can be discontinued with successful highly active antiretroviral therapy (HAART) and immune recovery
- Coccidiomycosis or blastomycosis: treatment for moderately or severely ill patients, those with prolonged disease, those with extrapulmonary infections, or those at risk for dissemination
  - Treatment is typically with itraconazole or fluconazole. Fluconazole has good CSF concentrations. Itraconazole is preferred for bone infections
  - Severe disease: amphotericin B, followed by azole therapy for consolidation

Cryptococcus

BASIC INFORMATION

- Disease is caused by *Cryptococcus neoformans* and *C. gattii*
- Risk of disease with defects in T-cell immunity: HIV/AIDS (with CD4 <100), malignancy, chronic steroid therapy, immunosuppressive therapy, organ transplantation, sarcoidosis
- Disease results from inhalation of organisms and subsequent dissemination
- Classically associated with pigeon excrement
- See also Nelson Textbook of Pediatrics, Chapter 235, "Cryptococcus neoformans."

CLINICAL PRESENTATION

- Pulmonary cryptococcosis: fever, cough, chest pain, shortness of breath, weight loss
  - CXR with pulmonary infiltrates, hilar adenopathy, effusion, and/or cavitation
- CNS cryptococcosis: most common presentation. May be subacute or indolent course, with progression of headache, fever, cranial nerve involvement, vision changes, and altered mental status, with increased intracranial pressure
  - CSF: increased opening pressure, increased protein, decreased glucose
- Skin or bone infection may be seen with disseminated disease
- Usually does *not* present with hepatosplenomegaly

DIAGNOSIS AND EVALUATION

- Cryptococcal antigen from blood, CSF, or urine
  - Serum cryptococcal antigen is typically negative in isolated pulmonary infection
- CSF India ink stain demonstrates the organisms, which have a characteristic "halo" due to their distinctive polysaccharide capsule
- May be isolated on culture

TREATMENT

- Combination therapy with amphotericin B and 5-FC for 2 weeks, followed by fluconazole for at least 8 weeks
- Urgent relief of increased intracranial pressure
- HIV-infected patients: fluconazole suppressive therapy. See pediatric opportunistic infection guidelines for considerations regarding discontinuation of secondary prophylaxis (available at http://aidsinfo.nih.gov/content files/lvguidelines/oi_guidelines_pediatrics.pdf)

Pneumocystis

BASIC INFORMATION

- Disease is caused by *Pneumocystis jirovecii*, formerly *P. carinii*. Genetic analyses point to *Pneumocystis* being a fungus; however, it has many features in common with protozoa
- Predominant opportunistic infection in immunocompromised patients: HIV/AIDS (typically with CD4 <200), severe combined immunodeficiency (SCID), malignancy, organ transplantation, chronic steroid therapy
- Disease may be seen in the setting of decreased adherence to prophylaxis in high-risk patients. Breakthrough cases also occur in patients who adhere to prophylaxis

CLINICAL PRESENTATION

- *Pneumocystis* pneumonia (PCP): fever, tachypnea, increased work of breathing, cough, hypoxia
  - "Quiet tachypnea" with apparently normal breath sounds on auscultation

- CXR: diffuse perihilar opacities that spread to the periphery—"batwing" appearance. (Can also demonstrate lobar consolidation or appear normal)
- Inflammatory response contributes to lung injury, decreased oxygenation, and mortality

DIAGNOSIS AND EVALUATION

- Identification of the organism on silver stain of induced sputum sample, BAL fluid, or pulmonary biopsy
- β-D-glucan and LDH are commonly used to support the diagnosis of PCP. However, these tests are not entirely specific for PCP (e.g. β-D-glucan can be elevated in certain endemic mycoses)

TREATMENT

- Trimethoprim-sulfamethoxazole (TMP-SMX) is the preferred treatment. Treatment course should be followed by prophylaxis
- Corticosteroid treatment should be initiated in moderate or severe disease
- Supportive care with supplemental oxygen; possible need for mechanical ventilation
- TMP-SMX is a superior choice for prevention of PCP. Alternatives: dapsone, aerosolized pentamidine, atovaquone

WORMS

Toxocara

BASIC INFORMATION

- Toxocariasis is caused by infection with *Toxocara canis* (found in dogs) or *T. cati* (found in cats). Along with pinworms, these are the most common helminth infections in the United States
- May be an important cause of asthma in high-risk populations in the United States
- Ingestion of eggs from contaminated soil, in the setting of pica. Larvae hatch in the small intestine, invade the intestinal wall, and disseminate to invade other organs: liver, lungs, CNS, eyes. Larvae induce hypersensitivity reaction and inflammation, eosinophilic granulomas
- Risk factors: poverty, pica, dog ownership (especially puppies)

CLINICAL PRESENTATION

- Visceral larva migrans: fever, bronchospasm/wheezing (mimicking asthma), hepatomegaly, peripheral eosinophilia, hypergammaglobulinemia. Can involve other organs as well
- Ocular larva migrans: unilateral vision changes resulting from invasion and granuloma formation within the retina. Can result in macular detachment and blindness

DIAGNOSIS AND EVALUATION

- Visceral larva migrans is suggested by multisystem disease, eosinophilia, and history of pica

- Antibodies to *T. canis* or *T. cati* may be detected
- Ocular disease is diagnosed clinically; serologies are not reliable for this diagnosis

TREATMENT

- Most patients recover without treatment
- Can treat with albendazole; may worsen inflammatory response
- Corticosteroids may be given to manage inflammatory manifestations

Ascaris lumbricoides

BASIC INFORMATION

- Most common helminth infection in the world. Seen in tropical settings and in the United States among immigrant, refugee, traveler, or internationally adopted children
  - Chronic childhood infection associated with stunting and impairments in cognitive development
- After ingestion of eggs from contaminated soil, larvae hatch in the small intestine, invade the intestinal wall, and enter the circulatory system. Larvae migrate from the portal vein to the liver, to the pulmonary vasculature, and invade into the alveoli, where they migrate up to the trachea and are swallowed back into the digestive system. This migration cycle causes physical destruction and inflammation in the lungs

CLINICAL PRESENTATION

- Löffler pneumonia: cough, wheeze, dyspnea, hemoptysis, "shifting" pulmonary infiltrates
- Abdominal pain and intestinal obstruction and perforation
- Malnutrition and malabsorption, impacting physical and cognitive development

DIAGNOSIS AND EVALUATION

- Peripheral eosinophilia and pulmonary infiltrates are suggestive. Eosinophils may be seen in sputum
- Ova seen on microscopic examination of stool

TREATMENT

- Albendazole or mebendazole. Alternatives: nitazoxanide, pyrantel pamoate

Enterobius vermicularis

BASIC INFORMATION

- Along with toxocariasis, most common helminth infections in the United States
- After ingestion of eggs, larvae hatch in the small intestine and migrate through the digestive tract. Adult females lay eggs in the perianal area, typically at night. Itching at the site of egg deposition leads to autoinoculation
- Risk factors: child care centers, elementary schools

CLINICAL PRESENTATION

- Intense perianal pruritus
- Can result in secondary bacterial infection. Can cause associated vaginitis and urinary tract infection (UTI) in girls

DIAGNOSIS AND EVALUATION

- Transparent tape applied to perianal area first thing in the morning and placed on a slide reveals the eggs

TREATMENT

- Mebendazole, pyrantel pamoate, or albendazole. It is recommended to repeat treatment 2 weeks later to eradicate all stages of infection
- Wash all linens
- Simultaneous treatment of all household members may be needed in the setting of repeated infections or infection in multiple household members

Necator americanus

BASIC INFORMATION

- Hookworm infections are a major cause of iron deficiency anemia and malnutrition worldwide
- *Necator americanus:* most common hookworm infection in the Western Hemisphere, Southeast Asia, and Africa
- Eggs deposited in soil hatch into larvae, which mature into a form that can penetrate skin. Humans become infected by walking barefoot on contaminated soil in rural areas. The larvae disseminate via lymphatics to the circulatory system and ultimately to the pulmonary vasculature, invade into the alveoli, and ascend upward to the trachea to be swallowed and enter the digestive system. In the small intestine, the larvae mature into adult worms, which attach to the intestinal mucosa and feed. The adult worms mate, and fertilized eggs are deposited in the intestinal lumen and excreted in the stool
- Young children and pregnant women are particularly vulnerable to iron deficiency anemia induced by hookworm infections

CLINICAL PRESENTATION

- Pruritus and characteristic rash at the site of hookworm entry in the skin
- Abdominal pain
- Anemia (can be severe), protein malnutrition, developmental delays

DIAGNOSIS AND EVALUATION

- Eggs may be identified on microscopic examination of stool

TREATMENT

- Albendazole or mebendazole

Cysticercosis

BASIC INFORMATION

- Cysticercosis is caused by infection with the tapeworm species *Taenia solium*
- Neurocysticercosis is a very common cause of adult-onset epilepsy in Latin America, sub-Saharan Africa, India, and Asia
- Ingested eggs (either from autoinoculation in an infected person or fecal-oral contamination) hatch in the intestine and release oncospheres that invade the intestinal wall and disseminate to muscles or organs, where they develop into cysticerci. Neurocysticercosis results from invasion of the CNS. Symptoms typically develop years later as a result of inflammatory response to the cysticerci

CLINICAL PRESENTATION

- Seizures (typically focal)
- Imaging demonstrates edema or enhancement at the location of the cysts
- Extraparenchymal lesions, depending on location, may obstruct CSF flow and present with signs of increased intracranial pressure or mass effect

DIAGNOSIS AND EVALUATION

- Brain imaging demonstrates characteristic cysts and can distinguish active or inactive (resolved) disease
- Serologies can support diagnosis

TREATMENT

- Corticosteroids to control inflammation
- Symptomatic management of seizures, cerebral edema, and increased intracranial pressure
- Anthelmintic treatment is somewhat controversial. Treatment decisions should take into account location and stage of infection
- Surgical intervention may be needed for some cysts

PROTOZOA

Toxoplasma

BASIC INFORMATION

- Infection is caused by *Toxoplasma gondii*
- Cats (definitive hosts) shed oocysts in their feces, which then persist in soil. Humans are infected either through ingestion of oocysts (e.g., after contact with cat litter or ingestion of contaminated produce) or through ingestion of tissue cysts in contaminated meat
- Human infection persists within tissue cysts in the brain, retina, cardiac, and skeletal muscles
- Reactivation occurs in the setting of immunosuppression (e.g., HIV/AIDS, bone marrow transplantation)
- Congenital toxoplasmosis: transplacental transmission occurs if mother becomes infected or has reactivation during pregnancy

CLINICAL PRESENTATION

- Primary infection:
  - Typically asymptomatic. Minority of patients experience nonspecific mononucleosis-like symptoms, such as fever, headache, sore throat, malaise, and lymphadenopathy
    - May have vision changes or eye pain. Retinal lesions may be seen in primary infection or in reactivation
- Congenital toxoplasmosis:
  - Symptoms of toxoplasmosis may not be apparent at birth; manifestations, including retinal lesions, may be identified years later
  - Symptoms at birth may include classic triad of hydrocephalus, chorioretinitis, and brain calcifications on imaging
    - Other possible symptoms: microcephaly, seizures, encephalitis, chorioretinitis, pericarditis, pneumonitis, hepatosplenomegaly, ascites, jaundice, thrombocytopenia, petechiae
  - Can be fatal
- Ocular toxoplasmosis:
  - Presents with vision changes, "floaters," scotoma, eye pain, chorioretinitis, vision loss. Can represent reactivation of congenital or postnatally acquired infection
- Reactivation in immunocompromised patients:
  - Encephalitis, brain abscesses, chorioretinitis, or pneumonitis

DIAGNOSIS AND EVALUATION

- Positive IgM indicates active infection. Serologic testing may be performed at the Palo Alto Medical Foundation Toxoplasma Serology Laboratory (http://www.pamf.org/serology/)
- Polymerase chain reaction (PCR)—for example, of amniotic fluid, blood, CSF, vitreous, or BAL fluid
- Toxoplasmic encephalitis: characteristic lesions on brain imaging. Response to therapy confirms diagnosis
  - Usually *Toxoplasma* is IgG positive and IgM negative
  - *Toxoplasma* PCR from CSF is helpful if positive
  - Histology from brain biopsy, if performed
- Ocular toxoplasmosis: characteristic retinal lesions, PCR of aqueous fluid, serologies from aqueous fluid and serum

TREATMENT

- Pregnant women may be given spiramycin to prevent congenital infection if amniotic fluid PCR is negative. If fetal infection is suspected or confirmed, the mother should be given combination of pyrimethamine, sulfadiazine, and leucovorin
- Congenital or postnatally acquired infection: treated with combination of pyrimethamine, sulfadiazine, and leucovorin. Steroids may be used if severe chorioretinitis or CNS disease with high CSF protein

Entamoeba histolytica

BASIC INFORMATION

- Amebiasis is caused by *Entamoeba histolytica*
  - By contrast, *E. dispar* and others in this genus are commensal organisms that do not cause disease

- Ingestion of cysts in contaminated food or water. Invasive disease: ulceration of colonic mucosa, hematogenous spread via portal vein
- Increased risk: history of residence in endemic areas, those living in institutional settings, men who have sex with men, and people with HIV/AIDS
- Severe disease in young children, pregnant women, older adults, and in the setting of malnutrition

CLINICAL PRESENTATION

- Progressive, bloody diarrhea and abdominal pain lasting weeks to months in some cases. May be associated with weight loss, stunting, and malnutrition
- Amebic liver abscess: fever, right upper quadrant abdominal pain, hepatomegaly, weight loss
- Amebiasis may be misdiagnosed as inflammatory bowel disease. Corticosteroid treatment may result in fulminant, fatal disease

DIAGNOSIS AND EVALUATION

- Liver abscesses may be seen on abdominal imaging
- Enzyme immunoassay (EIA) test of stool specimen is sensitive and specific
- Serologies support diagnosis

TREATMENT

- Asymptomatic infection: a luminal agent (paromomycin or diloxanide furoate)
- Amebic colitis or liver abscess: metronidazole or tinidazole, followed by a luminal agent

Giardia

BASIC INFORMATION

- *Giardia intestinalis* is the most common intestinal parasite diagnosed in the United States
- *Giardia* trophozoites attach to the intestinal wall via a sucking disk, damaging epithelial cells and brush border
- Risk factors are presented in Table 46.4

CLINICAL PRESENTATION

- Clinical presentation is discussed in Table 46.4

DIAGNOSIS AND EVALUATION

- *Giardia* trophozoites or cysts on microscopic examination of stool specimens
- *Giardia* antigens detected by EIA or by PCR
- Biopsy may be performed of small intestine in the setting of persistent symptoms with negative stool testing

TREATMENT

- Treatment is discussed in Table 46.4

Table 46.4. Comparison of Giardiasis and Cryptosporidiosis

Disease	Giardiasis	Cryptosporidiosis
Clinical presentation	Infection may be asymptomatic or may cause acute or chronic watery diarrhea. Chronic diarrhea may be associated with persistent abdominal cramps, bloating, flatulence, nausea, anorexia, and weight loss. Malabsorption or failure to thrive may occur.	Profuse, watery, nonbloody diarrhea. May be associated with abdominal pain, nausea, vomiting, fever, fatigue, anorexia, weight loss. Some patients have associated biliary tract disease. Severe, prolonged diarrheal disease in immunocompromised patients.
Epidemiology /risk factors	Child care center attendance, ingestion of contaminated water (e.g., ingestion of mountain stream water while hiking/camping, or recreational water exposures), travel to endemic areas, exposure to infected animals or persons, and men who have sex with men. Immunocompromising conditions: Common variable immunodeficiency, X-linked agammaglobulinemia.	Ingestion of contaminated water or food, or exposure to infected persons or animals. Outbreaks associated with recreational water parks or pools, child care centers, and hospitals. May be travel associated. Immunocompromising conditions: HIV/AIDS, malignancy, transplantation, or severe combined immunodeficiency (SCID), or malnourished children.
Treatment	Tinidazole, nitazoxanide, or metronidazole.	Immunocompetent patients: supportive care. Immunocompromised patients or severe disease: nitazoxanide.

Cryptosporidium

BASIC INFORMATION

- Infections are typically caused by *Cryptosporidium hominis* or *C. parvum*
- Risk factors are presented in Table 46.4
- Important cause of malabsorption, malnutrition, and developmental delays in children in developing countries

CLINICAL PRESENTATION

- Clinical presentation is discussed in Table 46.4

DIAGNOSIS AND EVALUATION

- May be detected by EIA or immunofluorescence assays (IFA)
- Oocysts seen on microscopic examination of stool specimens

TREATMENT

- Treatment is discussed in Table 46.4

Plasmodium (Malaria)

BASIC INFORMATION

- Human malaria disease is caused by *Plasmodium falciparum*, *P. vivax*, *P. ovale*, *P. malariae*, and *P. knowlesi*, with the most severe and fatal forms of the disease caused by *P. falciparum*
- In the United States, most cases are seen in patients with a history of travel to or residence in malaria-endemic areas. Diagnosis requires a high index of suspicion in patients with history of travel to areas of malaria endemicity
- More severe disease is seen in young children, persons without previous exposure to malaria, and persons who had moved away from an endemic area for a period of years
- Globally, most deaths occur in sub-Saharan Africa, predominantly among children <5 years of age
- *Plasmodium* sporozoites are transmitted by the bite of *Anopheles* mosquitoes. Asexual reproduction occurs in the liver. Resulting merozoites invade red blood cells to become trophozoite forms. These in turn develop into schizonts. Red cells ultimately rupture, releasing merozoites that go on to invade other red cells. Febrile episodes may cycle with the synchronized rupture of red cells and the release of merozoites; however, the classic description of cyclic fevers is not typical, particularly in children
- Sexual differentiation occurs within the red cells. Male and female gametocytes are taken up again by the bite of an *Anopheles* mosquito, and sexual reproduction stages occur within the mosquito

CLINICAL PRESENTATION

- Malaria is characterized by high fever, chills, headache, abdominal pain, nausea, vomiting, and diarrhea
  - Laboratory testing: Thrombocytopenia and hyponatremia may be seen
- Severe malaria: hyperparasitemia (≥5%), severe anemia, hypoglycemia, metabolic acidosis with respiratory distress, electrolyte disturbances, renal dysfunction, ARDS, hemoglobinuria, coagulopathy, hypotension
  - Cerebral malaria: altered mental status, seizures, coma
- Malaria can be rapidly fatal

DIAGNOSIS AND EVALUATION

- Recognition and testing for malaria is critical, as many malaria deaths in the United States are due to delays in diagnosis. *Any febrile patient with history of travel to or residence in an endemic area should be tested for malaria*
- Thick and thin blood smears should be performed; multiple smears may be needed if parasitemia is low

- Rapid diagnostic tests (RDTs), where available, are sensitive and specific for *P. falciparum* malaria, although sensitivity is reduced in low parasitemia and for non-*falciparum* species. RDTs may be particularly helpful where technical expertise in reading blood smears is limited; all RDTs should, however, be accompanied by blood smears

TREATMENT

- See treatment guidelines from the Centers for Disease Control and Prevention (CDC) for detailed management recommendations (available at https://www.cdc.gov/malaria/diagnosis_treatment/index.html)
- Children with suspected *P. falciparum* malaria should be hospitalized
- In cases of severe malaria or in those not tolerating oral therapy, patients should be treated intravenously with quinidine in combination with either doxycycline, tetracycline, or clindamycin
- Close monitoring is needed for cardiac status (QT prolongation, hypotension) due to quinidine, and for hypoglycemia, anemia, and electrolyte abnormalities
- Exchange transfusion may be needed for very high parasitemia or severe complications
- Blood smears should be repeated on treatment to monitor trend in parasitemia in response to therapy
- Oral treatment options for patients with uncomplicated malaria:
  - Artemether-lumefantrine, atovaquone-proguanil, or a combination of oral quinine sulfate and either doxycycline, tetracycline, or clindamycin

- Noncomplicated, non-*falciparum* malaria acquired in areas without chloroquine resistance may be treated with chloroquine
- If infection is due to *P. vivax* or *P. ovale*, additionally treat with primaquine to eradicate hypnozoite forms (liver stage) and prevent relapse

Review Questions

For review questions, please go to ExpertConsult.com.

Suggested Readings

1. American Academy of Pediatrics. *Pneumocystis jirovecii* infections. In: Kimberlin DW, Brady MT, Jackson MA, Long SS, eds. *Red Book: 2015 Report of the Committee on Infectious Diseases.* 30th ed. Elk Grove Village, IL: American Academy of Pediatrics; 2015:638–644.
2. Centers for Disease Control and Prevention. Malaria diagnosis and treatment in the United States. Available at https://www.cdc.gov/malaria/diagnosis_treatment/index.html.
3. Panel on Opportunistic Infections in HIV-Exposed and HIV-Infected Children. Guidelines for the prevention and treatment of opportunistic infections in HIV-exposed and HIV-infected children. Department of Health and Human Services. Available at: http://aidsinfo.nih.gov/contentfiles/lvguidelines/oi_guidelines_pediatrics.pdf.
4. Pappas PG, Kauffman CA, Andes DR, et al. Clinical practice guideline for the management of candidiasis: 2016 update by the Infectious Diseases Society of America. *Clin Infect Dis.* 2016;62(4):e1–e50.
5. Patterson TF, Thompson 3rd GR, Denning DW, et al. Practice guidelines for the diagnosis and management of aspergillosis: 2016 update by the Infectious Diseases Society of America. *Clin Infect Dis.* 2016;63(4):e1–e60.

47 Therapeutic Agents in Infectious Diseases

EVELYN LAI, RN, MSN, PNP-BC and BEATRIZ LARRU, MD, PhD

Antibacterial Drugs

PRINCIPLES OF ANTIINFECTIVE THERAPY

- Antibiotics should be used only when an infection is truly present or likely. Inappropriate use of antibiotics (i.e., for a viral infection) results in:
  - Exposing children to the adverse side effects of antibiotics
  - Selective pressure driving antibiotic resistance
  - Increases in health care cost
  - Possible delays in appropriate evaluation and treatment for the child's symptoms
- When selecting antimicrobial therapy, clinicians must consider:
  - Patient's characteristics (age, immune status, clinical severity, allergies, etc.)
  - Likely infectious organisms (use narrower-spectrum antibiotic)
  - Pharmacokinetic/pharmacodynamic (PK/PD) properties of the drug
  - Risk of drug toxicity in certain clinical scenarios (e.g., acute kidney injury [AKI])
  - See also Nelson Textbook of Pediatrics, Part 17, "Infectious Diseases."

ANTIINFECTIVE AGENT DOSING

- PK reflects the concentration of antibiotic over time
- PD describes the type of exposure needed for cure. It is usually described as:
  - Time dependent:
    - %T > minimum inhibitory concentration (MIC) = percentage of time in a 24-hour dosing interval that the antibiotic concentrations are above the MIC (MIC = the antibiotic concentration required for inhibition of growth of an organism)
  - Concentration dependent:
    - AUC = the area below the serum concentration versus time curve
    - C_{max} = maximal concentration of drug achieved at the tissue site
- Antibiotics that inhibit growth of the organism without killing it are termed *bacteriostatic* (minimum bactericidal concentration [MBC]/MIC ratio >4), whereas antibiotics that kill the organism are called *bactericidal*

MECHANISMS OF ANTIBIOTICS RESISTANCE

- Multiple mechanisms of antibiotics resistance are employed by bacteria. It should be noted that multiple mechanisms can be used by a single bacteria with an additive effect, particularly in Gram-negative bacilli (GNRs)
1. Enzymatic degradation or modification of the antibiotic
   - β-lactamases
     - Penicillinases inactivate penicillin in *Staphylococcus aureus*
     - A variety of enzymes do the same in GNRs (e.g., extended-spectrum β-lactamase [ESBL], klebsiella pneumoniae carbapenemase [KPC], cefotaximase [CTX-M], New Delhi metallo-beta-lactamase [NDM])
   - Acetyltransferases can inactivate aminoglycosides
   - Esterases can hydrolyze macrolides
2. Reduction in the bacterial antibiotic concentration
   - Cell wall permeability changes
     - Methicillin-resistant *S. aureus* (MRSA) has thickened cell wall requiring higher doses of vancomycin
   - Production of efflux pumps that actively pump tetracycline, macrolides, aminoglycosides, or fluoroquinolone in GNRs
   - Loss of porins in *Pseudomonas aeruginosa* that reduces carbapenem penetration
3. Modification of the antibiotic target site
   - Changes in target enzymes:
     - Lower affinity or decreased number of penicillin-binding proteins (PBPs) in penicillin-resistant *S. pneumoniae*
     - Low-affinity PBP2 encoded by *mecA* gene in MRSA
   - Alteration of cell wall precursors
     - Loss of terminal *D-ala* and *D-ala* in vancomycin-resistant *Enterococcus*
   - Alterations in ribosomal binding site
- Types of antibiotics resistance
  - Constitutively: expressed continuously
  - Inducible: expressed only when exposed to the antibiotic (i.e., β-lactamase activity encoded by *AmpC* in *Enterobacter* spp.)

INTERPRETATION OF SUSCEPTIBILITY RESULTS

- The MIC value at which an organism changes from susceptible to nonsusceptible is called *breakpoint*
- Absolute values of MIC for a single organism should not be compared across different drugs

Antibiotic Agents

- See Table 47.1 for details regarding pharmacology and side effects of antibacterial classes
- See Table 47.2 for details regarding spectrum of activity for individual antibacterial agents

Antiviral Agents (Other Than Antiretroviral Agents)

- Antiviral agents derive their effects by targeting specific functions during the virus life cycle (e.g., viral entry, transcription and replication, protein synthesis, viral assembly and release), often acting at a single step in viral replication
- As with antibacterial agents, resistance may develop to antiviral agents

- See Tables 47.3 and 47.4 for details regarding individual antivirals

Antifungal Agents

- Major sterol in fungi cell membranes is ergosterol (rather than cholesterol, as in human cells). This main difference has been exploited in antifungals development

Table 47.1. Antibacterial Classes by Mechanism of Action With Most Notable PK/PD Characteristics and Common Adverse Effects

Mechanism of Action	Antibacterial Class	PK/PD Characteristics	Toxicity/Monitoring
Cell wall synthesis	β-lactams PNCs Cephalosporins Monobactam Carbapenems	Time-dependent (%T > MIC) Bactericidal (maximum effect on rapid-growing bacteria) PNCs have very short half-life (<2 hours); ceftriaxone and doripenem can have once-daily dosing. Aztreonam has no cross-reactivity with other β-lactams (can be used in PNC-allergic for GNRs)	Hypersensitivity reactions (PNCs 1%–10% > cephalosporins 1%–3% > carbapenems) Seizures (PNC, Imipenem), biliary sludge (ceftriaxone), hepatitis (methicillin), nephrotoxicity, neutropenia (especially nafcillin and PNC G), hemolytic anemia, cephalosporins interfere vitamin K metabolism Avoid calcium-containing fluids concomitant with ceftriaxone. *Monitor CBC q 2–4 weeks* with PNC and cephalosporin
	Glycopeptides: Vancomycin, Dalbavancin, Oritavancin, Telavancin	AUC/MIC, bactericidal, vancomycin PO not absorbed, once-weekly dosing for dalbavancin and oritavancin	Nephrotoxicity, "Red man syndrome" due to histamine release (not hypersensitivity) *TDM essential*
Cell membrane	Lipopeptides: daptomycin	Concentration-dependent, prolonged PAE, bactericidal, cannot be used for pneumonia, synergy with β-lactams, aminoglycosides	Myopathy, neuropathy, eosinophilic pneumonia *Follow CPK q1–2 weeks*
	Polymyxins: polymyxin B, colistin	Concentration-dependent, use revisited for highly resistant GNRs	Nephrotoxicity, neurotoxicity
Protein synthesis (50S ribosome)	Macrolides/azalides Ketolides: telithromycin	AUC/MIC, Bacteriostatic, high intracellular concentrations	Gastrointestinal (erythromycin), rash, rare hepatotoxicity, prolongation QT
	Lincosamides: clindamycin	Bactericidal/bacteriostatic depending on site, bacteria, and drug concentration; 90% bioavailability, AUC/MIC	Diarrhea, rare hepatotoxicity
	Chloramphenicol	95%–100% bioavailability, rarely used	Irreversible bone marrow suppression
	Streptogramins: quinupristin-dalfopristin	Bactericidal	Phlebitis, myalgia, arthralgia
	Oxazolidinones: linezolid	Bacteriostatic, 95%–100% bioavailability	Bone marrow suppression, neuropathy, lactic acidosis *Monitor CBC q1–2 weeks*
Protein synthesis (30S ribosome)	Tetracycline Glycylcyclines: tigecycline	95%–100% bioavailability, absorption impaired by minerals, bacteriostatic low serum concentrations, bacteriostatic	Deposition into teeth and bones, photosensitivity, esophageal ulcers, pseudotumor cerebri Gastrointestinal
	Aminoglycosides	Concentration-dependent (C_{max}/MIC), prolonged PAE, bactericidal, synergistic killing of GP with cell wall agents, not active in low pH (pus) or low O_2	Nephrotoxicity, ototoxicity (permanent severe high-frequency bilateral sensorineural), neuromuscular blockade *Very low ratio of therapeutic benefit to toxic side effect; TDM essential*
DNA replication	Fluoroquinolones	Concentration-dependent (AUC/MIC) Prolonged PAE, 60%–100% bioavailability, absorption impaired by minerals, bactericidal	Gastrointestinal, prolongation QT, gastrointestinal, rupture of Achilles tendon, cartilage damage (in animal studies)
Nucleic acid structure	Nitroimidazoles: metronidazole	Concentration-dependent, prolonged PAE 95%–100% bioavailability, bactericidal	Peripheral neuropathy, encephalopathy, disulfiram reactions, gynecomastia
RNA polymerase	Rifamycins	Use in combination because mutations arise very rapidly, rifaximin not absorbed	Hepatotoxicity, bone marrow suppression, nephritis, colors body fluid, drug interactions
Folate metabolism	Sulfamethoxazole-trimethoprim	Concentration-dependent, 95%–100% bioavailability, bactericidal	Hypersensitivity reactions, bone marrow suppression, nephrotoxicity, hemolytic anemia

AUC, Area under the curve; *CBC,* complete blood count; *CPK,* creatine phosphokinase; *GNRs,* Gram-negative rods; *GP,* Gram-positive organisms; *MIC,* minimal inhibitory concentration; *PAE,* postantibiotic effect; *PD,* pharmacodynamic; *PK,* pharmacokinetic; *PNC,* penicillin; *PO,* oral route; *TDM,* therapeutic drug monitoring. Bioavailability: percent of a non-IV-administered drug that enters the bloodstream (i.e., PO) relative to an IV formulation of the same drug.

Table 47.2.   Antibacterial Classes by Spectrum of Activity

CELL WALL–ACTIVE AGENTS	
Penicillins	**Spectrum of Activity**
Natural PNCs: PO: penicillin V IV: penicillin V, penicillin G benzathine, penicillin G procaine, penicillin G benzathine plus procaine	*Gram-positive* (GAS, GBS, *S. viridans* group, *S. pneumoniae,* Enterococcus, Listeria) *Few Gram-negative* (*N. meningitidis,* Eikenella) *Anaerobes* (Clostridium, Actinomyces, Fusobacterium, Prevotella) *Other pathogens* (Treponema, Borrelia, Leptospira)
Penicillinase-stable PNCs: PO: dicloxacillin, cloxacillin IV: oxacillin, methicillin, nafcillin	*Gram-positive* (GAS, GBS, *S. pneumoniae* plus *S. aureus*—except MRSA) (drug of choice for MSSA)
Aminopenicillins: PO: amoxicillin IV: ampicillin	*Gram-positive* (as above for penicillins) (ampicillin is the drug of choice for susceptible Enterococci) *Gram-negative* (*E. coli, H. influenzae, N. meningitidis*) *Anaerobes* (as above for penicillins)
Carboxy/ureido PNCs: IV: ticarcillin, carbenicillin, piperacillin	*Gram-positive* (same Streptococci as penicillin) *Gram-negative* (*E. coli, H. influenzae,* Proteus, Klebsiella, Enterobacter, Serratia, *P. aeruginosa*) *Anaerobes* (Clostridium, Fusobacterium, Bacteroides, Prevotella)
β-Lactamase inhibitors PO: amoxicillin/clavulanate IV: ampicillin/sulbactam, ticarcillin/clavulanate, piperacillin/tazobactam, ceftazidime/avibactam	Adds β-lactamase-producing strains that the β-lactam in the combination has intrinsic activity. Avibactam has the broadest spectrum of activity.
Cephalosporins	**Spectrum of Activity**
First-generation: PO: cephalexin IV: cefazolin	*Gram-positive* (as above for Penicillinase-stable PNCs) *Gram-negative* (*E. coli,* Klebsiella, Proteus)
Second-generation: PO: cefaclor, cefprozil, cefuroxime IV: cefuroxime, cefoxitin, cefotetan (cephamycin)	*Gram-positive* (as above for first generation but weaker activity) *Gram-negative* (*E. coli, H. influenzae,* Klebsiella, Proteus, Salmonella, Shigella, Neisseria) *Few anaerobes* (cefoxitin/cefotetan)
Third-generation: PO: cefixime, cefdinir IV: cefotaxime, ceftriaxone, ceftazidime	*Gram-positive* (GAS, GBS, *S. viridans* group, *S. pneumoniae, S. aureus*—except MRSA) *Gram-negative* (*E. coli, H. influenzae, N. meningitidis,* Proteus) (For ceftazidime: *P. aeruginosa*)
Fourth-generation: IV: cefepime	*Gram-positive* (GAS, GBS, *S. viridans* group, *S. pneumoniae, S. aureus*—except MRSA) *Gram-negative* (as above for third generation, plus Enterobacter, Citrobacter, Serratia, *P. aeruginosa*)
Fifth-generation: IV: ceftaroline	As above for ceftriaxone/cefotaxime, plus MRSA (does not cover *P. aeruginosa*)
Carbapenems	**Spectrum of Activity**
IV: imipenem (+ cilastatin), meropenem, ertapenem, doripenem	*Gram-positive* (as above for fourth-generation cephalosporins, plus *Enterococcus faecalis*) *Gram-negative* (as above for fourth-generation cephalosporins, including ESBL-producing strains); *P. aeruginosa* except for ertapenem. Not Burkholderia or Stenotrophomonas *Anaerobes* (as extended-spectrum penicillins plus β-lactamase-producing strains) *Other pathogens* (nontuberculous Mycobacteria)
Monobactam	**Spectrum of Activity**
IV: aztreonam	*Gram-negative* (as third-generation cephalosporins, including *P. aeruginosa*)
Glycopeptides	**Spectrum of Activity**
Vancomycin, dalbavancin, oritavancin, telavancin	*Gram-positive* (GAS, GBS, *S. viridans* group, *S. pneumoniae, S. aureus*—including MRSA, Enterococcus, *S. epidermidis,* Listeria) *Anaerobes* (*Clostridium difficile*)
CELL MEMBRANE ACTIVE AGENTS	
Lipopeptides	**Spectrum of Activity**
Daptomycin	*Gram-positive* (GAS, GBS, *S. viridans,* *S.* pneumoniae, *S. aureus*—including MRSA, Enterococcus—including VRE)
Polymyxins	**Spectrum of Activity**
Colistin	*Gram-negative* (*E. coli, H. influenzae,* Klebsiella, Salmonella, Shigella, Enterobacter, Serratia, Citrobacter, Acinetobacter, *P. aeruginosa*)

Table 47.2.   Antibacterial Classes by Spectrum of Activity—cont'd

RIBOSOME ACTIVE AGENTS

Macrolides/Azalides/Ketolides	Spectrum of Activity
Erythromycin/clarithromycin, azithromycin/ telithromycin	*Gram-positive* (GAS, *S. pneumoniae, S. aureus*) *Gram-negative* (*H. influenzae*, Bordetella pertussis, Legionella, *Neisseria gonorrhoeae*, Bartonella (*Helicobacter pylori* for clarithromycin) *Other pathogens* (Chlamydia, Mycoplasma, Ureaplasma, for clarithromycin and azithromycin nontuberculous Mycobacteria)

Tetracyclines	Spectrum of Activity
Tetracycline, minocycline, doxycycline	*Gram-positive* (Actinomyces, Listeria) *Gram-negative* (Neisseria, Campylobacter, Brucella, Vibrio, Yersinia, Rickettsia) *Other pathogens* (Borrelia, Chlamydia, Entamoeba Mycoplasma, Ureaplasma, Treponema)

Glycylcyclines	Spectrum of Activity
Tigecycline	*Gram-positive* (GAS, GBS, *S. viridans* group, *S. pneumoniae, S. aureus*—including MRSA, Enterococcus, Listeria) *Gram-negative* (*E. coli, H. Klebsiella,* Shigella, Enterobacter, Serratia, Citrobacter, Acinetobacter, Pasteurella, Stenotrophomonas) Not *P. aeruginosa* *Other pathogens* (Chlamydia, Mycoplasma, Ureaplasma, nontuberculous Mycobacteria)

Lincosamides	Spectrum of Activity
Clindamycin	*Gram-positive* (GAS, GBS, *S. pneumoniae, S. aureus*—including MRSA), not Enterococcus *Anaerobes* (Actinomyces, Clostridium, Propionibacterium, Fusobacterium, Prevotella, Bacteroides) *Other pathogens* (Toxoplasma, Plasmodium, Pneumocystis in combination with other drugs)

Aminoglycosides	Spectrum of Activity
Gentamicin, tobramycin, amikacin	*Gram-positive* (*S. aureus,* synergy with PNC for Streptococci and Enterococcus) *Gram-negative* (*E. coli*, Klebsiella, Proteus, Enterobacter, Serratia, Citrobacter, Acinetobacter, Providencia, *P. aeruginosa*)
Streptomycin	*Gram-negative* (Brucella, Francisella) *Other pathogens* (*Mycobacterium tuberculosis*)
Paromomycin	*Other pathogens* (Entamoeba, Cryptosporidium)

Oxazolidinones	Spectrum of Activity
Linezolid, tedizolid	*Gram-positive* (GAS, GBS, *S. viridans, S. pneumoniae, S. aureus*—including MRSA; Enterococcus, including VRE)

Streptogramins	Spectrum of Activity
Quinupristin/dalfopristin	*Gram-positive* (GAS, GBS, *S. aureus* (including MRSA), *Enterococcus faecium* (including VRE)

NUCLEIC ACID ACTIVE AGENTS

Rifamycins	Spectrum of Activity
Rifampin	*Gram-positive* (*S. aureus*) *Gram-negative* (*Neisseria meningitides, H. influenzae*) *Other pathogens* (*Mycobacterium tuberculosis*, Mycobacterium avium complex)
Rifabutin, rifapentine	*Other pathogens* (*Mycobacterium tuberculosis*, Mycobacterium avium complex)
Rifaximin	*Gram-negative*, within gastrointestinal tract (*E. coli*, Campylobacter, Salmonella, Shigella, Vibrio, Yersinia)

Quinolones/Fluoroquinolones	Spectrum of Activity
Nalidixic acid	*Gram-negative* (*E. coli*, Proteus, Providencia, Morganella)
Ciprofloxacin	*Gram-positive* (GAS, *S. pneumoniae, S. aureus,* Enterococcus) *Gram-negative* (*E. coli*, Klebsiella, Campylobacter, Proteus, *H. influenzae,* Moraxella, Neisseria, Vibrio, Providencia, Campylobacter, Citrobacter, Serratia, Acinetobacter, Enterobacter, *P. aeruginosa*)
Levofloxacin, moxifloxacin, gatifloxacin	*Gram-positive* (GAS, *S. pneumoniae, S. viridans, S. aureus,* Enterococcus, Listeria) *Gram-negative* (*E. coli*, Klebsiella, Proteus, *H. influenzae,* Moraxella, Campylobacter, Citrobacter, Serratia, Acinetobacter, Enterobacter, *P. aeruginosa*) *Anaerobes* (Actinomyces, Bacillus, Clostridium) *Other pathogens* (Legionella, Chlamydophila, Mycoplasma)

Continued

Table 47.2. Antibacterial Classes by Spectrum of Activity—cont'd

Nitroimidazoles	Spectrum of Activity
Metronidazole	*Anaerobes* (Clostridium, Bacteroides, Fusobacterium, Peptococcus) *Other pathogens* (Giardia, Amoeba, Trichomonas)

Sulfonamides (Combined With Other Agents)	Spectrum of Activity
Sulfamethoxazole/trimethoprim	*Gram-positive* (S. pneumoniae, S. aureus—including MRSA, Nocardia) *Gram-negative* (E. coli, Klebsiella, H. influenzae, Proteus, Shigella, Morganella, Enterobacter, Stenotrophomonas, Burkholderia) *Other pathogens* (Pneumocystis jirovecii)
Sulfadiazine/pyrimethamine	*Other pathogens* (Toxoplasma gondii, Plasmodium)

GAS, Group A streptococcus; *GBS,* group B streptococcus; *ESBL,* extended-spectrum β-lactamase; *MRSA,* methicillin-resistant *Staphylococcus aureus; MSSA,* methicillin-sensitive *S. aureus; PNC,* penicillin; *VRE,* vancomycin-resistant Enterococcus.

Table 47.3. Anti–Herpes Virus Agents—Anti–DNA Virus Activity

Acyclovir	Nucleoside Analogue
Mechanism of action	Competitive inhibition of viral DNA polymerase; terminates DNA chain Dependent on phosphorylation by viral thymidine kinase (TK) for activation
Spectrum	Potent activity against HSV followed by VZV, moderate for CMV, minimal against EBV. Not effective against latent-state virus
PK	IV formulation with good tissue penetration and high concentrations (including CSF) PO poorly absorbed. Eliminated by kidneys and can crystallize in renal tubules
Adverse effects	Obstructive uropathy, interstitial nephritis, neurotoxicities with high doses, neutropenia, phlebitis
Resistance	▪ Primarily seen in immunocompromised patients with prolonged exposure ▪ Occurs via mutation in the *TK* gene, mutation of DNA polymerase less common
Indications (PO, IV, topical)	▪ Primary HSV infection, recurrent HSV disease, and severe HSV (including encephalitis, neonatal disease, mucocutaneous diseases) ▪ VZV infections ▪ Prophylaxis in immunocompromised patients (usually first 30 days post-HSCT) ▪ Prophylaxis of monkey bites for simian Herpes B virus
Others	▪ Valacyclovir (PO): prodrug of acyclovir, similar spectrum to acyclovir but 3–5× bioavailability ▪ Famciclovir (PO) and penciclovir (topical): similar spectrum to acyclovir
Ganciclovir	**Nucleoside Analogue**
Mechanism of action	Competitive inhibition of viral DNA polymerase, dependent on phosphorylation by viral kinase (encoded by *UL97* gene in CMV or *TK* in HSV and VZV)
Spectrum	Potent activity against CMV, active against all herpesviruses (active also against cellular DNA polymerases)
PK	Distributed to CSF and brain tissue, high concentrations in aqueous and vitreous humor and subretinal fluid; renally eliminated
Adverse effects	Significant myelosuppression, CNS effects, mild nephrotoxicities, hepatitis
Resistance	▪ Primarily seen in HIV patients with prolonged exposure ▪ Conferred by mutations of *UL97* (viral kinase, only affects ganciclovir, most common) or *UL54* (DNA polymerase, also affects cidofovir and foscarnet)
Indications (IV, intra-vitreous)	▪ CMV retinitis ▪ Severe CMV disease in neonates, immunocompromised patients ▪ Prophylaxis of CMV disease in high-risk populations ▪ Other: adenovirus infection
Others	▪ Valganciclovir (PO): prodrug of ganciclovir, absorbed in the intestine and converted to ganciclovir by intestinal and hepatic metabolism. Same spectrum as ganciclovir.
Foscarnet	**Pyrophosphate Analogue**
Mechanism of action	Noncompetitive inhibition via blocking of viral polymerase binding site—no phosphorylation required (active against HSV-TK and CMV-UL97)
Spectrum	Herpesviruses, HIV, HBV
PK	80% eliminated unmetabolized by kidneys; remaining 20% deposited in teeth and bones; CSF levels are 60% that of plasma
Adverse effects	Significant renal toxicities including renal tubular acidosis and interstitial nephritis, symptoms associated with electrolyte abnormalities (calcium, phosphate, magnesium, and potassium); some CNS effects
Resistance	Conferred by mutations of DNA polymerase

Table 47.3. Anti–Herpes Virus Agents—Anti–DNA Virus Activity—cont'd

Foscarnet	Pyrophosphate Analogue
Indications (IV, intravitreous)	■ CMV retinitis in patients with HIV ■ Acyclovir-resistant HSV, VZV infections ■ Ganciclovir-resistant CMV infections.

Cidofovir	Nucleotide Analogue
Mechanism of action	Selective inhibition of viral DNA polymerase—no phosphorylation required
Spectrum	Broad spectrum against DNA viruses (herpesviruses, papillomavirus, polyomavirus, adenovirus)
PK	Renal clearance by tubular secretion; no clear data on CNS penetration
Adverse effects	Significantly nephrotoxic (requires prehydration and coadministration with probenecid), Fanconi syndrome, ocular toxicities, neutropenia, reproductive toxicities, carcinogenesis, metabolic acidosis
Resistance	Conferred by mutations of DNA polymerase
Indications (IV)	■ CMV retinitis ■ Ganciclovir-resistant CMV disease. ■ Other uses in immunocompromised: BK hemorrhagic cystitis, Adenovirus ■ Intractable airway papilloma: HHV8 (intralesional)

CMV, Cytomegalovirus; *CNS*, central nervous system; *CSF*, cerebrospinal fluid; *EBV*, Epstein-Barr virus; *HBV*, hepatitis B virus; *HSCT*, hematopoietic stem cell transplantation; *HSV*, herpes simplex virus; *IV*, intravenous; *PK*, pharmacokinetics; *PO*, by mouth; *VZV*, varicella-zoster virus.

Table 47.4. Anti-Respiratory Viruses Agents—Anti-RNA virus activity

Ribavirin	Nucleoside Analogue
Mechanism of action	Interference with processing and translation of viral mRNA
Spectrum	Broad antiviral activity: RNA viruses >> DNA viruses—No resistance documented
PK	Primary renal elimination with hepatic metabolism, concentrates and persists in erythrocytes
Adverse effects	*Oral/IV:* hemolytic anemia, hyperbilirubinemia, teratogenic and embryocidal in animal studies; *Inhalation:* conjunctivitis, facial rash or bronchospasm
Indications (PO, IV, Inhalation)	■ Life-threating respiratory syncytial virus bronchiolitis (moderate effect, difficult to administer) ■ Hemorrhagic fevers (Lassa fever) ■ Combination therapy with interferon for treatment of chronic hepatitis C virus in adults

Amantadine and Rimantadine	Tricyclic amines
Mechanism of action	Blocks the H+ ion channel manufactured by viral M2 protein
Spectrum	Influenza A virus (influenza B lacks M2 protein—not susceptible)
PK	Well absorbed—Rimantadine is 10-fold more active
Adverse effects	Gastrointestinal and central nervous system disturbances—Amantadine more toxic
Resistance	Conferred by point mutations in M2 protein—cross- resistance occurs
Indications (PO)	Due to resistance is no longer recommended for treatment or prophylaxis of influenza virus

Oseltamivir and Zanamivir	Neuraminidase Inhibitors
Mechanism of action	Inhibition of viral neuraminidase preventing virus escape from cell
Spectrum	Influenza viruses (both A and B)
PK	■ *Oseltamivir*—high bioavailability, eliminated by kidneys ■ *Zanamivir*—renally eliminated, but minimal systemic absorption
Adverse effects	*Zanamivir:* bronchospasm; *Oseltamivir:* gastrointestinal upset
Resistance	Rare—Mutations in viral neuraminidase and/or hemagglutinin Oseltamivir >> Zanamivir; cross-resistance unusual
Indications (PO, Oseltamivir; inhalation, Zanamivir)	Treatment and prophylaxis of influenza A and B
Others:	Peramivir (IV): Inhibits influenza neuraminidase. FDA approved for uncomplicated influenza in adults.

PK, pharmacokinetics.

■ Fungi exist in two basic forms: *yeast*—unicellular forms (Candida, Cryptococcus)—and *molds*—branching hyphae (Aspergillus, Fusarium, Zygomycetes). *Dimorphic fungi* (Histoplasma, Blastomyces, Coccidioides) can exist in either form

■ See Tables 47.5 and 47.6 for details regarding antifungal agents

Table 47.5. Mechanism of Action of Antifungal Classes

Antifungal Class	Mechanism of Action
Polyene	Binds to ergosterol in cell *membrane,* causing cell lysis
Azole	Inhibits ergosterol production in *cell membranes*
Echinocandin	Inhibits *cell wall* β-1, 3-D-glucan production
Pyrimidine analogues	Inhibit RNA and *protein synthesis*
Allyamines	Inhibit cell membrane squalene epoxidase

Table 47.6. Antifungal Agents by Mechanism of Action With Spectrum of Activity, PK/PD Characteristics and Common Adverse Effects

Antifungal Agents	PK/PD Characteristics	Spectrum of Activity	Toxicity
Polyenes: Amphotericin B deoxycholate (IV) Lipid formulations of amphotericin B (IV) Nystatin (topical)	High serum concentrations (poor CSF) Very slow excretion by urine and bile (terminal half-life = 15 days) Fungicidal antifungal activity Concentration-dependent killing with prolonged postantifungal effect	*Candida* spp. and Aspergillus (salvage therapy), Cryptococcus, dimorphic fungi, Zygomycetes—not *C. lusitaniae, A. terreus,* Fusarium, Trichosporon Broadest-spectrum antifungal	Nephrotoxicity and electrolyte (K+, Mg+) wasting, anaphylaxis, infusion-related reactions (fever, rigors) Decreased nephrotoxicity with lipid formulations (with similar efficacy)
Pyrimidine analogues: Flucytosine (5-FC) (PO)	Resistance develops quickly—never use as monotherapy	Enhances antifungal activity of amphotericin in tissues with poor penetration (CSF, hear valves); Cryptococcal and Candida meningitis	Bone marrow suppression, gastrointestinal TDM indicated
Azoles: Imidazoles: miconazole, clotrimazole (topical), ketoconazole (topical, PO) Triazoles: fluconazole, itraconazole, voriconazole, posaconazole, isavuconazole (IV, PO)	▪ Fluconazole: 90% bioavailability, good CSF penetration, concentrates in urine, double loading dose ▪ Itraconazole: bioavailability capsules << solution (empty stomach) ▪ Voriconazole: linear PK in children, hepatic metabolism ▪ Posaconazole: food increases absorption, saturable kineticsAzoles are fungicidal against molds and fungistatic against yeast	▪ Fluconazole: Candida (not *C. krusei* or *C. glabrata*), Cryptococcus, Histoplasma, Coccidiomycosis—not active against molds ▪ Itraconazole: dimorphic fungi, Aspergillosis (mild diseases) ▪ Voriconazole: Aspergillus (drug of choice), Fusarium, Candida—not active in Mucormycosis- ▪ Posaconazole: Aspergillus, Candida, Mucormycosis, dimorphic fungi	▪ Fluconazole: hepatotoxicity, drug interactions ▪ Itraconazole: drug interactions, gastrointestinal, hepatotoxicity ▪ Voriconazole: hepatotoxicity, visual, photosensitivity, hallucinations, nephrotoxicity with IV formulation ▪ Posaconazole: hepatotoxicity, drug interactions Itraconazole, Voriconazole and Posaconazole—essential TDM
Echinocandins: Caspofungin, Micafungin, Anidulafungin (IV)	Fungicidal against Candida, fungistatic against Aspergillus Does not accumulate in urine, poor CSF penetration	Candida (critically ill patients), Aspergillus (alternative therapy), not active against Cryptococcus	Good safety profile; lower doses in severe hepatic dysfunction

CSF, Cerebrospinal fluid; *IV,* Intravenous route; *PD,* pharmacodynamic; *PK,* pharmacokinetic; *PO,* oral route; *TDM,* therapeutic drug monitoring.
Topical antifungals: Azoles: clotrimazole, miconazole, ketoconazole; Polyenes: Nystatin. Other: terbinafine (PO, topical) and griseofulvin (PO): approved for tinea capitis, metabolized in liver.

Review Questions

For review questions, please go to ExpertConsult.com

Suggested Readings

1. Bradley JS, Nelson JD. *Nelson's Pediatric Antimicrobial Therapy.* 22nd ed. American Academy of Pediatrics; 2011:1–20.
2. Gallagher JC, MacDouugall C. *Antibiotics simplified.* 3rd ed. Jones & Barlett Learning; 2014:1–253.
3. Long SS, Pickering LK. *Principles and Practice of Pediatric Infectious Diseases.* 4th ed. Philadelphia: Elsevier; 2012:1412–1517.
4. Southwick F. *Infectious Diseases; a clinician short course.* 3rd ed. McGraw Hill; 2014:1–59.

Metabolism

48 Clinical Approach to Suspected Metabolic Disorders

ALANNA STRONG, MD, PhD and REBECCA D. GANETZKY, MD

Approach to the Child with a Potential Inborn Error of Metabolism (IEM)

PHILOSOPHY

- IEMs are diverse and rare
- Most general pediatricians will see at most one case of any particular disease
- No single group of symptoms will capture every patient; a high index of suspicion is needed to make the diagnosis
- Prompt diagnosis is critical because some conditions are treatable and require genetic counseling for the family
- In this section, we focus on the patient with disorders of "intermediary" metabolism (fat, sugar, protein, mitochondrial metabolism) because of the critical nature of early diagnosis and management

GENERAL SYMPTOMS

- Always consider in patients with unexplained multiorgan system involvement
- Common symptoms include
  - Feeding aversion or specific food aversions (e.g., protein aversion)
  - Failure to thrive
  - Vomiting
  - Excessive fatigue
  - Developmental delay
  - Stepwise regression in the setting of fasting or illness
    - Hypoglycemia, metabolic acidosis, rhabdomyolysis
  - Dysfunction of organs with high energy demands and synthetic needs
    - Central nervous system (CNS)
    - Liver
    - Skeletal/cardiac muscle
    - Retinae
    - Proximal renal tubule
    - Auditory hair cells

IMMEDIATE WORKUP

- Blood for immediate management decisions
  - Blood gas (pH, acid-base balance)
  - Electrolytes (with anion gap calculation)
  - Glucose

- Lactate (very important to know if gap acidosis is lactic acidosis or not—other organic acids are more amenable to hemodialysis than lactate)
- Ammonia (guides immediate management)
- Plasma amino acids—if at a metabolic center, where results can be returned quickly—looking for amino acidopathies that need acute management (e.g., maple syrup urine disease [MSUD])
- Urine
  - Urinalysis
  - Urine organic acids
- Additional laboratory studies: used to validate presumptive diagnosis and to screen for additional, nonemergent complications
  - Creatinine kinase
  - Transaminases
  - Coagulation studies
  - 3-hydroxybutyrate
  - Acylcarnitine profile
  - Insulin
  - Cortisol
  - Lactate (n.b.: Lactate has poor sensitivity and specificity for metabolic disease but can be used as an adjunct to other tests. An acute lactate is helpful to guide acidosis management; when the child is stabilized, a repeat lactate is helpful to determine the likelihood of primary lactic acidosis.)

INTERVENTIONS

- Stop any potentially nontolerated food source (fat, protein)
- Dextrose infusion
  - High dextrose load provokes endogenous hyperinsulinism → prevents fat and protein breakdown and averts catabolic state
  - In the acute setting, the goal is to reach high euglycemia or even hyperglycemia
  - Exogenous insulin can be used in the acute setting once hyperglycemia is achieved
  - Dextrose converts to lactate in disorders of pyruvate and respiratory chain metabolism, and therefore dextrose concentration should be thoughtfully titrated in these patients (see Chapter 49 for details)
    - Dextrose must *never* be used in children with pyruvate dehydrogenase deficiency who are stabilized on the ketogenic diet; loss of ketosis can result in acute status epilepticus in these patients
- Tailor interventions to test results, once obtained

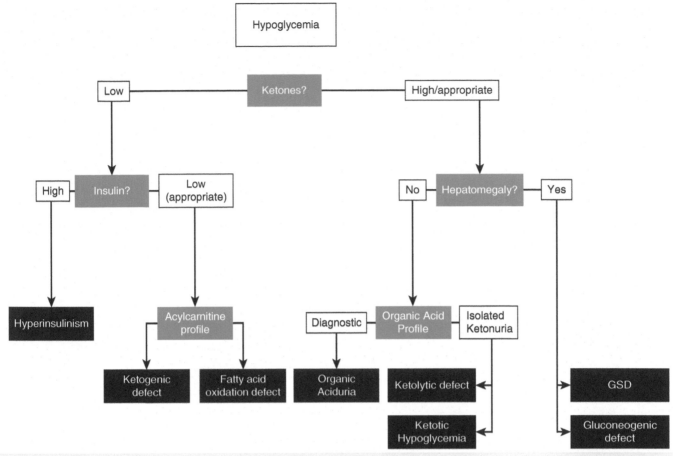

Fig. 48.1. Approach to hypoglycemia.

Disorders of Hypoglycemia (Fig. 48.1)

- Treat with glucose infusion
- Etiology differentiated based on ketones
  - Hypoketotic hypoglycemia
    - Low insulin: fatty acid oxidation defect, ketogenic defect (low insulin, increased free fatty acids)
    - High insulin: hyperinsulinism (increased insulin, decreased free fatty acids)
  - Ketotic hypoglycemia
    - Hepatomegaly absent: organic aciduria, ketolytic defect, ketotic hypoglycemia
    - Hepatomegaly present: glycogen storage disease, gluconeogenesis defect

Hyperammonemia (Fig. 48.2)

- Treat with protein restriction, ammonia removal (sodium benzoate and sodium phenylbutyrate, dialysis), and arginine to drive urea cycle, except in arginase deficiency (see Chapter 49)
- Differentiated based on height of ammonia and acidosis

- Acidosis present
  - Organic aciduria
  - Fatty acid oxidation defect
  - Defects in pyruvate metabolism (pyruvate dehydrogenase [PDH] or pyruvate carboxylase [PC] deficiency) or respiratory chain
- Acidosis absent
  - Measure citrulline
    Elevated
      Citrullinemia
      Argininosuccinate lyase deficiency
      Argininosuccinate synthase deficiency
    Normal or slightly increased
      Hyperornithinemia-hyperammonemia-homocitrullinuria (HHH) syndrome
      Arginase deficiency
      Fatty acid oxidation defect
    Low or absent
      Low orotic acid → carbamoyl phosphate synthetase I deficiency (CPSI) or N-acetylglutamate synthase deficiency (NAGS) deficiency
      Elevated orotic acid → ornithine transcarbamylase (OTC) deficiency

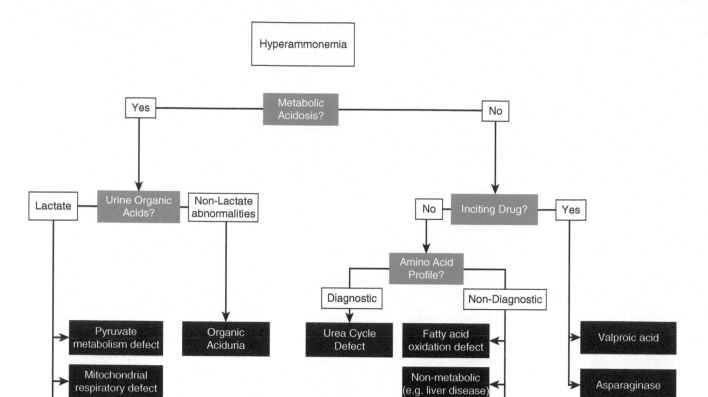

Fig. 48.2. Approach to hyperammonemia.

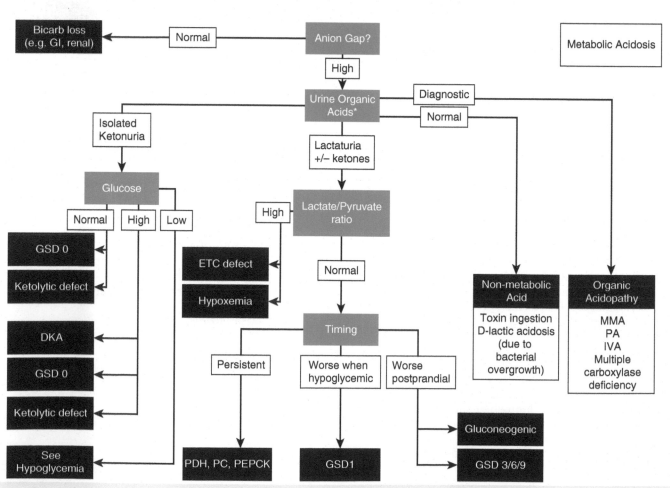

Fig. 48.3. Approach to acidosis.

Anion Gap Metabolic Acidosis (Fig. 48.3)

- Differentiated by lactate
  - Normal lactate → organic aciduria; differentiate based on organic acids
  - Elevated lactate
    - Secondary causes of lacticemia

      IEM
      - Organic acidopathies (diagnose on organic acids)
      - Fatty acid oxidation defects (diagnose on acyl-carnitine profile)

      Non-IEM
      - Multiorgan dysfunction (diagnose clinically)
      - Circulatory failure (diagnose clinically)
      - D-lacticemia (D-lactic acid is produced by gut bacteria; commonly elevated in bacterial overgrowth; diagnose by measuring D-lactate or enzymatic measurement of L-lactate)
    - Primary causes of lacticemia

      Measure pyruvate and pyruvate-to-lactate ratio
      - If normal/low pyruvate and L:P ratio increased → oxidative phosphorylation defect
      - If elevated pyruvate, differentiate based on clinical symptoms, genetic testing, or enzymology
      - Pyruvate dehydrogenase, pyruvate carboxylase deficiency (neurologic disease is predominant symptom, lacticemia is high and typically associated with acidosis; glucose provokes acute worsening of lacticemia)

      Phosphoenolpyruvate carboxykinase (PEPCK deficiency), fructose-1,6-bisphosphatase deficiency (hypoglycemia; lacticemia resolves with restoration of euglycemia)

      Glycogen storage disease (GSD) I (hepatosplenomegaly; lactate elevation decreases with glucose infusion; lacticemia)
- See also Nelson Textbook of Pediatrics, Part 11, "Metabolic Disorders."

Review Questions

For review questions, please go to ExpertConsult.com.

Suggested Readings

1. Ganetzky RD, Cuddapah SR. Neonatal lactic acidosis: a diagnostic and therapeutic approach. *Pediatr Rev.* 2017;18(4):e217–e227.
2. Levy PA. Inborn errors of metabolism. *Pediatr Rev.* 2009;30(4): 131–137.
3. Rice GM, Steiner RD. Inborn errors of metabolism. *Pediatr Rev.* 2016; 37(1):3–15.
4. Saububray JM, van den Berge G, Walter JH. *Inborn Metabolic Diseases: Diagnosis and Treatment.* Berlin, Germany: Springer; 2012.
5. Zschocke J, Hoffmann GF. *Vademecum Metabolicum.* 3rd ed. Friedrichsdorf, Germany: Milupa Metabolics GmbH and Company; 2011.

49 Review of Selected Metabolic Disorders

ALANNA STRONG, MD, PhD and REBECCA D. GANETZKY, MD

General Overview of Metabolism

BASIC INFORMATION

- Food consists of macromolecules
  - Carbohydrates (poly- and monosaccharides)
  - Proteins (amino acids)
  - Fats (fatty acids and triglycerides)
  - Nucleotides
- Metabolic processes are enzyme driven and take place in specific organelles
  - Macromolecules are metabolized to produce energy in the form of adenosine triphosphate (ATP)
  - Macromolecules are also synthesized by tissues for use (e.g., glycogen for energy storage, myelin for nerve conduction)
- Inborn errors of metabolism (IEMs)
  - Most IEMs are caused by enzyme deficiencies, with disease severity dictated by residual enzyme activity
  - Some are caused by receptor and transporter deficiencies
  - IEMs are usually autosomal recessive (except where noted otherwise)
- Disease in IEMs is caused by:
  - Toxicity of an accumulated intermediate
  - Deficiency of a required intermediate or product
  - Energy deficiency (ATP deficiency)
  - See also Nelson Textbook of Pediatrics, Part 11, "Metabolic Disorders."

Disorders of Amino Acid Metabolism

BASIC INFORMATION

- Amino acids are divided into essential (must be consumed in diet) versus nonessential
- Amino acids are converted into intermediates in the tricarboxylic acid (TCA) cycle and other metabolic pathways
- Defects in amino acid metabolism are divided into amino acidopathies and organic acidopathies
  - Amino acidopathies are diagnosed by plasma amino acids
  - Organic acidopathies are diagnosed by urine organic acids

Disorders of Branched-Chain Amino Acid (BCCA) Metabolism (Including Organic Acidurias)

BASIC INFORMATION

- BCAA = valine, isoleucine, leucine
- BCAA → propionyl-CoA → succinyl-CoA → TCA cycle and gluconeogenesis (Fig. 49.1)
- Defects impair energy generation and generate toxic metabolites
- Presentation typically occurs during neonatal period
- Exacerbations are triggered by:
  - Catabolism from illness
  - Protein intake
- General treatment approach involves protein restriction, essential amino acid supplementation, cofactor supplementation, and avoidance of catabolic state
  - Because these are intoxication disorders, hemodialysis can be used in severe, refractory cases
  - These metabolic pathways are primarily active in the liver; liver transplantation can benefit severe cases
- An overview of specific disorders is presented in Table 49.1

Maple Syrup Urine Disease (MSUD, BCKDH Deficiency)

BASIC INFORMATION

- Deficiency of any of the three subunits of the branched-chain ketoacid dehydrogenase (BCKDH) complex
- Pathology caused by accumulation of BCAAs and ketoacids

Isovaleric Aciduria (IVA, Isovaleryl-CoA Dehydrogenase Deficiency)

BASIC INFORMATION

- Disorder of leucine catabolism
- Deficiency → accumulation of isovaleric acid

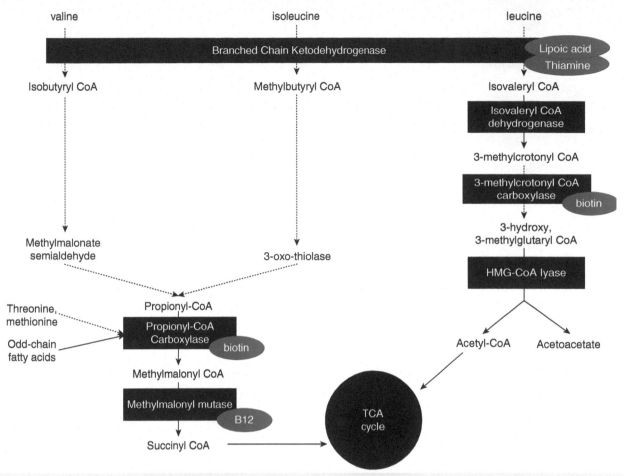

Fig. 49.1. Branched-chain amino acid metabolism.

Table 49.1. Clinical/Laboratory Features and Treatment for Disorders of Branched Chain Amino Acid Metabolism

	Maple Syrup Urine Disease	Isovaleric Aciduria	Propionic Aciduria	Methylmalonic Aciduria
Clinical presentation	Poor feeding, hyper- or hypotonia, lethargy, encephalopathy	Encephalopathy, or insidious psycho-motor retardation, decompensation with illness	Encephalopathy, lethargy, failure to thrive, seizures, pancreatitis, decompensation with illness, intellectual disability, hyperammonemia, metabolic stroke	Encephalopathy, lethargy, failure to thrive, seizures, pancreatitis, decompensation with illness, intellectual disability (typically more mild than propionic aciduria (PA)), hyperammonemia, osteopenia, anorexia, metabolic stroke
Distinct features	Maple syrup smelling urine/cerumen	Sweaty-feet odor	Dilated cardiomyopathy	Chronic kidney disease Post metabolic-crisis transient pancytopenia Autistic personality features
Screening laboratories	Ketones: ↑ Ammonia: normal/↑	Blood gas: anion gap metabolic acidosis Ketones: ↑ Ammonia: ↑	Blood gas: anion gap metabolic acidosis Ketones: ↑ Lactic acid: nl/↑ Ammonia: ↑ (initially 200–500)	Blood gas: anion gap metabolic acidosis Ketones: ↑ Lactic acid: nl/↑ Ammonia: ↑ (initially 150–400)
Diagnostic laboratories	Plasma amino acids: Presence of alloisoleucine; increased valine, leucine, and isoleucine; Urine organic acids: branched-chain oxo- and hydroxy acids	Urine organic acids: isovalerylglycine and 3-OH-oxovaleric acid Acylcarnitine: isovaleryl-carnitine (C5)	Plasma amino acids: Elevated glycine Urine organic acids: 3-hydroxypropionic acid, methylcitric acid, propionylglycine and tiglylglycine Acylcarnitine: propionylcarnitine (C3)	Plasma amino acids: ± Elevated glycine Urine organic acids: methylmalonic acid Acylcarnitine: propionylcarnitine (C3) ± methylmalonylcarnitine (C4DC)
Acute treatment	IV dextrose, branched-chain amino acid-free total parenteral nutrition (TPN), ± dialysis	Dextrose ± insulin, protein restriction	Dextrose, insulin, bicarbonate, nitrogen scavengers, ± dialysis; consider carglumic acid for hyperammonemia	Dextrose, insulin, bicarbonate, nitrogen scavengers, ± dialysis
Chronic Treatment	Branched-chain amino acid restriction, valine and isoleucine supplementation, trial of thiamine (rare forms are thiamine responsive), ± liver transplantation	Leucine restriction, glycine (binds isovaleric acid) ± carnitine	Isoleucine, valine, methionine, and threonine restriction; antibiotics to decrease gut flora; consider trial of biotin (rare forms are biotin responsive), ± liver transplantation	Trial of B₁₂; isoleucine, valine, methionine, and threonine restriction, ± liver transplantation, ± kidney transplantation
Genes	*BCKDHA, BCKDHB* more common than *DBT* and *DLD*	*IVD*	*PCCA, PCCB*	*MUT* more common than *MMAA, MMAB, MMACHC, MMADH, MCEE*

nl, normal.

3-Methylcrotonylcarboxylase Deficiency

BASIC INFORMATION

- Very common diagnosis on newborn screen, but most cases are asymptomatic
- Causes secondary deficiency of carnitine
- Acutely treat decompensation with intravenous (IV) dextrose

Propionic Aciduria (Propionic Acidemia, Propionyl-CoA Carboxylase Deficiency, PA)

BASIC INFORMATION

- Biotin-dependent
- Propionyl-CoA → methylmalonyl-CoA (final common pathway for branched chains, methionine, threonine, odd-chain fatty acid metabolism)
- Enables metabolite entry into the TCA cycle
- Accumulation of propionyl-CoA inhibits TCA cycle, gluconeogenesis, urea cycle (at N-acetylglutamate synthetase), and glycine catabolism

Methylmalonic Aciduria (MMA, Methylmalonic Acidemia, Mut0, Mut-, Methylmalonyl-CoA Mutase Deficiency)

BASIC INFORMATION

- Adenosylcobalamin (adenosyl B_{12})–dependent enzyme
- Mutation may be in enzyme itself or in B_{12} processing pathway
- May have elevations in homocysteine if methylcobalamin production is affected

Disorders of Phenylalanine and Tyrosine Metabolism

BASIC INFORMATION

- Phenylalanine is an essential amino acid (from diet or endogenous protein catabolism) that is irreversibly metabolized into tyrosine
- Catabolism requires tetrahydrobiopterin (BH_4) as a cofactor (Fig. 49.2)
- Disorders are summarized in Table 49.2

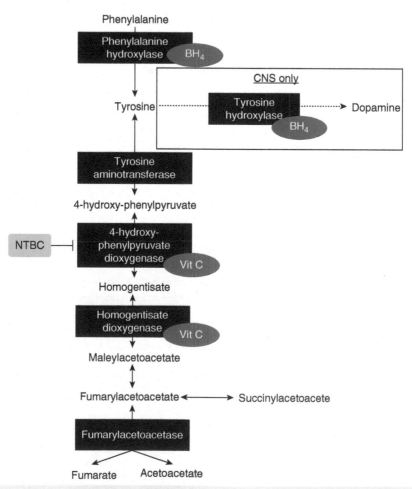

Fig. 49.2. Phenylalanine and tyrosine metabolism (BH_4 = tetrahydrobiopterin).

Table 49.2. Clinical/Laboratory Features and Treatment for Disorders of Phenylalanine and Tyrosine Metabolism

	Phenylketonuria	Tyrosinemia I	Transient Tyrosinemia of the Newborn	Alkaptonuria
Clinical presentation	Seizures, intellectual disability, fair skin and hair, movement disorder, spasticity	Hepatic dysfunction, can progress to cirrhosis; failure to thrive, porphyric crises, renal Fanconi	Asymptomatic	Black urine when alkaline; nail, skin, and scleral hyperpigmentation, arthritis, valvular disease, arteriosclerosis
Diagnostic laboratories	Plasma amino acids: increased phenylalanine "cofactor" testing (pterins, DHPR enzyme), gene testing	Plasma amino acids: increased tyrosine Urine organic acids: succinylacetone, (pathognomonic)	Plasma amino acids: very increased tyrosine ± methionine Urine organic acids: increased 4-OH phenylpyruvate, 4-OH phenyllactate, and 4-OH phenylacetate	Urine organic acids (increased homogentisic acid), gene testing
Treatment	Phenylalanine restriction, ± sapropterin, ± tyrosine supplementation Treatment completely ameliorates disease	Phenylalanine and tyrosine restriction, nitisinone (inhibits upstream metabolism) Treatment completely ameliorates disease	Vitamin C supplementation; most children do not require treatment	Vitamin C (enzyme cofactor), nitisinone (inhibit upstream metabolism)
Unique features	Mousy-odor urine			
Genes	PAH if pterins normal, else GCH1, PTS, QDPR, PCBD1 and SPR genes	FAH	None	HGD

Phenylketonuria (PKU)

BASIC INFORMATION

- Deficiencies cause phenylalanine accumulation
  - Inhibits myelination and neuronal growth
  - Competes with other large neutral amino acids for brain uptake → decreased neurotransmitter and catecholamine production
  - Impaired tyrosine generation → precursor for dopamine and melanin synthesis
- Usually caused by phenylalanine hydroxylase (PAH) deficiency → phenylalanine to tyrosine
- May also be caused by tetrahydrobiopterin (BH_4) biosynthesis defects (1%)
  - Does not respond clinically to dietary restriction alone
  - Manifestation includes movement disorders and seizures
  - Phenylalanine is lower than in PAH deficiency

NEWBORN SCREENING NOTES

- Almost all cases worldwide are now diagnosed by newborn screening
- Screening performed before a neonate has had a chance to receive protein (e.g., before feeding after birth) may be falsely negative

TREATMENT NOTES

- BH_4 metabolic defects are additionally treated with L-dopa, 5-hydroxytryptophan supplementation, and sapropterin; usually don't require dietary management
- Dietary control is critically important in pregnancy and 3 months preconception: high phenylalanine is teratogenic
  - Babies affected by maternal PKU: septal cardiac defects, microcephaly, intellectual disability

Tyrosinemia I (Hepatorenal Tyrosinemia, Fumarylacetoacetase Deficiency)

BASIC INFORMATION

- Very distal to tyrosine breakdown
- Because distal, elevated tyrosine is not a sensitive marker
- Results in accumulation of toxic metabolites
- Like all metabolic hepatopathies, it can progress to hepatocellular carcinoma if not treated

Transient Tyrosinemia of the Newborn

BASIC INFORMATION

- Asymptomatic elevation in tyrosine on newborn screen or amino acid testing in newborn
- Not a genetic disorder; more commonly seen in liver dysfunction, prematurity, or total parenteral nutrition (TPN)
- Tyrosine is not toxic, so no treatment is needed in most cases
- Resolves with time and cessation of TPN

Alkaptonuria

BASIC INFORMATION

- Homogentisate dioxygenase deficiency
- Leading to homogentisic acid accumulation and eventual metabolism into pigments that deposit within the connective tissue
- May present with black urine when alkalinized (e.g. "urine turns black when exposed to bleach/toilet bowl cleaner")

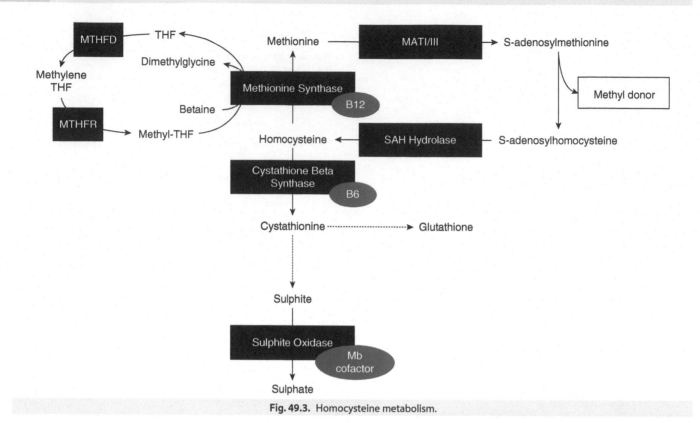

Fig. 49.3. Homocysteine metabolism.

Disorders of Methionine and Cysteine Metabolism

BASIC INFORMATION

- Defects → toxic metabolites, less protection from oxidative stress
- Methionine interconverts with homocysteine (remethylation; one carbon cycle; Fig. 49.3)
- Homocysteine toxicity: procoagulant
- Homocysteine → methionine dependent on B_{12} and tetrahydrofolate (B_{12}, folate deficiency, and IEMs are important differentials)

Cystathionine Beta Synthase Deficiency (CBS, Homocystinuria, Homocysteinemia)

BACKGROUND

- CBS deficiency
  - B_6-dependent enzyme
  - Homocysteine → cystathionine
- Homocysteine accumulation → endothelial damage → vascular compromise (central nervous system [CNS] especially) → intellectual disability
- Homocysteine interferes with coagulation → thromboembolic events
- Secondary cysteine depletion → abnormal connective tissue → eye and skeletal problems
- Most common metabolic cause of elevated homocysteine

CLINICAL PRESENTATION

- Marfanoid habitus
- Seizures
- Intellectual disability: distinguishes from Marfan
- Myopia
- Lens dislocation (downward)
- Osteoporosis
- Thromboembolic events
  - May be presenting symptom in milder forms of diagnosis
- Peripheral vascular disease
- Often pale for family

DIAGNOSIS

- Plasma amino acids (increased methionine and homocysteine, ± decreased cysteine)
  - Must be drawn on ice and processed immediately, or else homocysteine will bind to protein and be lost
- Gene testing (*CBS* gene)

TREATMENT

- Trial of pyridoxine (vitamin B_6) ± folate supplementation; B_{12} if deficient
- Betaine supplementation
  - Betaine = trimethylglycine; methyl donor encourages homocysteine conversion to methionine
- Methionine restriction

DISORDERS OF OTHER AMINO ACIDS

Glutaric Aciduria Type I (GA1)

BASIC INFORMATION

- Glutaryl-CoA dehydrogenase deficiency (mitochondrial enzyme, lysine and tryptophan catabolism)

CLINICAL PRESENTATION

- Macrocephaly (brain magnetic resonance imaging [MRI] usually shows benign extraaxial hydrocephalus and benign frontotemporal atrophy)
- Acute metabolic basal ganglia stroke with fever → extrapyramidal signs, or in severe form locked in
- Spontaneous subdural hemorrhage

DIAGNOSIS AND EVALUATION

- Urine organic acids (elevated glutaric acid and 3-hydroxyglutaric acid)
  - Low-excretor form can normalize glutaric acid in urine, but not 3-hydroxyglutaric acid
  - Free and total carnitine (decreased)
  - Acylcarnitine profile (elevated glutarylcarnitine = C5DC; can normalize in low-excretor form)
  - Gene testing (*GCDH* gene)

TREATMENT

- Strict and emergent avoidance of fever, using antipyretics and external cooling if necessary
- IV glucose when ill
  - Can prevent strokes and result in normal neurologic outcome
- Diet: lysine and tryptophan restriction
- Carnitine supplementation

Disorders of Amino Acid Transport

BASIC INFORMATION

- Amino acids are reabsorbed by intestine and kidney to prevent wasting
- In many cases same gene for jejunal absorption and renal reabsorption

Cystinuria

BASIC INFORMATION

- Autosomal recessive > autosomal dominant
- Basic amino acid transporter deficiency (renal and intestinal)
  - Impairs absorption of basic amino acids

- Increased urinary excretion, especially of cysteine. Cysteine → insoluble dimer → stone formation

CLINICAL PRESENTATION

- Late adolescence
- Renal staghorn calculi

DIAGNOSIS AND EVALUATION

- Urinalysis (flat hexagonal crystals in the urine)
- Abdominal x-ray (staghorn calculi)
- Urinary amino acids (increased cysteine > lysine, arginine, and ornithine; normal plasma amino acids)
- Gene studies (*SLC7A9* or *SLC3A1* genes)

TREATMENT

- Aggressive hydration
- Urine alkalinization
- Severe cases may require protein/sulfur-containing amino acid restriction

Urea Cycle Disorders

BASIC INFORMATION

- Most are autosomal recessive (ornithine transcarbamylase [OTC] is X-linked recessive)
- Amino acid catabolism generates free ammonia, which is converted to glutamine; both are neurotoxic
- Ammonia is converted to water-soluble urea by the urea cycle, allowing for clearance
  - Substrates: NH_3, ATP, and CO_2
  - Five-step pathway (Fig. 49.4)
  - Full cycle only occurs in liver
- Defects in this pathway lead to hyperammonemia in the neonatal period or with catabolic stress (see Table 49.3)
  - Lethargy, coma, death
  - Respiratory alkalosis (hiccupping or irregular breathing)
  - Cerebral edema → encephalopathy
- Milder patients may have protein aversion and intermittent psychiatric symptoms

DIAGNOSIS AND EVALUATION

- Plasma amino acids
- Urine orotic acid (alternate product of carbamoyl phosphate if urea cycle is blocked)

ACUTE TREATMENT

- Stop all protein intake
- Glucose infusion at high glucose infusion rate (GIR) to stop catabolism
- IV nitrogen scavengers (sodium phenylbutyrate, sodium benzoate)

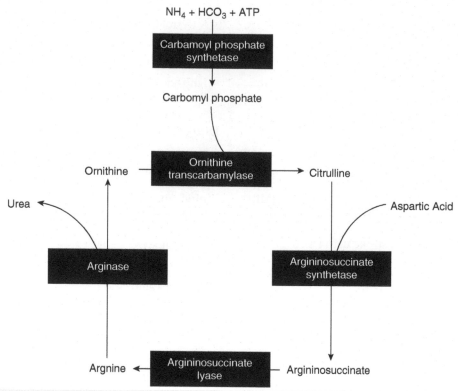

Fig. 49.4. Urea cycle.

Table 49.3. Clinical/Laboratory Features and Treatment for Urea Cycle Disorders

	Ornithine Transcarbamylase Deficiency	Argininosuccinate Synthetase Deficiency (Citrullinemia)	Argininosuccinate Lyase Deficiency	Arginase Deficiency
Mode of inheritance	X-linked recessive	Autosomal recessive	Autosomal recessive	Autosomal recessive

Diagnostic laboratories	Ammonia ↑
	Plasma Amino Acids:
	  ↓ citrulline,
	  ↑ glutamine)
	Orotic Acid: ↑
	Gene Testing (60% sensitive)
		Ammonia: ↑
		Plasma Amino Acids:
		  ↑ citrulline
		  ↓ arginine
		Orotic Acid: ↑
		Gene Testing
			Ammonia: ↑,
			  Plasma Amino Acids
			  ↑ citrulline
			  ↑ argininosuccinate
			  ↓ arginine
			Orotic Acid: ↑
			Gene Testing
				Ammonia: ↑
				Plasma Amino Acids:
				  ↑ arginine,
				Orotic Acid: ↑,
				Gene Testing

Acute treatment	Dextrose, insulin, nitrogen scavengers, protein restriction, dialysis, intravenous arginine			As others, but arginine contraindicated
Chronic treatment	Citrulline supplementation, protein restriction, oral ammonia scavengers, liver transplant	Arginine supplementation, protein restriction, oral nitrogenic scavengers, ± liver transplant	As citrullinemia, but nitrogen scavengers usually not required	Arginine restriction; nitrogen scavengers usually not required
Unique features	Most common urea cycle disorder, women can be symptomatic with hyperammonemic crises, often have psychiatric features at baseline		Hypertension (impaired nitric oxide generation), risk of hepatocellular carcinoma, attention-deficit hyperactivity disorder and learning difficulties (independent of ammonia control); hyperammonemia crises uncommon	Arginine supplementation contraindicated, ascending spasticity independent of ammonia control, hyperammonemic crises rare

- IV high-dose arginine (except in arginase deficiency)
- Dialysis may be needed to remove ammonia

CHRONIC TREATMENT

- Avoiding a catabolic state
- Protein restriction

- Arginine supplementation
- Replace amino acids in a disease-specific manner
- Nitrogen scavengers
- Replace relatively deficient amino acids in a disease-specific manner
- Avoid valproic acid → provokes hyperammonemia
- Consider liver transplantation in refractory cases

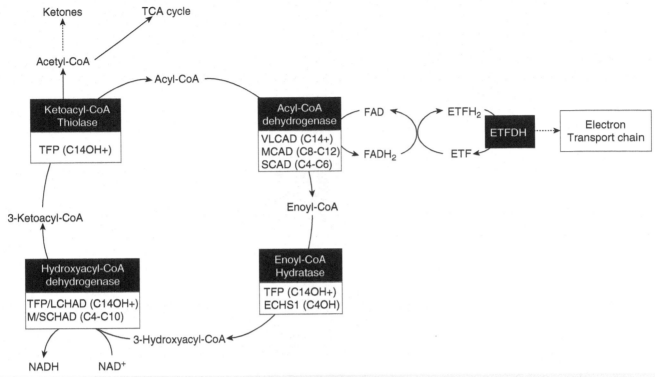

Fig. 49.5. Fatty acid oxidation spiral.

LONG-TERM SEQUELAE FROM HYPERAMMONEMIC CRISIS

- Stepwise regression after illnesses
- Spasticity, epilepsy, intellectual disability
- Risk is proportional to length of hyperammonemia in most disorders

DISORDERS OF FAT METABOLISM

Disorders of Mitochondrial Fatty Acid Oxidation

BASIC INFORMATION

- Energy during fasting generated from fatty acid beta-oxidation
- Provides ATP for gluconeogenesis
- Produces $FADH_2$ and NADH for the electron transport chain and acetyl-CoA for ketogenesis (Fig. 49.5)
- Long-chain fatty acids require transport across the mitochondrial membrane (Fig. 49.6)
- Defects in this pathway cause hypoketotic hypoglycemia and fasting intolerance
- Diagnosis through acylcarnitine profile and newborn screen
- Diseases are clinically similar (Table 49.4)
  - Autosomal recessive
  - Present with hypoketotic hypoglycemia

- Features of long-chain disorders
  - Intermittent rhabdomyolysis, especially with exertion or illness
  - Can have congenital or noncongenital dilated or hypertrophic cardiomyopathy ± arrhythmia
  - Severe neonatal forms have hyperammonemia and lactic acidosis

DIAGNOSIS

- Very important to do biochemical testing when ill → laboratory results can normalize when fed
- Urine organic acids show dicarboxylic aciduria but do not distinguish among long-chain fatty acid oxidation (FAO) disorders
- Acylcarnitine profile distinguishes among FAO disorders

GENERAL TREATMENT STRATEGY

- Avoid catabolism
  - High GIR when ill, neonatal presentations
    - Insulin may be required for severe presentations
  - Cornstarch at bedtime to provide overnight glucose source starting around 12 months
  - Fasting restriction
- Restrict long-chain fats (almost all naturally occurring dietary fats)
- Supplement with:
  - Medium-chain triglyceride oil to provide calories and source of fat (except MCAD)
  - Essential fatty acids
  - Carnitine to prevent secondary carnitine deficiency

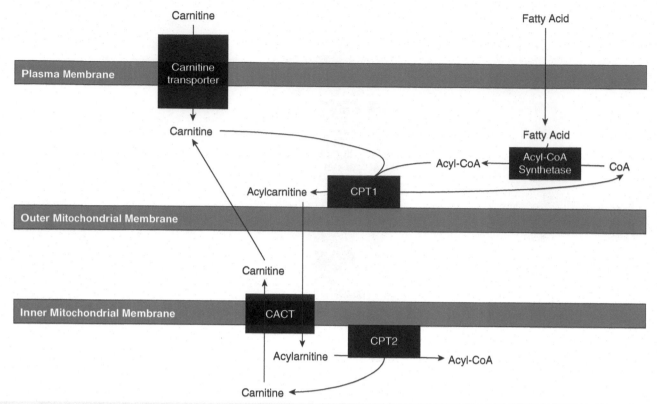

Fig. 49.6. Transport of long-chain fatty acids across the mitochondrial membrane for fatty acid oxidation.

Carnitine Transporter Deficiency

BASIC INFORMATION

- Carnitine transporter mutation → cannot bring carnitine into cells → insufficient carnitine to drive the carnitine shuttle → impaired FAO and ketogenesis

Carnitine Palmitoyltransferase Ii (CPT2) Deficiency

BASIC INFORMATION

- Converts long-chain acylcarnitines to long-chain acyl-CoAs (active form); frees carnitine
- Deficiency impairs long-chain fatty acid beta-oxidation and carnitine regeneration

CLINICAL PRESENTATION

- Most common: thermolabile variant
  - Intermittent rhabdomyolysis (often creatine kinase [CK] >100,000)
  - Hypertrophic or dilated cardiomyopathy can develop

DIAGNOSIS AND EVALUATION

- CK (intermittent elevation; may be persistent low-level elevation)

- Acylcarnitine profile (increased C16 and C18; decreased C2)
  - Biochemically identical to a rarer condition, carnitine-acylcarnitine translocase (CACT) deficiency
- Gene testing (*CPT2* gene)
- Enzyme assays

Very-Long-Chain Acyl-CoA (VLCAD) Deficiency

BASIC INFORMATION

- Initial step of long-chain fat beta-oxidation (C12–C22)
- Deficiency causes impaired ketogenesis (insufficient substrate generation) and beta-oxidation → fasting intolerance
- Heart and liver pathology
  - Energy deficiency → organs rely on fat for energy
  - Accumulating metabolites are cardiotoxic

Medium-Chain Acyl-CoA Dehydrogenase (MCAD) Deficiency

BASIC INFORMATION

- Involved in oxidation of medium-chain acyl-CoA fatty acids (C6-C12), which come from breakdown of longer-chain dietary fats

Table 49.4.   Clinical/Laboratory Features and Treatment for Fatty Acid Oxidation Disorders

	Carnitine Transporter Deficiency	Carnitine Transporter Protein II Deficiency	Very Long Chain Acyl-CoA Deficiency	Medium-Chain Acyl-CoA Dehydrogenase Deficiency	Short-Chain Acyl-CoA Dehydrogenase Deficiency	Short-Chain Hydroxyacyl-CoA Dehydrogenase Deficiency	Multiple Acyl-CoA Dehydrogenase Deficiency
Clinical presentation	Can be asymptomatic, may have cardiomyopathy and exertional rhabdomyolysis	Neonatal Form: Hypoketotic hypoglycemia, hyperammonemia, lactic acidosis, liver failure, cardiomyopathy, myopathy Thermolabile Form: Rhabdomyolysis, cardiomyopathy	Hypoketotic hypoglycemia, cardiomyopathy, rhabdomyolysis	Hypoketotic hypoglycemia, sudden neonatal death, arrhythmia, Reye-like syndrome	Usually asymptomatic, ± predisposition to hypoglycemia	Hypoketotic hypoglycemia, hyperinsulinism	Anion gap metabolic acidosis, hypoketotic hypoglycemia, ± hyperammonemia, ± cerebral malformations, ± cystic renal disease, ± cardiomyopathy
Screening labs	Creatine kinase (CK): nl/↑	CK: ↑ (may be chronic elevation)	CK: ↑ Glucose: ↓ Ketones: ↓	Glucose: ↓ Ketones: ↓		Glucose: ↓ Ketones: ↓	Glucose: ↓ Ketones: ↓ CK: ↑
Diagnostic labs	plasma carnitine: ↑ urine carnitine: ↓	Acylcarnitine profile: ↑C16, C18	Acylcarnitine profile ↑C16:0, C14:0, C14:1, C14:2	Urine organic acids: adipic, suberic, and sebacic acid, hexanoylglycine (pathognomonic), acylcarnitine profile: ↑C6, C8 and C10	Acylcarnitine profile: ↑C4 urine organic acids: ethylmalonic acid and methylsuccinate	Acylcarnitine profile: ↑ C_4OH urine organic acids: 3-hydroxybutyrate, 3-4-dihydroxybutyrate, and 3-hydroxyglutarate	Acylcarnitine profile: Like combined VLCAD, MCAD, and SCAD, plus glutarylcarnitine (C5DC), isovalerylcarnitine (C_5OH) Urine organic acids: as MCAD and SCAD, isovalerylglycine, glutaric acid, hydroxyglutaric acid
Treatment	Completely ameliorated by high-dose carnitine	Long-chain fat restriction, MCT oil	Long-chain fat restriction, MCT oil, carnitine supplementation	MCT supplementation contraindicated; breastfeeding must be supplemented with formula or expressed breast milk until well-established; ± carnitine	No treatment needed	As per hyperinsulinism	Long-chain fatty acid and protein restriction, riboflavin, CoQ
Distinct features		Neonatal form may have renal and brain cysts; thermolabile form may be missed on newborn screening	Range of phenotypes from severe neonatal presentation to late onset; may be missed on newborn screening	Does not have rhabdomyolysis		Hyperinsulinism	Rare adult-onset form has exertional rhabdomyolysis ± myopathy
Genes	SLC22A5	CPT2	ACADVL	ACADM	ACADS	HADHSC	ETFDH > ETFA, ETFB

CLINICAL PRESENTATION

- Because not involved in long-chain metabolism, does not get rhabdomyolysis
- Rarely hepatomegaly and steatosis
- Rarely hypotonia and developmental delay (from hypoglycemic insult)
- Sudden infant death syndrome (SIDS) was a common presentation pre-NBS
- Neonatal form: hypoglycemia, arrhythmia, cardiac arrest
  - Reported only in exclusively breastfed infants

TREATMENT

- Supplement breast milk with formula and/or expressed breast milk after feeds until supply is clearly established

Short-Chain Acyl-CoA Dehydrogenase (SCAD) Deficiency

BASIC INFORMATION

- Beta-oxidation of short-chain fatty acids (C4–C6)
- Once NBS started, found to be extremely common, not disease; many states no longer screen

Multiple Acyl-CoA Dehydrogenase Deficiency (MADD, Glutaric Aciduria Type 2)

BASIC INFORMATION

- Riboflavin-derived electron transport flavoprotein defect
- Compromises the transfer of electrons to the respiratory chain
- Compromises energy generation from FAO and amino acid metabolism

CLINICAL PRESENTATION

- Three clinical presentations
  - Type I: anion gap metabolic acidosis, hypoketotic hypoglycemia, hyperammonemia, cerebral malformations, cystic renal disease, "sweaty feet" odor, dysmorphic features, epilepsy, cardiomyopathy, myopathy
  - Type II: type I without dysmorphic features
  - Type III: rhabdomyolysis ± recurrent hepatic encephalopathy with metabolic stress

DIAGNOSIS AND EVALUATION

- Acylcarnitine profile (increase in C5, C5DC plus FAO metabolites, including C14, C16, C18 species [VLCAD], C6, C8, C10 species [MCAD], and C4 [SCAD])
  - Not all are always present
  - Shorter chains are more sensitive
- Urine organic acids (increased isovalerylglycine, isobutyryl dehydrogenase, glutaric acid, 3-methylglutaric, 3-hydroxyglutaric, 2-hydroxyglutaric, hexanoylglycine, suberylglycine, and ethylmalonic and dicarboxylic acids)
  - Not all are present all of the time
    - 2-hydroxyglutaric acid in combination with any other is pathognomonic
    - Any combination of an abnormal amino acid–derived organic acid (isovalerylglycine, isobutyrylglycine, glutarate species) and an abnormal fatty acid–derived organic acid (hexanoylglycine, suberylglycine, ethylmalonic, very high dicarboxylics) should raise concern

Short-Chain Hydroxyacyl-CoA Dehydrogenase (SCHAD) Deficiency

BASIC INFORMATION

- Disease is actually *not* due to impaired FAO
- Occurs because SCHAD is bifunctional and also regulates insulin release by inhibiting glutamate dehydrogenase (GDH)
- SCHAD deficiency → upregulated GDH → hyperinsulinism

Disorders of Ketone Metabolism

BASIC INFORMATION

- Ketones are glucose-sparing energy source, used after glycogen
- Ketogenesis occurs in liver
- Derived from fatty acid and amino acid metabolism
- Ketones are utilized (ketolysis) by brain, heart, and skeletal muscle (Fig. 49.7)
  - Heart preferentially uses ketones
  - Muscle preferentially uses ketones during exercise
- Generates acetyl-CoA for the TCA cycle
- Ketogenesis and ketolysis defects impair fasting tolerance → hypoglycemia
- Ketolysis defects → ketoacidosis even in the face of normal or high glucose; should be considered in differential for DKA, especially if ketones don't clear
- Ketogenesis defects → hypoketotic hypoglycemia

DISORDERS OF CARBOHYDRATE METABOLISM

Disorders of Galactose Metabolism

BASIC INFORMATION

- Galactose is a major dietary sugar in infancy (lactose = glucose + galactose)
- Used as a precursor for glycogen, glycoprotein, and glycolipid synthesis
- Typically converted to glucose (Fig. 49.8)
- Abnormal galactose metabolite galactitol is directly ophthotoxic

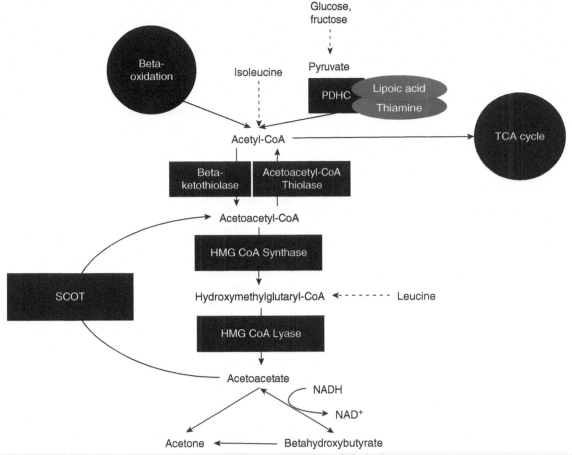

Fig. 49.7. Ketone generation and utilization.

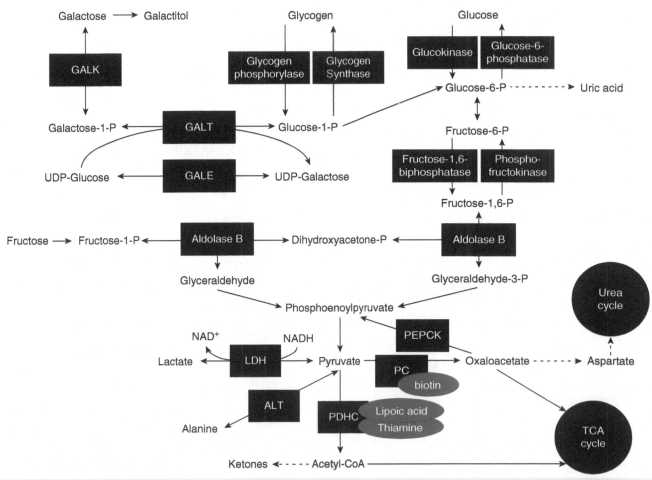

Fig. 49.8. Carbohydrate metabolism.

Galactose-1-Phosphate Uridyltransferase (GALT) Deficiency (Classic Galactosemia)

BASIC INFORMATION

- Symptoms secondary to accumulated galactose-1-phosphate, depleted glucose-1-phosphate, galactitol accumulation, and abnormal galactosylation of glycoproteins

CLINICAL PRESENTATION

- Vomiting/feeding intolerance, especially to lactose-containing foods
- Cataracts (50% congenital; typically responsive to diet)
- Liver failure
- Jaundice starting as unconjugated → conjugated
- Renal tubular acidosis
- *Escherichia coli* sepsis
- Poor growth
- Expressive language delay
- Premature ovarian insufficiency

DIAGNOSIS AND EVALUATION

- Blood total galactose and galactose-1-phosphate (elevated)
- Urine galactitol (elevated)
- Urine-reducing substances (elevated)
- Enzyme assays
- Gene testing (*GALT* gene)
- Variant galactosemia (most common is "Duarte") is an important consideration
  - High residual enzyme activity (approximately 20%–50%)
  - Galactose/gal-1-p may be elevated, but not to the same degree
  - Treatment is usually not needed

TREATMENT

- Galactose-free diet
- Still intellectual disability, growth retardation, and ovarian failure with treatment

Disorders of Fructose Metabolism

BASIC INFORMATION

- Fructose is a major sugar in Western diet (Sucrose = Glucose + Fructose; also in fruits and high fructose corn syrup (HFCS))
- Metabolized by the intestine, liver, and kidney (Fig. 49.8)

Hereditary Fructose Intolerance

BASIC INFORMATION

- Aldolase B deficiency
- Compromised gluconeogenesis (fructose-1,6-bisphosphate used in gluconeogenesis)
- Compromised glycogenolysis (accumulated fructose-1-phosphate inhibits glycogen phosphorylase)
- Inability to metabolize fructose-1-phosphate → phosphate sequestration and subsequent ATP depletion → increased adenine catabolism to generate ATP → increased uric acid

CLINICAL PRESENTATION

- Begins with introduction of fructose
  - Classically around 6 months with solids
  - Fructose, in the form of HFCS and/or sucrose, is in some infant formula
- Vomiting
- Lethargy
- Hepatosplenomegaly
- Liver failure
- Failure to thrive
- Renal tubular acidosis
- Spontaneous fructose aversion is common

DIAGNOSIS AND EVALUATION

- Screening laboratories: low blood glucose, combined anion gap and non-anion gap acidosis (lactic acidosis + renal tubular acidosis)
- Plasma amino acids (elevated methionine and tyrosine—nonspecific markers of liver dysfunction)
- Urine-reducing substances (elevated)
- Enzyme assays
- Gene testing (*ALDOB* gene)

TREATMENT

- Fructose restriction

Disorders of Gluconeogenesis

BASIC INFORMATION

- Gluconeogenesis = generation of glucose for maintenance of euglycemia and glycolysis during fasting (Fig. 49.8)
  - First common substrate is lactate
  - Produced also from glycerol and amino acids
  - Pathway overlaps glycogenolysis
- Defects present as hypoglycemia ± lactic acidosis ± ketosis
  - Lactic acid is the substrate for gluconeogenesis
  - Lactate and pyruvate elevations are proportional (differentiates from electron transport chain deficiency)
  - Lacticemia occurs during fasting and resolves with glucose administration
  - Ketosis is proportionate to hypoglycemia
- Diagnosis: metabolic derangements, enzyme assays, gene testing
- Treatment: carbohydrate-rich diet, fast avoidance

Table 49.5. Physical Examination and Laboratory Findings in Glycogen Storage Disorders

Type	Enzyme Deficiency	Primary Organ Involvement	Glucose	Lactate	Ketones*	Other Labs	Other Features
0	Glycogen Synthase	Liver	↓	↑	Appropriate-persistent	Hyperglycemia and lactic acidosis with feeds	No hepatomegaly
1	Glucose-6-phosphatase	Liver, kidney	↓	↑ (fasting)	↓	Increased uric acid and triglycerides	Severe hepatomegaly, doll face, gout, hepatic adenoma, neutropenia
2	Alpha glucosidase	Muscle and heart	Normal	Normal	Normal	Elevated CK	Short PR, cardiomegaly
3	Amylo-1, 6-glucosidase	Liver, muscle, heart	↓	↔/↑ (fed)	Appropriate-persistent	± elevated CK	Hepatomegaly, doll face, hepatic adenoma
4	Amylo-1,4 → 1, 6—transglucosylase	Muscle	↔	↔	↔	± elevated CK	Hepatomegaly, liver fibrosis
5	Phosphorylase	Muscle	↔	↔	↔	Elevated CK	Exercise intolerance with second wind phenomenon
6	Glycogen Phosphorylase	Liver	↓	↔/↑ (fed)	Appropriate-persistent	Mild hyperlipidemia transaminitis	Hepatomegaly, short stature
7	Phosphofructokinase	Muscle, red blood cells	↔	↔	↔	Elevated CK, LDH, reticulocytosis, hyperbili hyperuricemia	Exercise intolerance without second wind
9	Glycogen phosphorylase kinase	Muscle, liver	↓	↔/↑ (fed)	Appropriate-persistent	Mild hyperlipidemia transaminitis	± liver fibrosis

*Ketones in GSD0/3/6/9 usually occur only in the setting of hypoglycemia, but chronic ketosis may be seen in patients with poor metabolic control.

Glycogen Storage Disorders

BASIC INFORMATION

- Glycogen is made and stored in the liver and muscle
  - Liver glycogen is used as a first-line source of glucose/energy during fasting (Fig. 49.8)
  - Muscle glycogen is used for energy during exercise and does not provide circulating glucose
  - Glycogen storage disorders (GSDs) can be liver, muscle, or both
- Synthesized from the polymerization of glucose
- Defect can be in glycogenogenesis or glycogenolysis
- General symptoms (Table 49.5)
  - Hepatic glycogen metabolic defects
    - Hypoglycemia
    - Hepatomegaly
    - ± Lacticemia that varies with prandial state if gluconeogenesis is also affected
  - Myopathic glycogen metabolic defects
    - Exercise intolerance
    - Rhabdomyolysis
    - Cardiomyopathy
- Diagnosis: hypoglycemia, ketosis and lactic acidosis with fasting, liver/muscle histopathology, enzyme assays, gene testing
  - Fasting studies can be dangerous and should be done only in experienced metabolic centers. In other

institutions, enzymology, pathology, and genetic testing are first-line diagnostics

TREATMENT

- Chronic: low-glycemic-index diet prevents glycogen accumulation
- High-protein diet provides alternate energy source
- For hepatic GSDs
  - Acutely correct hypoglycemia
  - Overnight cornstarch
  - Small, frequent meals

Glycogen Storage Disease I (Von Gierke Disease)

BASIC INFORMATION

- Involved in hepatic gluconeogenesis and glycogenolysis (deficiency compromises both pathways)
- Inhibition of gluconeogenesis → lactic acidosis
- Subtypes
  - Type Ia (glucose-6-phosphatase deficiency) = 95%
  - Type Ib (endoplasmic reticulum glucose-6-phosphate transporter deficiency)
    - Glucose-6-phosphate → glucose occurs in the endoplasmic reticulum

- Like type Ia, **plus** neutropenia and Crohn-like bowel disease
- Accumulated glucose-6-phosphate perturbs many pathways
  - Pentose phosphate pathway → hyperuricemia
  - Hypertriglyceridemia

CLINICAL PRESENTATION

- Hepatomegaly
- Doll face
- Muscle weakness
- Failure to thrive
- Short stature
- Hypoketotic hypoglycemia
- Hypertriglyceridemia
- Gout from hyperuricemia
- Later-onset polycystic ovaries, renal disease, pancreatitis, hepatic adenoma, and pancreatitis

DIAGNOSIS AND EVALUATION

- Fasting study:
  - Blood sugar (decreased)
  - Lactate (elevated)
  - Triglycerides (elevated)
  - Uric acid (elevated)
  - Glucagon stimulation increases lactate but not glucose—do *not* give glucagon to a patient with known GSD I
- Enzyme studies
- Liver biopsy (glycogen accumulation)
- Gene testing (*G6PC* or *SLC37A4* gene)

TREATMENT

- Fructose, lactose, sucrose, and galactose restriction (cannot be converted to glucose)
- Type Ib: as above + granulocyte colony-stimulating factor (G-CSF)

Glycogen Storage Disease Ii (Pompe Disease, Acid Maltase Deficiency, Alpha-Glucosidase Deficiency)

BASIC INFORMATION

- Myopathic (cardiac, skeletal, and smooth)
- Lysosomal enzyme that hydrolyzes both the α-1,4- and α-1,6-bonds within glycogen to free glucose

CLINICAL PRESENTATION

- Infantile cardiomyopathic form
  - Hypertrophic cardiomyopathy
  - Short PR interval
  - Severe hypotonia
  - Failure to thrive (FTT)
  - Macroglossia
- Infantile noncardiomyopathic form
  - Benign cardiac hypertrophy without cardiomyopathy
  - ± Hypotonia
- Late-onset form
  - Progressive muscle weakness
  - Diaphragmatic failure is often life-limiting

DIAGNOSIS AND EVALUATION

- Added to recommended uniform screening panel for NBS in 2015; not yet screened in all states
- Glycogen-containing vacuoles on muscle biopsy
- Urine hex4 (tetrasaccharide) → level correlates with disease
- ECG (shortened PR, large QRS)
- Enzyme studies
- Gene studies (*GAA* gene)

TREATMENT

- Enzyme replacement therapy (Myozyme, Lumizyme)

Disorders of Glucose Transport

BASIC INFORMATION

- Glucose is the primary energy source of all cells
- Five channels each for different tissues
- Couple the transport of sodium along its concentration gradient to diffusion of glucose

GLUT1 Deficiency

BASIC INFORMATION

- Autosomal dominant
- GLUT1 is the glucose transporter for the brain and red blood cells
- Only insulin-independent glucose transporter
- Haploinsufficiency slows the rate of glucose diffusion into the brain

CLINICAL PRESENTATION

- Begins at 2 months of age when the brain is rapidly growing
- Neurologic symptoms: developmental delay and intellectual disability, seizures, microcephaly, hypotonia

DIAGNOSIS AND EVALUATION

- Normal blood sugar with relatively decreased CSF glucose and lactate
- Gene testing (*SLC2A1* gene)

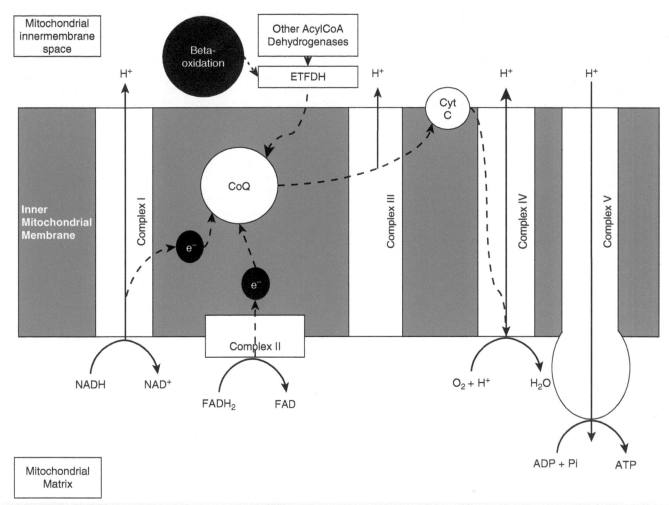

Fig. 49.9. Electron transport chain.

TREATMENT

- Ketogenic diet
- Carnitine supplementation because ketogenic diet uses high levels of carnitine

Disorders of Multiple Intermediary Metabolism (Cofactor Metabolic Defects)

- Overview
  - Many metabolic enzymes use dietary vitamins or minerals as cofactors
  - One cofactor is used by multiple enzymes, often related in function
  - Deficiency of vitamin (dietary or genetic transport or processing defects) results in multiple-enzyme deficiency
  - Treatable with high levels of active form of vitamin

DISORDERS OF ORGANELLE METABOLISM

Disorders of Mitochondrial Metabolism

BASIC INFORMATION

- The respiratory chain is the final system for energy generation (Fig. 49.9)
  - In mitochondria
  - Uses oxygen as a final electron acceptor
  - One glucose molecule → 38 ATP
- Defects
  - Compromised energy production
  - Excess reactive oxygen species
  - Increased NADH/NAD$^+$ and FADH$_2$/FAD ratios inhibit NAD$^+$ and FAD-dependent processes

Table 49.6. Clinical/Laboratory Features and Treatment of Selected Mitochondrial Respiratory Chain Disorders

	Hepatocerebral Depletion (*POLG*)	Leigh Syndrome	MELAS (*MT-TV*)	Leber Hereditary Optic Neuropathy	Pearson Syndrome	Kearns-Sayre Syndrome
Clinical presentation	Encephalopathy, liver failure (often precipitated by valproic acid), progressive external ophthalmoplegia, myopathy	Regression with illness	Stroke-like episodes, retinopathy, ataxia, ophthalmoplegia; same mutation can cause just diabetes and deafness at lower heteroplasmy levels	Sudden unilateral vision loss ± tremor and encephalopathy	Sideroblastic anemia, pancreatic insufficiency	Progressive external ophthalmoplegia, retinopathy, ataxia, cardiac conduction defects
Inheritance and genetics	Autosomal recessive, impaired mitochondrial DNA replication	Heterogeneous; autosomal recessive inheritance more common than maternal inheritance	Maternal inheritance	Complex I defects, maternal inheritance; not fully penetrant; penetrance higher in smokers and men	*De novo* mtDNA deletion	Maternal inheritance or *de novo*
Radiology	Cerebral atrophy Hepatic steatosis	Signal abnormalities in basal ganglia > other subcortical regions				
Treatment	For all mitochondrial diseases, a "cocktail" of vitamins may be used, but there is not clear evidence of efficacy					
			Arginine for stroke-like episodes; coenzyme Q and riboflavin	Idebenone (Europe only)		Spontaneously resolves, then may evolve into Kearns- Sayre

- Genetics
  - Mitochondrial genome contains 33 genes that are inherited maternally
    - There are multiple, nonidentical copies of the genome per mitochondria and multiple mitochondria per cell; "heteroplasmy" is the percentage of mitochondrial genomes in an organ containing a specific variant
  - The majority of pediatric mitochondrial disease is inherited in an autosomal recessive manner because nuclear genes encode proteins critical for mitochondrial function (e.g., all five respiratory chain complexes, import proteins) and maintenance (e.g., mitochondrial fission, fusion)

CLINICAL PRESENTATION (TABLE 49.6)

- Tissues with high energy requirements are most severely affected
  - Brain, eye, muscle, heart, liver, and kidney
  - General: failure to thrive, hypoglycemia, lactic acidosis
  - CNS: seizures, hypotonia, encephalopathy, regression (especially with fever), basal ganglia lesions/movement disorders, sensorineural hearing loss
  - Ophthalmologic: extraocular ophthalmoplegia, pigmentary retinopathy
  - Muscle: weakness, rhabdomyolysis
  - Cardiac: cardiomyopathy, hypertrophic or dilated
  - Endocrine: diabetes mellitus, thyroid dysfunction, primary adrenal insufficiency, short stature
  - GI: hepatic failure, especially precipitated by valproic acid
  - Renal: tubular acidosis

DIAGNOSIS AND EVALUATION

- Diagnosis of mitochondrial disorders requires an appreciation of the overall clinical presentation
- MRI findings
  - Basal ganglia and other deep brain lesions, bilaterally
  - Basal ganglia calcifications
- Lactate and pyruvate levels
  - Lactate will be elevated with relatively normal pyruvate because lactate → pyruvate is an NAD^+-dependent process
  - Not sensitive
- Because of genetic diversity, unbiased sequencing (e.g. exome)
  - mtDNA sequencing should be done on affected tissue if possible
- Muscle biopsy
  - Helpful, but invasive
  - Can perform respiratory chain analysis
  - Mitochondrial proliferation
    - Occurs in response to mitochondrial defect; more common in nuclear gene defects
  - Ragged red fibers = mitochondria accumulating in subsarcolemma; more common in mtDNA defects
  - Intracytoplasmic lipid droplets
  - "Ghost" mitochondria (with no cristae) or other structural differences
  - COX negative staining (fibers without complex IV)

TREATMENT

- Supportive; poor prognosis
- Mitochondrial cocktail is a scientifically reasonable collection of vitamins that are mitochondrial cofactors

Table 49.7. Laboratory Evaluation of Peroxisomal Disease

Disease	Very Long Chain Fatty Acids	Plasmalogens	Phytanic Acid	Pristanic Acid	Bile Acids
Zellweger disease	Elevated	Low or normal	Normal or high	Normal or high	Normal or high
Rhizomelic chondrodysplasia	Normal	Low	Normal or high	Low or normal	Normal
Adrenoleukodystrophy	High	Normal	Normal	Normal	Normal
Adult Refsum disease	Normal	Normal	High	Low	Normal

- No evidence supports use
- High variability in contents and dose
- Multiple named phenotypes exist, but presentations are variable (Table 49.6)
- Presentations
  - Mitochondrial depletion syndrome
    - Inability to make mtDNA due to nuclear mutation (autosomal recessive)
    - Symptoms include acute neurologic regression, classically accompanied by epilepsia partialis continua and fulminant liver failure (especially if treated with valproic acid)
    - Critical not to treat a patient with epilepsia partialis continua with valproic acid until mitochondrial disease ruled out
  - Leigh syndrome
    - Common phenotype with heterogenous genetics (recessive > mtDNA mutation)
    - Classic presentation: first fever → acute neurologic regression; MRI shows signal abnormalities in basal ganglia and other subcortical areas
    - Usually multiorgan involvement (most common: ophthalmoplegia, cardiomyopathy, renal tubular acidosis
  - Mitochondrial encephalopathy, lactic acidosis, and stroke-like episodes (MELAS)
    - Caused by mitochondrial DNA mutations in tRNA genes—most commonly *MTTL1* (m.3243A>G)
    - Lacticemia and stroke-like episodes that do not follow a vascular distribution
    - Acute treatment with arginine (NO donor) can reverse stroke-like episodes
  - Leber hereditary optic neuropathy (LHON)
    - Mitochondrial DNA mutations affecting complex I
    - Unilateral painless and sudden vision loss in adolescence
    - Contralateral disease classically follows in 2 to 3 months
  - Pearson syndrome
    - *De novo* mtDNA deletion
    - Sideroblastic anemia, which resolves with time if not fatal, and pancreatic insufficiency (exocrine > endocrine)
    - Typically will progress to Kearns-Sayre
  - Kearns-Sayre syndrome
    - Usually *de novo* mitochondrial DNA large deletion
    - Progressive external ophthalmoplegia, retinopathy, cardiac conduction block, and ataxia

Disorders of Peroxisomal Metabolism

BASIC INFORMATION

- Peroxisomes are derived from the endoplasmic reticulum and are responsible for:
  - Beta-oxidation of very-long-chain fatty acids (VLCFAs) to lengths usable by the mitochondria, pristanic acid, and bile acid intermediates
  - Alpha oxidation of phytanic acid
  - Ether phospholipid synthesis (plasmalogens)
  - Glyoxylate detoxification

DIAGNOSIS AND EVALUATION

- Typical elevation of peroxisome metabolites (Table 49.7)
- Liver function tests (LFTs; elevated)
- Measurement of peroxisomal products specific to suspected disease
  - VLCFAs
  - Plasmalogens
  - Phytanic acid
  - Pristinic acid
  - Bile acids
- Treatment → generally supportive care

Peroxisome Biogenesis Disorder (PBD) Spectrum (Zellweger Spectrum, ZS, Neonatal Adrenoleukodystrophy, and Infantile Refsum Disease)

BASIC INFORMATION

- Disorder of peroxisome biogenesis with loss of all peroxisome functions

CLINICAL PRESENTATION

- Dysmorphic features (high forehead, large fontanelle)
- Hypotonia, seizures, and sensorineural hearing loss
- Liver disease (jaundice, cholestasis)

DIAGNOSIS AND EVALUATION

- VLCFAs
- Gene testing (*PEX1* > *PEX6*, other *PEX* genes)

Rhizomelic Chondrodysplasia Punctata (RCDP)

CLINICAL PRESENTATION

- Rhizomelic limb shortening with striking epiphyseal stippling
- Dysmorphic features: broad forehead, contractures
- Intellectual disability
- Cataracts

DIAGNOSIS AND EVALUATION

- Low plasmalogens
- Epiphyseal stippling
- Gene testing (*PEX7*, *DHAPAT*, and *ADHAPS* genes)

X-Linked Adrenoleukodystrophy (XALD)

BASIC INFORMATION

- X-linked recessive deficiency in VLCFA transporter resulting in failure to import VLCFAs
- Only males are affected with the full phenotype; females may have adrenal insufficiency and/or myeloneuropathy

CLINICAL PRESENTATION

- Onset at 4 to 12 years old
- Developmental regression, classically starting with handwriting, accompanied by behavior deterioration (hyperactivity, attention-deficit hyperactivity disorder [ADHD])
- Neurologic deterioration, with ataxia, seizures, and paraplegia
- Adrenal insufficiency

DIAGNOSIS AND EVALUATION

- Elevated VLCFAs
- MRI shows an initially occipital demyelination with leading edge enhancement after gadolinium administration
- Gene testing (*ABCD1* gene)

TREATMENT

- Adrenal steroid hormone supplementation
- Bone marrow transplantation
- Lorenzo's oil has largely fallen out of favor due to difficulty of diet and minimal benefit

Lysosomal Storage Disorders (LSDs)

BASIC INFORMATION

- Intracellular organelle involved in macromolecule, organelle, and cell component catabolism
- Contain multiple hydrolytic enzymes
  - Synthesized in the Golgi
  - Delivered to the lysosome
  - Mannose-6-phosphate trafficking receptor is a common import pathway for many
- Disease caused by defects in lysosomal enzymes, enzyme activators, enzyme trafficking, or enzyme transport receptors
- Results in accumulation of metabolites → lysosomal swelling and dysfunction
- Affects organs where biosynthesis occurs
  - Specific to disease, but commonly liver, spleen, bone, and CNS
- Many families of disorders
  - Mucopolysaccharidoses (MPS)
  - Oligosaccharidoses
  - Sphingolipidoses
  - Mucolipidoses
  - Neuronal ceroid lipofuscinoses

MPS

BASIC INFORMATION

- Glycosaminoglycans (GAGs) accumulate
  - Localize to extracellular matrix
  - Composed of long polysaccharide chains
    - Keratan sulfate (cartilage, cornea, intervertebral disks)
    - Dermatan sulfate (heart, blood vessels, skin)
    - Heparan sulfate
  - Organ-specific accumulation results in symptoms
    - Liver and spleen → hepatosplenomegaly
    - Cornea → corneal clouding
    - Skeleton and joints → bone deformities, coarse facial features, joint stiffening/contractures, spinal cord compression, dysostosis multiplex, hydrocephalus due to foramen magnum narrowing
    - CNS → intellectual disability, behavior difficulties (hyperactivity, oppositional)
    - Other connective tissue → tonsillar hypertrophy, frequent otitis media due to inner ear obstruction, hernias, cardiac valvular thickening
      These symptoms may occur first
      Very important clinical consideration in the child with recurrent otitis, sleep apnea, and/or unexplained hernia
  - Table 49.8 outlines the clinical differences between the various MPSs
  - Diagnosis: urine glycosaminoglycans to differentiate between conditions, enzyme assays; gene testing
  - Treatment: enzyme replacement therapy for some; bone marrow transplant for some

MPS I (Hurler, Hurler-Scheie, and Scheie Syndromes; Alpha-L-Iduronidase Deficiency)

BASIC INFORMATION

- MPS 1 results from impaired dermatan and heparan sulfate metabolism

Table 49.8. Physical Examination and Laboratory Findings in Mucopolysaccharidoses

Disease	Enzyme Defect	Metabolite	Distinguishing Features
MPS I (Hurler and Scheie syndromes)	Alpha-L-iduronidase	Dermatan and heparan sulfate proteoglycans	Coarse features, intellectual disability, behavior difficulties, hepatosplenomegaly, obstructive sleep apnea (adenoid hypertrophy and macroglossia)
MPS II (Hunter syndrome)	Iduronate sulfatase	Dermatan and heparan sulfate proteoglycans	No corneal clouding
MPS III (Sanfilippo syndrome)	N-sulfatase Alpha-N-acetylglucosaminidase N-acetylglucosamine-6-sulfatase	Heparan sulfate proteoglycans	Minimal visceral findings (no corneal clouding, organomegaly, coarse features may be subtle or absent); severe behavior difficulties; insomnia
MPS IV (Morquio syndrome)	N-acetylgalactosamide-6-sulfatase Beta-galactosidase	Keratan sulfate and Chondroitin-6-sulfate proteoglycans	No intellectual disability, severe skeletal phenotype
MPS VI (Maroteaux-Lamy syndrome)	Arylsulfatase B	Dermatan sulfate proteoglycans	No intellectual disability, otherwise resembles MPS I
MPS VII (Sly syndrome)	Beta-glucuronidase	Dermatan, heparan, and chondroitin proteoglycans	Neonatal/fetal onset

- MPS 1 exists on a spectrum from Hurler syndrome (most severe) to Scheie syndrome (least severe)
  - Scheie features isolated corneal clouding, with minimal contractures and only subtly coarsened facial features

TREATMENT

- Hurler: fatal within 5 to 10 years if untreated
- Bone marrow transplantation may ameliorate disease
  - Must be done before CNS symptom onset
  - Usually <1 year of age
- Enzyme supplementation for non-CNS disease
  - Skeletal penetrance poor

MPS Ii (Hunter Syndrome; Iduronate-2-Sulfatase Deficiency)

BASIC INFORMATION

- X-linked recessive
- Impaired dermatan and heparan sulfate metabolism
- Females are **never** affected
- No eye involvement

TREATMENT

- Fatal within 10 to 20 years
- Enzyme replacement for non-CNS disease
- Bone marrow transplantation

MPS Iii (Sanfilippo Syndrome)

BASIC INFORMATION

- Caused by four different enzyme deficiencies, which are phenotypically identical
- Impaired heparan sulfate metabolism

CLINICAL PRESENTATION

- Intellectual regression (age 1–4) → behavioral worsening, intractable insomnia (lasts 3–4 years) → severe intellectual disability with relative resolution of behavioral problems and spasticity
- Likely underdiagnosed
- May have subtle additional features echoing MPS II

TREATMENT/PROGNOSIS

- Clinical trials of intrathecal enzyme replacement
- Death typically in 20s and 30s

Sphingolipidoses

BASIC INFORMATION

- Sphingolipid = modified phospholipids important for neuronal cell membranes
- Precursor accumulation → lysosomal swelling and dysfunction

CLINICAL FEATURES

- Regression
- Progressive psychomotor retardation
- Seizures
- Ataxia
- Hepatosplenomegaly
- ± Bilateral cherry red spot (normal macula surrounded by stored lipid appears red)
- Diagnosis → enzyme studies and gene testing

TAY-SACHS DISEASE (BETA-HEXOSAMINIDASE A DEFICIENCY)

- Onset 4 to 6 months of age
- Cognitive regression
- Hyperacusis

- No hepatosplenomegaly
- Bilateral cherry red spot
- Because of extensive targeted preconception screening since the 1970s, most modern cases are *not* Ashkenazi Jewish
- *HEXA* gene
- GM_2 ganglioside accumulation

NIEMANN-PICK A/B DISEASE (SPHINGOMYELINASE DEFICIENCY)

- Sphingomyelin accumulation
- *SMPD1* gene

NIEMANN-PICK C/D

- Sphingomyelin accumulation due to impaired lysosomal cholesterol transport (due to mutation in receptor *NPC1*, *NPC2*)
- Promising experimental treatment: cyclodextrin in clinical trials

GAUCHER DISEASE (GLUCOSYLCERAMIDASE DEFICIENCY, GLUCOCEREBROSIDASE DEFICIENCY)

- *GBA* gene
- Glucosylceramide (aka glucocerebroside) accumulation
- Three forms
  - Nonneuronopathic (type 1)
    - Most common
    - 1/850 of Ashkenazi Jews are affected
  - Neuronopathic
    - Type 2: severe, infantile onset
    - Type 3: juvenile onset
- Symptoms caused by storage ("Gaucher cells" with "crumpled silk")
  - Bone marrow
    - Bony pain and cortical expansion ("Erlenmeyer flask" deformation)
    - Bone marrow failure (pancytopenia)
  - Liver and spleen
    - Hepatosplenomegaly
    - Splenectomy causes acute decompensation
  - Neuronopathic forms
    - Seizures
    - Neurologic regression
    - Pyramidal signs
- Treatment with enzyme replacement therapy for type I

Neuronal Ceroid Lipofuscinoses

BASIC INFORMATION

- Class of ≥13 genetic entities with similar neurodegenerative phenotypes (epilepsy, developmental regression, vision loss)
- All are defects in one of three lysosomal enzymes

DIAGNOSIS AND EVALUATION

- Electron microscopy of tissue or blood shows classic "fingerprint" cells, "curvilinear bodies," and/or granular osmiophilic deposits

- Immunofluorescence (ceroid staining)
- Enzyme studies
- Gene testing
- Treatment → supportive; gene therapy in animal studies

DISORDERS OF GLYCOSYLATION

Congenital Disorders of Glycosylation

BASIC INFORMATION

- Many proteins (enzymes, receptors) require glycosylation for proper folding, cellular trafficking, and function (e.g., cell-cell recognition)
- There are various types of glycosylation (e.g., N-linked, O-linked, glycosylphosphatidylinositol [GPI] anchors) performed by a multitude of cellular enzymes
- The clinical presentation is highly variable with no single sensitive feature present in every glycosylation disorder. Some features include:
  - Child with unexplained multisystem disease
  - Child with developmental delay and one or more additional features
    - Inverted nipples
    - Abnormal fat pads (suprapubic fat pad with diminished buttock fat)
    - Strabismus
    - Mixed thrombophilic and coagulopathic profile (clotting factors and protein C and S are glycoproteins)
    - Hyperinsulinemic hypoglycemia
    - Cerebellar hypoplasia

DIAGNOSIS AND EVALUATION

- Carbohydrate-deficient transferrin analysis—analyzes for N-linked congenital disorders of glycosylations only
  - May be secondarily abnormal in disorders of sugar metabolism (galactosemia, hereditary fructose intolerance)
- N-glycan and O-glycan analysis
- Gene testing

TREATMENT

- Overall supportive with poor prognosis
- Rare forms respond to specific sugar supplementation

DISORDERS OF PURINE METABOLISM

Disorders of Purine Metabolism

BACKGROUND INFORMATION

- Purines are critical components of DNA
  - Primarily made via salvage pathway → free purines from dietary and metabolic sources
  - Second source *de novo*: generates purines from carbon dioxide, glutamine, and glycine

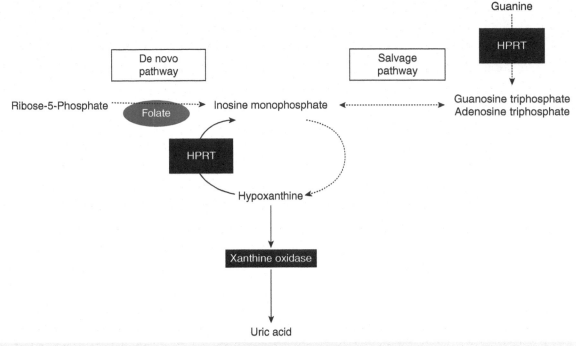

Fig. 49.10. Purine metabolism.

- Inosine monophosphate (IMP) is the key precursor in both pathways (Fig. 49.10)
- Purine catabolism generates uric acid

Lesch-Nyhan Syndrome

BACKGROUND INFORMATION

- X-linked recessive
- Deficiency of hypoxanthine guanine phosphoribosyl transferase (HPRT)
- Converts guanine and hypoxanthine to guanylic acid and IMP, respectively
- Consequent decreased recycling of guanine and hypoxanthine forces excess production of uric acid both through the activity of xanthine oxidase and increased dependence on *de novo* purine synthesis, which generates uric acid

CLINICAL PRESENTATION

- Motor delays are more significant initially followed by global developmental delay/regression starting at 4 to 8 months
- Gout
- Nephrolithiasis → renal failure
- Choreoathetosis
- Spasticity
- Dystonia
- Self-injurious behavior (self-mutilation, especially periorally)
- Megaloblastic anemia

- Milder forms exist
  - Isolated gout
  - Isolated nephrolithiasis
  - Female carriers have increased gout and nephrolithiasis

DIAGNOSIS AND EVALUATION

- Uric acid (increased plasma and urine)
- Urine uric acid to creatinine ratio (increased)
- HPRT enzyme activity (decreased or absent)
- *HPRT* sequencing

TREATMENT

- Allopurinol reduces gout and nephrolithiasis
- Restraints and tooth extraction for behavior

Review Questions

For review questions, please go to ExpertConsult.com

Suggested Readings

1. Saububray JM, van den Berge G, Walter JH. *Inborn metabolic diseases: diagnosis and treatment.* Berlin, Germany: Springer; 2012.
2. Sarafoglou K. *Pediatric endocrinology and inborn errors of metabolism.* New York: NY. McGraw Hill Medical; 2009.
3. Zschocke, Johannes, Hoffmann, Georg F. *Vademecum metabolicum.* 3rd ed. Friedrichsdorf, Germany: Milupa Metabolics GmbH and Company; 2011.
4. Levy PA. Inborn errors of metabolism. *Pediatr Rev.* 2009;30(4):131–137.
5. Rice GM, Steiner RD. Inborn errors of metabolism. *Pediatr Rev.* 2016;37(1):3–15.

Nephrology

50 Management of Fluids and Electrolytes

SHEENA SHARMA, MD, ABDULLA M. EHLAYEL, MD and
LAWRENCE COPELOVITCH, MD

Maintaining the proper fluid distribution and electrolyte composition in the extracellular and intracellular compartments is critical both for maintaining homeostasis and ensuring normal cellular function. The predominant electrolytes found in the intracellular fluid compartment are potassium and magnesium, whereas the predominant electrolytes found in the extracellular fluid compartment are sodium, chloride, and bicarbonate.

See also Nelson Textbook of Pediatrics, Part 7, "Fluid and Electrolyte Disorders."

Water Balance

BASIC INFORMATION

- Water comprises the majority of body weight and is represented by total body water (TBW). TBW is highest in a newborn (~75% of body weight) and decreases with age (~60% of body weight). See Fig. 50.1 details the distribution of TBW, including solute composition for each compartment.
- Two-thirds of TBW is found in the intracellular fluid (ICF) compartment and one-third in the extracellular fluid (ECF) compartment
- Three-fourths of the water in the ECF is interstitial, whereas one-fourth is intravascular.
- Water balance is the difference between intake (gastrointestinal, parenteral) and output (renal; gastrointestinal; insensible, such as skin; pulmonary)
  - Oral intake is primarily regulated by a thirst mechanism, when intact
  - Output is regulated by antidiuretic hormone
  - The majority of losses are urine, insensible (from breathing and skin), and stool
  - Insensible losses are a relatively greater proportion of total losses in newborns and younger children

Hypovolemia

BASIC INFORMATION

- Occurs due to a decrease in water intake or an increase in water loss. Causes of increased water loss are detailed in Table 50.1
- Impaired water intake is typically seen with altered mental status or in children with limited access to water (e.g., infants, children with developmental delay)

DIAGNOSIS

- Clinical manifestations of hypovolemia vary based on severity of dehydration (see Table 50.2)
- May show elevated hemoglobin and hematocrit due to hemoconcentration
- Disproportionately elevated blood urea nitrogen (BUN) compared with serum creatinine (SCr)
- Increased urine specific gravity >1.025
- With acute kidney injury (AKI), the fractional excretion of Na (FENa) can be helpful to distinguish prerenal versus intrinsic renal AKI

$$\text{FENa}\,(\%) = \frac{Urine\,Na \times serum\,Cr}{Serum\,Na \times urine\,Cr} \times 100$$

- FENa is <1% in prerenal AKI (e.g., hypovolemia, congestive heart failure [CHF]) and is >1% in intrinsic renal AKI (e.g., acute tubular necrosis). FENa can be calculated as above:

TREATMENT

- If pre-illness weight is available, calculate percent dehydration:

$$\% \text{ dehydration} = [(\text{Pre-illness weight} - \text{Current weight}) / \text{Pre-illness weight} \times 100$$

- If pre-illness weight is not available, percent dehydration can be clinically assessed, as in Table 50.2
- First restore intravascular volume with normal saline at 20 mL/kg. Repeat as needed until patient is no longer significantly dehydrated
- Calculate 24-hour fluid requirement: maintenance + remaining deficit
- May consider oral rehydration solution

MAINTENANCE FLUID ESTIMATION

- Maintenance fluid requirements can be estimated by the Holliday-Segar method. Daily water requirements are calculated based on body weight and on the assumption that each kilocalorie of energy metabolized results in the net consumption of 1 mL of water
  - See Table 50.3 for a method of calculation

365

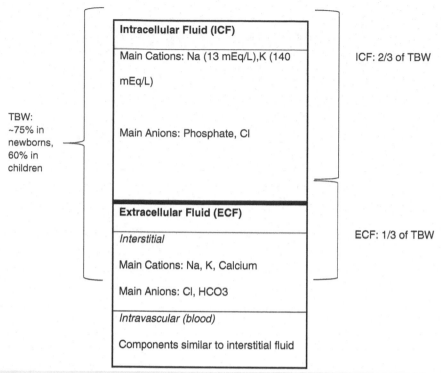

Fig. 50.1. Distribution of total body water (TBW), including solute composition for each compartment.

Table 50.1. Sources of Water Loss

System	Example
Gastrointestinal	Fluid losses with vomiting, diarrhea
Skin	Sweating, burns, ichthyosis
Respiratory	Tachypnea
Renal	Medication: diuretics Endocrine: diabetes mellitus, diabetes insipidus, adrenal insufficiency Renal: partial obstruction with aldosterone resistance Electrolyte: hypercalcemia, hypokalemia

- Calculation is based on the assumptions that all daily water losses occur as the result of either insensible or urine losses and that all homeostatic mechanisms are intact
- Holliday-Segar method may not be appropriate in children with urine outputs that are abnormally high (adrenal failure, diuretic exposure) or low (hypovolemia, syndrome of inappropriate antidiuretic hormone [SIADH], renal failure, CHF, nephrotic syndrome, cirrhosis)
- Insensible losses in the absence of conditions leading to increased fluid loss (e.g., fever, hyperventilation, prematurity and low birth weight, skin defects, burns) are usually 400 to 700 mL/m² body surface area (BSA; higher in neonates, up to 1150 mL/m²)

Hypervolemia

BASIC INFORMATION

- Occurs due to expansion of ECF, typically due to decreased urine output from renal failure, nephrotic syndrome, CHF, or liver failure

CLINICAL PRESENTATION

- Usually presents with generalized edema
  - May have pitting edema in the extremities, pleural effusion, and/or ascites
- Hypervolemia associated with CHF and liver cirrhosis has normal to low blood pressure
- Hypervolemia associated with renal failure is usually associated with hypertension and less pronounced edema

DIAGNOSIS

- Primarily dependent on history and physical examination, followed by focused evaluation based on the most likely underlying disorder (e.g., echocardiogram for CHF, ultrasound and serum laboratory testing for renal failure)

TREATMENT

- Treat the underlying disorder
- Sodium and fluid restriction
- Diuretics
- Renal replacement therapy may be necessary in the setting of anuria/oliguria with associated potentially life-threatening consequences if the volume not removed (e.g., pleural effusions leading to respiratory compromise). Examples include hemodialysis, peritoneal dialysis, and continuous renal replacement therapy

Sodium Balance

BASIC INFORMATION

- Sodium homeostasis in the body is maintained by a balance of intake (diet, medications) and output (urine losses, sweat)

Table 50.2. Clinical Manifestations of Hypovolemia

Symptom	Minimal or No Dehydration (<3% Loss of Body Weight)	Mild to Moderate Dehydration (3%–9% Loss of Body Weight)	Severe Dehydration (>9% Loss of Body Weight)
Mental status	Well, alert	Normal, fatigued or restless, irritable	Apathetic, lethargic, unconscious
Thirst	Drinks normally, might refuse liquids	Thirsty, eager to drink	Drinks poorly, unable to drink
Heart rate	Normal	Normal to increased	Tachycardia, with bradycardia in most severe cases
Quality of pulses	Normal	Normal to decreased	Weak, thready, or impalpable
Breathing	Normal	Normal, fast	Deep
Eyes	Normal	Slightly sunken	Deeply sunken
Tears	Present	Decreased	Absent
Mouth and tongue	Moist	Dry	Parched
Skinfold	Instant recoil	Recoil in <2 seconds	Recoil in <2 seconds
Capillary refill	Normal	Prolonged	Prolonged, minimal
Extremities	Warm	Cool	Cold, mottled, cyanotic
Urine output	Normal to decreased	Decreased	Minimal

Data from Duggan C, Santosham M, Glass RI. The management of acute diarrhea in children: oral rehydration, maintenance, and nutritional therapy. *MMWR*, 1992;41(No. RR-16):1–20; World Health Organization. The treatment of diarrhoea: a manual for physicians and other senior health workers. Geneva, Switzerland: World Health Organization, 1995. Available at http://www.who.int/child-adolescent-health/New_Publications/CHILD_HEALTH/WHO.CDR.95.3.htm.

Table 50.3. Holliday-Segar Method of Maintenance Fluid Calculation

Patient Weight	Maintenance per Hour (mL/hr)	Maintenance per Day (mL/day)
0–10 kg	4 mL/kg	100 mL/kg
10–20 kg	40 mL (for the first 10 kg) + 2 mL/kg for each kg >10	1000 mL (for the first 10 kg) + 50 mL/kg for each kg >10
>20 kg	40 mL (for the first 10 kg) + 20 mL (for the second 10 kg) + 2 mL/kg for each kg >20	1000 mL (for the first 10 kg) + 50 mL (for the second 10 kg) + 25 mL/kg for each kg >20

- Regulation of sodium is important to maintain the ECF volume
  - Complex mechanisms are involved; mainly rely on pressure receptors (i.e., baroreceptors), the juxtaglomerular apparatus, and hormone release (aldosterone, renin/angiotensin)

Hyponatremia

BASIC INFORMATION

- Definition: serum sodium concentration less than 135 mEq/L
- Etiology can be classified based on volume status (see Table 50.4)

CLINICAL PRESENTATION

- Anorexia, headache, nausea, vomiting, lethargy, muscle cramping
- Central nervous system (CNS): seizures, altered mental status, decreased reflexes
- Brainstem herniation due to cellular swelling and respiratory arrest is possible

Table 50.4. Etiologies of Hyponatremia

Euvolemia	Syndrome of inappropriate diuretic hormone (SIADH), hypothyroidism, psychogenic polydipsia, dilute infant formula
Hypervolemia	Congestive heart failure, nephrotic syndrome, cirrhosis, renal failure, pregnancy
	Salt poisoning
Hypovolemia	Gastroenteritis, diuretics, adrenal insufficiency, third-space losses (burns, pancreatitis, trauma)

TREATMENT

- Management should be based on the clinical presentation and underlying etiology
  - Acute symptomatic hyponatremia: hyponatremia that occurs <24 to 48 hours and is symptomatic (e.g., seizures): consider intravenous (IV) hypertonic saline (e.g., 2–6 mL/kg of 3% NaCl)
  - Chronic hyponatremia: occurs over >24 to 48 hours. In general, correct serum sodium at a rate of 0.5 mEq/L/hour or less, or 10 to 12 mEq/L in 24 hours. Rapid correction of hyponatremia (especially if chronic hyponatremia) can lead to central pontine myelinolysis
  - Hypovolemic hyponatremia: for hyponatremia with symptomatic hypovolemia, start with reexpansion of ECF volume with IV isotonic saline (e.g., normal saline solution 20 mL/kg over 30 to 60 minutes; may repeat as necessary)
  - Euvolemic hyponatremia: address underlying etiology (e.g., treat hypothyroidism)
    For SIADH: water restriction (25%–50% of daily maintenance requirement) with monitoring of serum sodium. Definitive management requires establishing the underlying etiology. Compare urine and serum osmolality to differentiate between SIADH and water intoxication. Withhold offending medications

■ Hypervolemic hyponatremia: treat underlying condition (renal, cardiac, hepatic). Consider fluid restriction

IATROGENIC HYPONATREMIA IN HOSPITALIZED CHILDREN

■ Hospitalized children may have various nonosmotic triggers for antidiuretic hormone (ADH) release, including nausea, emesis, pain, stress, postoperative state, CNS disorders (meningitis, encephalitis, tumors, head injury), pulmonary diseases (pneumonia, asthma, bronchiolitis), malignancies, and medications (morphine, cyclophosphamide, etc.)
■ Isotonic IV fluids (0.9% NaCl) are a reasonable option in children at risk for developing hyponatremia, although there is risk of hypernatremia
■ Slight fluid restriction may also be considered once the patient is euvolemic and hemodynamically stable

Hypernatremia

BASIC INFORMATION

■ Definition: serum sodium concentration greater than 145 mEq/L
■ Etiology can be classified based on volume status (see Table 50.5)

CLINICAL PRESENTATION

■ Irritability, muscle weakness, lethargy, restlessness, muscle twitching
■ CNS: altered mental status, seizures, coma

TREATMENT

■ Rapid correction of pronounced hypernatremia (especially if chronic hypernatremia) can result in life-threatening cerebral edema. In general, aim to lower serum sodium by 10 to 12 mEq/L every 24 hours
■ If patient is severely dehydrated, start with isotonic saline bolus (e.g., normal saline solution 20 mL/kg over 1 hour; may repeat) to restore circulation regardless of serum sodium level
■ Free water deficits (FWD) should be corrected over 24 to 48 hours. FWD can be estimated by 4 mL of free water (FW)/kg needed to reduce serum Na^+ by 1 mEq/L (for serum sodium <170 mEq/L). Choose a solution that is hypotonic but will not lower serum sodium too quickly. Remember to give maintenance fluid requirements as well. The formula that follows can be used to estimate FWD:

$$FWD\ (L) = 0.6 \times weight\ (kg) \times \frac{serum\ Na - 140}{140}$$

Potassium Balance

BASIC INFORMATION

■ Potassium is primarily an intracellular cation, with a small amount present within the extracellular space

Table 50.5.   Etiologies of Hypernatremia

Volume Status	Etiology	Clinical Scenarios
Hypovolemia	Diabetes insipidus (central or nephrogenic)	
	Insensible free water losses (e.g., burns)	
	Decreased water intake	Diarrhea and rehydration with inappropriately hyperosmolar formula Nonintact thirst mechanism in the context of inappropriately low free water administration
Hypervolemia	Hyperaldosteronism	
	Cushing syndrome	
	Salt poisoning	Medications (e.g., sodium bicarbonate, NaCl tablets) Seawater ingestion

■ The ratio of intracellular to extracellular potassium influences neuronal, muscular, and cardiovascular excitability. Therefore, any imbalances within potassium regulation could have potentially serious consequences.

Hypokalemia

BASIC INFORMATION

■ Etiology and differential diagnoses (see Table 50.6)

CLINICAL PRESENTATION

■ Nonspecific symptom of weakness or muscle cramps
■ Nephrogenic diabetes insipidus causing polyuria and polydipsia
■ Rarely, diaphragmatic paralysis leading to respiratory arrest
■ Ileus
■ Urinary retention
■ Cardiac arrhythmias

DIAGNOSIS AND EVALUATION

■ History and physical examination
■ ECG can show multiple changes, most commonly including flattened T waves and ST interval depression
■ U waves are less common and occur if hypokalemia is severe
■ Arrhythmias include sinus bradycardia, ventricular tachycardia or fibrillation, and torsade de pointes
■ Check for alkalosis because this may cause potassium to shift intracellularly
■ Check magnesium level because hypomagnesemia promotes renal potassium wasting, which may cause hypokalemia to become refractory to treatment

Table 50.6. Etiologies of Hypokalemia

Inadequate Intake	Less Common
Renal losses	■ Fanconi syndrome (proximal tubular dysfunction leading to hypokalemia, metabolic acidosis, hypophosphatemia, and glucosuria) ■ Bartter and Gitelman syndrome ■ Potassium-wasting diuretics (e.g., loop diuretics, thiazides) ■ Osmotic diuresis (e.g., hyperglycemia) ■ Primary aldosteronism ■ Congenital adrenal hyperplasia ■ Renal tubular acidosis (type I and type II) ■ Liddle syndrome, apparent mineralocorticoid excess (AME), glucocorticoid remediable aldosteronism (GRA) ■ Hypomagnesemia
Gastrointestinal losses	■ Emesis ■ Diarrhea ■ Gastric suctioning via nasogastric tube
Intracellular shift	■ Medication induced (e.g., insulin and albuterol) ■ Alkalosis ■ Catecholamine excess

TREATMENT

■ Treat the underlying cause if evaluation reveals a diagnosis
■ Oral potassium citrate/acetate, potassium chloride, or potassium phosphate if hypokalemia is mild
■ If patient is symptomatic, hypokalemia is severe, or patient cannot tolerate oral supplementation, IV potassium chloride can be given
  ■ There is increased risk of cardiac arrest from rapid administration of IV potassium
■ Ensure serum magnesium is replete

Hyperkalemia

BASIC INFORMATION

■ Etiology and differential diagnoses (see Table 50.7)

CLINICAL PRESENTATION

■ Nonspecific symptoms of weakness and paresthesias
■ Cardiac arrhythmias with ventricular fibrillation or asystole

DIAGNOSIS AND EVALUATION

■ History and physical examination
■ Free-flowing venipuncture is needed because hemolysis can occur with a tourniquet
■ ECG can show peaked T waves, PR-interval prolongation, widened QRS complexes, and shortened QT interval
■ Arrhythmias include sinus bradycardia, sinus arrest, ventricular tachycardia or fibrillation, and asystole

TREATMENT

■ Treat the underlying cause if evaluation reveals a diagnosis

Table 50.7. Etiology and Differential Diagnoses of Hyperkalemia

Increased intake (typically only problematic in the setting of renal failure)	■ IV fluids with potassium or total parenteral nutrition ■ Oral intake of high-potassium foods ■ Blood product transfusions
Decreased excretion of potassium by the kidneys	■ Angiotensin-converting enzyme inhibitors, angiotensin-receptor blockers, or potassium-sparing diuretics ■ Aldosterone deficiency or resistance ■ End-stage renal disease
Extracellular shift	■ Medication induced (e.g., beta-blockers) ■ Acidosis
Abnormal potassium release from cells	■ Tumor lysis syndrome (also with hyperuricemia, hypocalcemia, and hyperphosphatemia) ■ Rhabdomyolysis

■ Administer IV calcium gluconate to stabilize the cardiac membrane if ECG changes are present
■ Insulin/glucose, albuterol, and sodium bicarbonate all help shift potassium intracellularly but will not remove potassium from the body
■ Diuretics (e.g., loop diuretics if no renal failure), sodium polystyrene sulfonate, and dialysis are the methods that will remove potassium from the body
  ■ Sodium polystyrene sulfonate is not commonly used in neonates, especially those with reduced bowel motility for concerns of bowel necrosis

Calcium Balance

BASIC INFORMATION

■ Calcium is a cation found within the ECF
■ Calcium homeostasis is maintained through tight regulation with various hormones, most notably parathyroid hormone (PTH) and 1,25(OH)2D (the active form of vitamin D). Specific disorders will be detailed in Chapter 24
■ Calcium is needed for voltage-gated ion channels to function correctly, and therefore any imbalances may cause neuromuscular issues, neurologic symptoms (e.g. seizures), and/or cardiac dysrhythmias.

Hypocalcemia

BASIC INFORMATION

■ Etiology and differential diagnoses:
  ■ Hypoparathyroidism: familial, DiGeorge syndrome, idiopathic, postsurgical
  ■ Vitamin D deficiency: dietary deficiency, lack of sunlight, malabsorption
  ■ Vitamin D resistance: familial hypophosphatemic rickets
  ■ Other: chronic kidney disease, acute pancreatitis, magnesium deficiency, autosomal dominant hypocalcemic hypercalciuria

■ Neonatal hypocalcemia: prematurity, intrauterine growth restriction, infant of a diabetic mother

CLINICAL PRESENTATION

■ Nonspecific symptom of weakness
■ Neurologic symptoms including perioral numbness, paresthesia, carpal-pedal spasms, tetany, seizures, positive Chvostek sign, and positive Trousseau sign
■ Rickets if hypocalcemia is chronic

DIAGNOSIS AND EVALUATION

■ History and physical examination
■ Laboratory evaluation should include creatinine, phosphorus, magnesium, PTH, 25-OH vitamin D level, 1,25-OH vitamin D level, and urine calcium/urine creatinine
■ Albumin should always be assessed:
  ■ For every 1 g/dL that the serum albumin is below normal, 0.8 mg/dL should be added to the serum calcium
  ■ Ionized calcium is often a more reliable estimate of serum calcium level

TREATMENT

■ Treat the underlying cause if evaluation reveals a diagnosis
■ If severe (e.g., ECG changes showing prolonged QT interval) and/or symptomatic hypocalcemia, administer IV calcium gluconate
  ■ Consider ECG monitoring because there is a risk of cardiac arrest if infusion is too rapid
■ If the patient is stable and/or hypocalcemia is chronic, oral calcium should be initiated
■ Start cholecalciferol or calcitriol if values are noted to be low
■ Replete with magnesium if the patient is hypomagnesemic

Hypercalcemia

BASIC INFORMATION

■ Etiology and differential diagnoses:
  ■ Endocrine disorders: hyperparathyroidism, Addison disease, hyperthyroidism
  ■ Immobilization (especially after long-bone fracture)
  ■ Malignancy
  ■ Genetic conditions: Williams syndrome, *CYP24A1* gene mutations, familial hypocalciuric hypercalcemia
  ■ Granulomatous diseases (e.g., sarcoidosis, tuberculosis, Crohn disease)
  ■ Iatrogenic (e.g., excess vitamin D intake, total parenteral nutrition [TPN])
  ■ Pancreatitis

CLINICAL PRESENTATION

■ Nonspecific symptoms, including fatigue and lethargy
■ Neurologic symptoms, including muscle weakness, hyporeflexia, and impaired concentration
■ Gastrointestinal symptoms, including nausea, emesis, constipation, and abdominal pain
■ Hypertension may accompany hypercalcemia

■ Acquired nephrogenic diabetes insipidus will present with polyuria and polydipsia
■ Patients with chronic hypercalcemia may present with increased risk of nephrocalcinosis or nephrolithiasis

DIAGNOSIS AND EVALUATION

■ Similar to evaluation for hypocalcemia
■ History and physical examination
■ Laboratory evaluation should include creatinine, PTH, 25-OH vitamin D level, urine calcium/urine creatinine, and ionized calcium level
■ Additional specific workup should be obtained depending on clinical suspicion (e.g., thyroid function tests, angiotensin-converting enzyme level, renal/bladder ultrasound to assess for kidney stones)
■ ECG shows shortened QT interval

TREATMENT

■ Treat the underlying cause if evaluation reveals a diagnosis
■ Get an ECG to assess for shortened QT interval
■ Administer IV fluids with normal saline to increase excretion of calcium into the urine with or without loop diuretic
■ Bisphosphonates and calcitonin can be used but are more commonly used in adults
■ Cinacalcet is an allosteric activator of the calcium-sensing receptor that causes a decrease in PTH
■ Hemodialysis can be used in refractory cases

Review Questions

For review questions, please go to ExpertConsult.com.

Suggested Reading

1. Abdo A, Mohandas R, Wingo CS. A physiologic-based approach to the treatment of a patient with hypokalemia. *Am J Kidney Dis.* 2012;60(3):492–497.
2. Allon M. Disorders of calcium and phosphorus. In: Greenberg A, ed. *Primer on kidney diseases.* 5th ed. Philadelphia: Saunders Elsevier; 2009: 118–128.
3. Allon M. Disorders of potassium metabolism. In: Greenberg A, ed. *Primer on kidney diseases.* 5th ed. Philadelphia: Saunders Elsevier; 2009: 108–116.
4. Gillespie RS. Hyperkalemia. In: *Robert's Review of Pediatric Nephrology.* 2nd ed. Arlington: KidneyWeb Media; 2013:25–26.
5. Gillespie RS. Hypokalemia. In: *Robert's Review of Pediatric Nephrology.* 2nd ed. Arlington: KidneyWeb Media; 2013:25.
6. Gillespie RS. Hypocalcemia. In: *Robert's Review of Pediatric Nephrology.* 2nd ed. Arlington: KidneyWeb Media; 2013:27–28.
7. Gillespie RS. Hypercalcemia. In: *Robert's Review of Pediatric Nephrology.* 2nd ed. Arlington: KidneyWeb Media; 2013:28–29.
8. Greenbaum L. Maintenance and replacement therapy. In: Kliegman RM, St. Geme J, Stanton BMD, eds. *Nelson Textbook of Pediatrics.* 20th ed. Philadelphia: Elsevier; 2016.
9. Jain A. Body fluid composition. *PIR.* 2015;36(4):141–145.
10. Lehnhardt A, Kemper MJ. Pathogenesis, diagnosis and management of hyperkalemia. *Pediatr Nephrol.* 2011;26(3):377–384.
11. Lietman SA, Germain-Lee EL, Levine MA. Hypercalcemia in children and adolescents. *Curr Opin Pediatr.* 2010;22(4):508–515.
12. Moritz M, Ayus J. Disorders of water metabolism in children: hyponatremia and hypernatremia. *PIR.* Nov 2002;23(11):371–380.
13. Peacock M. Calcium metabolism in health and disease. *Clin J Am Soc Nephol.* 2010;5:S23–S30.
14. Viera AJ, Wouk N. Potassium disorders: hypokalemia and hyperkalemia. *Am Fam Physician.* 2015;92(6):487–495.

Clinical Approach to Acid-Base Disturbances

CELINA BRUNSON, BS, MD, CAROLINE GLUCK, MD, MTR and STEPHANIE CLARK, MD, MPH, MSHP

The human body requires careful maintenance of acid-base homeostasis. Normal serum pH ranges from 7.35 to 7.45. Derangements in the serum pH may lead to altered metabolic function and ultimately cell death. As such, the human body has a buffer system to maintain normal serum pH. The organs primarily responsible for maintaining this system are the lungs and the kidneys.

See also Nelson Textbook of Pediatrics, Chapter 55, "Electrolyte and Acid-Base Disorders."

Review of Acid-Base Physiology

- Definitions:
  - Acid = proton donor
  - Base = proton acceptor
  - Buffer = weak base, able to bind free protons
- The primary buffer in humans is the bicarbonate buffer system, which stabilizes serum pH
  - $H^+ + HCO_3^- \leftrightarrow H_2CO_3 \leftrightarrow H_2O + CO_2$
  - Henderson-Hasselbalch equation:
    - $pH = pKa + \log ([HCO_3^-]/[0.03 \times pCO_2])$
  - The bicarbonate buffer system stabilizes pH by accepting a proton and converting bicarbonate to carbon dioxide (via carbonic anhydrase)
- Other buffers include phosphate (bone), proteins, and phosphate (intracellular fluid)
- Lungs:
  - Carbon dioxide can be quickly eliminated through the lungs
  - Hyperventilation reduces carbon dioxide and increases serum pH; hypoventilation leads to increased carbon dioxide and lowers serum pH
- Kidneys:
  - Acid and base can be eliminated slowly through the kidneys
  - 80% to 90% of filtered bicarbonate is reabsorbed by the proximal tubule, and 10% of filtered bicarbonate is reabsorbed in the thick ascending limb of the loop of Henle
  - Acid (H^+) excretion, and to a lesser extent bicarbonate excretion, occurs in the collecting duct
  - Factors that affect proton excretion include:
    - Acidemia
    - Distal sodium delivery
    - Hyperkalemia
    - Aldosterone

Approach to Acid-Base Dysregulation

- Acidemia (serum pH lower than normal) or alkalemia (serum pH higher than normal) may be caused by:

- Metabolic acidosis
- Metabolic alkalosis
- Respiratory acidosis
- Respiratory alkalosis
- Combination of these processes
- Characterization of the underlying process can be achieved through the analysis of blood gas (pH, pCO_2, base deficit) and serum bicarbonate levels
  - Low pH = Acidemia
    - High pCO_2 → Respiratory acidosis
    - Low bicarbonate and base deficit → Metabolic acidosis
  - High pH = alkalemia
    - Low pCO_2 → Respiratory alkalosis
    - High bicarbonate and base excess → Metabolic alkalosis
- Acid-base compensation
  - To assess respiratory compensation in metabolic acidosis, Winters formula can be used:

$$pCO_2 = (1.5 \times HCO_3^-) + 8 +/- 2$$

  - If calculated pCO_2 equals measured pCO_2, there is an expected degree of respiratory compensation (i.e., Kussmaul breathing)
  - If measured pCO2 is higher than the calculated pCO2, there is a mixed metabolic and respiratory acidosis
  - If calculated pCO_2 is lower than measured pCO_2, there is a mixed respiratory and metabolic acidosis
  - Winters formula cannot be used to assess respiratory compensation for metabolic alkalosis
  - Formulas exist for expected compensation in other simple acid-base disorders as well (see Table 51.1)

Metabolic Acidosis

BASIC INFORMATION

- Metabolic acidosis is characterized on blood gas by acidemia (low pH), base deficit (>5 mEq/L), and low serum bicarbonate
- Metabolic acidosis may present in a myriad of ways dependent on the etiology of the acidosis. Deciphering the underlying etiology can best be achieved through careful history and physical examination, as well as serum and urine analysis
- Metabolic acidosis can be further characterized as increased anion gap (AG) or normal anion gap metabolic acidosis:
  - Anion gap = $Na^+ - (Cl^- + HCO_3^-)$
  - Normal anion gap = 8 to 12 mEq/L

Table 51.1. Appropriate Compensation During Simple Acid-Base Disorders

Disorder	Expected Compensation*
Metabolic acidosis	$P_{CO_2} = 1.5 \times [HCO_3^-] + 8 \pm 2$
Metabolic alkalosis	P_{CO_2} increases by 7 mm Hg for each 10-mEq/L increase in the serum $[HCO_3^-]$
RESPIRATORY ACIDOSIS	
Acute	$[HCO_3^-]$ increases by 1 for each 10-mm Hg increase in the P_{CO_2}
Chronic	$[HCO_3^-]$ increases by 3.5 for each 10-mm Hg increase in the P_{CO_2}
RESPIRATORY ALKALOSIS	
Acute	$[HCO_3^-]$ falls by 2 for each 10-mm Hg decrease in the P_{CO_2}
Chronic	$[HCO_3^-]$ falls by 4 for each 10-mm Hg decrease in the P_{CO_2}

*$[HCO_3^-]$ is expressed in mEq/L.

Table 51.2. Three General Mechanisms of Normal Anion Gap Metabolic Acidosis

Mechanism	Example	Urine Anion Gap	Urine Osmolal Gap
Increased loss of bicarbonate	Diarrhea Enterostomies Type II renal tubular acidosis	Negative	>150 mEq/L
Decreased acid excretion	Type I and type IV renal tubular acidosis Hypoaldosteronism	Positive	<50 mEq/L
Increased acid administration	Arginine chloride Total parenteral nutrition	Negative	>150 mEq/L

NORMAL ANION GAP ACIDOSIS

- Normal anion gap metabolic acidosis results from three general mechanisms (see Table 51.2):
  - Increased loss of bicarbonate
  - Reduced acid excretion
  - Increased acid administration
- Diagnostic tests for a normal anion gap acidosis:
  - Urine anion gap = $Na^+ + K^+ - Cl^-$
    - Normal urine anion gap = Zero to slightly positive (<10)
  - Urine osmolal gap = Measured urine osmolality – Calculated urine osmolality
    - Calculated Urine Osmolality = 2 x (urine Na+) + 2x (Urine K+) + (urinary urea nitrogen/2.8) + (urine glucose/18) where urea nitrogen and glucose are measured in mg/dL
    - Normal urine osmolal gap = 10 to 100 mEq/L

Increased Anion Gap Acidosis

- Increased anion gap metabolic acidosis results from:
  - Increased unmeasured anion (i.e., lactate) accumulation
  - Several mnemonics exist to facilitate recall of causes of increased anion gap metabolic acidoses (see Table 51.3)

Table 51.3. Mnemonics to Facilitate Recall of Causes of Increased Anion Gap Metabolic Acidoses

Mudpiles	Laaarrrk
Methanol poisoning	**L**actate
Uremia	**A**lcohols (methanol, ethanol, ethylene glycol)
Diabetic ketoacidosis	
Paraldehyde	**A**ldehydes (paraldehyde, formaldehyde)
Iron and **I**soniazid and Inborn Errors of Metabolism	**A**mino Acids
	Renal Failure
	Rhabdomyolysis
Lactic acidosis	**R**x (salicylates, oxoproline – metabolite of Tylenol, metformin, iron, INH)
Ethylene glycol poisoning	
Salicylate poisoning	**K**etoacids

- Osmolar gap = Measured serum osmolality – Calculated serum osmolality
  - Calculated serum osmolality = 2[Na+] + [Glucose]/18 + [BUN]/2.8 where [Glucose] and [BUN] are measured in mg/dL
  - Normal osmolar gap = 8 to 12 mOsm/L
  - Increased osmolar gap occurs with ingestion/production of small-molecular-weight compounds (e.g., alcohol ingestion as in ethylene glycol toxicity)
  - Determine the presence of a mixed increased anion gap and normal anion gap metabolic acidosis using the delta ratio:
    - Delta ratio = (Measured anion gap – Normal anion gap)/(Normal bicarbonate concentration – Measured bicarbonate concentration) = (Anion gap – 12 mmol/L)/(24 mmol/L – $[HCO_3^-]$)
    - Delta ratio ≥1 in pure increased anion gap acidosis
    - Delta ratio <1 in mixed increased anion gap and normal anion gap metabolic acidosis

Renal Tubular Acidosis (RTA)

- Renal tubular acidosis occurs because of a loss of bicarbonate through the urine or the inability to acidify the urine. There are four types of RTA, which can be distinguished by several features detailed in Table 51.4.

Type I (Distal) RTA

CLINICAL PRESENTATION

- Most commonly presents in infancy and early childhood with:
  - Failure to thrive
  - Hypercalciuria, nephrocalcinosis
  - Hypokalemia, muscle weakness
  - Osteopenia
- May be idiopathic or related to another inherited or acquired disease (i.e., sickle cell disease or Sjögren syndrome) or may be due to medications (i.e., amphotericin)
- Certain causal genetic mutations may have other associated symptoms:
  - Early deafness (seen with defect in *ATP6V1B1* gene)
  - Late deafness (seen with defect in *ATP6V0A4* gene)
  - Hemolytic anemia/spherocytosis (seen with defect in *SLC4A1* gene)

Table 51.4.   Renal Tubular Acidoses

Renal Tubular Acidosis	Mechanism	Urine pH	Serum Potassium	Urinary Anion Gap	Other Characteristics
Type I (Distal)	Inability to acidify the urine in the *distal* nephron	>5.5	Low	Positive	Commonly associated with hypercalciuria and nephrocalcinosis
Type II (Proximal)	Inability to reabsorb bicarbonate in the *proximal* tubule	<5.5 or normal	Low or normal	Negative or normal	May be associated with Fanconi syndrome due to inability of the proximal tubule to reabsorb other electrolytes, amino acids, and glucose
Type III (Mixed)	Defects in both reabsorption of bicarbonate in the *proximal* tubule and acid excretion in the *distal* nephron	>5.5	Low	Positive	This is very rare and usually associated with a defect in carbonic anhydrase II
Type IV	Aldosterone deficiency or resistance leads to hyperkalemia and decreased acid secretion in the distal nephron as well as reduced proximal tubule generation of ammonia	Variable	High	Positive	

DIAGNOSIS AND EVALUATION

- Clinical presentation
- Serum with low bicarbonate concentration and hypokalemia associated with high urinary pH
- Family history and genetic testing

TREATMENT

- Electrolyte repletion
  - In the acute presentation, hypokalemia must be corrected before acidemia is corrected
  - Young children will often require more alkali therapy (2–4 mEq/kg/day) than older children (1–3 mEq/kg/day)
- Monitor growth and bone health

Type II (Proximal) RTA

CLINICAL PRESENTATION

- Age of presentation: infancy and early childhood
- Failure to thrive
- Vomiting
- Polyuria and polydipsia
- Mild hypokalemia
- Rickets
- May have eye abnormalities
- Isolated proximal tubule defect in bicarbonate reabsorption (may be transient in the neonatal period) versus generalized proximal tubule dysfunction (Fanconi syndrome)
- Fanconi syndrome:
  - Characterized by glucosuria, phosphaturia, aminoaciduria, and bicarbonaturia
  - Idiopathic versus inherited versus acquired causes
    - Inherited: inborn errors of metabolism (cystinosis, tyrosinemia, galactosemia, hereditary fructose intolerance, Wilson disease, Lowe syndrome, mitochondrial disease)
    - Acquired: medications (i.e., aminoglycosides and alkylating agents) and toxins (i.e., glue sniffing [toluene], heavy metal poisoning)

DIAGNOSIS AND EVALUATION

- Clinical presentation
- Serum with low bicarbonate concentration ± hypokalemia, hypophosphatemia, volume contraction
- Urine with low-normal urinary pH with glucosuria, aminoaciduria, or phosphaturia
- Eye examination:
  - Cataracts (Lowe syndrome, galactosemia, autosomal recessive form of type II RTA)
  - Kayser-Fleischer rings (Wilson disease)
  - Cysteine crystals (cystinosis)
- Systemic involvement for inborn errors of metabolism

TREATMENT

- Alkali therapy 2 to 20 mEq/kg/day in small, frequent doses
- Electrolyte repletion
- Volume repletion (may require continuous large-volume feeds)
- Monitor growth and bone health
- Treat underlying inborn error of metabolism (i.e., cysteamine for cystinosis)

Type III (Mixed) RTA

CLINICAL PRESENTATION

- Osteopetrosis, mental retardation, and cerebral calcifications associated with a defect in carbonic anhydrase II

Type IV (Hyperkalemic) RTA

CLINICAL PRESENTATION

- Causes include:
  - Congenital adrenal hyperplasia (CAH)

- Pseudohypoaldosteronism I (epithelial sodium channel [ENaC] defect—autosomal recessive; aldosterone resistance—autosomal dominant)
  - Hyperkalemia and salt wasting
  - Newborns may have respiratory distress due to impaired salt and water reabsorption
- Pseudohypoaldosteronism II (Gordon syndrome)
  - Hyperkalemia and hypertension
- Obstructive uropathy and renal dysplasia
- Medications (i.e., angiotensin-converting enzyme [ACE] inhibition, tacrolimus, heparin)

DIAGNOSIS AND EVALUATION

- Clinical history is key to making diagnosis
- Serum with low bicarbonate concentration and high potassium concentration
  - Transtubular potassium gradient (TTKG) = ([Urine K^+] × Serum osmolality)/([Serum K^+] × Urine osmolality)
  - Low TTKG with hyperkalemia indicates aldosterone deficiency or resistance
- If indicated, serum renin and aldosterone levels

TREATMENT

- Alkali therapy
- Thiazide diuretics (Gordon syndrome)
- Glucocorticoid/mineralocorticoid repletion (CAH/Addison disease)
- Treatment of hyperkalemia with loop diuretics, low-potassium formulas/diets, and cation exchange resins (Kayexalate)

Metabolic Alkalosis

BASIC INFORMATION

- Metabolic alkalosis is identified by elevated pH on a blood gas and elevated serum bicarbonate. In response to metabolic alkalosis, the body compensates with hypoventilation, leading to increased pCO_2 and respiratory acidosis
- Metabolic alkalosis occurs when there is a loss of acid (more common) or accumulation of base from the extracellular fluid (ECF)
- The mechanisms include loss of NaCl leading to alkalosis by volume depletion (see Fig. 51.1) and loss of HCl/KCl causing increased secretion of HCO_3
- Causes and etiologies
  - Can divide metabolic alkalosis into chloride-responsive metabolic alkalosis and chloride-resistant metabolic alkalosis
  - Chloride-responsive metabolic alkalosis
    - Characterized by loss of chloride ions via the kidneys, gastrointestinal (GI) tract, or skin
      GI losses lead to decrease in volume of the ECF compartment; hypovolemia activates the renin-angiotensin system, leading to reabsorption of bicarbonate in the proximal tubules

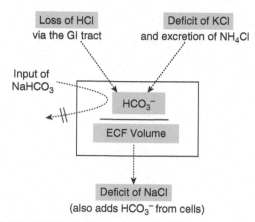

Fig. 51.1. Basis for a high concentration of HCO_3^- in the extracellular fluid (ECF) compartment. (From Halperin M, Kamel K, Goldstein M. *Fluid, Electrolyte, and Acid-Base Physiology.* Toronto: Saunders; 2010. Fig. 7.1)

Renal losses occur due to chronic diuretics, including furosemide and chlorothiazide
      Diuretics induce sodium delivery to the distal convoluted tubule, increasing sodium reabsorption and potassium secretion
      Low potassium levels stimulate bicarbonate reabsorption and ammonia production
  - Skin losses can be seen in patients with cystic fibrosis
  - Chloride-resistant metabolic alkalosis
    - Characterized by a combination of chloride and potassium depletion
    - Seen in several conditions:
      Conditions with excess mineralocorticoid activity such as Liddle syndrome (hyperactivity of sodium-chloride channels in the kidneys) or syndrome of apparent mineralocorticoid excess
      Bartter and Gitelman syndromes
      GI potassium loss associated with laxative use; however, this is a rare cause of metabolic alkalosis
  - Other causes
    - Milk alkali syndrome, characterized by net gain of bicarbonate and calcium in the setting of decreased glomerular filtration rate (GFR) and ECF volume, leading to decreased secretion of HCO_3 causing alkalosis

CLINICAL PRESENTATION

- Physical signs
  - Nonspecific symptoms that, when severe, include apathy, confusion, cardiac arrhythmias, and neuromuscular irritability
  - Symptoms usually not seen with a serum bicarbonate <40

DIAGNOSIS AND EVALUATION

- Initial evaluation includes measuring urine electrolytes, including urine chloride and potassium and sodium levels, which can allow differentiation between chloride-responsive and chloride-resistant metabolic alkalosis (see Fig. 51.2)

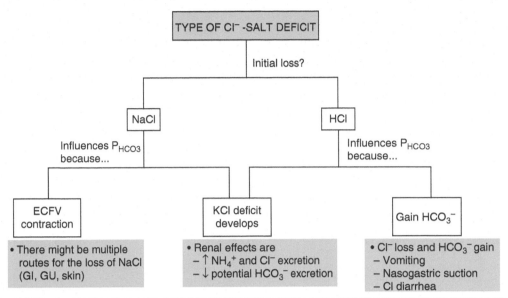

Fig. 51.2. Pathophysiology of metabolic alkalosis due to a deficit of Cl⁻ salts. (From Halperin M, Kamel K, Goldstein M. *Fluid, Electrolyte, and Acid-Base Physiology*. Toronto: Saunders; 2010. Flowchart 7.1)

- Urine chloride levels <25 mmol/L suggest chloride-responsive conditions
- Urine chloride levels >40 mmol/L suggest chloride-resistant conditions
- If chloride-resistant metabolic alkalosis is identified, examine the patient's extracellular volume (ECV) and blood pressure
  - Increased ECV and hypertension can be associated with conditions of excess mineralocorticoid activity
  - If the patient is normotensive, should consider conditions in the Bartter and Gitelman syndrome spectrum

TREATMENT

- Chloride-responsive metabolic alkalosis
  - Manage with administration of IV fluids with NaCl (± KCl) to expand the ECF, which counteracts renal sodium retention, allows bicarbonate excretion, and increases distal chloride secretion
- Chloride-resistant metabolic alkalosis
  - For patients with excess mineralocorticoid activity, treat underlying cause
  - Manage severe hypokalemia with oral potassium supplementation
  - In Bartter syndrome, correct alkalosis by limiting urinary potassium losses; manage with reduction of aldosterone with an aldosterone antagonist such as spironolactone; and decrease prostaglandin excretion with indomethacin
  - In Gitelman syndrome, limit urinary potassium losses and manage with potassium-sparing diuretics including spironolactone. May also require potassium supplementation
- Miscellaneous causes
  - Manage conditions with retention of HCO_3 by limiting bicarbonate ingestion (main source includes alkaline calcium salts)

Respiratory Acidosis

BASIC INFORMATION

- For a healthy individual, blood pCO_2 levels are maintained in the normal range by alveolar ventilation controlled by the central nervous system (CNS), in particular the pons and medulla oblongata, receiving information from various chemoreceptors in the body
- Respiratory acidosis occurs when there is an increase in pCO_2 concentration caused by increased production or decreased elimination
  - Rule of thumb: increase in $PaCO_2$ by 10 will decrease the pH by 0.08
- In response to respiratory acidosis, the body will retain HCO_3 to increase the pH; however, this compensation can take days as opposed to the faster rate of change seen in a primary metabolic disorder
- Causes and etiologies
  - Increased production of pCO_2
    - Increased cellular metabolic activity in conditions (i.e., infection, fever)
    - High carbohydrate load (i.e., patients on total parenteral nutrition)
    - These causes are rarely seen due to the body's ability to increase minute ventilation and eliminate pCO_2
  - Decreased elimination of pCO_2
    - Neurologic disorders that lead to CNS depression and decreased recognition of elevated pCO_2 levels (i.e., CNS trauma, seizures, narcotics)
    - Neuromuscular weakness/restrictive lung disease limiting chest expansion for ventilation (i.e., Flail chest, myasthenia gravis, pneumothorax)
    - Lung diseases limiting diffusion at the alveolus (i.e., pneumonia, pulmonary edema, interstitial lung disease)
    - Airway obstruction (i.e., obstructive sleep apnea, obesity-hypoventilation syndrome)

CLINICAL PRESENTATION

- Patients may present with anxiety and dyspnea and can progress to encephalopathy, delirium, and seizures in severe cases. This is known as carbon dioxide narcosis

DIAGNOSIS AND EVALUATION

- Thorough history and physical to determine acute versus chronic process (i.e., identifying the patient with chronic lung disease and chronic pCO_2 retention, which would not require acute management)
- Drug screen if patient presents with hypoventilation of unclear etiology
- Imaging, including chest x-ray (CXR) and chest CT, for evaluation of musculoskeletal or primary lung disorders

TREATMENT

- Increasing elimination of pCO_2 with increased ventilation either noninvasively with continuous positive airway pressure/bilevel positive airway pressure (CPAP/BiPAP) or invasively with intubation and mechanical ventilation

Respiratory Alkalosis

BASIC INFORMATION

- Respiratory alkalosis occurs when there is a decrease in pCO_2 concentration caused by excessive elimination
- In response to respiratory alkalosis, the body will eliminate HCO_3 to decrease the pH; however, this compensation can take days as opposed to the faster rate of change seen in a primary metabolic disorder
- Causes and etiologies
  - Can occur due to increased respiratory drive secondary to intoxication (i.e., salicylate toxicity), hyperammonemia, neurologic injury, pulmonary disease, anxiety, stress, pain

CLINICAL PRESENTATION

- Acute hyperventilation with decreased $PaCO_2$ causes a decrease in serum potassium and phosphate levels

due to intracellular shifts. Can also see decreased serum calcium due to increased binding to albumin in response to the change in pH
- Patients can present with paresthesias, circumoral numbness, chest pain, dyspnea, and tetany
- Neurologic symptoms can develop due to cerebral vasoconstriction in response to decreased $PaCO_2$, including seizures, dizziness, syncope, and confusion

DIAGNOSIS AND EVALUATION

- Thorough history and physical to determine acute versus chronic process
- Arterial blood gas, basic metabolic panel (BMP) for electrolyte derangements, drug screen
- Imaging of the lungs and/or CNS system to determine primary pulmonary process as guided by history and physical examination

TREATMENT

- Management of underlying disorder leading to alkalosis, which is unlikely life-threatening on its own

Review Questions

For review questions, please go to ExpertConsult.com

Suggested Readings

1. Berend K, deVries APJ, Gans ROB. Physiological approach to assessment of acid-base disturbances. *NEJM.* 2014;371(15):1434–1445.
2. Foreman JW. Renal tubular acidosis. In: Kher, Kanwal, eds. *Clinical Pediatric Nephrology.* 3rd ed. CRC Press; 2016:235–255. [Bookshelf Online].
3. Gluck S. Acid-base. *Lancet.* 1998;352(9126):474–479.
4. Halperin M, Kamel K, Goldstein M. Metabolic Alkalosis. In: *Fluid, Electrolyte and Acid-Base Physiology.* Toronto: Saunders; 2010:193–221.
5. Hsu B, Lakhani S, Wilhelm M. Acid-base disorders. *Pediatr Rev.* 2016;37(2):361–369.
6. Nesterova G, Gahl WA. Cystinosis: the evolution of a treatable disease. *Pediatr Nephrol.* 2013;28(1):51–59.
7. Quigley R. Acid-base homeostasis. In: Kher, Kanwal, eds. *Clinical Pediatric Nephrology.* 3rd ed. CRC Press; 2016. [Bookshelf Online].

52 Clinical Approach to Common Complaints in Nephrology

RADHA GAJJAR, MD, MSCE, DANIELLA LEVY EREZ, MD and ERUM A. HARTUNG, MD, MTR

In this chapter, we present a practical approach to the evaluation and management of common nephrology problems including hematuria, proteinuria, acute kidney injury (AKI), and chronic kidney disease (CKD).

Although hematuria and proteinuria are some of the most common reasons for referral to a nephrologist in an outpatient setting, the initial evaluation is often performed by the primary care provider. Some causes of hematuria and proteinuria are benign and may not require subspecialty referral, whereas others may require more urgent nephrology evaluation.

AKI is a common complication for many hospitalized children and may be caused by the underlying disease process or may be a consequence of medical therapies (such as nephrotoxic medications). CKD is a growing cause of morbidity in children and can arise from congenital abnormalities of the kidneys and urinary tract (CAKUT), acquired kidney diseases, or as part of other multisystem disorders.

Hematuria

BASIC INFORMATION

- Macroscopic hematuria is visible to the naked eye; microscopic hematuria is detected on urinalysis (dipstick) and/or urine microscopy only
  - Dipstick:
    - ≥1+ blood
    - Dipstick can also be positive in myoglobinuria or hemoglobinuria; presence of red blood cells (RBCs) must be confirmed on microscopy to diagnose hematuria
  - Urine microscopy:
    - >5 RBC/high-powered field in a fresh, centrifuged specimen from 10 mL of midstream urine
- Microscopic hematuria is often an incidental finding during workup of an unrelated symptom
  - Previously, screening urine dipstick was recommended for all patients at 5 years of age, but this is no longer recommended
- Other causes of red urine without hematuria (negative urine dipstick for blood and no RBCs):
  - Foods (beets, blackberries) and medications (rifampin, nitrofurantoin, metronidazole)
  - In infants, consider urate crystals with "brick dust" appearance

- As an outpatient, verify hematuria in two to three urine samples collected over several weeks. Thorough history and evaluation can help distinguish patients needing urgent evaluation versus those for whom outpatient workup is appropriate
- Hematuria includes a wide differential diagnosis (see Table 52.1); often no etiology is identified

CLINICAL PRESENTATION

- General description:
  - Microscopic: urine appears normal color
  - Macroscopic: urine color change visible with the naked eye
- Color:
  - Pink: small amount of blood mixed in urine
  - Bright red, cherry colored: fresh blood, lower urinary tract origin
  - Dark red: possibly stasis in bladder, or large volume of blood
  - Presence of clots: lower urinary tract origin
  - Brown, cola- or tea-colored: glomerular origin
- Pain:
  - Presence of pain usually indicative of nonglomerular source
    - Suprapubic pain associated with dysuria, flank pain: cystitis, pyelonephritis, hypercalciuria
    - Colicky flank or groin pain: nephrolithiasis, ureteropelvic junction (UPJ) obstruction
  - Painlessness: does not distinguish between upper or lower urinary tract
- Associated signs/symptoms:
  - Presence of hypertension and edema suggests glomerulonephritis (GN, see Chapter 53)
- Other distinguishing features:
  - Timing of hematuria:
    - Initial or early stream: urethral origin
    - Terminal: bladder or urethral origin
    - Throughout stream: nonspecific
  - Intermittent versus persistent
  - Menstrual

DIAGNOSIS AND EVALUATION

- Workup guided by presentation, clinical history, and distinction between:
  - Upper versus lower urinary tract origin
  - Glomerular versus nonglomerular origin

Table 52.1. Differential Diagnosis and Clinical Presentation of Hematuria

Diagnosis	Clinical Presentation/Clues
GLOMERULAR CAUSES OF HEMATURIA	
Postinfectious/poststreptococcal GN	Hypertension, tea- or cola-colored urine, edema, oliguria, proteinuria, RBC casts, AKI Recent infection, particularly Strep pharyngitis or skin infection; low C3 and normal C4 complement; elevated streptozyme/ASO
Lupus nephritis	Joint pain, alopecia, malar rash; low C3 and C4 complement; positive ANA and anti-ds-DNA± family history of autoimmune disease
Henoch-Schönlein purpura	Palpable purpura, joint pain, abdominal pain
IgA nephropathy	Gross hematuria concurrent with illnesses; acute GN uncommon ± Family history of hematuria
Membranoproliferative GN	Acute GN or indolent presentation; ± low C3 complement
Hereditary defects of GBM type 4 collagen	Family history of hematuria
Thin basement membrane nephropathy	Asymptomatic microscopic hematuria; ± gross hematuria with illness
Alport syndrome	Gross hematuria concurrent with illness, deafness, anterior lenticonus Family history of renal failure and deafness; usually X-linked; can see only microscopic hematuria in female carriers
Renal vasculitides	Usually ANCA positive; may present with rapidly progressive (crescentic) GN; fever, malaise, rash, sinusitis, pulmonary symptoms (e.g., hemoptysis)
Granulomatosis with polyangiitis	Usually PR3-ANCA positive
Microscopic polyangiitis	Usually MPO-ANCA positive
Anti-GBM (Goodpasture) disease	Rapidly progressive (crescentic) GN, pulmonary symptoms (e.g., hemoptysis)
Hemolytic uremic syndrome	Hemolytic anemia, thrombocytopenia; may be diarrhea associated (Shiga toxin–producing *E. coli* 0157:H7)
NONGLOMERULAR CAUSES OF HEMATURIA	
Infections	Dysuria, frequency, urgency, ± fever
Bacterial UTI	Suprapubic and/or flank pain; risk factors: abnormal urinary tract, sexually active
Viral cystitis	UTI symptoms with negative culture
Schistosomiasis	Travel to endemic areas
Tuberculosis	Travel to endemic areas, insidious onset
Crystalluria/stones	Dysuria, urgency, microscopic or gross hematuria; ± family history of stones or hematuria; increased risk from some medications (topiramate, excess vitamin D or calcium)
Hypercalciuria/crystalluria	May be asymptomatic
Kidney stones (nephrolithiasis)	Abdominal or flank pain Increased risk with abnormal urinary tract, recurrent UTI (struvite stones)
RENAL VASCULAR CAUSES	
Renal vein thrombosis	Gross hematuria, thrombocytopenia, ± flank pain or mass Risk factors: prematurity with history of umbilical vein catheter, newborns with poor feeding, hypercoagulable state, nephrotic syndrome
Nutcracker syndrome	Gross hematuria, left flank pain, compression of left renal vein between aorta and SMA
Intrinsic renal disease	
Renal papillary necrosis	Painless gross hematuria; due to infarcts/necrosis; risk factors: sickle cell trait, NSAID use
Renal cystic disease (autosomal dominant polycystic kidney disease)	Flank pain, palpable kidneys, gross hematuria, family history of cystic disease
Acute interstitial nephritis	Risk factors: NSAIDs, other medications
Urologic disease	
UPJ obstruction	History of unexplained abdominal pain and emesis
Bladder/urinary tract lesions (e.g., arteriovenous malformations)	Painless gross hematuria ± clots
Urethrorrhagia	Underwear spotting or terminal hematuria in males; idiopathic urethral inflammation, generally self-resolving
Tumors: nephroblastoma, Wilms tumor, rhabdomyosarcoma	Abdominal or flank mass, weight loss, hypertension
Miscellaneous	
Exercise-induced hematuria	Hematuria after vigorous exercise
Trauma	Gross hematuria after trauma
Hemorrhagic cystitis	Viral or medication-induced (cyclophosphamide)
Coagulopathy	Gross hematuria without precipitating event; other bleeding history (e.g., menorrhagia)
Non-urinary-tract causes	Perineal irritation, menstruation, STI

AKI, Acute kidney injury; *ANA*, antinuclear antibody; *ANCA*, antineutrophil cytoplasmic antibody; *anti-ds-DNA*, anti-double-stranded DNA antibody; *ASO*, antistreptolysin O; *GBM*, glomerular basement membrane; *GN*, glomerulonephritis; *MPO*, myeloperoxidase; *NSAID*, nonsteroidal antiinflammatory drugs; *PR3*, proteinase 3; *RBC*, red blood cell; *SMA*, superior mesenteric artery; *STI*, sexually transmitted infection; *UPJ*, ureteropelvic junction; *UTI*, urinary tract infection.

- Certain causes of hematuria are associated with particular clinical presentations (see Table 52.1).
- Diagnostic evaluation:
  - Algorithm for evaluation of hematuria—see Fig. 52.1
  - Urine: urine testing in all patients to confirm hematuria and test for proteinuria
    - Urine dipstick (urinalysis)
      False positive for blood with myoglobinuria
      False negative for blood with high ascorbic acid content
      False positive for protein with delayed testing, high specific gravity (SG)
    - Urine microscopic examination for urinary casts and morphology of RBCs
      RBC examination:
      Nondysmorphic: usually of nonglomerular origin
      Dysmorphic: glomerular origin
      Urinary casts:
      Casts are not detectable on urinalysis and rarely reported by central laboratory
      RBC casts: consistent with GN, always pathologic
      Hyaline casts: consistent with proteinuria; can be a normal finding
      Crystals:
      Some crystals (e.g., calcium oxalate, triple phosphate, uric acid) can be seen in normal urine, but large numbers may indicate stone-forming tendency; some crystals (e.g., cysteine) are always pathologic
  - Random urine calcium and urine creatinine to screen for hypercalciuria. Normal limits for urine calcium/creatinine ratio are age based:
    - <6 months: <0.8
    - 7 to 18 months: <0.6
    - 19 months to 6 years: <0.4
    - >6 years: <0.2
  - First morning urine protein and urine creatinine to screen for proteinuria. Normal limits for urine protein/creatinine ratio are age based (see Table 52.2)
  - Urine culture
  - Blood:
    - Basic metabolic panel (BMP): electrolytes, creatinine
    - Serum albumin
    - Complete blood count (CBC)
    - Hemoglobin electrophoresis if at risk for sickle cell disease/trait
    - Concern for postinfectious GN or poststreptococcal GN: complements (C3, C4), streptozyme (antistreptolysin O [ASO])
    - Concern for lupus, other nephritis: complements (C3, C4), antinuclear antibody (ANA), anti-double-stranded DNA (anti-ds-DNA) antibodies
    - Concern for vasculitides/renal-pulmonary syndromes: antineutrophil cytoplasmic antibodies (ANCA), anti–glomerular basement membrane (GBM) antibodies
  - Imaging:
    - Renal-bladder ultrasound (US) to evaluate for nephrolithiasis, mass/structural or vascular anomalies; consider cystoscopy for suspected lower urinary tract source

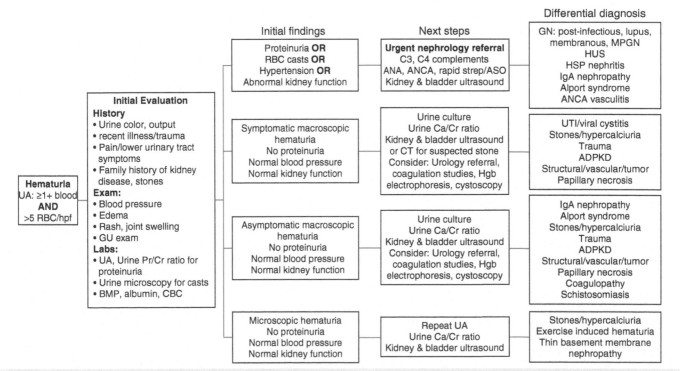

Fig. 52.1. Flowchart for evaluation of hematuria in children. *ADPKD,* autosomal dominant polycystic kidney disease; *ANA,* antinuclear antibody; *ANCA,* antineutrophil cytoplasmic antibody; *ASO,* antistreptolysin O antibody; *BMP,* basic metabolic panel; *Ca/Cr,* calcium/creatinine; *CBC,* complete blood count; CT, computed tomography scan; *GN,* glomerulonephritis; *GU,* genitourinary; *Hgb,* hemoglobin; *HSP,* Henoch-Schönlein purpura; *HUS,* hemolytic uremic syndrome; *MPGN,* membranoproliferative glomerulonephritis; *Pr/Cr,* protein/creatinine; *RBC,* red blood cells; *UA,* urinalysis; *UTI,* urinary tract infection.

Table 52.2. Definitions of Elevated Proteinuria by Age Group and Testing Method

| Age | Urine Dipstick | SPOT URINE PROTEIN/CREATININE RATIO | | 24-Hour Urine Collection |
		g/mmol	mg/mg	
Any age: significant proteinuria	≥1+			>4 mg/m²/hour OR >150 mg/1.73 m²/24 hours
6 months to 2 years		>0.06	>0.6	
>2 years		>0.02	>0.2	
Any age: nephrotic-range proteinuria		>0.2	>2	>40 mg/m²/hour OR >3 g/1.73 m²/24 hours

- Other:
  - Hearing test if family history is concerning for Alport syndrome
- Pathology:
  - Refer to pediatric nephrologist for consideration of biopsy if persistent hematuria and concern for significant renal pathology

TREATMENT

- Treatment based on etiology diagnosed by workup
- No etiology found in up to 80% of cases; treat underlying etiology if detected
- Referral to pediatric nephrologist:
  - Early referral if both hematuria and proteinuria, particularly if other signs of GN
  - If hematuria is persistent without clear cause after initial workup

Proteinuria

BASIC INFORMATION

- Proteinuria can be a common finding in children; up to 1.2% to 1.5% of school-age children with proteinuria on screening dipstick, but far fewer on repeat testing
- Urine dipstick errors:
  - False positive for protein:
    - Gross hematuria, pyuria or bacteriuria
    - concentrated specimen (SG > 1.025)
    - alkaline specimen (pH > 8.0)
    - If dipstick is kept in urine too long
    - specimen contaminated with antiseptic (e.g. benzalkonium chloride or chlorhexidine)
  - False negative for protein: dilute (SG <1.002) or acidic (pH <4.5) urine
  - Proteinuria can be transiently seen in the setting of fever, exercise, dehydration, and stress
  - If fixed/nephrotic range, can be suggestive of serious renal disease, especially if found in combination with hematuria (see Chapter 53)
  - Mechanisms of proteinuria:
  - Postural (orthostatic): benign, common in children/adolescents

- Glomerular proteinuria: glomerulopathies that compromise glomerular filtration barrier (i.e., glomerular capillaries, GBM, and/or podocytes)
- Tubular proteinuria: decreased tubular reabsorption of filtered proteins, usually low-molecular-weight

CLINICAL PRESENTATION

- Proteinuria is usually asymptomatic and incidentally discovered
- Nephrotic-range proteinuria may be associated with edema, weight gain, and oliguria
- Proteinuria can be a feature in other systemic disorders, therefore patients may have a variety of unique presentations. For instance:
  - In GN, patients may demonstrate edema, oliguria, hypertension, and macro- or microscopic hematuria
  - in Henoch Schonlein Purpura (HSP), proteinuria may be accompanied by a classic palpable purpuric rash
  - in Lupus nephritis, patients may have rash, joint findings, and/or alopecia
  - Recurrent UTI may be associated with proteinuria
  - Recent illness may suggest post-infecitous GN

DIAGNOSIS AND EVALUATION

- Clinical history is critical for evaluating proteinuria, as different histories may point towards different causes of proteinuria (see above)
- Family history: renal disease, dialysis, transplant, deafness, hypertension
- Physical examination
  - Vital signs:
    - Increased weight and hypertension can suggest GN
    - Growth failure can suggest CKD
  - Abdominal examination: abdominal masses can suggest hydronephrosis or polycystic kidney disease
  - Symptoms of fluid overload: periorbital edema, cardiac examination (gallop, murmur), lung examination (pleural effusions), hepatomegaly, periorbital or pretibial edema, ascites
  - Skin: alopecia may suggest lupus or rash—consider HSP, lupus, vasculitides
  - Joints: arthritis may suggest lupus or connective tissue disorder
- Laboratory testing
  - Urine:
    - If no suggestion of nephrotic syndrome or GN, repeat urinalysis (dipstick), urine protein, and urine creatinine (for protein/creatinine ratio) on first morning specimen twice, at least one week apart, to confirm presence of proteinuria
    - If 1+ protein or greater by dipstick and urine protein/creatinine ratio is elevated (see Table 52.2) on two repeat checks, further evaluation is needed
    - 24-hour urine collection is the preferred method for quantitation but is not always feasible in children. Spot urine protein/creatinine ratio is often more helpful for office evaluation and if not toilet-trained
  - Blood:
    - BMP: to assess electrolytes and creatinine
    - CBC: anemia and thrombocytopenia may suggest rheumatologic disease

Table 52.3. Differential Diagnosis of Proteinuria

Type of Proteinuria	Causes
Transient proteinuria	Idiopathic Fever, seizures, other illness Exercise, stress, dehydration
Orthostatic/postural proteinuria	Idiopathic
Glomerular proteinuria	Hyperfiltration injury (e.g., nephron loss due to reflux nephropathy) Minimal change disease Focal segmental glomerulosclerosis Congenital nephrotic syndrome Membranoproliferative glomerulonephritis Membranous nephropathy Infection-associated glomerulonephritis (e.g., hepatitis B and C, HIV) IgA nephropathy Lupus nephritis Henoch-Schönlein purpura Postinfectious or poststreptococcal glomerulonephritis Alport syndrome Diabetes mellitus Drugs/toxins (e.g., nonsteroidal antiinflammatory drugs [NSAIDs], heavy metals)
Tubular proteinuria	Acute tubulointerstitial nephritis (often drug-induced [e.g., NSAIDs], antibiotics) Chronic tubulointerstitial nephritis Acute tubular necrosis Proximal tubular dysfunction/Fanconi syndrome (e.g., Dent disease, cystinosis, galactosemia, tyrosinemia, hereditary fructose intolerance, Lowe syndrome, heavy metal poisoning, drugs such as aminoglycosides) Sickle cell disease Polycystic kidney disease Pyelonephritis Toxins (heavy metals)

- Serum cholesterol to confirm nephrotic syndrome if nephrotic-range proteinuria
- C3, C4 complements if concerned for postinfectious GN, lupus, or membranoproliferative GN (MPGN)
- Additional testing to consider:
  Hepatitis B, hepatitis C, HIV testing in the presence of risk factors and nephrotic-range proteinuria (focal segmental glomerulosclerosis [FSGS], membranous nephritis)
  Lupus panel (ANA, anti-ds-DNA antibodies) and ANCA if symptoms of connective tissue disorder are present
  Streptozyme (ASO) to evaluate for poststreptococcal GN
- Imaging:
  - Renal/bladder US to evaluate renal structure; consider Doppler if significant hypertension is present
  - Consider voiding cystourethrogram (VCUG) and dimercaptosuccinic acid (DMSA) scan if there is history of recurrent UTI suggestive of reflux and/or renal scarring
- Pathology:
  - Refer to pediatric nephrologist for consideration of biopsy if there is persistent proteinuria and concern for significant renal pathology
- Differential diagnosis of proteinuria (see Table 52.3)

TREATMENT

- Orthostatic proteinuria:
  - No treatment
  - Annual follow-up by primary care provider to confirm no progression

- Persistent proteinuria—refer to pediatric nephrologist
  - Low-grade (urine protein/creatinine ratio <0.5), asymptomatic proteinuria:
    - May not necessarily need kidney biopsy
    - Consider angiotensin-converting enzyme inhibitor (ACEi) or angiotensin receptor blocker (ARB) therapy to reduce proteinuria and for renal protective effect
- Nephrotic syndrome: see Chapter 53
- Urgent evaluation required for presentations concerning for nephritis or nephrotic syndrome.
- Nephritis:
  - Further evaluation needed: treatment based on etiology
- Recommended daily protein intake should be maintained

Acute Kidney Injury (AKI)

BASIC INFORMATION

- Definition
  - Abrupt decrease in kidney function within 7 days measured either by increased serum creatinine (SCr) or by decreased urine output
  - AKI stages: classified by Kidney Disease Improving Global Outcomes (KDIGO) guidelines (see Table 52.4)
- Epidemiology
  - 25% to 80% of patients admitted to the intensive care unit (ICU) are noted to have AKI
- AKI is an independent risk factor for mortality and a common complication of multiple systemic illnesses and therapeutic modalities

Table 52.4.   Stages of Acute Kidney Injury (AKI) by Kidney Disease Improving Global Outcomes (KDIGO) Classification

AKI Stage	Serum Creatinine (Cr)	Urine Output
Stage 1	Cr increase ≥0.3 mg/dL within 48 hours Or Cr increase to 1.5–1.9 times baseline	<0.5 mL/kg/h for 6–12 hours
Stage 2	Cr increase to 2–2.9 times baseline	<0.5 mL/kg/h for ≥12 hours
Stage 3	Cr increase to ≥4.0 mg/dL Or Cr increase to ≥3.0 times baseline Or Initiation of renal replacement therapy Or In patients <18 years, decrease in eGFR to <35 mL/min/1.73 m²	<0.5 mL/kg/h for ≥24 hours Or <0.3 mL/kg/h for ≥12 hours

eGFR, Estimated glomerular filtration rate.

- Causes
  - Prerenal: low effective circulating volume due to volume depletion (e.g., due to emesis or diarrhea), blood loss, or hypotension (e.g., due to heart failure/sepsis)
  - Intrinsic renal: acute tubular necrosis (ATN) due to shock or nephrotoxic agents (e.g., gentamicin, vancomycin, nonsteroidal antiinflammatory drugs [NSAIDs], calcineurin inhibitors [e.g., tacrolimus]), primary kidney disease (e.g., hemolytic uremic syndrome [HUS], rapidly progressive GN), rhabdomyolysis
  - Obstructive ("post"-renal): for example, due to posterior urethral valves (PUV), urine catheter obstruction, stones, or mass

CLINICAL PRESENTATION

- Signs/symptoms caused by AKI:
  - Oliguric/anuric AKI can present with signs of volume overload, such as peripheral edema, pulmonary edema, respiratory distress, and hypertension
  - Hypertension—if severe, can be symptomatic with encephalopathy and seizures
  - Severe hypocalcemia can present with tetany and muscle weakness

DIAGNOSIS AND EVALUATION

- Clinical history and physical exam are critical to determine the underlying etiology of AKI.
  - In prerenal AKI, may have signs/symptoms of volume depletion (e.g. dry mucous membranes, sunken eyes, poor skin turgor), heart failure (e.g. gallop, edema, hepatomegaly), or third-space losses (e.g. ascites in nephrotic syndrome or liver disease)
  - In intrinsic renal AKI, may have signs/symptoms of kidney-specific insults (e.g. polyuria in intersitital nephritis, hematuria and hypertension in GN, fever and flank pain in pyelonephritis) or systemic illnesses known to injury the kidneys (e.g. HUS, lupus, vasculitis)
  - In postrenal AKI, expect signs and symptoms of urinary obstruction (e.g. bladder fullness, flank pain)
- Additional attention should be paid to:
  - Blood pressure (hypertension is common in GN and other causes of AKI, while hypotension is causative of prerenal AKI)
  - exposure to potential nephrotoxins (e.g. NSAIDS)

- Assessment of fluid status by determining intake/output history and changes in weight
  - Weight gain in oliguric AKI from any cause; also in nephrotic syndrome and heart failure
  - Weight loss in prerenal AKI due to volume depletion
- Additional signs based on underlying cause:
  - Petechiae and pallor in HUS
  - Muscle tenderness in rhabdomyolysis
  - Poor perfusion or decreased capillary refill in shock
  - Rash, arthritis, or other extrarenal signs in lupus or vasculitis
  - Tremor in calcineurin inhibitor toxicity
  - Enlarged bladder in postrenal obstruction
- Laboratory testing:
  - BMP, phosphorus, albumin—to evaluate kidney function and look for electrolyte abnormalities (e.g., hyperkalemia, acidosis, hypocalcemia, hyperphosphatemia) and hypoalbuminemia
  - CBC—thrombocytopenia/anemia may suggest HUS or lupus; leukopenia may suggest lupus
    - Check markers of hemolysis for suspected HUS (e.g., schistocytes, elevated lactate dehydrogenase, low haptoglobin)
  - Drug levels as indicated (e.g., vancomycin, gentamicin, tacrolimus)
  - Urinalysis and urine microscopy—hematuria, proteinuria, and RBC casts in GN; granular or muddy brown casts in ATN; positive urine dipstick for blood without visible RBCs in rhabdomyolysis; high SG in prerenal state; pyuria in pyelonephritis
  - Urine culture
  - Urine osmolarity (UOsm) to assess urine concentration (high in prerenal state)
  - Urine sodium (UNa) and urine creatinine (UCr)
    - Used with SCr and serum sodium (SNa) to calculate fractional excretion of sodium (FeNa)
    - FeNa can help differentiate prerenal AKI from intrinsic renal process, such as ATN. In prerenal state (low effective circulating volume), kidneys will attempt to maximize reabsorption of sodium and water. Urine sodium and FeNa will therefore be low (<1%)

$$Fractional\ excretion\ of\ sodium\ (FeNa)$$
$$= \frac{U_{Na} \times S_{Cr}}{S_{Na} \times U_{Cr}} \times 100$$

  - FeNa is not reliable in patients on diuretics

Table 52.5. Differentiation Between Prerenal and Intrinsic Renal Causes of Acute Kidney Injury Based on Laboratory Results and Clinical Findings

Parameter	Prerenal AKI	Intrinsic Renal AKI
Urine osmolarity	>350 mOsm/kg	<350 mOsm/kg
Urine sodium	<20 mEq/L	>20 mEq/L
Fractional excretion of sodium (FeNa)	<1% (<2% neonates)	>2% (>2.5% neonates)
Urinalysis	SG >1.020 No hematuria/proteinuria	SG <1.010 in ATN, AIN Hematuria, proteinuria, RBC casts: glomerular disease (e.g., HUS, GN) Granular casts: ATN Eosinophiluria: AIN
Additional clues	Vomiting/diarrhea Cardiac disease (heart failure) Hypotension BUN/Cr ratio >20	Anemia/thrombocytopenia in HUS Low complement levels in GN/autoimmune disease Low serum albumin in GN, NS Elevated creatine kinase in rhabdomyolysis

AIN, Acute interstitial nephritis; *AKI*, acute kidney injury; *ATN*, acute tubular necrosis; *BUN*, blood urea nitrogen; *Cr*, creatinine; *GN*, glomerulonephritis; *HUS*, hemolytic uremic syndrome; *NS*, nephrotic syndrome; *RBC*, red blood cells; *SG*, specific gravity.

- Table 52.5: differentiation between prerenal and intrinsic renal causes of AKI based on laboratory results and clinical findings
- Imaging:
  - Renal bladder US
    - Kidneys can be either large (e.g., infiltrative process, acute interstitial nephritis) or normal size
    - Loss of corticomedullary differentiation in ATN
    - Bilateral hydronephrosis: suspect obstruction
    - Increased echogenicity: nonspecific finding in AKI
    - Doppler: evaluate renal vascular blood flow (unilateral thrombosis should not cause AKI if other side is normal)
  - Radionucleotide renal scan:
    - Not commonly used but can assist in evaluation and demonstrate decreased perfusion with delayed/absent function
- Pathology:
  - Biopsy may be performed if GN or interstitial nephritis is suspected

TREATMENT

- Prevention of AKI: close monitoring of SCr and urine output in patients at risk (e.g., patients in ICU, receiving nephrotoxic medications), monitoring nephrotoxic drug levels, close attention to body fluid balance
- General management of AKI:
  - Remove nephrotoxic drugs (e.g., NSAIDs, aminoglycosides) or drugs that affect renal perfusion (e.g., NSAIDs, ACEi). In prerenal state, kidney is dependent on vasodilatory prostaglandin synthesis to maintain perfusion; thus administration of NSAIDs or ACEi can augment renal injury
  - Adjust medication dosing depending on estimated glomerular filtration rate (GFR). The most commonly used pediatric formula is the modified (CKiD) Schwartz formula, based on height and SCr:

$$GFR = \frac{0.413 \times height\ (cm)}{S_{Cr}}$$

- Caution: formula provides accurate estimate of GFR only if SCr is in steady state—if SCr is rising in context of AKI, formula will overestimate GFR because Cr takes several days to peak
- No evidence that any medications can prevent or treat AKI (e.g., N-acetylcysteine, "renal-dose" dopamine)
- Fluid management:
  - If hypovolemic: fluid resuscitation (normal saline as first line to restore intravascular volume)
  - When euvolemic: maintain euvolemia by replacing insensible losses (generally about one-third maintenance fluid rate calculated by Holliday-Segar method) and measured losses (e.g., urine output, drains)
    - Holliday-Segar method for calculating maintenance fluids: 100 mL/kg/day for first 10 kg of body weight, plus 50 mL/kg/day for second 10 kg of body weight, plus 20 mL/kg/day for every kg thereafter
    - Insensible losses will be higher in patient who is febrile or tachypneic, lower if mechanically ventilated (lower respiratory losses with closed humidified circuit)
    - If volume overloaded: fluid restriction; consider diuretics (may need higher doses than usual in patients with AKI)
  - May need dialysis if severely volume overloaded
- Electrolyte/acid-base management:
  - Hyponatremia: may occur due to volume overload and may require fluid restriction or dialysis. Occasionally may occur due to urinary sodium losses (e.g., polyuric AKI in interstitial nephritis) and may require sodium supplementation.
  - Hyperkalemia: management discussed in Chapter 50
  - Hyperphosphatemia: patients generally require low-phosphorus diet/intake, can add phosphate binders to decrease absorption of phosphorus from foods (must be given with food, most commonly calcium carbonate)
  - Hypocalcemia: can be caused by impaired production of activated vitamin D (calcitriol) by the kidneys and by hyperphosphatemia
    - Correct hypocalcemia judiciously in patients with severe hyperphosphatemia—patients can develop calcium-phosphorus crystals

- Correct hypocalcemia before giving sodium bicarbonate, which can further depress ionized calcium levels
- Acidosis: treated by sodium bicarbonate supplementation
- Blood pressure management:
  - Hypotensive patients: inotropic agents or pressors to maintain adequate renal perfusion
  - Hypertension:
    - In severe hypertension, especially if long-standing, blood pressure should not be lowered too quickly to prevent cerebral hypoperfusion
      - Recommend no more than 25% decrease in blood pressure within the first 8 to 12 hours, then gradual normalization over next 48 to 72 hours
    - Antihypertensive therapies: if volume overloaded, may use diuretics; other options include short-acting IV agents as intermittent doses (e.g., labetalol, hydralazine) or continuous infusion (e.g., nicardipine, esmolol), or short-acting oral agents (e.g., nifedipine, clonidine). ACEi are generally avoided in AKI
- Diet:
  - May require fluid restriction if volume overloaded
  - Low-potassium/low-phosphorus diet as indicated
  - May need to dialyze if the volume restrictions interfere with nutritional needs
  - Maintain daily protein intake needs; children with AKI have high protein requirements (at least 2–3 g/kg/day) due to catabolic state; may need to increase further if on dialysis due to loss of amino acids
- Indications for renal replacement therapy (continuous renal replacement therapy [CRRT], intermittent hemodialysis [HD], or peritoneal dialysis [PD]). "AEIOU" mnemonic:
  - **A**cidosis refractory to medical therapy
  - **E**lectrolyte abnormalities refractory to medical therapy (e.g., hyperkalemia, severe hyperphosphatemia with hypocalcemia)
  - **I**ntoxications, ingestions, or inborn errors of metabolism
  - **O**verload (volume), particularly if interfering with ability to provide adequate nutrition
  - **U**remia (symptomatic) (e.g., uremic encephalopathy, platelet dysfunction, pericarditis)

Neonatal AKI

- Neonatal serum Cr at first day of life reflects maternal serum Cr and gradually decreases
- In term infants, GFR improves from 10 to 20 mL/min/1.73 m² during the first days of life to 30 to 40 mL/min/1.73 m² by 2 weeks of life. In premature infants, GFR at birth is even lower and increases more slowly than in term infants. GFR improves steadily over the first few months of life, reaching adult GFR (>90 mL/min/1.73 m²) by 2 years of age
- Classification:
  - Neonatal KDIGO classification: modified definition, based on an absolute rise from previous trough; should be used up until 120 days of age (see Table 52.6)
- Causes:
  - Perinatal asphyxia, nephrotoxic exposures (NSAIDs pre- or postnatally, gentamicin, vancomycin), sepsis (most common >70%)
- Evaluation:
  - Detailed history
    - Prenatal oligohydramnios or polyhydramnios, history of drug exposure, family history of renal failure, abnormal delivery and fetal distress, infections
  - Physical examination
    - Dysmorphic features, palpate abdomen (cysts/large bladder), hypotension/sepsis presentation, Potter syndrome features (abnormal facies/hypoplastic lungs), evaluation of fluid status
  - Laboratory results
    - Similar to pediatric AKI, except GN/autoimmune disease not common in this age group
- Management:
  - Similar to pediatric AKI; PD is generally the preferred dialysis modality

Chronic Kidney Disease (CKD)

BASIC INFORMATION

- Epidemiology
  - Increasing incidence and prevalence over the last several decades

Table 52.6. Stages of Neonatal Acute Kidney Injury (AKI) by Modified Kidney Disease Improving Global Outcomes (KDIGO) Classification (up to 120 Days of Age)

AKI Stage	Serum Creatinine (Cr)	Urine Output
Stage 0	No change in Cr or rise <0.3 mg/dL	≥0.5 mL/kg/h
Stage 1	Cr increase ≥0.3 mg/dL within 48 hours *Or* Cr increase to 1.5–1.9 times reference Cr* within 7 days	<0.5 mL/kg/h for 6–12 hours
Stage 2	Cr increase to 2–2.9 times reference Cr*	<0.5 mL/kg/h for ≥12 hours
Stage 3	Cr increase to ≥3.0 times reference Cr* *Or* Cr ≥2.5 mg/dL *Or* Initiation of renal replacement therapy	<0.3 mL/kg/h for ≥24 hours *Or* Anuria for ≥12 hours

*Reference Cr is defined as lowest previous Cr value.
Estimated glomerular filtration rate.

- Definition
  - Evidence of structural or functional kidney abnormalities persisting for over 3 months, with or without decreased GFR
  - CKD stages (applicable for >2 years old): see Table 52.7
    - Based on GFR calculated using modified (CKiD) Schwartz formula (see AKI section for GFR calculation)
- Causes:
  - Below 5 years of age: most common causes of CKD are CAKUT (e.g., dysplastic/hypoplastic kidneys, obstructive uropathy)
  - Above 5 years of age: glomerulopathies such as FSGS and GN; genetic kidney disease such as polycystic kidney disease and ciliopathies

CLINICAL PRESENTATION

- Symptoms arise when severity of CKD increases
- Failure to thrive: poor weight gain and linear growth (can be secondary to inadequate nutrition [e.g., due to poor appetite, vomiting], acidosis, lack of response to growth hormone, CKD–bone mineral disorder)
- May have bruising secondary to platelet dysfunction
- Decreased cognitive function
- Pruritus (due to calcium-phosphate crystal deposits in skin)
- Hypertension: if severe, can be symptomatic (e.g., visual changes, seizures, chest pain)
- Fatigue (due to anemia, uremia)

DIAGNOSIS AND EVALUATION

- Clinical history:
  - Birth history, antenatal US findings (e.g., oligohydramnios, hydronephrosis)
  - History of UTI
  - Symptoms of connective tissue disorder: joint pain, joint swelling, rash, alopecia
  - Family history: renal disease, dialysis, transplant, deafness, hypertension
- Physical examination
  - Vital signs:
    - Hypertension
    - Short stature, poor weight gain
    - May have weight gain if fluid overloaded
  - Signs of end-organ effects of hypertension: heart murmur, cotton wool changes in retina
  - Signs of symptomatic uremia: bruising, pericardial friction rub, cognitive dysfunction, fatigue
  - Signs of anemia of CKD: pallor, fatigue

Table 52.7. Stages of Chronic Kidney Disease (CKD)

CKD Stage	Glomerular Filtration Rate, mL/min/1.73 m^2
1	≥90
2	60–89
3	30–59
4	15–29
5	<15 or on dialysis

- Signs of CKD–bone mineral disorder: deformities due to rickets (renal osteodystrophy)—bowed legs, widened metaphyses
- Laboratory testing:
  - BMP, phosphorus: Cr to calculate GFR; assess for electrolyte abnormalities (acidosis, hyperkalemia, hyperphosphatemia, hypocalcemia)
  - CBC, ferritin, iron profile
    - Assess for anemia of CKD—due to decreased erythropoietin production in the kidney as well as decreased iron utilization
  - Intact parathyroid hormone (iPTH), 25-hydroxyvitamin D level
    - Secondary hyperparathyroidism develops due to inability to activate 25-hydroxyvitamin D into 1,25-hydroxyvitamin D in the kidneys; impaired phosphate excretion leads to hyperphosphatemia and hypocalcemia
- Imaging: kidney/bladder US
  - Kidneys can be small in chronic process or hypoplasia/dysplasia
  - May be enlarged/cystic in polycystic kidney disease
- Kidney biopsy
  - Can give additional information regarding etiology in earlier stages of CKD
  - Of limited utility in patients with CKD Stage 5 (end-stage kidney disease) because it generally shows generalized fibrosis

TREATMENT

- Kidney function: prevent further decline in kidney function through management of underlying disease:
  - Prevent UTIs and ensure adequate urinary drainage in patients with CAKUT
  - Treat autoimmune diseases, vasculitis, or GN with appropriate immune suppression
  - ACEi can be renoprotective
- Electrolyte derangements
  - Acidosis: may require chronic alkali therapy (e.g., sodium bicarbonate or citrate)
  - Hyperkalemia: low-potassium diet, sodium polystyrene sulfonate (Kayexalate)
  - Hypocalcemia: calcium supplementation (between meals to maximize absorption), activated vitamin D therapy (calcitriol)
  - Hyperphosphatemia: low-phosphate diet, phosphorus binders (calcium carbonate or noncalcium binders such as sevelamer, given with meals)
- Anemia
  - Maintain adequate iron levels
  - Erythropoietin as needed
- Hypertension
  - ACEi may have a benefit of slowing CKD progression in earlier stages; ACEi is also helpful for renin-mediated hypertension, which is common in many causes of CKD
  - Can also use other long-acting antihypertensives (e.g., calcium channel blockers, beta-blockers, diuretics)
  - Strict blood pressure control may slow CKD progression

- CKD-mineral bone disorder
  - Calcium supplementation (between meals), phosphate binders, and calcitriol (activated vitamin D) to help control secondary hyperparathyroidism
- Growth
  - Ensure adequate nutrition
    - Protein restriction is not recommended in children
    - Supplemental feeding is often needed (often via nasogastric or gastric tube)—renal formulas are available (low potassium, low phosphorus)
  - May need recombinant human growth hormone injections if poor growth despite adequate nutrition
- Treat proteinuria
  - Using ACEi or ARBs—may slow CKD progression
- Renal replacement therapy:
  - Dialysis: HD or PD
    - Indications similar to AKI, but also consider long-term factors such as poor growth and subtle developmental delay or decline in school performance attributed to uremia
  - Kidney transplant:
    - Provides best quality of life
    - Preemptive kidney transplant (i.e., without dialysis first) is usually preferable
    - Living donor or deceased donor transplants are possible. Living donor transplant has slightly better outcomes

ACKNOWLEDGEMENT

Drs. Gajjar and Levy Erez have contributed equally to this work.

Review Questions

For review questions, please go to ExpertConsult.com.

Suggested Readings

1. Becherucci F, Roperto RM, Materassi M, Romagnani P. Chronic kidney disease in children. *Clin Kidney J*. 2016;9(4):583–591.
2. Copelovitch L, Warady BA, Furth SL. Insights from the chronic kidney disease in children (CKiD) study. *Clin J Am Soc Nephrol*. 2011;6(8):2047–2053.
3. Fortenberry JD, Paden ML, Goldstein SL. Acute kidney injury in children: an update on diagnosis and treatment. *Pediatr Clin North Am*. 2013;60(3):669–688.
4. Kaddourah A, Basu RK, Bagshaw SM, Goldstein SL. AWARE Investigators. Epidemiology of acute kidney injury in critically ill children and young adults. *N Engl J Med*. 2017;376(1):11–20.
5. Leung AK, Wong AHC. Proteinuria in children. *Am Fam Physician*. 2010;82(6):645–651.
6. Massengill SF. Hematuria. *Pediatr Rev*. 2008;29(10):342–348.
7. Selewski DT, Charlton JR, Jetton JG, et al. Neonatal acute kidney injury. *Pediatrics*. 2015;136(2):e463–e473.

Nephritic and Nephrotic Syndromes

MELISSA R. MEYERS, MD and MADHURA PRADHAN, MD

This chapter will cover a practical approach to the evaluation, diagnosis, and basic management of nephrotic and nephritic syndromes in pediatric patients. The initial screening and evaluation of these syndromes are frequently performed in the outpatient setting by a patient's primary pediatrician before referral to a pediatric nephrologist.

See also Nelson Textbook of Pediatrics, Chapter 527, "Nephrotic Syndrome."

Nephrotic Syndrome

BASIC INFORMATION

- Nephrotic syndrome is defined by:
  - Hyperlipidemia
  - Edema
  - Hypoalbuminemia
  - Proteinuria
- Epidemiology
  - Incidence is 2/100,00 to 7/100,000 children
  - Prevalence is 16/100,000 children
- Causes and etiology
  - Most cases of childhood nephrotic syndrome are idiopathic
  - Etiology is thought to be a T-cell disorder that leads to glomerular podocyte dysfunction, causing increased glomerular permeability
- Types of primary nephrotic syndrome in children:
  - Most common cause: minimal change nephrotic syndrome (MCNS)
    - Typically presents in school-age children with 2:1 male predominance
  - Other causes:
    - Focal segmental glomerulosclerosis (FSGS)
    - Membranous nephropathy
    - Congenital (birth to 3 months) and infantile (3–12 months of age) nephrotic syndrome are commonly caused by genetic disorders or infections
- Secondary causes include:
  - Genetic disorders (*NPHS1*, *NPHS2*); many disorders lead to genetic FSGS
  - Medications (penicillamine, gold, nonsteroidal antiinflammatory drugs [NSAIDs], heroin, lithium)
  - Infections (hepatitis B and C, HIV)
  - Malignancy (leukemia/lymphoma)

CLINICAL PRESENTATION

- Periorbital edema is noticed in the morning as a first sign
- Pedal edema and abdominal distention (ascites) are noted over time
- Decreased urine output with weight gain
- Commonly preceded by a respiratory infection
- Often misdiagnosed as allergies and treated with antihistamines

DIAGNOSIS AND EVALUATION

- Urinalysis shows high-grade proteinuria
- On dipstick: proteinuria: 2+ or more
  - Urine protein/creatinine ratio: ≥2 mg/mg
  - 24-hr urine protein: 40 mg/m^2/hr
- Microscopic hematuria is seen in 20% of children with MCNS
- Serum albumin is low, generally <2.5 g/dL
- Serum cholesterol is elevated

DEFINITIONS USED IN NEPHROTIC SYNDROME

- Remission: urine protein trace or negative on dipstick for 3 consecutive days
- Relapse: urine protein 2+ or more on dipstick for 3 consecutive days
- Steroid resistance: failure to achieve remission during initial 8 weeks of corticosteroid therapy
- Steroid dependent: two consecutive relapses during steroid therapy or within 14 days of ceasing therapy

TREATMENT

- Glucocorticoids (prednisone) are first-line treatment
  - Prednisone is given for 4 to 6 weeks daily, followed by a taper for 4 to 6 weeks
- Low-salt diet
- Fluid restriction is not necessary in most children with nephrotic syndrome
- Furosemide with or without albumin is used in the acute setting for severe edema
- Steroid-sparing agents are used in frequently relapsing/steroid-dependent nephrotic syndrome:
  - Alkylating agents such as cyclophosphamide for 8 to 12 weeks
  - Calcineurin inhibitors such as cyclosporine and tacrolimus for 6 to 12 months
  - Newer agents such as mycophenolate mofetil and rituximab (anti-CD20 monoclonal antibody) have been used

NATURAL HISTORY AND PROGNOSIS

- 95% of children with MCNS respond to prednisone (75% by 2 weeks)

- Only 20% of children with FSGS respond to prednisone
- 80% of children who respond will develop one or more relapses
- Most children with MCNS attain long-term remission eventually (84% are relapse-free 10 years after onset)
- Steroid-resistant nephrotic syndrome has a poor prognosis, with most children eventually developing chronic kidney disease

COMPLICATIONS

- Infections
  - More common in nephrotic syndrome due to loss of urine proteins (immunoglobulins and properdin) and steroid therapy
  - Serious infections include spontaneous bacterial peritonitis and cellulitis
  - Pneumococcal vaccination (PPSV 23) is recommended in children with nephrotic syndrome
- Thromboembolic complications
  - Loss of coagulation factors increases risk of venous thrombosis
  - Deep vein thrombosis should be suspected with asymmetric edema and/or pain in extremities
  - Cerebral venous thrombosis should be suspected in a child with a severe headache or any neurologic symptoms

Focal Segmental Glomerulosclerosis (FSGS)

BASIC INFORMATION

- A form of steroid-resistant nephrotic syndrome
- More common in males and African-Americans
- Biopsy is indicated if proteinuria persists after 8 weeks of steroid therapy
  - Light microscopy shows sclerosis affecting portions (segments) of some glomeruli (focal)
  - Nonspecific immunofluorescence
  - Electron microscopy (EM) shows diffuse podocyte effacement; sometimes mesangial electron dense deposits are also noted
- Once diagnosed, treatment is focused on proteinuric control with angiotensin-converting enzyme inhibitors (ACEIs) or angiotensin receptor blockers (ARBs) and immunosuppression, typically calcineurin inhibitors and low-dose corticosteroid therapy; mycophenolate mofetil and rituximab have also been used as second-line agents
- Mycophenolate mofetil and rituximab have also been used as second line agents
- Prognosis is guarded with 25-50% of children with FSGS progressing to ESRD within 5-10 years
- Post-transplant course is complicated by recurrence in 30-40% of patients

Nephritic Syndromes

- Nephritic syndromes typically present with:
  - Hematuria
  - Hypertension
  - Proteinuria
- Acute kidney injury
- Oliguria
- Although there can be overlap between nephritic and nephrotic syndromes, gross hematuria is much more common in nephritis

Poststreptococcal Glomerulonephritis (PSGN)

BASIC INFORMATION

- More common in developing countries; annual incidence is 9.3/100,000 children
- Developed countries' annual incidence is 0.3/100,000 to 0.64/100,000 children
- Most common cause of glomerulonephritis (GN) in children, typically affecting school-age children
- Glomerular injury in PSGN is mediated by immune complex deposition in the glomeruli
- Caused by nephritogenic strains of group A streptococcus, which are subtyped by the surface M proteins
  - Nephritogenic strains of group A streptococci cause pharyngitis (M1, 4, 12, 25) or pyoderma (M2, 42, 49, 56)

CLINICAL PRESENTATION

- Classic triad of PSGN: hematuria, edema, hypertension
  - Painless gross hematuria ("cola-colored") is a common presenting symptom of PSGN
  - Hematuria is seen in all patients; one-third have gross hematuria
- History of preceding pharyngitis (1–2 weeks before presentation) or skin infection (3–6 weeks before presentation). This is in contrast to synpharyngitic syndromes in which nephritis can occur within 2 days after infection (e.g. IgA GN, Alport, MPGN; see below)
- Subclinical cases may have only microscopic hematuria with normal or mildly elevated blood pressure and may not come to medical attention
- Edema is secondary to fluid overload from oliguria; seen in 65% to 90% of all patients
  - Pulmonary edema and congestive heart failure are seen in severe cases
  - Hypertension is seen in 60% to 80% of patients
  - Cerebral symptoms and hypertensive encephalopathy are reported in some patients

DIAGNOSIS AND EVALUATION

- Nephritis preceded by group A streptococcal infection is strongly suggestive of PSGN
- Laboratory tests
  - Urine analysis: nonnephrotic proteinuria and large blood
    - Microscopy reveals dysmorphic red blood cells (RBCs) and RBC casts
    - May see leukocytes and white blood cell (WBC) casts as well
- Serologic evidence of recent streptococcal infection
  - Antistreptolysin (ASO) titers are commonly used but will be negative with skin infections
  - DNase B will be elevated with pharyngitis and skin infections

Table 53.1. Brief Overview of Glomerulonephritis by Complement Levels

LOW C3, NORMAL C4	LOW C3, LOW C4
■ Poststreptococcal glomerulonephritis ■ Dense deposit disease (formerly known as MPGN type II)	■ Lupus nephritis ■ Membranoproliferative glomerulonephritis (MPGN) ■ Shunt nephritis (or chronic bacteremia) ■ Postinfectious glomerulonephritis in infective endocarditis

NORMAL C3	
■ Henoch-Schönlein purpura nephritis ■ IgA nephropathy ■ Alport syndrome	■ Goodpasture syndrome ■ Antineutrophil cytoplasmic antibody vasculitides ■ Microscopic polyangiitis ■ Granulomatosis with polyarteritis

- Low C3 is seen in 90% of patients with PSGN and is of greatest diagnostic value
  - C4 is normal because alternate complement pathway is activated in PSGN
  - Hypocomplementemia is transient in PSGN (but may stay low for up to 2 months)
  - Acute GN can be classified on the basis of low or normal complement levels (see Table 53.1)
- Renal biopsy is not indicated in typical cases of PSGN
  - Renal biopsy is needed if there is a rapid rise in serum creatinine
  - Biopsy findings:
    - Light microscopy: increased cellularity and neutrophil infiltration in glomeruli
    - Immunofluorescence: IgG, C3
    - EM: hallmark finding of subepithelial immune deposits on electron microscopy. Crescents are seen in severe cases

TREATMENT

- Supportive treatment for manifestations of nephritis
  - Sodium and fluid restriction for edema and hypertension
  - Low-potassium diet and potassium binding exchange resins for hyperkalemia
  - No evidence for benefit of steroid therapy, even for crescentic PSGN
- Treatment of hypertension:
  - Diuretics: thiazides or loop diuretics are first line
  - Calcium channel blockers and beta blockers
  - ACEIs are effective but to be used with caution in the presence of hyperkalemia or elevated creatinine
- Natural history and prognosis
  - Edema and hypertension resolve in ~10 days
  - Gross hematuria resolves in ~10 days with rare instances of recurrence during febrile illnesses in subsequent weeks
  - Serum creatinine normalizes in 3 to 4 weeks
  - Proteinuria resolves in 4 to 5 weeks
  - Serum C3 level normalizes in 6 to 8 weeks
  - Microhematuria can persist up to a few years
  - Few patients have long-term sequelae such as:
    - Persistent hematuria/proteinuria (5%–20%)
    - Hypertension (3%)
    - Chronic kidney disease (1%)

Postinfectious Glomerulonephritis (PIGN)

BASIC INFORMATION

- 80% of PIGN is PSGN
- Infective endocarditis (IE) is responsible for an additional 10% of PIGN
- Other rarer forms of PIGN include:
  - Shunt nephritis (ventriculoatrial)
  - Syphilis
  - Methicillin-resistant *Staphylococcus aureus* (MRSA)–associated IgA-dominant GN
  - Other infections (viruses, fungi, and parasites)
- PIGN in IE:
  - Renal involvement is typically seen in 25% to 50% of IE; many cases are asymptomatic and often found at autopsy
  - Acute GN secondary to IE is typically diagnosed due to findings of microscopic hematuria and proteinuria (nonnephrotic)
  - Serum studies will note low C3 and C4
  - One-third of patients demonstrate mild azotemia (elevated blood urea nitrogen [BUN] and creatinine); even mild renal dysfunction is a poor prognosis
  - Biopsy findings on light microscopy note focal hypercellularity and a mixed or mononuclear leukocyte infiltration in glomeruli with granular IgG, IgM, and C3 immune complex deposition in peripheral glomerular capillary walls and subepithelial deposits (or "humps") on EM. Crescents are rare
    - About 25% of IE-related GN also show interstitial nephritis, which is not typically seen in PSGN
    - Embolic renal disease: localized embolic infarcts are found primarily in autopsies
- PIGN resolves with treatment of underlying infection
  - Antibiotic treatment for IE is typically 4 to 6 weeks

IgA Nephropathy

BASIC INFORMATION

- Most prevalent primary chronic glomerular disease in the world
  - Highest incidence in Asia and in individuals of Asian descent
    - Incidence ranges from 0.57/100,000 person-years in the United States to 4.5/100,000 person-years in Japan
    - 2:1 ratio of boys to girls in Western countries; 1:1 ratio in Asia
- Caused by abnormally glycosylated IgA immune complexes depositing in renal mesangium
  - Secondary causes of IgA (rare) include neoplasms, infections, chronic liver disease, and multisystem disease

CLINICAL PRESENTATION

- Painless gross hematuria concurrent with illness (e.g. upper respiratory infection); called a "synpharyngitic" presentation

- IgA nephropathy can also present with asymptomatic microhematuria and proteinuria; acute nephritis with crescentic GN, acute kidney injury, and hypertension; or nephrotic syndrome

DIAGNOSIS AND EVALUATION

- Urinalysis shows microscopic hematuria and proteinuria with RBC casts
  - Quantify urine protein (see nephrotic syndrome, described previously)
- Serologic evaluation
  - Basic metabolic panel: elevated creatinine seen with acute nephritic presentation and with crescentic IgA nephropathy
  - Normal complement (C3): distinguishes from PIGN
  - Serum IgA levels are not consistently elevated and hence not useful
- Definitive diagnosis is made on renal biopsy
  - Consider biopsy for nephritic syndrome, persistent proteinuria, or elevated creatinine at presentation
    - The hallmark of IgA nephropathy is mesangial proliferation on light microscopy with IgA deposition in the mesangium on immunofluorescence
    - Findings are identical to Henoch-Schönlein purpura (HSP) nephritis

TREATMENT

- Spontaneous remission is common in children
- ACEIs or ARBs are recommended if proteinuria is >1 g/day and should be considered for proteinuria >0.5 g/day
- Corticosteroids course for 6 months if there is an inadequate response to ACEI/ARB in decreasing proteinuria after 3 to 6 months
- Cyclophosphamide or azathioprine is used for rapidly progressive crescentic IgA nephropathy in addition to steroids
- Fish oil (polyunsaturated fatty acids) may reduce proteinuria and delay rise in creatinine
- Natural history and prognosis
  - Chronic persistent microscopic hematuria with periodic episodes of gross hematuria with respiratory infections is common
  - Often progresses to chronic kidney disease in adulthood (50% progress to end-stage renal disease [ESRD] in 25 years)
  - Poor prognostic signs: nephrotic-range proteinuria, hypertension, or renal dysfunction
  - Risk of recurrence posttransplant

Henoch-Schönlein Purpura (HSP) Nephritis

BASIC INFORMATION

- HSP is a small-vessel vasculitis composed predominantly of IgA immune complexes, with significant renal involvement
- Details for HSP are provided in Chapter 83
- Classically presents in school-age children with a nonthrombocytopenic palpable purpuric rash, nondeforming arthritis/arthralgia, gastrointestinal (GI) manifestations, and nephritis (in ~40% of all HSP cases)
- HSP nephritis
  - Presents later than other findings
    - HSP nephritis is more likely if age is >8 years and if there is abdominal pain and recurrent rash
  - Most cases (90%) present within the first 8 weeks
  - Ranges from microscopic hematuria or proteinuria to acute nephritis or nephrotic syndrome
- Serologic evaluation
  - Basic metabolic panel: elevated creatinine is seen with acute nephritic presentation and with crescentic nephropathy, as in IgA
  - Normal complement (C3): distinguishes from PIGN
  - Serum IgA levels are not consistently elevated and hence not useful
- Histologic evaluation:
  - Skin biopsy notes classic leukocytoclastic vasculitis (with neutrophils)
- Renal biopsy
  - The hallmark HSP nephritis is mesangial proliferation on light microscopy with IgA deposition in the mesangium on immunofluorescence
  - Findings are identical to IgA nephropathy

TREATMENT

- Often self-limited
- ACEI or ARBs are recommended if proteinuria is >0.5 g/day
- Use corticosteroids for persistent proteinuria on ACEI/ARB and for crescentic GN
  - Steroids given at onset of nephritis have not been shown to reduce duration of nephritis or progression to ESRD
- As in IgA nephropathy, cyclophosphamide or azathioprine can be used for rapidly progressive crescentic
- Natural history and prognosis
  - Long-term prognosis correlates with renal manifestations at onset
  - Rarely nephritis persists and can progress to ESRD, requiring kidney transplant or dialysis

Lupus Nephritis (LN, Also Known as Systemic Lupus Erythematosus [SLE] Nephritis)

BASIC INFORMATION

- More common in adolescents, females, Asians, and individuals of Afro-Caribbean descent
- Details for SLE are provided in Chapter 82
- Patients who have renal involvement at presentation have worse outcomes

CLINICAL PRESENTATION

- About 40% to 60% of children with lupus have renal manifestations at presentation including:
  - Microscopic hematuria (79%)
  - Proteinuria—may be nonnephrotic range to nephrotic range (43%–55%)

Table 53.2. Abbreviated International Society of Nephrology/Renal Pathology Society (ISN/RPS) Classification of Lupus Nephritis (2003)

Class I: Minimal mesangial lupus nephritis

Class II: Mesangial proliferative lupus nephritis

Class III: Focal lupus nephritis

Class IV: Diffuse segmental (IV-S) or global (IV-G) lupus nephritis

Class V: Membranous lupus nephritis[1]

Class VI: Advanced sclerosing lupus nephritis

[1]Class V may be combined with class III or IV.

- Hypertension (40%)
- Elevated creatinine (50%)
- Rarer presentations include gross hematuria and acute kidney injury (<2%)

DIAGNOSIS

- Definition: urine protein: creatinine ≥500 mg/24 hr or RBC casts
- Serum: positive antinuclear antibody (ANA) with double-stranded DNA (dsDNA)
  - Low C3 and C4 indicate active lupus activity
  - Anti-C1q antibodies predict more severe renal involvement
- Urine
  - Urinalysis: assess proteinuria and hematuria
    - Microscopy: evaluate for active sediment (dysmorphic RBCs, RBC casts, and WBC casts)
- Biopsy
  - Suspicion of LN should be confirmed by renal biopsy because histology guides treatment
    - Histology varies by class (see Table 53.2)
    - Classic description of lupus nephritis is called "full house" on immunofluorescence, referring to presence of IgG, IgM, IgA, C3, C4, and C1q; present in ~25% of patients with LN

TREATMENT

- Induction for class III/IV typically includes pulse corticosteroids followed by high-dose oral steroids and cyclophosphamide or mycophenolate mofetil for 6 months; maintenance therapy with mycophenolate or azathioprine is then continued for a minimum of 1 year
- Severe cases may benefit from plasma exchange and/or rituximab

Membranoproliferative Glomerulonephritis (MPGN)

BASIC INFORMATION

- Previously described as types I–III
- All forms are rare in children
- Presentation ranges from asymptomatic proteinuria to nephritic or nephrotic syndromes
- A new pathophysiology-based classification system was published in 2015 with two main types:
  1. Immunocomplex-mediated MPGN

- Caused by a trigger activating the classical complement pathway
  - Infections (hepatitis B, hepatitis C, and chronic infections)
  - Autoimmune diseases (cryoglobulinemia, lupus)
- Although rare, this is the most common MPGN in children
- Evaluation should focus on identifying the underlying cause and on assessment of complement levels (low C3, C4, and CH50)
- Biopsy:
  - Light microscopy will note double-contour "tram-tracking" between glomerular endothelium and basement membrane caused by mesangial cell migration and trapping of immune complexes between the endothelium and neo-basement membrane during the repair phase
  - Immunofluorescence: positive IgG, IgM, and C3
  - EM: mesangial subendothelial electron-dense deposits (immune complexes)
- Treatment is based on treating the underlying disease along with immunosuppressive agents to prevent cell proliferation agents (mycophenolate mofetil, cyclophosphamide, or rituximab)
  - ACEIs or ARBs are used as antiproteinuric therapy
  - Prognosis is guarded; 40% of patients progress to ESRD in 10 years
  2. Complement-mediated MPGN
- Caused by alternative complement pathway dysregulation, often from genetic mutations or autoantibodies leading to low C3 and positive C3 nephritic factor (C3NF)
- Two subtypes:
  - C3 glomerulopathy
  - Dense deposit disease (DDD), previously aka type II MPGN
    - Biopsy notes "tram-tracking" on light microscopy
      - Immunofluorescence: C3 glomerular staining
      - EM: continuous dense, ribbon-like deposits along the glomerular basement membrane (DDD)
    - Targeted treatment depends on underlying cause:
      - Plasma exchange (to remove C3NeF and replace missing or ineffective factor H)
      - Eculizumab, an anti-C5 monoclonal antibody, preventing formation of C5b (used off-label)
      - Very high risk of recurrence posttransplant despite immunosuppression

Alport Syndrome

BASIC INFORMATION

- Previously known as Hereditary Nephritis
- A form of familial glomerular hematuria caused by type IV collagen mutations (COL4A3, COL4A, and COL4A5) in the glomerular basement membrane
- Inheritance may be X-linked (80%), autosomal dominant, or autosomal recessive

- Associated with progressive sensorineural deafness by early adulthood, lens and retina anomalies, and esophageal/tracheobronchial leiomyomas
- Typically presents with episodic gross hematuria concurrent with an illness ("synpharyngitic")
- Urinary testing for microscopic hematuria and proteinuria is indicated
- Biopsy findings:
  - Light microscopy: presentation initially may appear to be mild (like MCNS); later presentation can demonstrate focal glomerulosclerosis, tubular atrophy, and interstitial fibrosis. If present, interstitial foam cells may also be seen
    - Immunofluorescence: positive collagen staining
    - Electron microscopy: diffuse thickening of glomerular capillary wall with "basket weave" transformation of lamina densa, attenuation of glomerular basement membrane scalloped edge, and loss of podocyte foot processes
- Treatment is based on proteinuric control with ACEI or ARBs
- Progression to ESRD is typically late adolescence or early adulthood for males and later for females
- Posttransplant, there is a risk of antiglomerular basement membrane nephritis

Review Questions

For review questions, please go to ExpertConsult.com.

Suggested Readings

1. Andolino TP, Reid-Adam J. Nephrotic syndrome. *Pediatr Rev.* 2015;36(3):117–126.
2. Eddy AA, Symons JM. Nephrotic syndrome in childhood. *Lancet.* 2003;362:629–639.
3. Kidney disease: improving global outcomes (KDIGO) glomerulonephritis work group. KDIGO clinical practice guideline for glomerulonephritis. *Kidney Int.* 2012;2(supp):139–274.
4. McCarthy HJ, Tizard EJ. Diagnosis and management of Henoch-Schönlein purpura. *E J Pediatr.* 2010;169(6):643–650.
5. Sethi A, Nester CM, Smith RJH. Membranoproliferative glomerulonephritis and C3 glomerulopathy: resolving the confusion. *Kidney Int.* 2012;81:434–441.
6. Van DeVoorde RG. Acute poststreptococcal glomerulonephritis: the most common acute glomerulonephritis. *Pediatr Rev.* 2015;36(1): 3–13.
7. Vogt B. Nephrology update: glomerular disease in children. *FP Essentials.* 2016;444(4):30–40.

54 Selected Topics in Nephrology

AADIL KAKAJIWALA, MBBS and KEVIN E.C. MEYERS, MBBCH

Infections of the Urinary Tract

BASIC INFORMATION

- If urinary tract infection (UTI) involves only bladder: cystitis (usually without fevers)
- If UTI involves kidney: pyelonephritis (usually with high fevers)

Epidemiology

- During first 3 months of life, most common in uncircumcised males, followed by female infants, and then circumcised males
- *After* 3 months of age, females are at higher risk
- More likely in white febrile infants
- Risk factors:
  - Uncircumcised male
  - At the time of toilet training
  - Sexual activity in females
  - Constipation
  - Dysfunctional elimination
  - Family history of recurrent UTI
  - Urinary bladder catheterization
- Vesicoureteral reflux increases risk of development of febrile UTI and pyelonephritis
- See also Nelson Textbook of Pediatrics, Chapter 538, "Urinary Tracts Infections."

Causes and Etiology

See Table 54.1.

CLINICAL PRESENTATION

- In infants: high fever without a source, irritability, emesis, poor feeding
- >2 years: abdominal/flank pain, fevers, dysuria, urgency, frequency, incontinence, hematuria, secondary enuresis
- "Foul-smelling urine" is not helpful
- On examination: suprapubic tenderness, costovertebral angle tenderness, uncircumcised male

DIAGNOSIS AND EVALUATION

- Urinalysis:
  - Performed within 1 hour at room temperature and 4 hours on refrigerated sample
  - High rates of false negative if urine is not in bladder for enough time
  - Presence of WBC (pyuria) and bacteria suggests UTI
  - Nitrites: specific but not very sensitive
  - Leukocyte esterase: sensitive but not very specific
- Urine culture:
  - Obtained ideally by catheterization/suprapubic aspiration (pre–toilet training) or midstream clean catch (after toilet training)
  - >50,000 CFU/mL of single pathogen is diagnostic (any positive for suprapubic is significant)
  - <10,000 CFU/mL is likely a contaminant
  - Causes of false negative: high urine volume, low osmolality, low pH
  - Bag specimen is unreliable for urine culture
- C-reactive protein (CRP) alone cannot differentiate lower UTI from pyelonephritis
- Blood culture is usually not helpful in UTI (unless <3 months of age)
- Follow-up studies with confirmed UTI (see Table 54.2)

TREATMENT

- Initiating treatment orally or parenterally is equally efficacious
  - Uncomplicated cystitis: 3 to 7 days of oral antibiotics
  - Uncomplicated pyelonephritis: 10 days of oral antibiotics
- Antibiotics used:
  - First choice:
    - Cephalosporins (e.g., third generation: cefixime, first generation: cephalexin)
  - If type 1 penicillin allergy/cephalosporin allergy:
    - Trimethoprim-sulfamethoxazole (increasing resistance)

Table 54.1. Various Causes of Urinary Tract Infection in Children

Clinical Scenario	Organism
Most common organism causing urinary tract infection	Escherichia coli
Associated with renal calculi (struvite stones)	Proteus mirabilis
Urinary tract infection in sexually active females	Escherichia coli Staphylococcus saprophyticus Chlamydia trachomatis
Nosocomial infections	E. coli Candida albicans Pseudomonas aeruginosa
Viruses causing hemorrhagic cystitis	Adenovirus BK virus (posttransplant)
Associated with instrumentation of the urinary tract	C. albicans
Predominantly seen in neonates	Group B streptococcus
Hematogenous spread	S. aureus

Table 54.2. Follow-Up Studies in Patients with Confirmed Urinary Tract Infection

Ultrasound (kidney and bladder): ■ Looks for structural abnormalities of the kidney and urinary tract, hydronephrosis, renal abscess, renal scarring, and sometimes pyelonephritis	Consider if: ■ Female less than 3 years old with first urinary tract infection (UTI) ■ Male any age with first UTI ■ Male or female any age with first febrile UTI ■ History of recurrent UTI ■ First UTI with family history of UTI Not helpful to diagnose reflux (will miss low-grade reflux)
Dimercaptosuccinic acid (DMSA) scan: ■ Looks for renal scarring	May consider in patients with a history of recurrent febrile UTI
Voiding cystourethrogram (VCUG)	No need for VCUG in most infants and young children with first febrile UTI Consider if: ■ Abnormal renal ultrasound/DMSA ■ After second UTI/recurrent UTI ■ Atypical/complex presentation ■ First UTI with family history of UTI

■ If sulfa allergy:
  ■ Ciprofloxacin (useful if recurrent UTI is resistant to other drugs, or allergies)
■ Other medications:
  ■ Amoxicillin (too much resistance when used as monotherapy), but used along with other medication or in treatment of Enterococcus UTI
  ■ Amoxicillin-clavulanate
  ■ Nitrofurantoin (good for prophylaxis)
■ Admission criteria: infants <3 months of age (due to risk of bacteremia), sepsis, acute kidney injury (AKI), poor hydration, failed outpatient treatment, renal abscess
  ■ Inpatient pyelonephritis: 10 to 14 days IV and PO antibiotics:
    ▪ Gentamicin/cefotaxime and ampicillin (enterococcal coverage)
    ▪ Tailor antibiotics based on culture results
  ■ Abscesses need antibiotics for 14 days and possible surgery
■ *Do not* treat asymptomatic bacteriuria (no symptoms of UTI and urinalysis showing *no* pyuria but positive urine culture)
■ Consult urology if structural abnormality, abscess, or dysfunctional elimination

UTI

Prophylaxis

■ The benefit of prophylactic antibiotics in patients with reflux is uncertain
■ Consider prophylactic antibiotics in patients with recurrent UTI
■ Postcoital UTI in females:
  ■ Single doses of Bactrim, nitrofurantoin, or cephalexin within 2 hours of intercourse
  ■ Use continuous prophylaxis if postcoital single dose fails (if no further UTIs, may discontinue after 6 to 12 months and watch)

Nephrolithiasis and Related Disorders

BASIC INFORMATION

■ Urolithiasis:
  ■ Stones at any location in urinary tract
■ Nephrolithiasis:
  ■ Stones exclusively in kidney
■ Nephrocalcinosis:
  ■ Calcium deposits in renal parenchyma

Epidemiology

■ Much lower incidence in children compared with adults, but rapidly rising in incidence (especially among adolescent females and African-Americans)
■ More common in males
■ More common in Caucasians compared with African-Americans

Causes and Etiology

■ Most common stones are calcium oxalate, followed by calcium phosphate
■ Most common metabolic abnormality associated with stone formation is hypercalciuria
■ Stone inhibitors in urine: citrate (hypocitraturia increases risk for stones), magnesium, potassium
■ Stone promotors in urine: calcium, sodium, oxalate, phosphate, uric acid
■ Risk factors for calcium stone development:
  ■ Hypercalcemia (elevated parathyroid hormone, vitamin D excess)
  ■ Hypercalciuria
  ■ Familial idiopathic hypercalciuria with normocalcemia
  ■ Immobilization
  ■ Loop diuretics
  ■ Intestinal malabsorption, such as in inflammatory bowel disease, cystic fibrosis, and celiac disease (oxalate stones)
  ■ Ketogenic diet
  ■ Certain renal diseases (Dent disease, distal renal tubular acidosis, medullary sponge kidney)
■ Struvite/triple-phosphate stones
  ■ Associated with proteus UTI and very alkaline urine (pH > 7)
  ■ Can present with large staghorn calculi
■ Uric acid stones
  ■ Uric acid is end product of purine metabolism
  ■ Associated with acidic urine (pH < 6), high protein diet, tumor lysis syndrome, and certain metabolic disorders (e.g. Lesch-Nyhan syndrome [see chapter 35 for details], idiopathic renal hypouricemia)
■ Urate crystals
  ■ May be seen in healthy infants
  ■ Particularly common among breastfed newborns in first few days of life when uric acid excretion is high and urine volumes are low
  ■ Pink granules seen in diaper
■ Cystine Stones
  ■ Abnormal transport of dibasic amino acids resulting in increased urine cysteine, ornithine, arginine, and lysine (mnemonic: "COAL") and consequent renal stones.

CLINICAL PRESENTATION

- Gross hematuria
- Pain that radiates from loin to groin
- Dysuria and frequency suggest hypercalciuria
- Passage of stone in urine
- Recurrent UTIs (Proteus UTI with struvite stones)
- Pertinent history:
  - Diet (calcium, dairy, sodium, and protein intake)
  - Medications
  - Family history of stones

DIAGNOSIS AND EVALUATION

- Initial studies (patients with acute stone):
  - Blood work:
    - Basic metabolic profile (BMP)

- Urinalysis:
  - pH less than 6 associated with uric acid stones
  - pH greater than 7 associated with calcium phosphate and struvite stones
  - Pyuria (WBC in urine)
  - Microscopic hematuria or gross hematuria
  - May consider evaluation of stones (see Fig. 54.1)
- Imaging:
  - Ultrasound
    Helpful to detect obstruction from stone
    May miss small stones
  - CT scan without contrast (if patient is symptomatic with pain)
    Radiodense: calcium oxalate and calcium phosphate
    Radiolucent: uric acid stones

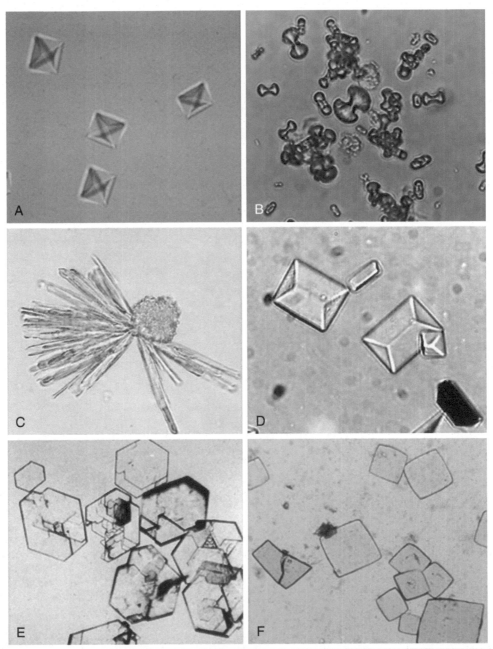

Fig. 54.1. Urine crystals: (A) calcium oxalate dihydrate "envelope shaped"; (B) calcium oxalate monohydrate "dumbbell shaped"; (C) calcium phosphate "needle/rosette shaped"; (D) triple phosphate (struvite) "coffin lid shaped"; (E) cystine "hexagon shape"; (F) uric acid crystals "rhomboid shaped."

- Additional workup:
  - Blood work:
    - Calcium, phosphorus
    - Uric acid
    - Vitamin D, parathyroid hormone
  - Hypercalciuria:
    - If >2 years old: urine calcium: creatinine ratio >0.25 or 4 mg/kg/day of calcium in urine
    - If <2 years old: urine calcium: creatinine ratio >0.6
  - Best test is 24-hour urine sample to assess risk factors for stone development
    - Look for total volume, hypercalciuria, hyperoxaluria, hypocitraturia, hyperuricosuria, and cystinuria

TREATMENT

- Dietary modifications: increase fluid intake and restrict sodium intake; however, continue normal recommended daily allowance for calcium and protein; restriction is not recommended in children
- Stone-specific treatments:
  - Potassium citrate if hypocitraturia
  - Hydrochlorothiazide to reduce urine calcium excretion
  - Antibiotics for struvite stones
  - Allopurinol (inhibitor of xanthine oxidase) for patients with recurrent uric acid stones
- Surgical options are presented in Chapter 84
  - Indicated if stone is >5 mm or obstructing
  - Options include nephrolithotomy, extracorporeal lithotripsy, or retrograde endoscopic lithotripsy

Hypertension

BASIC INFORMATION

- Diagnostic criteria for hypertension and followup as recommended by 2017 AAP guidelines are discussed in Chapter 5.
- Most common cause of hypertension is essential hypertension, associated with obesity, in the adolescent
- In pediatrics, the most common cause of *secondary* hypertension is renal parenchymal disease (acute glomerulonephritis plus chronic kidney disease) (see Table 54.4)
- Neonatal hypertension risk factors: bronchopulmonary dysplasia, prematurity, renal ischemia, caffeine therapy, history of umbilical artery catheter, maternal drug abuse, renal vein thrombosis

CLINICAL PRESENTATION

- Hypertension screening frequency and technique discussed in Chapter 5.
- Children are usually asymptomatic.
- Infants may demonstrate poor feeding and irritability.
- If severe hypertension, children may present with headaches, blurry vision, nosebleeds, and nausea
- Hypertensive emergency (see Table 54.3):
  - Central nervous system: altered mental status, seizures, edema, increased intracranial pressure , reversible posterior leukoencephalopathy syndrome (RPLS, see Chapter 56)

Table 54.3. Hypertensive Urgency vs. Emergency in Children

Stage	Definition
Hypertensive urgency	Severe hypertension, but no target organ damage
Hypertensive emergency	Severe hypertension and clinical signs/symptoms of target organ damage

Table 54.4. Secondary Causes of Hypertension

Renal parenchymal disease	■ Acute glomerulonephritis ■ Polycystic kidney disease ■ Chronic kidney disease, renal scarring
Renal artery stenosis	■ Fibromuscular dysplasia ■ Williams syndrome ■ Neurofibromatosis ■ Alagille syndrome ■ Takayasu arteritis
COARCTATION OF THE AORTA	
Endocrine causes	■ Hyperaldosteronism (includes Cushing syndrome, congenital adrenal hyperplasia) ■ Pheochromocytoma (seen in *NF1*, VHL, MEN) ■ Hyperthyroidism or hypothyroidism
Neurologic causes	■ Increased intracranial pressure
Medications	■ Oral contraceptive medications ■ Albuterol ■ Steroids ■ Over-the-counter decongestants (phenylephrine and pseudoephedrine) ■ Stimulant medications used for attention-deficit/hyperactivity disorder ■ Illicit drugs (cocaine, PCP, Ecstasy) ■ Caffeine

MEN, multiple endocrine neoplasia; *NF1*, neurofibromatosis 1; *VHL*, Von Hippel-Lindau.

- Heart: left ventricular hypertrophy and heart failure
- Eyes: papilledema/retinal hemorrhages

DIAGNOSIS AND EVALUATION

- A detailed history, including family history and medications, is very important in the evaluation of hypertension
- Blood pressure follow-up frequency is based on severity of hypertension (See Chapter 5)
- Four extremity blood pressures to assess for coarctation or midaortic syndrome
- Examination: eyes, heart for murmurs, skin (café-au-lait spots in neurofibromatosis)
- Initial workup of hypertension:
  - Basic metabolic panel:
    - Elevated creatinine suggests renal injury
    - Low potassium in patients with hyperaldosteronism or congenital adrenal hyperplasia with associated hypertension
  - Urinalysis to look for hematuria or proteinuria
  - Complete blood count (CBC):
    - Anemia will suggest chronic kidney disease
    - Anemia, thrombocytopenia, and elevated creatinine will be seen in hemolytic uremic syndrome

- Fasting lipid panel and hemoglobin A1c in obese children with concern for essential hypertension
- Echocardiogram to look for left ventricular hypertrophy
- Additional workup for secondary causes of hypertension:
  - Renal artery stenosis:
    - Listen for abdominal bruit
    - Ultrasound with Doppler
      - Looks at renal size, structure, scarring, and blood flow to the kidney
    - CT angiogram
    - Formal angiogram
  - MRI brain if there is concern for RPLS (white matter edema is parieto-occipital region)
  - Other tests for secondary hypertension:
    - Thyroid function test (thyroid-stimulating hormone [TSH] and free T4)
    - Urine drug screen
    - Renin and aldosterone levels
      - Both high in renal parenchymal disease and renal artery stenosis
      - Low renin in hyperaldosteronism
    - If concern for pheochromocytoma
      - 24-hour urine catecholamines (epinephrine, norepinephrine, vanillylmandelic acid (VMA), and homovanillic acid (HMA)) and plasma metanephrines
      - Metaiodobenzylguanidine scan
    - May consider polysomnography (sleep study) for obstructive sleep apnea, which is associated with hypertension

TREATMENT

- Lifestyle modifications, including diet, exercise, and weight loss, are the most important steps for essential hypertension
- Salt restriction in diet
- Chronic medications for hypertension:
  - Angiotensin-converting enzyme inhibitors (ACEI) or angiotensin receptor blockers (ARBs)
    - Best medication if renal scarring, chronic kidney disease with proteinuria, and unilateral renal artery stenosis
    - *Do not use* in bilateral renal artery stenosis
    - Side effects include elevated potassium, elevated creatinine, angioedema, and dry cough
    - Teratogenic; *do not use* in pregnancy
    - Used in neonatal hypertension
  - Calcium channel blockers
    - Considered first-line therapy in children along with ACEI/ARBs
    - Minimal side effects
  - Diuretics
    - Useful with acute glomerulonephritis or with hypertension secondary to corticosteroids
    - Spironolactone (potassium sparing) used in hyperaldosteronism
    - Avoid as chronic medication in athletes
  - Alpha-blockers
    - Central (e.g., clonidine) alpha-blockers have sedative side effects

- Peripheral (e.g., phenoxybenzamine) alpha-blockers are helpful as initial treatment in pheochromocytoma
  - Beta-blockers
    - Avoid in patients with diabetes on insulin (masks symptoms of hypoglycemia) and in asthmatics
  - Direct vasodilators
- Emergency medications (IV):
  - Goal is to reduce blood pressures gradually over 24 hours
    - Nicardipine
    - Enalaprilat
    - Sodium nitroprusside (watch for cyanide toxicity)
    - Labetalol
    - Esmolol
    - Hydralazine
- Surgical intervention may be required for coarctation of aorta/middle aortic syndrome (MAS)
- May need angioplasty for renal artery stenosis

Renal Vein Thrombosis

BASIC INFORMATION

Epidemiology

- Occurs in 2.2/100,000 live births
- 50% of newborns with renal vein thrombosis are premature

Causes and Etiology

- Most common cause of non-catheter-associated thrombosis in newborns
- Risk factors:
  - Prematurity
  - Maternal gestational diabetes
  - Perinatal asphyxia
  - Hypercoagulable (factor V Leiden, protein C deficiency, homocystinuria)
  - Polycythemia
  - Sepsis

CLINICAL PRESENTATION

- Flank mass
- Gross hematuria
- Hypertension
- AKI if bilateral

DIAGNOSIS AND EVALUATION

- Thrombocytopenia
- Elevated creatinine
- Renal ultrasound with Doppler will confirm diagnosis
  - Swollen echogenic kidney(s)
- CT angiogram is diagnostic

TREATMENT

- Consult hematology
- Heparin or low-molecular-weight heparin to prevent progression
- Nephrectomy is rarely required

CYSTIC KIDNEY DISEASES

Multicystic Dysplastic Kidney

BASIC INFORMATION

- Multiple "grape-like" clusters of noncommunicating cysts separated by dysplastic tissue, resulting in abnormal renal architecture and renal dysfunction.

Epidemiology

- Frequency: 1/2200 to 1/4300 live births
- Usually unilateral, more often on the left; bilateral involvement is life-threatening
- Usually sporadic; some reports of familial cases

Causes and Etiology

- Abnormal development of the kidney and urinary tract
  - Abnormal interaction between the metanephric mesenchyme and ureteric bud
  - Leads to urinary tract obstruction
- Teratogens (viral infections, medications)

CLINICAL PRESENTATION

- Prenatal
  - Cystic kidneys on ultrasound
  - Oligohydramnios
- Postnatal
  - Unilateral flank mass
  - Elevated blood pressures
  - By age of 10 years, compensatory hypertrophy of contralateral kidney occurs in 81% of patients
- Contralateral kidney may be associated with
  - Vesicoureteral reflux (~30% cases)
  - Urinary tract obstruction (~15% cases)
  - Ipsilateral internal genital anomalies (e.g., absent vas deferens, uterine abnormalities)
- Medullary cystic kidney disease (MCKD) may involute spontaneously

DIAGNOSIS AND EVALUATION

- Renal ultrasound
  - Look for multiple cysts in affected kidney
  - Contralateral kidney with compensatory hypertrophy
  - Affected kidney may shrink or disappear (involute) spontaneously
- Consider voiding cystourethrogram (VCUG) to evaluate contralateral kidney

TREATMENT

- Monitor renal function and creatinine closely
- Avoid nephrotoxic medications
- Consider prophylactic antibiotics to protect uninvolved kidney (if VCUG shows reflux)
  - Amoxicillin in the nursery
  - Switch to Bactrim (trimethoprim-sulfamethoxazole) at 2 months

- Refer to urology if:
  - Concern for outflow tract obstruction amenable to surgery
  - Patient has recurrent UTI
  - Increasing size of the kidney (concern for malignant transformation—extremely uncommon)
- It is generally advised that patients avoid contact sports to prevent injury to unilateral functional kidney (although it would be a rare occurrence)
- Patients with bilateral disease are at higher risk for chronic kidney disease and hypertension

Autosomal Dominant Polycystic Kidney Disease (ADPKD)

BASIC INFORMATION

- Considered to be an "adult-onset disease" because manifestations usually develop later in life, but disease can be seen in childhood
- Cysts develop anywhere along the nephron
- Associated with numerous large cysts in the kidney with loss of normal shape of the kidney (see Fig. 54.2)

Epidemiology

- 1/400 to 1/1000 of the general population
- Second most common genetic disease with autosomal dominant inheritance (after familial hypercholesterolemia)

Causes and Etiology

- Mutation of *PKD1* gene located on chromosome 16 (85% of cases) or *PKD2* gene located on chromosome 4 (15% of cases)
- Spontaneous mutations may occur frequently

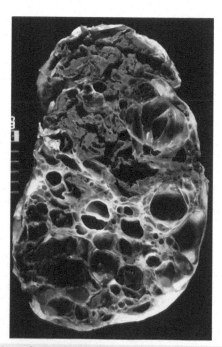

Fig. 54.2. Loss of normal kidney shape due to large cysts in autosomal dominant polycystic kidney disease.

CLINICAL PRESENTATION

- Rarely seen in neonates. Oligohydramnios is uncommon
- Usually includes a family history of adults with renal disease and/or cerebral aneurysms
- Classic triad of adult presentation is hypertension, hematuria, and flank pain; kidney may be enlarged on examination
- Cysts in other organs, including liver, pancreas, arachnoid membrane, ovaries, and seminal vesicle
- Cerebral vessel aneurysms
  - 5% prevalence in children and 20% in adults
  - Risk of rupture if >7 mm in size or poorly controlled hypertension
  - Familial predilection
- Mitral valve prolapse
- Colonic diverticula, abdominal wall and inguinal hernias
- May have recurrent UTIs
- End-stage kidney disease does not develop until 50 to 60 years of age (50% by 50 years of age)

DIAGNOSIS AND EVALUATION

- Evidence of kidney involvement may include elevation of blood urea nitrogen/creatinine (BUN/Cr) and hematuria
- Ultrasound:
  - Kidneys with macrocysts visible on ultrasound
  - Even a single cyst in a patient with a positive family history of ADPKD is diagnostic
  - Otherwise need one cyst in one kidney and at least two cysts in the other kidney
- Genetics testing
- Screen for aneurysms if:
  - Severe headaches
  - Previous rupture
  - Positive family history of cerebral aneurysm rupture or intracranial bleed/stroke
  - High-risk occupation

TREATMENT

- At least annual evaluation for proteinuria and hypertension
- Avoid caffeine and recommend adequate but normal fluid intake
- Management of hypertension and urinary tract infections
- Start ACEI if patient develops hypertension or proteinuria
- Statins may slow cyst enlargement and thereby preserve renal function
- Decision for surgical intervention for brain aneurysms depends on the balance of the risk for rupture versus the risk of surgery

Autosomal Recessive Polycystic Kidney Disease (ARPKD)

BASIC INFORMATION

- Cysts are initially dilated renal collecting ducts; later true cysts form

- Multiple minute cystic spaces throughout the medulla; kidney shape is maintained (see Fig. 54.3)
- Liver involvement (congenital hepatic fibrosis) due to malformation of the developing bile ducts

Epidemiology

- 1/20,000 live births

Etiology

- Mutations in *PKHD1* gene located on chromosome 6

CLINICAL PRESENTATION

- Degree of renal and hepatic involvement varies from patient to patient
- Bilateral flank masses may present at birth
- Prenatal findings include oligohydramnios during pregnancy (due to low urine output) and enlarged echogenic kidneys on screening ultrasound
- Potter syndrome:
  - Characteristic of neonate with oligohydramnios associated with:
    - Pulmonary hypoplasia
    - Facial flattening (pseudoepicanthus, low-set ears, flat nose, retracted chin)
    - Limb abnormalities (clubfoot and hip dislocation)
- Hepatomegaly, dilatation of the biliary duct (Caroli disease)
- Synthetic liver dysfunction and features of portal hypertension
  - Hematemesis, esophageal varices, thrombocytopenia, and/or splenomegaly
- High mortality in neonatal period usually due to severe pulmonary hypoplasia
- Lifetime will have progressive renal cyst enlargement, fibrosis, and insufficiency

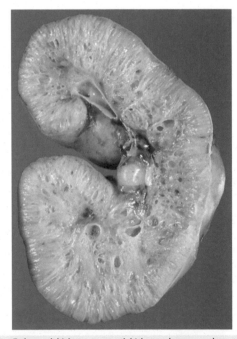

Fig. 54.3. Enlarged kidney, normal kidney shape, and small cysts in autosomal recessive polycystic kidney disease.

■ For those who survive the first year, there is a 50% chance of end-stage kidney disease by 10 years of age and 85% survival at 15 years of age

DIAGNOSIS AND EVALUATION

- Ultrasound:
  - Kidney: large echogenic kidneys—initially do *not* see macrocysts
  - Liver: hepatomegaly and increased echogenicity due to congenital hepatic fibrosis (CHF)
- CBC and liver function test: usually have normal liver enzymes, but have synthetic dysfunction
- BMP
- Genetic studies

TREATMENT

- Monitor renal function closely and manage abnormal electrolytes and azotemia
- Blood pressure control may require multiple medications (ACEI and loop diuretic)
- May need dialysis during childhood due to end-stage kidney disease
- Surgical interventions include nephrectomies, shunt procedures for portal hypertension, and potential kidney and/or liver transplants

Nephronophthisis

BASIC INFORMATION

- Genetically heterogeneous disorder
- Autosomal recessive inheritance
- Associated with reduced urinary concentration and chronic tubulointerstitial nephritis

Causes and Etiology

- Mutations in *NPH* gene
  - *NPH1:* juvenile (most common, 25% of cases)
  - *NPH2:* infantile
  - *NPH3:* adolescent
- Infantile and adolescent forms are rare

CLINICAL PRESENTATION

- Polyuria, enuresis, polydipsia
- Hyposthenuria (inability to concentrate urine; therefore urinalysis with low specific gravity)
- Bland urinalysis (no hematuria or proteinuria) on presentation, and slow progression to end-stage renal disease
- Anemia out of proportion to kidney disease
- Failure to thrive, short stature
- Retinitis pigmentosa: Senior-Loken syndrome
- May have ocular apraxia
- Cerebellar aplasia and coloboma of the eye: Joubert syndrome

DIAGNOSIS AND EVALUATION

- Monitoring renal function and CBC
- Renal ultrasound:
  - Normal or slight decrease in renal size and increased echogenicity

TREATMENT

- Often need erythropoietin for anemia
- Rarely have hypertension because they are salt-wasting
- Ophthalmology evaluation needed for risk of retinitis pigmentosa and apraxia

Meckel-Gruber Syndrome

- Autosomal recessive
- Associated with:
  - Cystic dysplasia of the kidney
  - Hepatic fibrosis
  - Brain: occipital encephalocele
  - Postaxial polydactyly

Bardet-Biedl Syndrome

- Autosomal recessive (numerous genes)
- Associated with:
  - Cystic dysplasia of the kidneys
  - Obesity
  - Retinitis pigmentosa
  - Hypogenitalism
  - Postaxial polydactyly
  - Cognitive delay

Review Questions

For review questions, please go to ExpertConsult.com.

Suggested Readings
1. American Association of Pediatrics. Urinary tract infection: clinical practice guideline for the diagnosis and management of the initial UTI in febrile infants and children 2 to 24 months. *Pediatrics.* 2011;128(3): 595–610.
2. Feld LG, Corey H. Hypertension in childhood. *Pediatr Rev.* 2007;28(8):283–297.
3. Feld LG, Mattoo TK. Urinary tract infections and vesicoureteral reflux in infants and children. *Pediatr Rev.* 2010;31(11):451–463.
4. Gillespie RS, Stapleton FB. Nephrolithiasis in children. *Pediatr Rev.* 2004;25(4):131–139.
5. Jackson EC. Urinary tract infections in children: knowledge updates and a salute to the future. *Pediatr Rev.* 2015;36(4):153–166.
6. McKay CP. Renal stone disease. *Pediatr Rev.* 2010;31(5):179–188.
7. Meyers KEC, Cahill AM, Sethna CS. Interventions for pediatric renovascular hypertension. *Curr Hypertens Rep.* 2014;16(4):422. 24522941.
8. Norwood VF. Hypertension. *Pediatr Rev.* 2002;23(6):197–209.
9. Verghese P, Miyashita Y. Neonatal polycystic kidney disease. *Clin Perinatol.* 2014;41(3):543–600.

Neurology

The neurological assessment begins with a framework of considering the differential diagnosis based on the chief presentation with then further localization determined by the history and neurological examination. In general, localization of a presenting symptom can be crudely divided into central versus peripheral, keeping in mind that this is an arbitrary line and that in clinical practice there may be overlap between the two, particularly in systemic illnesses and metabolic or genetic conditions. Central etiologies include cortical pathology that may be focal (such as tumors) or diffuse (such as cerebrovascular diseases). Peripheral etiologies can be subdivided by locations as well. Features that suggest a particular location are summarized in Table 55.1. The subsequent neurologic examination should then help direct this differential.

The neurologic examination in the pediatric population can be challenging; the younger the child, the more the examination will rely on observation and indirect tests of examination. For example, in a toddler presenting with a chief complaint of change in gait, direct confrontation testing of isolated muscle strength may be challenging. Observing a patient's spontaneous movements in the parent's lap, encouraging the patient to play with the examiner, and encouraging him or her to walk toward a parent may yield more information. The younger the child, the less sensitive the examination may be and in practice will rely on ancillary testing such as neuroimaging for further evaluation.

See also Nelson Textbook of Pediatrics, Chapter 590, "Neurological Evaluation."

Neurologic Assessment

ELEMENTS OF THE INTERVIEW

- History
  - Neurologic baseline: the differential diagnosis for a previously healthy child compared with that for a child with chronic or progressive static encephalopathy will differ significantly. Early on in the assessment, it is important to establish the child's cognitive, language, motor, and fine motor baseline and to determine how the child's presenting symptom represents a change from baseline
  - Presenting symptom: important features
    - Age of onset
    - Evolution and duration of symptoms—acute, subacute, or chronic
    - Focal or generalized
- Past medical history
  - Pregnancy history (including prenatal exposures)
  - Birth history (including any complications)

- Developmental history
  - Any note of regression should raise a red flag for an underlying metabolic, genetic, or progressive metabolic condition requiring further evaluation
- Family history
  - Any other family members with developmental delay, visual or sensorineural hearing loss as a child, metabolic or genetic diseases, or involvement of neurologic diseases such as epilepsy are important to elicit
- Prior testing
  - Newborn screening
  - Prior laboratory testing, including genetic testing
  - Prior neuroimaging evaluation

ELEMENTS OF THE NEUROLOGIC EXAM

- Vital signs
- Growth parameters: weight, length, head circumference
  - Presence of macrocephaly, microcephaly, or a plateau in head growth should be another red flag
- General examination
  - Presence of dysmorphic features may help direct toward a metabolic or genetic etiology
  - Presence of hepatosplenomegaly may direct considerations toward metabolic etiology
  - Skin findings: may be present in various genetic syndromes (e.g., the presence of multiple café-au-lait lesions may help with diagnosis of neurofibromatosis type 1)
  - Genitourinary (GU) findings: for example, abnormal genitalia such as ambiguous genitalia raises concern for underlying metabolic or genetic disorder
  - Muscle bulk: if primary presentation is chronic weakness, bulk should be examined to help with upper versus lower motor neuron pathology
- Neurologic examination
  - Mental status: this should be assessed throughout the examination
  - Cognitive testing: formal tests of cognition, such as attention, fund of knowledge, and memory tests, may be difficult to perform in a young child. It is important to adjust the examination to age-appropriate tasks such as naming colors for a 3-year-old or reading sentences for a second-grader
  - Cranial nerves: see Table 55.2 for appropriate assessment of cranial nerve function. A few clinical relevant pearls are included below
    - Cranial nerve II: a funduscopic examination should be attempted in pertinent clinical scenarios. For example, in an acute headache evaluation, presence of papilledema would urgently change management

Table 55.1. Localization Based on Presenting Neurologic Symptoms

Cortical	■ Presence of seizures ■ Presence of encephalopathy ■ Involvement of higher cognitive functions such as language or speech, reading, and extinction ■ Dysmorphic features
Brain stem	■ Cranial neuropathies: this may manifest as double vision, facial numbness, facial weakness, difficulty with swallowing or a hoarse voice ■ May have altered mental status with this as well
Spinal cord	■ Presence of a sensory level or weakness ■ Involvement of bowel or urinary incontinence
Cerebellar	■ Imbalance and incoordination of movements
Anterior horn cell	■ Presence of fasciculations
Peripheral nerve	■ Motor or sensory loss consistent with a peripheral distribution of a nerve
Neuromuscular junction	■ Can be difficult to distinguish between other peripheral causes but may have a fatigability characteristic or a waxing and waning pattern of motor weakness (particularly ptosis or extraocular muscles)
Muscle	■ Typically has a more proximal than distal muscle involvement—difficulty with raising arm above head to brush hair, for example, or to climb stairs

Table 55.2. Cranial Nerves

Number	Name	Function
I	Olfactory nerve	■ Sense of smell
II	Optic nerve	■ Visual acuity ■ Visual fields ■ Afferent limb of pupillomotor action (with cranial nerve III, dilates or constricts the pupil)
III	Oculomotor nerve	■ Most of the eye movements (except those controlled by cranial nerve IV and VI) ■ Efferent limb of pupillomotor action
IV	Trochlear nerve	■ Superior oblique muscle: depresses and intorts the eye ■ Afferent limb of corneal reflex
V	Trigeminal nerve	■ Facial sensation (divided into three divisions: V_1, V_2, and V_3) ■ Muscles of mastication
VI	Abducens nerve	■ Lateral rectus muscle: abducts the eye
VII	Facial nerve	■ Muscles of facial expression ■ Efferent limb of the corneal reflex ■ Sense of taste in anterior two-thirds of the tongue
VIII	Vestibulocochlear nerve	■ Sense of hearing ■ Vestibular organ: coordination of eye movements and equilibrium
IX	Glossopharyngeal nerve	■ Sense of taste and sensation in posterior two-thirds of the tongue ■ Afferent limb of the carotid baroreceptor and gag reflexes
X	Vagus nerve	■ Muscles of the palate ■ Efferent limb of the baroreceptor and gag reflexes ■ Provides parasympathetics to most organs
XI	Spinal accessory nerve	■ Sternocleidomastoids and trapezius are responsible for turning the head contralaterally and ipsilateral elevation of the shoulder, respectively
XII	Hypoglossal nerve	■ Muscles of the tongue

■ Cranial nerve III: observe for presence of ptosis because cranial nerve III (not VII) is responsible for levator palpebrae, which retracts and elevates the eyelid
■ Cranial nerves III, IV, and VI are responsible for all ocular movements. Cranial nerves IV and VI are each responsible for one muscle; the rest are due to cranial nerve III. Injury of any of these nerves can present as head tilt or double vision due to issues with eye alignment
■ Cranial nerve VII: differentiate between central versus peripheral
  Lesion in the facial nerve or nucleus will present with ipsilateral muscle weakness including deficits in forehead wrinkling and the lower face (Bell's palsy). Because the facial nerve also innervates the stapedius, patients may note unilateral hyperacusis
  Lesions centrally, such as in an arterial ischemic stroke, will spare the forehead and cause isolated contralateral lower facial weakness
■ Motor examination: typically graded on a MRC scale from 0 to 5
  ■ Grades 1–5
    Grade 5/5: strong resistance against examiner (normal)
    Grade 4/5: some resistance against examiner
    Grade 3/5: no resistance against examiner, but able to move extremity against gravity
    Grade 2/5: unable to move extremity against gravity but can move within plane of extremity
    Grade 1/5: flickers of movement
    Grade 0/5: no movement at all
  ■ Indirect tests of motor strength: observing a child's strength in reaching for interesting objects, observing

their walk including heel/toe walking, or ability to rise from a chair or crawl onto the examining table, or their gait in running can yield helpful information about major muscle groups that may be involved
■ Tone
  ■ Posture: observe how the patient is at rest. A term neonate will be comfortably flexed in the upper extremities and lower extremities. A hypotonic neonate will have a splayed position of the limbs
  ■ Test tone by passive movement through two joints of a limb; tone can be decreased or increased. If tone increases with velocity-dependent maneuvers, this is called *spasticity*
■ Sensory
  ■ Sensory deficits should be closely examined with multiple modalities (pinprick, vibration, light touch) and observed to see whether there is consistency across a dermatome
  ■ Assess for light touch, pinprick, and temperature (spinothalamic tracts)
  ■ Assess for proprioception and vibration (dorsal columns)

Table 55.3. Upper Versus Lower Motor Neuron Signs

	Upper Motor Neuron	Lower Motor Neuron
Deep tendon reflexes	Increased	Decreased
Babinski	Present (up-going)	Not present
Tone	Increased, may have spasticity	Decreased
Muscle fasciculation	Not present	Present

- Reflexes
  - Primitive reflexes are the neonatal reflexes that eventually disappear with brain maturation, which inhibits these reflexes. These include root, suck, palmar, plantar, Moro, and others
  - Babinski is an upward extension of the big toe with stroking of the lateral to medial plantar surface of the foot. This can be normal in a neonate, but if found after 1 year of life can be suggestive of a central pathology
  - Deep tendon reflexes
    - 4+: hyperreflexic, presence of clonus
    - 3+: hyperreflexic, crossed adductors may be present
    - 2+: normal
    - 1+: hyporeflexic
    - 0: no reflexes
- Coordination
  - Finger–nose–finger: to assess for dysmetria
- Gait
- Upper versus lower motor neuron localization (see Table 55.3)
  - Features that suggest an upper motor neuron lesion (spinal cord, brain stem, cortex) are "up"—increased reflexes, up-going Babinski, and increased tone or presence of spasticity
  - Lower motor neuron lesion (anterior horn, plexus, peripheral nerve, neuromuscular junction, muscle) where findings are "down"—decreased or absent reflexes and decreased tone
  - Atrophy typically is seen more commonly with lower motor neuron lesions, but "disuse" atrophy can also be seen with chronic upper motor neuron lesions such as those seen in a stroke

Approach to Neuroimaging

HEAD ULTRASOUND

- Advantages:
  - Portable, fast, noninvasive, and can provide immediate, actionable information
  - Head ultrasounds are sensitive for presence of hydrocephalus or intraventricular hemorrhages
- Disadvantages:
  - Dependent on presence of an open fontanelle
  - Less reliable for detecting posterior fossa injury or lesions in the periphery
  - Technician-dependent for quality
  - May have nonspecific hyperechogenic findings, which can represent ischemia, hemorrhage, or white matter injury or can be normal

Table 55.4. MRI Sequences

Sequence	Appearance			Clinical Utility
	Water (CSF)	Fat	Brain	
T1 weighted	Dark	Bright	Gray matter = gray White matter = white	Best for visualizing general anatomy
T2 weighted	Bright	Bright	Gray matter = white White matter = gray	Best for visualizing posterior fossa pathology and demyelinating lesions
T2 FLAIR	Dark	Bright	Gray matter = white White matter = gray	Particularly useful for detecting changes in the periventricular area (as CSF is now dark) and peripheral areas. Also good for visualizing cerebral edema
DWI	Dark	Dark	Gray matter = gray White matter = darker gray	Low-resolution images. The combination of DWI and ADC is useful for detecting acute pathology, particularly for ischemic stroke (within a 7–10 day window) or in cases of certain tumors or infections (abscesses)
ADC	Bright	Dark	Gray matter = gray White matter = lighter gray	

ADC, Apparent diffusion coefficient maps; *CSF,* cerebrospinal fluid; *DWI,* diffusion-weighted imaging; *FLAIR,* fluid attenuation inversion recovery; *MRI,* magnetic resonance imaging.

HEAD COMPUTED TOMOGRAPHY (CT)

- Advantages:
  - Sensitive and reliable indicator for acute presence of hemorrhage, large ischemia, hydrocephalus, and herniation
  - Superior to magnetic resonance imaging (MRI) for detecting bony changes such as fractures
  - Useful for urgent clinical situations in providing timely information because it requires less time to obtain
- Disadvantages
  - Radiation exposure
  - Not sensitive for most central nervous system (CNS) pathology such as inflammation, periventricular leukomalacia, or ischemia
  - May still require sedation for the younger population despite short time period required

MRI BRAIN

- Advantages:
  - Most sensitive for intracranial pathology
- Disadvantages:
  - Long duration often necessitates sedation of a young child to obtain high-quality images without motion artifact

- Multiple sequences are capable of portraying various information (see Table 55.4)
  - Hyperintense refers to areas that are lighter. A high-signal-intensity area is white
  - Hypointense refers to areas that are darker. A low-signal-intensity area is black
  - IV gadolinium is used after the above sequences have been obtained; if there are any disturbances to the blood-brain barrier, contrast will pass through and will cause areas of pathology to enhance, such as in cases of infection or tumors

VASCULAR IMAGING OPTIONS

- Computed tomography angiography (CTA) is used to assess arterial structures of the head or neck. The primary risk of this is the radiation exposure, but typically this is more sensitive than MRI-based techniques (see below) for detecting lesions such as arterial stenosis or aneurysm
  - This is the imaging of choice for patients who are unstable, have contraindications to MRI (such as metallic objects in body), or are within the window for urgent therapeutics, such as tPA in adults with acute arterial ischemic stroke
- Computed tomographic venography (CTV) is used to assess venous structures of the head or neck
  - Due to radiation, magnetic resonance venography (MRV) is typically preferred, except in urgent situations or where there are contraindications to MRI
- Magnetic resonance angiography (MRA) and MRV are used to assess arterial and venous anatomies of the brain, respectively, but can be less sensitive for many of the vascular findings compared with CT-based modalities. They do not carry risk of radiation

Suggested Readings

Caramant L, Diadori P. The neurologic examination. In: Maria BL, ed. *Current Management In Child Neurology.* 2nd ed. London: BC Dekker, Inc; 2002:28.

Swaiman KF. Neurologic examination of the older child. In: Swaiman KF, Ashwal S, Ferriero DM, eds. *Neurology. Principles and Practice.* 4th ed. Philadelphia: Mosby Elsevier; 2006:17.

56 *Altered Mental Status and Headache*

NAN LIN, MD

ALTERED MENTAL STATUS

Altered mental status or encephalopathy is a change or deviation from a child's cognitive, behavioral, or mental baseline. Presentation of encephalopathy can range from very subtle signs of irritability to coma. Because there is a wide range of causative factors, some with devastating consequences if untreated, early recognition, diagnosis, and appropriate management are crucial. Table 56.1 provides a differential diagnosis of encephalopathy but is by no means an exhaustive list; rather, it provides a framework for considering initial diagnoses for a child with an acute presentation of encephalopathy. The mnemonic VITAMINS can be helpful to avoid overlooking a category when pursuing this evaluation.

- **V**ascular
- **I**nfectious/inflammatory
- **T**raumatic/toxic
- **A**utoimmune
- **M**etabolic/malignancy
- **I**atrogenic/intussusception/idiopathic
- **N**eoplastic/neurologic
- **S**troke/seizure/structural

The differential diagnosis is quite large (see Table 56.1). Episodic or chronic forms of encephalopathy will not be discussed here.

GENERAL APPROACH

- A thorough history should be obtained including:
  - Age of child
  - Onset of symptoms
  - Rate of progression—rapid progression of symptoms suggests an acute vascular or traumatic cause, whereas a more gradual onset of symptoms favors metabolic or infectious causes
  - Exposures to environmental causes such as carbon monoxide or accidental ingestion of medications
  - Risk factors
- Physical examination
  - Vital signs are vital for a reason
    - Fever should not be missed as a potential sign of underlying infection or inflammation
    - Cushing triad is a late sign of increasing intracranial pressure, but its presence requires urgent evaluation for impending intracranial herniation
  - Mental status: levels of consciousness
    - Lethargy: patient can be awakened with moderate stimulation but then easily falls back to sleep

- Obtundation: similar to lethargy but requires more stimulation to be aroused
- Stupor: able to be awakened only with vigorous and painful stimulation but then promptly returns to sleep
- Coma: unable to be awakened, even with vigorous and painful stimulation
- The Glasgow Coma Scale (see Chapter 15) is an objective, quick measure of a level of consciousness for rapid triage and subsequent serial evaluations
  - A thorough physical examination should be performed because there may be clues on examination that offer an etiology such as the presence of meningismus for an infectious etiology
  - A new focal neurological finding should raise concern for an acute intracranial process
- Laboratory Evaluation
  - Serologic testing
    - Should be tailored to history and physical examination
    - If causation remains unclear, reasonable first-tier screening laboratories focus on reversible causes of encephalopathy including glucose, electrolytes, and basic infectious studies. Drug and urine studies should be sent as indicated
    - Electrocardiogram (ECG): some toxic etiologies of altered mental status can cause cardiac rhythm changes and should be performed in the appropriate context
  - Lumbar puncture (LP): this should be obtained in any patient with an unclear cause of encephalopathy, even without presence of fever, if there are no contraindications present
- Adjunctive Neurologic Studies
  - Neuroimaging
    - Depending on the patient's clinical status, head computed tomography (CT) versus magnetic resonance imaging (MRI) brain should be strongly considered, particularly if the etiology is unclear, prioritizing patient stabilization first
    - Head CT is preferred in scenarios where speed is of the utmost importance (e.g., rapidly declining patient due to a suspected bleed or with signs of increased intracranial pressure)
    - MRI brain provides the most sensitive detection of structural changes associated with any underlying disease and should be considered for any pediatric encephalopathy with focal findings or unclear etiology

Table 56.1. Differential Diagnosis for Acute Pediatric Encephalopathy

TOXIC-METABOLIC	VASCULAR	INFECTIOUS
Hypoglycemia	Diffuse anoxic injury	Sepsis
Hyper-/hyponatremia	Arterial ischemic stroke	Shock
Other electrolyte disturbances	Hemorrhagic stroke (subarachnoid, subdural, epidural)	Meningitis
Hepatic or uremic encephalopathy	Sinus venous thrombosis	Encephalitis
Hypercarbia	Reversible posterior leukoencephalopathy syndrome	HSV encephalitis
Endocrine disorders (such as diabetic ketoacidosis or thyroid dysfunction)		
Toxic ingestion		
Medication overdose		
Environmental exposure (such as carbon monoxide)		
Inborn errors of metabolism		

NEUROLOGIC	STRUCTURAL	TRAUMA
Acute demyelinating encephalomyelitis (ADEM)	Tumor or mass Hydrocephalus	Concussion Nonaccidental trauma
Seizures including postictal state	Cerebral edema	Diffuse axonal injury
Status epilepticus	Obstructed ventriculoperitoneal shunt	
Complicated migraine	Herniation	

IMMUNE-MEDIATED	PSYCHIATRIC	OTHER
Autoimmune encephalitis	Catatonia	Intussusception
Paraneoplastic encephalitis	Conversion	Malignancy

- Electroencephalogram (EEG): consider obtaining to evaluate for nonconvulsive status epilepticus, particularly if there is a history of seizures or epilepsy

TREATMENT

- Management of airway, breathing, and circulation should be foremost. Intravenous (IV) access should be established
- Low threshold for considering empiric antibiotic coverage; antiviral coverage (i.e., acyclovir) should also be considered for meningitis, infectious encephalitis, or unexplained encephalopathy in the very young because this is one of the few urgently treatable causes of pediatric encephalopathy
- Treatment should be tailored to suspected etiologies

Central Nervous System Infections—Meningitis and Encephalitis

BASIC INFORMATION

- There is significant morbidity and mortality associated with untreated infectious meningitis and encephalitis;

early recognition, management, and treatment are key, especially for bacterial and certain treatable viral pathogens including herpes simplex virus (HSV) encephalitis
- Overlap exists between presentation of meningitis and encephalitis
  - Encephalitis is defined as the inflammation of the brain parenchyma, whereas meningitis is inflammation of the covering meninges
  - Although differentiating between meningitis and encephalitis will help narrow the differential diagnosis and direct treatment (see later), some diseases can present with both, which is termed meningoencephalitis
- Differential diagnosis
  - Infectious causes of meningitis and encephalitis are the most common
    - Approximately 50% or more (depending on population) cases of encephalitis will not be able to be identified, although viruses are the most common cause of encephalitis among identified pathogens
    - Important risk factors for central nervous system (CNS) infections are listed in Table 56.2
  - Noninfectious differential diagnosis:
    - Postinfectious, encephalomyelitis (e.g., ADEM, see later)
    - Autoimmune process (e.g., anti-NMDA receptor encephalitis, see later)
    - CNS inflammation (e.g., Behçet, systemic lupus erythematosus [SLE], sarcoidosis)
      Chemical meningitis
      Malignancy
- Encephalopathy and encephalitis are not the same
  - Encephalopathy is a clinical presentation that may or may not be due to an underlying CNS inflammation
  - Encephalitis (Table 56.3) is defined by inflammation due to infectious or other processes of the CNS. Encephalitis will present with encephalopathy by definition

CLINICAL PRESENTATION

- Because of the meningeal inflammation around the brain and spinal cord in meningitis, patients will present with signs of meningeal irritation
  - In the older child, headaches, irritability, photophobia, nausea, vomiting, and stiff neck in the context of a fever develop over the course of hours to days
  - In the neonate or infant, symptoms are nonspecific and can range from subtle irritability to poor feeding, lethargy, or seizures
- Clinical presentation of encephalitis requires altered mental status for ≥24 hours and may include the features mentioned in Table 56.3.
- Physical examination:
  - Trend vital signs (e.g., fever) and head circumference in young infants (for signs of increased intracranial pressure or worsening hydrocephalus)
    - Cushing triad is a late sign of increased intracranial pressure
  - Neurologic signs can be nonspecific in the infant but may include irritability, lethargy, decrease in tone, or seizures
    - Concerning signs: bulging fontanelle, papilledema, or focal neurologic signs
    - Older children may demonstrate nuchal rigidity and other classic signs of meningeal irritation:

Table 56.2.   Central Nervous System Infectious Risk Factors

	Neonate		Children
Maternal factors	Perinatal infection	Immuno-deficiency	Primary immunodeficiency
	Maternal group B streptococcus colonization		Asplenia (anatomic or functional)
	Chorioamnionitis		HIV
	Endometritis		Sickle cell anemia
	Maternal sexually transmitted diseases (including herpes simplex virus)		Immunosuppressive agents
Delivery	Prolonged duration of intrauterine monitoring (>12 hours)	Exposure/ environmental	Day care attendance
	Prolonged rupture of membranes		Travel (to a wooded area or areas where certain diseases are endemic)
	Traumatic delivery		Exposure to cases of meningococcal or *Haemophilus influenzae* type B meningitis
			Tuberculosis exposure
Neonatal factors	Preterm birth		*Exposure to ticks, mosquitos, cats, bats, birds, or vectors
	Low birth weight (<2.5 kg)	Surgical/ trauma	Cochlear implant
	Galactosemia		Central nervous system shunts
	Urinary tract abnormalities		Dermal sinus tract of the spine
	Dermal sinus tract of the spine		Penetrating head injury
			Cerebrospinal fluid leak
		Medical history	Recent upper respiratory tract infection
			Lack of immunizations
			Recent antibiotic exposure

*Important for encephalitis.
Data from Mann K, Jackson MA. Meningitis. *Pediatr Rev.* 2008;29(12):417–429; Swanson D. Meningitis. *Pediatr Rev.* 2015;36(12):514–524.

Table 56.3.   Clinical Features in Encephalitis

Documented fever ≥38°C (100.4°F) within the 72 hr before or after presentation

Generalized or partial seizures not fully attributable to a preexisting seizure disorder

New onset of focal neurologic findings

Cerebrospinal fluid white blood cell count ≥5 mm³

Abnormality of brain parenchyma on neuroimaging suggestive of encephalitis that is either new from prior studies or appears acute in onset

Abnormality on electroencephalography that is consistent with encephalitis and not attributable to another cause

Data from Venkatesan A, Tunkel AR, Bloch KC, Lauring AS, Sejvar J, Bitnun A, et al. Case definitions, diagnostic algorithms, and priorities in encephalitis: consensus statement of the International Encephalitis Consortium. *Clin Infect Dis.* 2013;57(8):1114–1128.

- Kernig sign is present when the hip and knee are flexed at 90 degrees and the examiner is unable to extend one leg past 135 degrees due to pain, or if the patient flexes the opposite knee during the maneuver
- Brudzinski sign is present when active neck flexion by the examiner results in subsequent hip and knee flexion
- Kernig and Brudzinski signs have low sensitivity (but reasonable specificity)
- Infants often lack classic signs of meningismus; rather, they may demonstrate paradoxic irritability when held
- Systemic signs, including evaluating a patient's respiratory and cardiac system, are also crucial:

- Changes in respiratory pattern can be ominous (e.g., Cheyne-Stokes breathing, apnea) and require emergent management
- Hepatomegaly may suggest associated hepatitis or a hepatic encephalopathy
- Rashes may help direct diagnosis (e.g., petechiae and purpura for invasive meningococcal or pneumococcal disease, vesicles for HSV). Note that the lack of skin findings does not rule out presence of these diseases

DIAGNOSIS AND EVALUATION

- Initial evaluation should foremost consider patient stability with establishing venous access, close monitoring of vital signs and providing fluids, hemodynamic support, and respiratory support as indicated
- Evaluation for meningitis/sepsis in a young infant is detailed in Chapter 43
- Serologic testing for diagnosis and evaluation of CNS infections should include:
  - A complete blood count with differential
  - At least two separate blood cultures
  - Complete metabolic panel—syndrome of inappropriate antidiuretic hormone secretion (SIADH) can occur as a side effect of intracranial infections, and thus sodium should be closely monitored (see Chapter 26). It is also important to assess renal and liver function in the setting of sepsis or shock
  - Inflammatory markers such as C-reactive protein may be obtained to help trend patient's response to treatment

Table 56.4. CSF Normal Values by Age and Different CSF Infectious Profiles

WBC (cells/µL)		Infectious Cause	OP	WBC	Diff	Pro	Glu	Cx	Misc
Infants 0–28 days	0–19	Bacterial	↑	↑↑↑	S	↑	↓	+	
Infants 29–56 days	0–9	Viral	Nl	↑	L/M	Sl↑	Nl	−	
Child	0–7	Herpes simplex virus	↑	↑	L	↑	Nl	−	PCR
Glucose (mg/dL)		Tuberculosis	↑	Nl/↑	L	↑	↓		AFB
Infants 0–28 days	30–61	Mycoplasma	Nl	Nl	L	↑	Nl	−	Ab+
Infants 29–56 days	30–66	Sarcoid		↑↑	L	↑	Nl/↓	−	ACE
Child	40–80	Neurosyphilis		↑↑	L/M	↑	Nl		+VDRL/ FTA
Protein (mg/dL)		Lyme	Nl	↑↑↑	L	↑	Nl		+OCB
Infants 0–28 days	<115	Fungal meningitis	↑	↑↑↑	L	↑	Nl/↓	+	Ag
Infants 29–56 days	<89	Postinfectious		↑↑	L	Nl/↑	Nl	−	
Child	5–40								

Ab+, antibody positive; ACE, angiotensin-converting enzyme; AFB, acid-fast bacillus; Ag, antigen; CSF, cerebrospinal fluid; Cx, culture; Diff, differential; FTA, fluorescent treponemal antibody; Glu, glucose; L, lymphocytes; M, monocytes; Nl, normal; OCB, oligoclonal bands; OP, opening pressure, leave WBC alone; PCR, polymerase chain reaction; Pro, protein; *S, polymorphonuclear leukocytes; Sl, slightly; VDRL, Venereal Disease Research Laboratory; WBC, white blood cell.

- Coagulation markers are often obtained to monitor for coagulopathy
- For encephalitis specifically, serologic testing for Epstein-Barr virus (EBV) serology, *Mycoplasma pneumoniae* IgM/IgG, HIV, and rapid plasma reagin (RPR) can be sent (Venkatesan et al., 2013). Serum is often held for later testing
- Imaging
  - A CT of the head is warranted with any signs of increased intracranial pressure or with focal neurologic signs, presence of prior surgical instrumentation (such as cerebrospinal fluid [CSF] shunt), history of prior CNS conditions (such as tumor), or papilledema
  - MRI brain with and without contrast is indicated in cases of encephalitis and is often recommended for meningitis
- CSF
  - If there are no contraindications for a lumbar puncture (LP), this should be performed in suspected cases of meningitis or encephalitis
  - Contraindications for LP:
    - Patient instability
    - Severe coagulopathy
    - Skin infection over the site of the lumbar puncture
    - Concern for impending herniation
  - Imaging should be considered before a lumbar puncture if the following risk factors are present: immunocompromised or immunosuppressed patient, history of CNS disease, new-onset seizures, presence of a focal neurologic deficit or papilledema
  - CSF data:
    - Opening pressure, cell counts (white blood cell [WBC] with differential and red blood cell [RBC]), protein, glucose, Gram stain, and culture should be obtained
    - Saving CSF specimen for future testing is often useful as well
    - Polymerase chain reaction (PCR) testing for HSV in CSF should always be considered
  - Normal values for CSF parameters are listed in Table 56.4. Normal opening pressure is usually between 10 to 25 cm H_2O obtained when the patient is the lateral decubitus position

- Clinically differentiating between bacterial and viral meningitis can be difficult; some laboratory parameters can help elucidate this (see Table 56.4)
  - Bacterial meningitis will have a very elevated CSF WBC ranging from 1000 to 5000 cells/µL. The differential will generally favor neutrophils >80%. Glucose will be less than 40 mg/dL in about half of the patients. CSF protein will be elevated. A positive Gram stain will be helpful if positive, but if negative, does not rule out presence of bacterial infection
  - Viral meningitis can have CSF WBC from 50 to 1000 cells/µL with predominantly lymphocytes on differential (exceptions are Lyme and early tuberculous meningitis)
  - Typically CSF:serum glucose ratio (normal being ≥0.5) will be less than 0.5 for bacteria and greater than 0.5 for viral
- For encephalitis, a minimum of HSV and enterovirus in CSF should be sent along with other viral studies, dependent on clinical cases
  - Immunocompromised patients are susceptible to a wider range of infectious encephalitides (e.g., cytomegalovirus [CMV], HHV6/7, HIV, Cryptococcus, Toxoplasma, tuberculosis, fungus, West Nile virus)
  - Parechovirus is especially associated with encephalitis in children <3 years old
  - Travel or environmental factors may require additional testing (Table 56.5)
  - Guidance for additional testing based on history, laboratory features, and neuroimaging provided in Venkatesan et al. (2013)
- EEG testing should be performed for cases of severe encephalopathy and in most cases of encephalitis

TREATMENT

- Empiric antibodies should not be delayed (even for an LP!) Target treatment based on age, risk factors, testing results, and clinical context. Common bacterial pathogens based on age and empiric therapy are listed in Table 56.6

Table 56.5. Specific Considerations for Encephalitis

Geographic	Africa—malaria, trypanosomiasis, dengue
	Asia—Japanese encephalitis, dengue, malaria
	Central and South America—dengue, malaria
	North America—based on location, West Nile virus, Eastern equine encephalitis, Lyme, Powassan
Season/exposure	Summer/fall—tick-borne disease, arboviruses
	Cat—bartonella
	Tick exposure—tick-borne disease testing
	Animal bite or bat exposure—rabies
	Swimming in fresh water or use of nasal irrigation — *Naegleria fowleri*

Data from Venkatesan A, Tunkel AR, Bloch KC, Lauring AS, Sejvar J, Bitnun A, et al. Case definitions, diagnostic algorithms, and priorities in encephalitis: consensus statement of the International Encephalitis Consortium. *Clin Infect Dis.* 2013;57(8):1114–1128.

- Supportive treatment including hemodynamic and respiratory support may be needed. Admission to the intensive care unit is often indicated for close monitoring
- Role of steroids is controversial
  - In a metaanalysis performed, use of dexamethasone may help reduce hearing loss as a result of Hib-associated meningitis, but its use in other causes of bacterial meningitis remains highly controversial
- Chemoprophylaxis is indicated for close contacts for those exposed to meningococcal meningitis and may be indicated in specific cases for Hib meningitis. Rifampin, ciprofloxacin, or ceftriaxone is typically used

PROGNOSIS

- Mortality of meningitis ranges from 5% to 15%; this is influenced by multiple factors including the causative pathogen, patient risk factors, age of patient, and timing of antibiotic initiation
- Morbidity of bacterial meningitis includes hearing loss (in particular with meningococcal meningitis and Hib meningitis), cognitive and developmental disability, epilepsy, hydrocephalus, weakness, and endocrine dysfunction (diabetes insipidus [DI], hypothalamic dysfunction)

Reversible Posterior Leukoencephalopathy Syndrome (RPLS)

BASIC INFORMATION

- Also referred to as posterior reversible encephalopathy syndrome (PRES)
- Generally reversible and the posterior area, but there are cases where neither are true
- Pathogenesis is thought to be multifactorial and in part due to failure of cerebral regulation of the blood-brain barrier in the setting of hypertension and endothelial dysfunction with subsequent vasogenic edema

Table 56.6. Common CNS Bacterial Pathogens and Treatment by Age

Predisposing Factor	Common Bacterial Pathogen	Empiric Antibiotic Therapy
AGE		
<1 month	Group B streptococcus *Escherichia coli* *Listeria monocytogenes* *Klebsiella* species	Ampicillin plus cefotaxime or ampicillin plus gentamicin
1 to 3 months	Group B streptococcus Gram-negative bacilli° *Streptococcus pneumoniae* *Neisseria meningitides* *Listeria monocytogenes* *Haemophilus influenzae*	Third- or fourth-generation cephalosporin plus vancomycin
3 months to 3 years	*Streptococcus pneumoniae* *Neisseria meningitides* Group B streptococcus Gram-negative bacilli *Haemophilus influenzae*	Third- or fourth-generation cephalosporin plus vancomycin
3 to 10 years	*Streptococcus pneumoniae* *Neisseria meningitides* Other bacteria‡ Group B streptococcus	Third- or fourth-generation cephalosporin plus vancomycin
10 to 18 years	*Neisseria meningitides* *Streptococcus pneumoniae* Other bacteria‡ Group B streptococcus Gram-negative bacilli	Third- or fourth-generation cephalosporin plus vancomycin
HEAD TRAUMA		
Basilar skull fracture	*Streptococcus pneumoniae* *Haemophilus influenzae* Group A β-hemolytic streptococci	Third-generation cephalosporin plus vancomycin
Penetrating trauma	*Staphylococcus aureus* Coagulase-negative staphylococci (especially *Staphylococcus epidermidis*) Aerobic Gram-negative bacilli (including *Pseudomonas aeruginosa*)	Cefepime plus vancomycin or ceftazidime plus vancomycin or meropenem plus vancomycin
Postneurosurgery	Aerobic Gram-negative bacilli (including *Pseudomonas aeruginosa*) *Staphylococcus aureus* Coagulase-negative staphylococci (especially *Staphylococcus epidermidis*)	Cefepime plus vancomycin or ceftazidime plus vancomycin or meropenem plus vancomycin
Cerebrospinal fluid shunt	coagulase-negative staphylococci (especially *Staphylococcus epidermidis*) *Staphylococcus aureus* Aerobic Gram-negative bacilli (including *Pseudomonas aeruginosa*) *Propionibacterium acnes*	Cefepime plus vancomycin or ceftazidime plus vancomycin or meropenem plus vancomycin

°If there is high level of suspicion or evidence of Gram-negative bacilli, therapy should include a carbapenem plus gentamicin until the organism is identified.

‡Other bacteria = *Listeria monocytogenes*, group A streptococcus.

Data from McGuire JL, Greene AM. Central Nervous System Infections. In: Abend NS, Helfaer M, eds. *Pediatric Neurocritical Care.* New York: Demos; 2013; Tunkel AR, Hartman BJ, Kaplan SL, Kaufman BA, Roos KL, Scheld WM, Whitley RJ. Practice guidelines for the management of bacterial meningitis. *Clin Infect Dis.* 2004;39(9):1267–1284.

CLINICAL PRESENTATION

- Patients present with headaches, encephalopathy, visual disturbances, and/or seizures in setting of elevated blood pressure
  - Blood pressure may not be at "hypertensive emergency" criteria, but are generally increased above baseline.
- Provoking factor is typically a rapid increase in blood pressure, which may be due to a number of causes. Risk factors include:
  - Chemotherapy or cytotoxic drugs (tacrolimus is a common offending agent)
  - Kidney disease
  - Post organ transplantation
  - Autoimmune disease
  - Eclampsia

DIAGNOSIS AND EVALUATION

- Neurologic examination may reveal visual deficits such as hemianopia (field cut respecting vertical midline), visual neglect, or cortical blindness. Funduscopic examination can be normal or have presence of papilledema. Upper motor neuron signs such as hyperreflexia or presence of Babinski sign may be found
- Differential diagnosis based on clinical presentation can include stroke, ADEM, or encephalitis
- Neuroimaging is critical to making this diagnosis and ruling out others
  - Classic MRI findings are of symmetrical white matter changes in the posterior cerebral hemispheres
- EEG should be obtained if any concerns for seizures, clinical or subclinical

TREATMENT

- Hypertension should be urgently treated
- Treat underlying etiology (such as temporarily discontinuing any provoking medications or treating underlying disease)
- Antiepileptic agents are used to treat any symptomatic seizures

PROGNOSIS

- Generally favorable with full recovery, but there have been rare cases of significant morbidity and mortality as well as rare cases of recurrence

Acute Disseminated Encephalomyelitis (ADEM)

BASIC INFORMATION

- ADEM is an entity characterized by acute presentation of encephalopathy presumed to be due to a single demyelinating/autoinflammatory event
- Presentation may include several focal neurologic deficits, including motor deficits (e.g., hemiparesis), sensory deficits, brain stem dysfunction (e.g., oculomotor palsies, dysphagia, dysarthria), or ataxia. Seizures may be present
  - May present with or without a fever
  - May include other nonspecific symptoms (headache, vomiting, behavioral changes)
  - Cannot be due to an infection
  - LP findings may show lymphocytosis, but generally <100 WBC
- Common triggers are infections (classically a viral illness 1 to 8 weeks before neurologic symptoms) and, less commonly, immunizations
- Is associated with diffuse lesions seen on MRI, primarily in the cerebral white matter (but may include some gray matter as well)
- This typically occurs only once and is known as a monophasic illness
  - First-line therapy is steroids; IV immunoglobulin (IG) and plasmapheresis reserved for refractory cases
  - Confirmation that this is ADEM is retrospective after other causes have been ruled out
  - Diagnosis requires that no new clinical or MRI findings emerge 3 months or more after initial episode of ADEM
  - Complete recovery in 60% to 90% of cases
- An important differential diagnosis also includes the first presentation of pediatric multiple sclerosis (MS)
  - MS typically will not have presenting features of fever or encephalopathy
  - MS can have multiple episodes of symptoms, whereas ADEM is a single episode by definition
  - Neuroimaging for MS tends have more discrete white matter changes and will not involve gray or deep brain matter as it can for ADEM

Anti-NMDA Receptor Encephalitis

BASIC INFORMATION

- An autoimmune syndrome that can present acutely or subacutely with a wide range of symptoms including neuropsychiatric, catatonia, encephalopathy, refractory epilepsy, autonomic instabilities, speech disorder, and movement disorder
- This is associated with the presence of anti-N-methyl-D-aspartate (NMDA) receptor antibodies in serum and CSF
- Eighty percent of the patients with NMDA receptor encephalitis are female

DIAGNOSIS AND EVALUATION

- Serum and CSF should be sent for presence of anti-NMDA receptor antibodies. The sensitivity of testing is approximately 15% higher from the CSF than from serum
- Evaluation should include neuroimaging, lumbar puncture, and EEG studies
  - A mild CSF pleocytosis and increased protein can be present. Oligoclonal bands can be seen

- MRI brain is normal half of the time. Note that mild, typically transient MRI changes can be seen in the other 50%
- EEG should be obtained because it is usually abnormal. In addition to presence of seizures, EEG can sometimes show a characteristic pattern known as "delta brush"
- Evaluation for an underlying neoplastic etiology should be sought (but anti-NMDA receptor encephalitis can occur without underlying tumor). Most commonly this is an ovarian teratoma in women

TREATMENT

- Symptomatic seizures should be appropriately managed with antiepileptic medications
- First-line acute immunotherapy is usually IV steroids combined with IVIG or plasmapheresis
- Immunosuppressants such as rituximab are used to treat this disorder. Note that treatment should not be held pending confirmation of anti-NMDA receptor antibodies
- Any underlying neoplasm should be treated

PROGNOSIS

- Most have a good recovery, but this can be prolonged over 1 to 2 years. The rest can have severe disability. Estimated mortality is at 4%
- There is a risk of reoccurrence requiring further immunotherapy

Brain Death or Irreversible Cessation of All Brain Function

BASIC INFORMATION

- Must meet specific criteria established by the American Academy of Neurology, but actual practices can be institution dependent
- Institutional policy can differ for required observation period before performing the neurologic examination, the duration between examinations, and the role of addition of ancillary studies for children less than 1 year of age
- In addition, neurologic examination after an acute presentation concerning for irreversible cessation of brain function such as cardiac arrest or severe brain injuries is generally deferred for at least 24 hours

DIAGNOSIS AND EVALUATION

Note that all criteria must be met
- There must be an identified cause of irreversible cessation of all brain function
- No confounding factors for the neurologic examination can be present. This specifically includes:
  - Patient hypothermia
  - Sedation of the patient due to sedation medications or antiepileptic medications medications that are above the usual therapeutic range
  - Pharmacologic neuromuscular blockade
  - Injuries to the patient's face or eyes that preclude elements of the physical examination, as outlined later
  - Significant hypotension in the patient as judged by the attending physician (reference values for blood pressure vary by patient age and clinical circumstances)
  - Significant electrolyte, acid-base, or endocrine disturbances as judged by the attending physician
- Physical examination must be consistent with coma and cessation of higher cortical and brain stem functions
  - Patient must be in a coma—complete unconsciousness, no vocalization or volitional activity
  - Determine absence of brain stem reflexes
    - Pupils unreactive to light in the absence of drugs influencing pupillary activity
    - No spontaneous or induced (oculocephalic, oculovestibular) eye movements
    - No bulbar (facial or oral pharyngeal) muscle movement
    - Absence of the following reflexes: corneal, gag, cough, sucking, rooting
  - Flaccidity, with no spontaneous movements during any part of this examination; excluding reflex withdrawal or spinal myoclonus
    - If there is any question of abnormal movements, neurology should be consulted or ancillary studies should be considered
  - Apnea test
    - Generally performed after the second neurologic examination
    - Patient must have complete absence of documented respiratory effort by formal apnea testing demonstrating a $PaCO_2$ >60 mm Hg and >20 mm Hg increase above baseline
- Role of ancillary testing
  - Not indicated if patient fulfills previous criteria for irreversible cessation of brain function
  - Indications:
    1. If any of the previously described components cannot be performed (such as facial injury precluding cranial nerve examination) or if the apnea test cannot be performed safely
    2. If the neurologic examination is inconsistent or cannot exclude abnormal movements as spinal reflexes
    3. If one is unable to exclude pharmacologic confounding factors
    4. To reduce interexamination period
  - Types:
    - EEG: this is usually done via a protocol that is more sensitive to cerebral electrical activity than routine EEGs. Finding consistent with irreversible cessation of brain function would be complete electrocerebral silence
    - Cerebral blood flow: cerebral blood flow demonstrating no flow through the cerebral arteries would be consistent with brain death

Table 56.7. Indications for Neuroimaging in a Child With Headaches

- Abnormal neurologic examination or the development of focal symptoms/signs during a headache or aura (except classic visual symptoms of migriane).
- Seizures
- An acute secondary headache (i.e., headache with known underlying illness or insult)
- Headache in children younger than 6 years old or in any child who cannot adequately describe his or her headache
- Headache worst on first awakening or that awakens the child from sleep
- Migrainous headache in the child with no family history of migraine or its equivalent

PEDIATRIC HEADACHE

- Pediatric headaches are a common complaint but may still be underrecognized in the young. When undiagnosed or not properly managed, headaches can cause significant disability
- The first step is determining whether the headache is a primary headache (such as a migraine or tension headache) or a secondary headache (secondary to a specific organic cause)
  - Some secondary causes are especially important to consider and will require urgent, or even emergent, imaging. These "red flags" are listed in Table 56.7
- A thorough neurologic examination should be performed, including looking closely at the vital signs, obtaining head circumference, and performing a funduscopic examination
  - If there is an abnormal neurologic examination present such as focal weakness or papilledema, the child should be referred urgently for evaluation
- Imaging
  - MRI is generally the imaging of choice because it provides superior detail and better images of the posterior fossa
  - Head CT is generally reserved for any acute-onset headaches in which increased intracranial pressure and/or intracranial bleeding is suspected (e.g., subarachnoid hemorrhage/aneurysm)
- Secondary causes of headache are broad and complex (Tables 56.8 and 56.9)
- Here we will provide a review of primary headaches (guidelines for diagnoses per the International Headache Society, third edition) and some of the common secondary causes of pediatric headaches
- See also Nelson Textbook of Pediatrics, Chapter 595, "Headaches."

Migraines

BASIC INFORMATION

- Most common type of primary headache in the pediatric population

Table 56.8. Secondary Causes of Headaches

Systemic Diseases With Headaches	Neurologic Diseases With Headaches
INFECTIOUS	**INFECTIOUS**
Viral infection	Meningitis/encephalitis
Sinusitis	Intracranial abscess
HIV infection	Ventriculoperitoneal shunt infection
METABOLIC	Lyme disease
Hypoxia/hypercapnia	**DISORDERS WITH FOCAL SYMPTOMS OR SIGNS**
Hypothyroidism	
Hypoglycemia/fasting	Seizure
Hyperglycemia/diabetic ketoacidosis	Ischemic stroke
Rheumatologic disease	Intracranial hemorrhage
Systemic lupus erythematosus	Carotid or vertebral artery dissection
Kawasaki	Migraines
Rheumatoid arthritis	ADEM
Behçet disease	**DISORDERS WITH SYMPTOMS OF INCREASED INTRACRANIAL PRESSURE**
Sarcoidosis	
Polyarteritis nodosa	
CNS vasculitis	Brain tumor
OTHER	Idiopathic intracranial hypertension
	Cerebral venous sinus thrombosis
Pregnancy	Cerebral cysts (e.g., pineal, colloid, arachnoid)
Drug-induced headache	
Hypertension	

Data from McGuire JL, Greene AM. Central Nervous System Infections. In: Abend NS, Helfaer M, eds. *Pediatric Neurocritical Care*. New York: Demos; 2013.

Table 56.9. Classic Descriptions of Pain in Select Secondary Causes of Headaches

OCCIPITAL LOCATION
Cervicogenic
Arnold-Chiari malformation
Brain tumor
Vertebral artery dissection

PRECIPITATED BY VALSALVA/WORSE WHEN LYING DOWN
Arnold-Chiari malformation
All causes of increased cerebrospinal fluid pressure

WORSE WHEN UPRIGHT
Intracranial hypotension (e.g., cerebrospinal fluid leak)
Postural orthostatic tachycardia syndrome
Migraine

SUDDEN ONSET
Intracranial hemorrhage
Cerebral venous sinus thrombosis
Ischemic stroke
Cervical artery dissection
Colloid cyst
Spontaneous intracranial hypotension
Sinusitis
Meningitis/encephalitis

Data from McGuire JL, Greene AM. Central Nervous System Infections. In: Abend NS, Helfaer M, eds. *Pediatric Neurocritical Care*. New York: Demos; 2013.

CLINICAL PRESENTATION

- History of at least five episodes
- Pain lasts from 2 to 72 hours (either not treated or not successfully treated)
- Have at least two of the following features:

- Location: can be bilateral in children (as opposed to unilateral in adults) that generally transitions to a unilateral characteristic closer to adulthood
- Quality: pulsating or throbbing
- Severity: moderate to severe intensity
- Aggravated by routine physical activity
- Includes one of the associated features during headache:
  - Nausea and/or vomiting
  - Photophobia—note that this can be inferred by observation if the child prefers to lie in a dark room after onset of headache
  - Phonophobia
- If associated with aura, please see separate section on migraine with aura (later)

DIAGNOSIS AND EVALUATION

- History
  - Obtain standard clinical history with onset of symptoms, frequency and duration, associated symptoms and signs, alleviating and aggravating factors, response to treatment, and associated disability
  - Pediatric Quality of Life Inventory (PedsQL) and Pediatric Migraine Disability Assessment (PedMIDAS) are clinical tools used to assess disability
- General physical and neurologic examination should be normal
- Testing
  - No further testing is indicated if the history is consistent with primary headache and the neurologic examination is normal

TREATMENT

- Healthy habits or headache hygiene
  - Optimization of sleep, hydration, exercise, appropriate diet, and stress management
  - Avoidance of any identified triggers
  - Counsel on avoiding medication overuse headache
  - Counsel on treating headache at onset of headache
- Acute treatments
  - Outpatient abortive treatments
    - Nonsteroidal antiinflammatory drugs (NSAIDs) have demonstrated efficacy over acetaminophen and placebo
      - Avoid aspirin in pediatric population
    - Triptans are commonly used in acute treatment of migraines
      - Contraindicated in patients with cardiovascular disease
      - Avoid in patients with hemiplegic migraine
      - Side effects: worsened headache, flushing, nausea, chest pain, dizziness, fatigue
      - There are now four triptans approved for the pediatric population: almotriptan, sumatriptan/naproxen, zolmitriptan nasal spray, rizatriptan
- Antinausea medications: metoclopramide, promethazine, ondansetron
- If refractory to treatment described previously, consider referral to emergency department for further evaluation and IV medication treatment. This typically includes fluid optimization and an IV NSAID in combination with an IV antiemetic (such as IV metoclopramide or Compazine). Neurologic team consult and inpatient admission as indicated
- Preventative treatments
  - If headaches are consistently occurring more than once a week or if headaches have significant associated disability may consider ongoing headache therapies include cyproheptadine, amitriptyline, topiramate, propranlol, behavioral interventions (e.g. cognitive behavioral therapy) and/or nutraceuticals (Vitamin B2, magnesium). Neurology outpatient follow-up is recommended to manage these regimens.

Migraines with Aura

BASIC INFORMATION

- Up to 20% of children with migraines can have auras
- The most common aura is a change in vision.
  - "Positive" phenomena include the appearance of wavy lines or zig-zags.
  - "Negative" phenomena can be blurry vision or scotoma.
- The second most common auras are sensory changes (e.g. paresthesias, numbness).
- Auras can also involve difficulty speaking or brain stem symptoms (e.g. dizziness, diplopia).
- Migraine with any associated negative symptoms (e.g. sensory deficit, brain stem dysfunction) is a diagnosis of exclusion; other acute causes such as basilar stroke should be ruled out first
  - An entity called *confusional migraine* is a controversial diagnosis of exclusion after appropriate workup for stroke, seizure, toxic-metabolic, and other causes have been evaluated. Patients may present with higher cortical dysfunction, including speech difficulties, disorientation, agitation, or amnesia
  - If the aura involves motor weakness, this may be a hemiplegic migraine but other causes should be excluded first. Please see separate section on this (later)

CLINICAL PRESENTATION

- Meets criteria for migraine
- There can be more than one aura present concurrently
- Aura must resolve spontaneously and not last more than 60 minutes
- Aura should precede headache by window of less than 60 minutes (note that aura can start with timing of headache)

DIAGNOSIS AND EVALUATION

- Testing: to meet criteria for migraine with aura, other causes of secondary headache should first be ruled out
  - MRI brain: unlike migraines without aura, there is generally a low threshold for obtaining urgent neuroimaging, particularly if this is a headache accompanied by presence of negative symptoms such as weakness, sensory deficits, or brain stem symptoms
  - Lumbar puncture may be indicated depending on clinical presentation

TREATMENT

- Acute and preventative treatments are similar to those for migraines without aura
  - Exception: triptans should be avoided in patients with hemiplegic migraines due to theoretical risk of ischemia
- WHO recommends that women with migraine with aura avoid combination contraceptive use because it can increase risk of ischemic stroke

Hemiplegic Migraine

BASIC INFORMATION

- Must rule out other causes of migraine associated with weakness with appropriate investigations
- Divided into sporadic hemiplegic migraine (SHM) or familial hemiplegic migraine (FHM) with similar criteria, with the latter including one first-degree relative with identical attacks
- Patients present with not only motor weakness but also with other sensory, language, or visual changes concurrently preceding their headaches. During episodes, they may have motor deficits, Babinski sign, and unilateral hyperreflexia.
- Hemiplegic migraine is a diagnosis of exclusion after other causes have been ruled out in the acute presentation period
- Physical examination is usually normal between episodes.
- MRI brain, often done to rule out arterial ischemic stroke, is often normal but may have subtle findings beyond the scope of this review.
- Lumbar puncture is indicated if patient has altered mental status. Mildly elevated WBC in CSF can be seen in cases of hemiplegic migraine
- EEG is sometimes indicated if patient has altered mental status with this, which can show diffuse slowing in affected cerebral hemisphere
- Send the hemiplegic migraine genetic panel for further testing. Most commonly, this is in a calcium-channel, CACNA1A, mutation but can be seen in other genes such as *ATP1A2*, *SCN1A*, or *PRRT2*
- Treatment may involve acetazolamide for acute attacks. Beta blockers and triptans are avoided due ot theoretical risk of stroke.

Tension Headache

BASIC INFORMATION

- Incidence is less well defined in the pediatric population
- Can overlap with migraine

CLINICAL PRESENTATION

- At least 10 attacks over a month
- Pain lasts from 30 minutes to 7 days
- Have at least two of the following features:
  - Location: bilateral
  - Quality: pressing or tightening (not pulsatile)
  - Severity: mild to moderate
  - Not aggravated by routine physical activity
- Is not associated with:
  - Nausea and/or vomiting
  - No more than one of either photophobia or phonophobia
- Note that this phenotype can overlap with migraine and give a mixed type of headache

DIAGNOSIS AND EVALUATION

- History
  - Exclude secondary causes of headache
  - Obtain standard clinical history with onset of symptoms, frequency and duration, associated symptoms and signs, alleviating and aggravating factors, response to treatment, and associated disability
- Neurologic examination should be normal. Patients may have tenderness at sites of greater and lesser occipital nerves located in the posterior cranium
- Testing
  - Not indicated if history is consistent with tension headaches and patient's neurologic examination is normal

TREATMENT

- Generally acute treatment is similar to that of migraine headaches
- Less evidence of preventative treatment for tension-type headaches
- Preventative treatments
  - Medication: clinical consensus favors amitriptyline
  - Behavioral interventions

Pseudotumor Cerebri

BASIC INFORMATION

- Incidence of 1/100,000 to 2/100,000 population; rare in children younger than 3 years
- Previously called *idiopathic intracranial hypertension* or *benign intracranial hypertension*, but this term has fallen out of favor because secondary causes are often found and it is not necessarily a benign condition due to the risk of irreversible visual loss
- Can be divided into primary or secondary pseudotumor cerebri (PTC)

CLINICAL PRESENTATION

- Obesity is a significant risk factor
- See Table 56.10 for secondary causes of PTC
- Symptoms of presentation are similar to those of increased intracranial pressure (throbbing headache, which can be associated with nausea/vomiting and worsens with Valsalva maneuvers)
  - Other symptoms include transient decreased vision, pulsatile tinnitus, flashes of light (photopsia), and double vision
  - If untreated, this can lead to irreversible vision loss

DIAGNOSIS AND EVALUATION

- Criteria for definitive diagnosis of PTC (Friedman et al., 2013):
  - Ophthalmologic examination revealing papilledema
    - In absence of papilledema, the diagnosis can be made if criteria described later are fulfilled and patient has presence of cranial nerve VI palsy
  - Normal neurologic examination (other than cranioneuropathies, most commonly cranial nerve VI palsy)
  - Normal neuroimaging, including MRI brain with and without gadolinium, and magnetic resonance venography (MRV)
  - Normal CSF composition
  - Elevated opening pressure on lumbar puncture (≥ 250 mm H_2O CSF in adults; ≥ 250 mm H_2O CSF in children who are not sedated and not obese, otherwise ≥ 280 mm H_2O CSF in children)
- Probable PTC diagnosis can be made if papilledema or cranial nerve VI palsy is not present if previous criteria are otherwise fulfilled and at least three of the neuroimaging criteria are found:
  - Empty sella
  - Flattening of the posterior aspect of the globe
  - Distention of the perioptic subarachnoid space with or without a tortuous optic nerve
  - Transverse venous sinus stenosis
- In addition, visual acuity and formal visual field should be assessed and serially followed.

TREATMENT

- Discontinue any provoking medications, if present; weight loss is considered one of the first line treatments
- Medications
  - Acetazolamide is first-line treatment
- Close ophthalmologic surveillance to follow visual acuity, visual field testing, and funduscopic examinations
- Temporizing measures, such as trial of corticosteroids and serial lumbar punctures, are used if there is visual loss with presentation as a bridge to more definitive treatment
- Indications for surgery are if symptoms are refractory to medications, if visual loss worsens, if visual fields decrease, or if intractable headache is present
  - Optic nerve fenestration
  - CSF shunt
- Treat headaches per their phenotypes
  - Avoid medication overuse

PROGNOSIS

- Can have permanent visual loss if not diagnosed and treated
  - Risk factors include higher-grade papilledema and presenting symptom of visual loss
- Reoccurrence of symptoms; weight gain may precede this

Table 56.10. Secondary Causes of Pseudotumor Cerebri

Cerebral venous anomalies	Cerebral venous sinus thrombosis Bilateral jugular vein thrombosis or surgical ligation Middle ear or mastoid infection Increased right heart pressure Superior vena cava syndrome Arteriovenous fistula Decreased cerebrospinal fluid absorption from previous intracranial infection or subarachnoid hemorrhage Hypercoagulable states
Medications and exposures	Antibiotics: tetracycline, minocycline, doxycycline, sulfa drugs Vitamin A and retinoids Hormones: human growth hormone, thyroxine, anabolic steroids, levonorgestrel Withdrawal from chronic corticosteroids Lithium
Medical conditions	Endocrine: Addison disease, hypoparathyroidism Hypercapnia: sleep apnea, Pickwickian syndrome Anemia Renal failure Turner syndrome Down syndrome

Data from Friedman DI, Liu GT, Digre KB. Revised diagnostic criteria for the pseudotumor cerebri syndrome in adults and children. *Neurology.* 2013;81(13):1159–1165.

Review Questions

For review questions, please go to ExpertConsult.com.

Suggested Readings

Anttila P. Tension-type headache in childhood and adolescence. *Lancet Neurol.* 2006;5(3):268–274.

Asghar S, Milesi-Halle A, Kaushik C, Glasier C, Sharp GB. Variable manifestations of familial hemiplegic migraine associated with reversible cerebral edema in children. *Pediatr Neurol.* 2012;47(3):201–204.

Avner JR. Altered states of consciousness. *Pediatr Rev.* 2006;27(9):331–338.

Blume HK. Pediatric headache: a review. *Pediatr Rev.* 2012;(12):33.

Curtain RP, Smith RL, Ovcaric M, Griffiths LR. Minor head trauma-induced sporadic hemiplegic migraine coma. *Pediatr Neurol.* 2006;34(4):329–332.

Dalmau J, Lancaster E, Martinez-Hernandez E, et al. Clinical experience and laboratory investigations in patients with anti-NMDAR encephalitis. *Lancet Neurol.* 2011;10(1):63–74.

Ducros A, Denier C, et al. The clinical spectrum of familial hemiplegic migraine associated with mutations in a neuronal calcium channel. *N Engl J Med.* 2001;345(1):17–24.

Friedman DI, Liu GT, Digre KB. Revised diagnostic criteria for the pseudotumor cerebri syndrome in adults and children. *Neurology.* 2013;81(13):1159–1165.

Friedman DI. Papilledema and idiopathic intracranial hypertension. *Continuum.* 2014;20(4):857–876.

Fugate JE, Rabinstein AA. Posterior reversible encephalopathy syndrome: clinical and radiological manifestations, pathophysiology, and outstanding questions. *Lancet Neurol.* 2015;14:914–925.

Fugate JE, Wijdicks EF. Brain death, vegetative state, and minimally conscious states. In: Daroff RB, Jankovic J, Mazziotta JC, Pomeroy SL, eds. *Bradley's Neurology in Clinical Practice.* 7th ed. Philadelphia: Elsevier; 2016;6:51–56.e1.

Hershey AD. Pediatric headache. *Continuum.* 2015;21(4):1132–1145. International Headache Society. Guidelines. Available at: http://www.ihs-headache.org/ichd-guidelines.

Krupp LB, Tardieu M, Amato MP, et al. International Pediatric Multiple Sclerosis Study Group criteria for pediatric multiple sclerosis and immune-mediated sclerosis and immune-mediated central nervous system demyelinating disorders: revisions to the 2007 definitions. *Mult Scler J*. 2013;19(10):1261–1267.

Lewis DW. Headaches in children and adolescents. *Am Fam Physician*. 2002;65(4):625–633.

Mann K, Jackson MA. Meningitis. *Pediatr Rev*. 2008;29(12):417–429.

McGuire JL, Greene AM. Central nervous system infections. In: Abend NS, Helfaer M, eds. *Pediatric Neurocritical Care*. New York: Demos; 2013: 267–336.

Nakagawa TA, Ashwal S, Mathur M, et al. Guidelines for the determination of brain death in infants and children: an update of the 1987 Task Force recommendations. *Crit Care Med*. 2011;39(9):2139–2155.

Powers SW, Coffey CS, Chamberlin LA, et al. Trial of amitriptyline, topiramate and placebo for pediatric migraine. *NEJM*. 2017;376:115–124.

Russell MB, Ducros A. Sporadic and familial hemiplegic migraine; pathophysiological mechanisms, clinical characteristics, diagnosis and management. *Lancet Neurol*. 2011;10(5):457–470.

Singhi PD, Singh SC, Newton C, Simon J. Central nervous system infections. In: Nichols DG, ed. *Rogers' Textbook of Pediatric Intensive Care*. 4th ed. Philadelphia: Lippincott Williams & Wilkins; 2008.

Swanson D. Meningitis. *Pediatr Rev*. 2015;36(12):514–524.

Tunkel AR, Glaser CA, Bloch KC, et al. The management of encephalitis: clinical practice guidelines by the Infectious Diseases Society of America. *Clin Infect Dis*. 2008;47(3):303–327.d.

Tunkel AR, Hartman BJ, Kaplan SL, et al. Practice guidelines for the management of bacterial meningitis. *Clin Infect Dis*. 2004;39(9):1267–1284.

Venkatesan A, Tunkel AR, Bloch KC, et al. Case definitions, diagnostic algorithms, and priorities in encephalitis: consensus statement of the International Encephalitis Consortium. *Clin Infect Dis*. 2013;57(8):1114–1128.

Wijdicks EF, Varelas PN, Gronseth GS, Greer DM. Evidence-based guideline update: determining brain death in adults: report of the Quality Standards Subcommittee of the American Academy of Neurology. *Neurology*. 2010;74(23):1911–1918.

57 *Seizures*

DOUGLAS M. SMITH, MD

Basic Information

- Definition (International League Against Epilepsy [ILAE], 2014)
  - Seizure: transient occurrence of signs and/or symptoms due to abnormal excessive or synchronous neuronal activity in the brain
  - Epilepsy: any one of the following:
    - At least two unprovoked (or reflex) seizures occurring >24 hours apart
    - One unprovoked (or reflex) seizure and a probability of further seizures similar to that of the general recurrence risk (at least 60%) after two unprovoked seizures, occurring over the next 10 years
    - Diagnosis of an epilepsy syndrome
- Epidemiology
  - Highest incidence rate is in neonates and in the elderly
  - Lifetime incidence rate is 3% to 4%
  - Overall prevalence in United States is around 1%
- See also Nelson Textbook of Pediatrics, Chapter 593, "Seizures in Childhood."

Clinical Presentation and Evaluation

- Appearance depends on generalized versus focal seizure, and from which part of the brain the focal seizure arises
  - See Table 57.1 for descriptions of common (but not all) seizure types
  - Movements may be *clonic* (rhythmic, typically medium-amplitude twitches), *tonic* (sustained stiffness, typically in an extensor position), *myoclonic* (lightning-like high- amplitude individual twitch), *atonic* (sudden loss of tone), or *tonic-clonic* (evolving from stiff to rhythmically twitching)
  - Generalized seizures occur simultaneously throughout brain
    - Do not start in one place and spread
    - Only some medications work for generalized epilepsy (Table 57.2)

SIMPLE FEBRILE SEIZURE

- Diagnostic criteria:
  - Occurs between ages 6 months and 6 years in *developmentally normal* children with no prior history of afebrile seizures
  - One seizure in 24 hours that lasts less than 15 minutes, with no focal features to either seizure or postictal state
  - Fever of at least 38°C within 24 hours of seizure
- If back to baseline, management is based on fever only

- Consider lumbar puncture (LP) if under 12 months of age; LP recommended if under 6 months of age or unvaccinated
- No need for imaging or electroencephalogram (EEG), unless any features are atypical of a simple febrile seizure
- Although a common recommendation, round-the-clock antipyretics will not prevent febrile seizures; the only effective prophylaxis is antiepileptic drugs (AEDs), but these are not recommended for simple febrile seizures
- Generally do not recommend home seizure abortive medications (e.g., Diastat)
- Higher risk of recurrence if younger age and lower temperature at onset
- Long-term small increase in lifetime risk of epilepsy over general population
  - No increased incidence of sudden infant death syndrome (SIDS)

COMPLEX FEBRILE SEIZURE

- Febrile seizures are considered "complex" if longer than 15 minutes, *any* focal features present (including one-sided postictal paralysis), more than one in 24 hours, or in a developmentally abnormal child
- One factor above—2.5% risk of ultimately being diagnosed with epilepsy
- Two to three factors—5% to 10% risk of ultimately being diagnosed with epilepsy
- Management varies—consult your neurologist

EPILEPSY SYNDROMES

- Typical patterns of seizure types, ages at presentation, and comorbidities that enable some degree of prediction as to the course of their epilepsy
- Most children with seizures or epilepsy will *not* have an identifiable epilepsy syndrome
- Benign Rolandic epilepsy
  - Officially called "self-limited childhood epilepsy with centrotemporal spikes"
  - Childhood onset (4 to 8 years of age)
  - Rolandic seizures (see Table 57.1) during sleep; typically no generalized tonic-clonic seizures (GTCs)
  - EEG with classic finding (centrotemporal spikes that are very active while asleep)
  - Treatment is optional, but typically carbamazepine or oxcarbazepine is used
  - Typically outgrown by age 16 years
- Juvenile myoclonic epilepsy
  - Juvenile onset (8 to 20 years of age)
  - Morning myoclonus, absence seizures, eventually GTCs

Table 57.1. Typical Appearance (or Semiology) of Common Seizures Based on Location and Type

FOCAL SEIZURES

(All of these below may evolve into a *secondarily generalized tonic-clonic seizure*, or the classic "grand mal")

Frontal lobe	Primary motor cortex	Classic "Jacksonian march" of clonic movements
	Supplementary motor	Contralateral tonic posturing with "figure of four"
	Frontal operculum ("Rolandic")	Hemifacial clonus with potential spread to arm or leg, typically from sleep; prominent postictal drooling
	Dorsolateral frontal	Involves Broca area → aphasia
	Orbitofrontal cortex	Classic behavioral arrest and staring ± automatisms, autonomic changes, and olfactory hallucinations
	Nocturnal frontal lobe	Complex motor movements, including pelvic thrusting and bicycling; arise from sleep and often mistaken for parasomnias
Temporal lobe	Mesial temporal/ hippocampal	Rising epigastric sensation, déjà vu, strong sense of fear; smell and taste hallucinations (especially burning)
	Neocortical temporal	Simple auditory or complex visual hallucinations, typically with secondary generalization
Neonatal		Tend to be one or more limbs with nonsuppressible clonus or tonic movements; typically secondary to acute process; typically do not have generalized tonic-clonic seizures
		May be very subtle—vital sign derangements, breathing changes, eye movements

GENERALIZED SEIZURES

Absence	Staring and unresponsiveness lasting 5 to 10 seconds; typically will have oral automatisms, hand movements, or eye fluttering. Rarely staring alone. Happens many times a day. Associated with 3-Hz spike and wave on electroencephalogram (EEG).
	Compared with complex partial seizures, absence seizures are much shorter (5–10 seconds versus 1–2 minutes), are much more frequent (dozens to hundreds of times per day versus daily to weekly), have no postictal period, and very rarely have urinary incontinence.
Atonic	Sudden loss of tone, typically falling forward. Often seen in Lennox-Gastaut syndrome and myoclonic-astatic epilepsy of Doose.
Generalized tonic-clonic seizure	Typically no aura, followed by generalized stiffening and an "ictal cry," followed by generalized rhythmic clonic movements. Gradually these movements evolve to become higher amplitude and lower frequency.
Myoclonic	Brief, lightning-like movement. Classically part of juvenile myoclonic epilepsy that occurs early in the morning. Myoclonus is not always epileptic in origin (e.g., benign nocturnal myoclonus).
Epileptic (or infantile) spasm	Clusters of rapid bilateral upper-extremity extension or flexion with head drop. Each spasm lasts about a second with 5 to 10 seconds between spasms in a cluster. Associated with hypsarrhythmia on EEG and West syndrome.
Tonic seizure	Generalized stiffening, often occurring at night, typically lasting 5 to 10 seconds. Characteristic of Lennox-Gastaut syndrome, but not exclusive.

Table 57.2. Common Anticonvulsants, Treatment Indications, and Side Effects

Anticonvulsant	Indication	Side Effects and Notes
Adrenocorticotropic hormone (ACTH)	West syndrome	Hypertension, hyperglycemia, gastric ulcers, insomnia, irritability, immune suppression
Clonazepam (Klonopin)	All epilepsy types	Somnolence, irritability, ataxia, withdrawal seizures
Ethosuximide (Zarontin)	Absence seizures	Nausea and vomiting
Lacosamide (Vimpat)	Focal epilepsy; can be given intravenously (IV)	Dizziness, tremor, diplopia, **PR interval prolongation**
Lamotrigine (Lamictal)	Generalized epilepsy Absence seizures Focal epilepsy Safe in pregnancy	**Stevens-Johnson syndrome**, tremor, ataxia, insomnia Also effective for bipolar disorder and migraines May worsen myoclonic seizures
Levetiracetam (Keppra)	All epilepsy types Safe in pregnancy Can be given IV	Behavior changes/**aggression** Pyridoxine (vitamin B$_6$) may help behavioral side effect
Oxcarbazepine (Trileptal)	Focal epilepsy only	Somnolence, dizziness, diplopia, **hyponatremia,** leukopenia
Phenobarbital	Neonatal seizures All epilepsy types Can be given IV	Sedation, cognitive changes, behavior changes, irritability Strong P450 enzyme inducer, induces own metabolism
Phenytoin/ fosphenytoin (Dilantin/Cerebyx)	Mostly used in severe focal epilepsy Severe neonatal epilepsy Can be given IV	Stevens-Johnson syndrome, ataxia, **cerebellar degeneration, gingival hyperplasia,** dysarthria Phenytoin is highly toxic if extravasates when given IV (causes **purple glove syndrome**), which is why fosphenytoin is often used

Table 57.2.   Common Anticonvulsants, Treatment Indications, and Side Effects—cont'd

Anticonvulsant	Indication	Side Effects and Notes
Topiramate (Topamax)	All epilepsy types Third-line West syndrome	Word-finding difficulties, weight loss, anhidrosis, **kidney stones,** fatigue, **metabolic acidosis,** limb and perioral paresthesias
Valproic acid (Depakote)	All epilepsy types Absence seizures Can be given IV	Tremor, weight gain, lethargy, alopecia, nausea/vomiting, **hyperammonemia** (with or without transaminitis), decreases carnitine levels, **hepatotoxicity** (if under 2 years), pancreatitis, neutropenia, **polycystic ovarian syndrome** Contraindicated in liver failure, mitochondrial disease, and pregnancy
Vigabatrin (Sabril)	West syndrome Severe focal epilepsy	**Irreversible visual field deficit** (controversial), sedation, diplopia, ataxia
Zonisamide (Zonegran)	All epilepsy types	Same side effects as topiramate, only less frequent

- EEG with 4-Hz generalized spike and polyspike and wave, photosensitivity
- Treat with broad-spectrum drugs (levetiracetam, valproic acid)
- Typically lifelong
- West syndrome
  - Combination of infantile spasms, hypsarrhythmia on EEG, and developmental regression
  - Considered an "epileptic encephalopathy" with many causes
    - Down syndrome, tuberous sclerosis (TS), hypoxic-ischemic encephalopathy (HIE)
    - Peak incidence is 4 to 6 months of age
  - Classified as *cryptogenic* or *symptomatic*, which largely determines treatment
    - Cryptogenic spasms: normal preceding development, no abnormalities on metabolic screening or imaging
    - Symptomatic spasms: if abnormalities of above
  - Left untreated, 75% will develop intellectual disability and 50% will have lifelong epilepsy
    - Improved long-term outcomes if cryptogenic spasms are treated urgently (within 10 days)
  - Outcome improvements are less clear with symptomatic spasms
  - Treatment of symptomatic spasms is highly variable
  - Treat with adrenocorticotropic hormone (ACTH) or steroids
    - Use vigabatrin if caused by TS
- Childhood absence epilepsy
  - Childhood onset (ages 4 to 7 years)
  - Absence seizures only—may have dozens to hundreds of brief absence seizures per day
  - Normal development, normal cognition, normal examination
  - Classic 3-Hz generalized spike and wave pattern on EEG
  - Use ethosuximide, valproic acid, or lamotrigine
- Lennox-Gastaut syndrome
  - "Final common pathway" of a number of causes of epilepsy that results in severe, refractory, lifelong epilepsy
  - Associated with significant intellectual impairment
  - Multiple seizure types, usually daily
    - Tonic seizures while asleep; also myoclonic, atonic, and GTC seizures
  - Difficult to treat—clobazam, rufinamide, and cannabidiol (medical marijuana) are often used

Treatment

- In all cases, rule out provoked seizure—fingerstick glucose, screen electrolytes (including magnesium and phosphorus); consider lumbar puncture and brain imaging
- First afebrile seizure
  - Rule out provoked seizure foremost
  - If back to normal, management becomes establishing the risk of further unprovoked seizures (e.g., future risk of epilepsy)
  - If back to normal, emergent imaging likely is not necessary
  - Typical workup is magnetic resonance imaging (MRI) and EEG as outpatient (highly variable)
  - Typically do not start a medicine after first seizure unless it meets definition for epilepsy (defined previously)
- Status epilepticus
  - Definition
    - 5-minute GTC seizure
    - 10-minute complex partial or multiple seizures without returning to baseline
    - 10- to 15-minute absence status epilepticus
  - Treatment
    - First- and second-line: benzodiazepines
      Intravenous (IV) lorazepam 0.1 mg/kg (maximum 4 mg)
      Intramuscular (IM) or buccal midazolam 0.2 mg/kg (maximum 20 mg)
      PR diazepam 0.2 mg/kg (maximum 20 mg)
    - After benzodiazepines, phenytoin or fosphenytoin, valproic acid, or levetiracetam (choice depends on clinical scenario and local institution preferences)
  - Nonconvulsive status epilepticus (NCSE)
    - Typically presents with lack of return to baseline after convulsive seizures
    - Requires urgent EEG to diagnose
    - Treat with same medications as convulsive status epilepticus, with priority on avoiding endotracheal intubation if possible
- Neonatal seizures
  - Unlike most seizures, neonatal seizures tend to be symptomatic—need to rapidly establish a cause
    - Most often: HIE, infection
    - Also: intraventricular hemorrhage, stroke (recent or remote), hypoglycemia, hypocalcemia, metabolic disorders, and cerebral malformations

- Treat infection empirically while obtaining head imaging, LP, and metabolic screening
  - Seizures are very frequently subclinical—long-term EEG monitoring should be done if available
- Treatment: phenobarbital, levetiracetam, phenytoin
- Review of anticonvulsant medications (Table 57.2)
- Other treatment modalities
  - Ketogenic diet
    - High-fat, high-protein diet with almost no carbohydrates
    - Mechanism of efficacy is poorly understood
    - Avoid giving dextrose in fluids; avoid giving medicines in liquid form (almost always have sugar)
  - Vagus nerve stimulation (VNS)
    - "Pacemaker" in chest provides electrical stimulation to coil wrapped around vagus nerve
    - Mechanism of efficacy is poorly understood
    - Must be shut off before any magnetic resonance (MR) imaging
  - Responsive neurostimulation (RNS)
    - Implanted recording device detects focal seizures and administers "shock" when seizure is detected

Nonepileptic Events and Seizure Mimics

- Psychogenic
  - Typically affects teenagers; affects females more so than males
  - Frequently occurs in children who also have epileptic seizures
  - Longer than epileptic seizures (10 minutes or longer)
  - Partially responsive—flinch if pinched, dropped hand misses face
  - Asynchronous, high-amplitude movements and pelvic thrusting
  - Movements suddenly start and stop—no gradual resolution
  - Very brief or absent postictal phase
- Breath-holding spells
  - 6 months to 6 years
  - Sudden color change and loss of consciousness after painful stimulus or prolonged crying
- Syncope
  - Event preceded by tunnel vision and things sounding distant
  - Precipitated by hair traction, prolonged standing, sudden position change, high temperature, and painful stimuli (including blood draws and vaccines)
  - May convulse briefly after loss of consciousness
  - Rapid return to baseline—usually
- Nocturnal myoclonus
  - Random high-amplitude movements shortly after falling asleep
  - Like "popcorn popping"

Review Questions

For review questions, please go to ExpertConsult.com.

58 *Weakness and Ataxia*

RACHEL GOTTLIEB-SMITH, MD

General Approach to Weakness

Weakness may result if any part of the motor system is affected, from the upper motor neuron (UMN) to the lower motor neuron (LMN) to the nerve to the muscle. More specifically, localizations of weakness include areas of the central nervous system (CNS): motor cortex (where the UMNs sit), corticobulbar and corticospinal tracts containing descending axons passing through the internal capsule and brainstem, corticospinal tracts descending into the spinal cord, and anterior horn cells in the spinal cord (the lower motor neurons). In the peripheral nervous system (PNS), localizations of weakness include the spinal nerve root, the plexus, the peripheral nerve, the neuromuscular junction, and the muscle itself. Patterns and distributions of weakness can help you differentiate which part of the motor pathway is affected (Tables 58.1 and 58.2). Once you have a localization in mind, you can further narrow your differential diagnosis by the time course of the weakness (acute versus subacute versus chronic).

See also Nelson Textbook of Pediatrics, Chapter 597, "Movement Disorders."

LOCALIZATION: BRAIN

Arterial Ischemic Stroke

- Usually presents with acute onset of unilateral face/arm or face/arm/leg weakness, often with associated aphasia or neglect
- See Chapter 60 for additional details

Cerebral Palsy (CP)

BASIC INFORMATION

- Definition
  - Heterogeneous group of disorders due to a static insult to the developing brain leading to abnormal tone, posture, and movement
  - The disorder is not progressive, but the clinical manifestations may change over time as the child develops
- Causes (not just birth trauma)
  - Prematurity
    - Often associated with periventricular leukomalacia (PVL) or intraventricular hemorrhage
    - Perinatal infection is the most common risk factor for premature neonates developing CP
  - Perinatal hypoxic ischemic injury

- Prenatal/perinatal stroke
- Structural brain malformations (may be due to genetics, teratogens, or intrauterine infections)

CLINICAL PRESENTATION

- Types of CP
  - Spastic: most common (over half of cases); presents with UMN signs, contractures
    - Spastic hemiplegia
      - One side of the body is affected, typically an arm more so than a leg
      - Often due to prenatal/perinatal stroke
    - Spastic diplegia
      - Bilateral legs more affected than arms
      - Often associated with PVL
    - Spastic quadriplegia
      - All limbs affected
  - Dyskinetic: involuntary movements; think hypoxic/ischemic injury to basal ganglia
    - Choreoathetotic CP
      - Chorea: dance-like movements
      - Athetosis: writhing movements
      - May also be caused by kernicterus (high bilirubin leading to brain dysfunction)
    - Dystonic CP
      - Abnormal posturing
  - Ataxic CP: uncoordinated/clumsy, slow/jerky speech
- Associated conditions
  - Intellectual disability in 50% of patients
  - Other associated conditions: epilepsy, vision and hearing problems, speech disorders, orthopedic problems

EVALUATION

- Magnetic resonance imaging (MRI) brain: may see evidence of prior stroke, hypoxic ischemic injury, PVL, or cortical malformations
- May consider additional metabolic/genetic testing

Table 58.1. Upper Motor Neuron Versus Lower Motor Neuron Findings

	Lesion Location	
	Upper Motor Neuron	*Lower Motor Neuron*
Abnormal movements	None	Fasciculations
Muscle tone	↓ initially, then ↑	↓
Muscle bulk	Normal or ↓	↓
Strength	↓	↓
Deep tendon reflexes	↓ initially, then ↑	↓

Table 58.2. Additional Localization Clues

Lesion Location	UMN vs LMN	Typical Pattern of Weakness	Additional Clues
Brain (motor cortex or internal capsule)	UMN	Often unilateral (on the contralateral side)—typically face/arm or face/arm/leg	If cortical—may have other cortical signs (e.g., left brain: aphasia, right brain: neglect)
Brainstem	UMN	Crossed findings: ipsilateral face, contralateral arm/leg	The "d" symptoms: diplopia, dysarthria, dysphagia, dysphonia
Spinal cord (corticospinal tract)	UMN	Often bilateral arm and/or leg weakness, spares the face	May have associated sphincter dysfunction—bowel/bladder incontinence, often with associated sensory level
Spinal cord (anterior horn cell)	LMN	Often bilateral arm and/or leg weakness, spares the face	Typically no sensory changes
Nerve root/plexus/peripheral nerve	LMN	May see unilateral arm or leg weakness in a particular root/plexus/nerve distribution; many peripheral nerve processes (neuropathies) involve distal, symmetric weakness	Typically involves sensory changes in same distribution; nerve root lesions (radiculopathies) are often painful
Neuromuscular junction	N/A	Bilateral proximal, fatigable weakness	May also involve bulbar symptoms (dysarthria, dysphagia) and respiratory insufficiency, no sensory changes
Muscle	N/A	Bilateral proximal weakness	No sensory changes, high creatine kinase

LMN, Lower motor neuron; *UMN*, upper motor neuron.

TREATMENT

- Supportive: focus on maximizing communication, mobility, social/emotional development
- Physical and occupational therapy ± speech therapy
- Orthopedic: serial casting, muscle-tendon surgery
- For spasticity: botox, oral antispasmodics (e.g., baclofen, benzodiazepines), intrathecal baclofen

LOCALIZATION: SPINAL CORD

Transverse Myelitis

BASIC INFORMATION

- Neuroinflammatory problem of the spinal cord with rapid onset of weakness, sensory changes, and bowel or bladder dysfunction
- Causes
  - Postinfectious (e.g., West Nile virus, herpes viruses, HIV, Lyme disease, Mycoplasma, and syphilis)
  - CNS demyelinating disorder: multiple sclerosis (MS), neuromyelitis optica, acute disseminated encephalomyelitis
  - Associated with systemic autoimmune diseases (e.g., systemic lupus erythematosus, Sjögren syndrome, sarcoidosis)
  - Idiopathic

CLINICAL PRESENTATION

- Rapidly progressing bilateral weakness over hours to days—will typically involve legs and sometimes arms (if C-spine is involved)
- Most patients will have a sensory level
- Bowel/bladder dysfunction (often retention)
- UMN signs (Table 58.3): initially low tone and deep tendon reflexes (DTRs) that progress to increased tone and hyperreflexia

- If in C-spine may have respiratory arrest (remember, "C3-4-5 keep the diaphragm alive!")

INITIAL EVALUATION

- MRI with contrast of the spinal cord: look for inflammatory spinal cord lesion not due to compression, vascular process, nutritional deficiency, or neoplasm
- Also get an MRI with contrast of the brain to look for lesions suggestive of MS
- Cerebrospinal fluid (CSF) studies: lymphocytosis with elevated protein

TREATMENT

- Intravenous (IV) glucocorticoids, typically for 3 to 5 days

PROGNOSIS

- Usually at least partial recovery; may take months to years

Spinal Muscular Atrophy (SMA)

BASIC INFORMATION

- Cause: degeneration of the anterior horn cells (LMNs) of the spinal cord and motor nuclei (also LMNs) of the brainstem, resulting in symmetric flaccid weakness

CLINICAL PRESENTATION

- Diffuse symmetric weakness that is more proximal than distal and is typically more prominent in the lower limbs
- Restrictive, progressive respiratory insufficiency
- LMN signs: reduced muscle bulk, low tone, fasciculations (including tongue fasciculations), minimal to absent DTRs

Table 58.3.   Review

Diagnosis	Age of Onset	Pattern of Deficits	Buzz Words/Differentiating Features
Arterial ischemic stroke	Any age; in children most common in neonates	Acute onset of unilateral face/arm or face/arm/leg weakness ± cortical signs	*Acute* onset; unilateral
Cerebral palsy	Pre- or perinatal insult—present at birth, usually noted by age 2	Different forms: spastic vs dyskinetic vs ataxic, *not* progressive	Prematurity, kernicterus
Transverse myelitis	Any age; typically school age and older	Rapid onset of weakness, sensory changes, and bowel or bladder dysfunction over hours to days	Bilateral; bowel or bladder involvement; may be part of acute disseminated encephalomyelitis, neuromyelitis optica, or multiple sclerosis
Spinal muscular atrophy	Depends on type; type 1 is most common and presents in infancy	Diffuse symmetric weakness, proximal more than distal	Tongue fasciculations; minimal to absent DTRs; die from respiratory insufficiency
Acute flaccid myelitis	Any age	Rapid onset of focal limb weakness progressing over hours to days	Enterovirus D-68
Neonatal brachial plexopathy	Neonates	Unilateral arm weakness	Shoulder dystocia
Guillain-Barré syndrome	Any age	Progressive, symmetric ascending weakness with loss of DTRs	Absent DTRs; albuminocytologic dissociation; increased F wave latency on NCS
Tick paralysis	Any age	Lethargy and weakness → acute ataxia → ascending flaccid paralysis	Look for the tick
Charcot-Marie-Tooth disease	Often does not present until later in childhood	Slowly progressive, symmetric distal weakness with loss of distal sensation; lose distal DTRs	Hereditary; *PMP22*; autosomal dominant
Myasthenia gravis	Any age; typically school age and older	Fluctuating, fatigable weakness in proximal limb, neck, ocular (ptosis, ophthalmoplegia), bulbar, and respiratory muscles	Fatigable, fluctuating; Tensilon test; acetylcholine receptor antibody
Congenital myasthenic syndromes	Birth or early childhood	Fatigable weakness mainly affecting the ocular and bulbar muscles	Genetic defect
Transient neonatal myasthenia gravis	Neonates	Generalized weakness and hypotonia at birth with intact DTRs	Mother with myasthenia gravis; eye involvement less common
Infant botulism	2 to 8 months	Constipation → progressive hypotonia and weakness (may be descending) + cranial nerve dysfunction (including impaired pupillary response)	Honey, construction sites
Duchenne muscular dystrophy	2 to 3 years	Progressive proximal > distal weakness	Elevated creatine kinase; Gowers sign; X-linked; dystrophin mutation (disrupts reading frame); calf pseudohypertrophy; cardiomyopathy
Becker muscular dystrophy	Later presentation than DMD (preschool age and later)	Progressive proximal > distal weakness	Same as DMD except mutation doesn't disrupt reading frame; often ambulate until age 15+
Myotonic dystrophy	Depends on type; congenital = neonatal vs childhood vs classic = adult	Skeletal and respiratory muscle weakness, *myotonia*	Myotonia; trinucleotide repeat expansion; autosomal dominant; cataracts; cardiac arrhythmias
Acute cerebellar ataxia	Typically <6 years	Ataxia develops over hours to days after prodromal illness	Full recovery
Ataxia telangiectasia	2 to 3 years	Progressive ataxia	Cancer; elevated AFP; immunodeficiency
Friedreich ataxia	Adolescence	Progressive ataxia and sensory loss with eventual loss of DTRs	Posterior columns; hypertrophic cardiomyopathy; diabetes mellitus

AFP, Alpha fetoprotein; *DMD*, Duchenne muscular dystrophy; *DTR*, deep tendon reflex; *NCS*, nerve conduction studies.

- Types are classified by severity
  - SMA type 1: Werdnig-Hoffman disease—most severe, neonatal onset
    - Decreased fetal movement in utero
    - Weak cry, poor suck and swallow, aspiration, and tongue fasciculations
    - Typically have alert expression and normal eye movements
    - Majority die before 1 year from respiratory insufficiency
- SMA type 2: "sitters"
  - Able to sit without support when placed into seated position
- SMA type 3: "walkers"
  - Begins after child has started walking
  - Typically survive into adulthood and walk until 30s to 40s
- SMA type 4: adult onset

EVALUATION

- Electrodiagnostic studies (electromyography [EMG] and nerve conduction studies [NCS]) ± muscle biopsy
- Genetics: mutation in *SMN1* gene

TREATMENT

- Supportive: respiratory, nutrition, physical therapy, spinal bracing
- A biologic agent known as nusinersen that increases the level of SMN protein is now available!

Acute Flaccid Myelitis

BASIC INFORMATION

- Recent condition (recognized in 2014) of unknown etiology, but suspected to be caused by enterovirus D-68 (related to polio)
- Affects anterior horn cells (as in SMA and polio)

CLINICAL PRESENTATION

- Acute onset of focal limb weakness progressing over hours to days
  - Typically after respiratory illness 1 to 2 weeks prior
- Depending on level of spinal cord involved, may develop respiratory failure requiring mechanical ventilation
- Typically no altered mental status or seizures

EVALUATION

- MRI of the spinal cord: nonenhancing lesions largely restricted to the gray matter
- CSF studies: typically see a pleocytosis

TREATMENT

- Supportive
- Immunomodulatory therapies (steroids, intravenous immunoglobulin [IVIG], plasma exchange) have shown *no* benefit

PROGNOSIS

- Recovery is generally limited

LOCALIZATION: NERVE ROOT, PLEXUS, AND/OR PERIPHERAL NERVE

Neonatal Brachial Plexopathy

BASIC INFORMATION

- Cause: stretch of the shoulder during birth → stretch on the brachial plexus
- Major risk factor: shoulder dystocia

CLINICAL PRESENTATION

- Unilateral arm weakness presenting at birth
- Asymmetric Moro reflex
- C5 and C6 injury (+ sometimes C7) = Erb palsy
  - "Waiter's tip" posture: arm hangs by the side and is rotated medially; forearm is extended and pronated
- C8 and T1 injury: Klumpke palsy
  - Hand paralysis

EVALUATION

- If not classic: EMG/NCS, may consider C-spine imaging to look for proximal root avulsion

TREATMENT

- Observation and physical therapy initially—focus on range of motion
- If no functional recovery after 3 months: may consider surgical intervention

PROGNOSIS

- Most cases with spontaneous recovery within 1 to 3 months

Guillain-Barré Syndrome (GBS)

BASIC INFORMATION

- Acute paralyzing illness thought to be caused by an immune response against peripheral nerves leading to demyelination
- Triggering events
  - Infections, especially *Campylobacter jejuni*
  - Less commonly: immunizations (including influenza), surgery, trauma
- Polyradiculoneuropathy: multiple nerve roots and peripheral nerves are affected

CLINICAL PRESENTATION

- Classic GBS
  - Progressive, symmetric weakness that typically starts in the legs and ascends upward with loss of DTRs
  - Can cause severe respiratory muscle weakness requiring ventilatory support
  - Pain and paresthesias are common
  - Dysautonomia is also common
- Miller Fisher variant
  - Ophthalmoplegia with ataxia and areflexia
  - May or may not have weakness
  - Associated with GQ1b antibodies (ganglioside component of nerve)
- Timeline: typically progresses over 2 weeks

EVALUATION

- Clinical diagnosis: do not wait for tests to treat!
- CSF studies

- Albuminocytologic dissociation: elevated CSF protein with normal CSF white blood cell (WBC) count
- EMG/NCS
  - Show features of demyelination
  - Buzz word: "increased F wave latency"

TREATMENT

- Supportive care: respiratory support, treat autonomic dysfunction, pain control, rehabilitation
- Plasma exchange and IVIG hasten recovery
- Note: glucocorticoids are *not* effective for GBS

PROGNOSIS

- Recovery over weeks to months
- Most (up to 85%) eventually recover with minimal or no disability

Tick Paralysis

BASIC INFORMATION

- Caused by a neurotoxin released by a tick that has latched on
- In the United States, most commonly caused by Dermacentor ticks
  - Most cases occur April through June
  - Causes both decreased nerve conduction (localization: peripheral nerve) *and* presynaptic decrease in acetylcholine release (localization: neuromuscular junction)

CLINICAL PRESENTATION

- Typically starts with lethargy and weakness, followed by acute ataxia, progressing to ascending flaccid paralysis
- No sensory involvement

EVALUATION

- Look for the tick!
- CSF studies and neuroimaging will typically be normal

TREATMENT

- Remove the tick—patients typically recover within hours of removal

Charcot-Marie-Tooth (CMT) Disease

BASIC INFORMATION

- Hereditary neuropathy affecting both motor and sensory nerves
- Most common: type 1
  - Caused by *PMP22* gene duplication (PMP stands for "peripheral myelin protein")
  - Autosomal dominant inheritance

CLINICAL PRESENTATION

- Slowly progressive, symmetric distal weakness
  - Foot drop causing frequent tripping
- Atrophy of distal muscles
- Contractures of hands and feet due to weak distal muscles
  - Pes cavus: high-arched feet
  - Hammer toes
- Gradual loss of distal sensation

EVALUATION

- EMG/NCS

TREATMENT

- Supportive care: stretching, orthotics
- May require orthopedic foot surgery
- No disease-modifying treatment or gene therapy at this time

LOCALIZATION: NEUROMUSCULAR JUNCTION

Infant Botulism

BASIC INFORMATION

- Etiology
  - *Clostridium botulinum* colonizes the intestines → produces a neurotoxin that causes a neuromuscular blockade
- Risk factors
  - Living in areas where the spores can survive in the soil: Pennsylvania, Utah, California
    - Especially around construction sites
- Can also be foodborne: honey or canned foods

CLINICAL PRESENTATION

- Typical age range: 2 to 8 months
- Initial presentation: constipation and poor feeding
- Followed by progressive hypotonia and weakness (may be descending), as well as cranial nerve dysfunction
  - Ptosis, large pupils that do not constrict, ophthalmoparesis, diminished gag and suck
- Respiratory muscle weakness can lead to respiratory failure requiring ventilatory support

EVALUATION

- Clinical diagnosis: may proceed with treatment before confirmatory testing
- Stool testing for *C. botulinum* spores and the toxin (testing may be delayed due to constipation)
- May consider EMG/NCS

TREATMENT

- Botulism immune globulin (Baby BIG)
  - Administer as early as possible

- Reduces time spent in hospital and need for mechanical ventilation
- Supportive care: respiratory and feeding support

PROGNOSIS

- With supportive care, most patients make a full recovery, typically over months

Myasthenia Gravis

BASIC INFORMATION

- Cause: autoantibodies directed at acetylcholine receptors at the neuromuscular junction
- Associated with thymic hyperplasia or thymoma in some patients

CLINICAL PRESENTATION

- Fluctuating, fatigable weakness in proximal limb, neck, ocular, bulbar, and respiratory muscles
  - "Fatigable" weakness worsens with activity (e.g., by the end of the day) and improves with rest
    - Ocular symptoms
      - Ptosis
      - Binocular diplopia (double vision that goes away when the patient closes one eye)
  - Bulbar symptoms: dysarthria, dysphagia
  - Respiratory muscle weakness can lead to respiratory failure requiring ventilatory support ("myasthenic crisis")

EVALUATION

- Tensilon (Edrophonium) test
  - Tensilon: acetylcholinesterase inhibitor
  - Give Tensilon → positive test if immediate improvement in ptosis, ophthalmoparesis, or strength is observed
- Acetylcholine receptor antibody testing
- EMG/NCS
  - See decremental response with repetitive stimulation

TREATMENT

- Supportive: oral acetylcholinesterase inhibitors (pyridostigmine [Mestinon])
- Immunomodulatory therapies
  - For acute exacerbations: IVIG or plasma exchange
  - Chronic immunotherapies: steroids or steroid-sparing agents
- Some patients may benefit from thymectomy

Congenital Myasthenic Syndromes

BASIC INFORMATION

- Cause: genetic defects in the neuromuscular junction
- No immune system involvement

CLINICAL PRESENTATION

- Onset at birth or early childhood (lifelong)
- Fatigable weakness mainly affecting the ocular and bulbar muscles

EVALUATION

- EMG/NCS
- Genetic testing

TREATMENT

- Pyridostigmine can worsen certain subtypes
- Albuterol or fluoxetine may be beneficial for some subtypes

Transient Neonatal Myasthenia Gravis

BASIC INFORMATION

- Cause: maternal acetylcholine receptor antibodies are transferred to the fetus
- Only occurs in about 10% to 20% of infants born to mothers with myasthenia gravis

CLINICAL PRESENTATION

- Generalized weakness and hypotonia at birth with intact DTRs
- Bulbar weakness is common, but eye involvement (ptosis and ophthalmoplegia) is less common

EVALUATION

- Suspect based on clinical history
- If mother does not have known myasthenia gravis and diagnosis is unclear, can assess response to acetylcholinesterase inhibitor (like neostigmine or edrophonium)

TREATMENT

- Supportive: neostigmine

PROGNOSIS

- Most recover within a few weeks

LOCALIZATION: MUSCLE

Duchenne Muscular Dystrophy (DMD) and Becker Muscular Dystrophy (BMD)

BASIC INFORMATION

- DMD and BMD are caused by mutations in the gene for dystrophin

- Dystrophin is on the cell membrane of muscle fibers
- Gene is on the X chromosome → X-linked disorders
- Largest gene identified in humans
- DMD mutations disrupt reading frame → truncated protein
- BMD mutations maintain reading frame → semifunctional protein

CLINICAL PRESENTATION

- DMD
  - Onset of weakness between 2 and 3 years
  - Proximal > distal, lower extremities > upper extremities
  - Calf pseudohypertrophy (replacement with connective tissue and fat)
  - Gowers' sign: need to use hand support to get up from floor
  - Systemic manifestations
    - Cardiomyopathy presents ~15 years of age
    - Orthopedic: fractures, progressive scoliosis
    - Impaired pulmonary function
    - Decreased gastric motility
- BMD
  - Later onset and milder symptoms
  - Still has significant cardiac involvement

EVALUATION

- Creatine kinase (CK): elevated
- Genetic testing: look for dystrophin gene mutations
- May consider EMG/NCS and/or muscle biopsy if there is diagnostic uncertainty

TREATMENT

- Glucocorticoids
  - Used for patients with DMD aged 2 to 5+ years with plateaued or declining function
  - Benefits: increased motor function, increased pulmonary function, reduction of scoliosis, possibly delayed onset of cardiomyopathy
  - Mechanism unclear
- Multidisciplinary supportive management
  - Cardiac
    - Baseline assessment
    - May require angiotensin-converting enzyme (ACE) inhibitor or beta-blocker
  - Pulmonary
    - Baseline pulmonary function tests before wheelchair confinement
    - Sequentially increasing support (noninvasive ventilation as necessary)
  - Orthopedic
    - Physical therapy, stretching exercises, braces
    - Surgery: for contractures, spine surgery
    - Bone health: vitamin D supplementation
- Novel gene therapies are in development (e.g., exon skipping)

PROGNOSIS

- DMD
  - Patients typically confined to wheelchair by age 12 years

- Patients often die in late teens to 20s from respiratory insufficiency or cardiomyopathy
- BMD
  - Patients typically can walk past age 16 years
  - Patients usually survive beyond age 30 years

Myotonic Dystrophy

BASIC INFORMATION

- Myotonic dystrophy type 1 (DM1) is caused by expansion of a CTG-trinucleotide repeat
- Autosomal dominant inheritance
- Anticipation: trinucleotide repeat count increases over successive generations → next generation presents earlier

CLINICAL PRESENTATION

- Congenital DM1
  - Hypotonia, arthrogryposis, poor feeding, and respiratory failure in neonatal period
- Childhood DM1
  - First symptoms include cognitive and behavioral problems before age 10 years
  - Later development of skeletal and respiratory muscle weakness, myotonia, cataracts, and cardiac arrhythmias
    - Typical pattern of weakness: facial muscles, hand intrinsic muscles, ankle dorsiflexors
    - Myotonia: delayed relaxation after muscle contraction
- Classic DM1 and myotonic dystrophy type 2 (DM2) typically do not present until adulthood

EVALUATION

- Genetic testing
- EMG/NCS if there is diagnostic uncertainty
- CK is usually only mildly elevated

TREATMENT

- Supportive: no disease-modifying treatment is available

General Approach to Hypotonia

Tone is the resistance of muscles to passive stretch. Although hypotonia and weakness may go together at times, they are *not* the same thing. You can measure axial (neck and truncal) tone in infants by looking at their head control and holding them in vertical and horizontal suspension. Appendicular (extremity) tone can be assessed by passively moving the limbs. The resting posture of a hypotonic newborn is "frog-legged." If hypotonia *is* associated with significant weakness, it is generally due to a problem in the motor system at the level of or distal to the lower motor neuron (meaning at the anterior horn cell, nerve, neuromuscular junction, or muscle). You will typically see *reduced* or *absent* DTRs. If hypotonia is *not* associated with significant weakness, it is generally due to a problem diffusely impacting the CNS (think infection, hypoxic ischemic injury, metabolic disorders, and chromosomal abnormalities). You may see *normal* or *increased* DTRs.

Note that with diseases that more focally affect the motor system in the CNS, you typically instead see hypertonia as opposed to hypotonia (see Table 58.1)

General Approach to Ataxia

Ataxia is the lack of smooth, coordinated movements. A few buzz words for ataxia are "unsteady, wide-based gait." You may also see truncal titubation, uncoordinated limb movements, and dysarthria. Ataxia is generally caused by cerebellar dysfunction but can also be caused by problems in the motor and sensory networks that connect to the cerebellum to help with motor planning and feedback.

Acute Cerebellar Ataxia

BASIC INFORMATION

- Most common cause of ataxia in children
- Typically postinfectious

CLINICAL PRESENTATION

- Previously well children
- Ataxia develops over hours to days after prodromal illness
  - Nystagmus, slurred speech, difficulty with fine motor movements, truncal titubation, gait instability
- Should not have altered mental status, seizures, or meningismus

EVALUATION

- Clinical diagnosis
- Send toxicology screen to exclude ingestions
- If atypical features, consider lumbar puncture and/or neuroimaging

TREATMENT

- Supportive

PROGNOSIS

- Ataxia typically completely resolves within 2 to 3 weeks

Ataxia-Telangiectasia

BASIC INFORMATION

- Autosomal recessive disorder
- Defect in *ATM* gene involved in DNA repair

CLINICAL PRESENTATION

- At first, infants appear normal—may learn to walk on time
- By age 2 to 3 years, ataxia appears and then progresses, typically requiring wheelchair by age 15 years
- Oculomotor apraxia: patient cannot make fast voluntary eye movements, so he or she turns head instead
- Other systemic manifestations
  - Telangiectasias—on eyes and skin, typically appear after age 3 years

- Immunodeficiency: frequent upper and lower respiratory tract infections, with decreased levels of Ig and T-cell dysfunction
- Malignancy: increased risk of cancer (often leukemia or lymphoma)
- Progressive pulmonary disease: infection, interstitial lung disease

EVALUATION

- Serum alpha fetoprotein (AFP): elevated
- Serum IgA: reduced
- Genetic testing

TREATMENT

- Supportive—no disease-modifying treatment is available

PROGNOSIS

- Poor prognosis; median age of death in mid-20s

Friedreich Ataxia

BASIC INFORMATION

- Most common hereditary ataxia
- Usually autosomal recessive or sporadic
- Loss of function mutations in the frataxin gene, usually due to expansion of a GAA-trinucleotide repeat
- Atrophy of spinal cord and medulla

CLINICAL PRESENTATION

- Typically presents in adolescence
- Progressive ataxia of all extremities
- Dysarthria is common
- Sensory loss, particularly vibration and proprioception (posterior columns, dorsal root, and peripheral nerves are affected)
- Eventual loss of DTRs
- Other systemic manifestations
  - Hypertrophic cardiomyopathy
  - Kyphoscoliosis
  - Diabetes mellitus

EVALUATION

- Neuroimaging of brain and spinal cord to exclude other causes
- Genetic testing

TREATMENT

- Supportive: no disease-modifying treatment is available

PROGNOSIS

- Patients usually confined to wheelchair by late teens
- Age of death is usually in mid-30s from cardiac complications

Review Questions

For review questions, please go to ExpertConsult.com.

Suggested Readings

1. Caffarelli M, Kimia A, Torres A. Acute ataxia in children: a review of the differential diagnosis and evaluation in the emergency department. *Pediatr Neurol.* 2016;65:14–30.

2. Gilhus N. Myasthenia gravis. *N Engl J Med.* 2016;375:2570–2581.

3. Matthews E, Brassington R, Kuntzer T, et al. Corticosteroids for the treatment of Duchenne muscular dystrophy. *Cochrane Database of Syst Rev.* 2016;5:CD003725.

4. McAdams R, Juul S. Cerebral palsy: prevalence, predictability, and parental counseling. *NeoReviews.* 2011;12(10):e564.

5. Peredo D, Hannibal M. The floppy infant. *Pediatr Rev.* 2009;30(9): e66.

59 Congenital Malformations of the Central Nervous System

DOUGLAS M. SMITH, MD

An exhaustive review of all congenital malformations is beyond the scope of this chapter. Here we will briefly review the more common congenital malformations of particular significance to the general pediatrician. Also included are conditions (e.g., Chiari I malformation) that are not clearly congenital but are of clinical significance.

See also Nelson Textbook of Pediatrics, Chapter 591, "Congenital Anomalies of the Central Nervous System."

Failure of Caudal Neural Tube Closure

SPINA BIFIDA OCCULTA

- Spinal cord dysraphisms
- Failure of spinous processes to completely form or fuse
- Spinal canal and overlying skin remain intact
- May have tuft of hair over defect or dimple
- Very common—about 10% of the population has spina bifida occulta
- Usually of no neurologic consequence
- All other types of spinal cord dysraphisms have elevated alpha fetoprotein (AFP) on prenatal screening

MENINGOCELE

- Protrusion of meninges through a spinal defect, resulting in the appearance of a cyst over (typically) lumbar spine
- Spinal cord typically remains intact
- Usually neurologically asymptomatic

MYELOMENINGOCELE

- Protrusion of meninges and spinal roots through defect (cyst remains covered by meninges)
- Results in severe neurologic complications with variable loss of function below the spinal level of the defect
  - Strength and sensation are typically more affected than urinary and sexual function, although all are typically involved
  - Myeloschisis
    - Most severe form of spinal cord dysraphism
    - Protrusion of meninges and spinal roots through defect with an open lesion over the back, resulting in a direct communication between the spinal canal and the external environment
    - Carries a high risk of central nervous system (CNS) infection

- Complications of myelomeningocele and myeloschisis:
  - Chiari II malformations (see later)
  - Cognitive issues
    Disruptions in white matter tracts, including agenesis of corpus callosum
    Attention-deficit/hyperactivity disorder (ADHD), executive dysfunction
  - Latex allergy
    Up to 70% with some allergy to latex
    Severity varies from rash to anaphylaxis
  - Tethered cord
    Can occur with *any* type of spinal cord dysraphism
    Cord is "tethered" to base of spine as spinal column grows, pulling on cord
    Presents during periods of growth with subacute progression of gait abnormalities and urinary changes
    Treatment: surgical release if symptomatic
- Prevention: prenatal supplementation with folic acid
  - Exact quantity of folic acid is controversial, ranging from 1 to 5 mg daily
  - Higher risk of dysraphism if patient is taking anticonvulsants
- Treatment
  - Surgical intervention is generally reserved for symptomatic dysraphisms
  - In utero surgery is controversial, but a recent randomized controlled trial (RCT) suggests improved cognitive benefit and reduced need for shunt

Failure of Rostral Neural Tube Closure

- Encephalocele: defect of skull closure
  - Same spectrum of severity as spinal cord dysraphisms
  - May be bone-only defect or may have herniation of brain contents
  - Most frequently anterior (e.g., forehead) or posterior (e.g., occiput)
- Anencephaly
  - Failure of brain, skull, and scalp formation
  - Majority result in spontaneous abortion or die during delivery
  - No treatment available; incidence may be reduced by folic acid supplementation

Malformations of Cortical Development

- Focal cortical dysplasia
  - Isolated region(s) where neurons fail to segregate appropriately into six layers
    - Can occur anywhere, but is slightly more frequently found in frontal lobe
    - Magnetic resonance imaging (MRI) findings: loss of gray-white differentiation, a "tail" of T2 hyperintensity from cortex to lateral ventricle, or completely normal
    - Typically presents with epilepsy; often refractory to medical therapy
      - If asymptomatic or well controlled with antiepileptics, no further treatments are necessary
      - If refractory epilepsy, surgical resection may be indicated
- Polymicrogyria
  - More numerous, with much smaller gyri, resulting in a "cobblestone" appearance of cortex
  - May be focal or more diverse
  - Frequently perisylvian: involves much of the cortex around the lateral sulcus (sylvian fissure), bilaterally
  - May be congenital or due to prenatal CNS infection
  - Presents with variable severity ranging from mild neurologic deficits to severe intellectual deficiency, cerebral palsy, and epilepsy
  - Therapies are targeted at associated symptoms (e.g., seizures, cerebral palsy)
- Subcortical band heterotopia—"double cortex"
  - Some neurons appropriately migrate to cortex, whereas others fail, resulting in two distinct layers of neurons on imaging, often with malformed cortex
  - Occurs more often in girls
  - Presents nearly universally with severe neurologic impairment
- Lissencephaly—"smooth brain"
  - Failure to form typical gyri and sulci
  - May be primarily frontal, occipital, or diffuse
  - Presents nearly universally with severe neurologic impairment

Disorders of Midline Structure Formation

- Agenesis of the corpus callosum
  - Varies from dysgenesis (corpus callosum is present but abnormal) to partial agenesis (missing either anterior or posterior portion only) to complete agenesis
  - Has many causes, and presentations are variable, depending on the cause
  - Many have normal IQ with subtle cognitive impairments; thus it is often discovered incidentally
- Septo-optic dysplasia
  - Triad of absence of septum pellucidum, optic nerve hypoplasia, and pituitary dysfunction
  - Can have normal cognition, but about 50% demonstrate mild to moderate intellectual disability

- Can be discovered during neonatal period (poor transition, hypotonia), infancy (delayed visual milestones, congenital nystagmus, cerebral palsy), or later (endocrine dysfunction, especially growth hormone deficiency)
- Requires screening of pituitary function if imaging raises concern for both optic nerves and corpus callosum development
- Holoprosencephaly
  - Most severe form—alobar—usually includes single eye (cyclopia) and absent or misplaced nose (proboscis)
  - Semilobar holoprosencephaly—partial fusion of hemispheres
  - Lobar holoprosencephaly—partial interdigitation of hemispheres, typically frontally
  - Severity is variable based on extent of fusion, but generally severe intellectual disability, cerebral palsy, and epilepsy

Disorders of Posterior Fossa Formation

- Dandy-Walker malformation
  - Enlarged fourth ventricle, elevated torculum, agenesis of cerebellar vermis, and typically agenesis of much of the cerebellar hemispheres
  - Often associated with midbrain and pons malformation and hydrocephalus
  - Neurologic impairment primarily with fine-motor and gait impairment, but also with variable intellectual disability
- Joubert syndrome
  - "Molar tooth" appearance of midbrain on MRI
  - Severe developmental outcome with variable cranial nerve and bulbar symptoms
- Pontocerebellar hypoplasia
  - Underdevelopment of brain stem and cerebellum
  - Multiple genetic causes
  - Nearly universal poor neurologic outcome

Other Posterior Fossa Structural Disorders

- Chiari malformation type I
  - Herniation of cerebellar tonsils through foramen magnum >5 mm
  - Apparent obstruction of flow of cerebrospinal fluid
  - May be congenital or acquired
  - Acquired cases are usually due to trauma or connective tissue disorders (e.g., Ehlers-Danlos, Marfan)
  - Symptoms are usually attributed to obstruction of CSF flow or impingement of posterior fossa structures
    - Headaches are worse with Valsalva
    - Dysarthria, difficulty swallowing, ataxia
    - Majority are likely asymptomatic
  - Potential complications
- Syringomyelia
  - Enlargement of central canal of spinal cord

- Causes sensory loss and weakness in bilateral upper extremities and shoulder in a "cape-like" distribution
  - Scoliosis
  - Tethered cord
- Chiari malformation type II
  - Typically associated with myelomeningocele, described previously
  - Unlike Chiari malformation type I, associated with hydrocephalus and cognitive impairment
  - Radiographically unique compared with type I: fourth ventricle herniates through foramen magnum, "beaked" tectum, "kinked" medulla
- Chiari malformation type III
  - Rarest form of Chiari malformation
  - Radiographically resembles type II
  - Associated with occipital encephalocele or cervical spinal dysraphism

Review Questions

For review questions, please go to ExpertConsult.com

60 Selected Topics in Neurology

JULIE ZIOBRO, MD, PhD and PATRICK DONALD LEE MABRAY, MD, PhD

Pediatric stroke is remarkably common, occurring as frequently as pediatric brain tumors. Acute presentations are considered a neurologic emergency because early intervention may prevent significant morbidity and mortality.

See also Nelson Textbook of Pediatrics, Chapter 601, "Pediatric Stroke."

Pediatric Stroke

BASIC INFORMATION

Arterial ischemic stroke (AIS)

- Makes up 55% of pediatric strokes
- Localized AIS
  - Hypercoagulable state
  - Response to endothelial damage
  - Arterial dissection
  - Inflammation
  - Vasculopathy
    - Arteriopathy (genetic or acquired abnormality of the arteries) is found in half of all cases of AIS
    - Sickle cell disease (SCD) is one of the most common risk factors for stroke in children
      Ischemic stroke occurs in 11% of SCD patients by age 20 years
    - May cause microvascular occlusion
    - Endothelial damage may lead to arteriopathy (hyperplasia of the vessel wall with luminal narrowing)
      Moyamoya disease
        Narrowing of the distal internal carotid artery (ICA) or middle cerebral artery (MCA) with the appearance of compensatory collateral vessels (making a "puff of smoke" appearance on vessel imaging)
        May be idiopathic, but is more common in patients of East Asian descent
        Sickle cell disease, NF-1, trisomy 21, and history of radiation are risk factors
- Thromboembolic AIS
  - Embolus from a distant site that travels to a cerebral artery
  - Cardiac disease is second most common risk factor
    - Produces intracardiac thrombi or paradoxic embolisms via right-to-left shunts
    - Anticoagulation may increase risk of hemorrhagic stroke
    - Surgical repair requiring bypass also increases risk of stroke
  - Prothrombotic conditions
    - 13% of pediatric arterial stroke patients have a hereditary thrombophilia

- Also consider oral contraceptive pill (OCP) use, malignancy, and infection
- Vasculitis
  - Inflammation of blood vessels secondary to infection or autoimmune disorder, which may lead to localized or distant thromboembolus
- Arterial dissection
  - May occur after rapid torsion injury or in patients with connective tissue disorders. Disrupted laminar flow may lead to thromboembolus formation

Hemorrhagic stroke

- May be intraparenchymal or subarachnoid
- Risk factors: vascular anomalies or hemorrhagic conversion after ischemic stroke
  - Vascular anomalies account for 45% of nontraumatic hemorrhagic strokes in children

Cerebral sinovenous thrombosis (CSVT)

- Obstruction by clot of a major venous sinus draining the brain parenchyma, leading to infarct
- May lead to secondary hemorrhage

CLINICAL PRESENTATION

- Sudden-onset focal neurologic deficits occur in 85% of pediatric strokes
  - Anterior-circulation stroke (MCA or anterior cerebral artery [ACA])
    - Lateralized motor deficits, speech disturbance, or fixed gaze deviation
  - Posterior-circulation stroke
    - Altered mental status, dizziness, vomiting, ataxia, eye movement abnormalities
- 60% of children with stroke have generalized signs or symptoms that are not easily localized to a single vascular territory
  - Seizure is the sentinel sign of acute stroke in 31% of children
  - Postictal Todd paralysis is a diagnosis of exclusion
- Moyamoya or other vasculopathies:
  - May present with stroke or recurrent transient ischemic attack (TIA), especially after hyperventilation or dehydration

DIAGNOSIS AND EVALUATION

- Stroke suspected—onset within hours
  - Determine time of last known normal for appropriate management

Table 60.1. Mimics of Acute Ischemic Stroke

MELAS (mitochondrial encephalomyopathy, lactic acidosis, and stroke-like episodes)

Migraine with aura

Seizure (with Todd paralysis)

Tumor

Metabolic derangement

Pseudotumor cerebri

Demyelinating disease

Infection

Somatoform disorder

Table 60.2. Workup for Etiology of Arterial Ischemic Stroke

INITIAL LABORATORY TESTING

Complete blood count, erythrocyte sedimentation rate, C-reactive protein, thyroid-stimulating hormone, cholesterol panel, blood culture, beta–human chorionic gonadotropin, sickle cell preparation, prothrombin time/partial thromboplastin time/international normalized ratio, thrombin time, fibrinogen

Prothrombotic workup (before initiating anticoagulation): D-Dimer, protein C, protein S, antithrombin III, lupus anticoagulant, factor VIII activity

ADDITIONAL WORKUP

Prothrombotic: factor V Leiden mutation, prothrombin gene mutation, homocysteine, beta-2 glycoprotein antibody, lipoprotein A, anticardiolipin

Vasculopathy: varicella-zoster virus, HIV, cytomegalovirus, parvovirus, mycoplasma, Lyme, enterovirus, venereal disease research laboratory, C3/C4 complement, albumin, anti-double stranded DNA ab, ANCA, RF, ANCA, anti-SM ab

Metabolic disorders: serum amino acids, urine organic acids, mitochondrial DNA

- Urgent magnetic resonance imaging/angiography (MRI/MRA) if available
  - AIS will be noted as bright on diffusion-weighted imaging (DWI) and dark on apparent diffusion coefficient (ADC) imaging with no evidence of hemorrhage
  - Some AIS will also demonstrate vascular occlusion on MRA
- If MRI is not available or contraindicated, consider obtaining computed tomography (CT) of the brain with CT angiogram (CTA) of the head and neck
  - CT may be normal in acute period; thus a negative result does not necessarily rule out AIS (however, a CT might be used in an emergency department setting before an MRI to rule out other life-threatening causes of stroke symptoms)
  - If there is vascular occlusion on CTA, AIS is confirmed
- If AIS is not confirmed on imaging, consider alternatives: CSVT, hemorrhage, old stroke
- The differential diagnosis for AIS includes many disorders (see Table 60.1)

TREATMENT

- AIS
  - Consider thrombolytic or endovascular treatment if onset of symptoms is within 4.5 hours in select cases
  - Admit patient to intensive care unit (ICU) for neuroprotective care
    - Maximize cerebral perfusion and oxygenation
      Avoid hypotension
      Maintain head of bed flat with head midline
    - Minimize metabolic demands
      Maintain normothermia, normonatremia, and euglycemia
      Provide seizure precautions, and treat seizures aggressively
    - Start aspirin
    - Consider anticoagulation in arterial dissection or CSVT
    - Patients with SCD may require urgent exchange transfusion
  - New diagnosis of stroke often requires extensive laboratory testing to determine the etiology (e.g., thrombophilia, infection); see Table 60.2 for a sample workup
  - Echocardiogram with bubble study
- Hemorrhagic stroke: acute neurosurgical evaluation
  - Seizure prophylaxis
  - Monitor for signs of increased intracranial pressure (ICP) and manage appropriately
  - Treat cause of bleed because of high risk of rebleed
- Moyamoya: consult neurosurgery, and consider revascularization surgery when appropriate

Neonatal Stroke

BASIC INFORMATION

- Occurs as commonly as stroke in the elderly
- Defined as stroke occurring between 20 weeks' gestation and 28 days after birth
- 80% are ischemic, 20% hemorrhage or CSVT
- Results from multiple risk factors in the mother, fetus, and placenta during peripartum period that may lead to hypercoagulability
  - Major risk factors: congenital heart disease, meningitis
  - May co-occur with hypoxic ischemic encephalopathy

CLINICAL PRESENTATION

- Seizure at 24 to 72 hours of life
  - 70% to 90% of infants with stroke will present with seizure
- Encephalopathy
  - Irritable or lethargic with poor feeding
- May develop early hand preference or delayed motor milestones

DIAGNOSIS AND EVALUATION

- MRI with vessel imaging is optimal
- Echocardiogram with bubble study
- Thrombophilia evaluation

TREATMENT

- Anticoagulation is indicated only in CSVT that propagates or in some cases of cardiac disease

- Seizure prevention
- Prevention of stroke recurrence

Cerebral Sinovenous Thrombosis (CSVT)

BASIC INFORMATION

- Cerebral venous drainage is achieved by superficial and deep veins
- Thrombosis in the venous system results in outflow obstruction, venous congestion, and increase in hydrostatic pressure that ultimately compromises arterial flow, leading to ischemia
- 40% of childhood CSVT occurs in the neonatal period. Incidence after the neonatal period is 0.4/100,000 to 0.7/100,000 children per year

CLINICAL PRESENTATION

- Seizures are the most common presentation in neonates
- Focal and diffuse signs are more common in older infants and children
- Some symptoms may be nonspecific:
  - Impaired mental status, headache, nausea, vomiting, visual impairment, papilledema, hemiparesis, ataxia, cranial nerve palsies, sensory changes
- 95% with a predisposing comorbid condition
  - Risk factors: dehydration, infection (including meningitis, sinusitis, upper respiratory infection [URI]), head injury, anemia, autoimmune disorders, renal disease, cardiac disease, medications (steroids, oral contraceptives), metabolic conditions (diabetic ketoacidosis [DKA], homocystinuria)

DIAGNOSIS AND EVALUATION

- High index of suspicion is important for timely diagnosis and treatment
- CT venography or MR venography are the imaging of choice
  - CT with contrast but without dedicated venous imaging may miss diagnosis in up to 40% of cases
- Search for predisposing condition, including infection and prothrombotic conditions

TREATMENT

- Supportive treatment similar to that for AIS. In addition:
  - Monitor for signs of increased ICP, changes in mental status, seizures, and changes in visual fields and acuity
  - For unconscious patients: continuous electroencephalogram (EEG) monitoring and repeat neuroimaging. Consider ICP monitoring
- Ensure adequate rehydration, and treat underlying cause
- If neurologically stable, treat with intravenous (IV) heparin, subcutaneous heparin, or warfarin
  - Closely monitor levels and for signs of intracranial bleeding

- If unstable, consider neurosurgical or neurointerventional evaluation for thrombectomy or surgical decompression

Vascular Anomalies

BASIC INFORMATION

- Arteriovenous malformation (AVM)
  - Abnormal arteries connect directly to draining veins without a capillary bed
- Vein of Galen malformation
  - Dilation of the vein of Galen secondary to a mass of dilated vessels and an enlarged artery or an arteriovenous fistula connected directly to the vein
- Cerebral aneurysm
  - Associated with genetic conditions
    - Aortic coarctation
    - Polycystic kidney disease
    - Sickle cell disease
    - Ehlers-Danlos type IV
    - Fibromuscular dysplasia

CLINICAL PRESENTATION

- Seizures, headache, focal neurologic deficits, or hemorrhage
- Hemorrhage risk for a known AVM is 2% to 4% per year
- Vein of Galen malformation may present in infancy with high-output heart failure and hydrocephalus

DIAGNOSIS AND EVALUATION

- MRI and MRA, CTA, or conventional angiogram
- Consider underlying genetic condition

TREATMENT

- Close neurosurgical monitoring and intervention based on risk/benefit if no bleeding is present
  - May consider embolization, surgical resection, or radiosurgery

Multiple Sclerosis (MS)

BASIC INFORMATION

- Chronic, autoimmune, inflammatory, demyelinating disease of the central nervous system (CNS)
- Etiology is still unknown, although autoimmune, genetic, and environmental factors play a role
  - May have a geographic distribution—50% of all MS patients are from Europe
- Two types based on clinical course: relapsing-remitting MS or primary progressive MS
  - Pediatric cases are almost always relapsing-remitting at first
- Pediatric patients may have more relapses than adults but have faster recovery and slower disease progression compared with adults

CLINICAL PRESENTATION

- First attack may be any neurologic symptom without encephalopathy and may include vision change, focal weakness, focal sensory change, ataxia, and so forth
- Most frequently begins between the second and fourth decades of life
  - First attack occurs at younger than 18 years of age in only 2.7% to 5.4% of all MS patients
  - Average age of pediatric MS onset is 15 years old, but onset can be as young as 2 years old
  - Positive family history in 6% to 20%
- Differential Diagnosis:
  - Other demyelinating diseases: acute disseminated encephalomyelitis (ADEM) or neuromyelitis optica (NMO)
  - Autoimmune disease: neurosarcoidosis, systemic lupus erythematosus (SLE), CNS vasculitis, myasthenia gravis, and so forth
  - Vascular diseases: stroke, arteriopathy
  - Infections: viral encephalitis, neuroborreliosis, neurosyphilis
  - Metabolic disease: mitochondrial disease, vitamin B deficiency
  - Tumors or paraneoplastic process
- Fatigue, depression, and cognitive deficits are often associated with MS but may not be present at initial diagnosis

DIAGNOSIS AND EVALUATION

- MRI with and without contrast has a high sensitivity in the detection of disease activity
- Diagnostic criteria for MS:
  - Two or more nonencephalopathic clinical events with presumed inflammatory cause, involving more than one region of the CNS, which are separated by more than 30 days, *or*
  - One clinical event plus findings on MRI that establish demyelinating events separated by time and space, *or*
  - First event that does not satisfy criteria for ADEM and whose MRI findings were in accordance with the revised McDonald criteria in 2010 (only in children 12 years and older)
    - McDonald criteria include MRI findings with at least one T2 change in two of four typical regions for MS (periventricular, juxtacortical, infratentorial, spinal cord)
  - ADEM with recurrent event at least 3 months later, without encephalopathy and with new lesions on MRI
- Clinically isolated syndrome (CIS)
  - Single demyelinating event without evidence of dissemination in time or dissemination in space
  - Increased risk of developing MS
  - Presents with encephalopathy in 15% to 20% and may be difficult to distinguish from ADEM
    - Serial MRI imaging may determine whether there is progression
- Cerebrospinal fluid (CSF) may reveal oligoclonal bands, elevated IgG index, or pleocytosis
  - CSF is not necessary for diagnosis of MS but may be useful to rule out other disorders

TREATMENT

- Immunomodulatory therapy
  - Should be discussed with a pediatric neurologist once the diagnosis of MS has been made
  - Goal of reducing clinical and MRI disease activity
  - Studies in the pediatric population are scarce, and none have been FDA approved in children (e.g., interferon beta-1a/1b, glatiramer acetate, dimethyl fumarate, natalizumab)
- Treatment of relapses: tailored to severity of deficit and response to previous treatments
  - High-dose steroids for 3 to 5 days
  - IV immunoglobulin (IVIG)
  - Plasmapheresis
- Additional therapies
  - Vitamin D may play a role in modulating the course of MS, but this is still being researched
  - Symptomatic treatment for pain, anxiety, depression, fatigue, urinary dysfunction, and so forth
  - Physical therapy as needed

PEDIATRIC MOVEMENT DISORDERS

Pediatric movement disorders are remarkably common, and making the diagnosis can be tricky. Once the diagnosis is made, oftentimes benign disorders can simply be monitored and the families counseled regarding expectations.

Hypokinetic Movement Disorders

BASIC INFORMATION

- Parkinsonism: extremely rare in children
  - Causes and etiology
- Drug-induced parkinsonism—most common cause
  - Neuroleptic medications (dopamine antagonists), calcium channel blockers, antiemetics (metoclopramide)
- Infectious and autoimmune encephalitis
- Primary Parkinson disease (juvenile Parkinson disease if onset is before 20 years of age)
  - Typically due to single gene mutations
  - Loss of dopaminergic neurons from substantia nigra
- Neurodegenerative disease, including mitochondrial disorders, Wilson disease, or lysosomal storage disease, may have parkinsonism

CLINICAL PRESENTATION

- Parkinsonism
  - Acute onset to subacute onset after starting a new medication
  - Reduced amplitude and speed of movements
  - May have difficulty with more frequent falls
- Parkinson disease:
  - Characterized by the triad of bradykinesia, akinesia, cogwheel rigidity, and resting tremor (often not seen in pediatrics)

DIAGNOSIS AND EVALUATION

- Detailed history and physical examination, including medication history
- Genetic evaluation for Parkinson disease if idiopathic
- MRI of the brain and imaging of dopamine metabolism may be helpful in some cases

TREATMENT

- Parkinsonism
  - Stop offending medications
- Parkinson disease
  - Dopamine and dopamine agonists have been the mainstay of therapy
  - Other agents include glutamate antagonists, anticholinergics, catechol-O-methyltransferase (COMT) inhibitors, and monoamine oxidase (MAO) inhibitors

HYPERKINETIC MOVEMENT DISORDERS

Dystonia

BASIC INFORMATION

- Defined as concurrent activation of agonist and antagonist muscle groups, resulting in abnormal twisting and posturing movements
- Causes and etiology
  - Acute dystonic reactions
    - Secondary to dopamine antagonists, including metoclopramide, prochlorperazine, and neuroleptics
  - Chronic dystonias
    - Primary dystonias:
      There are 12 types currently diagnosed by causative gene mutation (DYT 1–12) as well as dopamine-responsive dystonia
      Typically have their onset in the teens with focal dystonia that tends to generalize, limiting function
      In most cases the patients have normal cognitive functioning
    - Secondary dystonias
      Cerebral palsy: most common and can overlap with spasticity
      Normally these patients will have damage to their basal ganglia on neuroimaging
      Neurodegenerative disease or malformations of cortical development

CLINICAL PRESENTATION

- May be focal (such as cervical dystonia) or generalized
- Typically provoked by activity and may be task specific (e.g., a writer's cramp)
- Acute dystonic reactions are typically focal with cervical dystonia, blepharospasm, opisthotonus, tongue, trunk, extremity spasms or laryngospasms

- Patients may develop a sensory trick to alleviate the dystonic posturing

DIAGNOSIS AND EVALUATION

- Detailed history, including family history
- Genetic evaluation may help
- An MRI of the brain may be useful in acute-onset dystonias

TREATMENT

- Acute dystonic reactions respond to antihistamines, anticholinergics, and benzodiazepines
- Stop any offending agents that caused the dystonic reaction
- Chronic dystonia treatments:
  - Botulinum toxin injections for focal dystonias
  - Baclofen (oral or intrathecal) or trihexyphenidyl for generalized dystonia
  - Deep brain stimulation may be pursued in certain patients
  - Dopamine may work for dopamine-responsive dystonia with dramatic improvements in quality of life

Chorea/Athetosis

BACKGROUND

- Chorea is defined as near-continuous irregular movements of a dancelike or writhing quality, neither rhythmic nor stereotyped
- Athetosis is same as chorea, just higher amplitude
  - Often occurs with cerebral palsy with basal ganglia injury co-occurring with dystonia
  - Physiologic chorea occurs at 6 months of age in healthy children
  - Juvenile Huntington disease
    - Autosomal dominant neurodegenerative disease due to a CAG repeat expansion in the *huntingtin* gene on chromosome 4
    - The longer the repeat, the earlier the onset of disease (normal is 20 repeats and juvenile onset typically with >80 repeats)
- Chorea from metabolic causes
  - Can be secondary to hypo- or hyperglycemia, hypo- or hypernatremia, hypocalcemia, or hyperthyroidism
  - May occur after cardiopulmonary bypass and is known as postpump chorea

CLINICAL PRESENTATION

- Sydenham chorea
  - Molecular mimicry with antistreptolysin O (ASO) antibodies cross-reacting with basal ganglia antigens
  - Develops 1 to 2 months after infection
  - Typically bilateral, but can be unilateral
  - Can occur with facial dystonia, hypotonia, dysarthria, and milkmaid grip
  - Emotional lability and some obsessive compulsive disorder (OCD) behaviors may occur
  - Recurs in 20% of patients within 2 years
  - Associated with rheumatic carditis and arthritis

- Huntington chorea
  - Very rare in children
  - Presents with rigidity, speech disorder, seizures, and cerebellar signs
  - Should have a family history with 90% paternal inheritance and may experience anticipation

DIAGNOSIS AND EVALUATION

- Thorough history and physical
- Evaluate for any medication changes correlated with chorea
- A brain MRI may prove useful
- Testing for ceruloplasmin, copper, and lysosomal storage diseases based on history and physical
- ASO titers are typically back to normal by the time Sydenham chorea manifests
- Genetic evaluation if family history is concerning for Huntington disease

TREATMENT

- Sydenham chorea
  - Treat with IVIG, steroids, or plasma exchange
  - Patients may need prophylaxis for rheumatic fever if Jones criteria are met
- Symptomatic chorea responds best to tetrabenazine (although this is off-label except for in Huntington chorea)

Tics

BACKGROUND

- Involuntary, sudden, rapid, abrupt, repetitive, recurrent, and nonrhythmic movement or vocalization
- Common comorbidities include attention-deficit/hyperactivity disorder (ADHD), OCD behaviors, anxiety, and depression

CLINICAL PRESENTATION

- Occur in up to 20% of children at some point in life with a 4:1 male-to-female predominance
- Typical age of onset is 4 to 8 years of life
- Motor tics
  - Simple motor tics are single muscle group, such as eye blinking, shoulder shrugging, neck extension, or abdominal flexion
  - Complex motor tics involve groups of muscles and can have dystonic posturing with writhing movements; examples include jumping, abdominal flexion, and foot shaking/tapping; these are usually accompanied by simple motor tics
- Vocal tics
  - Simple vocal tics include repetitive sniffing, throat clearing, barking, snorting, and blocking tics that stop sounds and can be confused with stuttering
  - Complex vocal tics commonly include echolalia (repeating others' words) and palilalia (repeating one's own words), whereas coprolalia (repeating obscenities) is much more rare

- Typically a waxing/waning course
- 90% of adults and 40% of children will describe a premonitory urge
- Tics are suppressible and suggestible
- Tourette syndrome is a subset of tic disorders
  - Requires both motor and vocal tics
  - Minimum of 1 year of duration
  - Onset before 18 years of age

DIAGNOSIS AND EVALUATION

- Clinical history and examination, during which the behaviors often can be observed in the office
- Examination of recordings of movements can be helpful

TREATMENT

- Observation: tics should be treated only if causing psychosocial impairment, pain, or interfering with activities
- Comprehensive behavioral intervention for tics
  - Therapy to recognize premonitory urges and to sublimate a competing movement for the tic
  - Is as effective as first-line medications
- Pharmacotherapy
  - Alpha-2 adrenergic agonists (clonidine, guanfacine)
  - Neuroleptics, including the typical agents (fluphenazine and pimozide) or atypical agents (risperidone and aripiprazole)
  - Topiramate

Stereotypies

BACKGROUND

- Consistent, rhythmic, repetitive movements without a clear purpose but done on purpose
- Comorbidities include learning disabilities, ADHD, depression, and anxiety

CLINICAL PRESENTATION

- Typical age of onset is 1 to 3 years of life
- Examples include hand flapping, rocking back and forth, mouth posturing, vocalizing, and head shaking
- Often seen in patients with autism spectrum disorders or Rett syndrome
- May occur when children are excited or in other heightened states of arousal
- Most are with the natural history is for a gradual reduction in frequency tend to gradually reduce in frequency and severity as children reach school age

DIAGNOSIS AND EVALUATION

- Clinical history and examination
- Examination of recordings of movements can be helpful

TREATMENT

- May respond to neuroleptics
- Habit reversal therapy may be effective

Tremor

BACKGROUND

- Rhythmic oscillating movement with a fixed frequency
- Everyone has a low-amplitude inherent physiologic tremor that can be exacerbated by anxiety, excitement, stress, caffeine, steroids, thyroid-stimulating hormone (TSH), and so forth

CLINICAL PRESENTATION

- Essential (familial) tremor
  - Is an enhanced physiologic tremor that can occur as early as 2 years of age
  - Presents in limbs in use; may include the head
  - Typically between 4 and 8 hertz
  - Tremor increases with the precision required for a movement
  - Typically presents first in the hands
  - Should be rhythmic and not dysmetric (will not get worse at the distal end of a movement)

DIAGNOSIS AND EVALUATION

- Essential tremor does not require any imaging or laboratory work
- Electromyogram (EMG) studies may be helpful in diagnosing tremor
- Thorough evaluation if any signs of hyperthyroidism, including TSH and T4
- May need to evaluate for Wilson disease (copper and ceruloplasmin) or heavy metal toxicity

TREATMENT

- Essential tremor
  - Propranolol or primidone
  - Deep brain stimulation

Ataxia (covered in Chapter 58)

PEDIATRIC SLEEP DISORDERS

Sleep is an integral physiologic function that impacts growth and development in children. By some estimates, up to 50% of children will have some sleep disorder during their lifetime, which can often impact the health of the patient and of his or her family.

Narcolepsy

BASIC INFORMATION

- Shorter latency to REM sleep can occur (<20 minutes compared with 90 minutes normally)
- Loss/deficiency of orexin-producing neurons in the hypothalamus

CLINICAL PRESENTATION

- Typical onset is between 20s and 30s, but can occur in childhood
- Clinical features include:
  - Narcolepsy: three to four short sleep attacks during the day
  - Cataplexy: a sudden loss of muscle tone can be induced by heightened emotions or startle that typically occur in the afternoons
  - Sleep paralysis: when transitioning from sleep to wakefulness, the patient is aware but unable to move
  - Hypnagogic hallucinations: vivid visual and auditory hallucinations occurring during the transition from wakefulness to sleep
  - Disturbed nighttime sleep: usually with some repetitive behaviors, such as speaking or writing gibberish without any recollection of the activity

DIAGNOSIS AND EVALUATION

- Detailed clinical history
- Multiple sleep latency test

TREATMENT

- Scheduled naps can be helpful
- Excessive sedation can be treated with modafinil as first line, followed by stimulants, including methylphenidate
- Cataplexy may respond to selective serotonin reuptake inhibitors (SSRIs)

Sleep Terrors and Sleepwalking

BASIC INFORMATION

- A parasomnia likely due to partial arousal from non-REM sleep

CLINICAL PRESENTATION

- Typically begins between 4 and 6 years of age
- The episode occurs 2 hours after sleep initiation and can last from 5 to 60 minutes
- Characterized by screaming inconsolably or by hypermotor behaviors such as trying to run or kick
- The child will return to sleep afterward with no memory of the event
- 50% will stop by 8 years of age, and 30% will continue into adolescence

DIAGNOSIS AND EVALUATION

- Family history is positive in many cases
- A sleep study or overnight EEG can differentiate complex partial seizures or OSA causing the awakenings

TREATMENT

- Scheduled awakenings before the events may help to extinguish them
- Benzodiazepines at bedtime for children at risk of injury

Review Questions

For review questions, please go to ExpertConsult.com.

Suggested Readings

1. Belman AL, Krupp LB, Olsen CS, et al. Characteristics of children and adolescents with multiple sclerosis. *Pediatrics.* 2016;138(1):e20160120.
2. Bernson-Leung ME, Rivkin MJ. Stroke in neonates and children. *Pediatr Rev.* 2016;37(11):463–477.
3. Bhargava S. Diagnosis and management of common sleep problems in children. *Pediatr Rev.* 2011;32(3):91–98.
4. Elbers J, Wainwright MS, Amlie-Lefond C. The pediatric stroke code: early management of the child with stroke. *J Pediatr.* 2015;167(1):19–24.
5. Fenichel G. Movement disorders. In: Fenichel GM, *Clinical Pediatric Neurology: A Signs and Symptoms Approach.* 6th ed. Philadelphia: Elsevier Saunders; 2009:293–312.
6. Jacic J, Nikolic B, Ivancevic N, et al. Multiple sclerosis in pediatrics: current concepts and treatment options. *Neurol Ther.* 2016;5:131–143.
7. Kirton A, deVeber G. Paediatric stroke: pressing issues and promising directions. *Lancet Neurol.* 2015;14:92–102.
8. Kruer MC. Pediatric movement disorders. *Pediatr Rev.* 2015;36(3):104–115.
9. Nevsimalova S. The diagnosis and treatment of pediatric narcolepsy. *Curr Neurol Neurosci Rep.* 2014;14(8):469.

Oncology

61 *Hematologic Malignancies*

SNEHA RAMAKRISHNA, MD

This chapter will review key concepts of hematologic malignancies. Specifically, this will review major clinical presentations, initial approaches to diagnosis and evaluation, differential diagnoses, and treatment options. It will also highlight some of the major difference between each of these malignancies. The chapter specifically focuses on Acute Lymphoblastic Leukemia (B and T cell), Acute Myelogenous Leukemia, Chronic Myeloid Leukemia, Juvenile Myelomonocytic Leukemia, Hodgkin Lymphoma, and Non-Hodgkin Lymphoma.

Acute Lymphoblastic Leukemia (ALL)

BASIC INFORMATION

- Epidemiology:
  - Most common childhood cancer
  - Peak onset in children is 2 to 5 years old; more commonly occurs in males
  - Down syndrome patients are 10 to 20 times more likely to develop leukemias (ratio of acute myelogenous leukemia [AML] to ALL 1:1 due to FAB M7 AML) and are more likely to have treatment-related issues, including infections and sensitivity to chemotherapy; trisomy 21 patients are generally treated on protocols with additional supportive therapies
- Major types include B and T lymphoblastic leukemia
  - Pre-B-cell ALL
    - Risk stratification (Table 61.1) is a mainstay of childhood ALL therapy with lower risk resulting in less toxic regimens
  - T-cell ALL
    - Comprises 10% to 15% of pediatric ALL
    - Called "terrible T cell" because it historically has had lower cure rates, but with more aggressive therapies, survival rates approach B-precursor ALL
    - See also Nelson Textbook of Pediatrics, Chapter 495, "The Leukemias."

CLINICAL PRESENTATION

- Most common presenting symptoms:
  - Fevers (approximately 60%)
  - Bruising, epistaxis (approximately 50%)
  - Bone pain (approximately 20%)
  - Pallor, anorexia, fatigue
- Physical examination findings:

- Hepatosplenomegaly (approximately >60%) and lymphadenopathy (approximately 50%)
- Petechiae
- Other important physical examination locations: testes (essential to examine in boys because this can be a sanctuary site and changes the treatment plan)

DIAGNOSIS AND EVALUATION

- Laboratory studies:
  - Complete blood count (CBC) + differential with peripheral blood smear
    - Often low platelets and low hemoglobin due to crowding of bone marrow with leukemic cells
    - White blood cell (WBC) count can be elevated, normal, or low. High WBC count may be a medical emergency due to concern for leukocytosis (see Chapter 64)
  - Peripheral blood flow cytometry
    - Could provide diagnosis earlier and allow for initiation of therapy sooner
  - Complete metabolic panel (CMP), including magnesium, phosphorus, uric acid, and lactate dehydrogenase (LDH)
    - Markers of tumor lysis syndrome (see Chapter 64)
    - Look for hyperkalemia, hyperphosphatemia, hyperuricemia, and hypercalcemia, which must be addressed swiftly
    - Elevated LDH is a marker of high cell turnover (but not a value worth treating, itself)
  - Coagulation studies
    - Coagulopathy can add to the risk of bleeding in early stages of diagnosis (larger concern in AML than in ALL)
  - Type and screen
    - Obtain at initial laboratory testing due to need for early and continued transfusion support
  - Urinalysis
- Imaging studies:
  - Chest x-ray
    - Evaluate for mediastinal mass because this will affect the patient's ability to undergo anesthesia for procedures and may affect potential immediate airway risk
- Bone marrow biopsy and aspirate:
  - 5% lymphoblasts is highly suggestive for leukemia, but for diagnosis, >25% of bone marrow with blasts is required. If between 5% and 25%, consider diagnosis of lymphoma

Table 61.1.   Risk Stratification for Acute Lymphoblastic Leukemia

	Favorable Risk	High Risk
Age	Between 1 and 10 years old	<1 year old ≥10 years old
White blood cell count at presentation	<50,000/μL	>50,000/μL
Exposure		Corticosteroid exposure before diagnostic workup
Sanctuary sites		Central nervous system (blasts on cytospin or >5 leukocytes/μL on cerebrospinal fluid count) Testicular involvement
Genetic mutations	TEL-AML1 (or ETV6-RUNX1) Hyperdiploid	BCR-ABL1 (Philadelphia chromosome) Mixed-lineage leukemia rearranged Hypodiploid
Response to induction	Negative for minimal residual disease	Induction failure or positive minimal residual disease

- Lumbar puncture:
  - To evaluate for central nervous system (CNS) disease; generally done with intrathecal injection of chemotherapy if diagnosis of leukemia is clear from peripheral blood

DIFFERENTIAL DIAGNOSIS

- Nonmalignant conditions:
  - Systemic lupus erythematosus: less likely to present with thrombocytopenia than leukemia
  - Viral suppression sometimes can cause single, but not multiple, cell lines to reduce counts.
  - Idiopathic thrombocytopenic purpura: can cause low platelets, but is less likely to cause low hemoglobin or changed WBC/differential
  - Infectious mononucleosis: both have atypical lymphocytes, cytopenias, joint pain, and splenomegaly, but ALL has more pronounced cytopenia and circulating blasts (>25% of bone marrow)
  - Aplastic anemia: bone marrow will be empty as opposed to being full of blasts. Additionally, unlike in leukemia, aplastic anemia usually does not cause hepatosplenomegaly and lymphadenopathy
  - Juvenile rheumatoid arthritis: also presents with joint pain, fever, hepatosplenomegaly, and pallor. Consider doing bone marrow evaluation before using steroids in suspected cases
  - Hypereosinophilic syndrome: consider doing bone marrow evaluation for assessment; look for blasts and genetic markers of abnormalities
- Malignant conditions: rare, but think solid tumors that can involve the bone marrow:
  - Neuroblastoma
  - Retinoblastoma
  - Rhabdomyosarcoma

TREATMENT

- Pre-B-cell ALL and T-cell ALL
  - Hyperhydration, alkalinization, allopurinol; watch for TLS (see Chapter 64)
  - If febrile, evaluate for occult infection and administer antibiotics
- Induction:
  - 28 days of therapy, with remission induction rates of 95%
  - Usually includes steroids, vincristine, intrathecal methotrexate, and peg-asparaginase. Daunomycin is added for high-risk and very-high-risk populations
  - CNS space can be a sanctuary site and must be treated with intrathecal chemotherapy
- Consolidation:
  - Includes consolidation, interim maintenance, and delayed intensification
  - Intensity and duration are dependent on risk stratification
- Maintenance:
  - Maintenance is a combination of daily oral 6-mercaptopurine, weekly oral methotrexate, monthly pulses of steroid and vincristine, and quarterly intrathecal methotrexate
  - Duration is 2 years for girls and 3 years for boys
- Other considerations:
  - Ph-like ALL with BCR-ABL genetic findings—consider adding tyrosine kinase inhibitor
- Relapse
  - Most common sites of recurrence: CNS and testes
  - If relapse, treatment often progresses to bone marrow transplant
  - Likelihood of CR after first remission reduces from >90% to 30% and decreases with each subsequent relapse
  - New therapies with immunotherapy are on the horizon, including chimeric antigen receptor T-cell therapies (FDA approved for CD19 CAR therapy), bispecific T-cell engaging antibodies (BiTE such as blinatumomab – anti-CD19/CD3 antibody), and immunotoxins

Acute Myelogenous Leukemia

BASIC INFORMATION

- Epidemiology:
  - Can be associated with Down syndrome, Fanconi anemia, Kostmann syndrome, or neurofibromatosis
  - Has an overall more aggressive and poorer prognosis compared with ALL
- Better prognostic indicators:
  - Genetic: core-binding factor (CBF) mutations [inversion16 (p13;1q22), t(16;16)(p13;q22), t(8;21) (q22;q22), or AML/ETO], CEBPα, NPM1
  - Down syndrome: 30% risk of acute megakaryocytic leukemia (M7), presenting around 2 years old. Much better prognosis with less need for chemotherapy and excellent response; however, there are increased treatment-related issues, including infections and sensitivity to chemotherapy, so generally this is treated on protocols with additional supportive therapies

- Worse prognostic indicators:
  - Monosomy 5, monosomy 7
  - Infant AML
  - AML arising from myelodysplastic syndrome (MDS)
  - FLT-3/ITD, although improving in the setting of directed therapy and bone marrow transplant options, still portends a poorer prognosis
- Transient myeloproliferative disorder (TMD): a preleukemic disorder that arises during fetal development and hematopoiesis in Down syndrome patients
  - Detectable in 10% to 30% of Down syndrome neonates; only ~10% are clinically evident, and 20% have silent cases
  - Generally diagnosed by presence of megakaryoblasts in peripheral smear
  - Majority (~80%) of cases spontaneously regress by 3 to 7 months of life
  - 20% to 30% of TMD cases will develop AML by 4 years of age (same morphology as AMKL, M7 AML)

CLINICAL PRESENTATION

- Most common presenting symptoms (similar presentation to ALL):
  - Fevers
  - Bone pain
  - Bruising, epistaxis
  - Pallor, anorexia, fatigue
- Physical examination findings:
  - Hepatosplenomegaly
  - Pallor
  - Petechiae
  - Uncommon, but unique association: gingival hypertrophy

DIAGNOSIS AND EVALUATION

- Laboratory studies and imaging:
  - Laboratory evaluation and need for chest x-ray are the same as previously described for ALL
  - Of note, in AML:
    - High WBC count in AML is much more conducive to effects of hyperviscosity and should be considered with WBC >150,000
    - There is a higher risk of bleeding with coagulopathy in AML than ALL
- Bone marrow biopsy and aspirate:
  - For leukemia, >25% of bone marrow with blasts is required. If between 5% and 25%, consider diagnosis of lymphoma. Look for Auer rods in blasts
- Lumbar puncture:
  - To evaluate for CNS disease; generally done with intrathecal injection of chemotherapy if diagnosis of leukemia is clear from peripheral blood

DIFFERENTIAL DIAGNOSIS

- Similar to ALL differential diagnosis, described previously

TREATMENT

- General principles:
  - Hyperhydration, alkalinization, allopurinol, watch for TLS
  - If febrile, evaluate for occult infection and administer antibiotics
  - Coagulopathy: correct coagulation abnormalities and DI
  - Generally includes 6 months of intensive chemotherapy. Each cycle is profoundly immunosuppressive and requires hospitalization until count recovery
- Unique complications:
  - Hyperleukocytosis: occurs in 5% to 22% AML patients
    - Symptoms include changes in mental status, headache, blurry vision, dizziness, stroke, seizure, cerebral hemorrhage, retinal vessel distention, dyspnea, hypoxia, priapism, or acidosis
    - Treatment requires pheresis if >200,000 or if symptoms are life-threatening
  - Neutropenia: more risk of prolonged neutropenia with AML
    - Opportunistic infections are the most common cause of death
  - Mediastinal mass: avoid sedation
    - If there are respiratory or cardiovascular symptoms, swiftly administer IV methylprednisolone and consider radiation therapy
- Chemotherapy pearls:
  - Induction chemotherapy includes daunomycin/cytarabine/etoposide
    - Remission induction rate of 70% to 85%
    - For acute promyelocytic leukemia, treat with all-trans retinoic acid (ATRA) with 80% survival
  - Due to daunomycin exposure, monitoring cardiac status is essential, especially for Down syndrome patients
  - Due to risk of relapse, there is a higher likelihood of requiring bone marrow transplant compared with ALL patients
- Relapse:
  - Predictors of relapse include karyotype, FLT2 status, and response to induction therapy
  - In relapse, salvage chemotherapy regimens are poor at providing second remission
  - Best hope of a cure remains bone marrow transplant, but patients should try to achieve a minimal residual disease negative complete remission before attempting because transplant-related toxicity remains high

Chronic Myeloid Leukemia (CML)

BASIC INFORMATION

- 3% of all pediatric leukemia; slight male predominance
- Translocation associated with disease is *BCR-ABL* fusion gene (Philadelphia chromosome)

CLINICAL PRESENTATION

- Most common presenting symptoms:
  - Asthenia (45%)
  - Splenic discomfort (20%–30%)
  - Weight loss (18%)
  - Bleeding (18%)
- Physical examination findings:
  - Palpable spleen (70%)
  - Palpable liver (15%)
  - Lymphadenopathy (10%)

DIAGNOSIS AND EVALUATION

- Laboratory studies:
  - Same studies as for acute leukemias, listed previously
- Bone marrow: evaluation recommended in almost all cases at diagnosis
- Evaluation of translocation:
  - Peripheral blood equivalent to bone marrow
    - Fluorescence in situ hybridization (FISH): fastest method to detect Philadelphia chromosome
    - Polymerase chain reaction (PCR): ensures detectable translocation present for monitoring
  - Bone marrow better than peripheral blood (easier to grow)
    - Karyotype: can detect Ph+ translocation not seen in FISH/PCR
    - Flow cytometry: least helpful for ruling in CML because it would show myeloid maturation, but good for quantifying blasts
- Classification of CML
  - Chronic phase:
    - No features of accelerated phase or blast crisis
  - Accelerated phase:
    - 15% to 29% blasts, ≥30% blasts + progranulocytes, basophilia ≥20%, platelets <100,000/µL, and cytogenetic clonal evolution
  - Blast crisis:
    - ≥30% blasts, extramedullary disease with localized immature blasts

TREATMENT

- Curative options:
  - Allogeneic transplant is the only proven curative option
  - Utilize tyrosine kinase inhibitors such as imatinib as a first-line agent
- Supportive principles:
  - Hyperviscosity: treat if symptomatic or if WBC is >100,000 and rising
  - Tumor lysis syndrome:
    - Allopurinol: maintain for 1 to 2 months after initiation of tyrosine kinase inhibitor or until sustained normalization of WBC count
    - Rasburicase: use if there is renal insufficiency

Juvenile Myelomonocytic Leukemia (JMML)

BASIC INFORMATION

- Considered an aggressive pediatric mixed MDS/myeloproliferative disorder (MPD)
- Epidemiology:
  - Constitutes 30% of MDS and 1% to 3% of childhood leukemia
  - Median age at presentation is 2 years old; most patients present by 6 years of age
  - Male predominance
- Genetics:
  - 70% to 85% of cases involved in RAS/MAPK pathway
  - 11% have NF1

- Poor prognostic factors:
  - Age >2 years
  - Thrombocytopenia (<33,000)
  - Elevated fetal hemoglobin levels (>15%)

CLINICAL PRESENTATION

- Most common presenting symptoms:
  - Pallor
  - Fever
  - Infection
  - Skin rash
  - Cough, diarrhea (secondary to infiltration into lungs and gastrointestinal tract)
- Physical examination findings:
  - Marked splenomegaly, moderate hepatomegaly
  - Lymphadenopathy

DIAGNOSIS AND EVALUATION

- Laboratory studies:
  - CBC + differential with peripheral blood smear
    - Look for anemia and thrombocytopenia (common)
  - Complete metabolic panel, including magnesium, phosphorus, uric acid, and LDH
- Lumbar puncture:
  - CNS involvement is rare
- Bone marrow:
  - Nonspecific findings, but consistent with myeloproliferative disease with hypercellularity; granulocytic and monocytic forms are predominant
- Diagnostic criteria:
  - Requires all of the following:
    - Absence of Philadelphia chromosome (BCR/ABL rearrangement)
    - Absolute monocyte count >1000/µL
    - <20% blasts in bone marrow
    - Splenomegaly
  - Requires at least one of the following:
    - Somatic mutation in PTPN11, K-RAS, or N-RAS
    - Clinical diagnosis of NF-1 or germline NF1 mutation
    - Germline CBL mutation and loss of heterozygosity of CBL
  - Or at least two of the following:
    - Monosomy 7 or other chromosomal abnormality
    - Increased fetal hemoglobin for age
    - Myeloid precursors on peripheral blood smear
    - Granulocyte-macrophage colony-stimulating factor (GM-CSF) hypersensitivity in colony assay
    - Hyperphosphorylation of STAT5

TREATMENT

- Chemotherapy is ineffective
- 13-Cis retinoic acid
  - Disease stabilizing; can lead to partial remission but not complete remission
- Hematopoietic stem cell transplant
  - 50% curative
  - However, 30% to 40% relapse rate, with median time to relapse of 4 to 6 months
  - Second transplant is of some benefit in this group

Table 61.2.	Summary of Pediatric Lymphomas	
	B-Cell	**T-Cell**
Immature	B lymphoblastic lymphoma	T lymphoblastic lymphoma
Mature	Hodgkin lymphoma Burkitt (and Burkitt-like) lymphoma Diffuse large B-cell lymphoma Primary mediastinal lymphoma Follicular lymphoma	Anaplastic large-cell lymphoma Peripheral T-cell lymphoma

LYMPHOMA

See Table 61.2

Hodgkin Lymphoma

BASIC INFORMATION

- Epidemiologic groups:
  - Hodgkin lymphoma is more common than non-Hodgkin lymphoma in pediatric patients >10 years old
  - Age: bimodal distribution of presentation; first peak in 20s and second peak in >50s
  - Associated with Epstein-Barr virus (EBV) infections
- Biology:
  - Origin: germinal center B-cell, clonal Ig gene rearrangement
  - Classic Hodgkin lymphoma (cHL):
    - Tumor cell: Reed-Sternberg cells
  - Nonlymphoproliferative Hodgkin disease (NLPHD):
    - Tumor cell: lymphocytic-histiocytic popcorn cells

CLINICAL PRESENTATION

- General presenting symptoms:
  - Painless, slow-growing, fixed, firm lymphadenopathy (classically supraclavicular)
  - Mediastinal involvement >65%
  - Horner syndrome, proptosis
  - Cough, orthopnea
  - Testicular or vaginal mass
  - Prognostic symptoms: systemic (B) symptoms (20%–30%)
    - Fever >38°C for 3 days, weight loss >10% within 6 months, drenching night sweats
  - Nonprognostic symptoms: anorexia, fatigue, pruritic, pain after drinking alcohol
  - Less common symptoms: abdominal symptoms, jaw symptoms, superior vena cava (SVC) syndrome, airway obstruction, tonsil and adenoids
- Physical examination findings:
  - Hepatosplenomegaly
  - Lymphadenopathy concerning for malignancy:
    - Cervical/axillary: >1 cm
    - Inguinal: >1.5 cm
    - Epitrochlear: >0.5 cm
    - Supraclavicular: any size
    - Abdominal/pelvic mass

DIAGNOSIS AND EVALUATION

- Laboratory studies:
  - CBC: may find leukocytosis with relatively low lymphocyte count
  - CMP: look at albumin for staging criteria
  - Erythrocyte sedimentation rate (ESR) and C-reactive protein (CRP): signs of inflammation; can be used to trend relapse later in monitoring
- Staging workup (Fig. 61.1):
  - Imaging: computed tomography (CT) of chest, abdomen, and pelvis; chest x-ray; positron emission tomography (PET) scan
  - Bilateral bone marrow biopsies: as with diagnosis of lymphoma, <25% bone marrow involvement is required
  - Staging:
    - 1: localized disease (single lymph node region or single organ)
    - 2: two or more lymph node regions on the same side of the diaphragm
    - 3: two or more lymph node regions both above and below the diaphragm
    - 4: widespread disease (multiple organs, with or without lymph node involvement)

DIFFERENTIAL DIAGNOSIS

- Infection:
  - Lymphadenitis
  - Viral infections (cytomegalovirus, EBV/infectious mononucleosis, HIV)
  - Bacterial infections (syphilis, toxoplasmosis, atypical and typical tuberculosis)
- Malignancy:
  - Non-Hodgkin lymphoma
  - Rhabdomyosarcoma
  - Other solid tumors
- Rheumatologic / Autoimmune Disease:
  - Sarcoidosis
  - Systemic lupus erythematosus
  - Kawasaki disease
  - Serum sickness
  - Immunodeficiencies

TREATMENT

- Chemotherapy
- Involved-field radiation therapy
- Relapse:
  - Consider autologous or allogeneic bone marrow transplantation
- Targeted therapies: brentuximab may be a useful targeted therapy for patients due to expression of CD30
- Prognostic scoring:
  - Childhood Hodgkin International Prognostic Score (CHIPS)
    - One point for each of the following:
      - Stage IV
      - Bulky disease (mediastinal mass >⅓ of thoracic cavity or >6 cm in length)
      - Albumin <3.5
      - Fever

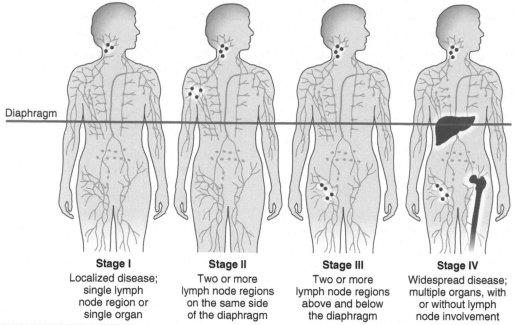

Fig. 61.1. Staging for Hodgkin lymphoma.

Stage I	Stage II	Stage III	Stage IV
Localized disease; single lymph node region or single organ	Two or more lymph node regions on the same side of the diaphragm	Two or more lymph node regions above and below the diaphragm	Widespread disease; multiple organs, with or without lymph node involvement

- CHIPS 0–1 → event-free survival 90%
- CHIPS 2 → event-free survival 78%
- CHIPS 3 → event-free survival 62%

Non-Hodgkin Lymphoma

BASIC INFORMATION

- Non-Hodgkin lymphoma is more common than Hodgkin lymphoma in pediatric patients <10 years old
- Major types include:
  - Burkitt lymphoma
  - lymphoblastic lymphoma (T-cell or B-cell), or
  - large-cell lymphoma diffuse large B-cell lymphoma, anaplastic
  - large-cell lymphoma
- Other rare lymphomas: follicular lymphoma, mucosa-associated lymphoid tissue lymphoma, nodal marginal zone lymphoma, primary cutaneous T-cell lymphoma, subcutaneous panniculitis-like T-cell lymphoma, mediastinal B-cell lymphoma
- Overall survival:
  - Non-Hodgkin overall: 70% to 95% depending on stage and histology
  - Lymphoblastic lymphoma: 90% overall survival for low-stage disease and 80% for high-stage disease
  - Burkitt lymphoma: 85% for all (lower with CNS disease)
  - Diffuse large B-cell lymphoma: >90% overall survival
  - Anaplastic large-cell lymphoma 70% to 85% overall survival
- Pathogenesis:
  - Immunodeficiencies: ataxia-telangiectasia, Wiskott-Aldrich syndrome, X-linked lymphoproliferative disease, AIDS, post-hematopoietic stem cell transplant, autoimmune lymphoproliferative syndrome (ALPS)
  - Infection: EBV (EBV-associated and Burkitt lymphoma account for 50% of all childhood cancers in equatorial Africa), human T-cell leukemia virus (HTLV)
  - Radiation
  - Post-therapy Hodgkin disease
  - Toxic: organic solvents, insecticides

CLINICAL PRESENTATION

- Burkitt lymphoma
  - Rapid growth, abdomen (intussusception), lymphadenopathy (retroperitoneal, mesentery), head and neck (jawbone/orbit—more so in endemic population), marrow/CNS
- Diffuse large B-cell lymphoma
  - Head and neck, mediastinum, lymphadenopathy, soft tissue (skin, bones, gastrointestinal tract), CNS (rare)
- Anaplastic large-cell lymphoma
  - 70% present in stages III–IV
  - Extranodal sites (skin, nodes, bones), primary systemic and primary cutaneous variants, much less likely to have systemic B symptoms (weight loss, fever, night sweats), CNS and marrow involvement are uncommon
- Lymphoblastic lymphoma
  - Lymphadenopathy (neck, supraclavicular, axillary), anterior mediastinum, effusions (pleural, pericardial), hepatosplenomegaly, marrow/CNS involvement

DIAGNOSIS AND EVALUATION

- General laboratory studies:
  - Due to rapid growth, watch for tumor lysis syndrome: CBC, CMP, magnesium, phosphorus, uric acid, LDH
- Burkitt lymphoma:
  - Phenotype: mature B cell
  - Histology: "starry sky" vacuoles
  - Unique features: EBV positive in endemic forms

- Diffuse large B-cell lymphoma: short, intensive chemotherapy
  - Phenotype: B-cell
  - Histology: large cells, increased cytoplasm
- Anaplastic large-cell lymphoma:
  - Phenotype: T-cell and null cell
  - Histology: "hallmark" cells have horseshoe- or kidney bean–shaped nucleus with prominent nucleoli, abundant cytoplasm, and prominent eosinophilic Golgi
  - Unique features: ALK positive
- Lymphoblastic lymphoma:
  - Phenotype: T cell > B cell
  - Histology: sheets of lymphoblasts

DIFFERENTIAL DIAGNOSIS

- Similar to Hodgkin lymphoma

TREATMENT

- Burkitt lymphoma: short, intensive chemotherapy with CNS prophylaxis

- Diffuse large B-cell lymphoma: short, intensive chemotherapy
- Anaplastic large-cell lymphoma: 2 to 6 months of therapy based on stage
- Lymphoblastic lymphoma: ALL-like therapy with induction, consolidation, intensification, and prolonged maintenance and CNS prophylaxis
- Targeted therapies: rituximab may be a useful targeted therapy for patients with mature B-cell phenotype, due to expression of CD20

Review Questions

For review questions, please go to ExpertConsult.com.

Suggested Reading

Hunger SP, Mullighan CG. Acute lymphoblastic leukemia in children. *N Engl J Med.* 2015;373:1541–1552.

Neuroblastoma and brain tumors encompass the most common solid tumors encountered in pediatric patients. Symptoms are dependent on the location of the tumor, and treatment varies based on the specific tumor type and stage. The role of the pediatrician in initial diagnosis and evaluation is paramount.

See also Nelson Textbook of Pediatrics, Chapter 498, "Neuroblastoma."

Neuroblastoma

BASIC INFORMATION

- Most common extracranial solid tumor in children
- Most common solid tumor of infancy
  - Median age: 18 months; 90% occur at age <10 years
  - Age <18 months portends better prognosis because many will spontaneously regress
- Genetic predisposition: rare, 1% to 2% of cases
  - *ALK* gain of function mutation in the majority of familial cases
  - *PHOX2B* mutation in cases associated with Hirschsprung disease and central hypoventilation
- Pathophysiology: arises from sympathetic nerve progenitor cells
  - 50% arise from the medulla of adrenal gland, but neuroblastomas can arise anywhere along the sympathetic nerve chain (e.g., paraspinal, mediastinum, neck)
- Staging: depends on age of diagnosis, location of disease, and genetic markers
- 50% to 70% of patients will have metastatic disease at diagnosis
  - Common sites of metastases include:
    - Regional lymph nodes
    - Bone marrow
    - Bone (e.g., orbits)
    - Liver and skin sites are more common in young infants with disease that regresses on its own
  - Genetic markers associated with poor prognosis: MYCN amplification, chromosome 11q loss, *ATRX* and *TERT* mutations

CLINICAL PRESENTATION

- Dependent on location/stage of tumor
  - Low-risk disease: often asymptomatic, and abdominal masses may be found incidentally
  - High-risk disease: fever, weight loss, abdominal distention, bone pain
  - Location of tumor/metastases can cause specific findings:

- Abdominal organ compression:
  - Bowel: constipation
  - Urinary system: retention, urinary tract infection (UTI)
  - Renal artery: hypertension
- Orbital lesion: proptosis or raccoon eyes
- Paraspinal with nerve root invasion: weakness/paraplegia
- Cervical chain: Horner syndrome
- Mediastinal: respiratory symptoms, laryngeal nerve compression/hoarseness
- Large liver metastases: respiratory distress (from abdominal competition), coagulopathy, renal impairment
- Paraneoplastic syndromes:
  - Opsoclonus-myoclonus syndrome
    - Opsoclonus: rapid involuntary conjugate movement of eyes in all directions
    - Myoclonus: irregular jerking of limbs/trunk
    - Ataxia and irritability are common
    - Caused by antineural antibodies attacking cerebellum
    - Usually associated with low-risk tumors
  - High-volume secretory diarrhea secondary to excessive vasoactive intestinal polypeptide (VIP) secretion
  - Secretion of catecholamines may cause flushing, headaches, palpitations, and hypertension

DIAGNOSIS AND EVALUATION

- Supportive laboratory findings
  - Complete blood count (CBC): often shows anemia, thrombocytopenia, or pancytopenia from metastatic disease
  - Liver function test (LFT) and coagulation studies: can be abnormal if liver metastases are present
  - Elevated ferritin
  - Elevated lactate dehydrogenase (LDH)
- Specific diagnostic testing
  - Urine or serum catecholamines (homovanillic acid [HVA], vanillylmandelic acid [VMA])
  - ^{123}I-metaiodobenzylguanidine (MIBG) scan
    - Radiolabeled MIBG—similar in structure to noradrenaline and taken up by tumor
    - 90% of neuroblastomas are MIBG avid
  - Biopsy of primary tumor
- Additional staging workup
  - Imaging:
    - Computed tomography (CT)/magnetic resonance imaging (MRI) of primary site, chest, abdomen, and pelvis
    - MIBG or PET scan if MIBG is nonavid
  - Bone marrow biopsy to evaluate for metastatic disease

TREATMENT

- Low-risk disease: patients <18 months of age without worrisome genetic findings
  - Can often observe only for regression
  - Occasionally need small amount of chemotherapy due to symptoms from primary tumor
    - Opsoclonus-myoclonus is treated with immuno-suppression: intravenous immunoglobulin (IVIG), rituximab, and steroids
  - If localized tumor and easily resectable, can also use surgery
  - Excellent overall survival
- Intermediate disease: large primary tumors, certain metastatic disease in age <18 months
  - Limited chemotherapy, and surgery if able
- High-risk disease: metastatic MYCN amplification
  - Intensive regimen involving chemotherapy, surgery, radiation, autologous stem cell transplant, and immunotherapy with GD2-directed antibody (dinutuximab)
  - High rate of relapse: up to 50%

Neuro-oncology

BASIC INFORMATION

- Pediatric brain tumors are a diverse group of tumors that occur in the central nervous system (CNS). Together they comprise the most common solid tumor in pediatrics and the second most common type of cancer overall (behind leukemia).
- 2016 update in World Health Organization classification
  - Generally divided by cell of origin
    - Neuroepithelial: gliomas, ependymomas
    - Embryonal
    - Meningeal
    - Cranial and paraspinal nerve tumors
    - Choroid plexus tumors
  - New classification includes not only histology (cell type of origin) but also molecular and genetic information
- Classically tumors also described based on location
  - Supratentorial: above the tentorium. Includes cerebrum, lateral and third ventricles, choroid plexus, hypothalamus, pineal gland, and optic nerve
  - Infratentorial: below the tentorium. Includes cerebellum, midbrain, pons, and medulla. Majority of pediatric tumors are infratentorial
  - Parasellar: around pituitary
  - Spinal: involving the spinal cord
- Predisposing conditions with increased risk of brain tumor:
  - Genetic predisposition syndromes (see Table 62.1)
  - Exposure to radiation
  - Immunodeficiency (either congenital or acquired) increases risk of primary CNS lymphoma

CLINICAL PRESENTATION

- Headache

Table 62.1. Genetic Predisposition Syndrome for Brain Tumors

Genetic Syndrome	Brain Tumors	Other Features of Syndrome
Neurofibromatosis (NF) 1	Optic pathway and other low-grade gliomas, malignant peripheral nerve sheath tumors	Café-au-lait spots, axillary and groin freckling, neurofibromas on skin, Lisch nodules on iris
NF2	Acoustic schwannomas, meningiomas, ependymomas	Juvenile cataracts
Tuberous sclerosis	Subependymal nodules and giant-cell astrocytomas	Ash leaf spots and shagreen patches on skin, angiofibromas on the face, angiomyolipomas in kidney, developmental issues, seizures
Turcot	Most often gliomas, but can also have medulloblastomas, ependymomas, astrocytomas	Polyps in colon
Gorlin	Medulloblastomas	Increased risk of basal cell carcinoma, pits in palms and soles, skeletal abnormalities, macrocephaly
Li Fraumeni	Astrocytomas, glioblastomas, medulloblastomas, choroid plexus carcinomas	Increased risk of breast cancer, osteosarcoma and other sarcomas, leukemia, and adrenocortical carcinoma
von Hippel-Lindau	Hemangioblastomas	Pancreatic and genitourinary tract cysts, increased risk of renal cell carcinoma and pheochromocytoma

- Nausea and vomiting, classically in the morning
  - Related to vasodilation of cerebral vessels overnight; leads to increased cerebral blood volume, followed by increased cerebrospinal fluid (CSF) production
- Macrocephaly in infants/toddlers
- Irritability
- Obstructive hydrocephalus (papilledema, vomiting, obtundation)
- Neurologic symptoms based on location:
  - Supratentorial
    - New seizure
    - Visual changes
      - Visual field defect: involvement of optic nerves or tracts
    - Diencephalic syndrome: severe emaciation and failure to thrive in an otherwise happy infant
      - From tumors in hypothalamus
  - Infratentorial
    - Ataxia, gait abnormalities
    - Nystagmus, especially with cerebellar tumors

- Parinaud syndrome: paralysis of up-gaze, pupils that are mid-dilated and poorly reactive to light, convergence or retraction nystagmus, and eyelid retraction
  - From pineal or dorsal midbrain tumors
  - Tumors compress the rostral interstitial nucleus of medial longitudinal fasciculus (riMLF) on the mesencephalic tectum
- Head tilt
- Obstructive hydrocephalus
- Resection of infratentorial tumors often leads to cerebellar mutism syndrome
  - After surgery, patients have mutism, irritability, ataxia, and hypotonia that last a few weeks to 6 months, followed by a period of dysarthria that eventually self-resolves
  - Occurs in up to 24% of patients with infratentorial resections, most commonly in medulloblastoma
- Parasellar
  - Endocrine dysfunction: either underproduction or overproduction of hormones
  - Visual field defects from growth upward into optic nerve
- Spinal
  - Weakness, pain

DIAGNOSIS AND EVALUATION

- Brain and spinal MRI
- CSF evaluation to look for metastatic cells
- Laboratory testing to work up secondary findings
  - Basic metabolic panel (BMP) and urinalysis (UA) to evaluate for diabetes insipidus
  - Thyroid-stimulating hormone (TSH), growth hormone (GH), prolactin, and other hormone levels if pituitary is involved
  - Alpha-fetoprotein (AFP) and beta–human chorionic gonadotropin (HCG) to evaluate for germ cell tumor
- Biopsy for definitive diagnosis

OVERVIEW OF SPECIFIC TUMORS

- Low-grade gliomas
  - Most common brain tumor in children
  - Neuroepithelial cell of origin
  - Generally slow growing, but based on location, can cause significant symptoms
    - Pilocytic astrocytoma:
      - Infratentorial, usually arising in cerebellum
      - Most common glioma in children
    - Optic nerve gliomas: associated with NF1
    - Diffuse fibrillary astrocytomas
- High-grade gliomas
  - Neuroepithelial cell of origin
  - Infratentorial: most often diffuse intrinsic pontine glioma (DIPG)
  - Supratentorial: anaplastic astrocytoma, glioblastoma multiforme (GBM)
- Medulloblastomas
  - Most common malignant (high-grade) brain tumors in children
  - Embryonal cell of origin

- Arise in cerebellum
- Can be metastatic to bone marrow (bone marrow biopsy required as part of workup)
- Parasellar tumors
  - Craniopharyngioma:
    - Arise from ectodermal remnants or Rathke cleft
    - In region of pituitary and hypothalamus
      - Endocrine issues are common
      - Visual findings if optic chiasm is involved
    - Skull film can show calcification in the sella turcica
    - Excellent prognosis: >90% survival
  - Pituitary adenoma
    - Anterior pituitary gland tumor
    - Benign
    - Microadenoma is <1 cm, and macroadenoma is >1 cm diameter
    - Nonsecreting tumors: 30%
      - Can be completely asymptomatic
      - May cause hypopituitarism from compression
    - Hormone-secreting tumors: 70%
      - Prolactinomas cause milk production and inhibit GnRH, resulting in diminished testicular/ovarian function
      - Gigantism/acromegaly from GH
      - Cushing disease from adrenocorticotropic hormone (ACTH)
      - Hyperthyroidism from TSH
- Germ cell tumors
  - Germinomas: most common, good prognosis
  - Nongerminomas
    - Some can produce hormones
      - Choriocarcinoma: beta-HCG (b-HCG)
      - Yolk sac tumor: AFP
- Ependymoma
  - Derived from ependymal cells that secrete CSF
  - 65% to 75% are infratentorial in childhood
  - Can be low grade or high grade
- Choroid plexus carcinoma
  - Mass in region of choroid plexus
  - Often causes hydrocephalus because it arises in ventricles
  - High-grade tumor, poor prognosis
- Atypical teratoid/rhabdoid tumors (ATRT)
  - Aggressive tumor that can arise anywhere in the CNS, usually in patients less than 3 years old
  - Caused by mutations in *SMARCB1*
    - Germline mutations in *SMARCB1* often result in multifocal tumors both inside the CNS and in the body (most commonly renal tumors)

TREATMENT

- Dexamethasone is used to relieve symptoms/brain edema
- Surgical resection when able
  - For low-grade tumors, resection alone may be curative
  - Ventriculoperitoneal (VP) shunts or ventriculostomies are often necessary
- Chemotherapy
- Radiation
- Notable exception:
  - Pituitary adenoma

- No need to treat microadenoma if not symptomatic
- Medical management of prolactinomas
  - Dopamine agonist: decreases size of adenoma and decreases prolactin
  - If prolactin levels do not normalize, proceed to surgical debulking

Review Questions

For review questions, please go to ExpertConsult.com

Suggested Readings

1. Maris JM. Recent advances in neuroblastoma. *N Engl J Med*. 2010;362:2202–2211.
2. Matthay KK, Maris JM, Schleiermacher G, et al. Neuroblastoma. *Nat Rev Dis Primers*. 2016;10(2):16078.
3. Segal D, Karajannis MA. Pediatric brain tumors: an update. *Curr Probl Pediatr Adolesc Health Care*. 2016;46(7):242–250.
4. Wells EM, Packer RJ. Pediatric brain tumors. *Continuum (Minneap Minn)*. 2015;21 (2 Neuro-oncology):373–396.

63 *Solid Tumors*

JESSICA FOSTER, MD

KIDNEY AND LIVER NEOPLASMS

Wilms Tumor (WT)

BASIC INFORMATION

- Also known as *nephroblastoma*
- Accounts for 95% of pediatric renal tumors
- Male-to-female ratio is 1:1
- Average age of presentation is 44 months for unilateral and 31 months for bilateral; usually does not present in neonates
- 10% of Wilms patients have a congenital anomaly or associated syndrome
  - Sporadic aniridia
  - Genitourinary (GU) malformation (e.g., cryptorchidism, hypospadias, horseshoe kidney)
  - Hemihypertrophy
  - Associated genetic syndromes and predisposition
    - See Table 63.1
    - Require monitoring ultrasounds every 3 months for development of WT starting at birth until at least age 8 years
  - See also *Nelson Textbook of Pediatrics*, Chapter 499, "Neoplasms of the Kidney"

CLINICAL PRESENTATION

- Typically presents as a painless abdominal mass incidentally found during a bath or at a pediatrician visit
  - 90% to 95% are unilateral (with increased incidence of bilateral tumors in predisposition syndromes)
  - Mass does not cross midline but often will penetrate renal capsule
- Other symptoms may include:
  - Abdominal pain (40%)
  - Blood in urine (18% gross, 24% microscopic)
  - Hypertension (25%)
  - Acquired von Willebrand disease (1%–8%)
    - Due to von Willebrand multimers binding to the tumor, reducing circulating amount
  - Inferior vena cava (IVC) obstruction
    - May present with varicocele (especially if spermatic vein compression) and prominent abdominal wall vessels
- Metastatic disease may occur in regional abdominal lymph nodes, lungs, or liver (rarely)
- Differential diagnosis
  - Other abdominal tumors: neuroblastoma, hepatoblastoma, sarcoma, lymphoma, germ cell tumor
  - Nephroblastomatosis: nonmalignant nephrogenic rests
    - Can be premalignant and eventually develop into Wilms tumor
    - Patients are monitored with serial imaging

OTHER RENAL TUMORS

- See Table 63.2
  - Mesoblastic nephroma: benign hamartoma that is the most common renal tumor in infants <3 months of age
    - Abdominal mass found incidentally on prenatal ultrasound or examination, hematuria. Less often can present with hypertension or anemia
    - Nephrectomy is usually curative
  - Clear-cell sarcoma: second most common pediatric renal tumor (~1–6 years old)
    - Aggressive cancer requiring surgery, chemotherapy, and radiation
    - Propensity to metastasize to bone and brain
  - Rhabdoid tumor:
    - Extremely aggressive, occurring in young children (mean age is 11 months)
    - Can also occur in the brain (called *atypical teratoid/rhabdoid tumor* [ATRT])
  - Renal cell carcinoma: most common renal tumor in adolescents
    - Presents with gross hematuria, flank pain, and/or mass
    - About half of patients present with metastases: nodes, lungs, liver

DIAGNOSIS AND EVALUATION

- Imaging
  - Renal/bladder ultrasound is the usual initial test
    - Should include Doppler to evaluate for vascular extension of the tumor because tumors can invade renal vessels and IVC
  - Computed tomography (CT) or magnetic resonance imaging (MRI) of the abdomen for definitive imaging
    - Solid, intrinsic renal mass that displaces normal renal parenchyma toward its rim = "claw sign"
    - Usually no calcifications, in contrast to neuroblastoma
  - Chest x-ray (CXR) and/or chest CT to evaluate for pulmonary metastases
  - Positron emission tomography (PET) imaging is usually not needed because disease is unlikely to spread outside the abdomen or chest
- Laboratory testing
  - Catecholamines to rule out neuroblastoma
  - Von Willebrand factor studies
- Biopsy
  - Usually attempt full excision/nephrectomy initially to ensure no tumor spillage if the tumor appears to be localized (stages 1–2)
  - Histologic subtypes

Table 63.1. Heritable Conditions Associated With Wilms Tumor

Syndrome/Condition Associated With Wilms	Genes Involved	Additional Clinical Manifestations	Overgrowth Phenotype
WAGR	*WT1*/del chromosome 11p13	**W**ilms tumor, **A**niridia, **G**enitourinary anomaly, mental **R**etardation	No
Denys-Drash	*WT1*	Genitourinary anomalies, pseudo-hermaphroditism, and/or renal disease	No
Beckwith-Wiedemann	*WT2*/chromosome 11p15 uniparental disomy	Hemihypertrophy, large tongue, omphalocele or umbilical hernia at birth, creases or pits in the skin near the ears, kidney abnormalities, and neonatal hypoglycemia	Yes
Perlman	*DIS3L2*/autosomal recessive chromosome 2q37	Fetal gigantism, renal dysplasia and nephroblastomatosis, islet cell hypertrophy, multiple congenital anomalies, and mental retardation	Yes
Familial Wilms tumor	*FWT1* (17q12-q21) and *FWT2* (19q13.4)/autosomal dominant	Genitourinary tract malformations	No

Table 63.2. Renal Tumors

Tumor Name	Age of Presentation	Presenting Symptoms	Metastatic Sites	Treatment Strategy
Wilms	2–5 years	Painless abdominal mass	Regional nodes, lungs, liver	Surgery and chemotherapy, with radiation if advanced
Mesoblastic nephroma	<1 year, median age 1–2 months	Abdominal mass (can be noted prenatally), hematuria	None/benign	Nephrectomy alone
Clear-cell carcinoma	1–6 years	Abdominal mass	Lungs, brain, bone	Surgery, chemotherapy, and radiation
Rhabdoid tumor	<3 years	Fever, hematuria	Lungs, brain (atypical teratoid/rhabdoid tumor)	Surgery, chemotherapy, and often radiation
Renal cell carcinoma	Adolescents	Hematuria, flank pain, abdominal mass	Regional nodes, lung, liver	Complete surgical resection including affected nodes

- Favorable histology: mimics triphasic development of a normal kidney, including blastemal, epithelial, and stromal cell types
- Anaplastic: polypoid mitotic figures, nuclear enlargement, and/or hyperchromasia
   Can be focal or diffuse, with diffuse conferring a worse prognosis

TREATMENT

- Staging and treatment are dependent on the degree of tumor extension beyond the kidney, the presence of metastatic disease, tumor histology, and the presence of bilateral tumors
   - Nephrectomy is usually indicated in WT, with the addition of chemotherapy (commonly vincristine and actinomycin, with doxorubicin, cyclophosphamide, and etoposide for higher stages)
   - Radiation therapy is also indicated in higher-stage disease
- Overall survival: 80% to 90% for favorable histology of any stage and as low as 30% to 40% for anaplastic stage IV

Hepatoblastoma

BASIC INFORMATION

- Most common pediatric liver malignancy; third most common abdominal tumor
- Usually presents before age 3 years; median age is 18 months
- Associated syndromes are detailed in Table 63.3

Table 63.3. Liver Tumor Associations

Hepatoblastoma	Hepatocellular Carcinoma
Beckwith-Wiedemann/hemihypertrophy	Chronic hepatitis B and C
Very low birth weight/prematurity	Alagille syndrome
Glycogen storage diseases	Glycogen storage diseases
Familial adenomatous polyposis	Tyrosinemia
Trisomy 18	Progressive familial intrahepatic cholestasis
	Wilson disease
	Hemochromatosis
	Autoimmune hepatitis

CLINICAL PRESENTATION

- Most commonly presents as abdominal distention and incidental mass
   - Rarely with nonspecific symptoms: weight loss, abdominal pain, decreased appetite, fever, vomiting, jaundice
- If hemorrhage or tumor rupture, can present with acute abdominal symptoms such as severe pain, vomiting, and anemia
- Very rarely precocious puberty or virilization from beta–human chorionic gonadotropin (beta-HCG) production in the tumor

DIAGNOSIS AND EVALUATION

- Laboratory testing
   - Liver enzymes and function

- Complete blood count (CBC) to evaluate for anemia
- Elevated alpha-fetoprotein (AFP) in >90% of tumors
- Beta-HCG may also be elevated
- Imaging
  - Ultrasound will reveal mass centered in the liver
  - CT or MRI is most useful
    - Determines pretreatment extent of disease (PRE-TEXT) staging
      - Liver is divided into four sections, and tumors are graded I–IV depending on how many sections are involved
    - CT of chest to evaluate for metastatic disease
- Biopsy
  - Pure fetal histology—excellent prognosis
  - Various mixed subtypes—majority of tumors
  - Small-cell undifferentiated—poor prognosis

TREATMENT

- Surgery is preferred for lower stages (I or II), but higher stages may require neoadjuvant chemotherapy before resection
- Chemotherapy regimens commonly include cisplatin, doxorubicin, vincristine, and 5-fluorouracil (5FU)
- Liver transplant is necessary for nonresectable tumors

Hepatocellular Carcinoma

BASIC INFORMATION

- Second most common liver tumor
- Usually occurs in older children/adolescents
- Associated with various liver diseases (see Table 63.3)

CLINICAL PRESENTATION

- Abdominal mass with pain
- Early satiety
- If extension of tumor into hepatic or portal veins: arteriovenous shunting and gastrointestinal (GI) bleeding
- With advanced disease: jaundice, weight loss, fever
- Hepatic failure is usually reflective of underlying liver disease (if present)
  - Coagulopathy, ascites, encephalopathy
- Can also present with paraneoplastic syndrome
  - Hypoglycemia
  - Erythrocytosis
  - Hypercalcemia
  - Watery diarrhea
  - Various cutaneous manifestations

DIAGNOSIS AND EVALUATION

- Laboratory testing:
  - Liver function and enzymes
  - AFP is elevated in 55% to 65% of cases
- Imaging:
  - Abdominal ultrasound is usually performed first
  - CT/MRI of abdomen is preferred

TREATMENT

- Surgery: complete resection is essential
- Chemotherapy: cisplatin and doxorubicin are often used adjuvantly/neoadjuvantly
- Antiviral therapy for tumors arising from hepatitis B

Germ Cell Tumors

BASIC INFORMATION

- Can occur in gonads or extragonadal
  - Two-thirds of cases occur outside of gonads
- Gonadal tumor predisposition:
  - Klinefelter syndrome
  - Turner syndrome
  - Cryptorchidism
- Divided into:
  - Teratoma
    - Mature
    - Immature
  - Malignant germ cell tumors
    - Seminomas/dysgerminomas (testes/ovary)
    - Yolk sac tumor
    - Choriocarcinoma
    - Gonadoblastoma
    - Mixed

CLINICAL PRESENTATION

- Gonadal: abdominal pain, mass, swelling
- Extragonadal: usually occur in the midline (sacrococcygeal, mediastinal, retroperitoneal) with symptoms from mass effect

DIAGNOSIS AND EVALUATION

- Laboratory testing: lactate dehydrogenase (LDH), AFP, beta-HCG
- Imaging: MRI of pelvis, CT of chest, PET to evaluate for distant metastasis

TREATMENT

- Surgical resection
- Chemotherapy: cisplatin, etoposide, bleomycin

MESENCHYMAL TUMORS (BONE AND MUSCLE)

Osteosarcoma

BASIC INFORMATION

- See Table 63.4
- Most common malignant bone tumor
- More common in males than in females
- Slightly more common in African-Americans than in Caucasians

Table 63.4. Comparison of Bone Tumors

	Osteosarcoma	Ewing Sarcoma
Age	Adolescent	10–20-year-olds
Location	Femur > tibia > humerus	Lower extremity > pelvis > chest wall
Area of bone	Metaphysis (with "sunburst" appearance)	Diaphysis (with "onion skin" appearance)
Classic genetic finding	None	EWSR1-FLI1 fusion (t11,22)
Treatment	Surgery and chemotherapy	Surgery or radiation, and chemotherapy

- Bimodal age distribution
  - Peak incidence is during adolescence/time of growth spurt
  - Second peak occurs in adulthood around sixth decade
- Most commonly occurs in metaphysis of long bones
  - Distal femur > proximal tibia > humerus
  - 50% occur around the knee

CLINICAL PRESENTATION

- Unilateral bone pain
  - This is in contrast to "growing pains," which are usually bilateral and occur at night
- Pathologic fracture
- Palpable hard mass/swelling
- Rarely erythematous (mimicking infection)

DIAGNOSIS AND EVALUATION

- Imaging
  - X-ray: periosteal new bone formation (described as a "sunburst")
  - MRI of affected bone
  - CT of chest to evaluate for metastatic spread
    - Lung is most common site of metastasis; 15% at time of diagnosis
  - Bone scan/PET to evaluate for other metastatic disease
    - Other bones are second most common site
- Biopsy is required for diagnosis

TREATMENT

- Surgical resection is required
  - Amputation or limb-sparing surgery
  - Radiation is not effective in fully eradicating
- Neoadjuvant and adjuvant chemotherapy are also necessary for cure because 80% of patients have micrometastatic disease
  - Methotrexate, doxorubicin, and cisplatin

Ewing Sarcoma

BASIC INFORMATION

- Second most common bone tumor
  - Lower extremity > pelvis > chest wall
  - Can also arise outside of bone

- Peaks in second decade of life
- Nine times more common in Caucasians than in African-Americans
- Caused by translocation of *EWS* gene
  - 85% include *EWSR1-FLI1* fusion from t(11,22)

CLINICAL PRESENTATION

- Pain, dependent on site
- Pathologic fracture
- Constitutional symptoms are more common in metastatic disease
- Due to marrow involvement, can have pancytopenia

DIAGNOSIS AND EVALUATION

- Laboratory testing
  - LDH is important because it offers prognostic information
- Imaging
  - X-ray: destructive diaphyseal bone lesion sometimes accompanied by periosteal reaction (described as "onion skinning")
  - MRI of involved area
  - CT of chest
  - PET scan for evaluation of distant metastasis
- Bone marrow aspiration and biopsy
  - To evaluate for metastatic disease

TREATMENT

- Local control
  - Surgery is preferred
  - Radiation therapy is also effective; used in patients with unresectable disease
- Chemotherapy is necessary because all patients are assumed to have micrometastatic disease
  - Vincristine, doxorubicin, cyclophosphamide, ifosfamide, and etoposide
- Prognostic factors
  - Improved outcomes in the young, in females, and for extraskeletal tumors
  - Elevated LDH—worse prognosis

Osteoid Osteoma

BASIC INFORMATION

- Common benign bone tumor
- Usually long bones of the lower extremity
- More common in boys than in girls

CLINICAL PRESENTATION

- Pain that is usually worse at night

DIAGNOSIS AND EVALUATION

- X-ray reveals central radiolucent area surrounded by thick sclerotic bone
- MRI is necessary to fully characterize
- Biopsy for definitive diagnosis and to rule out malignancy

TREATMENT

- Most resolve on their own but may take several years
- For painful lesions
  - Analgesics: nonsteroidal antiinflammatory drugs (NSAIDs), Tylenol
  - CT-guided radiofrequency ablation

Rhabdomyosarcoma

BASIC INFORMATION

- Most common soft tissue sarcoma
- Derived from primitive mesenchymal cells
  - Cells that normally develop into muscle, fat, fibrous tissue, bone, or cartilage
- Usually occurs within first decade of life
- Can occur anywhere in the body
  - Most common sites include head/neck, GU tract, and extremities
- Genetic predisposition to develop rhabdomyosarcoma
  - Li-Fraumeni (p53)
  - Neurofibromatosis (NF) 1
  - Pleuropulmonary blastoma (*DICER1* mutations)
  - Beckwith-Wiedemann syndrome
    - WT and hepatoblastoma are more common
  - Costello syndrome
  - Noonan syndrome

CLINICAL PRESENTATION

- Mass effect from location of the tumor
- Sometimes pain, depending on location
- Location varies with age
  - Infants can have botryoid variant, which arises in mucous membranes
    - Often vaginal: looks like "cluster of grapes"
  - School-age children will most often have orbital tumors: head or neck
  - Adolescents/older children often have extremity lesions: hand or foot

DIAGNOSIS AND EVALUATION

- Imaging
  - MRI of primary site
    - Certain sites are considered favorable and have better prognosis
      - Orbit
      - Nonparameningeal head and neck
      - GU tract other than kidney, bladder, and prostate
      - Biliary tract
  - CT of chest and PET scan for metastatic disease
- Biopsy: histology and molecular characterization ("fusion negative," "fusion positive") guide therapy and prognosis

TREATMENT

- Surgery: often done first if feasible
- Chemotherapy
  - Intensity depends on staging
- Radiotherapy
  - Most patients require radiation for additional local control, unless a patient has localized fusion-negative/embryonal tumor that is fully resected

Review Questions

For review questions, please go to ExpertConsult.com.

Suggested Readings
1. Aronson DC, Meyers RL. Malignant tumors of the liver in children. *Semin Pediatr Surg.* 2016;25(5):265–275.
2. Lowe LH, et al. Pediatric renal masses: Wilms tumor and beyond. *RadioGraphics.* 2000;20:1585–1603.
3. Williams RF, Fernandez-Pineda I, Gosain A. Pediatric sarcomas. *Surg Clin North Am.* 2016;96(5):1107–1125.

64 *Selected Topics in Oncology*

JESSICA B. FOSTER, MD, ARUN GURUNATHAN, MD and
MALA K. TALEKAR, MD

In this chapter, we will review complications that can be encountered during the presentation, progression, and treatment of childhood cancers. Many of these complications are considered "oncologic emergencies," requiring prompt institution of treatment and fastidious monitoring. Consequently, a key factor in the treatment of such emergencies is their prompt recognition, which may depend on facets of the patient's medical history (Table 64.1).

COMPLICATIONS IN THE EARLY COURSE OF THE MALIGNANCY

Superior Vena Cava Syndrome (SVCS) and Superior Mediastinal Syndrome (SMS)

BASIC INFORMATION

- SVCS refers to signs and symptoms resulting from compression, obstruction, invasion, or thrombosis of superior vena cava (SVC) precluding the venous blood return
- When tracheal compression also occurs, the term SMS is used
- Airway obstruction complicates pediatric mediastinal masses frequently (60%); children are at increased risk because their tracheas and bronchi are compressible with smaller intraluminal diameters
- Mediastinal masses in children can cause simultaneous compression/obstruction of vasculature as well as airway; hence SVCS and SMS are often used interchangeably

ETIOLOGY

- Most common primary cause: malignant mediastinal masses
  - Leukemia, lymphoma, rhabdomyosarcoma, neuroblastoma, and germ cell tumors are most common diagnoses
- Most common secondary cause: thrombotic complications of cardiovascular surgery and occlusion of central venous catheters

CLINICAL PRESENTATION

- Symptoms can be gradual or sudden and depend on the level of obstruction

- Signs/symptoms of vascular involvement:
  - Facial edema, plethora; cyanotic facies with venous engorgement of the neck, arms, and chest; and development of collateral blood vessels in the upper part of the body
  - In sudden cases of SVCS, a child could present with shock caused by reduced ventricular volume from decreased venous return
- Signs/symptoms of airway compromise:
  - Stridor indicates upper airway obstruction (i.e., extrathoracic involvement)
  - Lower airway obstruction is heralded by cough, wheezing, dyspnea, and orthopnea
- Pleural and/or pericardial effusion(s) may be present

DIAGNOSIS AND EVALUATION

- In children with palpable lymph nodes who present with tachypnea, malignancy (mediastinal mass) should be considered if symptoms worsen with bending or supine position
- Plain chest radiographs (CXRs) can confirm a mediastinal mass in 97% of cases; lateral CXRs show anterosuperior mediastinal widening, often with tracheal compression or deviation
- Computed tomography (CT) and/or magnetic resonance imaging (MRI) scan of the chest can characterize the mass and may be useful in assessing the airway and extent of thrombosis and collateral circulation; however, imaging may be difficult to obtain in a child with positional respiratory compromise, especially if sedation is required

Table 64.1. Historical Information Contributing to Diagnosis and Management of Oncologic Emergencies in Children

Historical Information	Helpful for
The type of cancer	Can point to specific anticipated complications
Last chemotherapy received	Specific anticipated side effects of the chemotherapy received
Time since last chemotherapy	Duration of expected neutropenia, likelihood of infection
Presence of indwelling central/peripheral lines, port, other catheters	Blood cultures and other blood tests; risk of central line-associated bloodstream infection, risk of thrombosis
Previous complications, surgeries	Risk of recurrent complications
Most recent blood counts	Anticipation of cytopenias

- Imaging also helps in detection of concomitant pleural and/or pericardial effusions
- Complete blood count (CBC) with differential might help with diagnosis as two-thirds of children presenting with mediastinal masses have leukemia or lymphoma
- Other supportive blood and urine tests:
  - Chemistry panel, uric acid, lactic dehydrogenase (LDH), and erythrocyte sedimentation rate (ESR) can point toward a malignancy diagnosis
  - Alpha-fetoprotein (AFP) and beta-human chorionic gonadotropin (β-HCG) are elevated in germ cell tumors
  - Urine catecholamines are elevated in neuroblastoma

TREATMENT

- Principles of management:
  - Three main principles of management of SVCS/SMS:
    - Prompt diagnosis
    - Prevention of progression to respiratory distress (Table 64.2)
    - Definitive treatment of primary cause

Spinal Cord Compression (SCC)

BASIC INFORMATION

- In childhood cancers, SCC can be a presenting symptom of a malignancy, a result of late metastases, or an isolated recurrence of a previous tumor

Table 64.2. Prevention of Progression to Respiratory Distress

- Elevation of head of the bed/keep patient in sitting/upright position
- Keep the child calm, apply supplemental oxygen, and may consider gentle diuresis
- Achieve IV access; obtain blood for laboratory tests (as noted previously), hydration with IV fluids
- Avoid sedation
- Endotracheal intubation may be required in the event of a life-threatening obstruction; however, the obstruction may be beyond the reach of the endotracheal tube; therefore these patients require preemptive emergency planning for the event of respiratory or cardiac collapse
- In case of thrombosis- related SVCS remove intravascular device; consider anticoagulation, stenting where necessary
- Pleurocentesis/pericardiocentesis for immediate (short-term) therapeutic relief and diagnostic material
- Monitoring for and management of tumor lysis syndrome (see details under section Tumor Lysis Syndrome)
- Tissue diagnosis: should be made as soon as possible; assess risk for anesthesia and if low, proceed with biopsy (bone marrow aspiration and biopsy/peripheral lymph node biopsy/thoracocentesis of mediastinal mass); if high risk, proceed with temporizing empiric chemotherapy and/or radiation therapy (pending stability for anesthesia)
  - Empiric chemotherapy usually comprises a combination of steroids with drugs such as vincristine and cyclophosphamide commonly referred to by the acronym COP [cyclophosphamide, oncovin (vincristine), prednisone]
  - Important to note: prebiopsy empiric chemotherapy and/or radiotherapy may render subsequent histologic specimens uninterpretable

IV, Intravenous; *SVCS,* superior vena cava syndrome.

- SCC can result in permanent neurologic impairment if treatment is delayed even by a few hours
- SCC has been seen in about 10% of pediatric patients with solid tumors

ETIOLOGY

- SCC related to solid tumors (e.g., neuroblastoma) and soft tissue tumors (e.g., Ewing sarcoma, rhabdomyosarcoma) are usually extradural
- Other tumors that can cause SCC include osteosarcomas, Hodgkin disease, non-Hodgkin lymphoma, germ cell tumors, and hepatoma (rarely)
- In most cases of malignancy-related SCC, cord compression occurs because of local extension of disease from paravertebral tumor sites
- The soft tissue tumor invades the spinal canal via the neural foramina, compressing the spinal cord in a circumferential manner
- Rarely, primary astrocytoma and ependymomas can present as intramedullary lesions
- Compression of vertebral vasculature by epidural location of a tumor can lead to vasogenic cord edema, venous hemorrhage, loss of myelin, and ischemia

CLINICAL PRESENTATION

- The most common presenting symptom of SCC is back pain, which could be localized or radicular and occurs in 80% of children with SCC
  - A child with cancer, presenting with back pain, even in the absence of neurologic findings, should be presumed to have SCC until proven otherwise
  - The pain may be aggravated by movement, neck flexion, straight-leg raising, or Valsalva maneuver
- Other symptoms:
  - Lower extremity weakness
  - Urinary retention and incontinence
  - Gait anomalies, sensory deficits, and pain that increase with percussion of the vertebral bodies might be difficult to elicit in a preverbal/preambulatory child

DIAGNOSIS AND EVALUATION

- When SCC is suspected, a thorough neurologic examination and immediate imaging is warranted
- Weakness, if present, is usually symmetric
- MRI is the preferred imaging modality; the entire spine should be imaged irrespective of the clinically suspected level of SCC to localize the cause and to determine and characterize the current extent of the tumor and further potential invasion
- Although plain films may show lytic/sclerotic lesions in adjacent bones, enlargement of neural foramina, and/or calcifications within a mass around the spine, they are only diagnostic in about 30% to 35% of cases
- Examination of cerebrospinal fluid (CSF) provides nonspecific information (cell count is usually normal), and lumbar puncture (LP) may involve the risk of coning and further neurologic deterioration and should be performed under very close monitoring

TREATMENT

- Neuronal ischemia can result in irreversible loss of function; treatment of SCC should not be postponed awaiting diagnostic certainty
- On suspicion of SCC, intravenous (IV) dexamethasone, 1 to 2 mg/kg may be immediately administered followed by emergent MRI study
  - If lymphoproliferative disease is suspected as the likely etiology, then local radiation may be preferred
- Decompressive laminectomy is an effective surgical approach depending on imaging characteristics and also provides tissue for diagnosis
- Chemotherapy initiation in chemosensitive tumors such as neuroblastoma, non-Hodgkin and Hodgkin lymphoma, and Ewing sarcoma is also helpful
- Prognosis for neurologic recovery depends on the extent of disability at presentation which, in turn, depends on duration of symptoms and time to diagnosis from symptom onset

COMPLICATIONS ON TREATMENT INITIATION

Tumor Lysis Syndrome (TLS)

BASIC INFORMATION

- TLS refers to a group of electrolyte and metabolic derangements resulting from the rapid release of intracellular ions (potassium, phosphorus, etc.), nucleic acids, proteins, and their metabolites into the extracellular space from lysed malignant cells
  - Common metabolic derangements in TLS include hyperuricemia, hyperkalemia, hyperphosphatemia, hypocalcemia, and uremia

- TLS can lead to renal insufficiency, cardiac arrhythmias, seizures, and neurologic complications and potentially be fatal; anticipation, prevention, early recognition, and prompt aggressive management are essential

ETIOLOGY

- TLS is most prevalent in malignancies that are highly proliferative and have a high tumor burden (e.g., leukemia, lymphoma)
  - Especially prevalent in B-cell acute lymphoblastic leukemia (ALL), T-cell leukemia, and Burkitt lymphoma
  - It has been documented rarely with solid tumors such as stage IV neuroblastoma and medulloblastoma
- Predisposing risk factors are preexisting renal impairment, elevated pretreatment uric acid levels, elevated levels of LDH, SVCS, pleural effusions, ascites, and cerebral edema

CLINICAL PRESENTATION

- Commonly present within 12 to 72 hours of initiation of cytotoxic therapy but might also manifest spontaneously (before start of cytotoxic therapy)
- Common symptoms/signs and specific abnormalities with their causes, recommended monitoring, and management are outlined in Table 64.3

Febrile Neutropenia

BASIC INFORMATION

- Fever defined as a single temperature greater than 38.3°C or sustained temperature greater than 38°C for 1 hour (Infectious Diseases Society of America)
  - Note: do not use rectal thermometer in neutropenic patients because trauma to mucosa can increase risk of infection

Table 64.3. Signs and Symptoms of Tumor Lysis Syndrome in Children

General symptoms/signs: abdominal pain, distension, anorexia, nausea, vomiting, lethargy, back pain, edema, fluid overload, congestive heart failure, cardiac dysrhythmias, seizures, muscle cramps, spasms, tetany, altered mental status, syncope, and sudden death

	Specific Abnormalities		
Abnormality	Symptoms/causes	Laboratory data/monitoring	Management
Renal insufficiency	Reduced/absent urine output, dysuria/hematuria, hypertension, altered mental status Cause: precipitation of uric acid and calcium phosphate crystals in renal tubules and microvasculature of kidneys leading to acute renal failure/renal insufficiency	Monitor urine output every 4–8 hours, urine pH, blood gases, serum chemistries, ionized calcium	■ Avoid nephrotoxic medications ■ Adjust dosages of renally excreted drugs ■ Fluid and electrolyte management ■ Hydration and alkalinization: IV D5 1/2NS + 40 mEq $NaHCO_3$ at two to four times the maintenance rate ■ Goal urine pH: 7–8 ■ Dialysis, hemofiltration may be necessary, especially if the patient becomes anuric ■ Consider diuretics (e.g., furosemide, mannitol)
Hyperphosphatemia	Pruritus, arthritis, iritis Cause: release of intracellular phosphate from malignant cells (which can contain up to 4x more phosphate then normal cells); worsened by acidosis	Moderate >5 mg/dL Severe usually associated with hypocalcemia	Moderate: ■ Avoid IV phosphate administration ■ Phosphate binders (e.g., aluminum hydroxide, sevelamer) Severe: ■ Dialysis, continuous renal replacement therapy (CRRT)

Continued

Table 64.3.   Signs and Symptoms of Tumor Lysis Syndrome in Children—cont'd

	Specific Abnormalities		
Abnormality	*Symptoms/causes*	*Laboratory data/monitoring*	*Management*
Hyperkalemia	Weakness, ECG changes Cause: rapid release of intracellular contents from malignant cells, exacerbated by renal insufficiency and acidosis	Moderate: >5.5 to 6.0 mmol/L Severe: >6.0 to 7.0 mmol/L; or symptomatic	Moderate and asymptomatic: ■ ECG and cardiac rhythm monitoring ■ Sodium polystyrene sulfonate ■ Consider loop diuretics Severe and/or symptomatic: ■ Same as previously mentioned, plus ■ Calcium gluconate 100–200 mg/kg IV and/or ■ D25 (2 mL/kg) IV with regular insulin (0.1 unit/kg) IV ■ Albuterol ■ Dialysis/CRRT
Hypocalcemia	Vomiting, cramps, carpopedal spasm, tetany, seizures Cause: calcium phosphate crystal precipitation in microvasculature	<6 mg/dL	Asymptomatic: ■ No therapy Symptomatic: ■ Calcium gluconate 50–100 mg/kg IV
Hyperuricemia	Lethargy, nausea, vomiting Cause: breakdown of intracellular components	Serum creatinine > 1.5x ULN *or* Uric acid >7 mg/dL	Allopurinol: ■ PO 300 mg/m^2/day or 10 mg/kg/day ■ IV: 200 mg/m^2/day (maximum 600 mg/day) Rasburicase: ■ 0.15–0.2 mg/kg/day IV daily up to 5 days (alkalinization not required, expensive; contraindicated in glucose 6-phosphate dehydrogenase deficiency)
Hyponatremia	SIADH	Na: <130 mEq/L Serum osmolality: <280 mOsm/L Urine osmolality: >500 mOsm/L	Fluid restriction Consider loop diuretics
Hypercalcemia	—	Mild: >10.5–11.9 mg/dL Moderate: >12–13.9 mg/dL Severe: >14 mg/dL	Monitor ionized calcium, serum pH, potassium, magnesium and phosphorus; obtain ECG; IVF; bisphosphonate (pamidronate, zoledronate)

CRRT, continuous renal replacement therapy; *ECG*, electrocardiogram; *IV*, intravenous; *IVF*, Intravenous Fluids; *NS*, normal saline; *po*, by mouth; *SIADH*, syndrome of inappropriate antidiuretic hormone secretion; *ULN*, upper limit of normal.

■ Neutropenia defined as absolute neutrophil count (ANC) less than 1500
  ■ <500 is severe and highest risk for complications
  ■ Patient also considered neutropenic if ANC is falling and expected to fall below 500 within 48 hours
■ Life-threatening complication because of high risk of bacteremia and infectious complications
  ■ Prolonged neutropenia >7 days or recurrent neutropenia are at highest risk

ETIOLOGY

■ Direct effect of chemotherapy on the immune system and mucosal barriers
■ Most common cause is thought to be translocation of bacterial flora from gastrointestinal (GI) tract
  ■ Other sources include cellulitis, pneumonia, or other focal infection
  ■ Indwelling central line also a common nidus for infection
■ Infectious source identified only 10% to 40% of the time
  ■ 10% to 25% of patients show documented bacteremia
  ■ Gram-positive slightly more common than Gram-negative
  ■ See Table 64.4 for pathogens

Table 64.4.   Common Pathogens in Febrile Neutropenia

Bacterial Gram-positive Gram-negative	Staph epidermidis Staph aureus (including methicillin resistant) Streptococci (including viridans streptococcus) Enterococci
	Pseudomonas Enterobacteriaceae (including *Escherichia coli* and *Klebsiella* species)
Fungal	*Candida* *Aspergillus* Mucormycosis *Pneumocystis jirovecii*
Viral	Human herpesviruses (including HSV, VSV, CMV, and EBV) Respiratory viruses (including influenza)

CMV, Cytomegalovirus; *EBV*, Epstein–Barr virus; *HSV*, herpes simplex virus; *VSV*, vesicular stomatitis virus.

CLINICAL PRESENTATION

■ Fever
■ Can progress rapidly to sepsis
  ■ Tachycardia, tachypnea, hypotension, delayed capillary refill, and end-organ damage
■ Evidence of local infection, if present

DIAGNOSIS AND EVALUATION

- Laboratory tests
  - CBC with differential
  - Blood culture
  - Comprehensive metabolic panel (CMP) to evaluate renal and hepatic function
  - Additional testing based on signs/symptoms
    - Viral polymerase chain reaction (PCR)
    - Stool studies including *Clostridium difficile* toxin assay
    - Culture of any drainage or purulence
- Imaging as needed based on symptoms
  - CXR if hypoxic or respiratory symptoms
  - Abdominal films for belly pain
  - CT sinus, chest, abdomen, and pelvis if concerned for fungal infection
- Biopsy of suspicious lesions may be indicated to rule out fungal disease

TREATMENT

- Acute management
  - Broad-spectrum antibiotics to cover Gram-positive and Gram-negative bacteria
    - Prompt administration improves outcomes
    - Continue therapy until neutrophil count is recovered or until treatment of identified source of infection is complete (whichever is longer)
    - Most patients will be admitted for IV antibiotic therapy (e.g., vancomycin and cefepime)
    - Some patients deemed to be low risk can be treated as outpatient with oral antibiotics
      Low-risk criteria includes well appearing, expected neutropenia will be <7 days, no comorbid conditions, no renal or hepatic impairment, and no dehydration or vital sign changes
  - Antifungal agent added if clinical symptoms suspicious, or fever persistent >5 days after initiation of antibiotics
  - Antiviral agents added if clinical concern
  - Management of sepsis or other complications as needed
  - Use of granulocyte colony-stimulating factor (G-CSF) acutely is controversial, but may be indicated for prolonged or complicated febrile neutropenia
- Prophylaxis
  - G-CSF administered with most chemotherapy regimens to reduce duration of chemotherapy-induced neutropenia
  - Patients anticipated to have prolonged neutropenia are treated empirically with bacterial and fungal prophylaxis at the time of neutropenia
    - Acute myeloid leukemia (AML)
    - Bone marrow transplant
  - Bactrim typically administered for *Pneumocystis jiroveci* pneumonia (PJP) prophylaxis in all patients

Typhlitis

BASIC INFORMATION

- Also called neutropenic enterocolitis
- Microbial infection leading to necrosis of the bowel wall

- Usually starts at the cecum and extends to the ileum and up the ascending colon, although all parts of the large and small intestine can be involved

ETIOLOGY

- Exact pathogenesis unknown
  - Multiple factors contribute including:
    - Mucosal damage from chemotherapeutic agent
    - Impaired host immune system with profound neutropenia
- Often polymicrobial infection:
  - Gram-negative bacilli
  - Gram-positive cocci
  - Anaerobes
  - *Candida*
- Predilection for cecum likely caused by relatively decreased vascular supply compared with other parts of the colon, and increased distensibility

CLINICAL PRESENTATION

- Occurs in the setting of severe neutropenia: ANC < 500
  - Typically 1 to 2 weeks after chemotherapy
- Common symptoms include fever and abdominal pain
  - Can mimic appendicitis
  - Other symptoms may include abdominal distension, diarrhea, nausea, vomiting, and hematochezia
- Peritoneal signs indicate bowel perforation
- May see evidence of widespread mucositis in the mouth and throat

DIAGNOSIS AND EVALUATION

- While abdominal X-rays are often obtained to screen for typhlitis, CT of the abdomen is the gold standard for diagnosis
  - Shows bowel-wall thickening
  - Can also show mesenteric stranding, bowel dilatation, mucosal enhancement, and pneumatosis
- Obtain blood cultures because bacteremia from gut microbial translocation is common
- Obtain stool cultures including *C. difficile* toxin assay

TREATMENT

- Uncomplicated enterocolitis can be managed conservatively
  - Bowel rest, nasogastric (NG) sump, broad-spectrum antibiotics, fluid resuscitation, and nutrition support
  - Antibiotics typically used include piperacillin-tazobactam, imipenem, or ceftazidime/cefepime plus metronidazole
  - Include metronidazole or vancomycin to cover *C. difficile* until ruled out
  Antifungal coverage added if patient remains febrile/ill after 72 hours of antibacterial coverage
  - G-CSF can be added to improve neutropenia in severely ill patients
    - Use is controversial because data are lacking
  - Complicated enterocolitis may need surgical intervention

■ Perforation, abscess formation, or excessive bleeding not resolving with blood product replacement
■ If surgery is indicated, all necrotic bowel must be removed

Mucositis

BASIC INFORMATION

■ Sloughing of epithelial lining that occurs as a side effect after chemotherapy administration
■ Can occur anywhere along the GI tract from mouth to anus
■ Increased risk of infection caused by disruption of barrier and immunocompromised host

ETIOLOGY

■ Chemotherapy targets all rapidly dividing cells, including healthy tissue
  ■ Breakdown of epithelium from death of rapidly dividing mucosal epithelial cells
  ■ Certain chemotherapeutic agents more likely to cause mucositis
    ▪ Alkylating agents
    ▪ Anthracyclines
    ▪ Antimetabolites

Radiation Therapy Induces Local Trauma

CLINICAL PRESENTATION

■ Usually 5 to 10 days after chemotherapy regimen
■ Within weeks of starting irradiation
■ Ranges from redness to discrete ulcerations
■ Very painful, limiting oral intake

DIAGNOSIS AND EVALUATION

■ Diagnosis usually made based on history and physical examination
  ■ Oral/rectal lesions evident on physical examination
  ■ Abdominal pain
  ■ Poor appetite

TREATMENT

■ Supportive care
  ■ Pain medications
    ▪ Systemic opioids often necessary
    ▪ Topical analgesics
  ■ Nutritional support
  ■ Basic oral care
    ▪ Soft toothbrushes
    ▪ Oral rinses for decontamination
■ Prevention
  ■ H_2 blocker or proton pump inhibitor (PPI) for gastric protection

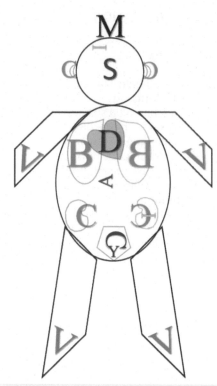

Fig. 64.1. The Chemo-Tox man. A = asparaginase = pancreatitis; B = bleomycin, busulfan = pulmonary fibrosis; C = cisplatin, carboplatin = ototoxicity, nephrotoxicity; Cy = cyclophosphamide = hemorrhagic cystitis; D = daunorubicin, dactinomycin = cardiac toxicity; I = ifosfamide = hemorrhagic cystitis, neurotoxicity; M = intrathecal methotrexate toxicity = neurologic symptoms; S = steroids = facial puffiness; V = vincristine = peripheral neuropathy.

■ G-CSF to prevent neutropenia
■ Cryotherapy (e.g., eating popsicle) during drug administration can help for short infusions such as 5-FU
  ■ Decreases blood flow to oral epithelium, decreasing exposure to drug

Chemotherapy Complications

BASIC INFORMATION

■ Chemotherapeutic agents are associated with a host of adverse effects; although it is beyond the scope of the pediatric board examiner to be familiar with the complete list of adverse effects for each agent, some are associated with "classic" side effects (Fig. 64.1 and Table 64.5)

COMPLICATIONS SPECIFIC FOR HEMATOPOIETIC STEM CELL TRANSPLANT

Graft-versus-Host Disease (GvHD)

BASIC INFORMATION

■ GvHD occurs when donor immune cells recognize and damage the tissues in the immunocompromised recipient

Table 64.5. Chemotherapies and Their Common Side Effects

Drug/MOA	Common Indications	Unique Toxicities	Other Side Effects
Anthracyclines (doxorubicin, daunorubicin, idarubicin) MOA: antibiotic, intercalation of dsDNA	Leukemia (ALL, AML), Ewing sarcoma, NBL, NHL, Wilms	Cardiac toxicity: cardiomyopathy, LV dysfunction, arrhythmias Red urine (without kidney injury) Secondary malignancy (AML)	Hepatotoxicity Vesicant
Antithymocyte globulin	Conditioning agent for HSCT	Allergic reaction, anaphylaxis	Chills/rigors, fever, headaches, rash, hypotension, anaphylaxis Hemolysis Serum sickness
Asparaginase (PEG-Asp, *Erwinia*)	ALL	Pancreatitis	Hypersensitivity: allergic reactions, anaphylaxis CNS thrombosis/bleed Coagulopathy Hyperglycemia
Bleomycin	Hodgkin lymphoma Osteosarcoma	Pulmonary toxicity: pneumonitis, fibrosis	Hyperpigmentation Hypersensitivity Raynaud syndrome Delayed myelosuppression
Busulfan MOA: alkylating agent	CML, Stem cell toxin, conditioning agent for HSCT	Pulmonary fibrosis	Hyperpigmentation Gonadal dysfunction Delayed myelosuppression
Carboplatin/cisplatin MOA: platinum (heavy metal) containing DNA alkylating agent	Solid tumors: Wilms, osteosarcoma, NBL, retinoblastoma	Nephrotoxicity Ototoxicity Secondary malignancy (AML)	Hepatotoxicity Hypersensitivity Highly emetogenic
Cyclophosphamide (Cytoxan) MOA: alkylating agent	Leukemia, lymphomas, NBL, retinoblastoma, iii	Hemorrhagic cystitis Cardiotoxicity Secondary neoplasm	SIADH Pulmonary fibrosis Infertility Hepatotoxicity
Cytarabine (Ara-C) MOA: antimetabolite; interferes with DNA synthesis	ALL AML Lymphomas	Ocular: conjunctivitis (high dose) CNS: cerebellar toxicity High-dose Ara-C: neurocognitive deficits or leukoencephalopathy	Fever Hepatotoxicity Rash
Dactinomycin MOA: polypeptide antibiotic, binds to DNA and interferes with cell replication	Wilms, Ewing sarcoma, RMS, osteosarcoma	Hepatotoxicity	Radiation recall Photosensitivity Acne Highly emetogenic
Etoposide (VP-16) MOA: topoisomerase II inhibitor	AML, Ewing sarcoma, lymphomas, Wilms, NBL, osteosarcoma, retinoblastoma	Hypotension Secondary malignancy: AML	Fever Hypersensitivity Highly emetogenic
Fluorouracil (5-FU)	—	Diarrhea: severe, may be dose limiting Cardiotoxicity: angina, ischemia, arrhythmias	Photosensitivity Rash Thrombophlebitis Encephalopathy
Ifosfamide	—	Neurotoxicity Hemorrhagic cystitis	Nephrotoxicity SIADH Highly emetogenic
Mercaptopurine (6-MP) MOA: antimetabolite, interferes with DNA synthesis	ALL, NHL	Hepatotoxicity	—
Methotrexate (MTX)	—	Mucositis Hepatotoxicity Neurotoxicity (when administered intrathecally) Nephrotoxicity	Highly emetogenic
Mitoxantrone	—	Cardiotoxicity Blue discoloration of secretions	—
Paclitaxel	—	Hypotension Cardiotoxicity	Peripheral neuropathy
Thioguanine (6-TG)	—	Hepatotoxicity (VOD)	Photosensitivity Rash Stomatitis
Vinblastine	Lymphoma Brain tumors	Peripheral Neuropathy Constipation	Phlebitis, vesicant Photophobia Rash
Vincristine	Leukemia Lymphoma NBL Wilms tumor RMS	Peripheral Neuropathy Constipation SIADH Fatal if administered intrathecally	Vesicant

ALL, acute lymphoblastic leukemia; *AML*, acute myeloid leukemia; *CML*, chronic myelogenous leukemia; *CNS*, central nervous system; *ds*, double stranded; *HSCT*, hematopoietic stem cell transplant; *LV*, left ventricular; *MOA*, mechanism of action; *NBL*, neuroblastoma; *NHL*, non-Hodgkin lymphoma; *RMS*, rhabdomyosarcoma; *SIADH*, syndrome of inappropriate antidiuretic hormone secretion; *VOD*, venoocclusive disease.

- Occurs in allogeneic (a different individual serves as the donor) hematopoietic stem cell transplant (HSCT), generally does not occur in autologous (patient's own hematopoietic stem cells are collected and then given back after bone marrow-ablative chemotherapy) HSCT
- GvHD is a major cause of morbidity and mortality after allogeneic HSCT
- Although clinically this is not always the case, for the purposes of the board acute GvHD occurs within the first 100 days post-HSCT, whereas chronic GvHD occurs after 100 days from HSCT
- Incidence of acute GvHD varies greatly based on donor-specific and patient-specific factors, but mean incidence is around 35% to 50%

ETIOLOGY

- Donor T cells cause GvHD; therefore, patients who receive T-cell–depleted products generally do not get GvHD
- Factors that increase risk of GvHD: higher human leukocyte antigen (HLA) disparity between donor and recipient, peripheral blood stem cell product, higher intensity pre-HSCT conditioning chemotherapy, increased age of the donor and recipient, sex-mismatched donor (especially female multiparous donor for a male recipient)

CLINICAL PRESENTATION

- Acute GvHD: skin, GI tract, and liver are most likely to be affected
  - Skin (most common): erythematous rash often involving the palms and soles
  - GI: most common GI manifestation is diarrhea (can be bloody); other findings include abdominal cramping and pain, malabsorption, and nausea/vomiting
  - Liver: cholestasis with jaundice, hepatomegaly, and right upper quadrant pain
  - Less commonly affects eyes, oral mucosa, and lungs
- Chronic GvHD
  - Most often but not always occurs in patients who have had acute GvHD
  - Essentially every organ system can be affected by chronic GvHD, which is generally a fibrotic/sclerotic process

DIAGNOSIS AND EVALUATION

- Acute GvHD:
  - GvHD can be confirmed via biopsy, although this is not always necessary (more likely to be done to confirm GI GvHD)
  - Skin, GI, and liver GvHD are staged from 0 to 4 based on extent of rash (skin GvHD), amount of stool output (GI GvHD), or bilirubin (liver GvHD). Based on these stages acute GvHD is given a grade from I to IV
- Chronic GvHD: no specific staging/grading criteria; diagnosis generally made on the basis of clinical presentation, and sometimes with confirmatory biopsy

TREATMENT

- Generally, immunosuppressive agents (especially to suppress T cells)

- High-dose corticosteroids are generally the first-line choice for acute GvHD
- Often, the clinical presentation may resemble an infection (e.g., *C. difficile* colitis), which may warrant investigation before initiating immunosuppression

Sinusoidal Obstruction Syndrome (SOS)

BASIC INFORMATION

- Also known as venoocclusive disease (VOD)
- Ranges from a mild, reversible process to a life-threatening syndrome with multiorgan failure
- Mean incidence of SOS in pediatric patients undergoing HSCT is 25%

ETIOLOGY

- Arises from damage to the epithelial cells of the sinusoids and to hepatocytes during HSCT
- Risk factors include liver dysfunction before HSCT, active viral hepatitis, or cytomegalovirus (CMV) before HSCT, history of prior abdominal radiation or prior HSCT, higher HLA incompatibility between donor and recipient, and certain pre-HSCT conditioning chemotherapeutics

CLINICAL PRESENTATION

- SOS is characterized by weight gain, fluid retention with ascites, tender hepatomegaly, and hyperbilirubinemia
- Coagulopathy, renal failure, pleural effusions, and encephalopathy can occur in severe cases
- Generally occurs between the day of transplant (day 0) and day +30 post-HSCT

DIAGNOSIS AND EVALUATION

- Diagnosed when the previously mentioned clinical features develop relatively quickly with no other identifiable cause for liver dysfunction
- Hepatic ultrasound with Doppler showing reversal of portal vein flow also aids in diagnosis
- Most commonly used diagnostic criteria are the Baltimore and Modified Seattle criteria, but the specifics of these are beyond the scope of the boards

TREATMENT

- Supportive care: diuresis, fluid and salt restriction, correction of coagulopathies, paracentesis to relieve discomfort from ascites and improve ventilation, and analgesia
- Defibrotide and/or high-dose corticosteroids

Thrombotic Microangiopathy (TMA)

BASIC INFORMATION

- TMA is the major cause of kidney disease after HSCT
- Occurs in 10% to 25% of transplant recipients

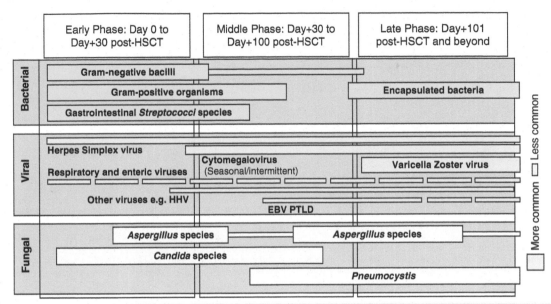

Fig. 64.2. Infectious risks associated with hematopoietic stem cell transplant (HSCT). Day 0 indicates day of transplant. *EBV*, Epstein–Barr virus; *PTLD*, posttransplant lymphoproliferative disorder. Modified from Tomblyn, M., Chiller, T., Einsele, H., et al. Guidelines for preventing infectious complications among hematopoietic cell transplant recipients: a global perspective. *Biol Blood Marrow Transplant.* 2009;15(10):1143–1238.

ETIOLOGY

- Is caused by endothelial injury causing platelet aggregation and erythrocyte fragmentation, leading to fibrin deposition and thrombosis in the microcirculation of the kidney and other organs
- Risk factors include radiation and certain types of chemotherapy during pre-HSCT conditioning, and GvHD prophylaxis with calcineurin inhibitors (e.g., cyclosporine) and/or mTOR inhibitors (e.g., sirolimus)

CLINICAL PRESENTATION

- Signs/symptoms include rising creatinine, hypertension, hemolytic anemia, thrombocytopenia, and proteinuria

DIAGNOSIS AND EVALUATION

- TMA can be diagnosed via biopsy, but this rarely needs to be done
- In addition to the previously mentioned signs/symptoms, schistocytes are often noted on blood smear, and complement studies show complement hyperactivation

TREATMENT

- Dose reduction or withdrawal of offending agent (e.g., calcineurin inhibitor) when possible
- Some centers use eculizumab (blocks terminal complement)

Infectious Complications and HSCT

BASIC INFORMATION

- Major cause of morbidity and mortality in children undergoing HSCT
- Infection can impair the management of other HSCT-induced complications, such as GvHD

ETIOLOGY

- Bacterial, viral, and fungal infections can occur
  - Early phase of HSCT (day of transplant to day +30 post-HSCT): bacterial infections are the most common
  - Middle phase (day +30 to day +100 post-HSCT): bacterial infections become less common, but there is a rise in fungal infections and CMV reactivation
  - Late phase (later than day +100 post-HSCT): encapsulated bacteria, PJP, *Aspergillus*, and varicella-zoster virus (VZV) are the most common pathogens encountered (Fig. 64.2)
- HSCT-related complications that require use of immunosuppressive medications (especially GvHD) increase the risk of infection
- Infectious prophylaxis
  - Environment: preventing dust accumulation, positive pressure rooms with air filtration, and hand hygiene
  - Antibacterial, antiviral, and antifungal prophylaxis agents are often used, especially during periods of profound myelosuppression

Review Questions

For review questions, please go to ExpertConsult.com.

Suggested Readings

1. Baeksgaard L, Sørensen J. Acute tumor lysis syndrome in solid tumors—a case report and review of the literature. *Cancer Chemother Pharmacol.* 2003;51(3):187–192.
2. Brown VI, ed. *Hematopoietic Stem Cell Transplantation for the Pediatric Hematologist Oncologist.* Cham, Switzerland: Springer International; 2018:215–282.
3. Byrne TN. Spinal cord compression from epidural metastases. *N Engl J Med.* 1992;327(9):614–619.
4. Cairo MS, Bishop M. Tumour lysis syndrome: new therapeutic strategies and classification. *Br J Haematol.* 2004;127(1):3–11.
5. Cairo MS, Coiffier B, Reiter A, Younes A. Recommendations for the evaluation of risk and prophylaxis of tumour lysis syndrome (TLS) in adults and children with malignant diseases: an expert TLS panel consensus. *Br J Haematol.* 2010;149(4):578–586.

6. D'Angio GJ, Mius A, Evans AE. The superior mediastinal syndrome in children with cancer. *Am J Roentgenol Radium Ther Nucl Med.* 1965;93:537–544.

7. Fisher M, Rheingold S. *Oncologic Emergencies. Principles and Practices of Pediatric Oncology.* 6th ed. Philadelphia: Lippincott Williams and Wilkins; 2011:1125–1151.

8. Guilcher GMT. Hematopoietic stem cell transplantation in children and adults. *Pediatr Rev.* 2016;37(4):135–144.

9. Hain RD, Rayner L, Weitzman S, Lorenzana A. Acute tumour lysis syndrome complicating treatment of stage IVS neuroblastoma in infants under six months old. *Pediatr Blood Cancer.* 1994;23(2):136–139.

10. Harris GJ, Harman PK, Trinkle JK, Grover FL. Standard biplane roentgenography is highly sensitive in documenting mediastinal masses. *Ann Thorac Surg.* 1987;44(3):238–241.

11. Higdon ML, Higdon JA. Treatment of oncologic emergencies. *Am Fam Physician.* 2006;74(11).

12. Hogarty M, Lange B. *Oncologic Emergencies. Textbook of Pediatric Emergency Medicine.* 4th ed. Philadelphia: Lippincott Williams & Wilkins; 2000:1169–1170.

13. Ingram L, Rivera GK, Shapiro DN. Superior vena cava syndrome associated with childhood malignancy: analysis of 24 cases. *Pediatr Blood Cancer.* 1990;18(6):476–481.

14. Kalemkerian GP, Darwish B, Varterasian ML. Tumor lysis syndrome in small cell carcinoma and other solid tumors. *Am J Med.* 1997;103(5):363–367.

15. Kelly KM, Lange B. Oncologic emergencies. *Pediatr Clin North Am.* 1997;44(4):809–830.

16. Klein SL, Sanford RA, Muhlbauer MS. Pediatric spinal epidural metastases. *J Neurosurg.* 1991;74(1):70–75.

17. Kramer ED, Lewis D, Raney B, Womer R, Packer RJ. Neurologic complications in children with soft tissue and osseous sarcoma. *Cancer.* 1989;64(12):2600–2603.

18. Lee D, Margolin J. *Emergencies in Pediatric Cancer Patients.* Waltham, MA: UpToDate; 2013.

19. Lewis DW, Packer RJ, Raney B, Rak IW, Belasco J, Lange B. Incidence, presentation, and outcome of spinal cord disease in children with systemic cancer. *Pediatrics.* 1986;78(3):438–443.

20. Loeffler JS, Leopold KA, Recht A, Weinstein HJ, Tarbell NJ. Emergency prebiopsy radiation for mediastinal masses: impact on subsequent pathologic diagnosis and outcome. *J Clin Oncol.* 1986;4(5):716–721.

21. Manabe S, Tanaka H, Higo Y, Park P, Ohno T, Tateishi A. Experimental analysis of the spinal cord compressed by spinal metastasis. *Spine.* 1989;14(12):1308–1315.

22. Nathan D, Oski F. *Hematology of Infancy and Childhood.* Philadelphia: WB Saunders Company; 1993:1187–1188.

23. Neville KA, Steuber CP. *Clinical Assessment of the Child with Suspected Cancer.* Waltham, MA: UpToDate; 2013.

24. Parish JM, Marschke Jr R, Dines D, Lee R, eds. *Etiologic Considerations in Superior Vena Cava Syndrome.* Mayo Clinic Proceedings; 1981.

25. Posner JB, Howieson J, Cvitkovic E. "Disappearing" spinal cord compression: oncolytic effect of glucocorticoids (and other chemotherapeutic agents) on epidural metastases. *Ann neurol.* 1977;2(5):409–413.

26. Prusakowski MK, Cannone D. Pediatric oncologic emergencies. *Emerg Med Clin.* 2014;32(3):527–548.

27. Rheingold S, Lange B. *Oncologic Emergencies. Principles and Practice of Pediatric Oncology.* 5th ed. Philadelphia: Lippincott Williams & Wilkins; 2006:1202–1230.

28. Rodrigues FG, et al. Neutropenic enterocolitis. *World J Gastroenterol.* 2017;23(1):42–47.

29. Sanderson I, Pritchard J, Marsh HT. Chemotherapy as the initial treatment of spinal cord compression due to disseminated neuroblastoma. *J neurosurg.* 1989;70(5):688–690.

30. Seth R, Bhat AS. Management of common oncologic emergencies. *Indian J Med Sci.* 2011;78(6):709–717.

31. Tomblyn M, Chiller T, Einsele H, et al. Guidelines for preventing infectious complications among hematopoietic cell transplant recipients: a global perspective. *Biol Blood Marrow Transplant.* 2009;15(10):1143–1238.

32. Truini-Pittman L, Rossetto C, eds. *Pediatric Considerations in Tumor Lysis Syndrome. Seminars in Oncology Nursing.* Elsevier; 2002.

33. U.S. Department of Health and Human Services, National Institutes of Health, National Cancer Institute. *Common Terminology Criteria for Adverse Events (CTCAE). Version v4.03*; 2010.

34. White L, Ybarra M. Neutropenic fever. *Hematol Oncol Clin North Am.* 2017;31(6):981–993.

35. Wright CD, Mathisen DJ. Mediastinal tumors: diagnosis and treatment. *World J Surg.* 2001;25(2):204–209.

36. Zimmerman R, Bilaniuk L. Imaging of tumors of the spinal canal and cord. *Radiol Clin North Am.* 1988;26(5):965–1007.

Ophthalmology

Essentials in Funduscopy

- Instruments
  - Direct ophthalmoscope
    - Handheld instrument with an eyepiece and light source capable of magnification (15×)
    - Provides monocular view to the fundus but lacks depth perception
  - Ophthalmologists frequently use dilating eye drops to enhance viewing abilities of all instruments, as well as other ophthalmoscopes (e.g., monocular indirect ophthalmoscope, binocular indirect ophthalmoscope)
- The following can be evaluated with a direct ophthalmoscope:
  - Corneal light reflex, centration, clarity, red reflex, symmetry
  - Posterior segment evaluation (may have limited view with direct ophthalmoscope and without dilating drops; see Fig. 65.1)
    - Vitreous
    - Optic nerve (A)
    - Macula, fovea (B)
    - Vessels
    - Peripheral retina

Leukocoria (White Pupil)

BASIC INFORMATION

- Commonly used to describe a difference in color of the red reflex between the two eyes
  - Pupils normally have a dark or red-orange reflex; the affected eye(s) appear white or lighter in color
- Requires evaluation for a varied differential diagnosis
  - Strabismus
    - Physically interferes with normal reflection of light
    - See Chapter 66
  - Cataract
    - Physically interferes with or blocks normal reflection of light
    - See Chapter 67
  - Uveitis
    - Produces light scattering, making reflex appear dull
    - See Chapter 67
  - Vitreous hemorrhage
    - Blocks reflection of light from the retina

- Coloboma
  - Failure of embryonic fissure to close, producing defect that may be chorioretinal and/or involve only the optic nerve
  - Not progressive; can be associated with retinal detachments
  - Physically interferes with normal reflection of light
- Retinoblastoma (life- and vision-threatening)
  - Physically interferes with normal reflection of light
  - See Chapter 68
- Retinopathy of prematurity
  - Physically interferes with normal reflection of light or produces differences in axial length between the two eyes
  - See Chapter 68
- Toxocariasis
  - Retinal granuloma caused by *Toxocara canis*
  - Usually unilateral; can cause macular traction
  - Physically interferes with normal reflection of light
- Other causes
  - Persistent fetal vasculature
  - Coats disease
  - Anisometropia

DIAGNOSIS AND EVALUATION

- History: age of onset, family history of similar issues, birth/pregnancy history, postnatal course
- Examination
  - Compare reflection from both eyes by looking with broad light beam of direct ophthalmoscope simultaneously at both eyes from a distance
  - Vision, pupils, alignment, motility, and external examination are necessary
  - Ophthalmologists may perform slit-lamp examination, dilated fundus examination, and retinoscopy
- Leukocoria always requires ophthalmology consultation to rule out life- and vision-threatening causes

TREATMENT

- Treatment is guided by etiology (see corresponding chapters mentioned previously)
- Coloboma
  - Glasses, patching
  - Close observation for retinal detachments
- Toxocariasis
  - Varies with location and structural damage

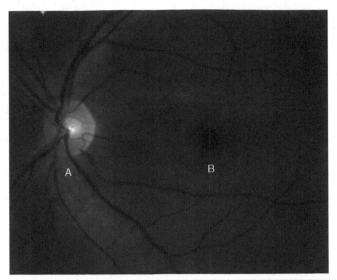

Fig. 65.1. Photograph of the posterior pole demonstrating normal retinal anatomy. (A) Optic nerve with a cup-to-disk ratio of 0.2. (B) Macula with foveal center apparent as a reflective just inferior and temporal to the optic nerve.

- Observation for peripheral lesions without macular traction
- Use systemic steroids if lesions are posterior/vision-threatening or if endophthalmitis is suspected
- Surgery for retinal traction or secondary issues such as glaucoma, cataract, or cyclitic membranes
- Systemic anthelmintics are not helpful
- Vitreous hemorrhage
  - Observation for resolution or surgery for clearing
  - Must address the cause of hemorrhage

Traumatic Eye Injuries

BASIC INFORMATION

- Accounts for 30% of blindness in children
- More common in boys than girls
- Causes and etiologies (see Table 65.1)

Open Globe Injury

- History
  - Usually high-velocity projectile without eye protection
  - Determine what material might have been involved in injury in case of retained object (see later)
- Symptoms
  - Blurry vision and pain when opening/moving eye or with looking at light
- Clinical signs
  - Decreased vision; relative afferent pupillary defect (RAPD); eccentric pupil; deepening or shallowing of anterior chamber; vitreous, uveal, or other extrusion of ocular contents; tenting of cornea/sclera; Seidel sign (leaking of intraocular fluid observed with fluorescein staining)

Intraocular Foreign Body

- History
  - Similar to open globe

Table 65.1. Causes and Etiologies of Eye Injury

Traumatic Force	Common Examples
Blunt force	Ocular compartment syndrome
	Orbital blowout fracture
	Hyphema
Penetrating/perforating injury	Open globe ± intraocular or intraorbital foreign body
	Hyphema
Burns	Chemical
	Fireworks
Lacerations (partial or full thickness)	Corneal laceration
	Scleral laceration
	Eyelid laceration
Tractional injury	Eyelid laceration

- Symptoms
  - Similar to open globe.
- Signs
  - Similar to open globe injury, foreign body may be visible on inspection
  - Microcystic corneal edema
  - Intraocular inflammation varies with composition:
    - Significant inflammatory reaction
      Magnetic: iron, steel
      Nonmagnetic: copper and vegetable matter
    - Mild inflammatory reaction
      Magnetic: nickel
      Nonmagnetic: aluminum, mercury, zinc, vegetable matter
  - Inert: carbon, gold, coal, glass, lead, plaster, platinum, silver, stone, rubber, brass

Orbital Compartment Syndrome

- Mechanism
  - Traumatic intraorbital hemorrhage and elevation of intraorbital pressure
  - Pressure builds up in the retroorbital space because no outflow passage is available
  - Pressure on optic nerve can result in ischemia and vision loss
- History
  - Blunt trauma, bleeding disorder, or anticoagulant use
- Symptoms
  - Decreased vision, periorbital pain, ocular pain, distorted color vision
- Signs
  - Tight eyelids, swelling, erythema, ocular proptosis, vision loss, abnormal color vision, RAPD, elevated intraocular pressure (IOP), subconjunctival hemorrhage and conjunctival chemosis, restricted extraocular motility (EOM), vascular and optic disk edema

Chemical Eye Exposures

- History
  - Type of agent may determine damage (alkaline exposures penetrate deeper and cause more damage than acidic)
  - Type and amount of irrigation used to wash out eye prior to arrival (see Fig. 65.2)

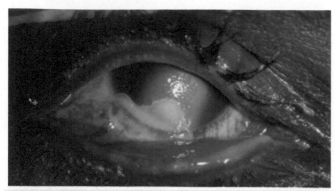

Fig. 65.2. Alkaline corneal burn. (Photo courtesy Dr. Jeffrey Goshe, MD.)

- Symptoms
  - Blurry vision, pain, discomfort with eye opening, sensitivity to light
- Signs
  - Decreased vision, blepharospasm, conjunctival injection, photophobia, alkaline or acidic pH

Hyphema:

- History
  - Blunt or penetrating trauma
    - Also associated with sickle cell disease and use of anticoagulant medications or history of coagulopathy blood in the anterior chamber of the eye
- Symptoms
  - Pain, blurry vision, loss of vision, light sensitivity
- Signs
  - Decreased vision, blood or clot in the anterior chamber, elevated IOP, other signs of trauma

Orbital Blowout Fracture

- History
  - Blunt trauma to face
- Symptoms
  - Pain with eye movements, periorbital pain, swelling which can worsen after nose blowing or valsalva maneuver, double vision, numbness on cheek
- Signs
  - Decreased vision, restricted EOM, air underneath skin/conjunctiva, hypesthesia in V2 distribution, enophthalmos, eyelid edema, erythema and ecchymosis, step-off fracture of orbital rim
  - Children can present with "white-eyed blowout fractures": paucity of clinical signs except motility restriction (especially with upgaze)

Subconjunctival Hemorrhage

- Mechanism
  - Bleeding between the conjunctiva and sclera
  - Appears bright red initially and can change colors as blood is reabsorbed (Fig. 65.3)
- History
  - Trauma, foreign body in the eye, use of anticoagulation, history of coagulopathy, history of vomiting, coughing, straining, or lifting weights
- Symptoms
  - Usually asymptomatic but can cause mild irritation
- Signs

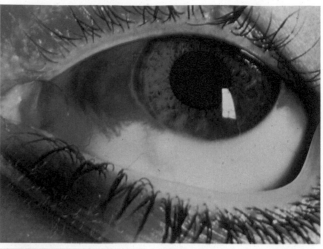

Fig. 65.3. Subconjunctival hemorrhage. (Photo courtesy Dr. Monte Del Monte, MD.)

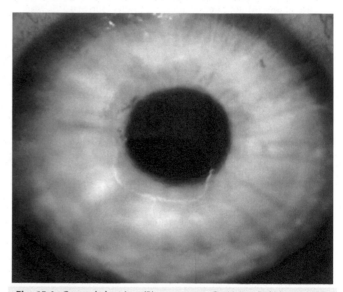

Fig. 65.4. Corneal abrasion. (Photo courtesy Dr. Monte Del Monte, MD.)

  - Dispersed blood under the conjunctiva
  - Look for other signs of injury, such as conjunctival laceration, foreign body, or ruptured globe

Corneal Abrasion

- Mechanism
  - Disruption of the corneal epithelial layer and exposure of corneal nerves (Fig. 65.4)
- History
  - Mechanism of injury, specifically if any soil material or dirt may be in the wound (i.e., dirty stick, fingernail, etc.)
  - History of contact lens use
- Symptoms
  - Pain, foreign body sensation, light sensitivity, pain with blinking or eye movement
- Signs
  - Decreased vision, blepharospasm, photophobia, injection, eyelid swelling
  - Defect stains yellow-green with fluorescein when viewed under a blue light (Fig. 65.5)

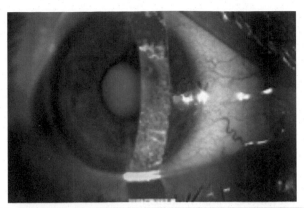

Fig. 65.5. Fluorescein staining of corneal abrasion. (Photo courtesy Dr. Monte Del Monte, MD.)

Corneal or Conjunctival Foreign Body

- Foreign body embedded in tissue, not penetrating injury
- History
  - Usually particulate matter (such as dust or debris) gets trapped in the eye, commonly while patient isn't wearing eye protection
  - Composition of foreign body
- Symptoms
  - Pain, photophobia, foreign body sensation, tearing, redness
- Signs
  - Foreign body embedded in cornea or conjunctiva
  - Metallic foreign bodies in cornea develop a rust ring
  - Conjunctival injection, epiphora, eyelid edema, ptosis or guarding, anterior chamber cell or flare, corneal infiltrate, staining of corneal surface with fluorescein dye

Traumatic Iritis:

- History
  - Blunt trauma up to 3 days before symptoms intraocular inflammation after nonpenetrating trauma
- Symptoms
  - Pain, light sensitivity, tearing, blurry vision
- Signs
  - Anterior chamber white blood cells, red blood cells, and/or flare; photophobia; pain; low IOP; anisocoria (with poor pupillary response in affected eye); decreased vision; conjunctival injection

Eyelid Laceration

- History
  - Direct laceration or tractional injury
- Symptoms
  - Tearing, pain, ptosis, or other malposition of eyelid
- Signs
  - Eyelid defect (partial or full thickness), epiphora, ptosis, fat prolapse
  - May involve lacrimal drainage system

Retinal Detachment

- Mechanism
  - Neurosensory retina lifts up from retinal pigment epithelium

- History
  - Prior retinal tears/detachment, myopic correction, Stickler syndrome, family history
- Symptoms
  - Flashing lights, floaters, decreased vision, curtain or shadow over part of the visual field; deficits can be in central or peripheral field
- Signs
  - Retina is elevated due to a tear in the neurosensory retina (can be seen on dilated exam or ocular ultrasound)

DIAGNOSIS AND EVALUATION

Physical Examination

- If there is suspicion of open globe injury, do not manipulate globe. Please place shield over globe and call ophthalmology immediately
- Clinical triage
  - Life-threatening injuries need to be identified and stabilized before assessing the eyes
  - Sight-threatening injury identified by targeted history: chemical eye exposure, orbital compartment syndrome, open globe injury with or without intraocular foreign body
- External appearance
  - Periorbital swelling, ecchymosis, erythema
  - Orbital bony deformity
  - Eyelid laceration, ptosis, or avulsion
    - Gently open eyelid with a retractor or by pulling upward from the orbital rim. Never put pressure on the globe
  - Other facial lacerations/deformities
- "Eye vitals": vision, pupils, EOM
  - Open eyelids (use a paper clip or eyelid retractor if necessary)
  - Vision may be decreased or normal
  - Pupils
    - Dilated or constricted, nonreactive
    - Asymmetric in appearance or reactivity
    - RAPD
  - EOM
    - Restriction in up or lateral gaze
    - Nausea, vomiting, bradycardia, or severe pain with EOM
- Anterior segment
  - Look for protrusion of intraocular contents from eye
    - Vitreous is a clear, jelly-like substance
    - Uveal tissue is dark
    - Lens is clear/slightly opaque and firm
  - Foreign body in the fornices (under the upper and lower eyelids)
  - Conjunctival injection, laceration, hemorrhage, or foreign body
  - Corneal abrasion, foreign body, laceration
    - Fluorescein can stain denuded tissues, which appears yellow-green under blue light
  - Anterior chamber
    - Look for foreign body
    - Check for depth; if shallow, suspect open globe
    - Compare view to the iris: unobstructed view to the iris when clear; can appear hazy with inflammatory cells or opaque/hazy with hyphema

Table 65.2. Clinical Signs of Ocular Trauma Requiring Urgent Ophthalmology Referral

Irregular pupil

Decreased vision

Orbital fracture with persistent nausea, vomiting, bradycardia, severe pain, or incarcerated extraocular muscle on imaging

Deep, complex margin–involving or canalicular-involving eyelid laceration

Sudden gush of fluid from the eyes

Injury with high-velocity projectile

Corneal abrasion with history of contact lens use

Suspicion for open globe or intraocular foreign body

Chemical injury

- With both eyes open, check red reflex for symmetry between the two eyes
- Ophthalmology consult for complete ocular examination, including dilation and ocular pressure testing

MANAGEMENT

- Table 65.2 depicts clinical signs of ocular trauma requiring urgent ophthalmology referral
- Open globe injury with or without intraocular foreign body
  - Before calling ophthalmology:
    - Do not apply pressure to the eye
    - Do not place medications into the eye
    - Do not remove any foreign bodies
    - Make patient NPO (nothing by mouth); usually requires surgical correction within 24 hours of injury
    - Place a *shield only* (no patch) over the eye
    - Keep patient on bed rest with elevated head of bed
    - Control emesis to avoid increasing intraorbital pressure
    - Control pain
    - Acquire computed tomography (CT) of orbits (small cuts)
    - Intravenous (IV) antibiotics: vancomycin plus ceftazidime or fluoroquinolone (if age allows)
  - Surgical exploration, closure of the globe, and removal of any foreign bodies are necessary

Orbital Compartment Syndrome

- Emergent lateral canthotomy and inferior cantholysis may be necessary (do *not* wait for ophthalmology)
- Otherwise, provide routine management of coagulopathy (if present) and minimize IOP (elevate head of bed, avoid pain/cough/emesis)

Chemical Eye Exposure

- Before calling ophthalmology:
  - Check pH and begin copious irrigation with normal saline until pH is neutralized
  - Sweep fornices with cotton swab to eliminate any particulate matter
- Post-irrigation care usually includes artificial tears, prednisolone eye drops, and antibiotics
  - Severe cases may require surgical intervention (e.g., tarsorrhaphy to prevent exposure)

Hyphema

- Before calling ophthalmology:
  - Shield over affected eye (no patch!)
    - Minimize IOP (elevate head of bed, avoid pain/cough/emesis)
    - Correct coagulopathy and avoid NSAIDs or aspirin-containing products
    - Obtain a sickle cell screen if status is unknown
- Eye drops may reduce discomfort (e.g., atropine, cyclopentolate) and decrease inflammation (prednisolone)
- Requires close monitoring by ophthalmology for elevated IOP, corneal stromal blood staining, and prolonged hyphema clearing
- May require anterior chamber washout if IOP remains elevated for an extended period of time or patient has sickle cell disease

Orbital Fracture

- Before calling ophthalmology:
  - Minimize IOP (elevate head of bed, avoid pain/cough/emesis)
    - Ice packs may provide comfort and decrease swelling
    - Start broad-spectrum oral antibiotics
    - Obtain CT of orbits (3-mm cuts); if roof fracture, consult neurosurgery
- Small fractures without enophthalmos or muscle entrapment may be observed
- Urgent surgical management is required for muscle entrapment (e.g., incarcerated or "missing" inferior rectus muscle on CT), bradycardia, persistent emesis, or syncope with trapdoor fracture
- Follow-up is necessary within 1 to 2 weeks to evaluate for persistent diplopia in primary gaze

Subconjunctival Hemorrhage

- Rule out serious causes (foreign body, open globe)
- Observe, with artificial tears if there is any discomfort
- If recurrent, work up for coagulopathy

Corneal Abrasion

- Before calling ophthalmology:
  - Examine for and attempt to remove any foreign body
  - Stain the cornea with fluorescein dye and look with a blue light
  - If patient is a contact lens user, remove and save contact lens and lens case for possible cultures. Avoid contact lens wear until fully healed
  - Start antibiotics
    - If vegetable matter or injury was with fingernail/dirty object: erythromycin, bacitracin, Polysporin or polymyxin
    - If contact lens user: pseudomonas coverage with tobramycin, gatifloxacin, moxifloxacin, or ciprofloxacin
- Monitor for traumatic iritis
- Avoid patching in children
- Reasons for ophthalmology consult
  - Defect not healed in 48 to 72 hours
  - Contact lens user
  - History of ocular herpetic disease

Corneal or conjunctival foreign body

- Evert eyelids to ensure no other foreign bodies noted
- Additional imaging may be necessary to rule out additional foreign bodies (e.g., CT orbits)
- Often requires ophthalmology consultation for removal

Traumatic iritis

- Medical management is first-line, including:
  - Cycloplegic agent (to decrease pain and prevent intraocular scarring)
  - Steroid drop (if no corneal epithelial defect) with slow taper

Eyelid laceration

- Surgical repair is required for most eyelid lacerations (with the exception of superficial lacerations), especially if there is deep/complex laceration, lacrimal system involvement, or ptotic eyelid in children <7 years of age

- Additional management
  - Consider CT scan brain/orbits to rule out an orbital foreign body, orbital fracture, or ruptured globe
  - Broad-spectrum oral antibiotics and tetanus prophylaxis

Retinal detachment

- Usually requires ophthalmology consultation and intervention

Review Questions

For review questions, please go to ExpertConsult.com.

Suggested Reading

1. Ehlers JP, Shah CP. *The Wills Eye Manual: Office and Emergency Room Diagnosis and Treatment of Eye Disease*. 5th ed. Philadelphia: LWW; 2008:12–48; 167–169.

66 Disorders of Eye Alignment and Motility

CATHERINE CHOI, MD

Esotropia (Inward Deviation of Eyes)

BASIC INFORMATION

Causes

- Congenital esotropia
  - Manifests within first 6 months of life
  - Deviation is usually large (40–50 prism diopters) and constant
  - Associated with latent nystagmus and dissociated vertical deviation
- Duane syndrome, Type I
  - Congenital malformation of cranial nerve VI nucleus resulting in esotropia
  - Associated with abduction deficit
  - Differentiated from cranial nerve VI palsy by straight alignment in primary position
  - Globe retraction and palpebral fissure narrowing on attempted adduction
- Accommodative esotropia
  - Usually occurs in patients with moderate to high hyperopia, resulting in excessive convergence driven by the accommodative reflex
  - Manifests around ages 2 to 3 years
- Cranial nerve VI palsy
  - Esotropia associated with abduction deficit (unilateral or bilateral)
  - Constant eye turn (not usually intermittent) that is incomitant (varying angle of deviation depending on direction of gaze)
- Sensory deprivation esotropia
  - Secondary to very poor vision in one eye (i.e., dense amblyopia)
- Pseudoesotropia
  - Secondary to appearance of wide nasal bridge and/or epicanthal folds
  - No actual deviation based on cover testing
- Esophoria
  - Latent esodeviation that manifests only when fusion is disrupted
  - Alignment is straight under binocular conditions
  - See also Nelson Textbook of Pediatrics, Chapter 623, "Disorders of Eye Movement and Alignment."

CLINICAL PRESENTATION

- One or both eyes are turned inward

- Can be associated with poor vision in one eye secondary to amblyopia from strabismus

DIAGNOSIS AND EVALUATION

- History: age of onset, frequency of episodes, prior treatments
- Visual acuity of each eye (while patching fellow eye to prevent peeking)
- Motility examination—check for restriction
- Cover testing
- Ophthalmology examination includes cycloplegic refraction (using dilating drops), slit lamp, and fundus evaluation

TREATMENT

- Congenital
  - Strabismus surgery (usually bilateral medial rectus recessions)
- Duane syndrome, Type I
  - If eyes are straight in primary position, can be monitored
  - Patching for amblyopia component
  - Surgery for deviation in primary position, significant anomalous head position, and/or increased symptoms in lateral gaze
- Accommodative
  - Full-time wear of glasses to correct the hyperopia
  - Patching for any amblyopia component
  - Surgery for residual deviation despite proper spectacle correction and patching
- Cranial nerve VI palsy
  - Urgent imaging to rule out intracranial mass and elevated intracranial pressure; if imaging is normal, monitor closely for resolution
  - Patching for amblyopia
  - If deviation persists greater than 6 months, consider surgical correction
- Sensory deprivation esotropia
  - Surgery for cosmesis
- Pseudoesotropia
  - Reassure parents and monitor until appearance improves
- Esophoria
  - No acute intervention, just monitoring over time
  - Phoria may decompensate into tropia over time, which may require surgery

Exotropia (Outward Deviation)

BASIC INFORMATION

Causes and Etiology

- Intermittent exotropia
  - Most common outward deviation in children; usually manifests before age 5 years
  - Significant amblyopia is rare
- Convergence insufficiency
  - Usually affects patients >10 years old
  - Blurred near vision, eyestrain, or diplopia when reading
- Cranial nerve III palsy
  - Limited eye movements superiorly, medially, and inferiorly
  - Often associated with ptosis ± anisocoria
- Duane syndrome, Type II
  - Congenital malformation of cranial nerve III nucleus
  - Associated with adduction deficit
  - Globe retraction and palpebral fissure narrowing on attempted adduction
- Sensory exotropia
  - Secondary to poor vision (i.e., dense amblyopia) in one eye
- Pseudoexotropia
  - Secondary to wide interpupillary distance, positive angle kappa, and temporal macular dragging (secondary to retinopathy of prematurity)
  - No actual deviation measured on cover testing
- Exophoria
  - Latent exodeviation that manifests only when fusion is disrupted
  - Alignment is straight under binocular conditions

CLINICAL PRESENTATION

- One or both eyes are turned outward
- Can be associated with poor vision in one eye secondary to amblyopia from strabismus

DIAGNOSIS AND EVALUATION

- Same as for esotropia

TREATMENT

- Intermittent exotropia
  - Over-minus glasses, alternate patching, close monitoring if control is good to fair
  - Strabismus surgery for very poor control (near constant deviation)
- Convergence insufficiency
  - Correction of refractive error (if present)
  - Convergence exercises (i.e., pencil push-ups)
  - Base-out prisms
- Cranial nerve III palsy
  - If acute or new, urgent imaging to rule out intracranial mass
  - Patching for amblyopia
  - If imaging is normal, monitor closely for resolution
  - If deviation persists greater than 6 months, consider surgical correction
- Duane syndrome, Type II
  - If eyes are straight in primary position, can be monitored
  - Patching for amblyopia component
  - Surgery for deviation in primary position, significant anomalous head position, and/or increased symptoms in lateral gaze
- Sensory deprivation exotropia
  - Surgery for cosmesis
- Pseudoexotropia
  - Reassurance of parents and monitoring until appearance improves
- Exophoria
  - No acute intervention, just monitoring over time
  - Phoria may decompensate into tropia over time, which may require surgery

Hypertropia or Hypotropia (Vertical Misalignment)

BASIC INFORMATION

Causes and Etiology

- Monocular elevation deficiency (congenital)
  - Unilateral limitation of elevation (poor function of superior rectus and inferior oblique muscles)
  - Often associated with ptosis and chin-up position to maintain fusion
  - Amblyopia often occurs in affected eye
- Brown syndrome
  - Limitation of elevation in adduction
  - Often congenital but can be acquired secondary to trauma, surgery, or inflammation in trochlea
  - Alignment is usually straight in primary position
- Cranial nerve III palsy
  - Limited eye movements superiorly, medially, and inferiorly
  - Often associated with ptosis ± anisocoria
- Thyroid eye disease
  - Uncommon in children but common etiology of vertical deviation in adults

CLINICAL PRESENTATION

- One eye is higher or lower than the fellow eye
- Can be associated with poor vision in one eye secondary to amblyopia from strabismus

DIAGNOSIS AND EVALUATION

- Same as for esotropia

TREATMENT

- Monocular elevation deficiency
  - Patching to treat amblyopia
  - Ptosis surgery
  - Strabismus surgery

- Brown syndrome
  - Surgery is not often indicated, unless Brown syndrome causes abnormal head position and/or misalignment in primary position
- Cranial nerve III palsy
  - If acute or new, urgent imaging to rule out intracranial mass
  - Patching for amblyopia
  - If imaging normal, monitor closely for resolution
  - If deviation persists greater than 6 months, consider surgical correction

Suggested Readings

1. Bell AL, Rodes ME, Kellar LC. Childhood Eye Examination. *Am Fam Physician.* 2013;88(4):241–248.
2. Ehlers JP, Shah CP. *The Wills Eye Manual: Office and Emergency Room Diagnosis and Treatment of Eye Disease.* 5th ed. Philadelphia: LWW; 2008:173–178.
3. Wright KW, Strube YNJ. *Pediatric Ophthalmology and Strabismus.* 3rd ed. Oxford University Press, Inc; 2012.

67 External Disorders of the Eye

CATHERINE CHOI, MD

Ptosis

BASIC INFORMATION AND CLINICAL PRESENTATION

Ptosis (Fig. 67.1) is often described as a "drooping" of the upper eyelid. Etiologies include both congenital and acquired disorders, which are able to be distinguished based on clinical findings associated with the ptosis.

See also Nelson Textbook of Pediatrics, Chapter 624, "Abnormalities of the Lids."

- Causes
  - Congenital ptosis
    - Due to abnormal function of levator muscle
    - Ptosis accompanied by poorly formed upper eyelid crease
    - Often associated with anisometropia (astigmatism) and possible amblyopia on affected side
  - Blepharophimosis
    - Inherited disorder (autosomal dominant) in which ptosis is associated with telecanthus (wide-set eyes) and epicanthal folds
  - Cranial nerve dysinnervation syndrome (i.e., Marcus Gunn jaw winking)
    - A form of congenital ptosis in which a unilateral upper lid droop occurs with contraction of muscles of mastication, leading to "winking" while chewing or smiling
    - Upper eyelid crease intact
  - Horner syndrome
    - A congenital or acquired disorder in which ptosis can be associated with iris heterochromia (difference in iris coloration between eyes), anisocoria (smaller pupil on side of lid droop), and/or anhidrosis
    - Secondary to disruption of or damage to the sympathetic innervation to the eye and adnexal structures (i.e., brachial plexus injury/birth trauma, neuroblastoma, apical lung tumors)
  - Myasthenia gravis
    - Fluctuating pattern of ptosis and strabismus
    - Rare in children
  - Cranial nerve III palsy (see Chapter 66)
  - Monocular elevation deficiency (see Chapter 66)

DIAGNOSIS AND EVALUATION

- Patients with ptosis deserve assessment of visual acuity, motility, and pupil measurements of each eye
- Measurement of position and depth of the upper eyelid crease is useful for differential diagnosis
- Measurement of marginal reflex distance (between corneal light reflex and upper eyelid margin)
- Measurement of levator function
- Ophthalmologist may evaluate cycloplegic refraction (using dilating drops) and perform slit-lamp and fundus evaluations

TREATMENT

- Congenital
  - If mild, observation
  - Patching for amblyopia
  - Glasses for anisometropia
  - Surgery if lid droop is severe and causes significant deprivation amblyopia
- Blepharophimosis
  - Ptosis surgery (frontalis sling procedure)
- Cranial nerve dysinnervation syndrome
  - Usually no treatment if mild
  - Jaw winking usually improves over time
- Horner syndrome
  - Magnetic resonance imaging (MRI) of the brain/chest/abdomen to rule out neuroblastoma
- Myasthenia gravis
  - Check serum acetylcholine receptor antibodies
  - Tensilon or ice test
  - Could consider single-fiber electromyography (EMG) studies
- Cranial nerve III palsy (see Chapter 66)
- Monocular elevation deficiency (see Chapter 66)

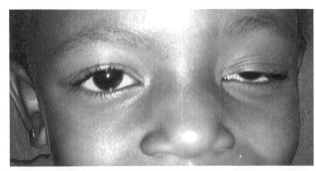

Fig. 67.1. Patient with congenital ptosis of the left upper eyelid. Note the poorly formed upper eyelid crease indicating weak adhesions of the levator muscle to the external skin.

Hordeolum/Chalazion

BASIC INFORMATION

- Causes and etiology
  - Hordeolum: abscess/acute infection of gland of Zeis (external) or meibomian gland (internal)
    - Usually associated with *Staphylococcus aureus* infection
  - Chalazion: chronic focal inflammation secondary to obstruction of meibomian gland

CLINICAL PRESENTATION

- Acute or chronic eyelid lump/swelling and tenderness, ± erythema

DIAGNOSIS AND EVALUATION

- History: previous trauma or ocular surgery, recurrences, duration
- Slit-lamp examination to evaluate for meibomian gland dysfunction (blepharitis)

TREATMENT

- Warm compresses and massage
- Lid scrubs with baby shampoo
- Topical antibiotic-steroid combination
- If there is no improvement with conservative measures, refer patient to ophthalmology for incision and drainage of lesion

Periorbital Cellulitis

BASIC INFORMATION

- Causes and etiology
  - Sinusitis, local skin trauma or abrasion, hordeolum, insect bites

CLINICAL PRESENTATION

- Tenderness, erythema, swelling of eyelid and periorbital skin
- May be associated with fever
- May also have conjunctival injection

DIAGNOSIS AND EVALUATION

- Diagnosis is often clinical, relying on the history and physical examination
- History: recent sinus infection, local skin trauma, hordeolum, insect bite
  - Ensure the presentation is inconsistent with orbital cellulitis, which requires additional imaging and definite inpatient admission for intravenous (IV) antibiotics
- Palpate head and neck for enlarged lymph nodes
- Culture and Gram stain any open wound or drainage

- If extent of disease is unclear, may pursue computed tomography (CT) scan of brain and orbits to rule out orbital cellulitis/subperiosteal abscess
- Complete blood count (CBC) with differential and blood cultures can be sent if patient is toxic with fever

TREATMENT

- If mild, > 5 years of age, and afebrile, may try outpatient treatment with oral antibiotics that have staphylococcal and streptococcal coverage (e.g. amoxicillin-clavulanate, clindamycin, cefaclor).
- If moderate to severe disease, toxic appearance, poor tolerance, <1 year of age, or no improvement after few days of oral antibiotics, then admit for IV antibiotics (e.g., ampicillin-sulbactam, ceftriaxone, vancomycin if methicillin-resistant *S. aureus* [MRSA] colonized)
- Bacitracin ointment to lid three to four times daily
- Nasal decongestants if sinusitis is present
- Incision and drainage of abscess with cultures
- Daily follow-up until clinical improvement is noted

Orbital Cellulitis

BASIC INFORMATION

- Causes and etiology
  - Sinusitis (usually ethmoiditis), focal periorbital infection (i.e., dacryocystitis), dental infection
  - Less likely to be spread hematogenously from intracranial venous system
  - Exacerbated clinical presentation in immunocompromised or diabetic patients

CLINICAL PRESENTATION

- Appears similarly to periorbital cellulitis, but also often has:
  - Proptosis
  - Restricted ocular motility
  - Pain with eye movements
  - Conjunctival infection and chemosis
  - Decreased visual acuity/afferent pupillary defect (APD)
- More likely than periorbital cellulitis to be associated with fever

DIAGNOSIS AND EVALUATION

- Complete ocular examination is necessary for orbital cellulitis, including evaluation of motility (to rule out restriction), proptosis, elevated intraocular pressure, color vision deficits, and APD
- Facial sensation in V1 and V2 distributions may be affected
- Palpate head and neck for enlarged lymph nodes
- Unlike cases of periorbital cellulitis, cases with suspicion for orbital cellulitis require CT scan of brain and orbits (+ paranasal sinuses)
- CBC with differential and blood cultures
- Culture and Gram stain any open wound or drainage

TREATMENT

- Hospital admission for IV broad-spectrum antibiotics covering Gram-positive (including staphylococcus), Gram-negative, and anaerobes for a course of 14 to 21 days. Courses include ampicillin-sulbactam, clindamycin, or in severe cases, vancomycin with a third-generation cephalosporin
- Consultation of ophthalmologist is necessary for complete ophthalmologic assessment; ear-nose-throat (ENT) consultation is necessary if there is evidence of sinus involvement
- Possible emergent canthotomy/cantholysis if orbit is tight and optic neuropathy is present
- Surgical drainage of orbital abscesses may be necessary

COMPLICATIONS

- Due to the valveless venous system, orbital cellulitis can lead to intracranial extension and subsequent cavernous sinus thromboses and abscess formation.

Nasolacrimal Duct Obstruction

BASIC INFORMATION

- Causes and etiology
  - Imperforate membrane at distal end of nasolacrimal duct over valve of Hasner

CLINICAL PRESENTATION

- Frequent tearing since birth
- Matting of lashes and mucoid discharge/crusting around eye
- Reflux of mucoid discharge from punctum when pressure is applied over lacrimal sac
- Firm, bluish mass inferior to medial canthus may occur (dacryocystocele; Fig. 67.2) from proximal obstruction of duct
- Erythematous tender swelling occurs over nasal aspect of lower eyelid in cases with dacryocystitis

DIAGNOSIS AND EVALUATION

- Palpation over lacrimal sac (Fig. 67.3) to see whether mucoid discharge refluxes through punctum
- Palpation for dacryocystocele, which is often associated with nasal cysts

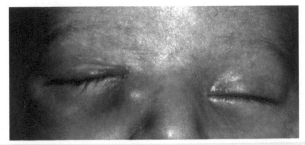

Fig. 67.2. Dacryocystocele below inner canthus of the right eye.

TREATMENT

- Tear duct massage along distal aspect of duct
- Topical antibiotics if mild conjunctivitis is also suspected
- Systemic antibiotics if dacryocystitis (red, inflamed lacrimal sac) is also present
- Probing procedure if not resolved by 1 year of age
- More urgent probing is required if dacryocystocele is present; may require joint procedure with ENT for endoscopic nasal cyst marsupialization (if present)

CORNEAL AND ANTERIOR SEGMENT DISORDERS

Conjunctivitis

BASIC INFORMATION

- Causes and etiology
  - Viral: usually adenovirus (epidemic keratoconjunctivitis); can be associated with pharyngitis and fever
    - Coxsackie and enterovirus infections can cause acute hemorrhagic conjunctivitis (tropical regions)
  - Bacterial: usually *S. aureus*, *S. epidermidis*, *Haemophilus influenzae*, *Streptococcus pneumoniae*, or *Moraxella catarrhalis*
  - Allergic: systemic allergies, environmental allergens
  - Ophthalmia neonatorum
    - Within 24 hours of birth: chemical-induced from silver nitrate
    - Within 4 days of birth: gonorrhea (copious, thick discharge)
    - Within 5 days to 3 weeks: chlamydia (often associated with pulmonary and/or nasopharyngeal infections)

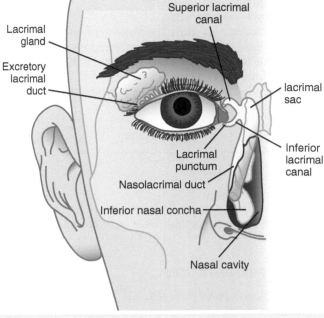

Fig. 67.3. The lacrimal apparatus.

CLINICAL PRESENTATION

- Tearing, ocular injection, eyelid crusting, watery or mucopurulent discharge
- Itchiness, corneal changes with allergic presentation
- Recent upper respiratory infection (URI) or sick contacts
- Pseudomembranes or true membranes in viral conjunctivitis

Diagnosis and Evaluation

- History: duration of symptoms, concurrent URI symptoms
- Complete ocular examination: look for membranes/pseudomembranes on palpebral conjunctiva, follicles (viral) versus papillae (allergic, bacterial), and corneal opacities (infiltrates)
- Conjunctival cultures

Treatment

- Viral: counseling on self-limited course within 7 to 14 days and highly contagious nature
    - Frequent hand-washing
    - Artificial tears, cool compresses
    - Peeling of membranes/pseudomembranes, if present, ± topical steroids
    - If herpes simplex virus (HSV) is suspected, adding an oral acyclovir is necessary
    - Keep out of school/day care for 48 hours after onset (most highly contagious period)
- Bacterial: topical antibiotics (moxifloxacin), oral amoxicillin/clavulanate for *H. influenzae* causes
    - If gonococcal in etiology, treat with systemic ceftriaxone or fluoroquinolone, and treat with azithromycin for presumed chlamydial coinfection
- Allergic: frequent artificial tears, cool compresses, topical antihistamine (i.e., Patanol), topical steroid (severe cases), and oral antihistamine
- Ophthalmia neonatorum
    - Chemical: discontinue offending agent, artificial tears
    - Gonococcal: hospital admission, systemic ceftriaxone, antibiotic ointment, concurrent coverage for chlamydia (see later)
    - Chlamydial: oral and topical erythromycin

Corneal Abrasion/Ulcer

BASIC INFORMATION

- Causes and etiology
    - Trauma, foreign body, contact lens wear, exposure keratopathy from lagophthalmos (incomplete closure of eyelid)

CLINICAL PRESENTATION

- Ocular injection and pain, tearing
- Decline in vision

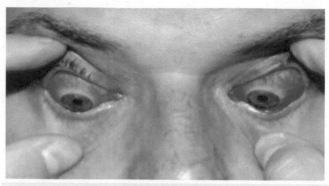

Fig. 67.4. Episcleritis.

DIAGNOSIS AND EVALUATION

- Complete ocular examination—check for epithelial defect (with fluorescein staining) and possible infiltrate, and rule out anterior segment inflammation/hypopyon
- Referral to ophthalmology for culturing of ulcers >1 mm in size (Gram stain, chocolate/thioglycolate/blood agar cultures)

TREATMENT

- Frequent topical antibiotics (fluoroquinolone such as moxifloxacin)
- If anterior segment inflammation is present, topical cycloplegic drop will help prevent symptomatic photophobia and iris adhesions
- Daily follow-up with an ophthalmologist

Episcleritis/Scleritis

BASIC INFORMATION

- Causes and etiology
    - Inflammation of episcleral or scleral vessels (Fig. 67.4)
    - Seen in autoimmune disease (i.e., rheumatoid arthritis [RA], systemic lupus erythematosus [SLE], polyarteritis nodosa [PAN])

CLINICAL PRESENTATION

- Ocular injection, boring eye pain (scleritis), or a milder ocular irritation (episcleritis)
- Bluish hue of sclera in scleritis
- Scleral nodules

DIAGNOSIS AND EVALUATION

- History: duration of symptoms, history of autoimmune disease, associated joint pains, fevers, rash, and so forth
- Complete ocular examination: check to rule out intraocular inflammation
- Referral to ophthalmology for further workup and treatment
- First-time episcleritis does not require additional laboratory workup

- Scleritis should be worked up with CBC, erythrocyte sedimentation rate (ESR), rapid plasma reagin (RPR), fluorescent treponemal antibody absorption (FTA-Abs), rheumatoid factor (RF), antinuclear antibodies (ANA), angiotensin-converting enzyme (ACE), and antineutrophil cytoplasm antibodies (ANCA)

TREATMENT

- Episcleritis: artificial tears (mild), topical steroid ± oral nonsteroidal antiinflammatory drugs (NSAIDs; moderate to severe)
- Scleritis: oral NSAIDs (ibuprofen, naproxen) ± oral steroids or immunosuppressive therapy if systemic cause is identified

Iritis/Uveitis

BASIC INFORMATION

- Causes and etiology
  - Inflammation of anterior or posterior segment or both
  - Autoimmune disease (i.e., RA, SLE, PAN, juvenile idiopathic arthritis [JIA])
  - Trauma
  - Infection (syphilis, tuberculosis, sarcoidosis)

CLINICAL PRESENTATION

- Ocular pain and injection, photophobia, decreased vision

DIAGNOSIS AND EVALUATION

- History: duration of symptoms, history of autoimmune disease, recent trauma or infection, associated joint pains, fevers, rash, and so forth
- Referral to ophthalmologist for complete ocular examination
- In bilateral or recurrent cases, obtain CBC, ESR, RPR, FTA-Abs, RF, ANA, ACE, lysozyme, ANCA, and HLA-B27

TREATMENT

- Topical steroids (prednisolone) and cycloplegics (atropine)
- May require oral steroids ± immunomodulatory therapy, especially if autoimmune

Herpetic Keratitis

BASIC INFORMATION

- Causes and etiology
- Usually HSV or herpes zoster virus (HZV)

CLINICAL PRESENTATION

- Ocular injection and pain, photophobia, decreased vision

- Vesicular rash in dermatomal distribution (HZV)
- Cold sores (HSV)

DIAGNOSIS AND EVALUATION

- History: duration of symptoms, history of chicken pox infection, recent cold sores
- Complete ocular examination: fluorescein stain to check for dendritic epithelial defect of cornea; check for cell and flare in anterior chamber
- Could consider viral culture with swab from cornea if dendrite is present

TREATMENT

- Oral antiviral agent (i.e., acyclovir)
- Topical antibiotics for epithelial defects
- May require topical steroids if intraocular inflammation or corneal stromal inflammation is present—needs to be managed closely by ophthalmologist

Congenital Cataracts

BASIC INFORMATION

- Causes and etiology
  - 60% are idiopathic and 10% to 35% are genetic (usually autosomal dominant)
  - May be related to Toxoplasmosis, Other, Rubella, Cytomegalovirus, Herpes [TORCH] infections (i.e., rubella)
  - Metabolic storage disorders (i.e., galactosemia)
  - May be present in Wilms tumor, Aniridia, Genitourinary anomalies, mental Retardation [WAGR] syndrome, which also presents with multisystem abnormalities

CLINICAL PRESENTATION

- Poor visual behavior (bilateral or unilateral)
- Could present with nystagmus and/or strabismus

DIAGNOSIS AND EVALUATION

- History: family history of cataracts, infections during pregnancy, immunization records, changes in visual behavior, presence of strabismus or nystagmus
- Complete ocular examination: retinoscopy to check for symmetric red reflex before evaluation

TREATMENT

- Observation if not visually significant
- Glasses for induced refractive errors
- Cataract surgery for visually significant cases, with possible aphakic contact lens and amblyopia treatment

Review Questions

For review questions, please go to ExpertConsult.com.

Suggested Readings

1. Bell AL, Rodes ME, Kellar LC. Childhood Eye Examination. *Am Fam Physician*. 2013;88(4):241–248.
2. Ehlers JP, Shah CP. *The Wills Eye Manual: Office and Emergency Room Diagnosis and Treatment of Eye Disease*. 5th ed. Philadelphia: LWW; 2008:173–178.
3. Wright KW, Strube YNJ. *Pediatric Ophthalmology and Strabismus*. 3rd ed. Oxford University Press, Inc.; 2012.

68 Disorders of the Posterior Segment

MARINA EISENBERG, MD

Childhood Glaucoma

BASIC INFORMATION

- Causes and etiology
  - Congenital (infantile)
    - Sporadic is most common but can be inherited (usually autosomal recessive [AR])
    - Usually bilateral
    - Usually not associated with other conditions
  - Juvenile
    - Usually autosomal dominant (AD)
  - Anterior-segment dysgenesis syndromes
    - Usually AD
  - Other associated conditions: Sturge-Weber syndrome, Lowe syndrome, rubella, aniridia

CLINICAL PRESENTATION

- Classic triad: photophobia, tearing, blepharospasm (involuntary eyelid closure)
  - All three signs do not need to be present to suspect the diagnosis
- Buphthalmos (enlargement of the eyeball), corneal enlargement, conjunctival injection, and corneal clouding
- Poor vision

DIAGNOSIS AND EVALUATION

- History
  - Family history of congenital glaucoma/vision loss in young family members
  - History of cloudy cornea or large eyes from early childhood
- Complete ocular examination should include visual acuity and funduscopic examination (e.g., corneal haze, increased cup-to-disk ratio [see Fig. 68.1])
- Formal ophthalmology examination will reveal other signs of glaucoma

TREATMENT

- Medical
  - Typically not effective for infantile glaucoma
  - Juvenile and secondary glaucoma are sometimes responsive to medical therapy—either ophthalmic drops (e.g., beta-blocker, carbonic anhydrase inhibitors) or oral medications (e.g., acetazolamide)
- Surgical options include trabeculotomy, goniotomy, glaucoma drainage devices, and/or cycloablative procedures

Papilledema

BASIC INFORMATION

- Swelling of the optic disk due to increased intracranial pressure
- Causes and etiology
  - Pseudotumor cerebri (see Chapter 56)
  - Hydrocephalus
  - Mass lesions (i.e., tumors)
  - Arteriovenous malformation
  - Meningitis/encephalitis/brain abscess
  - Central venous sinus thrombosis

CLINICAL PRESENTATION

- Symptoms
  - Headaches, nausea, vomiting, transient visual obscurations, diplopia
  - Pulsatile tinnitus, color vision deficits, visual field defects
  - Can get transient CN6 palsy
- Signs
  - Acute papilledema: optic disks appear swollen and hyperemic with blurred disk margins and blood vessel obscuration at the margins (see Fig. 68.2), retinal peripapillary hemorrhages, loss of venous pulsations, dilated tortuous vessels, enlarged blind spot
  - Chronic: pale optic disk and narrowed vessels, color vision impairment, and central and peripheral visual field defects

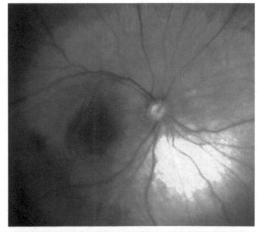

Fig. 68.1. Posterior pole in a patient with infantile glaucoma showing enlarged cup-to-disk ratio. (Photo courtesy Dr. Marina Eisenberg, MD.)

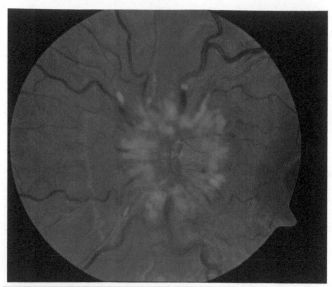

Fig. 68.2. Papilledema. (Photo courtesy Dr. Elias Traboulsi, MD.)

DIAGNOSIS AND EVALUATION

- Ophthalmology and neurology examination
- Workup may involve imaging (magnetic resonance imaging/magnetic resonance venography [MRI/MRV]) and lumbar puncture (LP) with measurement of opening pressure and cerebrospinal fluid (CSF) analysis

TREATMENT

- Address the underlying cause of papilledema

Optic Neuritis

BASIC INFORMATION

- Inflammation of the myelin sheath of the optic nerve
- Causes and etiology
  - Typically, the cause is unknown, but it commonly occurs after viral infections (e.g., mumps, measles, chicken pox, other viruses), immunizations, and bee stings
  - Can be isolated or associated with multiple sclerosis (MS), disseminated encephalomyelitis, or neuromyelitis optica (NMO)
  - Association between optic neuritis and MS/NMO is not as strong as in adults

CLINICAL PRESENTATION

- Symptoms
  - Severe vision loss, headache, nausea, vomiting, lethargy, and pain with eye movements
- Signs
  - Bilateral or unilateral severely decreased vision
  - More common to have optic disk swelling, but can have retrobulbar optic neuritis that does not have any visible optic disk swelling

DIAGNOSIS AND EVALUATION

- Complete ocular examination, including vision, pupils, motility, intraocular pressure, color vision, peripheral vision, and anterior- and posterior-segment examination
- MRI of brain/orbits may provide insight into underlying cause
- LP with fluid analysis to rule out infectious causes and NMO antibody
- Blood work to check for infectious and autoimmune causes

TREATMENT

- Controversial: IV steroids can be considered if vision loss is bilateral

Retinitis Pigmentosa (RP)

BASIC INFORMATION

- Heterogenous group of inherited rod-cone dystrophies
- Causes and etiology
  - Can be isolated to the eye or can be associated with other syndromes (e.g., Usher syndrome, Bassen-Kornzweig syndrome)
  - Inheritance pattern varies: AR is most common; AD (least severe), sporadic, and X-linked (most severe and rarest)

CLINICAL PRESENTATION

- History
  - History of poor night vision; family history of RP
- Signs and symptoms
  - Night blindness, visual field defects, tunnel vision with eventual central vision loss
  - Bilateral or asymmetric in presentation

DIAGNOSIS AND EVALUATION

- Complete ocular examination: vitreous cells, waxy optic disk pallor, pigment clumps in peripheral retina (perivascular) eventually developing into a bone spicule appearance
- Formal ophthalmologic examination and testing will find additional signs of RP
- Genetic testing and counseling

TREATMENT

- Ultraviolet (UV) protection glasses
- Cataract extraction
- Carbonic anhydrase inhibitors (oral and/or topical) and steroids for macular edema
- Low vision evaluation
- Lutein and vitamin A supplementation
- Argus retinal implant for patients with very advanced disease

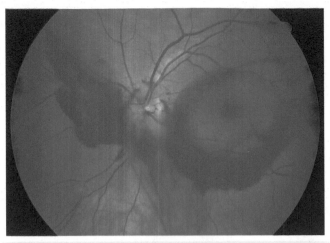

Fig. 68.3. Diffuse multilayered hemorrhage suggestive of nonaccidental trauma. (Photo courtesy Dr. Monte Del Monte, MD.)

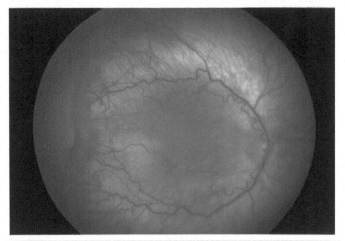

Fig. 68.4. Retinopathy of prematurity, Stage 3, Zone 2, plus disease. (Photo courtesy Dr. Cagri Besirli, MD, PhD.)

Shaken Baby Syndrome/ Nonaccidental Trauma

BASIC INFORMATION

- See Chapter 90 for details
- Combination of retinal hemorrhages, intracranial hemorrhages, and other injuries due to violent shaking
- Hemorrhages in multiple retinal layers (preretinal, intraretinal, subretinal [see Fig. 68.3]). Additional findings may include external ecchymosis, subconjunctival hemorrhage, hyphema, corneal burns, lacerations, cataract/lens dislocation, and retinal detachments
- 20% of survivors have vision loss

Retinopathy of Prematurity (ROP)

BASIC INFORMATION

- Abnormal vascular proliferation of the retina occurring after birth that can result in vision impairment and blindness
- Causes and etiology
  - Birth <32 weeks completed gestational age (GA) (last menstrual period [LMP])
  - Birth weight <1500 g
  - Supplemental oxygen, hypoxemia, hypercarbia, severe illness

CLINICAL PRESENTATION

- Signs: classically characterized by inappropriate vessel growth and neovascularization (see Fig. 68.4), avascular peripheral retina, extraretinal fibrovascular proliferation, and vitreous hemorrhage; may present with retinal detachment in severe cases

DIAGNOSIS AND EVALUATION

- Serial dilated fundus examinations with scleral depression
- Formal ophthalmology examination will reveal other signs of ROP

- Screening recommendations:
  - Screening provides a mechanism for identifying and following babies at risk for developing vision-threatening stages of ROP
  - Criteria:
    - Body weight (BW) <1500 g; GA ≤32 weeks, or any GA/BW with unstable clinical course
  - Timing of first examination:
    - At 31 to 32 weeks' GA (by LMP) or 4 weeks of age (whichever is later)
- Classification (see Fig. 68.5)
  - Stage:
    - 0: Immature vessels
    - 1: Demarcation line between vascular and avascular retina
    - 2: Ridge at demarcation line
    - 3: Extraretinal fibrovascular proliferation—neovascular tissue extends from the ridge into the vitreous
    - 4: Partial retinal detachment
    - 5: Total retinal detachment
  - Location: Zone 1–3
    - 1: Encompasses area centered on the optic disk with a radius of twice the distance from the optic disk to the macular center
    - 2: Extends from the edge of Zone 1 to the nasal ora serrata (has a disk shape)
    - 3: Temporal area extending from the edge of Zone 2 to the temporal ora serrata
  - Extent: clock hours
  - Plus disease: presence of increased venous dilation and arterial tortuosity

TREATMENT

- Close follow-up is necessary for early detection and intervention to prevent vision-threatening stages of ROP (Table 68.1)
- Treatment
  - Within 72 hours of examination
  - Modalities:
    - Laser
    - Cryotherapy

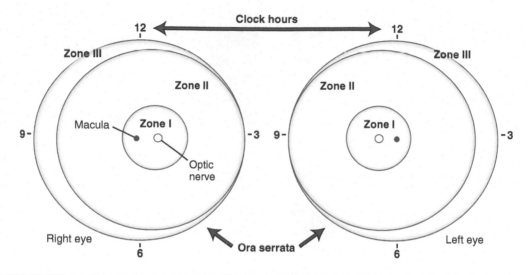

Fig. 68.5. Stages of retinopathy of prematurity.

Table 68.1. Timing of Retinopathy of Prematurity Follow-up Examinations

Follow-up Timing	Disease Severity
Within 1 week	Zone 1: Stage 1 or 2
	Zone 2: Stage 3
1–2 weeks	Zone 2: Stage 2
	Zone 1: Regressing ROP or immature vessels
2 weeks	Zone 2: Stage 1 or regressing ROP
2–3 weeks	Zone 2: Immature vessels
	Zone 3: Stage 1, 2, or regressing ROP

ROP, Retinopathy of prematurity.

- Intraocular bevacizumab injections
- Surgery
- Criteria for treatment:
  - Zone 1: any stage with plus disease
  - Zone 1: Stage 3, no plus
  - Zone 2: Stage 2 or 3, with plus disease

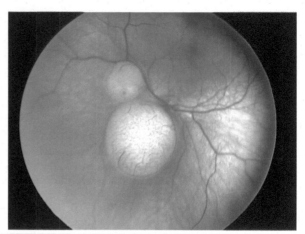

Fig. 68.6. Retinoblastoma. (Photo courtesy Dr. Elias Traboulsi, MD.)

- Vision loss, red eye, periocular swelling/redness (Fig. 68.6)
- Signs:
  - Leukocoria (most common), strabismus
  - Pineal gland involvement in cases of bilateral retinoblastoma (trilateral)

Retinoblastoma

BASIC INFORMATION

- Most common ocular malignant tumor in children
- Causes and etiology
  - Sporadic or hereditary
  - *RB* gene on 13q14
  - Usually noted by 1 year of age in familial cases; 1 to 3 years of age in sporadic cases; rare after 5 years of age

CLINICAL PRESENTATION

- History
  - Family history of ocular tumor, loss of vision or loss of the eye at a young age
- Symptoms

DIAGNOSIS AND EVALUATION

- Complete ocular examination: one or multiple white masses, vitreous hemorrhage/haze (if endophytic growth) versus retinal detachment (if exophytic growth); may be associated with ocular or periocular inflammation
- Formal ophthalmology examination will reveal other signs of retinoblastoma
- Ocular ultrasound to check for extent and presence of calcification
- MRI brain and orbits
  - Computed tomography (CT) can provide useful information, but it is not recommended in these patients due to susceptibility to radiation

TREATMENT

- Collaborative approach involving multiple services (ophthalmology, hematology/oncology, etc) to determine appropriate therapy on a case by case basis. Options include external beam radiotherapy, primary enucleation of eyes, chemotherapy, and other local therapies
- Monitoring for nonocular tumors is essential:
  - Osteogenic sarcoma, soft tissue sarcoma, cutaneous melanoma, breast cancer, lung cancer, brain tumors, Hodgkin lymphoma

- Genetic counseling for assessing risk for future family members
  - Examine other family members
  - Hereditary cases: patient and siblings examined every 4 months until 3 to 4 years old; every 6 months until 6 years old

Suggested Reading

Ehlers JP, Shah CP. *The Wills Eye Manual: Office and Emergency Room Diagnosis and Treatment of Eye Disease*. 5th ed. Philadelphia: LWW; 2008:169–171, 184–186.

Otorhinolaryngology

69 Disorders of the Ear and Audition

CHRISTOPHER LIU, MD

Pediatric Hearing Loss

BASIC INFORMATION

- Etiology
  - Incidence: 1 to 2 per 1000 infants are diagnosed with hearing loss
  - Congenital hearing loss
    - 50% due to environmental/acquired causes
      Viruses: cytomegalovirus (CMV), rubella, measles, mumps
      Kernicterus: up to 20% will develop high-frequency hearing loss
      Syphilis
    - 50% due to genetic factors
      70% of genetic hearing loss is nonsyndromic
      30% of genetic hearing loss is associated with a syndrome
    - Inheritance patterns of common genetic hearing loss disorders
      75% to 80% autosomal recessive (AR)
        Connexin 26
          Most common nonsyndromic genetic cause of congenital hearing loss
        Usher syndrome
          Most common AR syndromic hearing loss
          Sensorineural hearing loss (SNHL)
          Retinitis pigmentosa
        Jervell and Lange-Nielsen syndrome
          Profound SNHL
          Prolonged QT: often treated with beta-blockers
      20% autosomal dominant
        Waardenburg syndrome
          Most common cause of autosomal dominant (AD) congenital deafness
          Variable degrees of SNHL
          Also: white forelock, heterochromatic iris, premature graying, vitiligo
        Branchio-oto-renal syndrome
          Variable forms of hearing loss
          Also: branchial tags/fistulas and renal abnormalities
        Stickler syndrome
          SNHL or mixed hearing loss
          Also: craniofacial abnormalities
        Treacher Collins syndrome
          Conductive hearing loss (ossicular chain anomalies)
          Also: craniofacial abnormalities
      1% to 3% X-linked

Alport syndrome
  Defect in Type IV collagen found in the basement membrane
  Progressive SNHL
  Also: renal failure with hematuria
  See also Nelson Textbook of Pediatrics, Chapter 637, "Hearing Loss."

DIAGNOSIS AND EVALUATION

- Newborn hearing screening (based on Joint Committee on Infant Hearing Statement 2007)
  - All neonates should be screened within the first year of life
  - Identification of permanent hearing loss should occur by 3 months of age
  - Screen with auditory brainstem response (ABR) or otoacoustic emission (OAE) testing
  - Neonates with risk factors should be reevaluated with ABR at least once before 30 months of age (see Table 69.1)
  - Bilateral failed hearing screen requires urgent evaluation and treatment
    - Less likely to be a false-positive test
    - Refer to an otolaryngologist and offer genetics consultation
    - Application of hearing aids by 2 months of age
  - Unilateral hearing loss
    - Reduced sound localization and hearing discrimination in noise
  - Does not affect speech and language development but puts patients at risk for poor school performance

Table 69.1. Neonatal Hearing Loss Risk Factors

- Prolonged neonatal intensive care unit admission
- In utero infection
  - Toxoplasmosis
  - Other (syphilis, varicella, parvovirus)
  - Rubella
  - Cytomegalovirus
  - Herpes
- Strong family history of hearing loss in childhood
- Craniofacial abnormalities
- Neurodegenerative disorders
- Trauma
- Extracorporeal membrane oxygenation
- Chemotherapy
- Cranial irradiation
- Hyperbilirubinemia
- Persistent pulmonary hypertension

- Screening tests
  - ABRs
    - Use electroencephalogram (EEG) to measure electrical activity from the auditory nerve to the midbrain when sound stimulus is presented; it is unaffected by ambient noise
    - Objective test that does not depend on behavioral response of subject; therefore it is best for patients who cannot participate in pure tone audiometry testing (e.g., newborns, young age, developmental delay) or even for evaluation of malingerers
    - For accurate thresholds, child must either be asleep or sedated
    - Unreliable if child is awake
    - Unsedated sleep ABR testing is possible in children <6 months old
    - Auditory thresholds can be estimated based on ABR results
    - OAEs
    - Measures sound generated by mechanical activity of outer hair cells in the cochlea when a sound stimulus is presented
    - Absent in ears with >30-dB hearing loss
    - Presence of OAEs suggests normal cochlear sensitivity
    - Does not predict perception of sound because OAEs do not measure transmission of neural signal from cochlea to the brain
    - Relatively simple to administer. Does not require electrode placement. Can be used for several applications
    - Used for newborn hearing screening, evaluation of malingering, and monitoring of cochleotoxic medications.
- Diagnostic tests
  - Pure tone audiometry
    - Sound stimulus delivery
      As a sound field if child is too young to participate (i.e., <2 years old)
        Hearing thresholds to this type of stimulus reflect performance of the better-hearing ear and cannot rule out unilateral hearing loss
        Older patients undergo testing of air conduction thresholds via headphones and bone conduction thresholds via bone oscillators on the skull
    - Method depends on the age and cooperation of the child
      Behavioral observation audiometry (0 to 5 months)
        Observe changes in behavior that reflect perception of sound stimulus presented as a sound field; ear-specific information is unavailable
        Results depend on skill of tester
      Visual reinforcement audiometry (6 months to 2 years)
        If child looks up or to the side of sound stimulus presented as a sound field, he or she is rewarded with a lighted toy or video clip; ear-specific information is unavailable
        Results depend on skill of tester
      Conditioned play audiometry (2 to 5 years)
        Child shown how to listen and perform a repetitive play task whenever a sound stimulus is perceived

Table 69.2. Causes of Hearing Loss

Sensorineural Hearing Loss	Conductive Hearing Loss
Ototoxic drug exposure	Cholesteatoma
Aminoglycosides (gentamicin, tobramycin)	Craniofacial
	Cleft palate
Chemotherapeutics (cisplatin, carboplatin)	Goldenhar syndrome
	Treacher Collins syndrome
Loop diuretics (furosemide, ethacrynic acid)	Eustachian tube dysfunction
	External auditory canal obstruction
Nonsteroidal antiinflammatory drugs (salicylates)	Atresia
	Cerumen impaction
Infectious	Foreign body
Bacterial meningitis	Tumor
Cytomegalovirus	Middle ear effusion
Measles	Ossicular chain abnormality
Mumps	Otosclerosis
Rubella	Tympanosclerosis
Syphilis	Congenital malformation
Toxoplasmosis	Disruption of the ossicles
Genetic	Erosion from chronic infection
Alport syndrome	Trauma
Connexin 26 mutation	Tympanic membrane perforation
Jervell and Lange-Nielsen syndrome	
Neurofibromatosis	
Pendred syndrome	
Stickler syndrome	
Usher syndrome	
Waardenburg syndrome	
Developmental	
Cochlear malformation	
Enlarged vestibular aqueduct	
Tumor	
Cerebellopontine angle mass	

    Ear-specific information available because headphones and bone oscillators can be used at this age
    Thresholds obtained via this method are as reliable as those from conventional audiometry
  Conventional audiometry (>5 years old)
    Gold standard test
    Child raises hand or pushes button whenever he or she hears the sound stimulus
  - Interpretation of audiometric testing
    Degrees of hearing loss
      0–20 dB: normal
      21–40 dB: mild
      41–55 dB: moderate
      56–70 dB: moderately severe
      >70 dB: severe to profound
    SNHL
      Both bone conduction and air conduction thresholds are increased
      No air conduction–bone conduction gap is present
      Differential diagnosis (Table 69.2)
    Conductive hearing loss
      Normal bone conduction threshold, but air conduction threshold is elevated
      Air-bone gap: difference between air and bone threshold measurements
      Differential diagnosis (Table 69.2)
    Mixed hearing loss
      Bone conduction and air conduction thresholds are both elevated but not equal, suggesting

presence of both sensorineural and conductive hearing loss
- Tympanometry
  - A probe is inserted into the ear canal, and an airtight seal is created. A sound is introduced into the canal while a pump generates negative and positive pressure. A microphone detects the returned sound energy
  - Measures tympanic membrane mobility and middle ear function
    - Type A: normal tympanic membrane mobility and middle ear function
    - Type B: flat line reflecting little to no mobility of the tympanic membrane
      - Middle ear fluid
      - Cholesteatoma
      - Middle ear tumor
      - Scarring in the middle ear
      - Tympanic membrane perforation
    - Type C: negative middle ear pressure
      - Eustachian tube dysfunction

TREATMENT

- Additional nonauditory testing may be considered for those with congenital hearing loss, including ophthalmic examination, ECG, and thyroid function testing. It often prompts referral to genetics for guidance regarding additional imaging
- Referrals to otolaryngology, speech-language pathology, and early intervention programs are critical for follow-up
- Interventions include assistive learning devices, preferential seating in the classroom, and hearing aids
- Bone-anchored hearing aid (BAHA)
  - Indicated for conductive hearing loss and unilateral SNHL
  - Implant osseointegrates into the skull and amplifies sound via bone conduction by vibrating the skull
  - Minimum age for BAHA surgery is 5 years old
    - Thinness of temporal bone in young children leads to higher rate of failure
    - In the meantime, can use softband bone conduction hearing aid
- Cochlear implantation
  - Indicated for profound SNHL
  - Immunization for *Streptococcus pneumoniae* is strongly recommended before implantation
  - Early implantation yields the best result
  - Can implant as early as 1 year old

Otalgia

BASIC INFORMATION

- The differential diagnosis for otalgia is large and may be related to a variety of etiologies related to the external ear, external auditory canal, and inner/middle ear. The pain may also be referred. Table 69.3 lists potential causes

Table 69.3.   Differential Diagnosis: Otalgia

External Ear	Inner/Middle Ear
Autoimmune	Acute otitis media
Relapsing polychondritis	Mastoiditis
Cellulitis	Petrous apicitis
Contact dermatitis	Cholesteatoma
Herpes zoster oticus	Chronic otomastoiditis
Insect bite	Penetrating Trauma
Trauma	Temporal bone fracture
Auricular hematoma	Tympanic membrane perforation
	Tumor
	Langerhans cell histiocytosis
	Rhabdomyosarcoma
	Lymphoma
EXTERNAL AUDITORY CANAL	**REFERRED PAIN**
Cerumen impaction	Cervical spine injury
Contact dermatitis	Dental pain
Foreign body	Eagle syndrome
Herpes zoster oticus	Lymphadenitis (preauricular lymph nodes)
Otitis externa	
Fungal	Nasopharyngeal tumor
Bacterial	Oropharyngeal infection
Skull base osteomyelitis	Postsurgical pain
Trauma	Tonsillectomy and adenoidectomy
Tumor	Parotitis
Langerhans cell histiocytosis	Sinusitis
Rhabdomyosarcoma	Temporomandibular joint pain
Lymphoma	Trigeminal neuralgia

DISORDERS OF THE EXTERNAL EAR

Microtia and External Auditory Canal Atresia

BASIC INFORMATION

- Affects 1 in 7000 births; more common in males
- Associated with external auditory canal atresia and conductive hearing loss

CLINICAL PRESENTATION

- Small, malformed ear, most commonly presenting as absence of the external ear (with only vestigial structures present) with absence of the external auditory canal and tympanic membrane (Grade III). Other grades exist with variable development of the auricle and auditory canal
- Affects the right ear more frequently than the left ear
- Bilateral microtia suggests craniofacial syndrome
- Absence of lobule is uncommon and is associated with CHARGE Syndrome (Coloboma of the eye, Heart defects, Atresia of the choanae, Retardation of growth, Genitourinary defects, Ear anomalies)

DIAGNOSIS AND EVALUATION

- Thorough physical examination to rule out potential syndromic diagnosis
- Ear-specific audiologic assessment as soon as possible
- High-resolution temporal bone computed tomography (CT) scan to evaluate inner and middle ear structures

TREATMENT

- Monitor speech and language development; referral to otolaryngology and plastic surgery
- Hearing amplification as soon as possible
  - Children with bilateral atresia should receive bone conduction hearing aids
  - Children with unilateral atresia and one normal-hearing ear do not usually require amplification or special education for speech development
- Reconstruction of auricle when child is at least 5 years old
- Atresia repair should be delayed until microtia surgery is complete

Preauricular Pits and Sinuses

BASIC INFORMATION AND CLINICAL PRESENTATION

- Sinus or pit usually is found near the root of the helix. However, it can be found anywhere on the external ear
- Incidence is higher in children of African and Asian descent
- Diagnostic imaging and testing are not necessary
- Most are asymptomatic and remain untreated unless they become infected or drain
- Incision and drainage may be required if there is no improvement with antibiotic therapy and obvious presence of abscess
- Patients with pits that persistently drain or become infected should be referred to otolaryngologist for surgical excision

Auricular Hematoma

BASIC INFORMATION

- Trauma to the ear causing accumulation of blood in the subperichondrial space of the auricular cartilage
- Loss of vascular supply to the underlying cartilage leads to cartilage destruction and deformity

CLINICAL PRESENTATION

- Common injury in sports, especially wrestling
- Swelling of the auricle with effacement of landmarks
- Additional testing and imaging are unnecessary

TREATMENT

- Counsel patient on use of headgear during sports participation
- Incision and drainage of the hematoma and placement of compression bandage or bolster to prevent reaccumulation
- Undrained hematoma can cause permanent deformity—"cauliflower ear"

Table 69.4. Differential Diagnosis of Otorrhea

External Auditory Canal	Middle Ear
Bacterial otitis externa	Cerebrospinal fluid leak
Cerumen impaction	Congenital
Contact dermatitis	Traumatic
First branchial cleft cyst	Cholesteatoma
Foreign body	Infectious/Inflammatory
Keratosis obturans	Acute otitis media with tympanic
Otomycosis (fungal otitis externa)	membrane perforation
Skull base osteomyelitis	Chronic suppurative otitis media
	Myringitis
	Tuberculous otitis
	Tympanostomy tube otorrhea
	Neoplasm
	Langerhans cell histiocytosis
	Rhabdomyosarcoma

Perichondritis

BASIC INFORMATION AND CLINICAL PRESENTATION

- Inflammation or infection of the perichondrium of the auricle, which can be seen related to trauma, insect bites, systemic inflammatory conditions (relapsing polychondritis), and infections

DIAGNOSIS AND EVALUATION

- Erythema, pain, and swelling of the affected ear
- Lobule is spared in cases of systemic inflammatory conditions

TREATMENT

- Antibiotic therapy
  - Fluoroquinolones are first line because of cartilage penetration
    - Potential for musculoskeletal complications when used in children
  - Chosen antibiotic should cover *Staphylococcus aureus*, *S. pyogenes*, and *Pseudomonas aeruginosa*
    - Incision and drainage if abscess is present
    - Remove any foreign objects, including earrings
- Warm compresses for comfort

DISORDERS OF THE EXTERNAL AUDITORY CANAL

Otorrhea

BASIC INFORMATION

- Ear discharge of a variety of characteristics: serous, sanguinous, exudative
- A common complaint in the pediatric population, with a myriad of disorders of the external auditory canal and middle ear (see Table 69.4)

Cerumen Impaction

CLINICAL PRESENTATION

- Hearing loss (often presenting with failed hearing screen)
- Pain and sensation of fullness

DIAGNOSIS AND EVALUATION

- Otoscopy reveals cerumen occluding the external auditory canal

TREATMENT

- Saline or water irrigations
- Cerumenolytics (carbamide peroxide, hydrogen peroxide, mineral oil)
- Manual removal with curette, forceps, or suction
- If unable to remove, may need referral to otolaryngologist

Otitis Externa (OE)

BASIC INFORMATION

- Infection and inflammation of the external auditory canal
- Prolonged exposure to water (e.g., in swimmers) or injury to ear canal lining (e.g., infected hair follicle, ear trauma, foreign body) impairs immunologic defense and alters pH so that pathogenic organisms are allowed to grow
- Common bacterial pathogens: *P. aeruginosa* and *S. aureus*
- Common fungal pathogens: Aspergillus and Candida
- Other infectious and autoimmune conditions and malignancies can cause OE but are beyond the scope of this review

CLINICAL PRESENTATION

- Fever
- Otorrhea
- Otalgia, including pain with manipulation of the tragus
- Hearing loss due to obstruction of canal by debris and soft tissue edema
- May see signs of extension beyond the ear canal (e.g., soft tissue cellulitis of the auricle and surrounding tissue, cervical lymphadenopathy)
- Cranial nerve deficits can be seen in cases of necrotizing OE
- Gray and black fungal elements seen in ear canal in cases of otomycosis

DIAGNOSIS AND EVALUATION

- Physical examination demonstrates erythema, edema, and narrowing of the external auditory canal
  - Rule out otitis media with tympanic membrane perforation
- Cultures and laboratory studies typically not necessary unless symptoms persist or patient is immunocompromised; routine imaging studies are not indicated

TREATMENT

- Pain management (acetaminophen or ibuprofen)
- Topical medications for 7 to 10 days, such as acetic acid in aluminum acetate, ofloxacin otic, ciprofloxacin/dexamethasone otic
  - Can be given even if antibiotic resistance is detected in cultures. The antibiotic concentration in ototopical preparations far exceeds the minimal inhibitory concentrations of resistant organisms
- Otomycosis can be treated with topical antifungals such as otic clotrimazole solution and nystatin powder
- Systemic antibiotics are indicated only if there is extension beyond the ear canal or if there is history of immunodeficiency
- Severe cases may require debridement of the external auditory canal and placement of ear wick
- Prevention
  - Acidification of ear canal with boric acid or acetic acid drops before and after water exposure
  - Dry ear precautions
  - Earplugs

Ear Foreign Body

BASIC INFORMATION

- Oftentimes found incidentally in the pediatric population
- 75% of ear foreign bodies are found in children <8 years old

CLINICAL PRESENTATION

- Symptoms mimic otitis media and OE
  - Otalgia
  - Otorrhea
  - Hearing loss
  - Sensation of fullness
- Common foreign bodies: beads, plastic toys, pebbles, popcorn

DIAGNOSIS AND EVALUATION

- Otoscopy reveals foreign body in the external auditory canal
- Multiple foreign bodies are common, especially in young children. Inspect contralateral ear and nasal cavities

TREATMENT

- Restraint or sedation may be necessary if child is uncooperative
- Method of removal depends on the foreign body
  - Most can be removed with water irrigations or microinstruments (alligator forceps, cerumen loops, right-angle ball hooks, suction)
  - Special cases:
    - Live insects can be killed with alcohol, lidocaine, or mineral oil first before removal
    - Button batteries should not be irrigated but should be removed as soon as possible and have otolaryngology consult, even if removed successfully

- Organic matter should not be irrigated because it may expand and become lodged
- Consider otolaryngology referral if:
  - Failed multiple attempts
  - Object is medial and/or resting against the tympanic membrane
  - Sharp objects (glass)
  - Button batteries
- After removal, inspect for tympanic membrane perforation, OE, or canal laceration
- Audiogram if there is concern for hearing loss or tympanic membrane injury

DISORDERS OF THE MIDDLE EAR

Otitis Media with Effusion (OME)

BASIC INFORMATION

- Defined as middle ear effusion without signs or symptoms of acute inflammation
- Associated conditions:
  - Eustachian tube dysfunction
  - Allergic rhinitis
  - Adenoidal hypertrophy

CLINICAL PRESENTATION

- Hearing loss concerns
- Speech delay
- Aural fullness
- Symptoms suggesting infection, such as fever and otalgia, are absent

DIAGNOSIS AND EVALUATION

- Otoscopy
  - Dull tympanic membrane
  - Presence of fluid behind the tympanic membrane
  - Air-fluid levels
- Pneumatic otoscopy—decreased or no movement suggesting middle ear effusion
- Tympanometry
- Audiogram

TREATMENT

- Observation
  - Indicated for children who are not at risk for learning disabilities
  - Reevaluate at 3- to 6-month intervals until fluid resolves
  - Audiogram if effusion persists for >3 months or if hearing loss/speech delay becomes apparent
- Referral for myringotomy and tympanostomy tube placement if:
  - Persistent OME for >3 months
  - Speech delay
  - Children at risk for learning disabilities
  - Hearing loss on audiogram
- Routine use of antibiotics, decongestants, and antihistamines are not indicated

Acute Otitis Media (AOM)

BASIC INFORMATION

- Most common bacterial infection treated by pediatricians in the United States
- Accounts for up to 25% of office visits in children <3 years old
  - Highest incidence occurs between ages 6 and 11 months
- Infants and young children are at higher risk because eustachian tubes are shorter, wider, and more horizontal
  - By 7 years of age, the eustachian tube has developed into an adult configuration, and the prevalence of otitis media decreases
- Common pathogens: *S. pneumoniae*, nontypeable *Haemophilus influenzae*, *Moraxella catarrhalis*
  - Frequency of *S. pneumoniae* is decreasing due to pneumococcal vaccination
- See Table 69.5 for risk factors

CLINICAL PRESENTATION

- Fever
- Irritability or feeding difficulties
- Otalgia and ear tugging
- Hearing loss
- Sensation of aural fullness

DIAGNOSIS AND EVALUATION

- Otoscopy similar to otitis media with effusion but with the following additions:
  - Bulging or fullness of the tympanic membrane
  - Erythema of the tympanic membrane
  - Acute perforation with otorrhea
- Pneumatic otoscopy
  - Absence of or decreased mobility suggests perforation or middle ear effusion
- Tympanometry
- Audiometry if there is concern for hearing loss

TREATMENT

- Address pain with acetaminophen or ibuprofen
- Consider outpatient observation for 48 to 72 hours in the following cases:
  - Young children (6–23 months) with nonsevere unilateral AOM

Table 69.5. Risk Factors for Acute Otitis Media

Host	Environmental
Age	Cigarette smoke exposure
Cleft palate	Day care attendance
Ethnicity (Native American, Alaskan Eskimo)	Lack of breastfeeding
Immunoglobulin deficiency	Pacifier use
Male gender	
Prematurity	

- Children >2 years old with nonsevere unilateral or bilateral AOM
  - Nonsevere AOM: AOM with mild otalgia and temperature <39°C
- Otherwise, consider antibiotic therapy—10-day course
  - High-dose amoxicillin is the most common first-line agent
  - Add β-lactamase coverage if:
    - Amoxicillin use in the last 30 days
    - Concurrent purulent conjunctivitis
    - History of recurrent AOM unresponsive to amoxicillin
  - Cephalosporin or macrolide antibiotic if penicillin allergy
  - Refer to ear, nose, and throat (ENT) if second-line therapies fail
  - Antihistamines and decongestants are not recommended

Recurrent Otitis Media (ROM)

BASIC INFORMATION

- Most commonly occurs in children <2 years old, with highest incidence in children 6 to 12 months of age
- Defined as >3 episodes of AOM in 6 months or >4 episodes of AOM in 12 months
- Treat each episode as you would AOM
- Prophylactic antibiotics are not indicated
- Referral for tympanostomy tubes
  - Decreases frequency of AOM
  - Episodes of infection can be treated effectively with topical antibiotics

Chronic Suppurative Otitis Media

BASIC INFORMATION

- One of the most common causes of preventable hearing loss
- Perforated tympanic membrane with persistent drainage from the middle ear lasting greater than 6 weeks
- Compare with chronic serous otitis media, which is persistent middle ear effusion without perforation
- Results from inadequately treated AOM that progresses to tympanic membrane perforation and contamination by external auditory canal
- Common pathogens:
  - *P. aeruginosa*
  - *S. aureus*
  - Proteus
  - *Klebsiella pneumoniae*
  - Diphtheroids

CLINICAL PRESENTATION

- Persistent otorrhea lasting greater than 6 weeks

DIAGNOSIS AND EVALUATION

- Otoscopy demonstrates purulent otorrhea with tympanic membrane perforation

- Differential diagnosis includes cholesteatoma, which must be ruled out
- Audiogram

TREATMENT

- Aural toilet: may require debridement under a microscope by an otolaryngologist
- Ototopical antibiotics (fluoroquinolone)
  - Ofloxacin otic solution
  - Ciprofloxacin-dexamethasone otic solution
- Routine use of systemic antibiotics is not recommended

Mastoiditis

BASIC INFORMATION

- Suppurative infection of the mastoid; severe cases may have destruction of the mastoid air cells with extension into surrounding tissues
- Most often occurs secondary to extension of middle ear infection into the mastoid cortex; most common intratemporal complication of AOM
- Highest incidence in children <2 years old

CLINICAL PRESENTATION

- Fever
- Ear pain
- Postauricular tenderness, erythema, swelling (fluctuance if subperiosteal absence present)
- Protrusion of the auricle
- Otorrhea if tympanic membrane perforation is present

DIAGNOSIS AND EVALUATION

- Otoscopy may demonstrate bulging tympanic membrane with middle ear effusion or tympanic membrane perforation; absence of middle ear effusion does not exclude mastoiditis
- Diagnostic tests
  - Laboratory findings are nonspecific and do not make the diagnosis
    - Elevated white blood cells (WBCs) with left shift
    - Elevated C-reactive protein (CRP) and erythrocyte sedimentation rate (ESR)
  - Culture of middle ear or abscess fluid (if purulent)
  - Consider blood cultures if temperature >39°C
  - CT temporal bone with contrast is recommended
    - Fluid or mucosal thickening in the middle ear/mastoid
    - Loss of bony septae (coalescent mastoiditis)
    - Loss of definition of the mastoid cortex
    - Subperiosteal abscess

COMPLICATIONS

- Extracranial complications include those related to destruction of the auditory system (e.g., hearing loss, labyrinthitis), nearby nerves (e.g., facial paralysis), and bony structures (e.g., acute petrositis, subperiosteal abscess)

- Intracranial complications include invasion into the central nervous system (e.g., meningitis, subdural/extradural abscess) and venous sinus (e.g., sigmoid sinus thrombosis)

TREATMENT

- Consultation with an otolaryngologist
- Uncomplicated acute mastoiditis (without sepsis, intracranial involvement, or abscess) can be initially managed with broad-spectrum intravenous (IV) antibiotics that cross the blood-brain barrier
  - Antibiotic therapy should be directed at common organisms of AOM and Pseudomonas
    - Vancomycin and cefepime
    - Vancomycin and piperacillin-tazobactam
- Ototopical antibiotics can be used if there is a tympanic membrane perforation or after ear tube placement
- Surgical management (e.g., incision and drainage, mastoidectomy, tympanostomy) is indicated in cases with suppurative complications or if there is failure to improve with conservative therapies

Cholesteatoma

BASIC INFORMATION

- Presence of squamous epithelium in the middle ear and/or mastoid
- Causes
  - Acquired: severe tympanic membrane retraction or epithelial migration into the middle ear
  - Congenital: epithelial rests in the middle ear
- Associated complications
  - Untreated cholesteatoma will continue to grow and may become secondarily infected. Complications are related to erosion of bone overlying important structures
  - Hearing loss
  - Cranial nerve palsy
  - Vertigo
  - Intracranial infections

CLINICAL PRESENTATION

- Congenital cholesteatomas are often found incidentally on routine physical examination
- Acquired cholesteatomas present with recurrent/persistent otorrhea and hearing loss that fail to respond to antibiotic treatment
  - Erosion of the ossicles and tympanic membrane perforation/retraction contribute to conductive hearing loss

DIAGNOSIS AND EVALUATION

- Physical examination—most important
  - Congenital cholesteatoma
    - White mass behind an intact tympanic membrane
    - May or may not have hearing loss
  - Acquired cholesteatoma

- Retraction of the pars flaccida or tympanic membrane perforation with squamous debris tracking into the middle ear
- Purulent otorrhea
- Granulation tissue and polyps
- Hearing loss
- Diagnostic tests
  - Audiogram
  - CT temporal bone without contrast
    - Presence of soft tissue and fluid in the middle and mastoid
    - Determines extent of bony erosion
    - Assists with surgical planning

TREATMENT

- Removal of debris from the ear canal
- Dry ear precautions
- Ototopical antibiotics
- Referral to otolaryngologist for surgical removal

Tympanostomy Tubes (Ear Tubes)

BASIC INFORMATION

- A tube is inserted into an incision in the tympanic membrane by an otolaryngologist
  - Ear tubes typically last 6 to 18 months
- Indications for placement
  - Chronic bilateral OME for >3 months and documented hearing loss
  - Chronic unilateral or bilateral OME for >3 months, and symptoms attributable to OME are present
    - Balance disturbances
    - Ear discomfort
    - Poor school performance
    - Behavioral problems
    - Reduced quality of life
  - ROM with presence of middle ear effusion at time of assessment for ear tubes
  - Bilateral or unilateral OME in at-risk children
    - Permanent hearing loss independent of middle ear effusion
    - Suspected speech and/or language delay
    - Autism spectrum disorders
    - Developmental delay
    - Craniofacial disorders (especially cleft lip/cleft palate)
    - Syndromes associated with speech/language delays (Down)
    - Blindness
- Potential complications
  - Inadvertent placement of ear tube into the middle ear
  - Persistent otorrhea
  - Blockage of the tube after placement
  - Premature extrusion of the ear tube
  - Myringosclerosis or atrophy of the eardrum at the site of tube placement
  - Persistent perforation after tube extrusion (1% to 2% of cases)
    - Repair with paper patch or formal tympanoplasty

- Special considerations
  - Routine use of earplugs while swimming is not necessary but can be considered in the following situations:
    - Pain/discomfort when water enters ear canal
    - Otorrhea
    - Swimming in >6 feet of water
    - Swimming in lakes or nonchlorinated pools
  - Tympanostomy tube otorrhea—suggests active infectious process
    - Dry ear precautions
    - Ototopical antibiotics (ofloxacin or ciprofloxacin-dexamethasone)
  - Avoid drops containing ototoxic antibiotics (gentamicin, neomycin)
  - Recurrent AOM or persistent OME in children >4 years old
    - Adenoidectomy at time of repeat ear tube placement may reduce risk of recurrent infections and need for more surgeries

DISORDERS OF THE INNER EAR

Benign Paroxysmal Vertigo of Childhood (BPV)

BASIC INFORMATION

- Although dizziness is uncommon, there are many different causes in the pediatric population (Table 69.6)
- BPV is of unclear etiology but is thought to be associated with migraine disorders
- Migraine-associated vertigo and benign paroxysmal vertigo of childhood may account for up to half of cases. The diagnosis and evaluation of dizziness in the pediatric population are especially challenging because children are oftentimes unable to describe their symptoms

CLINICAL PRESENTATION

- Recurrent episodes of brief disequilibrium in children 2 to 7 years old
  - Episodes last <1 minute
  - Recurs in clusters, remitting for several weeks at a time
- Family history of migraines
- Symptoms
  - Episodes of rapid-onset vertigo
  - Child appears frightened and off-balance
  - No alteration of consciousness
  - Nystagmus
  - Diaphoresis
  - Nausea/vomiting

DIAGNOSIS AND EVALUATION

- BPV is a diagnosis of exclusion:
  - Comprehensive neurologic examination will be otherwise nonfocal
  - Diagnostic testing will be normal
    - Vestibular function testing
    - Electronystagmography

Table 69.6. Differential Diagnosis of Pediatric Dizziness

OTOLOGIC

Benign paroxysmal positional vertigo
Cholesteatoma
Congenital inner ear malformations
Drug exposure
   Aminoglycosides
   Chemotherapeutics
   Salicylates
Meniere disease
Middle ear effusion
Perilymphatic fistula
Superior canal dehiscence syndrome
Usher syndrome
Vestibular neuritis/acute labyrinthitis

NEUROLOGIC

Benign paroxysmal vertigo of childhood
Chiari malformation
Head trauma
Intracranial infection
Migraine-associated vertigo
Motion sickness
Multiple sclerosis
Neoplasm
   Cerebellopontine angle—vestibular schwannoma
   Posterior fossa—cerebellar astrocytoma, ependymoma, glioma, medulloblastoma
Paroxysmal torticollis of infancy
Seizure disorder
Stroke

MISCELLANEOUS

Anemia
Autonomic dysfunction
Cardiac disease
Familial periodic ataxia/vertigo
Peripheral neuropathy
Pseudovertigo
Psychogenic
Thyroid dysfunction

- Balance assessment
- Audiogram
- CT/MR imaging if there is concern for head trauma or tumor

TREATMENT

- Reassurance: symptoms are usually self-limited and resolve spontaneously within 2 years
- BPV of childhood differs from adult benign positional paroxysmal vertigo; Epley maneuver is unlikely to be successful in ameliorating symptoms

Inner Ear Infections

BASIC INFORMATION

- Vestibular neuritis: auditory function preserved, and symptoms are primarily vestibular related
- Acute labyrinthitis: hearing loss is present
- Etiology is suspected to be a viral or postviral inflammatory disorder affecting cranial nerve VIII. Could also be a manifestation of AOM

CLINICAL PRESENTATION

- Acute onset of hearing loss and/or vertigo, nausea, vomiting, and gait impairment
- Rarely seen in young children. Typically occurs in the adolescent age group

DIAGNOSIS AND EVALUATION

- Diagnosis is based on clinical examination and history
- Physical examination
  - Nystagmus
  - Positive head thrust test
  - Gait instability
  - Absence of other neurologic symptoms
- Audiogram
- Consider MR imaging to rule out intracranial process

TREATMENT

- Symptoms are self-limited and will diminish over the course of several weeks
- Treatment during the acute phase:
  - Corticosteroids

- Short-term treatment of symptoms with antiemetics, antihistamines, anticholinergics, and benzodiazepines
  - Prolonged use can suppress vestibular activity and impair long-term compensation
- Vestibular rehabilitation

Review Questions

For review questions, please go to ExpertConsult.com.

Suggested Readings

1. Harlor Jr AD, Bower C, et al. Hearing assessment in infants and children: recommendations beyond neonatal screening. *Pediatrics.* 2009; 124(4):1252–1263.
2. Lieberthal AS, Carroll AE, Chonmaitree T, et al. The diagnosis and management of acute otitis media. *Pediatrics.* 2013;131(3):e964–e999.
3. Potsic WP, Lando T. Introduction to pediatric otology. In: Wetmore RF, Muntz HR, McGill TJ, eds. *Pediatric otolaryngology: principles and practice pathways.* 2nd ed. New York: Thieme Medical Publishers; 2012:196–209.
4. Rosenfeld RM, Schwartz SR, Cannon CR, et al. Clinical practice guideline: acute otitis externa executive summary. *Otolaryngol Head Neck Surg.* 2013;150(2):161–168.
5. Rosenfeld RM, Schwartz SR, Pynnonen MA, et al. Clinical practice guideline: tympanostomy tubes in children—executive summary. *Otolaryngol Head Neck Surg.* 2013;149(1):8–16.

70 Disorders of the Nose and Sinuses

ELEANOR PITZ KIELL, MD

NOSE

Upper Respiratory Infection (URI)

BASIC INFORMATION

- Most common illness seen by the primary care physician
- Characterized by nasal discharge and nasal congestion with variable components of cough, conjunctivitis, sore throat, and constitutional symptoms; usually self-limited
- Caused by viral infection, typically from four groups: (1) myxovirus and paramyxovirus groups (influenza, parainfluenza, respiratory syncytial viruses [RSV]), (2) adenoviruses, (3) picornavirus groups (enteroviruses and rhinoviruses), (4) coronaviruses
- Common for children to experience 10 URIs/year, whereas adults experience 2 to 3 URIs/year; varies based on child's age, number of siblings, and day care
- Seasonal variation is common; URIs are least common in summer, except croup from parainfluenza; rhinovirus is most common in fall/spring; coronaviruses, influenza viruses, and RSV are most prevalent in winter
- Spread of virus is difficult to control; can be spread via inhalation of small or large airborne particles and most commonly contamination of hands through the environment or other contact, which then inoculates mucosal surfaces (mucosa or conjunctiva)

CLINICAL PRESENTATION

- Typically last 5 to 7 days, but can last 10 to 14 days
- Symptoms:
  - Vary among patients
  - Nasal congestion
  - Nasal discharge (serous, mucoid, purulent)
  - Sneezing
  - Cough
  - Conjunctival inflammation
  - Sore throat
  - Constitutional symptoms (fever, malaise, myalgias)
- Physical findings:
  - Erythematous nasal and pharyngeal mucosa
  - Lymphoid hyperplasia in posterior pharynx
  - Possibly tonsil and adenoid hypertrophy
  - Mildly enlarged and tender cervical adenopathy
  - Irritated skin around nasal ala and upper lip

DIAGNOSIS AND EVALUATION

- Rarely necessary to diagnose the precise viral cause; a notable exception is when the clinical scenario warrants testing for influenza virus
- Consider nasopharyngeal or nasal cavity swab for viral studies

TREATMENT

- Supportive treatment is key (e.g., nasal saline spray, increased fluid intake, antipyretics)
- The following therapies don't affect disease course; rather, they provide only symptomatic relief at best and are generally avoided in young patients:
  - Mucolytics
  - Topical decongestants
  - Antihistamines or antihistamine-decongestant combinations: act by competitively blocking the histamine receptor site; relieve symptoms of sneezing, nasal itchiness, and watery rhinorrhea
- Antiviral therapy may be indicated for certain viruses and clinical scenarios

Rhinitis

BASIC INFORMATION

- Rhinitis describes inflammation within the nasal cavity, without regard to specific etiology
- Rhinitis is clinically diagnosed as the onset of at least two of the following:
  - Nasal discharge
  - Sneezing
  - Nasal itching
  - Nasal congestion
- Commonly separated into three categories: allergic, infectious, and chronic rhinitis
- Allergic rhinitis is a chronic inflammatory disorder induced by IgE-mediated mechanisms secondary to allergen exposure (see Chapter 2 for details; only nonallergic rhinitis will be covered here)
- Nonallergic rhinitis can have a clinical presentation surprisingly similar to that of allergic rhinitis, but no IgE-mediated trigger will be identified
  - Common triggers include environmental temperature changes, air pollution, and environmental irritants

(e.g., tobacco smoke); can be treated with similar therapies despite the unknown underlying mechanism
- Infectious rhinitis is most commonly viral in nature
- Bacterial rhinitis is most commonly caused by *Streptococcus pyogenes* (group A streptococcus)
- See also Nelson Textbook of Pediatrics, Chapter 143, "Allergic Rhinitis"

CLINICAL PRESENTATION

- Infectious rhinitis:
  - Viral: most common cause of infectious rhinitis
    - Characterized by sudden onset of symptoms (clear or mucoid rhinorrhea, nasal congestion, sneezing, and sore throat); may develop cough or fever
    - Young children (less than 4–5 years) may have high fever without superimposed bacterial infection
    - Physical examination may show red and inflamed nose, throat, and tympanic membranes
    - Average duration of symptoms is 1 week
    - Nasal secretions tend to become thicker and more purulent after day 2
    - May experience persistent mild cough for 2 to 3 weeks
  - Bacterial: most commonly group A streptococcus, but the most common clinical manifestation of group A streptococcus is pharyngitis (fever, tender anterior cervical lymphadenopathy)
    - Common in 5- to 15-year-old children
    - Persistent rhinitis in infants or toddlers (children <3 years) suggests possibility of streptococcal rhinitis
    - Presents with protracted cold with low-grade fever
- Chronic rhinitis: see chronic rhinosinusitis

DIAGNOSIS AND EVALUATION

- Diagnosis is primarily established by history and physical examination
  - Culture of nasopharynx with growth of group A streptococcus; may see complications of *S. pyogenes*

TREATMENT

- Infectious rhinitis:
  - Viral rhinitis—supportive; over-the-counter cough and cold medications have been shown not to be effective in children and may cause adverse events
  - Bacterial rhinitis—antibiotics with activity against group A streptococcus, such as amoxicillin may be considered; may consider culture-directed antibiotics, especially if persistent symptoms despite antibiotic therapy
- Chronic rhinitis: see chronic rhinosinusitis

Choanal Atresia

BASIC INFORMATION

- Nasal choana is the "doorway" from the nasal cavity to the nasopharynx
- Choanal atresia is the failure of this doorway to form
- Occurs in approximately 1/5000 to 1/8000 live births
- Twice as common in girls

Table 70.1. Abnormalities Associated With Choanal Atresia

Syndromic Associations	ENT Anomalies	Non-ENT Anomalies
CHARGE syndrome ■ C: coloboma ■ H: heart anomalies ■ A: choanal atresia ■ R: growth or mental retardation ■ G: genitourinary anomalies ■ E: ear abnormalities Crouzon syndrome	Facial asymmetry Cleft palate Hypertelorism Nasal deformities Auricular deformities	Polydactyly Craniosynostosis Microcephaly Meningocele

ENT, ear-nose-throat.

- Occurs unilaterally (65%–75% of cases) more commonly than bilaterally
- Up to 70% of children with choanal atresia have associated anomalies (see Table 70.1)
  - Bilateral disease is associated with other congenital abnormalities in 50% of patients

CLINICAL PRESENTATION

Bilateral

- Presents at birth with airway obstruction
- *Paradoxical cyanosis:* episodes of respiratory distress with cyanosis (especially during feeding) that is relieved with crying

Unilateral

- Presents with unilateral rhinorrhea and persistent obstruction between 2 and 5 years

DIAGNOSIS AND EVALUATION

Appropriate Evaluation

- Mirror under nose to evaluate for fogging with expiration
- Attempt to pass an 8 French catheter (if it will not pass >3.5 cm from anterior nose, concern should be raised)
- Nasal endoscopy (with or without nasal topical decongestion) can confirm atresia
- Computed tomography (CT) scan to evaluate the thickness of atresia plate, lateral bony involvement, and for surgical planning

Associated Congenital Anomalies

- Given the frequency of associated abnormalities, additional investigation is often pursued upon diagnosis of choanal atresia, including evaluation for CHARGE syndrome (see Chapter 35 and Table 70.1)

TREATMENT

- McGovern nipple (standard nipple with a large hole) or oral airway
- Surgical repair is dependent on severity of symptoms and severity of symptoms is often less with unilateral choanal atresia:
  - Unilateral choanal atresia: surgical repair can often be postponed until the child is older, unless there are

severe symptoms such as inability to feed or respiratory distress

- Bilateral choanal atresia: must occur early in life (first week of life) as neonates are obligate nasal breathers; neonates may require orotracheal intubation to maintain airway before surgical correction
- Surgical approach may be transnasal, transpalatal, or endoscopic transnasal; stenting after choanal atresia repair is controversial
- Revision surgery may be required and can occur early in recovery or later in life

Epistaxis

BASIC INFORMATION

- Over 90% of bleeds can be visualized anteriorly, with the most common site for bleeding being the anterior septum, called Little's area, which overlies Kiesselbach's plexus
- Causes can be from local or systemic pathology
  - Local etiology:
    - Trauma (digital, foreign body, fracture, surgery)
    - Desiccation
    - Drug induced (cocaine, nasal steroids)
    - Infectious (bacterial sinusitis or rhinitis)
    - Inflammatory (allergic rhinitis, granulomatous disease)
    - Neoplastic (angiofibroma, papilloma, carcinoma)
  - Systemic etiology:
    - Intrinsic coagulopathy (von Willebrand disease, hemophilia, hereditary hemorrhagic telangiectasia)
    - Drug-induced coagulopathy (acetylsalicylic acid [ASA], nonsteroidal anti-inflammatory drugs [NSAIDs], antiplatelet therapy)
    - Hypertension (HTN)
    - Neoplastic

CLINICAL PRESENTATION

- Acute hemorrhage—rarely-life threatening in children, but must evaluate airway, breathing & circulation (ABCs) and stabilize before considering underlying pathology
- Recurrent bleeds
  - Often at night
  - Parents report large amount of blood
  - Frequently self-limiting

DIAGNOSIS AND EVALUATION

- Clinical examination focuses on evaluating nasal septum, looking for scabbing, crusting, or visible vessels
- Consider consult with an ear, nose, throat specialist (ENT) in the acute setting if bleeding is persistent despite medical treatment, or if there is significant blood loss with persistent bleeding
- May consider CT scan in a patient with unilateral bleeding and obstruction or other visualized abnormalities

TREATMENT

- Acute bleed:
  - Stabilization of patient—ABCs

- Pressure pinching anterior (soft tissue of nose) between two fingers
- Visualization with good headlight
- Consider nasal decongestant (phenylephrine or oxymetazoline, topical)
- Manage blood pressure or underlying coagulopathy (if possible)
- Consider nasal packing (Merocel pack, Rhino Rocket, other inflatable devices) if there is persistent oozing despite treatments noted previously or if there is an anticipated delay to definitive treatment (i.e., transfer of treating facility, correction of coagulopathy)
- Recurrent bleeding:
  - Humidification (humidifier at night, nasal saline sprays, emollient to anterior vestibule at least daily)
  - Discourage nose picking and home "packing" of nose
  - If persistent after these measures, consider referral to specialist (otolaryngologist, hematologist, etc.)
    - In-office versus operative treatment of prominent vessels in anterior septum
    - Coagulopathy workup

Polyps

BASIC INFORMATION

- Polyps are an abnormal growth from the nasal or paranasal sinus mucosa, most often the result of an inflammatory process of varying etiology
- May be identified as unilateral or bilateral; single or multiple
- Overall incidence in children is 0.1% in the United States; in children with cystic fibrosis, incidence in children ranges from 6% to 48%

CLINICAL PRESENTATION

- Nasal obstruction
- Rhinorrhea
- Decreased sense of smell
- Headaches/facial pain
- Snoring/sleep apnea
- Postnasal drainage
- Visible "mass" in the child's nose

DIAGNOSIS AND EVALUATION

- All children with multiple polyps/bilateral polyps should have thorough evaluation for cystic fibrosis and asthma
  - Sweat test and pulmonary function tests; consider evaluation by pulmonologist
  - Nasal polyps, asthma, and aspirin/NSAID sensitivity comprise "Samter's Triad" and are suggestive of "aspirin-exacerbated respiratory disease"
  - The differential diagnosis includes additional etiologies to consider as well (see Table 70.2)
- Nasal examination using good lighting and nasal speculum
- Consider nasal endoscopy with rigid or flexible scopes (or refer to specialist)
- Consider imaging of face/sinuses/brain (CT vs magnetic resonance imaging [MRI]) depending on suspected diagnosis

Table 70.2.   Differential Diagnosis for Nasal Polyps

Bilateral Nasal Polyps	Unilateral Nasal Polyps
Chronic sinusitis	Antrochoanal polyp
Allergic rhinitis	Benign massive polyp
Cystic fibrosis	Benign tumor
Allergic fungal sinusitis	■ Encephalocele
	■ Glioma
	■ Dermoid
	■ Nasolacrimal duct cyst
	■ Hemangioma
	■ Papilloma
	■ Inverting papilloma
	■ Juvenile nasopharyngeal angiofibroma
	Malignant tumor
	■ Rhabdomyosarcoma
	■ Lymphoma
	■ Neuroblastoma
	■ Sarcoma
	■ Chordoma
	■ Nasopharyngeal carcinoma
	■ Inverting papilloma

TREATMENT

- Unilateral polyp identified as antrochoanal polyp or massive benign polyp should be referred to otolaryngology for evaluation and surgical management
- Bilateral polyps are often an indication of underlying chronic inflammatory disorder and usually require medical management initially
  - Medical management often include nasal rinses, steroid nasal sprays, antihistamine nasal sprays, and consideration of short course of antibiotics or systemic steroids
  - May consider referral to allergist or pulmonologist, depending on associated diagnosis
  - Referral to otolaryngology for surgical management may decrease disease burden and allow medical treatments to be more effective, but are generally not curative
- Polyps identified as other unilateral masses should be treated according to diagnosis; however, this will likely include referral to specialist (otolaryngologist, neurosurgeon, ophthalmologist, interventional radiologist), imaging (CT vs MRI), and surgical intervention

Juvenile Nasopharyngeal Angiofibroma

BASIC INFORMATION

- Rare but locally destructive vascular tumor in the nasopharynx, but can extend to surrounding structures, including the orbit and skull base
- Almost exclusively identified in adolescent males
- Commonly presents with unilateral nasal obstruction and/or epistaxis; less commonly, facial swelling, visual changes, or altered mental status can be presenting symptoms
- Diagnosis based on history, endoscopic findings, and imaging (CT and/or MRI); biopsy is not recommended
- Treatment is surgical resection with preoperative embolization to reduce blood loss
- More invasive tumors may require postoperative treatment with radiation or stereotactic radiosurgery; hormone therapy and chemotherapy are ineffective

Nasal Trauma

BASIC INFORMATION

- Commonly encountered nasal trauma includes nasal fracture, epistaxis, and septal hematoma
- Nose is the most commonly fractured bone in the face
- Frequency of nasal bone fractures increases with age; teenagers are far more likely to suffer facial fractures than are school-age children
  - Reasons for fewer fractures in children include comparatively more compliant bones in children than adults and thicker adipose and muscle in children's faces
- Nearly one-third of children who sustain facial trauma also have a concussion
- Septal hematoma is a concerning complication of nasal trauma:
  - Children are at especially high risk for septal hematoma due to the immature cartilage of the nose and its propensity for buckling without obvious fracture
  - The cartilage is separated from its blood supply in the overlying perichondrium; necrosis can result in septal perforation or saddle nose deformity
  - Management of septal hematoma requires evacuation by needle aspiration or incision and drainage
- Nasal trauma also uncommonly associated with:
  - Cerebrospinal fluid (CSF) leak
  - Other maxillofacial injuries (e.g., eye injury)
  - Intracranial injury
  - Maxillomandibular injury

CLINICAL PRESENTATION

- History is usually suggestive—commonly sports-related mechanism with blow to nose by ball or another athlete
- Visible nasal deformity, especially before swelling sets in
- Often accompanied by epistaxis

DIAGNOSIS AND EVALUATION

- Diagnosis is usually made by history and physical examination
- If evaluation is more than several hours after injury, visualization of deformity may be difficult; *must* palpate nasal bones for step-off deformity or crepitus
- If there is concern for additional facial injuries, one may consider imaging to include CT scan of the facial bones; there is limited role for plain film radiographs
- Must evaluate for septal hematoma by visualization and/or palpation: appears as a bulging bluish mass in the nasal septum; can use gloved finger to palpate for thickening of nasal septum as well
- Also ensure clinical evaluation of mandible and eyes to identify any associated injuries
- If CSF leak is suspected, consider testing beta-2 transferrin from fluid for confirmation

TREATMENT

- Initial management includes controlling any associated bleeding, managing soft tissue injuries (laceration), and pain control

- Patients with nasal fractures without obvious external deformity, adequate nasal airway, and no other injuries warranting surgery can be referred for outpatient ENT evaluation within 3 days of injury for reevaluation (postinjury edema will be resolving)
- Indications for surgery include unacceptable deformity and nasal obstruction
- Timing of surgery is crucial in children due to rapid healing: ideally between 3 and 5 days from injury, so they must be referred to surgical team (plastic surgery or ENT) *early*
- Patients should be counseled that of those who pursue surgical treatment, as many as half may desire future rhinoplasty

Nasal Foreign Body

BASIC INFORMATION

- Most common in children ages 2 to 5 years
- Involves any small object small enough to fit up the nostril (food, buttons, toys, erasers, etc.)
- Makes up to 0.1% of emergency department visits
- Special consideration for button batteries and magnets (when one is in each nasal cavity)

CLINICAL PRESENTATION

- "My child put something in his or her nose"
- Pain or discomfort
- Unilateral foul-smelling discharge
- Recurrent epistaxis
- Rhinorrhea/congestion
- Complications: local irritation, pain, ulceration, infection, epistaxis, septal perforation

DIAGNOSIS AND EVALUATION

- Visualization of foreign body with good headlight and possible use of nasal decongestant
- High index of suspicion when there is unilateral foul-smelling nasal discharge

TREATMENT

- Positive pressure: using pressure to "blow" the object out
  - Child blows while obstructing the other nostril (or releasing obstruction of the side with foreign body after pinching both and instructing child to blow)
  - Use a topical vasoconstrictor (phenylephrine or oxymetazoline) before attempts at removal
  - "Parent's kiss": patient's parent is instructed to blow into the child's mouth while occluding the unaffected nostril, thereby increasing pressure and in essence blowing the child's nose for him or her
  - Sterile saline to flush out the foreign body via the opposite side—harder to tolerate
  - These maneuvers do carry risk of foreign body aspiration if the foreign body is displaced posteriorly instead of anteriorly
- Mechanical extraction is indicated for objects refractory to the previous maneuvers
  - If not familiar with techniques, consider consultation of ENT for removal (can be done in emergency department or commonly done in the office)

SINUSES

Acute Sinusitis

BASIC INFORMATION

- Inflammation of sinonasal mucosa and obstruction of the sinus drainage pathways can lead to acute obstruction on a sinus with resultant acute sinusitis
- Obstruction may be the result of anatomic, mucosal, microbial, and immune factors or some combination of these factors
- Viral and bacterial infections likely play a large role in the pathogenesis of acute sinusitis
  - Viral infection may cause mucosal injury and swelling, resulting in sinus outflow obstruction, decreased ciliary activity, and increased production of mucus
  - Common bacterial pathogens include: *Streptococcus pneumoniae*, *Haemophilus influenzae* (nontypeable), *Moraxella catarrhalis*, and beta-hemolytic streptococcus
- Complications of acute sinusitis include:
  - Involvement of the orbit: may occur due to thin walls of the ethmoid sinus, resulting in subperiosteal abscess, orbital cellulitis, or orbital abscess
  - Involvement of the central nervous system (CNS): may occur from dissemination of frontal sinus via shared venous drainage with intracranial structures, resulting in meningitis, intracranial abscess, and venous sinus thrombosis
  - Involvement of the frontal bone: frontal sinusitis may lead to osteomyelitis and/or subperiosteal abscess

Clinical Presentation

- Symptoms include nasal drainage, nasal congestion, facial pressure/pain, postnasal drainage, hyposmia or anosmia, fever, cough, fatigue, maxillary dental pain, and ear pressure or fullness
- Symptom onset may be gradual or sudden
- "Classic" presentations include:
  - Prolonged nasal congestion/discharge after URI without improvement for >10 days
  - Sudden onset of fever and purulent nasal discharge for >3 days
  - Biphasic "double-sickening" with onset of symptoms 3 to 7 days after initial improvement after a URI

Diagnosis and Evaluation

- Physical examination is rarely helpful because the findings can rarely be distinguished from a typical viral URI; imaging is not indicated for diagnosis of acute bacterial sinusitis

- Consider referral to otolaryngology in patients who have complicated medical history or who are immunocompromised because sinus cultures may be helpful
  - Nasal swab cultures and throat cultures do not correlate with sinus cultures, so they are not used to dictate treatment
- Consider blood cultures if patient is hospitalized for acute sinusitis
- CT or MRI is indicated when there is concern for complication in an acute illness, such as periorbital or orbital cellulitis/abscess, intracranial extension, or venous sinus thrombosis

Treatment

- Symptom management using nasal saline irrigations or sprays, topical decongestant (oxymetazoline or phenylephrine), oral decongestants, and/or antihistamines can be considered
  - Topical decongestants should not be used >3 days due to physiologic dependence and rebound congestion
  - Oral decongestants are not advised in children <6 years of age and have not been proven to be definitively beneficial in children
- If symptoms have not improved after 10 days, consider 3 more days of observation versus initiation of antibiotic therapy
  - First line: The American Academy of Pediatrics (AAP) and Infectious Diseases Society of America (IDSA) differ in their recommendations, with the former preferring amoxicillin (with children in communities with resistant streptococcus requiring high-dose amoxicillin [80–90 mg/kg/day]); the IDSA prefers high-dose amoxicillin with clavulanate as first line, whereas the AAP reserves this for children who have moderate to severe illness, who are less than 2 years old, who attend day care, or who have received another antimicrobial within the prior 4 weeks
  - Penicillin allergy: cefuroxime, cefpodoxime, or cefdinir (children <2 years old may require a combination of clindamycin/linezolid and cefixime)
  - If there is suspicion for resistant *S. pneumoniae* or *H. influenzae*: clindamycin, linezolid, or quinolones can be used
  - Duration of therapy should be 14 to 21 days
  - Avoid trimethoprim-sulfamethoxazole and azithromycin due to high resistance of common organisms
- Failure to improve after 48 to 72 hours or worsening symptoms may be signs of antibiotic resistance
- Development of symptoms such as proptosis, changes in vision, restricted ocular motility, altered mental status, and worsening headache are concerning for complication of an acute sinusitis that requires workup, most likely through emergency department evaluation

Chronic Rhinosinusitis

BASIC INFORMATION

- Factors that may contribute to the development of chronic rhinosinusitis include allergies, anatomic variation, and impaired host immunity

Table 70.3. Criteria for Diagnosing Chronic Rhinosinusitis

Twelve weeks (or longer) of at least two of the following clinical findings:	AND	Inflammation documented by at least one of the following:
■ Mucopurulent drainage (anterior, posterior, or both) ■ Nasal obstruction or congestion ■ Facial pain-pressure-fullness ■ Decreased sense of smell-		■ Purulent (not clear) mucus or edema visualized in the middle meatus or anterior ethmoid region (by anterior rhinoscopy or rigid endoscopy) ■ Polyps in the nasal cavity or the middle meatus ■ Radiographic imaging showing inflammation of the paranasal sinuses

- The unified airway theory suggests that the nose, paranasal sinuses, larynx, trachea, bronchi, and lungs are a single functional unit of the respiratory system
- Children with diseases of the nose and paranasal sinuses should be closely evaluated for diseases of other parts of the respiratory system
- Allergic rhinitis or nonallergic rhinitis are commonly implicated in the development of chronic rhinosinusitis; less commonly, anatomic variations (septal deviation, nasal polyp) or gastroesophageal reflux have been implicated
- Allergic nasal polyps are uncommon in children under 10 years of age; therefore polyps in children less than 10 years old should prompt a workup for cystic fibrosis
- Recurrent purulent pansinusitis in a child should be suspicious for underlying host abnormality, such as immune disorder, primary ciliary dyskinesia, or cystic fibrosis
- Common organisms in chronic rhinosinusitis include staphylococcal organisms and anaerobes

CLINICAL PRESENTATION

- See diagnostic criteria in the following section.

DIAGNOSIS AND EVALUATION

- Diagnosed when a patient experiences clearance of acute bacterial sinusitis in 10 days, but occurs at least four times in a year *or* when symptoms persist for more than 12 weeks without progression to acute complications
- Criteria for diagnosis in Table 70.3

TREATMENT

- Medical therapy:
  - Antibiotic therapy with duration of 3 to 4 weeks
  - Antibiotic coverage should include antistaphylococcal coverage
  - Nasal saline irrigations
  - Intranasal steroid sprays
- Surgical options for those experiencing significant complications include antral lavage, adenoidectomy, endoscopic sinus surgery, and external drainage

Sinus Trauma

BASIC INFORMATION

- Frequency of facial fractures increases with age; teenagers are far more likely to suffer facial fractures than are school-age children
  - Facial fractures in toddlers have nearly equal male-to-female distribution but shift to 2:1 male predominance by early school age
  - Reasons for fewer fractures in children include comparatively more compliant bones in children than adults and thicker adipose and muscle in children's faces
- Nearly one-third of children who sustain facial trauma also have a concussion
- Midface fractures
  - Le Fort fractures—varying degrees of craniofacial separation caused by trauma
  - Zygomaticomaxillary complex fractures
- Frontal sinus fractures
  - Anterior table, posterior table, or combined

CLINICAL PRESENTATION

- History of trauma
- Physical signs

DIAGNOSIS AND EVALUATION

- Physical examination focusing on palpation of bony anatomy, mobility of bones especially palate, septal hematoma, widening of the nasal bridge, and dental occlusion
- CT scan of the facial bones

TREATMENT

- Referral to pediatric facial trauma specialist; may include plastic surgery, otolaryngology, or oromaxillofacial surgery
- Conservative management and a soft diet
- Surgical intervention including open reduction and internal fixation of fractures

Review Questions

For review questions, please go to ExpertConsult.com

Suggested Readings

1. Carpenter RJ, Neel III HB. Correction of congenital choanal atresia in children and adults. *Laryngoscope.* 1977;87:1304–1311.
2. Myer III CM, Cotton RT. Nasal obstruction in the pediatric patient. *Pediatrics.* 1983;72:766–777.

71 *Disorders of the Oropharynx and Neck*

CAROL NHAN, MD, FRCSC and CONOR M. DEVINE, MD

DISORDERS OF THE ORAL CAVITY AND OROPHARYNX

Cleft Lip and Palate

BASIC INFORMATION

- Approximately 1/1000 births
  - More common in Native American and Asian children
- Cleft lip ± palate more common than isolated cleft palate
  - 50% isolated cleft palate associated with syndromes/sequences (e.g., Stickler, 22q11 deletion, CHARGE)
  - 30% cleft lip ± palate associated with syndromes
- Pierre Robin sequence: micrognathia, glossoptosis, U-shaped cleft palate

CLINICAL PRESENTATION

- Present at birth; findings may be unilateral, bilateral, complete, incomplete
- Bifid uvula may be sign of submucous cleft, which occurs when the palate mucosa is intact but underlying palatal musculature is dehiscent
- Cleft palate presents with difficulty feeding, velopharyngeal insufficiency

TREATMENT

- Multidisciplinary management for velopharyngeal insufficiency, feeding, speech, recurrent otitis media, audiology, genetic consultation
  - Specialized bottles and nipples may be necessary for feeding with cleft palate (e.g., Pigeon, Haberman, Mead Johnson)
- Cleft lip repair at 3 months (Rule of 10's: >10 weeks, >10 lb, Hb >10), with cleft palate repair occurring closer to 12 months

Ankyloglossia

BASIC INFORMATION

- Short or tight lingual frenulum impairing the ability to raise the anterior of the tongue up to the palate or to protrude the tongue beyond the lower incisor
- May cause latching/feeding problems (related to inability to raise the tongue) and speech difficulties

- Frenotomy/frenuloplasty may be indicated depending on the functional impairment caused by the ankyloglossia

Tonsillar and Adenoid Hypertrophy

BASIC INFORMATION

- Tonsils and adenoids increase in size starting at 6 months to 3 years and peak at 7 years old, after which they begin to involute
- See also *Nelson Textbook of Pediatrics*, Chapter 383, "Tonsils and Adenoids"

CLINICAL PRESENTATION

- Snoring, obstructive sleep apnea (OSA)
- Tonsillar hypertrophy: may also cause dysphagia to solids
- Adenoid hypertrophy: nasal obstruction, hyponasal "pinched nose" voice, mouth breathing, rhinorrhea, sinusitis
  - Adenoidal hypertrophy is also associated with increased otitis media, not by physical obstruction, rather by acting as reservoir of bacteria protected by biofilm

DIAGNOSIS AND EVALUATION

- Lateral neck plain film: assess size of adenoids, tonsils, and airway
- Nasopharyngoscopy: direct visualization of adenoids and airway
- Polysomnography (sleep study): to assess for OSA

TREATMENT

- Elective tonsillectomy and adenoidectomy
  - Common indications include: OSA or sleep-disordered breathing, recurrent tonsillitis, recurrent sinusitis/acute otitis media (adenoidectomy), significant dysphagia, abnormal appearance of tonsil (i.e., concern for malignancy)
  - Postoperative complications include:
    - Velopharyngeal insufficiency, characterized by a hypernasal voice
    - Post–tonsillectomy and adenoidectomy (T&A) bleed: 1% to 3% incidence. Increased risk in older children, children with known bleeding disorder, acutely

infected at time of operation. Consider hematology consultation in children with family history of bleeding disorder for consideration of further testing and perioperative aminocaproic acid/desmopressin/factor replacement
- Postobstructive pulmonary edema: rare postoperative complication in children with severe OSA and/or obesity. Treat with positive pressure ventilation and diuresis
- In acute respiratory distress due to obstruction: nasal trumpet, corticosteroids, repositioning
- Topical nasal steroids may reduce adenoid hypertrophy

Other Causes of Oropharyngeal Airway Obstruction

- Glossoptosis
  - Mandibular hypoplasia (e.g., Pierre Robin sequence), macroglossia (e.g., Beckwith-Wiedemann syndrome, trisomy 21)
    - Severe cases may require surgical management (e.g., mandibular distraction osteogenesis, tongue-lip adhesion, lingual tonsillectomy, partial glossectomy, tongue suspension, tracheostomy)
  - Oral mass (e.g., tumor, Ludwig angina as an acute cause)
    - Surgical resection of tumor
    - Ludwig angina requires urgent attention of otolaryngology and anesthesiology to secure the airway (nasotracheal intubation or tracheostomy), followed by incision and drainage
- Neoplasms (e.g., teratomas can grow rapidly, requiring surgical excision)
- Pharyngomalacia (e.g., hypotonia) managed with positive pressure ventilation
- Some conditions may present with prenatal evidence of potential airway obstruction, requiring careful planning by multiple fetal specialists regarding delivery (e.g., EXIT [EXtrauterine Intrapartum Treatment] procedure; see later under Teratoma)

Infectious Pharyngitis and Stomatitis

BASIC INFORMATION

- Pharyngitis is often characterized by oropharyngeal erythema and tonsillar hypertrophy
- Viral upper respiratory infection (URI) is the most common cause (adenovirus, rhinovirus, echovirus, respiratory syncytial virus [RSV], influenza, parainfluenza, coxsackie virus), presenting with milder symptoms (sore throat, fever, dysphagia) than bacterial etiologies
- May also present with cough, rhinorrhea, sneezing, oropharyngeal ulcers

SPECIFIC VIRAL ETIOLOGIES

- Epstein-Barr virus (EBV) or cytomegalovirus (CMV; mononucleosis)
  - EBV is more common cause (responsible for 90%)
  - Transmitted through oral secretions
  - Presents with sore throat, odynophagia, and tonsillitis
    - Classically features gray-white tonsillar exudate
    - May also have petechiae at the junction of the hard and soft palate
  - Accompanied by fevers, fatigue, malaise, and hepatosplenomegaly
  - For details regarding EBV diagnosis and treatment, see Chapter 45
- HSV-1 or HSV-2 (herpes simplex)
  - HSV-1 more frequently presents with oral lesions than HSV-2
  - Presentation is described as a gingivostomatitis
    - Painful crops of vesicles on any mucosal surface including gums and vermilion border of lips, followed by gray ulcers with erythematous borders
    - Lesions may or may not be exudative
    - Primary episodes also have fever, malaise, headache, lymphadenopathy
    - Secondary (recurrent) episodes stimulated by stress/fatigue/trauma/immunosuppression
  - Diagnosis may be confirmed with tissue culture or polymerase chain reaction (PCR)
  - Treatment: supportive. Antivirals such as acyclovir may be used for immunosuppressed patients because disseminated disease in immunocompromised host can be fatal
- Coxsackie A virus (herpangina)
  - Ulcerative vesicles with erythematous base on posterior pharynx, tonsillar pillars, palate
  - Odynophagia, high fever, malaise, headache
  - Treatment: supportive

SPECIFIC BACTERIAL ETIOLOGIES

- Group A β-hemolytic streptococcus (GAS, *Streptococcus pyogenes*)
  - Primarily affects children >5 years old
  - Presents with sore throat, odynophagia, pharyngitis with exudate, cervical lymphadenopathy, fever
  - Diagnosis: test is indicated if clinical suspicion for bacterial pharyngitis (exudate, cervical adenopathy, absence of cough, or fever), but not if suspicious for viral etiology (cough, rhinorrhea, or ulcers)
    - Rapid antigen detection test is highly specific
    - Throat culture, antistreptococcal antibody titers will be positive if infection (does not confirm acute infection)
  - Complications and treatment of GAS detailed in Chapter 44
  - In the event of chronic, recurrent infections, some may consider elective tonsillectomy
- *Staphylococcus aureus*
  - Purulence, tonsillar pustules
  - Increased risk of methicillin-resistant *S. aureus* (MRSA) in infants <2 years old
  - Treatment: cultures and sensitivities helpful. Clindamycin or vancomycin if suspect MRSA
- *Corynebacterium diphtheriae*
  - Unvaccinated children
  - Exotoxin acts locally to cause inflammation and necrosis
    - Gray adherent pseudomembranes on tonsils/pharynx, bleeds when scraped
    - Can spread to larynx with airway compromise

- Dissemination of toxin causes circulatory collapse
- Diagnosis: culture and Gram stain (Gram + aerobic bacillus)
- Treatment: antitoxin within 48 hr of symptoms, high-dose penicillin

GRISEL SYNDROME

- Subluxation of atlantoaxial joint caused by inflammation in prevertebral ligaments, resulting in laxity and presenting as torticollis
- Can occur as a rare complication of adenoidectomy or pharyngitis/retropharyngeal infection
- Treatment: consultation to neurosurgery or orthopedic spine specialist for spine immobilization

SPECIFIC FUNGAL ETIOLOGIES

- *Candida Albicans* (Thrush)
  - Cheesy white plaques that scrape off an erythematous base
  - Increased risk when immunocompromised (e.g., corticosteroids, HIV, diabetes), on long-term antibiotics, malnutrition, poor oral hygiene
  - Diagnosis: confirmed by culture
  - Treatment: oral hygiene, topical antifungal (e.g., nystatin); if severe disease or compromised host, may consider systemic antifungals

Noninfectious Pharyngitis and Stomatitis

LARYNGOPHARYNGEAL REFLUX (LPR)

- Reflux of stomach acid up to the larynx and sometimes oropharynx and nasopharynx
- Variable presentation: regurgitation, laryngomalacia, failure to thrive, chronic cough, sore throat, throat clearing, voice complaints, halitosis, globus sensation, heartburn
- Is diagnosed clinically, but can be aided by laryngoscopy and reflux studies (24-hour pH probe is considered the gold standard)
- Treatment:
  - Lifestyle modification: elevate head of bed and stay upright after feeds, avoid foods that cause reflux (fatty, spicy, caffeinated, carbonated, minty, acidic) and avoid large meals and meals before bedtime
  - Medical: H2 antagonists, proton pump inhibitors (PPI); if there is delayed gastric emptying may consult gastrointestinal (GI) and consider promotility agent
  - Surgical: Nissen fundoplication ± G-tube in extreme circumstances

APHTHOUS STOMATITIS

- Idiopathic painful white ulcers with red rim on oral mucosa
- Often recurrent and may be exacerbated by stressors or trauma
- Variable types that may be distinct disorders

- Minor (85% of cases): small ulcers on labial and buccal mucosa, lateral tongue, or floor of mouth lasting 7 to 10 days and healing without scarring
- Major: large ulcers >1 cm on surface of tongue or gums with deeper ulcer that takes >20 days to heal and may leave scar
- Herpetiform: many small ulcers occurring in crops that may coalesce and last >20 days
- Self-limited
- Diagnosis: clinical
- Treatment: supportive (topical analgesic or anesthetics, antiseptics or rarely topical corticosteroids). Oral hygiene to prevent secondary infections
- Aphthous-like ulcers may occur in certain diseases (Crohn, celiac, Behçet, PFAPA [see later], HIV)

COLD-INDUCED PANNICULITIS

- Most often presents in infants (<1 year old) 1 to 2 days after cold exposure (e.g., Popsicle) as a "tender red nodule on the cheek"
  - Subcutaneous fat is more likely to be affected in infants than in adults
- May persist for several weeks, but no treatment is necessary (heals without scarring)

PEDIATRIC NECK MASSES

While pediatricians are most likely to encounter cervical lymphadenitis as the cause of a pediatric neck mass, there are several etiologies that one must consider in the differential diagnosis. Categorizing pediatric neck masses by location can greatly facilitate your differential diagnosis. Anatomically, neck masses are subdivided into midline and lateral (see Table 71.1). A supraclavicular lymph node is highly suggestive of malignancy with reported rates of up to 75%

Midline Neck Masses

Thyroglossal Duct Cyst

BASIC INFORMATION

- Failure of involution of the embryologic tract that forms as the thyroid gland descends from the foramen cecum at the base of tongue, down through the hyoid bone, to its final position
- Most common congenital neck mass (70%)

Table 71.1. Categorizing Pediatric Neck Masses by Location

Midline	Lateral
Thyroglossal duct cyst	Branchial cleft anomaly
Dermoid cyst	Lymphadenitis
Teratoma	Lymphatic or venous malformation
Plunging ranula	Thymic cyst
Thymic cyst	Thyroid malignancy
Thyroid malignancy	Other malignancy (e.g., lymphoma)

CLINICAL PRESENTATION

- Painless midline neck mass, classically described as "moving with swallowing"
  - >50% around the level of the hyoid
  - ~25% between the base of tongue and hyoid
  - ~13% between the hyoid and pyramidal lobe
  - ~3% lingual
- May present with acute enlargement in the setting of a URI
- Otherwise, may present with erythema and pain if superinfected

DIAGNOSIS AND EVALUATION

- Ultrasound (US) neck to show cystic structure (can also be seen on magnetic resonance imaging [MRI] and computed tomography [CT] scan)
  - Must also ensure that there is a separate thyroid gland before resection to ensure not removing only thyroid tissue
  - If no normal thyroid gland found, radioisotope thyroid scan to find ectopic thyroid tissue
- Thyroid function tests are indicated if thyroid pathology suspected

TREATMENT

- Surgery: Sistrunk procedure provides the best chances to prevent recurrence by completely excising cyst, its tract, and the midportion of the hyoid bone
  - Infections of a thyroglossal duct cyst should be treated before surgical management proceeds
- ~1% lifetime risk of malignancy

Dermoid and Epidermoid Cyst

BASIC INFORMATION

- Results from entrapped ectodermal and mesodermal cells along embryonic fusion lines
- Comprises 25% of midline neck masses
- Most present before 5 years of age with a slow-growing, nontender, well-circumscribed, superficial, mobile suprahyoid mass
- US is the usual diagnostic imaging modality (can also be seen on MRI and CT scan)
- Treatment: surgical excision

Teratoma

BASIC INFORMATION

- Neck, oral cavity, nasopharynx, nasal or orbital mass
- Contains tissue from all three germ layers

CLINICAL PRESENTATION

- Presents at birth and often is rapidly enlarging
  - Maternal polyhydramnios in 30%
- Can compromise airway and feeding

DIAGNOSIS AND EVALUATION

- Detected on prenatal US
- Evaluate with fetal MRI
- Raised maternal alpha-fetoprotein, elevated amniotic fluid alpha-fetoprotein and acetylcholinesterase

TREATMENT

- A multidisciplinary plan is required to secure the airway at birth
- Consider EXIT procedure (keeping baby attached to umbilical cord during partial delivery through cesarean section allows time to secure airway by relying on continued fetomaternal circulation)
- Once airway is secured, complete surgical resection

Cervical Thymic Cyst

BASIC INFORMATION

- Failure of obliteration of the tract formed from embryologic descent of the thymus from the pharynx down to the mediastinum. Usually presents as a slowly enlarging painless mass near the thoracic inlet, anterior or deep to the sternocleidomastoid
  - More commonly left midline
  - Can cause dysphagia, dyspnea, hoarseness, drainage if there is a sinus. Can become infected
  - Diagnosed by US, CT, or MRI showing a cystic mass
- Treatment is usually by surgical excision

Laryngocele

BASIC INFORMATION

- Uncommon cause of an asymptomatic cyst that can extend from the larynx through the thyrohyoid membrane to present on the external neck at the level of the hyoid bone
  - Described as increasing in size with Valsalva and decreasing with palpation
    - A laryngocele with a laryngeal component may present with hoarseness, dyspnea, dysphagia
    - Can become infected
- Diagnosed on anteroposterior (AP) and lateral plain film on inspiration and expiration (also seen on CT scan) as well as laryngoscopy
- Treatment is usually via surgical excision

Lateral Neck Masses

Cervical Lymphadenitis

VIRAL CERVICAL ADENITIS

- Most cases of viral adenitis are reactive and associated with URI (rhinovirus, adenovirus, enterovirus, coronavirus)

- This usually presents with bilateral, nontender, self-limiting lymph node enlargement that may persist for up to 2 weeks
- Special cases (see Chapter 45 for details):
  - EBV (infectious mononucleosis)
    - Bilateral posterior cervical adenopathy
  - CMV
    - Symptoms resemble EBV infection
  - HIV
    - Generalized lymphadenopathy, most commonly posterior cervical triangle
    - Acute infection may present similarly to EBV infection

BACTERIAL CERVICAL ADENITIS

- Usually presents with erythematous, enlarged, tender lymph node, most often unilateral
- Etiology is often polymicrobial, most commonly streptococcal species and *S. aureus*
- First-line antibiotics include clindamycin or amoxicillin-clavulanate/ampicillin-sulbactam, depending on local susceptibilities
  - Also consider the source of infection, which may include an adjacent GAβHS pharyngitis or salivary gland infection when choosing an antimicrobial agent
- Consider imaging for palpable fluctuance, failure to improve with antibiotic therapy, or development of fluctuance while on therapy (US, CT with contrast, or MRI)
  - A phlegmon or small abscess should be started with IV antibiotics and close observation
  - A significant abscess should be drained surgically with specimens sent for culture
    - Tissue can be considered to detect mycobacterial or Bartonella infections, or underlying malignancy

LESS COMMON CAUSES OF CERVICAL ADENITIS

- Atypical mycobacterium
  - Single, nontender, gradually enlarging node, violaceous overlying skin in late phase
  - Most commonly submandibular or upper cervical
  - Affects children <5 years old, more common in females
- *Mycobacterium tuberculosis*
  - Uncommon in children, with increased risk if immunocompromised or from endemic areas
- Cat-scratch disease
  - *Bartonella henselae* infection
  - Unilateral lymphadenopathy after cat bite or scratch to the ipsilateral side
  - Self-limited with resolution in months; rarely causes persistent draining lesion
  - Diagnosis: IgM titers to Bartonella
  - Treatment: observation may be considered for mild to moderate cases in immunocompetent hosts. Otherwise, first-line antimicrobial most often consists of macrolides (e.g., azithromycin)
- Lemierre syndrome (also called postanginal shock/sepsis)
  - Thrombophlebitis of the internal jugular vein as a complication of local invasion from nearby tonsillitis/pharyngitis or, less frequently, otitis, mastoiditis, sinusitis
  - *Fusobacterium necrophorum* is the most common causative organism

- Presents approximately a week after tonsillitis with cervical tenderness on the side of the thrombus, with picket-fence fevers (septic thrombophlebitis). May be complicated by pulmonary embolic infections
  - Treatment: IV antibiotics; address any drainable abscess that is the source of thrombophlebitis if one exists
    - If complicated by septic emboli, may consider ligation of the affected internal jugular vein
    - There is no clear evidence for or against anticoagulation
- PFAPA syndrome
  - **P**eriodic **f**ever, **a**phthous stomatitis, **p**haryngitis, **a**denitis syndrome
  - Recurrent symptoms for 3 to 7 days at regular 3- to 6-week intervals (fever with 1+ other symptoms), whereas asymptomatic between episodes
  - Usually spontaneously resolves; thus provide supportive treatment (acetaminophen, ibuprofen, corticosteroids to break fever) to reduce severity of episodes
    - May consider tonsillectomy for symptom reduction or resolution

Noninfectious, Nonneoplastic Lymphadenopathy

KAWASAKI DISEASE

- Nontender, nonfluctuant, cervical lymph node(s) ≥15 mm, often unilateral
- See Chapter 83 for details

KIKUCHI DISEASE

- Self-limiting benign condition with lymphadenopathy (often unilateral posterior cervical triangle), fever, fatigue, rarely hepatosplenomegaly
- Diagnosis: lymph node biopsy
  - Unlike in systemic lupus erythematosus (SLE), antinuclear antibodies (ANA), antiphospholipid antibodies, anti-dsDNA, and rheumatoid factor (RF) negative
- Treatment: supportive with NSAIDs and corticosteroids for severe generalized disease

KIMURA DISEASE

- Idiopathic unilateral adenopathy, most commonly submandibular
- More common in Asian males
- Associated with high IgE and eosinophilia, suggesting it is a hypersensitivity reaction

SARCOIDOSIS

- Lymphadenopathy may also involve cervical and paratracheal nodes

ROSAI-DORFMAN DISEASE

- Idiopathic histiocytosis with massive lymphadenopathy that can involve cervical lymph nodes
  - Self-limited, nonprogressive disease; rarely presents with autoimmune hemolytic anemia

Cervical Malignancies

BASIC INFORMATION

- Comprise <15% of neck masses
- Examination findings and components of the history that should raise concern:
  - Asymptomatic, painless mass
  - Unilateral symptoms of nasal obstruction, otalgia, hearing loss, middle ear effusion
  - Rapid growth of mass or bulky disease
  - History of radiation exposure or family history of thyroid disease
- Most common causes:
  - Lymphoma (comprises 50% of cervical malignancies, usually non-Hodgkin lymphoma)
  - Rhabdomyosarcoma (~20%)
  - Nonrhabdomyosarcoma soft tissue sarcoma (8%)
  - Thyroid malignancy (8%)
  - Others: nasopharyngeal carcinoma, neuroblastoma, salivary gland tumors

Branchial Cleft Anomalies

BASIC INFORMATION/CLINICAL PRESENTATION

- Second most common (20%–30%) congenital neck mass
- Anomaly of embryologic development of the branchial pouch or cleft (see Table 71.2)
- Can present as a cyst, a sinus (opening to the skin or internally), or a fistula (opening to both the skin and internally)
- Often presents with URI or when becomes infected as a draining sinus or swelling and erythema of the cyst

DIAGNOSIS AND EVALUATION

- Imaging is not required for second branchial anomalies
- CT with contrast or MRI for first, third, and fourth branchial anomalies

- Gas bubbles in a cyst are diagnostic of a third or fourth branchial anomaly

TREATMENT

- If infected, first treat with antibiotics and allow infection and inflammation to resolve
  - Antimicrobial coverage is provided against *S. aureus* (including MRSA), respiratory anaerobes
- Treatment typically is surgical (see Table 71.2)

Lymphatic Malformation

BASIC INFORMATION

- Also called lymphangioma or, formerly, cystic hygroma
- Dilated lymphatic vessels due to failure of flow into the downstream jugular sacs or failure of the jugular sacs to flow into the venous system
- May be focal, multifocal, or diffuse

CLINICAL PRESENTATION

- 50% apparent at birth, 90% present by 2 years
- Soft, compressible mass, most often in the posterior triangle of the neck
- Usually asymptomatic; however, may cause compressive symptoms such as pain, dysphagia, or stridor due to airway compromise
- May present with enlargement with URI
- If mass gets infected or hemorrhages, it could enlarge rapidly

DIAGNOSIS AND EVALUATION

- US or MRI
- May be detected in prenatal US in the second or third trimester

Table 71.2. Anomaly of Embryologic Development of the Branchial Pouch or Cleft

Branchial Cleft Cyst	Associated Artery and Nerve	Presentation/Location	Incidence	Treatment
First	Trigeminal nerve, maxillary artery	Work Type I presents as duplication cyst of external auditory canal, lateral to facial nerve. Draining pit or recurrent infections adjacent to EAC. Work Type II presents as draining pit or recurrent cyst/infection anywhere from EAC to angle of mandible. Course is variable in relation to facial nerve.	5%	Surgical excision. May require superficial parotidectomy due to proximity to facial nerve
Second	Facial nerve, stapedial artery	Most frequently presents as cyst anterior to sternocleidomastoid muscle and inferior to mandible. May also present as draining pit or fistula. Tracks up to ipsilateral tonsillar fossa, passes between internal and external carotid arteries.	Up to 93%	Surgical excision of entire tract up to pharynx.
Third/Fourth	Glossopharyngeal nerve, common carotid and internal carotid; superior laryngeal nerve and right subclavian/aortic arch	Most frequently presents as cyst in lower part of neck, anterior to sternocleidomastoid muscle or recurrent thyroid infections. More common on the left. Tracks to pyriform sinus.	2%–3%	Surgical excision or cautery to pit in pyriform sinus

EAC, external auditory canal.

- Those detected early (before the third trimester) are often associated with chromosomal anomalies (e.g., Turner, trisomy 21/18/13, Klinefelter, Noonan syndrome)

TREATMENT

- If diagnosed prenatally, fetal and ear-nose-throat (ENT) specialists are involved to develop a plan for potential airway obstruction upon delivery (see Teratoma, above)
- In acute airway compromise may decompress by needle aspiration until the airway can be secured
- Asymptomatic and small lesions may be observed up to 24 months; otherwise may consider sclerotherapy or surgical resection

Infantile Hemangioma

BASIC INFORMATION

- The most common soft tissue tumor of childhood, it is a benign vascular anomaly composed of endothelial cells with a multitude of clinical presentations, including hemangiomas that can obstruct the airway
- For details regarding infantile hemangioma, see Chapter 12
- A hemangioma with a segmental facial distribution (along dermatome of V1, V2, or V3) needs evaluation for PHACES syndrome (Posterior fossa abnormalities, Hemangioma, Arterial abnormalities, Cardiac abnormalities, Eye abnormalities, Sternal cleft/defect), which is associated with subglottic hemangiomas. Hemangiomas in the "beard" distribution require similar vigilance for airway obstruction
- Treatment depends on the size and location of the hemangioma, the impairment it causes, and the trajectory of the usual hemangioma growth stage (because most begin involution at ~12 months of age)

Fibromatosis Colli

BASIC INFORMATION

- Rare (0.4%), more common in males
- Also called "pseudotumor of infancy"
- Fibrotic change of the sternocleidomastoid (SCM) muscle causing contracture
  - Conjectured to be the result of birth trauma or malposition leading to vascular compression, ischemia, and necrosis of the SCM
  - Is associated with difficult labor, forceps delivery, breech, and primiparous birth
- Presents usually by 6 weeks of age as a firm, nontender mass of the mid/lower SCM muscle, more frequently on the right
- May cause torticollis, with a head tilt toward the affected side and chin to the opposite side
- Diagnosed by physical examination and follow-up US
- Treatment:
  - Physiotherapy for passive range of motion
  - For persistence beyond 12 months, consider surgical transection to prevent development of facial hemihypoplasia

DISORDERS OF THE SALIVARY GLANDS

Sialolithiasis

BASIC INFORMATION

- Caused by calculi or sludge obstructing salivary gland ducts, submandibular > parotid
- Often presents at >10 years of age (sometimes in the setting of dehydration) with postprandial glandular swelling/pain
- Upon palpation, may appreciate calculi in affected duct and decreased ability to express saliva
- Diagnostic approach includes US and dental plain films; CT scans have higher sensitivity and are sometimes required
- Initial treatment of small stones includes conservative measures: hydration, massage, warm compresses, sialogogues
- Refractory sialoliths may require sialolithotomy (excision of calculi from duct), sialoendoscopy with stone removal, or excision of gland if stone is proximal and cannot be removed otherwise

Sialadenitis

BASIC INFORMATION

- May have viral or bacterial etiology

VIRAL SIALADENITIS/PAROTITIS

- Most commonly affects preschool- and school-age children
- Usually causes swelling and erythema around the opening of Stensen duct, but without pus or overlying erythema
- Causes include mumps (see later), EBV (mononucleosis), influenza (especially influenza A), parainfluenza, and enteroviruses
- Generally requires supportive therapy including hydration, massage, warm compresses, sialogogues
- Special cases:
  - Mumps
    - Immunization gives incomplete protection
    - 95% bilateral parotid and submandibular
    - Diagnosis: primarily a clinical diagnosis, but may confirm with mumps IgM serology
  - HIV
    - Characterized by bilateral chronic, nontender glands, usually parotid > submandibular or sublingual glands
    - May become superinfected and require antibiotics or drainage
    - Risk of lymphoma or Kaposi sarcoma with HIV; therefore consider CT or MRI and biopsy for suspicious or rapidly growing salivary lesions

ACUTE BACTERIAL SIALADENITIS

- Etiologies include *S. aureus, S. viridans, Haemophilus influenzae, S. pneumoniae, Moraxella catarrhalis, Bacteroides melaninogenicus, Escherichia coli*
- Presents with pain, edema, erythema, purulent drainage from duct
  - Parotid > submandibular, unilateral
  - Can be associated with sialolithiasis
  - Patients often toxic-appearing with high fever
- Treatment:
  - Antibiotics (culture pus)
  - Supportive measures including hydration, massage, warm compresses, sialogogues
  - Surgical drainage may be required if there is abscess formation
  - If recurrent, consider sialoendoscopy and duct dilation to address scarring from chronic inflammation. For refractory cases, consider elective surgical excision of the affected gland.
  - For submandibular sialadenitis, assess and monitor for Ludwig angina (see later)

Juvenile Recurrent Parotitis

BASIC INFORMATION

- Idiopathic, nonobstructive, nonsuppurative parotid inflammation in children
  - Unilateral > bilateral
  - Bimodal presentation at 3 to 6 years and 6 to 10 years with resolution by puberty
- Diagnosed by history and US, MRI, sialography or sialoendoscopy (also therapeutic)
- Treatment often involves conservative management: hydration, massage, warm compresses, sialogogues, nonsteroidal antiinflammatory drugs (NSAIDs)
  - Ductal dilatation (including that which occurs during sialoendoscopy or during sialography) is therapeutic

OTHER INFECTIOUS DISORDERS

Ludwig Angina

BASIC INFORMATION

- Rapidly progressive cellulitis of floor of mouth, causing tongue to be pushed up and back and obstructing airway
  - Tongue swelling may prevent laryngeal exposure by a laryngoscope for intubation
- Most commonly caused by infections of the teeth anterior to the second mandibular molar tooth (i.e., from the first molar forward)
- Most common organisms: *Staphylococcus, Streptococcus, Bacteroides*

CLINICAL PRESENTATION

- "Wooden"/indurated floor of mouth, tongue and neck swelling, drooling
- Progresses rapidly to respiratory obstruction and distress

DIAGNOSIS AND EVALUATION

- Primarily a clinical diagnosis, requiring rapid intervention

TREATMENT

- Initial focus should be on safely securing the airway (e.g., awake fiber-optic nasotracheal intubation)
- Incision and drainage (usually expressive of weeping serous fluid) with aggressive antibiotic management (coverage includes Gram positives, Gram negatives, and anaerobic organisms)
- Consider airway dose intravenous (IV) steroids to decrease swelling

Peritonsillar Abscess

BASIC INFORMATION

- Presents >3 days after tonsillitis/pharyngitis with odynophagia, neck tenderness, "hot potato voice," and often referred ipsilateral otalgia
- Presents with trismus, bulging of the ipsilateral soft palate above the tonsil, and deviation of the uvula to the opposite side
- Caused by GAS or, less commonly, anaerobes
- Diagnosis: clinical; presence of drainable abscess may be confirmed by CT
- Treatment: first line is IV ampicillin-sulbactam or clindamycin; proceeding to drainage in the event of a significant mature abscess
  - In patients with recurrent abscesses, consider elective tonsillectomy

Retropharyngeal Abscess (RPA)

BASIC INFORMATION

- Necrotic degeneration of infected retropharyngeal lymph nodes present only in young children (these nodes drain the pharynx, nasopharynx, nasal cavity, paranasal sinuses, and middle ears)
  - RPA is seen in children <6 years old (most commonly 2–4 years old)
- Caused by mixed bacteria, most commonly streptococcal species, *S. aureus, H. influenzae,* or anaerobes (*Bacteroides, Peptostreptococci, Fusobacteria*)
- Presents with fever, sore throat, decreased PO intake, cervical pain, decreased neck range of motion, adenopathy
  - Examination of the oropharynx may reveal a bulge in posterior pharyngeal wall
- Diagnosis provided by clinical examination; lateral neck plain film shows thickening of prevertebral tissues (greater than half the width of the C2 vertebral body, or >7-mm diameter at C2, or >14-mm diameter at C6)
  - CT scan or MRI is often performed to confirm the diagnosis
- Treatment:
  - Empiric therapy is often with IV clindamycin or ampicillin-sulbactam; vancomycin may be considered for MRSA coverage

- Surgical drainage may be indicated in the event of mature abscess or failure to improve
- Complications include airway compromise, sepsis, mediastinitis (spread via danger space), jugular vein thrombosis, septic emboli, aspiration, atlantoaxial instability, vertebral osteomyelitis

Parapharyngeal Abscess

BASIC INFORMATION

- May vary in presentation depending on affected compartment
  - Anterior compartment: classically presents with odynophagia, trismus, and ipsilateral neck/jaw pain
  - Posterior compartment: classically has minimal symptoms, but concern for sepsis
- Similar in presentation to RPA; however, may be seen in older children as well

- Will not show prevertebral thickening unless retropharyngeal space also involved

Review Questions

For review questions, please go to ExpertConsult.com.

Suggested Readings

1. Baugh RF, Archer SM, Mitchell RB, et al. Clinical practice guideline: tonsillectomy in children. *Otolaryngol Head Neck Surg.* 2011;144(suppl 1): S1–S30. NB: this guideline is currently undergoing update.
2. Darrow DH, Greene AK, Mancini AJ, et al. Diagnosis and management of infantile hemangioma. *Am Acad Pediatr.* 2015;136(4): e1060–e1104.
3. Meier JD, Grimmer JF. Evaluation and management of neck masses in children. *Am Fam Physician.* 2014;89(5):353–358.
4. Shulman ST, Bisno AL, Clegg HW, et al. Clinical practice guideline for the diagnosis and management of group A streptococcal pharyngitis: 2012 update by the Infectious Diseases Society of America. *Clin Infect Dis.* 2012;58(10):1496.

Orthopedics

72 Common Orthopedic Injuries

ANDREW J. GAMBONE, MD, NEIL S. SHAH, MD and
JOHN T. LAWRENCE, MD, PhD

Fractures, sprains, and contusions are common orthopedic injuries seen in the pediatric population. Most of the time it is the emergency department clinician, pediatrician, or the family practitioner that is the first to encounter these patients. Understanding the anatomy and pathophysiology of these common orthopedic injuries is essential for their proper diagnosis and treatment. A detailed history, careful physical examination, obtaining appropriate additional imaging/testing, and knowing when to consult an orthopedic surgeon will maximize clinical outcome and limit deleterious sequelae such as growth disturbance, deformity, and neurovascular injury. This chapter, although not exhaustive, presents some of the more commonly encountered pediatric orthopedic injuries.

Fractures Involving the Physis

BASIC INFORMATION

- Anatomy
  - The major anatomic regions of growing bone include the diaphysis (shaft region with thick cortex), metaphysis (shaft side of the growth plate with flared and thin cortex), physis (growth plate), and epiphysis (end of the bone near the joint) (Fig. 72.1)
- Causes and epidemiology of physeal injuries
  - The physis may be weaker than surrounding ligamentous structures, making it more susceptible to traumatic injuries
    - Certain physes are more susceptible to injury, such as the proximal femur and radius
  - Injuries result from high- and low-energy mechanisms
  - Account for 15% to 18% of all pediatric fractures
  - Physeal injuries have the potential for growth arrest and subsequent deformity
    - Clinical significance depends on remaining growth and the location of the fracture
- Salter-Harris classification (Fig. 72.2) is based on location and prognosis:
  - Type I fracture
    - Extends directly through the growth plate, resulting in the separation of the epiphysis from the metaphysis
    - More common in younger patients with thicker physes
    - Nondisplaced fractures require a high index of suspicion and careful physical examination (pain with palpation on the physis and pain with stress or weight-bearing)

- Type II fracture
  - Most common type, accounting for 74% of all physeal fractures
  - Fracture line enters in the plane of the physis and exits through the metaphysis
    - Separate metaphyseal fragment is known as the Thurstan-Holland fragment
- Type III fracture
  - Similar to type II, the fracture line enters in the plane of the physis, but it exits instead through the epiphysis
  - Increased potential for growth arrest due to disruption of blood supply to the physis and for posttraumatic arthritis, given its intraarticular nature
- Type IV fracture
  - Fracture line crosses the physis, extending through both the metaphysis and epiphysis
  - Unstable fracture pattern that has increased potential for growth arrest and posttraumatic arthritis
- Type V fracture
  - Crush injury to the physis
  - Can be the result of an acute compressive force or chronic repetitive loading such as seen in gymnasts

CLINICAL PRESENTATION

- Pain and swelling at the site of injury with difficulty bearing weight and limited range of motion
  - Limb deformity depending on the fracture pattern and severity of displacement
- Open fractures normally dictate more emergent/urgent care, along with additional treatment measures
  - All temporary splints should be removed to evaluate the skin for a possible open fracture
- Possible neurovascular compromise

DIAGNOSIS AND EVALUATION

- History
  - Collect history of injury
    - Important to ascertain mechanism of injury and helps focus examination
    - High-energy versus low-energy injuries require different treatment and monitoring considerations
  - Maintain suspicion for contributing factors
    - Prior fractures may indicate underlying metabolic bone disease (e.g., vitamin deficiency, osteogenesis imperfecta [OI])

- Certain fractures may be consistent with nonaccidental trauma (see Chapter 90)
- Bony pain without trauma may indicate malignancy or infection
- Physical examination
  - Inspect for swelling, ecchymosis, and deformity
  - Evaluate neurovascular status
  - Tenderness over the physis is particularly important when assessing/diagnosing nondisplaced Salter-Harris type I fractures
  - Pain out of proportion to the injury or increasing analgesic requirements may indicate compartment syndrome
    - Increasing analgesic requirement is usually the first sign of a developing compartment syndrome
- Imaging
  - X-rays are the initial imaging modality of choice
    - At least two orthogonal radiographic views of the injured joint in question should be obtained for proper diagnosis and fracture characterization
    - Oblique radiographs greatly aid in the diagnosis of physeal fractures
  - Advanced imaging such as computed tomography (CT) or magnetic resonance imaging (MRI) is rarely needed and is reserved for better fracture characterization and preoperative planning

TREATMENT

- Any nondisplaced fracture should be immobilized with either a splint or cast, swelling permitting
  - Failure to properly immobilize a nondisplaced or minimally displaced fracture may result in further displacement
  - Displaced fractures should be emergently reduced to near-anatomic parameters, particularly if there are signs of neurovascular compromise
  - It is important to perform a postimmobilization physical examination
    - Worsening of the neurovascular examination should prompt removal of the immobilization and an orthopedics consultation
  - Postreduction radiographs should accompany any reduction attempt and splint/cast application
  - Open fractures are generally operative and should be treated as emergencies
    - Administration of antibiotics as soon as an open fracture is identified decreases infection risk
    - All fractures should be immobilized before transfer
    - This will help with pain management and avoid further injury to the extremity
  - Non-weight-bearing along with extremity elevation
  - All fractures should be referred to an orthopedic surgeon for further follow-up and management
  - Report abuse to appropriate agencies, required by law; all cases of abuse with fractures warrant hospital admission with multidisciplinary evaluation and Child Protective Services consultation

Buckle (Torus) Fractures

BASIC INFORMATION

- Anatomy
  - Buckle fractures occur in the metaphysis or at the junction between the metaphysis and diaphysis
  - Result from axial compressive forces directed onto the long bones
  - Appears as a disruption in the normal contour of the bone with a buckling/bulging at the metadiaphyseal junction (Fig. 72.3)

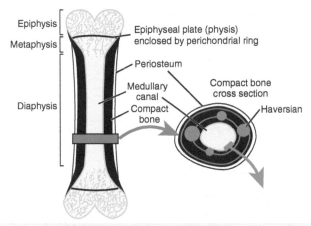

Fig. 72.1. Anatomy of the growing bone.

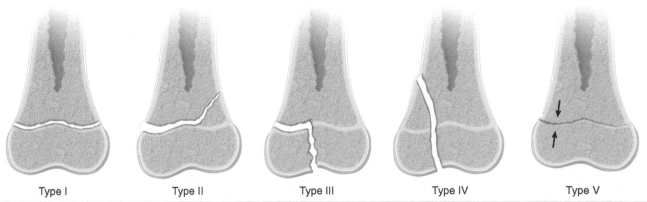

Fig. 72.2. Salter-Harris classification. (From Herring JA: Tachdjian's Procedures in Pediatric Orthopaedics. Philadelphia, Elsevier, 2017.)

- Buckle fractures commonly occur at the distal radius and distal tibia, but can occur anywhere
- Buckle fractures are stable injuries with little to no risk of displacement unless additional traumatic-level force is applied to the bone

CLINICAL PRESENTATION

- History
  - Recent trauma such as fall
  - Difficulty with weight-bearing or use of extremity
- Physical examination
  - Pain with range of motion
  - Swelling with little to no deformity
  - Tenderness to palpation at the fracture site
  - Although rare, neurovascular injury and compartment syndrome should always be ruled out
  - Assess for other injuries (the second injury is often the easiest injury to miss)
- Imaging
  - Anteroposterior (AP)/lateral radiographs of bone or joint in question
  - Buckling may be very subtle and evident on only one view
  - Radiographs of the contralateral extremity may be helpful for comparison

TREATMENT

- Immobilization for 2 to 4 weeks (e.g., casting)
  - Follow-up radiographs are not usually necessary because most of these injuries heal reliably and decision-making for removal of immobilization is based on being pain-free

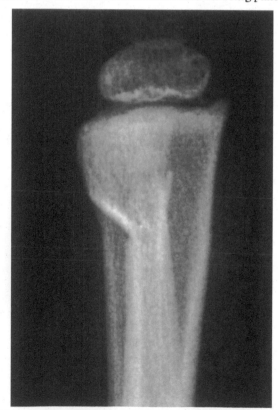

Fig. 72.3. Lateral radiograph of the distal radius showing a buckle fracture (From Herring JA: Tachdjian's Procedures in Pediatric Orthopaedics. Philadelphia, Elsevier, 2017.)

SHOULDER AND CLAVICLE INJURIES

Clavicle Fractures

BASIC INFORMATION

- Anatomy
  - The clavicle is an S-shaped bone that connects laterally to the scapula at the acromioclavicular joint and medially with the sternum at the sternoclavicular joint
  - It serves to provide stability to the shoulder girdle as well as to protect underlying neurovascular structures
  - 80% of clavicle fractures occur midshaft
- Epidemiology
  - Represents 10% to 15% of all pediatric fractures
  - Occurs in children of all ages through a variety of injury mechanisms
    - Birth trauma in infants
    - Fall onto an outstretched arm or direct blow in children and adolescents

CLINICAL PRESENTATION

- Swelling and ecchymosis over the supraclavicular region after a direct fall on an outstretched extremity
- Patients usually present with their arms adducted by their sides while being supported by the uninjured extremity and have pain with shoulder range of motion
- Deformity may be present

DIAGNOSIS AND EVALUATION

- Physical examination
  - Assess for any skin tenting
  - Although rare, cardiovascular as well as pulmonary status should be evaluated in cases of posterior sternoclavicular dislocation
  - Neurovascular status to the ipsilateral upper extremity should be assessed due to the proximity of the brachial plexus and subclavian vessels
- Imaging
  - Standard clavicle series radiographs (Fig. 72.4) will confirm location of fracture and displacement, if any
  - CT may help evaluate displacement, shortening, comminution, articular extension, and nonunion
    - Useful for medial physeal fractures and sternoclavicular injuries

TREATMENT

- Most pediatric clavicle fractures can be treated with sling immobilization or figure-of-eight bracing for 2 to 4 weeks, depending on pain
  - Recent studies have found no difference between either immobilization technique

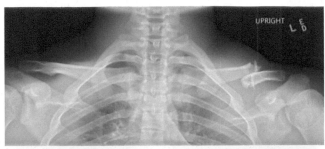

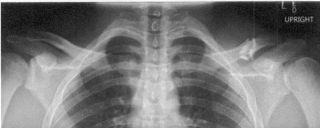

Fig. 72.4. Radiographs demonstrating midshaft clavicle fracture.

- Gentle range of motion within the limits of pain may be initiated when pain allows
- Emergent surgical intervention for:
  - Open fractures or a danger of impending open fracture (skin tenting)
  - Posterior sternoclavicular dislocation (which is more common in medial clavicle fractures)
  - Neurovascular compromise (e.g., distal clavicle fractures are more likely to have brachial plexus injury and nonunion)
- Clavicle fractures with significant displacement and shortening should be referred to an orthopedic surgeon for further evaluation and treatment

Acromioclavicular (AC) Sprain/ Separation

BASIC INFORMATION

- Anatomy
  - The distal clavicle physis is one of the last to close in the body and may persist into the late teens or early 20s
  - The AC joint is a plane synovial joint
  - Injury to this area may be to the joint or the physis
  - Primarily stabilized by the acromioclavicular and coracoclavicular ligaments

CLINICAL PRESENTATION

- Tenderness over the distal clavicle and AC joint, usually after direct trauma to the shoulder or fall onto an outstretched adducted arm
- Limited shoulder range of motion
- Deformity depending on degree of displacement

DIAGNOSIS AND EVALUATION

- Physical examination
  - Assess neurovascular status

Table 72.1. Acromioclavicular Separation Rockwood Classification

Type	Acromioclavicular Ligament	Coracoclavicular Ligament	Description	Management
I	Sprain	Intact	Nondisplaced	Sling
II	Torn	Sprain	Vertical separation of AC <25%	Sling
III	Torn	Torn	CC distance increased 25% to 100% compared with contralateral side	Controversial
IV	Torn	Torn	Clavicle is displaced posteriorly through trapezius	Surgery
V	Torn	Torn	Clavicle 100% displaced. Rupture of deltopectoral fascia	Surgery
VI	Torn	Torn	Clavicle inferiorly displaced behind coracobrachialis and biceps tendon	Surgery

- Palpate for AC joint tenderness
- Pain with shoulder forward flexion and abduction or adduction (e.g., "AC crossover test")
- Asymmetric step-off at AC joint
- Imaging
  - Bilateral AP shoulder views
    - Assess for widening of the AC joint (normal: 5–8 mm)
    - Greater than 2 to 4 mm asymmetry (compared with contralateral side)
  - Axillary lateral view
    - Assesses for posterior displacement of the clavicle
    - Required if shoulder dislocation is suspected
  - Zanca views
    - Better at visualizing the AC joint by eliminating overlying structures
    - Performed by tilting the x-ray beam 10 to 15 degrees toward the cephalic direction

TREATMENT

- Will depend on type of injury (see Table 72.1)
- Short period of immobilization in a sling (3–7 days) for type 1 and type 2 injuries followed by gradual return to activities
- Types III to VI injuries should be referred to an orthopedic surgeon for operative consideration

Shoulder Dislocation

BASIC INFORMATION

- Traumatic shoulder dislocations are commonly seen in teenagers

- Epidemiology
  - High recurrence rate (80%–90%) in pediatric population

CLINICAL PRESENTATION

- Swelling and ecchymosis over the shoulder after an acute traumatic injury
- Shoulder is typically in an abducted, externally rotated position when additional posteriorly directed force is placed on the arm, causing anterior humeral head dislocation
- Deformity may be present

DIAGNOSIS AND EVALUATION

- Physical examination
  - Deformity with fullness at the anterior shoulder will be noted when the joint is dislocated
  - Painful shoulder range, feeling of instability
  - Neurovascular status should be assessed, especially axillary nerve distribution
  - Apprehension sign with arm abducted and externally rotated once the joint is reduced
- Imaging
  - Shoulder trauma series including true AP, scapular Y, and axillary views
    - The axillary view is the most useful for detecting anterior or posterior shoulder dislocations that are not evident in the AP view
  - Additional imaging to be considered includes a CT to help evaluate bony injury and an MRI arthrogram for labral tears

TREATMENT

- Closed reduction is typically performed under procedural sedation in the emergency department setting
  - Postreduction x-rays, especially axillary view, to confirm reduction
- High rate of dislocation recurrence in adolescents
- Some evidence suggests that early surgical repair improves long-term outcomes
- Refer to orthopedic sports specialist for further evaluation

Proximal Humeral Epiphysiolysis

BASIC INFORMATION

- Known as "Little League shoulder," it affects primarily 11- to 16-year-olds engaged in repetitive overhead arm motions (e.g., pitching)
- Diagnosis: based on clinical examination and x-ray imaging (widened proximal humeral epiphysis); sometimes MRI may be indicated if equivocal x-ray or suspicion for tendon injury
- Treatment: rest from overhead activities, and return to play when pain-free (physical therapy may help muscle development)

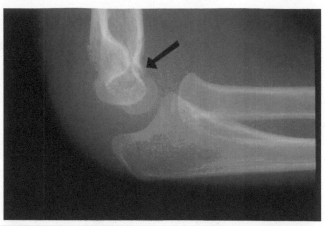

Fig. 72.5. Supracondylar fractures. (From Goodwin RC, Kuivila TE. Pediatric elbow and forearm fractures requiring surgical treatment. *Hand Clin,* 2002;18(1):135–148, Fig. 1.)

UPPER-EXTREMITY INJURIES

Supracondylar Humerus Fracture

BASIC INFORMATION

- Most common type of elbow fracture in the pediatric population
- Normally occurs in children 5 to 7 years of age
- Fractures broadly classified into extension versus flexion type (see Fig. 72.5)
  - Extension type fractures account for 98% of supracondylar humerus fractures

CLINICAL PRESENTATION

- Pain and swelling about the elbow, usually after a fall on an outstretched hand with the elbow fully extended (extension type) or direct blow with the elbow flexed (flexion type)
- Gross deformity of the arm with displaced fractures
  - Rule out other soft tissue and bony injuries
- There is risk of neurovascular injury with these fractures

DIAGNOSIS AND EVALUATION

- Physical examination
  - Limited elbow range of motion
  - Critical to evaluate neurovascular status
    - Higher risk of compartment syndrome with ipsilateral forearm fractures
    - Nerve injury occurs in approximately 11% of supracondylar humerus fractures
      - Extension type
        - Anterior interosseous nerve > median > radial > ulnar nerve
      - Flexion type
        - Ulnar nerve
    - Posterolateral displacement of the distal fragment is associated with vascular injury

- Imaging
  - AP/lateral radiographs of the injured elbow (see Fig. 72.5)
    - Anterior and posterior fat pad signs may be present with occult supracondylar fractures

Treatment

- Any supracondylar humerus fracture should be immobilized before transferring the patient to avoid further fracture displacement and soft tissue or neurovascular injury
  - Closed reduction in an emergency department setting is not recommended
- All treatment decisions should be made by an orthopedic surgeon and generally determined by displacement (nondisplaced often with casting; displaced fractures with closed/open reduction and pinning)
- A pink and pulseless hand is a surgical emergency

Lateral Condyle Fracture

BASIC INFORMATION

- Second most common elbow fracture (10%–20%) in pediatrics
- Occurs in an age distribution similar to that of supracondylar humerus fractures: 5- to 7-year-olds
- Most common fracture pattern is a Salter-Harris type IV
  - The intraarticular nature increases the risk of malunion/nonunion

CLINICAL PRESENTATION

- Lateral elbow pain with mild swelling, usually after a fall onto an outstretched hand, with the radial head impacting into the lateral condyle or through a varus or valgus stress on the elbow
- Limited elbow range of motion

DIAGNOSIS AND EVALUATION

- Physical examination
  - Limited elbow range of motion
  - Tenderness over lateral elbow
  - Critical to evaluate neurovascular status
- Imaging
  - AP, lateral, and oblique radiographs of the elbow
  - Advanced imaging such as CT and MRI rarely indicated

TREATMENT.

- Nondisplaced fractures (<2 mm displacement) are treated with long arm casting for 6 weeks with follow-up radiographs; displaced fractures usually require operative management
- Long-term follow-up is necessary to monitor for nonunion, avascular necrosis, physeal arrest, cubitus valgus, and ulnar nerve palsy

Nursemaid's Elbow

BASIC INFORMATION

- Interposition of the annular ligament into the radiocapitellar joint over the head of the proximal radius. Often referred to as a radial head "partial dislocation" or subluxation
- Seen more commonly in the younger pediatric population (ages 2–5) and in patients with ligamentous laxity
- Caused by traction on an extended and pronated forearm (e.g., swinging a child by the arms) pulling the radius distally from the elbow joint

CLINICAL PRESENTATION

- Patient holds the elbow in protective position (flexed and pronated) by side with refusal to move elbow
- Often accompanied by pain and swelling about the lateral elbow with tenderness at the radial head

DIAGNOSIS AND EVALUATION

- Imaging
  - With a classic history and physical examination, radiographs are not necessary
  - Radiographs of the injured elbow may not show abnormality

TREATMENT

- Closed reduction can be performed in the office or emergency department setting for most cases
  - Common technique is to apply pressure on the subluxed radial head while manually supinating the forearm and then maximally flexing the elbow
  - An audible and/or palpable "click" indicates successful reduction
  - Patients are often pain-free and using the elbow relatively normally within a short time
  - If patient is not using the arm fully after the injury, consider radiographs; if still not using the arm in 24 hours, then reevaluation is recommended
- Do not immobilize the elbow because it will cause unnecessary stiffness and may result in loss of elbow range of motion
- Recurrence may occur but is rare after age 5; chronic cases may require operative treatment

Medial Epicondyle Apophysitis

BASIC INFORMATION

- Known as "Little League elbow," this overuse injury associated with repetitive throwing motion results in inflammation of the growth plate on the medial aspect of the distal end of the humerus
- X-ray may show widening of the apophysis
- A rest period of 4 to 6 weeks is generally recommended for patients diagnosed with this condition

- This condition has led to suggested restrictions for the number of pitches per week (75 to 125 depending on age) and number of rest days between pitching appearances; young pitchers should play only three to four innings per game

Forearm Diaphyseal Fracture

BASIC INFORMATION

- Forearm fractures are common in the pediatric population, making up almost half of all pediatric fractures
- Mechanism of injury is typically a fall on an outstretched extremity resulting in fracture of the radius and/or ulna
- May vary in angulation (dorsal or volar), displacement (vs nondisplacement), and pattern (greenstick vs complete fracture, simple vs comminuted)
- Diagnosis via AP/lateral radiographs of the forearm; elbow and wrist radiographs help to rule out concomitant fractures or dislocations
- Treatment is often via closed reduction in the emergency department setting with sedation
- Operative indications include unstable fractures, open fractures, compartment syndrome, neurovascular compromise, significant displacement, fracture deformity, and/or angulation
- Any displaced or angulated fracture needs orthopedic consultation. All fractures require close early follow-up with weekly radiographs to ensure maintenance of the reduction

Distal Radius and Ulna Fracture

BASIC INFORMATION

- Distal radius and ulna fractures are common in the pediatric population
- Mechanism of injury is typically a fall on an outstretched extremity
- Can be categorized with the Salter-Harris classification or with descriptive terms
  - Angulation
  - Displacement
    - Dorsal (Colles fracture)
    - Volar (Smith fracture)
  - Fracture type: buckle/torus (incomplete metaphyseal fracture) versus complete fracture, simple transverse versus comminuted or intraarticular
  - Location
    - Physeal (Salter-Harris) versus metaphyseal
    - Intraarticular versus extraarticular
    - Involvement of radial styloid (Chauffeur fracture)
    - Involvement of dorsal rim of radius (dorsal Barton fracture)
    - Involvement of volar rim of radius (volar Barton fracture)

CLINICAL PRESENTATION

- Pain and swelling about the wrist, usually after acute trauma to the upper extremity
- Deformity of wrist indicates angulation or displacement

DIAGNOSIS AND EVALUATION

- Imaging
  - AP/lateral radiographs of the injured wrist
  - Elbow and forearm radiographs to rule out concomitant fractures or dislocations

TREATMENT

- With a displaced or angulated fracture, closed reduction can be performed in the emergency department setting
- Portable fluoroscopy can be very helpful while performing reductions
- Physeal fractures can be associated with growth arrest, especially when they involve the distal ulnar physis
  - Patient and parents should be counseled regarding importance of long-term follow-up even after fractures have healed
- Operative indications include unstable fractures, open fractures, compartment syndrome, neurovascular compromise, significant displacement, fracture deformity, and/or angulation

Monteggia and Galeazzi Fracture

BASIC INFORMATION

- Monteggia and Galeazzi injuries are less common, but commonly undiagnosed initially and important to recognize to provide proper treatment and avoid long-term problems
- Monteggia fracture involves most commonly an ulna fracture in association with proximal radioulnar joint dislocation
- Galeazzi fracture involves most commonly a radius fracture in association with distal radioulnar joint dislocation
- Mechanism of injury is typically a fall on an outstretched extremity
- Once diagnosed with radiographic studies, treatment involves caring for the fracture as well as the dislocation/instability

Carpal Fracture

BASIC INFORMATION

- Carpal fractures are rare in the pediatric population, but there must be a high index of suspicion for an adolescent with scaphoid fracture
- Scaphoid (carpal navicular) fractures are the most common carpal fractures
- Most scaphoid fractures occur at the waist or proximal poles of the scaphoid, which have significantly less vascularity than the distal pole; thus scaphoid fractures carry a high risk of nonunion and posttraumatic osteonecrosis

CLINICAL PRESENTATION

- Pain and swelling about the radial wrist that may be mistaken for a sprain or distal radius fracture after a fall on an outstretched hand with hyperextension and radial deviation of the wrist

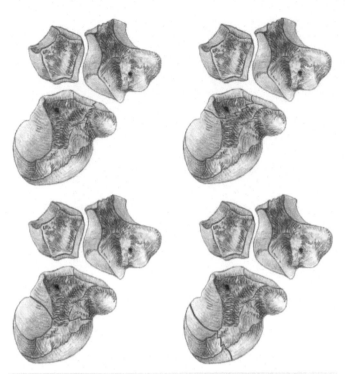

Fig. 72.6. Scaphoid fracture. (From Rao N, Hrehorovich P, Mathew M: Musculoskeletal Imaging. Philadelphia, Elsevier, 2015.)

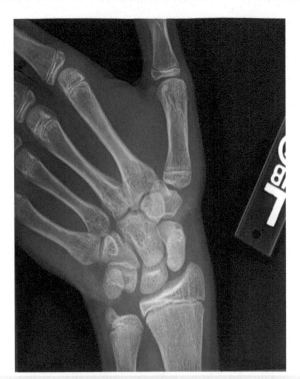

Fig. 72.7. Scaphoid view.

- Classic presentation includes "numbness over the anatomic snuffbox"
- May have limited thumb or wrist range of motion

DIAGNOSIS AND EVALUATION

- Imaging
  - PA/lateral radiographs of the injured wrist
  - Scaphoid view (slight wrist extension and ulnar deviation) places in profile (Figs. 72.6 and 72.7)
  - Note that x-rays are initially negative in one-third of cases
  - MRI has high accuracy in earlier diagnosis, though bone scan, CT, and ultrasound can also be used

TREATMENT

- Any suspected scaphoid fracture, even if x-rays are negative, should be treated with immobilization
  - Neglected injuries are at high risk of nonunion
- In patients with clinical suspicion of a scaphoid fracture but negative initial radiographs, immobilization with repeat clinical examination and x-rays out of the cast in 2 weeks is acceptable
- Immobilization has classically been described as thumb spica casting or bracing, but recent evidence demonstrates no difference in outcome with standard or thumb spica, long or short arm
- More proximal fractures are immobilized longer due to blood supply being tenuous
- Operative indications include displacement, fracture deformity, or dislocation and should be referred for definitive specialist management because posttraumatic arthrosis can result

Metacarpal Fracture

BASIC INFORMATION

- Majority can be treated with immobilization rather than surgery, especially in the fourth and fifth metacarpals, because those carpometacarpal (CMC) joints are more mobile and can compensate for fracture deformity
- "Boxer fracture" is a metacarpal neck fracture of the small finger resulting from a punch and is the most frequent type of metacarpal fracture

CLINICAL PRESENTATION

- Pain and swelling about the hand after a direct blow to the metacarpal head
- Limited finger range of motion

DIAGNOSIS AND EVALUATION

- Physical examination
  - Evaluate for open injury (all "fight bite" marks should be considered open and contaminated)
  - Assess for malrotation of digits or scissoring
    - Have the patient gently flex the digits, and they should all point toward the scaphoid tubercle with a smooth cascade; also compare with contralateral hand
- Imaging
  - PA/oblique/lateral radiographs of the injured hand centered over the metacarpals (Fig. 72.8)

TREATMENT

- Splint in intrinsic plus position
  - Wrist in extension

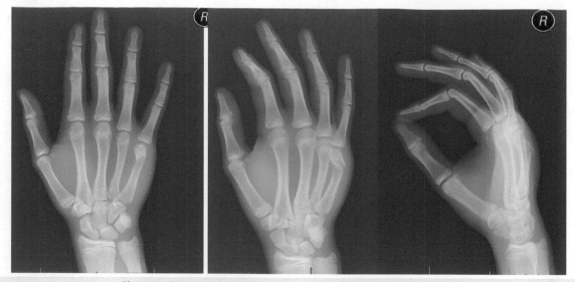

Fig. 72.8. Posteroanterior/oblique/lateral radiographs of a boxer's fracture.

- Metacarpophalangeal joints in 70 to 90 degrees of flexion
  - Interphalangeal joints neutral (fingers straight)
- Immobilize for 3 to 4 weeks, with the goal of early active range of motion
- Operative indications include open injuries (including "fight bite" wounds), multiple metacarpal fractures, digit malrotation, and significant displacement, shortening, and/or deformity
- Special considerations: thumb metacarpal intraarticular base fractures (Bennett, Rolando), which require specialized techniques to reduce and potentially operatively treat

LOWER-EXTREMITY INJURIES

The Limping Child

BASIC INFORMATION

- The inability to bear weight or a limp is a common pediatric problem
- Etiologies vary and can include:
  - Trauma
    - Sprain/contusion
    - Fracture
    - Vascular compromise
    - Compartment syndrome
    - Nonaccidental trauma
  - Overuse injuries
    - Osgood-Schlatter disease
    - Sever disease
  - Infection and inflammatory conditions
    - Septic arthritis
    - Toxic synovitis
    - Osteomyelitis
    - Juvenile idiopathic arthritis (JIA)
  - Developmental causes
    - Developmental dysplasia of the hip (DDH)
    - Legg-Calvé-Perthes disease

- Slipped capital femoral epiphysis (SCFE)
  - Leg length discrepancy
- Neoplasms
  - Benign tumors
  - Malignancies
- Proper and timely diagnosis will limit deleterious sequelae

Diagnosis and Evaluation

- History
  - Birth and developmental history
  - History of recent trauma
  - Ability to bear weight
  - Pattern of limp
    - Antalgic or nonantalgic?
  - Associated fever or chills
  - Presence or absence of night pain
  - Recent viral or bacterial infection
  - Recent bug bite or rash
  - Recent travel outside the United States
- Physical examination
  - Start with examination of the unaffected limb
  - Assess gait pattern
  - Examine entire body for evidence of rash or abnormal skin lesions
    - Presence may indicate Lyme disease, reactive arthritis, or a dermatologic condition
  - Examine spine for tenderness or step-off
    - Positive findings may point to a spinal etiology
  - Examine affected limb
    - Observe how child positions affected leg while at rest
      - Obligatory external rotation at the hip with pain and limited internal rotation may indicate a slipped capital femoral epiphysis
    - Assess neurovascular status
    - Evaluate the extremity for any swelling, warmth, or joint effusion
    - Palpate for any tenderness along joint line, growth plate, or diaphysis

Joint line tenderness along with painful range of motion may be a sign of septic arthritis

In the absence of trauma, tenderness along metaphysis and/or diaphysis may point to osteomyelitis or neoplasm

Tenderness along physis may indicate nondisplaced fracture

- All joints should be examined so as to rule out referred pain
  - Knee pain can be the result of a hip etiology and vice versa
  - For developmental hip disorders, see Chapter 73
- Imaging
  - Radiographs are initial image modality of choice
    - AP/lateral x-rays of affected bone or joint
      Recommend AP pelvis/lateral views of the hip in cases of knee pain to rule out SCFE
      Look for evidence of fracture, periosteal reaction, or joint effusion
  - MRI may be indicated in cases where:
    - SCFE is clinically suspected but radiographic results are equivocal
    - Osteomyelitis or neoplasm is suspected
  - Ultrasound is normally reserved for evaluation for joint effusion in cases of suspected hip septic arthritis
- Laboratory studies
  - In cases of suspected infection, appropriate laboratory tests are critical
  - Probability of septic arthritis ranges to 99.6% when all of the following criteria are met:
    - White blood cells (WBC) >12,000 cells/μL
    - Inability to bear weight
    - Fever >101.3°F (38.5°C)
    - Erythrocyte sedimentation rate (ESR) >40 mm/hr
    - C-reactive protein (CRP) >2 mg/dL
  - Joint aspiration will help confirm diagnosis if ultrasound notes an effusion
    - Cell count with differential
    - Gram stain, culture, and sensitivities
    - Glucose and protein levels
      A septic joint aspirate will typically show
      High WBC count (>50,000/mm³ with >75% polymorphonuclear leukocytes [PMNs])
      Glucose 50 mg/dL less than serum levels
  - Blood cultures
  - Lyme titers in cases of suspected Lyme disease

TREATMENT

- Treatment varies depending on etiology of limp
- Evaluation by musculoskeletal specialist or orthopedic surgeon usually recommended

Femoral Shaft Fractures

BASIC INFORMATION

- Represent 1% to 2% of all pediatric fractures
- Suspect child abuse in children younger than walking age
- In older children, usually the result of high-energy trauma

CLINICAL PRESENTATION

- Patients present with pain, swelling, and inability to ambulate
- Possible deformity
- Other injuries may be present in cases of high-energy trauma

DIAGNOSIS AND EVALUATION

- History
  - Suspect pathologic fracture in low-energy injuries
  - Suspect nonaccidental trauma in any patient who is not walking
- Physical examination
  - All high-energy trauma should be given full trauma evaluation
  - Assess neurovascular status
  - Monitor pulmonary status for signs of fat embolism
- Imaging
  - AP/lateral radiographs of the femur
    - Designated radiographs of the hip and knee should also be obtained to rule out concomitant injury
    - Trauma series radiographs should be obtained when appropriate
  - Advanced imaging is indicated if occult or pathologic fracture is suspected
    - CT angiogram for vascular injury

TREATMENT

- Urgent evaluation by orthopedics
- Immediate immobilization with splinting or traction
- Definitive treatment will vary based on age, fracture pattern, and patient factors

Ankle Sprains

BASIC INFORMATION

- Anatomy
  - Ligaments are fibrous connective tissues that connect two bones together
  - Injury occurs when force exceeds the ligament's tensile strength
  - The ligament itself and the ligament-to-bone interface may be stronger than the bone and the physis in children, so children with a "sprain" should be assessed for any underlying fracture
    - Avulsion fractures are common in children and occur when ligaments or tendons forcefully pull away from a bone, thereby causing a fragment or chip of bone to remain still attached to the ligament
    - Physeal fractures, especially Salter-Harris type I injuries, are also common and occur when ligaments pull on an epiphyseal bony fragment hard enough to cause an injury to the adjacent physis
- Grades of ligamentous sprains
  - Grade 1
    - Stretching of the ligament without a tear; usually with mild soft tissue swelling/pain and no joint laxity

- Grade 2
  - Partially torn ligament; soft tissue swelling or effusion, with more joint laxity than contralateral side, but with definite end point
- Grade 3
  - Completely torn ligament; grossly lax, with only a soft end-point

CLINICAL PRESENTATION

- Pain and swelling, with possible joint effusion
- Difficulty with weight-bearing
- Restricted or painful joint range of motion

DIAGNOSIS AND EVALUATION

- History
  - Twisting injury with possible audible "pop"
  - Inversion
    - Injury to the lateral ankle structures including the anterior talofibular ligament
  - Eversion
    - Injury to the medial ankle structures including the deltoid ligament
  - Dorsiflexion and eversion
    - Injury to the syndesmosis (high ankle injury)
  - Recurrent ankle sprains with painful flat feet should be evaluated for tarsal coalition (fusion of tarsal bones via fibrous or bony bridges, resulting in decreased mobility and inversion difficulty)
- Physical examination
  - Examination should include palpation of the medial and lateral malleoli and evaluation for any joint laxity
    - Comparison to contralateral side may be helpful
  - Tenderness over physis without clear radiographic evidence of fracture clinically indicates a Salter-Harris Type I fracture
  - Tests to assess for ligamentous stability
    - Anterior drawer: anterior talofibular ligament
    - Talar tilt test: calcaneofibular ligament
    - Eversion of heel: deltoid ligament
    - Tibia-fibula squeeze test: syndesmosis
  - Although less common, injury to the Achilles tendon should be ruled out
- Imaging
  - Use the Ottawa ankle rules for decision to obtain radiographs (applicable for children greater than 6 years of age)
  - X-rays should include AP, lateral, and ankle mortise views
  - Little indication for advanced imaging such as MRI and CT unless in cases with equivocal examination findings
    - Chronic ankle instability
    - Occult fractures
    - Osteochondral defects
- Ultrasound is increasing in popularity, but use is limited to centers with musculoskeletal radiologists

TREATMENT

- Rest, Ice, Compression, Elevation (RICE) has been the historical recommendation, although early introduction of range-of-motion exercises and progression to weight-bearing as tolerated are important
- Braces may help prevent reinjury
  - Crutches may be necessary during the acute painful stage; grade 3 sprains may require short period of immobilization
  - Structured rehabilitation programs have been shown to improve range of motion and to help reduce future injury
- Return to sports after demonstration of full range of motion, full strength, no swelling, no pain, and no joint instability
- Referral to orthopedic surgeon for
  - Chronic ankle instability
  - Worsening pain
  - Any concern for a high ankle sprain

Anterior Cruciate Ligament (ACL) Injury

BASIC INFORMATION

- ACL is one of the cruciate ligaments, along with the posterior cruciate ligament (PCL)
  - A primary static stabilizer of the knee joint by resisting anterior translation and medial rotation of the tibia
    - Is one of the commonly injured ligaments in the knee (see Table 72.2)
  - Acute ACL injuries may be associated with meniscal tears and chondral injury
  - Chronic deficiency results in degeneration of menisci and articular cartilage leading to arthritis

CLINICAL PRESENTATION

- Acute swelling and knee pain, usually with deceleration, hyperextension, and rotation about the knee (the majority of these are from noncontact injuries)
- May be accompanied by an audible pop with immediate knee pain
- Feeling of knee instability with pivoting and rotating movements once initial swelling and pain subside

DIAGNOSIS AND EVALUATION

- Physical examination
  - Assess for knee effusion
  - Often without tenderness on examination unless associated injuries are present; tenderness over medial or lateral joint line may indicate meniscal tear
    - Lateral meniscal tear associated more with acute ACL tears
    - Medial meniscal tears are associated more with subacute/chronic ACL tears
      - Absence of ACL transfers force to medial meniscus, which is a secondary stabilizer to anterior tibial translation
  - Assess for ligamentous laxity
    - Lachman: anterior force on the tibia performed with knee flexed at 30 degrees

Table 72.2. Isolated Ligamentous Knee Injuries

Injury	Mechanism	Presentation	Diagnostic Maneuver
Anterior cruciate ligament	Noncontact pivoting injury characterized by deceleration, hyperextension, or a rotational component	Acute pain and swelling along with knee instability	Lachman, anterior drawer, pivot shift
Posterior cruciate ligament	Direct blow to proximal tibia with a flexed knee (dashboard injury) Noncontact knee hyperflexion with a plantar-flexed foot Hyperextension injury	Posterior knee pain and Knee instability	Posterior drawer, posterior sag sign
Medial collateral ligament	Valgus and external rotation force to the lateral knee, or direct trauma	Medial joint line pain and difficulty ambulating	Valgus stress at 30 degrees knee flexion
Lateral collateral ligament	Varus and external rotation force to the medial knee, or direct trauma	Lateral joint line pain with instability in full extension	Varus stress at 30 degrees knee flexion
Meniscal injury	Twisting injury accompanied by axial load	Pain localizing to medial or lateral side of the knee with or without mechanical symptoms such as "locking and catching"	Thessaly test, McMurray test

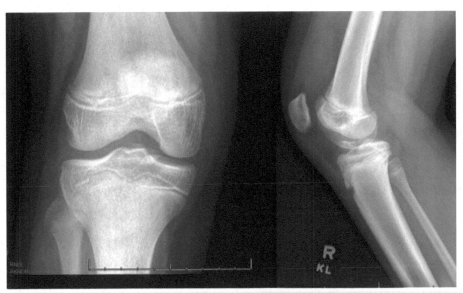

Fig. 72.9. Anteroposterior/lateral view of tibial spine fracture.

- Anterior drawer: anterior force on the tibia with the knee flexed 90 degrees
- Pivot shift: difficult to perform in office setting
- McMurray test: evaluate for meniscal tear
■ Imaging
- MRI is the imaging modality of choice to confirm the diagnosis
- Initial knee x-rays are normally readily obtainable and are appropriate to rule out fracture
  - Must distinguish from a tibial spine fracture, which is more common in skeletally immature patients (Fig. 72.9)

TREATMENT

- Rest, ice, compression, elevation with a period of knee immobilization
- Abstain from sports and activities that require cutting or pivoting
- Referral to orthopedic surgeon

Patellar Instability

BASIC INFORMATION

- Occurs more commonly in older children and adolescents
  - May be a predisposition to dislocation such as shallow femoral groove, ligamentous laxity, or other anatomic factors
- Congenital dislocation of patella is rare and often irreducible
  - Associated with conditions including Down syndrome, Larsen syndrome, arthrogryposis, diastrophic dysplasia

CLINICAL PRESENTATION

- Acute pain and swelling over the knee, often a "pop" related to traumatic event such as impact or a noncontact pivoting injury

- Patients may "self-reduce" due to the strong contractive pull of quadriceps
- Lateral dislocations with medial patellofemoral ligament tears are more common than medial dislocations

DIAGNOSIS AND EVALUATION

- Physical examination
  - Examine entire extremity including hip and ankle
  - Patellar apprehension or obvious abnormally positioned kneecap
  - Acute development of swelling/large effusion
  - Painful limited range of motion of knee
- Imaging
  - AP, lateral, and sunrise/Merchant radiographs of the knee should be obtained in the acute setting to evaluate for fracture
  - MRI should be considered on an outpatient basis for most patellar dislocations that still have an effusion 24 to 48 hours after the injury because a significant proportion of these patients have large chondral or osteochondral injuries that may benefit from early surgical intervention
  - In the chronically unstable patella, MRI can help diagnose medial patellofemoral ligament attenuation or tears, cartilage or osteochondral defects, and other anatomic factors that aid in surgical decision-making

TREATMENT

- In the emergency department setting, muscle relaxation to allow for extension of the knee is usually enough to reduce the patella. Occasionally, gentle medially directed pressure to the patella can reduce it
- Immobilization in extension (knee immobilizer), gentle compression, antiinflammatories, crutches, and activity modification may help for a few weeks to allow for ligamentous healing and to decrease pain. Early mobilization and weight-bearing are encouraged once the presence of a significant chondral or osteochondral defect is ruled out
- Lateral patellar support braces can help patients feel more stable
- For very large effusions limiting motion, consider aspiration to decrease pain and improve function
- Physical therapy may assist with range of motion and strengthening to prevent future recurrence
- Chronic dislocations may benefit from operative intervention such as arthroscopy or patellofemoral ligament reconstruction

Toddler's Fracture

BASIC INFORMATION

- Spiral, oblique, nondisplaced fracture of the tibial shaft (Fig. 72.10)

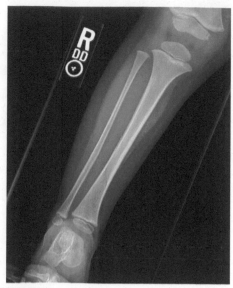

Fig. 72.10. Toddler's fracture. (From Nelson Textbook of Pediatrics, 20th ed. Philadelphia, Elsevier, 2016.)

- Fibula is normally intact
- Occurs in ambulatory children under the age of 3
- Result of low-energy trauma with a rotational component

CLINICAL PRESENTATION

- Afebrile with pain and swelling over the tibia
- Limp/inability to bear weight
- No signs or symptoms of infection

DIAGNOSIS AND EVALUATION

- History
  - Acute injury (i.e., witnessed fall or foot caught while sliding) with refusal to bear weight
- Physical examination
  - Examine entire extremity for hip, knee, or ankle pathology
  - Must rule out compartment syndrome
  - Localized tenderness over tibia
  - Warmth over the tibia
  - Painful dorsiflexion
  - Inability/refusal to bear weight (most sensitive test)
- Imaging
  - AP and lateral radiographs of the tibia/fibula
  - Additional views or advanced imaging is unnecessary and would not alter initial management
  - The use of advanced imaging should be reserved for patients who are febrile, lack a clear trauma history, or have elevated serum inflammatory markers

TREATMENT

- Long leg walking cast for 2 to 3 weeks
- Follow-up radiographs are unnecessary unless otherwise clinically indicated

LOWER-EXTREMITY OVERUSE INJURIES

Patellofemoral Dysfunction

BASIC INFORMATION

- Characterized by anterior knee pain during loaded flexion of the knee
- Can be the result of trauma, overuse, and/or abnormal patellar tracking
- Should be a diagnosis of exclusion and distinguished from adult anterior knee pain etiologies such as chondromalacia
- A comprehensive knee examination will help localize points of tenderness and assess for any ligamentous laxity or patellar maltracking
  - Important also to rule out any etiologies that may refer pain to the knee, such as from the hip or spine
- Preliminary x-rays should include AP, lateral, and sunrise views
  - Long leg standing films may be needed to assess overall alignment
- In the absence of fracture or clear anatomic derangement, initial treatment should include activity modification, oral antiinflammatory medications, and physical therapy
- Refer to an orthopedic surgeon for any further evaluation and treatment as needed

Osgood-Schlatter Syndrome

BASIC INFORMATION

- Characterized as a traction apophysitis of the tibial tubercle due to repetitive strain and chronic avulsion of the secondary ossification center of the tibial tuberosity
- Pain is localized to the tibial tubercle and may radiate along the patellar tendon
- Normally presents in males between the ages of 12 and 15 years and in females between the ages of 8 and 12 years
- Bilateral symptoms are observed in 20% to 30%
- Pain is exacerbated after activity involving jumping (basketball, volleyball, running) and/or on direct contact (e.g., kneeling)
- X-rays may show irregularity of the apophysis with separation from the tibial tuberosity in early stages and fragmentation in later stages
- Initial treatment may include application of ice, limitation of activities, oral antiinflammatory medications, protective knee padding, and physical therapy
- Usually self-limiting but may take 12 to 24 months to resolve
- A persistent bony ossicle may be visible on future x-rays

Sinding-Larsen-Johansson Syndrome

BASIC INFORMATION

- Analogous to Osgood-Schlatter syndrome, except that Sinding-Larsen-Johansson syndrome is a traction apophysitis of the inferior patellar pole
- Presentation is between ages of 10 and 12 years
- Physical examination normally demonstrates swelling and point tenderness over the inferior pole of the patella
- X-rays may show separation and elongation or calcification of the inferior patellar pole on the lateral view of the knee
- Normally responds to nonoperative management such as ice, limitation of activities, oral antiinflammatory medications, protective knee padding, and physical therapy

Iliotibial Band Syndrome

BASIC INFORMATION

- Common overuse injury typically seen in runners, cyclists, and military recruits
- Caused by repetitive anterior-posterior friction of the iliotibial band over the lateral femoral epicondyle
- Predisposing factors include genu varum, excessive internal tibial torsion, foot pronation, and hip abductor weakness
- Diagnosis is usually made based on history and physical examination
- Patients often have tenderness over the distal iliotibial band at the level of the lateral femoral epicondyle, radiating to Gerdy tubercle
- Imaging studies are usually reserved to rule out other pathologic entities
- Nonoperative management includes physical therapy programs focusing on stretching of the iliotibial band
- Recalcitrant cases should be referred to an orthopedic surgeon

Review Questions

For review questions, please go to ExpertConsult.com.

Suggested Readings

Caird MS, Flynn JM, Leung YL, et al. Factors distinguishing septic arthritis from transient synovitis of the hip in children: a prospective study. *J Bone Joint Surg [Am]*. 2006;88-A:1251–1257.
Egol Kenneth. *Handbook of Fractures*. Wolters Kluwer; 2018.
Green David P, et al. *Greens Operative Hand Surgery*. Elsevier; 2017.
Herring John A, Tachdjian Mihran O. *Tachdjians Pediatric Orthopaedics*. Saunders Elsevier; 2013.
Rang Mercer, et al. *Rangs Childrens Fractures*. Lippincott Williams & Wilkins; 2006.

73 Selected Topics in Orthopedics

SUSAN E. NELSON, MD, MPH and DANIEL J. MILLER, MD

Musculoskeletal (MSK) concerns in children are common presentations seen by the primary care pediatrician. Knowledge of hip, lower extremity, and spine conditions is essential for recognition of when a child can be observed and when referral to a specialist is required. Orthopedic concerns may be the presenting complaint of the child or parents, or MSK conditions may also be found on routine well-child examination, as may be the case with hip dysplasia, scoliosis, or leg length discrepancy. This highlights the importance of thorough MSK physical examination and a high index of suspicion. This chapter outlines a diversity of select important and common orthopaedic conditions to recognize, and will guide distinguishing those that require only reassurance and observation from those requiring prompt referral or urgent management.

Compartment Syndrome

BASIC INFORMATION

- A devastating complication in which elevated tissue pressures within a closed fascial compartment compromise tissue perfusion, resulting in muscle ischemia and necrosis
- Caused by increased compartment inflow (e.g., edema, hemorrhage) and/or decreased outflow (e.g., venous obstruction, constrictive dressings)
- Compartment syndrome is a surgical emergency
- See also *Nelson Textbook of Pediatrics*, Chapter 687, "Management of Musculoskeletal Injury"

CLINICAL PRESENTATION

- Can be seen after
  - Fracture
  - Crush injuries
  - Vascular injuries
  - Bleeding disorders
  - Constrictive dressings or casts

DIAGNOSIS AND EVALUATION

- Should be suspected after an extremity injury in which the child exhibits:
  - Increasing pain out of proportion to the injury
  - Increasing analgesia requirements
  - In young children this may be manifested as increasing anxiety or agitation
- Physical examination
  - Tense muscle compartment to palpation
  - Pain with passive stretch of the joints
  - Late findings include decreased sensory motor examination, decreased pulse, and pallor

TREATMENT

- Remove constrictive dressings or casts
- Limb should be placed at the level of the heart to optimize tissue perfusion (not above the heart)
- Suspicion of compartment syndrome should be emergently referred for evaluation
- Emergency surgical treatment with fasciotomies

HIP

Hip disease in children will commonly present to a primary care pediatrician. Thorough history and physical examination are important to detect hip disorders that can affect the acute and long-term function of the hip. Because of the long-term morbidity associated with certain hip disorders, a high index of suspicion should be maintained.

Developmental Hip Dysplasia (DDH)

BASIC INFORMATION

- Previously called "congenital dysplasia of the hip" or "congenital hip dislocation"
- Developmental dysplasia of the hip is a spectrum ranging from acetabular dysplasia, to hip subluxation, to hip dislocation
- Risk factors include female gender, first-born, breech position, and positive family history
- Most commonly involves the left hip

CLINICAL PRESENTATION

- Associated with intrauterine positioning deformities
  - Torticollis (20%)
  - Metatarsus adductus (10%)
- DDH is distinguished from teratologic hip dislocations (fixed dislocations at birth)
  - Teratologic hip dislocations occur in association with disorders or syndromes such as:
    - Larsen syndrome
    - Arthrogryposis
    - Myelomeningocele
    - Chromosomal abnormalities

DIAGNOSIS AND EVALUATION

- Physical examination
  - Early diagnosis in newborns can be made mainly with Barlow and Ortolani testing

- Infant should be placed on a firm surface with hips flexed to 90 degrees
- Barlow
  - Depression and adduction dislocates a reduced hip that is unstable
- Ortolani
  - Elevation and abduction to *relocate a dislocated hip*
- Hip clicks without instability are not clinically significant
- In older infants (>3 months), soft tissue contracture limits diagnosis with Ortolani and Barlow testing; therefore other signs include:
  - Limitation of abduction
  - Galeazzi sign: appearance of foreshortening of femur on affected side
- In children of walking age, findings include:
  - Limp and leg length discrepancy for unilateral dislocation
  - Waddling gait and hyperlordosis for bilateral dislocations
- Periodic hip surveillance with physical examination is essential because most children with DDH do not have risk factors
- Radiographic evaluation
  - Hip ultrasonography (US) is best for evaluation of the cartilaginous infant hip <4 to 6 months of age
  - US is useful for screening in infants with risk factors and normal physical examination and for evaluating treatment
  - USs performed before 6 weeks of age have a higher rate of false positives (so US after 6 weeks is ideal)
  - Anteroposterior (AP) pelvis x-ray may be obtained >4 to 6 months of age (Fig. 73.1)
    - An abnormal x-ray will show
      - Disruption of Shenton line (inferior border of superior pubic ramus)
      - Asymmetric ossific nuclei of the femoral head

The proximal medial metaphysis of the femoral neck is outside the inferior medial quadrant as divided by Perkin and Hilgenreiner lines
  - Hilgenreiner line is horizontal through the triradiate cartilage
  - Perkin line is perpendicular to Hilgenreiner line at the lateral edge of the acetabulum

TREATMENT

- Referral to a pediatric orthopedist for hips unstable on clinical examination, other concerning physical examination findings as outlined, or dysplastic on screening US
- Birth to 6 months old
  - Pavlik harness
  - Abduction brace
- >6 months
  - Operative treatment with closed or open reduction
- >18 months
  - Operative treatment may also include osteotomies of the pelvis and femur

Slipped Capital Femoral Epiphysis (SCFE)

BASIC INFORMATION

- Slipped capital femoral epiphysis is a condition in which the epiphysis is posteriorly displaced off the femoral metaphysis (Fig. 73.2)
- Occurs most often in obese young adolescent males (13–15 years); affected females tend to be younger (11–13 years)
  - Polynesian > Black > Hispanic > Caucasian > Indo-Mediterranean
- Most often occurs in the left hip

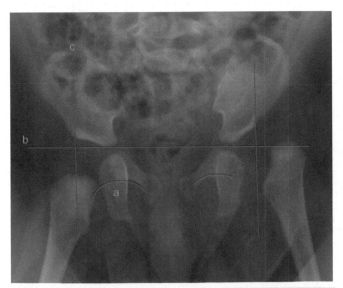

Fig. 73.1. Anteroposterior pelvis shows left developmental hip dysplasia with dislocated hip. Shenton line (a) is broken on the left, with the left hip lying outside the inferior medial quadrant of the intersection of Hilgenreiner (b) and Perkin (c) lines.

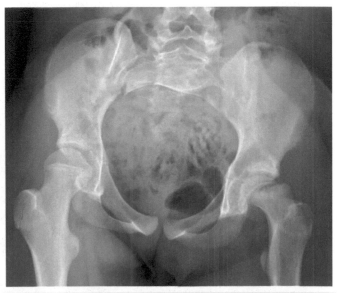

Fig. 73.2. Anteroposterior pelvis of an 11-year-old showing left hip slipped capital femoral epiphysis. The epiphysis is posterior and inferior to the femoral metaphysis.

- This is associated with mechanical factors and endocrine abnormalities (Table 73.1)
  - Mechanical factors make the hip more susceptible to shear forces, increasing the risk for slip
  - Endocrine abnormalities cause abnormality of the physis, which places it at risk for slip
- More severe slips have a worse prognosis regarding
  - Osteoarthritis
  - Decreased future range of motion (ROM)
  - Complications such as avascular necrosis (AVN) and chondrolysis

CLINICAL PRESENTATION

- Knee pain or groin pain on the affected side
  - The hip should always be included in evaluation when the presenting complaint is knee pain
  - May be acute (<3 weeks), chronic (>3 weeks), or acute on chronic in presentation
- Gait
  - Antalgic
  - Trendelenburg
  - Unable to weight bear
- Restricted flexion, abduction, and internal rotation
- Obligate external rotation with hip flexion

DIAGNOSIS AND EVLAUATION

- If the patient is unable to bear weight, the slip is unstable and at higher risk of AVN
- X-rays
  - AP pelvis and frog leg lateral (Fig. 73.3)
    - Frog-leg lateral will best show a subtle slip

Table 73.1. Etiological Factors in Slipped Capital Femoral Epiphysis

Femoral retroversion	Hypothyroidism
Increased obliquity of the physis	Growth hormone deficiency
Obesity	Chronic renal failure (secondary to hyperparathyroidism)

- Klein's line is drawn on the AP pelvis along the superior femoral neck
  - Normally this line intersects the epiphysis

TREATMENT

- Admission to hospital and bed rest
- Urgent surgical stabilization to prevent further slip
  - Most often via in situ pinning with a cannulated screw

Legg-Calvé-Perthes Disease (LCP)

BASIC INFORMATION

- Legg-Calvé-Perthes disease is idiopathic avascular necrosis of femoral epiphysis
- It is a diagnosis of exclusion and rarely bilateral
  - Differential diagnosis includes:
    - Skeletal dysplasia
    - Sickle cell
    - Hematogenous malignancy
    - Hypothyroidism
    - Gaucher disease
- Typically affects young children (~4–8 years old) and predominantly males over females (~5:1)
- Has been associated with
  - Attention-deficit/hyperactivity disorder
  - Delayed bone age
- Natural history
  - Age at onset and shape of the femoral head at skeletal maturity are important prognostic factors
  - <6 years and a spherical, congruent hip at maturity are good prognostic factors

CLINICAL PRESENTATION

- Insidious onset
- May present with a limp which can be
  - Painless
  - Antalgic
  - Trendelenburg

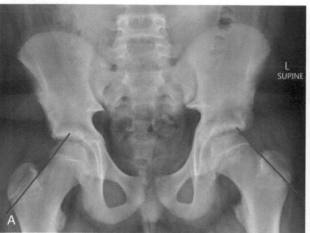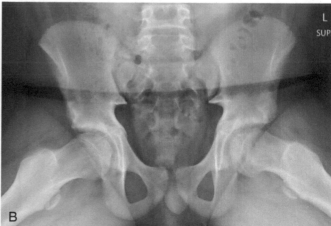

Fig. 73.3. (A) Anteroposterior pelvis with left hip mild slipped capital femoral epiphysis. Klein's line does not intersect the left femoral epiphysis as is seen on the right. (B) Frog-leg lateral of left mild slip.

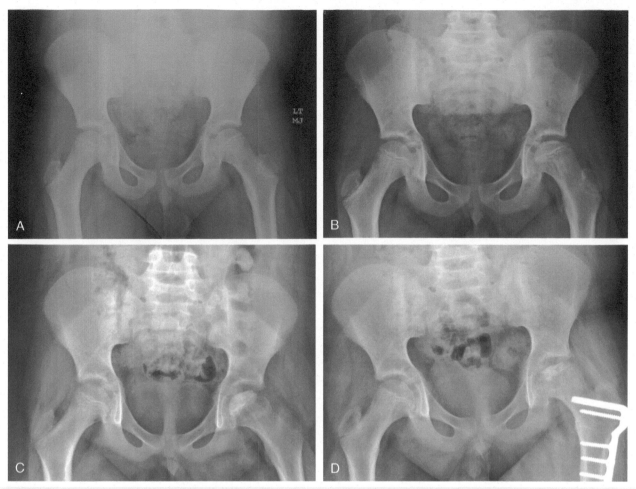

Fig. 73.4. An 8-year-old male presented with left hip pain with Legg-Calvé-Perthes. Initial x-rays (A) were normal. 4 months later (B) the left femoral head is flattened and progressed with sclerotic and cystic changes (C). The patient went on to have a proximal femoral varus osteotomy (D).

- Decreased ROM especially in
  - Internal rotation
  - Abduction

DIAGNOSIS AND EVALUATION

- AP pelvis and frog-leg lateral x-rays should be obtained
- X-rays vary depending on stage (Fig. 73.4)
  - Initial stage: x-ray may appear normal
  - Early findings: medial joint space widening, irregular femoral head ossification, crescent fracture
  - Fragmentation stage: collapse of the femoral epiphysis (average duration: 8 months)
  - Reossification: appearance of new bone (may last up to 18 months)
  - Remodeling: occurs through skeletal maturity
    - Shape of the femoral head and congruity within the acetabulum have implications for prognosis
    - An aspherical head that is incongruent will predispose to early osteoarthritis

TREATMENT

- The principle of treatment for LCP is to contain the hip within the acetabulum
  - This can be accomplished via nonoperative and operative means depending on the age and stage of presentation

- Nonoperative containment
  - Maintaining ROM is important
    - Activity modification and physical therapy
    - Abduction bracing/casting
- Operative containment (Fig. 73.4d)
  - Proximal femoral osteotomy
  - Pelvic osteotomy

LOWER-EXTREMITY ALIGNMENT/ DEFORMITY

Normal lower-extremity alignment varies throughout childhood. It is important to be familiar with physiologic alignment at various stages of growth because parents often present with complaints regarding their child's lower-extremity profile. Being able to identify deviations from normal physiologic alignment will guide further investigation and referral if necessary.

Angular Deformity

BASIC INFORMATION

- Normal physiologic lower-extremity alignment varies throughout development
  - Maximal genu varum (commonly referred to as an outward "bowing" of the knees) is reached from 6 to 12 months

Table 73.2. Differential Diagnosis of Angular Limb Deformities

Genu Varum	Genu Valgum
Physiologic	Physiologic
Metabolic bone disease	Metabolic bone disease
Rickets	Rickets
Renal osteodystrophy	
Osteogenesis imperfecta	
Skeletal dysplasia	Skeletal dysplasia
MED	MED
SED	SED
Focal fibrocartilaginous dysplasia	Pseudoachondroplasia
	Mucopolysaccharidoses
	Chondroectodermal dysplasia
Blount disease	Cozen fracture
Physeal injury	Physeal injury
Infection	Infection
Trauma	Trauma
Radiation	Radiation

MED, multiple epiphyseal dysplasia; *SED*, spondyloepiphyseal dysplasia.

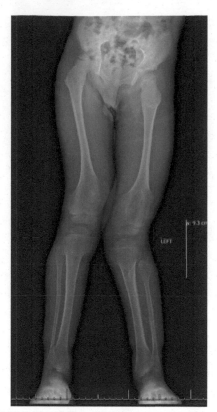

Fig. 73.5. Full-length standing lower-extremity x-rays reveal angular deformity and leg length discrepancy secondary to multiple hereditary exostosis.

- Neutral by 18 to 24 months
- Maximal genu valgum is reached by 4 years
- Normal adult lower-extremity alignment is approximately 6 degrees of *valgus*
  - Reached by approximately 11 years
- Genu varum
  - Most commonly physiologic up to age 2 years (Table 73.2)
- Genu valgum
  - Physiologic valgus should not increase past age 7 years (Table 73.2)

DIAGNOSIS AND EVALUATION

- A thorough history is important to help narrow the differential for angular deformities
  - Developmental history
  - Nutritional history
  - History of infection or trauma/previous fractures
  - Family history
- Full-length standing lower-extremity x-rays should be obtained for suspected pathologic angular deformity (Fig. 73.5)
  - Evidence of short stature
  - Asymmetry
  - Pain
  - Gait abnormality
  - History of infection, fracture, trauma
  - Other concerning physical examination findings
  - Genu varum past 2 years of age, excessive genu valgum in adolescence

Tibia Vara (Blount Disease)

GENERAL INFORMATION

- Blount disease (tibia vara) is progressive genu varum resulting from a pathologic proximal tibia physis that results in early growth arrest

- Infantile <3 years
  - 50% are bilateral
  - Risk factors: early walkers, obesity, Hispanic or African-American ethnicity
- Adolescent >10 years
  - More commonly unilateral and may be accompanied by distal femoral varus
  - Risk factors: obesity

CLINICAL PRESENTATION

- Commonly obese male
- Varus alignment
- Lateral thrust
- Internal tibial torsion

DIAGNOSIS AND EVALUATION

- Infantile
  - X-rays may not show irregularities until 18 months
  - Full-length lower-extremity x-rays show (Fig. 73.6)
    - Varus angulation at the proximal medial tibial metaphysis
    - Widened and irregular physis medially
    - Medially sloping and irregular wedge shape of the epiphysis
    - Medial "beaking" at the metaphysis
    - Lateral subluxation
- Adolescent
  - Standing full-length AP x-rays of the lower extremities should be obtained
    - The physeal appearance is less severe than in infantile Blount

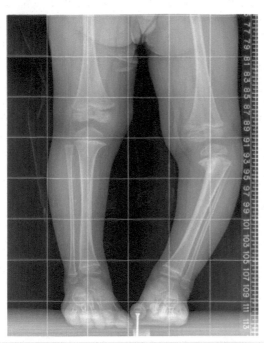

Fig. 73.6. Infantile tibia vara (Blount disease). Characteristic medial beaking is seen with varus alignment of the left.

- Narrowing of the tibial epiphysis with widening of the medial physis may be seen
- Medial beaking is less common

TREATMENT

- Suspected cases of Blount disease should be referred to a pediatric orthopedic specialist
- Infantile Blount disease
  - Nonoperative treatment
    - Children 3 years of age or younger with milder stages can be braced with a knee ankle foot orthosis (KAFO)
  - Operative treatment
    - Children over 3 years of age and those with more severe disease should be considered for early surgical management
      Goal to prevent joint incongruity, limb shortening, and persistent angular deformity
      Best results with intervention before age 4 years
- Adolescent Blount disease
  - Treatment is primarily surgical

Post-Traumatic Tibia Valga (Cozen Fracture)

BASIC INFORMATION

- In children, undisplaced proximal metaphyseal tibia fractures are often referred to as Cozen fractures. These commonly result in post-traumatic proximal tibia valgus deformity that may persist up to 1 year after injury and spontaneously improve
- After sustaining such a fracture, the patient should be observed and the family counseled regarding the possibility of tibia valga

- Rarely are there long-term functional deficits or symptoms; operative intervention is indicated only for cases of severe deformity, symptoms, or functional deficit

Rotational Deformities

BASIC INFORMATION

- In-toeing or out-toeing can originate from the rotational profile of the femur, the tibia, or both
  - The normal femoral neck is anteverted
    - At birth anteversion is 40 degrees and decreases to 15 degrees in adulthood
  - The tibia is rotated internally in children, which can be seen by looking at the thigh-foot angle
    - In children internal rotation is normal, changing to external rotation in adulthood
  - Most rotational deformity is physiologic and will resolve as the child grows

In-Toeing

BASIC INFORMATION

- Common in children
- Usually benign and can be observed
- See previous section for concerning features

CLINICAL PRESENTATION

- May present with parental complaints of tripping, awkward gait, and "W" sitting
  - Concerning history features
    - Developmental delay
    - Prematurity
    - Progressive deformity
    - Recent or acute onset
    - Pain
    - Persistent functional deficit
  - Concerning physical examination features
    - Short stature
    - Asymmetry
    - Syndromic features
    - Abnormal hip and foot examination
    - Abnormal neurologic examination

DIAGNOSIS AND EVALUATION

- Benign differential diagnosis
  - Internal tibial torsion
    - Most common
    - Usually present 1 to 3 years
    - Examine thigh-foot angle (Fig. 73.7)
      >15 degrees of internal rotation
  - Femoral anteversion
    - Usually present >3 years
    - Examine hip rotation (Fig. 73.7)
      >70 degrees internal rotation with <20 degrees external rotation
  - Metatarsus adductus
    - Usually presents in infancy
    - Lateral border of the foot is curved

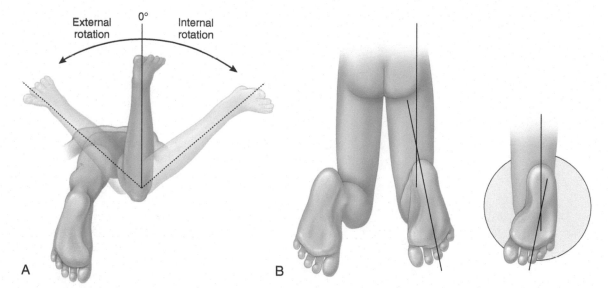

Fig. 73.7. Torsional profile examination with the patient prone. The examiner can expediently assess the thigh-foot axis to estimate tibial torsion and examine the shape of the lateral border of the foot to assess for the presence of metatarsus adductus (A) and to determine the amount of internal and external rotation of the hip as an indication of the amount of femoral anteversion (B). (From Herring JA. *Tachdjian's Pediatric Orthopaedics.* 5th ed. Philadelphia: Elsevier; 2014: Fig. 4.5.)

- Examine the heel bisector angle (Fig. 73.7)
  - Medial deviation of the forefoot with normally aligned hindfoot
- Pathologic differential diagnosis
  - Cerebral palsy (CP)
  - DDH
  - Clubfoot
  - Cavovarus foot
  - Skewfoot
  - Hallux varus

TREATMENT

- For benign causes, observation with reassurance that most will resolve
- Persistent deformity and functional deficit warrant orthopedic referral
  - Internal tibial torsion
    - Persistent deformity and functional deficit >6 years old
  - Femoral anteversion
    - Persistent deformity and function deficit >8 years old
  - Metatarsus adductus
    - Early mild deformities can be observed or stretched
    - For moderate deformities, one may consider serially casting
    - Failure to resolve, rigid deformity, or problems with shoe wear warrant referral for possible treatment

Leg Length Discrepancy

BASIC INFORMATION

- Up to two-thirds of the population will have a minor leg length discrepancy that causes no functional deficit (up to 2 cm may be well tolerated)
- Leg length inequality can be structural or functional (postural)

Table 73.3. Differential Diagnosis of Leg Length Discrepancy

Congenital	Acquired
Limb deficiency	Physeal growth arrest
Proximal femoral focal deficiency	Trauma/fracture
Congenitally short femur	Infection
Fibular deficiency/hemimelia	Radiation
Tibia deficiency/hemimelia	Blount disease
Tibial Bowing	Asymmetric Neurologic Conditions
Posteromedial bowing associated with calcaneovalgus foot	Hemiparesis
Anterolateral bowing associated with NF-1	Polio myositis
	Tumor
	Enchondroma
	Osteochondroma
	UBC
	Hemihypertrophy
	NF
	Klippel-Trenaunay syndrome
	Beckwith-Wiedemann syndrome
	Proteus syndrome
	Malunion
	Post slipped capital femoral epiphysis or Legg-Calvé-Perthes
	Inflammatory arthritis

NF, neurofibromatosis; *UBC,* unicameral bone cyst.

- The differential diagnosis is broad (Table 73.3), necessitating a thorough history and physical examination
- Leg length discrepancy can be quantified on physical examination using a tape measure (from anterior superior iliac spine to medial malleolus) or blocks of different heights under the short leg until the pelvis is level
- Full-length standing lower-extremity x-rays should be obtained to radiographically quantify the deformity and as part of the evaluation for underlying cause

- Treatment will vary widely depending on the etiology of the leg length discrepancy
- Referral to an orthopedic specialist is appropriate for most leg length inequality in the skeletally immature patient
- Leg length inequality that is <2 cm and stable with no functional deficit may be observed

Toe Walking

BASIC INFORMATION

- Painless toe walking may be seen most commonly in toddlers (ages 1–3 years); children should develop a normal heel strike and push off by approximately 3 years of age
- Parents may notice toe walking as their child begins to walk, or it may present later if the toe walking persists
- Differential diagnosis
  - Idiopathic
  - Mild spastic diplegia
  - Hereditary spastic paraparesis
- Perinatal history and developmental history can give clues to an underlying neurologic cause for toe walking
- A thorough physical examination includes gait examination, neurologic examination, and focused examination of the foot and ankle for rigidity and tight Achilles tendon
- Idiopathic toe walking that persists after 3 years of age can be treated with stretching of the Achilles tendon or serially casting

FOOT AND ANKLE

The appearance of the foot is variable, and this is often normal; flat feet and high arches are not necessarily pathologic. In newborns especially, many variations of normal can be seen. Intrauterine crowding or "packaging"-associated deformities like metatarsus adductus and calcaneovalgus are usually flexible and resolve spontaneously. It is important to recognize when the foot is not within normal limits and when further investigation and treatment are required.

Talipes Equinovarus (Clubfoot)

BASIC INFORMATION

- Clubfoot is a relatively common disorder affecting 1/1000 newborns
- Treatment should begin within the first few weeks of life
- 50% of cases are bilateral
- Genetic predisposition

CLINICAL PRESENTATION

- Characteristic foot deformity can be recognized using the acronym "CAVE" (Fig. 73.8)
  - **C**avus midfoot
  - **A**dductus of the forefoot
  - **V**arus hindfoot
  - **E**quinus (deficit in dorsiflexion at ankle)

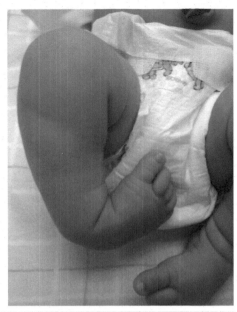

Fig. 73.8. Talipes equinovarus in a newborn. Clinical appearance of an untreated clubfoot. (From Herring JA. *Tachdjian's Pediatric Orthopaedics*. 5th ed. Philadelphia: Elsevier; 2014: Fig. 23.42.)

- A medial crease and posterior heel crease are evident
- In addition to the characteristic deformity, the affected foot will be smaller with a smaller calf

DIAGNOSIS AND EVALUATION

- May be diagnosed in utero by US
- Imaging is not necessary for diagnosis
- Look for associated conditions:
  - Arthrogryposis
  - Larsen syndrome
  - Torticollis
  - Hip dysplasia
  - Myelodysplasia
- Once the deformity is recognized, prompt referral to an orthopedic specialist should be made so that treatment can begin

TREATMENT

- Ponseti casting (serial long leg casting) has supplanted surgery as the primary treatment in North America
  - 85% to 90% will require a percutaneous Achilles tenotomy
  - Bracing is used after casting to age 4 years to prevent recurrence
- Surgical treatment is reserved for feet resistant to serial casting and is often required in clubfoot associated with another syndrome/disorder

Polydactyly

BASIC INFORMATION

- Most common congenital toe deformity, affecting 1.7/1000; associated with a syndrome in 10% to 20% of cases
- Bilateral in 50%

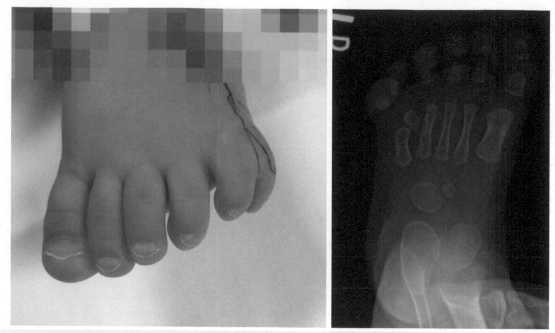

Fig. 73.9. 12-month-old with polydactyly. X-rays help guide decision-making regarding excision.

- Postaxial (fifth toe) duplication most common
- Duplicated toes may be well formed (Type A) or vestigial in nature (Type B)
- Look for polydactyly of the hands (associated with toe polydactyly 30% of cases)

DIAGNOSIS AND EVALUATION

- X-rays can be helpful to define the bony anatomy of the duplicated toe and to identify any other abnormalities (Fig. 73.9)

TREATMENT

- Polydactyly may interfere with shoe fitting and cause cosmetic concerns
- Referral for consideration of excision should be made before 1 year of age

Pes Planovalgus (Flatfoot)

BASIC INFORMATION

- A flexible flatfoot is a common finding associated with hypermobility in children and adolescents
- Distinguishing between a flexible flatfoot and a rigid flatfoot is important for guiding management
- Keep in mind that flatfoot may be associated with other conditions such as:
  - Peripheral neuropathy
  - Duchenne muscular dystrophy
  - CP

CLINICAL PRESENTATION

- The appearance of the foot with weight bearing is characterized by:
  - A valgus heel
  - A flat medial longitudinal arch
  - An abducted forefoot
- The foot may be symptomatic or asymptomatic

DIAGNOSIS AND EVALUATION

- History of pain or functional disability
- Flexible flatfoot
  - Arch reconstitutes in non-weight-bearing position
  - Arch reconstitutes with active muscle function such as standing on tiptoe
  - May be associated with a tight Achilles tendon
- Rigid flatfoot
  - If the arch does not reconstitute with tiptoe or non-weight-bearing, further investigation is warranted
  - Differential diagnosis:
    - Tarsal coalition
    - Congenital vertical talus
    - Juvenile idiopathic arthritis
    - Osteoid osteoma
    - Accessory navicular
- Imaging
  - X-rays are not required if history and physical examination confirm an idiopathic flexible flatfoot
  - Standing x-rays can help determine the diagnosis in a rigid flatfoot and help guide referral

TREATMENT

- No treatment is needed for an asymptomatic flexible flatfoot
- If there is contracture of the Achilles tendon, a stretching program should be initiated
  - Heel should be inverted and knee straight during stretching
- Symptomatic painful flatfoot: activity modification, physical therapy, shoe wear modification, and/or orthotics; surgery is the last line of therapy

Table 73.4. Differential Diagnosis of Cavovarus Foot

NEUROMUSCULAR

Hereditary Sensory Motor Neuropathy (Charcot-Marie-Tooth)
Friedreich ataxia
Spinal muscular atrophy
Myelomeningocele
Polio myositis
Cerebral palsy

ACQUIRED

Post compartment syndrome
Peripheral nerve injury
Burns

CONGENITAL

Residual clubfoot

Cavovarus Foot

BASIC INFORMATION

- Unlike pes planovalgus, which often requires no treatment and reassurance only, a cavovarus foot (elevated medial longitudinal arch, varus heel) should be investigated because the etiology is neurologic in most patients (Table 73.4)
- Patients may complain of painful calluses due to increased pressure under the first and fifth metatarsal and increased medial heel pressure
- A Coleman block test (placement of a block under the lateral border of the foot) helps establish the flexibility of the hindfoot varus (a flexible hindfoot will correct to neutral or valgus)
- A neurologic examination is essential to uncover any association with neurologic disorders, with referral to a neurologist for new presentations of unknown etiology
- Diagnosis: standing foot x-rays AP and lateral
- Referral to an orthopedic surgeon is appropriate for symptomatic feet; surgeon will help determine nonoperative versus operative treatment

NECK AND SPINE

Congenital Muscular Torticollis (CMT)

BASIC INFORMATION

- A painless rotational deformity of the head/neck caused by contracture of the sternocleidomastoid muscle
- Presents in the neonatal period
- Most likely caused by fibrosis of the sternocleidomastoid muscle in the prenatal or perinatal period

CLINICAL PRESENTATION

- Presents with the infant's head tilted toward the ipsilateral contracted sternocleidomastoid muscle and the chin rotated toward the contralateral shoulder
- In the first 3 months of life, an olive-shaped mass may be palpable within the midsubstance of the affected sternocleidomastoid
- In older infants (>3 months) a tight fibrous band is palpable over the length of the muscle

DIAGNOSIS AND EVALUATION

- In infants, CMT can be diagnosed based on clinical presentation
- In the absence of classic physical examination findings of CMT, alternative sources of torticollis should be considered, including:
  - Ocular torticollis: abnormal head tilting secondary to strabismus or eye muscle weakness
  - Sandifer syndrome: spasmodic torsional dystonia secondary to gastroesophageal reflux or esophagitis
  - Atlantoaxial rotatory displacement: rotational subluxation or dislocation of C1 vertebra on C2 vertebra secondary to spinal trauma or oropharyngeal inflammation (aka Grisel syndrome)
  - Infectious causes such as retropharyngeal abscesses or pyogenic cervical spondylitis
- CMT is associated with DDH and metatarsus adductus. Infants should be screened with physical examination of the feet and hip US

TREATMENT

- Physical therapy along with a home program of massage and stretching. Usually successful when initiated within the first 6 months of life
- If no response to therapy, plain radiographs should be taken to rule out cervical spine anomaly
- Torticollis refractory to prolonged and persistent therapy is managed with release/lengthening of the sternocleidomastoid muscle

Scoliosis

- Defined as a lateral deviation of the spine in the coronal plane greater than 10 degrees as measured using the Cobb method (Fig. 73.10).
- However, scoliosis represents a complex three-dimensional deformity with axial (rotational) and sagittal plane abnormalities as well.
  - Rotational deformity of the vertebra (and associated ribs) is the basis for the Adam's forward bend test.
- Scoliosis is classified and treated based on age of presentation and underlying etiology of spinal deformity.
  - Scoliosis in the young child (e.g., <8 years old) can have adverse effects on thoracic growth and pulmonary maturation.
  - Mild, stable scoliosis in the skeletally mature child or adult is well tolerated with minimal effect on function.
  - Severe scoliosis may be associated with cardiopulmonary compromise, back pain, adverse cosmesis, and poor sitting balance.
- Treatment (both operative and nonoperative) is based on patient age, skeletal maturity, severity of deformity, medical comorbidities, and family dynamics.

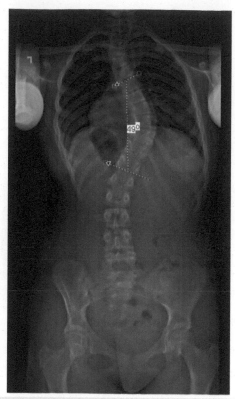

Fig. 73.10. The Cobb method is used to quantify the degree of spinal deformity in scoliosis and kyphosis. It is the angle subtended by a line drawn along the end plates of the most tilted vertebrae on the top and bottom of a curve. Standard measurement error for the Cobb method is approximately 5 degrees. Scoliosis x-rays are routinely viewed and measured as if the view is looking at the patient's back (i.e., opposite orientation of a chest x-ray).

Adolescent Idiopathic Scoliosis

BASIC INFORMATION

- Scoliosis in an otherwise healthy child >10 years old without identifiable cause
- Usually asymptomatic and without pain or neurologic deficit (patient or caregiver may notice asymmetry of back or rib prominence in bathing suit)
  - A child presenting with pain should prompt evaluation for another cause of pain
  - Presence of abnormal neurologic examination, foot deformity (e.g., cavus foot), or abdominal reflex asymmetry warrants MRI of neural axis to evaluate for syrinx or Chiari malformation
- Physical examination findings include asymmetric shoulder height, scapular prominence, and/or flank crease asymmetry
  - Adam's forward bend test is used to evaluate rib hump. To perform, view patient from behind with the back exposed. Have patient bend forward at the waist with knees extended and hands together. Observe for presence of a rib hump or lumbar paraspinal prominence. An inclinometer (manual or digital) may be used to quantify the degree of axial rotation. Greater than 7 degrees of rotation as measured by inclinometer is an indication for radiographic evaluation

- Diagnosis is confirmed with upright spine x-rays
- Mild/moderate curves tend not to progress at skeletal maturity, whereas severe curves tend to progress, even after skeletal maturity
- Treatment: observation for mild curves (<25 degrees) and for moderate curves (25–45 degrees) in patients with no growth remaining; spinal bracing may prevent/slow curve progression in skeletally immature patients with moderate deformity (20–45 degrees); spinal fusion surgery (Fig. 73.11) is considered for severe deformity (>50 degrees)

Congenital Scoliosis

BASIC INFORMATION

- Spinal deformity secondary to defect(s) in vertebral formation and/or segmentation during weeks 4 to 8 of gestation. Abnormalities in other mesenchymal organ systems (e.g., cardiac, renal) that are developing at the same time are common
- Most occur spontaneously but may be associated with parental maternal exposure (e.g., alcohol, valproic acid)
- Genetic causes/associations are rare (e.g., VACTERL [vertebral anomalies, anal atresia, cardiac defects, tracheo-esophageal fistual, renal anomalies, limb abnormalities])
- May be associated with chest wall abnormalities such as fused ribs

DIAGNOSIS AND EVALUATION

- May present at any age; often picked up incidentally on chest imaging
- Physical examination findings may include asymmetry of shoulder height difference, scapular prominence, and/or flank crease asymmetry
- Diagnosis confirmed on plain radiographs of the spine. Advanced imaging (e.g., computed tomography (CT) or MRI) may provide finer anatomic detail (Fig. 73.12)
- Due to association with VACTERL anomalies, patients should be *screened with renal ultrasonography and cardiac echocardiogram* for associated abnormalities; physical examination may uncover other aspects of the syndrome
- *Spinal MRI is mandatory before surgical intervention* to evaluate for associated neuraxial lesions
- Chromosome analysis, ophthalmologic evaluation, and head US are not routinely indicated

TREATMENT

- Curve progression is highly variable and difficult to predict
- Close observation with serial imaging by a pediatric spine surgeon is critical
- Bracing of congenital scoliosis has poor efficacy
- Surgical treatment is considered in the setting of progressive deformity. May include:
  - Hemivertebra excision
  - Limited spinal fusion
  - Nonfusion growing spinal constructs (e.g., growing rods)

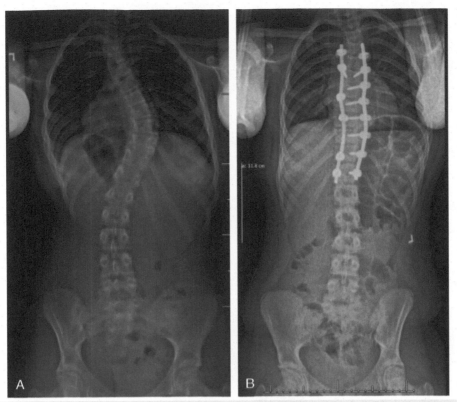

Fig. 73.11. Preoperative (A) and postoperative (B) x-rays of a patient with adolescent idiopathic scoliosis treatment with spinal fusion.

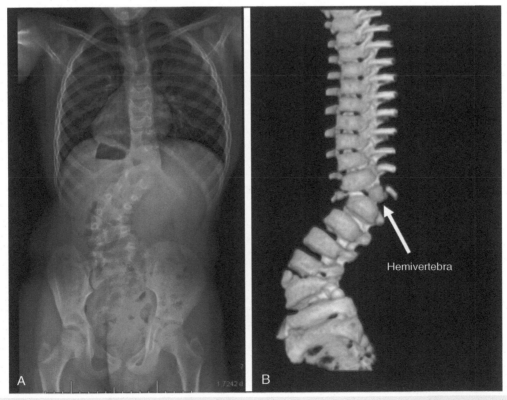

Hemivertebra

Fig. 73.12. X-ray (A) and three-dimensional reconstruction (B) of a patient with significant spinal deformity secondary to a congenital hemivertebra.

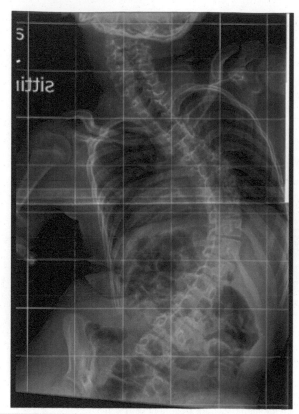

Fig. 73.13. Curves in neuromuscular spinal deformity are larger in magnitude, involve a greater portion of the spine, and are more likely to be associated with pelvic obliquity/tilt.

Neuromuscular Scoliosis

BASIC INFORMATION

- Spinal deformity secondary to disorders of the brain (e.g., CP), spinal cord (e.g., spinal muscular atrophy), or muscle (e.g., Duchenne muscular dystrophy)
- Neuromuscular scoliosis is generally more severe than idiopathic spinal deformities (Fig. 73.13), often resulting in severe symptoms and functional impairment, including pain, seating imbalance, and/or cardiopulmonary deterioration
- Assessing goals of treatment with caregivers is critical:
  - Bracing is not effective for preventing curve progression but may be used to facilitate upright posturing and seating
  - Spinal fusion indicated for severe, progressive deformities (~>50 degrees) in older children (e.g., >10 years old)
  - Spinal instrumentation without fusion (e.g., growing rods) may be utilized to control spinal deformity in patients who are young (<8 years old) to avoid premature arrest of spinal/thoracic growth

Kyphosis

- Kyphosis represents a convex spinal curvature in the sagittal plane (e.g., hunchback), typically in the thoracic spine. Normal thoracic kyphosis measures between 20 and 45 degrees via the Cobb method (Fig. 73.14)

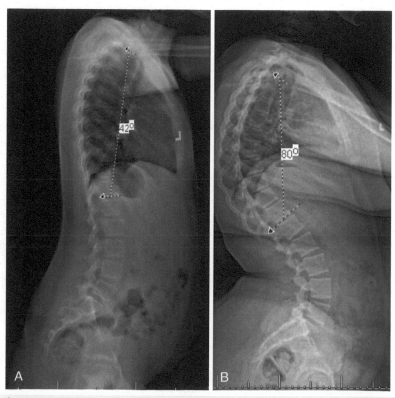

Fig. 73.14. Lateral spine x-ray of a patient with (A) normal thoracic kyphosis and (B) structural thoracic kyphosis consistent with Scheuermann disease.

Postural Kyphosis

BASIC INFORMATION

- Postural kyphosis refers to a kyphotic/round-back appearance that is passively correctable (either by the patient or a provider)
- Postural kyphosis is not a structural deformity and as such requires no specific treatment apart from symptomatic care (e.g., physical therapy for core strengthening)

Structural Kyphosis

BASIC INFORMATION

- Due to sagittal deformity secondary to structural abnormalities in the spinal vertebra
- The deformity cannot be corrected by asking the patient to "stand up straight"
- Structural kyphosis can be secondary to Scheuermann disease, congenital vertebral anomalies, or secondary to spinal injury (e.g., fracture). Numerous syndromes such as achondroplasia and the mucopolysaccharidoses are associated with kyphosis as well
- Similar to scoliosis care, treatment of kyphosis includes observation and nonoperative measures with surgery reserved for severe, progressive deformities

INFECTION

Osteomyelitis

BASIC INFORMATION

- Osteomyelitis is an infection of bone with potential associated soft tissue inflammation, abscess formation, osseous necrosis, and/or reactive bone formation
- Three main methods of spread:
  - Hematogenous spread: spread of infectious organisms to bone via bloodstream
  - Contiguous-focus: spread of infection/bacterial contamination from adjacent contamination (e.g., a surgical implant)
  - Direct-inoculation: contamination secondary to a penetrating injury (e.g., stepping on dirty nail) that deposits contaminated material directly into bone
- Pathophysiology
  - Osteomyelitis has predilection for young children in the first decade of life due to the sluggish metaphyseal blood flow in the skeletally immature child combined with a relatively immature immune system
- Annual incidence is ~1/5000 in children <13 years old, with half of all cases occurring in children <5 years of age
  - More common in males than in females (2.5:1 ratio)
- Osteomyelitis can be caused by a variety of organisms depending on age (Table 73.5)
  - *Staphylococcus aureus* is the most common overall
  - Unique situations include:
    - Patients with sickle cell anemia: Salmonella
    - After puncture wound to foot: Pseudomonas

Table 73.5. Causative Organisms of Osteoarticular Infections in Children

Age Group	Common Organisms
Neonates	Nosocomial: *S. aureus*, streptococcus species, Enterobacteriaceae, Candida Community: GBS, *S. aureus*, *E. coli*, Klebsiella
Infants and young children	*S. aureus*, Kingella kingae, *S. pneumoniae*, *Neisseria meningitides*, HIB (non-immunized)
Children (3–12 years)	*S. aureus*, GABHS
Adolescence (12–18 years)	*S. aureus*, GABHS, *N. gonorrhoeae* (sexually active)

GABHS, Group A beta hemolytic Step; *GBS*, Group B Step.

- Chronic osteomyelitis is characterized by focal areas of bone ischemia leading to necrosis (sequestrum) and adjacent areas of sclerotic new bone formation (involucrum)

CLINICAL PRESENTATION

- Variable combination of pain, immobility, and dysfunction involving the affected area
- May have associated systemic symptoms such as fever, malaise, anorexia, and/or emesis
- A history of trauma is common
- Symptoms/laboratory indices in chronic osteomyelitis are often milder and/or less constant compared with acute osteomyelitis

DIAGNOSIS AND EVALUATION

- Physical examination findings are variable and may include tenderness, swelling, erythema, limited ROM, and/or gait disturbance
- Physical examination findings are more focal for distal lesions
- Laboratory evaluation
  - Complete blood count (CBC) with differential
  - C-reactive protein (CRP) assay
  - Erythrocyte sedimentation rate (ESR)
  - Blood cultures
- X-rays
  - Normal early in course of infection
  - Soft tissue changes (muscle swelling and obliteration of the fat planes) are seen at 3 to 7 days
  - Osteolysis and reactive bone formation may be seen at 5 to 20 days
- MRI is the most sensitive imaging modality and may demonstrate bone marrow edema, soft tissue inflammation, and abscess formation. MRI may help guide aspiration or surgical intervention

TREATMENT

- Aspiration of infected tissue should be attempted for Gram stain and culture when readily accessible
- Intravenous antibiotic therapy is indicated for treatment of early osteomyelitis without associated abscess, necrotic bone, or foreign bodies

- Empiric antibiotic selection should be based on the child's age, medical history, allergies, and local infectious epidemiology
- Antibiotic therapy generally continues for 4 to 6 weeks based on response to treatment as assessed by symptoms, physical examination findings, and laboratory indices
- Surgery (irrigation and debridement) should be considered in instances of prolonged symptoms, failure of antibiotic therapy, persistent bacteremia, or in the presence of an abscess, sinus tract, or foreign body

Septic Arthritis

BASIC INFORMATION

- Septic arthritis is an infection of a joint that *requires urgent/emergent treatment* to prevent permanent, irreparable damage to joint cartilage
- Three main methods of spread are similar to those in osteomyelitis (see previous discussion)
- Annual incidence is ~5/100,000 to 37/100,000 children, with half of all cases occurring in children <2 years of age
- Septic arthritis is most common in joints with an intraarticular metaphysis (hip, shoulder, elbow, ankle); approximately one-third of cases involve the hip joint
- Septic arthritis can be caused by a variety of organisms similar to osteomyelitis (Table 73.5)

CLINICAL PRESENTATION

- Present with acute-onset combination of pain, immobility, and dysfunction involving the affected joint
- Limb typically is held in position to maximize joint volume
  - For example, flexion, abduction, and external rotation for the hip
- Pain *may be referred to the knee in instances of septic arthritis of the hip*. In these cases, pain may be exacerbated by hip ROM
- May have associated systemic symptoms such as fever, malaise, anorexia, and/or emesis
- Gonococcal arthritis usually characterized by multiple-joint involvement, tenosynovitis, and dermatitis

DIAGNOSIS AND EVALUATION

- Physical examination findings are variable and may include tenderness, swelling, effusion, erythema, limited ROM, gait disturbance, and refusal to bear weight
- Laboratory evaluation is helpful but not definitive
  - CBC with differential
  - CRP assay
  - ESR
  - Blood cultures
- Antistreptolysin O titers may be helpful in cases of suspected poststreptococcal reactive arthritis
- A Lyme disease titer may be helpful in endemic areas in patients with suspected Lyme arthritis. Lyme arthritis typically has a less severe presentation with improved joint ROM compared with septic arthritis
- X-rays
  - Normal early in course of infection
  - May show evidence of an effusion, joint space widening, joint subluxation, or adjacent osteomyelitis

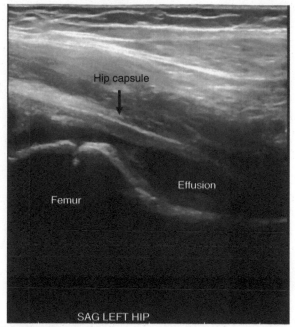

Fig. 73.15. Ultrasound of a hip demonstrating large effusion.

- Ultrasound
  - Confirms the presence of an effusion and helps guide arthrocentesis (Fig. 73.15)
- MRI is sensitive for detecting a joint effusion and/or adjacent osteomyelitis but may be difficult to obtain expeditiously and should not delay treatment
- Workup should include arthrocentesis and joint fluid analysis in equivocal cases
  - Typical joint fluid analysis findings in bacterial septic arthritis include elevated white blood cell (WBC) count (>50,000) and decreased glucose (less than 60% of serum glucose)
  - Gram stain of synovial fluid is positive in 33% to 50% of cases

TREATMENT

- For large joints (e.g., hip, shoulder, knee), urgent surgical irrigation and drainage of the joint combined with intravenous antibiotics
- Smaller joints (e.g., wrist) may be managed with serial joint aspiration and lavage
- Surgical debridement is not required in instances of Lyme arthritis or gonococcal arthritis
- After initiation of empiric antibiotics, culture-directed antibiotic therapy generally continues for 4 to 6 weeks. Duration is based on patient clinical response to treatment and trend in inflammatory markers

Transient Synovitis of the Hip

BASIC INFORMATION

- Also known as toxic synovitis of the hip, it is the most common cause of acute hip pain in children
- A benign, noninfectious, self-limiting condition that may be difficult to distinguish from septic arthritis of the hip

- Annual incidence is ~0.2% with a male to female ratio of ~2:1
- Children with prior history of transient synovitis are at higher risk for relapse (annual incidence 4%)

CLINICAL PRESENTATION

- Presents with acute onset of hip, groin, thigh, or knee pain associated with a limp or an unwillingness to bear weight
- Typically preceded by viral illness, upper respiratory infection, and/or gastrointestinal symptoms
- Bilateral involvement may occur but is rare (~1%–4% of cases)

DIAGNOSIS AND EVALUATION

- Transient synovitis should be a *diagnosis of exclusion*
  - More severe, time-sensitive pathologies (most notably septic arthritis of the hip) should be ruled out before initiating treatment for transient synovitis
- As with septic hip, the joint is frequently held in position of mild flexion, abduction, and external rotation to minimize intracapsular pressure
- Active and passive ROM are limited secondary to pain, but to a lesser degree in general compared with patients with septic arthritis
- It is often challenging to distinguish between transient synovitis and septic arthritis of the hip
  - The Kocher criteria were developed to help predict the probability of septic arthritis on the basis of four clinical and laboratory variables:
    1. Fever (>38.5°C)
    2. Inability of child to bear weight on limb
    3. Serum WBC >12.0 × 10^6 cells/L
    4. ESR >40 mm/h

- The predicted probability of septic arthritis on the basis of one, two, three, and four positive criteria in a large series was 3.0%, 40.0%, 93.1%, and 99.6%, respectively
- CRP >20 mg/L is an additional strong independent risk factor for septic arthritis over transient synovitis

TREATMENT

- Observation and supportive therapy (nonsteroidal anti-inflammatory drugs [NSAIDs], physical therapy)
- Symptoms should resolve over the course of 3 to 10 days; if no or little improvement is observed, alternative diagnoses should be investigated

Review Questions

For review questions, please go to ExpertConsult.com.

Suggested Readings

1. Arkader A, Brusalis C, Warner Jr WC, Conway JH, Noonan K. Update in pediatric musculoskeletal infections: when it is, when it isn't, and what to do. *J Am Acad Orthop Surg.* 2016;24(9):e112–e121.
2. Conrad DA. Acute hematogenous osteomyelitis. *Pediatr Rev.* 2010;31(11):464–471.
3. Herman MJ, Martinek M. The limping child. *Pediatr Rev.* 2015;36(5):184–195.
4. Kuo AA, Tritasavit S, Graham Jr JM. Congenital muscular torticollis and positional plagiocephaly. *Pediatr Rev.* 2014;35(2):79–87.
5. Lincoln TL, Suen PWJ. Common rotational variations in children. *Am Acad Orthop Surg.* 2003;11(5):312–320.
6. Nemeth BA, Narotam V. Developmental dysplasia of the hip. *Pediatr Rev.* 2012;33(12):553–561.
7. Rosenberg JJ. Scoliosis. *Pediatr Rev.* 2011;32(9):397–398.

Pulmonology

74 Clinical Approach to Common Pulmonologic Complaints

CASANDRA AREVALO-MARCANO, MD and PI CHUN CHENG, MD, MS

Respiratory illnesses are a prevalent and common problem during childhood. Accounting for almost 7 million emergency department (ED) visits in 2010, respiratory disorders were the second most common cause of ED visits. Consequently, the astute clinician must be able to evaluate common symptoms in the context of specific descriptions and clinical histories to arrive at the correct diagnosis. We provide here an overview of some commonly encountered pulmonologic complaints.

See also Nelson Textbook of Pediatrics, Chapter 384, "Chronic or Recurrent Respiratory Symptoms."

Cough

BASIC INFORMATION

- Cough is the most common complaint in children presenting for medical evaluation
- The cough reflex attempts to remove an airway irritant
  - Cough receptors are located anywhere from the pharynx to the terminal bronchioles
  - Afferent paths are the glossopharyngeal and vagus nerves
  - Efferent paths are the vagus, phrenic, and spinal motor nerves to the larynx, diaphragm, and abdominal and chest wall muscles
- Cough stimuli can be derived centrally or peripherally (airway, pulmonary parenchyma, pleura, or Arnold nerve in the external ear canal)
- Phases of cough
  - Deep inspiration
  - Glottic closure and expiratory muscles contraction
  - Forced exhalation followed by immediate opening of the glottis

EVALUATION

- Characterize the cough (wet, dry, barking, etc.)
  - Productive sputum is uncommon in young children
  - Productive purulent and foul-smelling sputum indicates cellular debris and does not suggest bacterial infection or acute viral infection exclusively
- Timing of cough and associated symptoms are useful criteria to help in narrowing the differential diagnosis (Tables 74.1 and 74.2)

- If there are no associated symptoms, one may consider a trial of bronchodilators if there is supicion for cough variant asthma (Fig. 74.1)

Noisy Breathing (Upper Airway Obstruction)

BASIC INFORMATION

- Breathing that is audible to most parents
- It is usually due to flow turbulence through narrowed airways, including the following:
  - Nasal vestibule
  - Posterior nasal orifices
  - Glottis
- Stridor: a high-pitched respiratory sound, most often inspiratory, due to an extrathoracic obstruction (e.g., croup)
  - Biphasic stridor may be present with glottic obstruction
  - Expiratory stridor can be seen with subglottic obstruction (e.g., tracheomalacia)
- Stertor: usually a mid- to low-pitched, snoring-like respiratory sound due to nasopharyngeal or oropharyngeal obstruction; may occur during inspiration or expiration

EVALUATION

- Parental description of their perception of noisy breathing, including phase of respiration and exacerbating/alleviating factors, is critical to narrow the differential diagnosis
- Parents or relatives might have a video or recording of the sounds
- Additional helpful history includes:
  - Common causes of stridor vary per age group (Table 74.3)
  - Acuity or chronicity of symptoms and evolution over time
  - Associated symptoms
- Timing of the noise may also narrow the differential diagnosis
  - While asleep: sleep disorder breathing
  - With exercise: vocal cord dysfunction
  - After feeding: gastroesophageal reflux
  - Sputum production: bronchitis
  - Dyspnea: lower respiratory problems

Table 74.1. Differential Diagnosis of Cough with Associated Symptoms

Associated Symptoms	Differential Diagnosis	Evaluation
Atopy, wheezing	Asthma	Allergy tests, pulmonary function tests and bronchial hyper-responsiveness, trial of asthma treatment
Clearing throat, worse when recumbent, allergic salute	Allergic rhinitis, postnasal drip	Trial of antirhinitis treatment
New onset of choking episode	Foreign body	Neck x-ray, bronchoscopy
Productive cough	Persistent endobronchial infection, bronchiectasis, foreign body, recurrent pneumonia, cystic fibrosis, primary ciliary dyskinesia, immunodeficiency	Sweat test, High-resolution computed tomography (CT), chest x-ray, bronchoscopy, ciliary function test, sputum culture, bronchoalveolar lavage, immune evaluation
Paroxysmal cough	Pertussis	Cultures, polymerase chain reaction, convalescent serology
Choking with feeds	Recurrent aspiration	Modified barium swallow
Neonatal onset	Tracheobronchomalacia, tracheoesophageal fistula, laryngeal cleft, neurologic disorder, cystic fibrosis, ciliary dyskinesia	Sweat test, barium esophagogram, bronchoscopy, immune evaluation
Brassy, barking cough	Tracheomalacia, bronchomalacia, foreign body	Bronchoscopy
Honking cough, disappears when asleep	Tic cough	Observe patterns, trial of suggestion therapy, diagnosis of exclusion
Dry cough, breathlessness	Interstitial lung disease	Spirometry, high-resolution CT, autoimmune markers, lung biopsy
Progressive cough, weight loss, fever	Chronic infection: tuberculosis, chronic retention of foreign body, mycoses, parasites	Mantoux test, chest x-ray, bronchoscopy
Hemoptysis	Bronchiectasis, cavitary lung disease, (tuberculosis or bacterial abscesses), congestive heart failure, hemosiderosis, foreign bodies, vascular lesions, endobronchial lesions, clotting disorders	Purified protein derivative and rule out tuberculosis Chest radiography Chest tomography Bronchoscopy
Failure to thrive, steatorrhea, recurrent lower airway infections	Cystic fibrosis	Sweat test, consider sending genetic evaluations

Table 74.2. Cough Diagnoses with Particular Onsets

While or after feeding	Aspiration, tracheoesophageal fistula, laryngeal clefts
Seasonal cough	Allergic rhinitis, postnasal drip, allergen exposure
Acute onset, choking risk	Foreign body aspiration
Productive morning cough	Bronchiectasis, sinusitis, aspiration, reflux, foreign body, recurrent pneumonia, cystic fibrosis, primary ciliary dyskinesia, immunodeficiency
Barking cough that is present while awake and absent while asleep	Psychogenic cough, behavioral
Exercise-induced cough, postexercise cough	Air hyperreactivity, vocal cord dysfunction
Neonatal onset	Tracheobronchomalacia, tracheoesophageal fistula, laryngeal cleft, neurologic disorder, cystic fibrosis, Primary ciliary dyskinesia. Infectious causes
Nighttime cough	Asthma (classically late at night), gastroesophageal reflux disease (when lying down)/postnasal drip (classically early at night)

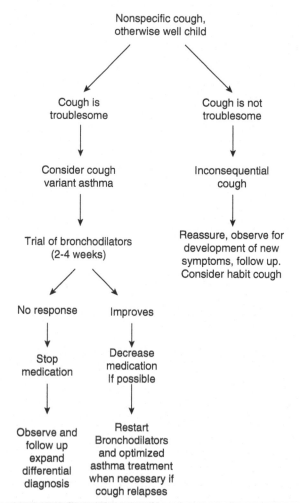

Fig. 74.1. Algorithm to guide the approach to cough without identifiable associated symptom.

- Common radiologic findings of frequent causes of noisy breathing in children include:
  - Croup (Fig. 74.2)
  - Foreign body aspiration (Fig. 74.3)
  - Tracheomalacia
  - Tracheobronchomalacia (Fig. 74.4)
  - Airway compression

Wheezing

BASIC INFORMATION

- Wheeze: musical, high-pitched sound caused by oscillation of the airway
- Very common presenting symptom in the asthmatic population; however, not all asthmatic patients wheeze
- One in three children will experience a wheezing episode by 4 years of age
- Two types of wheezes:
  - Polyphonic wheezing: multiple tones due to widespread narrowing of multiple airways
    - Differential diagnosis includes asthma, bronchiolitis, aspiration

Table 74.3. Common Causes of Stridor by Age Group

Neonatal period	Congenital anomalies such as rings and slings Subglottic stenosis Tracheal rings Proximal tracheomalacia Vocal cord paralysis or paresis Laryngomalacia Gastroesophageal reflux disease Laryngeal hemangiomas
Infants and toddlers	Laryngotracheitis (viral or bacterial) Foreign body aspiration Gastroesophageal reflux disease Retropharyngeal or peritonsillar abscesses Laryngeal papilloma Acute anaphylaxis Croup
Adolescents	Vocal cord dysfunction Laryngeal papilloma

- Monophonic wheezing: single tone due to intrathoracic large airway narrowing
  - Differential diagnosis includes tracheo-/bronchomalacia, foreign body, or anatomic compression asthma, bronchiolitis, or aspiration
- Differential diagnosis can be significantly narrowed depending on:
  - Acuity or chronicity of symptoms
    - Chronic conditions with the potential for wheeze include cystic fibrosis, Primary ciliary dyskinesia (PCD)
  - Associated symptoms
  - Evolution of symptoms over time
  - Age of patient (Table 74.4)

Cyanosis

BASIC INFORMATION

- Bluish coloration of the skin and membranes due to deoxyhemoglobin accumulation
  - Approximately 4 to 6 mg/100 mL of blood of deoxyhemoglobin is necessary to show cyanosis; consequently, children with polycythemia may demonstrate cyanosis more easily than those with anemia

Etiology

- Cyanosis can be caused by a broad list of differential diagnosis:
  - Respiratory causes are the most likely for an otherwise normal child
  - Cardiac causes (congenital heart and vascular malformations) are important to consider
- Causes for hypoxemia due to lung/respiratory pathology are often divided into five causes (Table 74.5):
  - Alveolar hypoventilation (air trapping, consolidations, pulmonary embolism, airway obstruction, impaired chest wall lung expansion due to trauma, stiff chest wall, etc.)
  - Diffusion impairment (thickening of the alveolar membrane or interstitial lung disease resulting in impaired oxygen exchange, also seen in pulmonary edema)

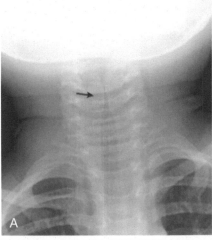
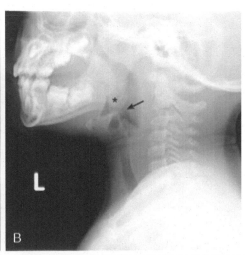

Fig. 74.2. (A) Radiography of the airway showing a tapared narrowing of the immediate subglotic airway characteristic of tracheitis. (B) Lateral view of the subglotic narrowing.

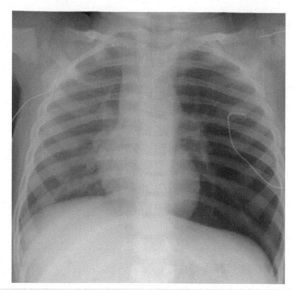

Fig. 74.3. Anteroposterior chest radiograph showing the characteristic findings on a foreign body aspiration with left hemithorax hyperinflation and left-side shifted mediastinum.

- Right to left shunt (shunting of nonoxygenated blood to systemic circulation, pulmonary hypertension, cardiac malformations atrioventricular canal, single-ventricle heart, etc.)
- Mismatch of ventilation and perfusion (pneumonia, pulmonary hemorrhage, pulmonary embolism, etc.)
- Low atmospheric pressure with decreased inspired oxygen (exposure to house fires, usually accompanied by carbon monoxide toxicity)

Physical Examination

- Peripheral cyanosis (acrocyanosis): skin of hands and feet
- Central cyanosis: tongue and mucous membranes
- Differential cyanosis: affecting only lower part of the body (indicative of congenital heart diseases such as PPH)

DIAGNOSIS AND EVALUATION

- Arterial blood gas will confirm clinical suspicion
- Pulse oximetry is unreliable in cases of inadequate perfusion of the extremity being sampled (e.g. extreme cold, hypotension) and/or hemoglobin poisonings (e.g. methemoglobinemia).

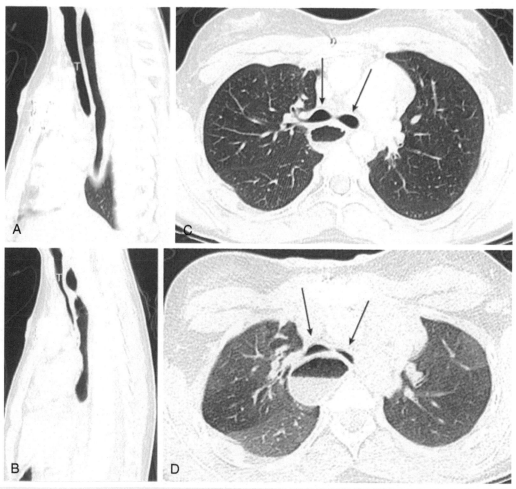

Fig. 74.4. Tracheobronchomalacia. (A and C) Inspiratory and (B and D) expiratory sagittal and axial computed tomography images show diffuse narrowing of the trachea (T) and main stem bronchi *(arrows)* on expiration in patient with tracheobronchomalacia. Homophonous wheeze is usually appreciated.

Table 74.4. Causes of Wheezing in Children by Age Group

Infancy	Bronchiolitis
	Asthma
	Laryngotracheobronchitis
	Vascular compression (rings and slings)
	Tracheal stenosis
	Tracheal webs
	Pulmonary edema
	Interstitial lung disease
	Recurrent aspiration
Infants and toddlers	Asthma
	Bronchitis
	Bronchiolitis obliterans
	Pulmonary edema
	Foreign body
	Interstitial lung disease
	Recurrent aspiration
	Tumors and lymphadenopathy
Adolescents	Asthma
	Vocal cord dysfunction
	Bronchitis
	Bronchiolitis obliterans
	Pulmonary edema
	Interstitial lung disease
	Tumors and lymphadenopathy

- Chest radiography to better assess pulmonary parenchyma and airway
- Specific laboratory testing to investigate suspected causes (i.e., methemoglobinemia)

Vocal Cord Dysfunction

BASIC INFORMATION

- Functional disorder characterized by inappropriate motion of the true vocal cords
  - Normal motion of the vocal cords includes abduction during inspiration and adduction during expiration
    - Normal adduction also occurs with phonation, coughing, and Valsalva maneuvers
    - Normal abduction of the cords occurs during sniffing and panting
  - Vocal cord dysfunction is usually characterized by episodic adduction of the true vocal cord during inspiration
  - Paradoxical motion will lead to abnormal constriction of the airway, leading to wheezing, stridor, or respiratory distress
- Differential diagnosis:
  - Asthma
  - Airway compression
  - Vocal cord paresis
  - Angioedema
  - Laryngomalacia
  - Laryngospasm
  - Tracheomalacia
- Triggers:
  - Asthma
  - Exercise
  - Postnasal drip
  - Mechanical ventilation

Table 74.5. Characteristics and Differential Diagnosis of Hypoxemia

Hypoventilation - Responds to oxygen therapy - P(A-a) O_2 is usually normal - $PaCO_2$ is high - PaO_2 and $PaCO_2$ move in opposite directions	Pump failure (impairment of chest wall movement or respiratory muscles weakness) Impaired central drive: - Drug overdose: opioids, benzodiazepines, alcohol - Brainstem hemorrhage, infarction - Primary alveolar hypoventilation Spinal cord injury: - Amyotrophic lateral sclerosis - Cervical spinal cord injury Nerve injury respiratory muscle: - Guillain–Barré syndrome Neuromuscular junction impairment: - Myasthenia gravis - Lambert–Eaton syndrome Respiratory muscles: myopathy Chest wall defects: - Kyphoscoliosis - Thoracoplasty - Fibrothorax
Ventilation perfusion (V/Q) mismatch - Normal V/Q = 0.8 - Easily corrected by supplemental oxygen therapy - Widened A-a oxygen gradient	Asthma Upper airway obstruction Secretions Pneumonia Pulmonary embolism Bronchiectasis Cystic fibrosis Interstitial lung diseases Pulmonary hypertension
Decreased diffusion capacity - Hypoxemia shows good response to oxygen therapy - P(A-a) O_2 is elevated - $PaCO_2$ is usually normal	Asthma Vocal cord dysfunction Bronchitis Bronchiolitis obliterans Pulmonary edema Interstitial lung disease Tumors and lymphadenopathy
Shunt - P(A-a) O_2 is elevated - Poor response to oxygen therapy - PCO_2 is normal	Pneumonia Pulmonary edema Acute respiratory distress syndrome (ARDS) Alveolar collapse Pulmonary arteriovenous communication
Decreased inspired oxygen (low atmospheric pressure or low FiO_2)	Smoke inhalation Altitude

- Psychosocial disorders/stress
- Gastroesophageal reflux

CLINICAL PRESENTATION

- Most common in females, athletes, and highly competitive personalities; affects all ages
- Patients present with:
  - Loud stridor
  - Respiratory distress
  - Sensation of choking and shortness of breath usually localized to the neck area

DIAGNOSIS AND EVALUATION

- Laryngoscopy is the gold standard

- Chest radiograph can rule out airway compression or anatomic anomalies
- Exercise provocation test with pulmonary function
- Pulmonary function test
  - Truncated flow over the inspiratory loop (Figs. 74.5, 74.6, 74.7, and 74.8)

TREATMENT

- Acute episode:
  - Patient and family education of the diagnosis and appropriate reassurance
  - Noninvasive positive airway pressure and endotracheal intubation, although unusual, might be necessary depending on the severity of the event
- Long-term management warrants a multidisciplinary approach:
  - No specific medical therapy other than controlling the insult to the airway (gastroesophageal reflux disease [GERD], asthma, postnasal drip, stress, etc.)

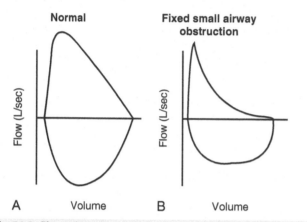

Fig. 74.5. Flow volume loops showing (A) normal pulmonary function and (B) expiratory loop concavity toward the volume axis, characteristic of asthma or obstructive pulmonary diseases.

- Behavioral and speech therapy
- Respiratory retraining, relaxation, and vocal hygiene

Reflux and Aspiration

BASIC INFORMATION

Etiology

- Retrograde flow of gastric contents that access the airway, causing respiratory irritation
- Common in neurologically impaired patients
  - Decreased tone of the esophageal sphincter
  - Highly susceptible to reflux due to horizontal position of infants until 9 months of age
  - Immature peristalsis of the gastrointestinal tract
  - Immature airway protection leading to reflux penetration and aspiration
- Aspiration content can be food (liquid and solids), gastric content, or saliva and upper airway secretions

Differential Diagnosis

- Airway reactivity
- Recurrent viral illnesses
- Tracheoesophageal fistula
- Peptic ulcer
- Cyclic vomiting
- Gastritis
- Irritable bowel syndrome
- Hiatal hernia
- Laryngeal clefts

CLINICAL PRESENTATION

Physical Signs

- Physical examination varies according to the age of presentation

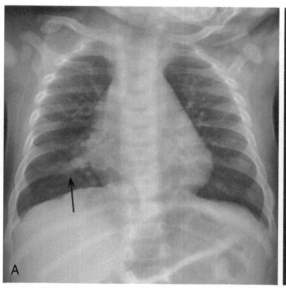
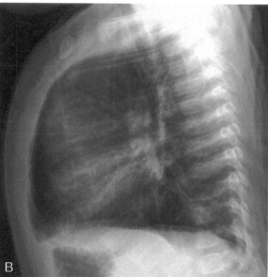

Fig. 74.6. (A) Frontal view shows increased perihilar markings and bandlike density in right middle lobe, representing subsegmental atelectasis. (B) Lateral view shows marked hyperinflation with flattened hemidiaphragms, increased anterior-to-posterior diameter of the chest, and barrel shape of chest.

- Atypical crying and irritability
- Sandifer syndrome (spasmodic torsional dystonia; opisthotonic posturing, mainly involving the neck, back, and upper extremities, associated with gastroesophageal reflux)

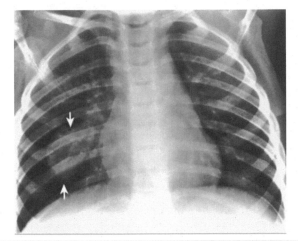

Fig. 74.7. Round pneumonia. Frontal chest radiograph demonstrating a well-circumscribed, rounded opacity in the right mid to lower lung *(arrows)*.

- Apnea and bradycardia
- Vomiting and wet burping
- Cough is the most common presenting symptom (present in 65% of the patients)
- Upper airway and laryngeal inflammation (stertor and noisy breathing associated with feeds)
- Intermittent wheezing
- Older children: chest pain, sore throat, epigastric pain, and halitosis
- Neurologically impaired patients present with recurrent lower airway infections

DIAGNOSIS AND EVALUATION

- Often diagnosed by history and physical examination
- Chest radiography can show some changes indicative of recurrent parenchymal damage (Fig. 74.9)
- Video barium swallow (VBS) is the gold standard
- Milk scan is less specific but more sensitive than VBS
- Salivagram is of use for patients in whom upper airway secretion–related aspiration is suspected
- More aggressive measures such as bronchoscopy with bronchoalveolar lavage (lipid-laden macrophages are indicative of aspiration)

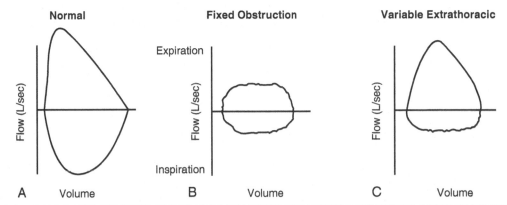

Fig. 74.8. Flow volume loops showing (A) normal pulmonary function; (B) truncated flow on both inspiratory and expiratory loop, indicative of a fixed obstruction; and (C) truncated flow appreciated over the inspiratory loop, indicative of a variable extrathoracic obstruction, as seen in vocal cord dysfunction.

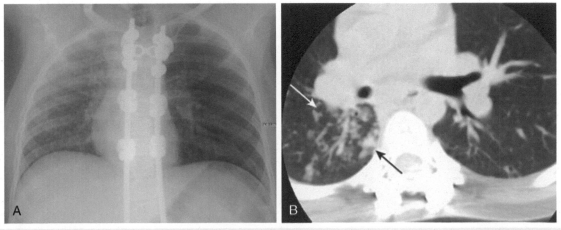

Fig. 74.9. (A) Radiograph in a child suspected of having aspiration shows increased nodular opacities in the right lung. (B) High-resolution computed tomography shows multiple nodular opacities *(arrows)* with tree-in-bud appearance.

TREATMENT

- Upright positioning after feeding (elevate the head of the bed and prone positioning)
- Pharmacologic treatment with proton pump inhibitor to decrease gastric acidity
- Symptomatic despite medical therapy
  - Motility agents (bethanechol, erythromycin, etc.)
  - Surgical evaluation for gastric fundoplication

Review Questions

For review questions, please go to ExpertConsult.com.

Suggested Readings

1. Academy of Pediatrics. Chlamydia (Chlamydophila) pneumoniae. In: Pickering LK, ed. *Red Book: 2003 Report of the Committee on Infectious Diseases*. 26th ed. Elk Grove Village, IL: American Academy of Pediatrics; 2003:235–237.
2. Ali S, Klassen T. Infections of the respiratory tract: bronchiolitis. In: Wilmott RW, Boat TF, Bush A, Deterding RR, Ratjen F, eds. *Kendig and Chernick's Disorders of the Respiratory Tract in Children*. 8th ed. Philadelphia: Elsevier Saunders; 2012:443–454.
3. Asher I, Twiss J, Ellwood E. Asthma: the epidemiology of asthma. In: Wilmott RW, Boat TF, Bush A, Deterding RR, Ratjen F, eds. *Kendig and Chernick's Disorders of the Respiratory Tract in Children*. 8th ed. Philadelphia: Elsevier Saunders; 2012:647–676.
4. Bradley J, Byington C, Shah S, et al. The management of community-acquired pneumonia in infants and children older than 3 months of age: clinical practice guidelines by the Pediatric Infectious Diseases Society and the Infectious Diseases Society of America. *Clinical Infectious Diseases Advance Access*. 2011;53(7):e25–76.
5. Donnelly L. Airway. In: Donnelly L. *Pediatric Imaging: The Fundamentals*. 1st ed. Philadelphia: Elsevier; 2009:25–28.
6. Donnelly L. Chest. In: Donnelly L. *Pediatric Imaging: The Fundamentals*. 1st ed. Philadelphia: Elsevier; 2009:326–361.
7. Marostica P, Stein R. Infections of the respiratory tract: community-acquired bacterial pneumonia. In: Wilmott RW, Boat TF, Bush A, Deterding RR, Ratjen F, eds. *Kendig and Chernick's Disorders of the Respiratory Tract in Children*. 8th ed. Philadelphia: Elsevier Saunders; 2012:461–471.
8. Pasterkamo H. General clinical considerations: the exam and history examination. In: Wilmott RW, Boat TF, Bush A, Deterding RR, Ratjen F, eds. *Kendig and Chernick's Disorders of the Respiratory Tract in Children*. 8th ed. Philadelphia: Elsevier Saunders; 2012:110–130.
9. Salpeter SR, Buckley NS, Ormiston TM, Salpeter EE. Meta-analysis: effect of long-acting beta-agonists on severe asthma exacerbations and asthma-related deaths. *Ann Internal Medicine*. 2006;144(12):904–912.
10. Shields MD, Bush A, Everard ML, McKenzie S, Primhak R. BTS guidelines: recommendations for the assessment and management of cough in children. *Thorax*. 2008;63. (Suppl 3):iii1–iii15.
11. Walters M, Robertson R. Chest imaging. In: Walters M, Robertson R. *Pediatric Radiology: The Requisites*. 4th ed. Philadelphia: Elsevier; 2016:26–61.

75 Neonatal Lung Disorders

JULIE L. FIERRO, MD, MPH

Respiratory disorders are the most common cause for neonatal intensive care unit admissions. Failure of adequate gas exchange at birth may be due to several factors, including prematurity, meconium aspiration, and congenital malformations. Infants have a highly compliant chest wall, the functional significance of which becomes apparent in the setting of neonatal lung disease. It is also important to consider that nonrespiratory pathology can also present with respiratory distress, including infection, asphyxia at birth, drugs that depress the respiratory status, metabolic disorders, and congenital cardiac disease.

See also Nelson Textbook of Pediatrics, Chapter 101, "Respiratory Tract Disorders."

Apnea of Prematurity

BASIC INFORMATION

- Defined as cessation of air flow for 20 seconds or an apneic event of less than 20 seconds associated with either bradycardia or cyanosis. Apneic events can be central, obstructive, or mixed. The majority of apneic events in premature infants are mixed
- The incidence and severity of apnea of prematurity (AOP) increase with earlier gestational age
- Attributed to immaturity of ventilatory control and the respiratory system
- AOP can occur spontaneously but may also be provoked or worsened by other processes, including infection, electrolyte abnormalities, or intracranial disease
- Events resolve on average by 36–40 weeks' postmenstrual age

DIAGNOSIS AND EVALUATION

- Rule out other etiologies associated with apnea in infants, including:
  - Infection
  - Central nervous system disorders
  - Gastroesophageal reflux
  - Metabolic disorders
  - Temperature instability
  - Drugs including narcotics and anticonvulsants

TREATMENT

- First-line treatment is a methylxanthine—specifically caffeine. Caffeine levels may be monitored at the beginning of treatment
  - Theophylline had previously been first line; however, caffeine is just as effective and is less likely to cause tachycardia or poor feeding

- Infants who do not respond to a methylxanthine can trial high-flow nasal cannula or continuous positive airway pressure (CPAP)
- An apnea monitor may be prescribed to premature infants having apnea until they are 43 weeks' postmenstrual age due to the potential increased risk of extreme apnea episodes. If an infant has frequent apneas lasting longer than 20 seconds beyond 43 weeks' postmenstrual age, monitoring for a longer duration may be required
- There are no data to suggest that AOP is associated with an increased risk of sudden infant death syndrome (SIDS)

Bronchopulmonary Dysplasia

BASIC INFORMATION

- Bronchopulmonary dysplasia (BPD) is a chronic lung disease of prematurity. It occurs in roughly 10,000 to 15,000 infants per year in the United States, with the incidence reported to be as high as 85% in neonates born between 500 and 699 g
- The histologic pattern of the "new BPD," which is seen in the postsurfactant era, consists of developmental arrest and impaired alveolar development. Alveolar numbers are reduced, and the alveoli that are present are larger than normal. This is in contrast to the "old BPD," seen during the presurfactant era, which was characterized by prominent interstitial fibrosis, areas of alternating atelectasis and hyperinflation, and airway smooth muscle hyperplasia
- Infants most at risk for developing BPD:
  - Premature infants
  - Infants undergoing prolonged mechanical ventilation
  - Infants with low birth weight
- Comorbidities associated with BPD:
  - Growth failure due to increased caloric needs
  - Pulmonary hypertension
  - Poor neurodevelopmental outcomes
  - Increased risk of respiratory infections
  - Decreased pulmonary function

CLINICAL PRESENTATION

- Generally defined as the need for supplemental oxygen for at least 28 days after birth and at 36 weeks' postmenstrual age
  - The definition of BPD attempts to categorize BPD severity according to the level of respiratory support required (Table 75.1)

Table 75.1.   NIH Consensus Conference: Diagnostic Criteria for Establishing and Classifying Disease Severity in BPD

	Gestational age	
	<32 Weeks	*>32 Weeks*
Time point of assessment	36 weeks' PMA or discharge to home, whichever comes first	>28 days but <56 days postnatal age or discharge to home, whichever comes first
Treatment with oxygen >21% for at least 28 days		
Mild BPD	Breathing room air at 36 weeks' PMA or discharge, whichever comes first	Breathing room air at 56 days postnatal age or discharge, whichever comes first
Moderate BPD	Need for <30% O_2 at 36 weeks' PMA or discharge, whichever comes first	Need for <30% O_2 at 56 days postnatal age or discharge, whichever comes first
Severe BPD	Need for >30% O_2 ± PPV or CPAP at 36 weeks' PMA or discharge, whichever comes first	Need for >30% O_2 ± PPV or CPAP at 56 days postnatal age or discharge, whichever comes first

BPD, Bronchopulmonary dysplasia; *CPAP*, continuous positive airway pressure; *PMA*, postmenstrual age; *PPV*, positive pressure ventilation.
From Abman SH. *Kendig and Chernick's Disorders of the Respiratory Tract in Children.* 8th ed. Philadelphia, PA: Elsevier; 2012, p. 388, Table 23.2.

- Physical examination findings include increased work of breathing (tachypnea, retractions, shallow breathing) and a variety of adventitious lung sounds (rhonchi, crackles, wheezing)

DIAGNOSIS AND EVALUATION

- Diagnosed in infants that meet the clinical definition
- Chest x-ray findings:
  - Nonspecific with small lung volumes and hazy lung fields
  - May also have areas of cystic changes and linear interstitial opacities
- Pathophysiologic characteristics: diffuse airway inflammation, decreased alveolarization, altered pulmonary vascular development, increased lung fluid

TREATMENT

- Management of BPD is focused on symptomatic therapy
- The use of chronic supplemental oxygen or noninvasive ventilation may be necessary
  - Various ventilator strategies and devices are being assessed regarding their ability to reduce the incidence of BPD
  - Supplemental oxygen is provided to target optimal oxyhemoglobin saturations without causing hyperoxic damage
- Diuretics, including furosemide and chlorothiazide, can be used to decrease pulmonary edema, thus improving pulmonary compliance and airway resistance
- Systemic steroids may be used to decrease airway inflammation, but use is limited due to the risk of poor neurodevelopmental outcomes

- Inhaled bronchodilators may be used in situations of airway hyperreactivity
- Monitoring weight gain and ensuring adequate nutrition are important in improving pulmonary outcomes
- Immunizations are important in infants with BPD due to an increased risk of recurrent respiratory tract infections and rehospitalizations.
  - Prophylaxis with respiratory syncytial virus (RSV) immunoglobulin is recommended for infants with BPD
- Infants with BPD are at an increased risk for rehospitalization in early childhood for respiratory distress because they have little respiratory reserve and are susceptible to common upper respiratory infections (URIs)
  - Illnesses often require escalation of respiratory support, including mechanical ventilation
  - They also have an increased incidence of wheezing and airway hyperreactivity, often needing additional inhaled therapies and airway clearance

Neonatal Respiratory Distress Syndrome

BASIC INFORMATION

- Respiratory distress syndrome (RDS), also known as hyaline membrane disease, is seen primarily in premature infants. There is increasing incidence of RDS with decreasing gestational age.
- Pathophysiology:
  - Occurs due to immaturity of the lung resulting in surfactant deficiency. Surfactant is produced by type 2 pneumocytes from the 24th week of gestation, and levels increase with increased gestational age.
  - Infants with RDS have less compliant lungs
  - Reduced surfactant levels result in increased surface tension of the alveoli, increased effort to expand the lung on inspiration, and an increased likelihood of alveolar collapse with expiration
- Incidence of disease and mortality is inversely proportional to gestational age
- There is also an increased risk for RDS in infants of a diabetic mother

CLINICAL PRESENTATION

- Physical examination findings:
  - Premature infant
  - Increased work of breathing: tachypnea, retractions, grunting, nasal flaring
- Signs of respiratory distress are usually present soon after birth. The respiratory distress worsens over the first 2 to 3 days of life
- Complications of RDS include air leaks and pulmonary hemorrhage

DIAGNOSIS AND EVALUATION

- Chest x-ray findings: poorly inflated lungs with a fine granular opacification of the lung fields ("ground glass" appearance) and air bronchograms (Fig. 75.1)
- An arterial blood gas will show hypercarbia and hypoxia

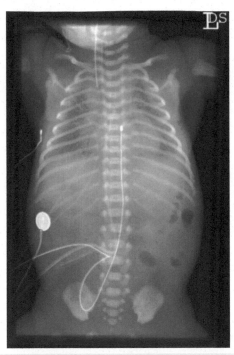

Fig. 75.1. Chest x-ray of an infant with neonatal respiratory distress syndrome with a diffuse reticulogranular appearance and an air bronchogram. (From Greenough A, Murthy V, Milner A. *Kendig and Chernick's Disorders of the Respiratory Tract in Children.* 8th ed. Philadelphia, PA: Elsevier; 2012, p. 364, Fig. 22.1.)

- Clinical picture is similar to sepsis
  - Infants should also be evaluated for early-onset septicemia and treated appropriately

TREATMENT

- Addressing the infant's respiratory needs, including supplemental oxygen, noninvasive ventilation, or intubation, if necessary
- Exogenous surfactant can be administered to the infant via endotracheal tube
- Preventive strategies include the administration of antenatal corticosteroids to the mother to mature the fetal lung before delivery
  - Routinely administered to women at risk for preterm delivery before 34 weeks' gestation
  - Treatment with antenatal corticosteroids is associated with a reduction in perinatal death, neonatal death, RDS, intraventricular hemorrhage, necrotizing enterocolitis, need for mechanical ventilation, and systemic infections in the first 48 hours of life
- Recovery from RDS is dependent on its severity, which is affected by gestation and birth weight

Pulmonary Interstitial Emphysema

BASIC INFORMATION

- Pulmonary interstitial emphysema (PIE) usually occurs in neonates with RDS supported by mechanical ventilation. The incidence is inversely related to birth weight

- It is due to the rupture of small airways resulting in gas in the interstitium. The trapped gas interferes with gas exchange
- Most commonly seen in a critically ill infant with hypoxemia and hypercarbia
- Chest x-ray findings include hyperinflation and a characteristic cystic appearance throughout the lung fields. Mediastinal compression may also be seen
- If PIE is localized, the infant should be placed with the affected lung dependent. Selective intubation to bypass the affected lung can be attempted for a short duration
- If there is widespread PIE, ventilator pressures should be reduced, and the infant may require paralysis to avoid extension of the air leak. Other modes of ventilation may be needed
- Pneumatoceles, pneumothorax, or pneumomediastinum can occur as a result of PIE

Neonatal Pneumonia

BASIC INFORMATION

- Early-onset pneumonia is diagnosed if clinical presentation is in the first 48 hours after birth. It is acquired transplacentally or during labor or delivery
  - Risk factors:
    - Prolonged rupture of membranes
    - Premature labor
    - Chorioamnionitis
    - Organisms present in the vaginal canal
  - Transplacental organisms that cause pneumonia include *Listeria monocytogenes, Mycobacterium tuberculosis, Treponema pallidum,* rubella, cytomegalovirus, herpes simplex virus, and adenovirus
  - Ascending infection is primarily due to group B streptococcus (GBS), which is the most common organism responsible for early-onset pneumonia. *Escherichia coli* is the second most common cause
- Late-onset pneumonia can be due to a variety of etiologies often dependent on the clinical scenario
  - A ventilated premature infant is prone to coagulase-negative Staphylococci, *S. aureus,* and Gram-negative organisms
  - Atypical pathogens, including *Chlamydia trachomatis,* can occur if there is a history of maternal colonization
  - Viral pneumonia is also a common cause of late-onset pneumonia

CLINICAL PRESENTATION

- Progressive respiratory distress
- Signs of systemic infection (i.e., temperature instability)
- Nonspecific signs, including irritability and poor feeding
- Infants with congenitally acquired Listeria may have hepatomegaly, diarrhea, an erythematous skin rash, and small pinkish-gray cutaneous granulomas

DIAGNOSIS AND EVALUATION

- Chest x-ray findings: an area of consolidation

- A pleural effusion may be present, which would be atypical in RDS and meconium aspiration syndrome (MAS)
- A complete blood count (CBC) with differential count and a blood culture should be obtained

TREATMENT

- Infants with respiratory distress should receive appropriate antimicrobial treatment, including a combination of ampicillin and an aminoglycoside; vancomycin may be considered based on age and local methicillin-resistant *S. aureus* (MRSA) prevalence
- Chlamydial pneumonia is treated with 2 weeks of oral erythromycin
- Intrapartum antibiotics (ampicillin or penicillin) can be given to the mother to prevent vertical transmission of GBS if a woman has been identified as being a carrier of GBS
- Supportive interventions, including oxygen or mechanical ventilation, may be required

Meconium Aspiration Syndrome

BASIC INFORMATION

- 5% of babies born through meconium-stained amniotic fluid will develop MAS
- This is a disease of term or postterm neonates because meconium does not proceed to the descending colon until 34 weeks' gestational age
- Pathophysiology:
  - Meconium creates a ball-valve mechanism in the airway, causing gas trapping and lung overdistention. This can cause air leaks
  - Meconium is an irritant and can cause pneumonitis as well as infection
  - The resulting inflammatory reaction can block small airways, impair gas exchange, and result in pulmonary hypertension

CLINICAL PRESENTATION

- Infants with MAS typically present in the first 12 hours after birth with varying degrees of respiratory distress
- Physical examination findings:
  - Tachypnea, retractions, accessory muscles use, hypoxia
  - Diffuse crackles and rhonchi
- Infants can also develop signs of pulmonary hypertension

DIAGNOSIS AND EVALUATION

- Chest x-ray findings: diffuse patchy infiltration and overexpansion that is classically "asymmetric" in appearance (Fig. 75.2)
- Air leaks, including pneumothorax and pneumomediastinum, are common and can be seen on chest x-ray

TREATMENT

- Follow Neonatal Resuscitation Program (NRP) guidelines regarding delivery room management

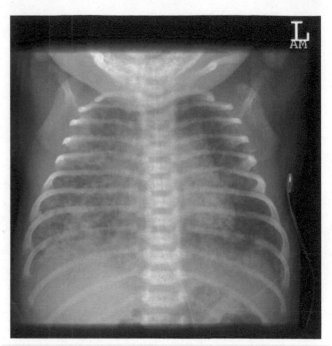

Fig. 75.2. Chest x-ray of an infant with meconium aspiration syndrome showing diffuse patchy infiltrates. (From Greenough A, Murthy V, Milner A. *Kendig and Chernick's Disorders of the Respiratory Tract in Children.* 8th ed. Philadelphia, PA: Elsevier; 2012, p. 371, Fig. 22.7.)

- Support the infants' respiratory needs with supplemental oxygen, noninvasive ventilation, and intubation with mechanical ventilation if necessary
- Antibiotics are routinely given due to the increased risk of infection
- Treat pulmonary hypertension if medically indicated
- In severe cases of MAS, extracorporeal membrane oxygenation (ECMO) may be necessary when other treatments have failed

Persistent Pulmonary Hypertension of the Newborn

BASIC INFORMATION

- Infants with persistent pulmonary hypertension of the newborn (PPHN) fail to adapt to the ex utero environment after birth. They have persistent right-to-left shunting at the level of the ductus arteriosus and the foramen ovale due to persistently high pulmonary vascular resistance
- May be primary or secondary due to infection, pulmonary hypoplasia, underlying lung disease, or congenital heart disease. Classically associated with MAS

CLINICAL PRESENTATION

- Physical examination findings:
  - Cyanosis
  - Mild respiratory distress
  - Loud second heart sound due to increased pulmonary arterial pressure
  - Hypoxemia

DIAGNOSIS AND EVALUATION

- PPHN is often difficult to differentiate from cyanotic heart disease. An echocardiogram is important to exclude cyanotic heart disease and also to estimate pulmonary arterial pressure
- Chest x-ray changes are often minimal in primary PPHN (secondary PPHN may have residual findings from the primary insult [e.g., MAS])
- Preductal saturations will be significantly higher than postductal oxyhemoglobin saturations

TREATMENT

- Support the respiratory needs of the infant with mechanical ventilation if necessary
- Pulmonary vasodilators are widely used:
  - Including inhaled nitric oxide (iNO)
  - Phosphodiesterase inhibitors (e.g., milrinone, sildenafil)
  - Endothelin receptor antagonists (e.g., bosentan)
- Infants with PPHN are fragile and intolerant of stimulation
  - Minimal handling, sedation, and paralysis may be necessary
- ECMO may be necessary in severe cases
- Treat the underlying pathology

Surfactant Protein Deficiency

BASIC INFORMATION

- Surfactant is a mixture of proteins and phospholipids that prevents collapse of alveoli at the end of expiration
- Two types of surfactant protein deficiency are surfactant protein B deficiency and surfactant protein C deficiency
- Newborns with type B surfactant deficiency, an autosomal recessive disorder, are typically full-term infants that present within the first few hours of life with rapidly progressive respiratory failure and hypoxemia
- Infants with type C deficiency, an autosomal dominant disorder or a sporadic mutation, can have a variable presentation, presenting in infancy similar to newborns with type B surfactant deficiency, but the deficiency can also present later in life
- Chest x-ray findings are nonspecific and include diffuse haziness and air bronchograms
- Genetic testing is necessary to identify a mutation. A lung biopsy may be necessary for further determination of disease process
- Lung transplantation is the only treatment for surfactant protein B deficiency. Treatment ranges from supportive care with supplemental oxygen to lung transplantation in children with protein C deficiency

Tracheoesophageal Fistula

BASIC INFORMATION

- There are several types of tracheoesophageal fistula (TEF) (see Fig. 75.3)
  - The fistula can connect the trachea to the proximal portion, distal portion, or both portions of the esophagus
  - The distal TEF accounts for the majority of cases
  - The H-type fistula occurs when there is a connection between the esophagus and trachea without esophageal atresia
- Most cases of TEF are sporadic
  - It can also occur in association with chromosomal abnormalities including trisomy 18, trisomy 21, and DiGeorge
  - It is also associated with several syndromes including VATER, VACTERL, and CHARGE syndrome

CLINICAL PRESENTATION

- Examination findings at birth:
  - Choking
  - Frothing
  - Coughing
  - Aspiration during feeding
  - Excessive salivation
- May have maternal polyhydramnios
- H-type fistulas may not present until a child is several months of age and is noted to have a chronic cough, choking with feeds, recurrent pneumonia, and/or failure to thrive

DIAGNOSIS AND EVALUATION

- A prenatal ultrasound may show polyhydramnios and a small stomach
- If there is suspicion for TEF, a nasogastric tube should be passed
  - A chest radiograph will show the tip of a nasogastric tube curled upward in the upper pouch of the esophagus
- An H-type fistula is diagnosed with a barium study with contrast material infused through a nasogastric tube
- The infant should be evaluated for other associated anomalies if this condition is suspected

TREATMENT

- Definitive management is by surgical correction
- Postoperative complications include:
  - Tracheomalacia
  - Gastroesophageal reflux
  - Dysphagia

Transient Tachypnea of the Newborn

BASIC INFORMATION

- Transient tachypnea of the newborn (TTN) occurs in 4/1000 to 6/1000 at-term infants (37–42 weeks' gestation)
- Due to delayed fetal lung fluid clearance

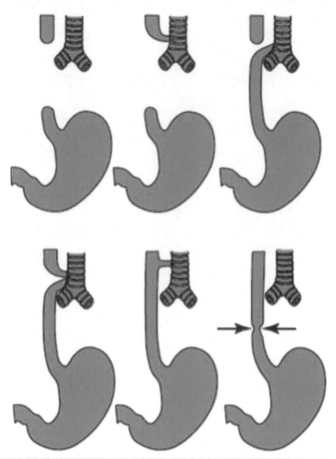

Fig. 75.3. Types of tracheoesophageal fistula. (From Abel RM, Bush A, Chitty LS, Harcourt J, Nicholson AG. *Kendig and Chernick's Disorders of the Respiratory Tract in Children.* 8th ed. Philadelphia, PA: Elsevier; 2012, p. 344, Fig. 21.26.)

- Risk factors:
  - Delivery by caesarean section without labor
  - Maternal diabetes
  - Maternal asthma
  - Male sex
  - Low birth weight
  - Macrosomia

CLINICAL PRESENTATION

- Physical examination findings:
  - Tachypnea often with a respiratory rate over 100 breaths/min
  - Grunting, retractions, and nasal flaring

DIAGNOSIS AND EVALUATION

- Chest x-ray findings (Fig. 75.4):
  - Hyperinflation
  - Prominent perihilar vascular markings
  - Fluid in the fissures
- Infant should be evaluated for infection and treated appropriately

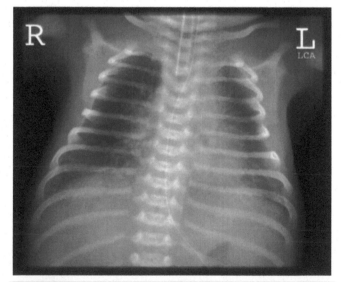

Fig. 75.4. Chest x-ray of an infant with transient tachypnea of the newborn showing areas of consolidation. (From Greenough A, Murthy V, Milner A. *Kendig and Chernick's Disorders of the Respiratory Tract in Children.* 8th ed. Philadelphia, PA: Elsevier; 2012, p. 368, Fig. 22.2.)

TREATMENT

- Self-limited condition often has a good prognosis. Infants often recover within a few days of birth

- Supportive care with supplemental oxygen, if needed, on average for 2 to 3 days
- Feeds may need to be withheld pending improvement in the infant's respiratory rate

CONGENITAL LUNG MALFORMATIONS

Congenital Cystic Adenomatous Malformation/Congenital Pulmonary Airway Malformation

BASIC INFORMATION

- Congenital pulmonary airway malformation (CPAM) is a multicystic mass of pulmonary tissue in which vascular supply is from the pulmonary circulation
  - There are five types of CPAMs that are classified based on the location of the malformation in the airway
- Associations with other congenital malformations have been described, including congenital cardiac disease and congenital diaphragmatic hernia (CDH)

CLINICAL PRESENTATION

- There is a spectrum of clinical presentations ranging from asymptomatic infants to infants in respiratory failure due to the mass effect of a large lesion
- May present as an incidental finding, unresolving pneumonia, or a pneumothorax
- There is a risk of superinfection in these lesions
- There is also a risk of tumor formation in certain types of CPAMs, specifically the formation of pleuropulmonary blastoma

DIAGNOSIS AND EVALUATION

- Frequently diagnosed prenatally on ultrasound
- Can also be diagnosed incidentally on routine imaging

TREATMENT

- Surgery is indicated if there is recurring infection, compression of nearby structures, or an increased familial cancer risk
- Management of an asymptomatic CPAM is controversial

Congenital Lobar Emphysema

BASIC INFORMATION

- The exact cause of congenital lobar emphysema (CLE) is unknown
- Microscopic evaluation of excised lobes shows one of two patterns:
  - Hyperexpanded lobe with a normal number of enlarged alveoli
  - Enlarged lobe containing an increased number of alveoli
- Pathophysiology:
  - The affected lobe cannot deflate
  - It overdistends, displacing adjacent lobes and mediastinal structures

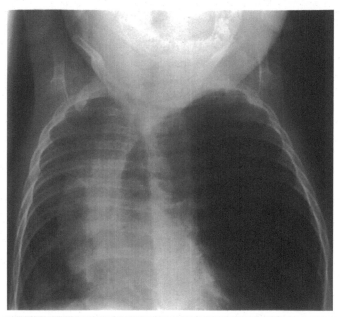

Fig. 75.5. Chest x-ray of an infant with congenital lobar emphysema demonstrating a large hyperlucent lobe. (From Abel RM, Bush A, Chitty LS, Harcourt J, Nicholson AG. *Kendig and Chernick's Disorders of the Respiratory Tract in Children*. 8th ed. Philadelphia, PA: Elsevier; 2012, p. 342, Fig. 21.23.)

CLINICAL PRESENTATION

- Can present in the newborn period with tachypnea, decreased breath sounds on the affected side, and wheezing. The child may also have failure to thrive
- More than 80% of cases will present by 6 months of age

DIAGNOSIS AND EVALUATION

- Can be diagnosed prenatally
- Chest radiograph shows (Fig. 75.5):
  - Hyperinflation of a lobe
  - Compression of the ipsilateral lung
  - Herniation of the emphysematous lung across the mediastinum, with compression of the contralateral lung

TREATMENT

- A lobectomy is the treatment of choice in the event of respiratory distress

Bronchopulmonary Sequestration

BASIC INFORMATION

- The classical type of bronchopulmonary sequestration consists of an isolated segment of lung tissue fed by the systemic circulation (different vascular supply compared with a CPAM). The blood supply is from the thoracic or abdominal aorta in most cases. Venous drainage is usually to the right atrium, creating a left-to-right shunt
  - It can be located within the lung parenchyma (intrapulmonary variant) or isolated from and accessory to the lung (extralobar variant)

- Usually left-sided and found between the lower lobe and diaphragm
- An extralobar sequestration is generally detected in infancy because of associated congenital malformations
- A bronchopulmonary sequestration can be an incidental finding on routine imaging. It can also present with respiratory distress in the newborn period due to mass effect, high-output cardiac failure, or other associated anomalies
- There is an increased risk of infection of the lesion
- A chest x-ray may show the lesion in the retrocardiac area. A chest computed tomography (CT) and magnetic resonance imaging (MRI) allow for better characterization of the lesion and its associated blood supply
- Surgical resection is the standard treatment for symptomatic lesions

Bronchogenic Cyst

BASIC INFORMATION

- Formed when a piece of bronchial tissue separates from the developing airway, resulting in an epithelium-lined sac that contains cartilage in the wall
- In most cases, there is no connection between the bronchogenic cyst and the normal airway, and most remain asymptomatic and are detected incidentally later in life
- If there is a connection between the bronchogenic cyst and the normal airway, a patient can develop recurrent or chronic infections of the cyst
- About 50% are in the mediastinum close to the carina. The degree of symptoms depends on the location of the cyst
  - If the lesion is in the peritracheal area, it can cause airway narrowing and noisy breathing
  - If there is associated compression of the esophagus, it can also cause feeding difficulties
- Evaluation of bronchogenic cysts includes a barium esophagram and CT scan
- Surgical removal of the bronchogenic cyst is necessary if it is causing symptoms. Management for asymptomatic lesions is controversial

Congenital Diaphragmatic Hernia

BASIC INFORMATION

- A developmental failure of the diaphragm during its formation allows herniation of abdominal organs into the chest, affecting lung growth
- The extension of abdominal viscera into the thoracic cavity results in lung hypoplasia. Vascular abnormalities also occur, increasing the risk of pulmonary hypertension
- The classic CDH is through a posterolateral defect in the diaphragm (Bochdalek hernia)
- The majority of hernias are left-sided
- There is increased frequency in premature infants and male infants

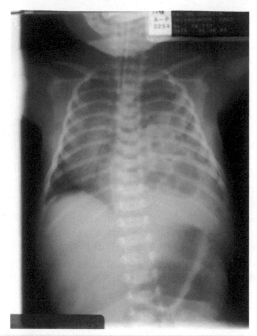

Fig. 75.6. Chest x-ray of an infant with a left-sided congenital diaphragmatic hernia. Note the loops of bowel in the chest. (From Abel RM, Bush A, Chitty LS, Harcourt J, Nicholson AG. *Kendig and Chernick's Disorders of the Respiratory Tract in Children.* 8th ed. Philadelphia, PA: Elsevier; 2012, p. 351, Fig. 21.35.)

- The incidence of associated anomalies is approximately 30% and includes skeletal and cardiac abnormalities
- CDH also occurs in several syndromes, including trisomies 21, 18, 13; Beckwith-Wiedemann syndrome; and Goldenhar syndrome

CLINICAL PRESENTATION

- Physical examination findings:
  - Respiratory distress at birth
  - A scaphoid abdomen if a significant amount of abdominal viscera is displaced into the thorax
  - Bowel sounds over the thorax and the absence of breath sounds on the affected side

DIAGNOSIS AND EVALUATION

- Typically made on prenatal ultrasound
- After birth, a chest radiograph will show bowel in the chest cavity and deviation of the mediastinum toward the unaffected side (Fig. 75.6)

TREATMENT

- Initial management includes stabilization of the infant's respiratory status with endotracheal intubation and placement of a nasogastric tube to decompress the stomach and small bowel of swallowed air
- Surgery to close the diaphragmatic defect is necessary

Pulmonary Hypoplasia

BASIC INFORMATION

- Generalized pulmonary hypoplasia is associated with several intrauterine insults:
  - Hydrops fetalis
  - Renal anomalies
  - CDH
  - Omphalocele
  - Skeletal abnormalities
  - Small chest syndromes (i.e., Jeune syndrome)
  - Oligohydramnios
- The most severe form of oligohydramnios and pulmonary hypoplasia is Potter syndrome
  - The absence of urine production due to renal agenesis leads to severe oligohydramnios with associated defects including a flattened facies, clubfeet, intrauterine growth retardation, and pulmonary hypoplasia

CLINICAL PRESENTATION

- Mild hypoplasia can present with tachypnea
- More severe hypoplasia can present as respiratory failure in the neonatal period
- Chest wall is disproportionately small with respect to the abdomen

DIAGNOSIS AND EVALUATION

- Underlying etiologies of pulmonary hypoplasia are often diagnosed prenatally on ultrasound
- Postnatally, a chest x-ray may demonstrate features of the infant's underlying condition

TREATMENT

- Addressing the underlying condition
- Providing ventilator support if needed
- Treating underlying pulmonary hypertension if present

Pulmonary Agenesis and Pulmonary Aplasia

BASIC INFORMATION

- Complete pulmonary agenesis, or agenesis of both lungs, is incompatible with life. Lesser degrees of agenesis can be seen, including agenesis of one lung or of one or more lobes of a lung
- Pulmonary aplasia is defined as an absent lung, typically with a mainstem bronchial stump and absence of the distal lung. Secretions can pool in the stump and become infected
- Pulmonary agenesis and aplasia are often associated with other congenital abnormalities including cardiac defects
- Infants can present with neonatal respiratory distress
- Pulmonary agenesis and aplasia are often diagnosed on prenatal ultrasound. A chest x-ray can show hemithorax white-out or ipsilateral loss of lung volume dependent on the degree of agenesis. There can also be ipsilateral mediastinal shift
- Treatment is supportive care of the infants' respiratory needs. It is also essential to assess for and treat other congenital anomalies

Pulmonary Lymphangiectasia

BASIC INFORMATION

- Characterized by dilatation of pulmonary lymphatic vessels and disordered drainage leading to the accumulation of lymph within the lungs. Secondary pulmonary lymphangiectasia usually involves congenital cardiac diseases that obstruct pulmonary venous flow or lymphatic drainage
- Usually presents during the neonatal period with respiratory distress progressing to respiratory failure. Chylous effusions may also be present
- A chest x-ray may show interstitial infiltrates and hyperinflation, with or without pleural effusions. A chest CT may show thickening of peribronchovascular septa and septa surrounding lobules
- The gold standard for diagnosis, which is a lung biopsy, will show dilated lymphatic vessels located in the interlobular septa. There may also be thickening and widening of interlobular septa
- Treatment is supportive. Pulmonary lymphangiectasia carries a high rate of mortality when diagnosed in the neonatal period

Review Questions

For review questions, please go to ExpertConsult.com.

Suggested Readings

1. Abel RM, Bush A, Chitty LS, Harcourt J, Nicholson AG. Congenital lung disease. In: Wilmott RW, et al., eds. *Kendig and Chernick's disorders of the respiratory tract in children.* 8th ed. Philadelphia: Elsevier Saunders; 2012:317–357.
2. Abman SH. Bronchopulmonary dysplasia. In: Wilmott RW, et al., eds. *Kendig and Chernick's Disorders of The Respiratory Tract in Children.* 8th ed. Philadelphia: Elsevier Saunders; 2012:386–398.
3. Eichenwald EC, Committee on Fetus and Newborn. Apnea of Prematurity. *Pediatrics.* 2016;137(1):1–7.
4. Gallacher DJ, Hart K, Kotecha S. Common respiratory conditions of the newborn. *Breathe.* 2016;12(1):30–42.
5. Greenough A, Murthy V, Milner AD. Respiratory disorders in the newborn. In: Wilmott RW, et al., ed. *Kendig and Chernick's disorders of the respiratory tract in children.* 8th edn. Philadelphia: Elsevier Saunders; 2012:358–385.
6. O'Sullivan B, Kinane TB. Congenital lung anomalies. In: Light MJ, ed. *Pediatric Pulmonology.* 1st ed. *American Academy of Pediatrics.* 2011:277–307.
7. Warren JB, Anderson JM. Newborn respiratory disorders. *Pediatri Rev.* 2010;31(12):487–496.

76 Disorders of the Upper and Lower Airways

NICHOLAS L. FRIEDMAN, DO and JASON Z. BRONSTEIN, MD

UPPER RESPIRATORY TRACT DISORDERS

The upper airway (upper respiratory tract) is comprised of the parts of the respiratory system that are outside of the thoracic cavity (i.e. extrathoracic). Obstructive congenital lesions of the upper airway produce turbulent airflow. This turbulent airflow through the narrowed segment of the upper airways produces some distinctive sounds, which are diagnostically useful. Stridor is a high-pitched inspiratory sound that is generated from obstruction in the extrathoracic airway. Stertor is a low-pitched inspiratory snoring sound produced by obstruction in the nasal or nasopharyngeal passages. Upper airway obstruction is commonly caused by either congenital abnormalities or infectious processes.

Laryngomalacia

BASIC INFORMATION

- Prolapse of the supraglottic structures into the laryngeal airway on inspiration
- Unclear etiology, possibly due to incomplete integration of laryngeal sensation with brain stem–mediated reflexes
- Most common congenital anomaly of the upper airway
- Most frequent congenital cause of stridor in infants
- 80% of children with laryngomalacia have esophageal and laryngopharyngeal reflux
- Reflux of gastric contents causes inflammation and edema of the laryngeal mucosa, which can worsen laryngomalacia

CLINICAL PRESENTATION

- Stridor developing in the first 2 weeks of life (not present at birth)
- Stridor is most pronounced at 2 to 4 months of life
- Despite stridor, most children are nontoxic-appearing and in no distress
- Stridor often changes with position
  - Worse with feeding, when lying supine, and during periods of agitation
  - Improved with lying prone
- Hoarseness is not a symptom of laryngomalacia and may be suggestive of a vocal cord abnormality
- 5% to 10% of patients with laryngomalacia have severe laryngomalacia resulting in respiratory distress, failure to thrive, cyanotic episodes, acute life-threatening

events, or an inability to tolerate oral feeds; these patients should be evaluated for concurrent airway lesions (up to 20% have other airway anomalies)

DIAGNOSIS AND EVALUATION

- Diagnosis is confirmed by direct visualization on flexible transnasal fiber-optic laryngoscopy
- Laryngoscopy can be performed while the patient is awake, at bedside, or in the clinic
- Findings of laryngomalacia on laryngoscopy (Fig. 76.1):
  - Omega-shaped epiglottis, which may be retroflexed
  - Short, vertical aryepiglottic folds
  - Redundant arytenoid mucosa
  - Prolapse of redundant tissue overlying the arytenoid cartilage
  - May be inflammation and edema of laryngeal mucosa, secondary to reflux

TREATMENT

- Most often self-resolves between the ages of 12 and 18 months
- Management of gastroesophageal reflux disease (GERD) with histamine 2 blockers or proton pump inhibitors
- Children with severe laryngomalacia may require surgical intervention—supraglottoplasty. In supraglottoplasty, redundant tissue over the arytenoids is removed, and both aryepiglottic folds are divided

Vocal Cord Paralysis (VCP)

BASIC INFORMATION

- May be unilateral or bilateral (40% of cases)
- Unilateral VCP:
  - Usually caused by a nonfunctioning peripheral nerve (recurrent laryngeal nerve), most often secondary to iatrogenic injury (e.g., surgical repair of a tracheoesophageal fistula [TEF] or a congenital cardiac anomaly, internal trauma from an endotracheal tube). May also result from birth trauma or great vessel abnormalities
  - Unilateral VCP is more common on the left due to the longer course of the recurrent laryngeal nerve
- Bilateral VCP:
  - More often associated with a central nervous system abnormality (i.e., myelomeningocele, Arnold-Chiari malformation, and hydrocephalus)

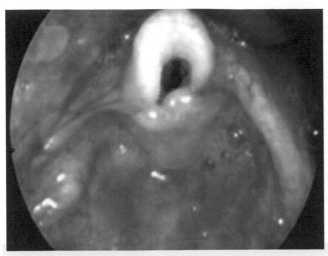

Fig. 76.1. Laryngomalacia. (From Goldsmith JP, et al. *Assisted ventilation of the neonate.* 6th ed. Philadelphia: Elsevier; 2017, p. 120, Fig. 13.2 [Left].)

CLINICAL PRESENTATION

- Unilateral VCP:
  - Hoarseness of voice; a weak, breathy cry; and aspiration leading to cough
  - Airway obstruction and stridor are less common in unilateral VCP because the paralyzed vocal cord remains fixed in a lateral position
- Bilateral VCP:
  - High-pitched inspiratory stridor and respiratory distress
  - Inspiratory stridor in children with bilateral VCP is relieved with endotracheal intubation

DIAGNOSIS AND EVALUATION

- Both unilateral and bilateral VCP are diagnosed by endoscopic airway evaluation
- Once VCP is diagnosed and determined to be unilateral or bilateral, further imaging may be required to assess for cardiac or neurologic abnormalities

TREATMENT

- Acquired VCP usually resolves in 6 to 12 months. If there is no resolution of VCP by 2 years of life, it is unlikely to improve spontaneously
- Unilateral VCP may be managed with observation, temporary injection medialization (to decrease aspiration), and speech therapy. If there is no resolution of paralysis in 1 year after initial interventions, more permanent interventions (reinnervation or long-term injection medialization) may be considered
- In cases of bilateral VCP, tracheostomy placement while awaiting possible spontaneous resolution of the VCP is the traditional treatment. Otherwise, treatment of any underlying neurologic abnormality will promote resolution of bilateral VCP
- If there is no spontaneous resolution of bilateral VCP, surgical interventions by otorhinolaryngologists may be considered, including laryngotracheal reconstruction (LTR)

Subglottic Stenosis (SGS)

BASIC INFORMATION

- Estimated that 40% of SGS cases are congenital, with the rest being acquired
- Congenital SGS is defined as a tracheal lumen with a diameter of ≤4.0 mm at the level of the cricoid cartilage (2–3 mm below the vocal cords)
- Congenital SGS results from failure of the laryngeal lumen to recanalize and is often associated with other congenital head and neck lesions and syndromes (i.e., Down syndrome)
- Acquired SGS is most often caused by prolonged endotracheal intubation, particularly in the neonatal period
- GERD is a cofactor in the development of acquired SGS

CLINICAL PRESENTATION

- Presentation is based on the degree of SGS severity (Fig. 76.2)
- Severe congenital SGS may present with biphasic stridor (fixed obstruction) and respiratory distress in the neonatal period, whereas children with mild SGS (congenital or acquired) may be asymptomatic or minimally symptomatic, demonstrating stridor and respiratory distress only during periods of upper respiratory tract infections (URIs)
- Children with SGS may present with recurrent pneumonias or prolonged tracheobronchitis due to an inability to clear increased respiratory secretions during periods of illness
- Children with more severe SGS often have tracheostomy dependency

DIAGNOSIS AND EVALUATION

- Diagnosed by direct endoscopic visualization
- Initial anteroposterior (AP) and lateral soft-tissue neck radiographs may help raise suspicion for SGS; however, they do not take the place of endoscopic visualization and measurement of the airway diameter
- Severity of SGS is graded using the Cotton-Myer grading scale, which is based on the percentage of tracheal lumen obstruction

TREATMENT

- Children with grade 1 or 2 SGS (congenital or acquired) may only require antibiotics during URIs, management of GERD, and observation of their respiratory status; tracheostomy is necessary in more than half of children with severe SGS (grades 3 and 4)
- After tracheostomy placement, serial airway dilations under general anesthesia often result in improvement in the SGS and eventual tracheostomy decannulation. Some patients may require more complicated surgical reconstruction

Tracheomalacia

BASIC INFORMATION

- Dynamic tracheal collapse during respiration, more commonly of the intrathoracic trachea. This causes

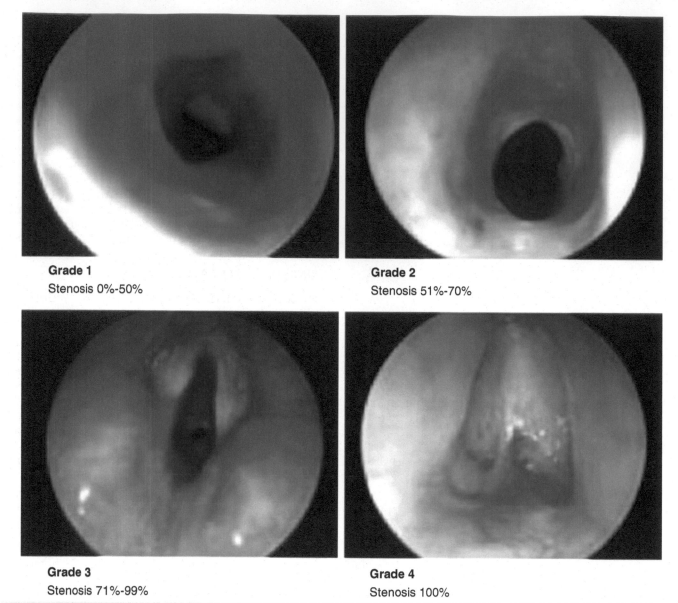

Grade 1
Stenosis 0%-50%

Grade 2
Stenosis 51%-70%

Grade 3
Stenosis 71%-99%

Grade 4
Stenosis 100%

Fig. 76.2. Examples of subglottic stenosis. (From Goldsmith JP, et al. *Assisted ventilation of the neonate.* 6th ed. Philadelphia: Elsevier; 2017, p. 120, Fig. 13.2.)

obstruction when the intrathoracic pressure is positive relative to the tracheal lumen (i.e., during expiration)
- Can result from an intrinsic defect in the cartilaginous tracheal rings (primary tracheomalacia) or from extrinsic compression of the trachea (secondary tracheomalacia)
- Three categories of tracheomalacia:
  - Type 1: congenital, due to weakness in the tracheal rings; may be associated with TEF or polychondritis of the tracheobronchial tree
  - Type 2: caused by extrinsic tracheal compression secondary to vascular or lymphatic malformations or neoplasms
  - Type 3: acquired from prolonged inflammation or irritation (e.g., prolonged intubation or irritation from GERD or local infection)

CLINICAL PRESENTATION

- Homophonous wheezing (from intrathoracic central airway collapse). Extrathoracic (cervical) tracheomalacia may present with inspiratory stridor
- Recurrent barking cough
- Frequent respiratory infections or reactive airway disease that is refractory to standard medical therapy, particularly bronchodilators
- Rarely, brief resolved unexplained event (BRUE) or respiratory distress may be due to tracheomalacia
- Severity of presentation depends on the degree of tracheal collapse

DIAGNOSIS AND EVALUATION

- Definitive diagnosis is obtained during bronchoscopy performed with the child breathing spontaneously (Fig. 76.3)
- Static radiographs have little role in evaluating tracheomalacia, unless to assess for possible secondary tracheomalacia due to extrinsic airway compression
- Airway fluoroscopy can be considered for identifying tracheomalacia (not definitive)

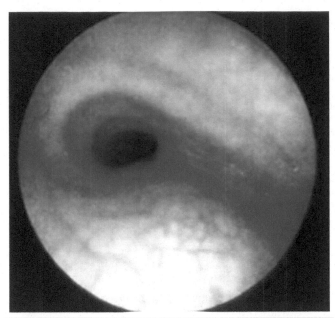

Fig. 76.3. Tracheomalacia. (From Goldsmith JP, et al. *Assisted ventilation of the neonate.* 6th ed. Philadelphia: Elsevier; 2017, p. 399, Fig. 36.7.)

TREATMENT

- Most patients with tracheomalacia outgrow it in the first 2 years of life
- Bethanechol, a cholinergic agent that can increase smooth muscle tone in the trachea, may improve tracheomalacia
- Inhaled ipratropium bromide can also be used to increase tracheal smooth muscle tone
- Beta-2 agonists (e.g. albuterol) can theoretically cause decrease of tracheal tone and may worsen tracheomalacia
- Management of GERD is critical because it can worsen tracheomalacia
- Severe tracheomalacia (which can result in severe obstructive symptoms, failure to thrive, BRUEs, or respiratory distress) may require noninvasive positive pressure ventilation or surgical intervention
- If the tracheomalacia is secondary to extrinsic airway compression, removal of the compression may not immediately correct the tracheal weakness

Vascular Rings

BASIC INFORMATION

- Anomalous formations of the great vessels that cross over or encircle the trachea and esophagus
- Multiple varieties of vascular rings:
  - Double aortic arch
  - Right aortic arch with left ductus arteriosus or ligamentum arteriosum
  - Anomalous innominate artery
  - Pulmonary artery sling
- "Rings" encircle both the trachea and esophagus
- "Slings" encircle one or the other

CLINICAL PRESENTATION

- Usually presents in the first few months of life as biphasic stridor and/or a barking cough
- May develop dysphagia when transitioning to solid foods if there is esophageal compression
- Often misdiagnosed as GERD, laryngomalacia, tracheomalacia, or reactive airway disease

DIAGNOSIS AND EVALUATION

- Initial evaluation is performed with barium esophagography to assess for vascular indentation on the esophagus
- Contrast computed tomography (CT) or magnetic resonance imaging (MRI) to assess the exact location and anatomy of the vascular malformation
- Bronchoscopy should be performed to dynamically evaluate the tracheobronchial tract and to assess the degree and location of dynamic compression

TREATMENT

- Surgical intervention for correction of the vascular lesion
- A residual tracheal deformity and tracheomalacia will persist postoperatively
- Stridor may remain for 6 to 24 months after surgical repair

Croup (Viral Laryngotracheobronchitis/Viral Laryngotracheitis)

BASIC INFORMATION

- Acute inflammation of the glottis and subglottis
- Inflammatory edema results in the characteristic barking cough and stridor
- Most common infectious cause of upper airway obstruction in children
- Most commonly due to parainfluenza virus type 1
  - Other viral etiologies are parainfluenza types 2 and 3, adenovirus, respiratory syncytial virus (RSV), rhinovirus, measles, and human metapneumovirus
- Bacterial secondary infection is possible (commonly *Staphylococcus aureus, Streptococcus pyogenes, and S. pneumonia*) but uncommon

CLINICAL PRESENTATION

- Most commonly occurs in children 6 to 36 months of age
- Slight male predominance (1.4:1)
- Most commonly occurs in fall and winter months
- Children often have a viral prodrome with cough and coryza 12 to 24 hours before the onset of barking cough, stridor, hoarseness, and respiratory distress in moderate to severe cases
- Table 76.1 classifies the severity of croup based on clinical presentation and provides management strategies

Table 76.1. Severity of Croup With Clinical Features and Management

Clinical Feature	Mild	Moderate	Severe
Appearance	Nontoxic, mild hoarseness, will still eat and drink	Mild respiratory distress, mild tachypnea, worsened hoarseness, will drink	Increasing respiratory distress, moderate-severe tachypnea, tired-appearing, will not take per os (PO)
Cough	Intermittent barking	Frequent barking	Incessant cough
Stridor	None at rest, may develop with agitation	Audible at rest	Pronounced and prominent
Retractions	None at rest	Mild-moderate	Severe
Agitation	None	Little to none	Significant
Management	Largely supportive; antipyretics, fluids, humidification, and a single dose of oral corticosteroids	Oral or intravenous (IV) corticosteroids, nebulized racemic epinephrine or epinephrine, close observation	Intramuscular (IM) or IV corticosteroids, supplemental O_2 if hypoxemia, multiple doses of nebulized racemic epinephrine or epinephrine, Heliox, consideration of endotracheal intubation if impending respiratory failure

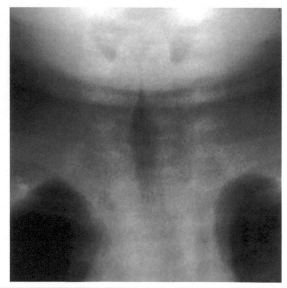

Fig. 76.4. Croup (laryngotracheobronchitis): steeple sign. (From Zitelli BJ, et al. *Zitelli and Davis' atlas of pediatric physical diagnosis.* 6th ed. Philadelphia: Elsevier; 2012, p. 627, Fig. 16.17)

DIAGNOSIS AND EVALUATION

- Croup is primarily diagnosed clinically
- AP and lateral airway radiographs may reveal the trachea terminating into a narrowed subglottis—"steeple sign" (Fig. 76.4)

TREATMENT

- Treatment is based primarily on the severity of symptoms (Table 76.1)
- Regardless of the severity, it is essential to keep the child calm and comfortable because agitation and anxiety can worsen respiratory distress
- Supportive care for mild croup—fluids, antipyretics, and humidification (humidification is largely anecdotal with no supportive evidence)
- Corticosteroids are used for all levels of croup severity—decrease airway inflammation (may administer orally if the child can tolerate per os [PO] intake; otherwise, give intramuscularly [IM] or intravenously [IV])

- Dexamethasone is most commonly used (0.6 mg/kg/dose PO, IV, or IM); lower doses (0.15 mg/kg/dose) have also been shown to be effective
  - Dexamethasone lasts 12 to 24 hours
  - Prednisolone is also effective; however, it has a shorter half-life than dexamethasone
- Nebulized epinephrine/racemic epinephrine provides decrease in airway wall edema and bronchodilation
  - Rapid onset of action (within 30 minutes); lasts for 2 to 3 hours
  - Can be readministered every 15 to 20 minutes as necessary
  - Must observe the patient for 3 to 4 hours after administration because rebound mucosal edema may occur
  - If more than two doses of nebulized epinephrine/racemic epinephrine are administered, hospitalization should be considered
- Heliox (combination of helium and oxygen) can be considered in severe cases
  - Low-density helium (vs nitrogen present in air) converts turbulent airflow to laminar flow
- Supplemental oxygen may be used for patients with hypoxemia (unlikely)
- Intubation in the case of respiratory failure—approximately 1% of patients with croup
  - Intubation of a child with croup may predispose the child to developing SGS after extubation

Spasmodic Croup (Recurrent Croup)

BASIC INFORMATION

- Noninfectious variant of croup
- Most likely allergic in etiology, may be related to GERD

CLINICAL PRESENTATION

- Frequent nocturnal barking cough and stridor without a viral prodrome
- Rapid onset and resolution
- No viral prodrome

DIAGNOSIS AND EVALUATION

- Evaluation for allergic etiologies
- Evaluation for GERD
- Consider AP and lateral neck radiographs
- If persistent, referral to ear, nose, and throat (ENT) for evaluation for airway abnormalities

TREATMENT

- Reassurance
- Management of allergies (antihistamines)
- Management of GERD

Epiglottitis

BASIC INFORMATION

- Acute inflammation of the epiglottis and adjacent supraglottic structures
- Infection causes edema of the supraglottic airway that results in airway narrowing and curling of the epiglottis into the airway
- Potentially life-threatening infection that can cause fatal airway obstruction and cardiorespiratory arrest if treatment is delayed
- Historically caused by *Haemophilus influenzae* type B (HIB); however, since the initiation of the HIB vaccination, epiglottitis has become quite rare
- HIB is still the most common cause of epiglottitis (unvaccinated children, immunocompromised state, and trisomy 21)
  - Several other causative organisms have been identified: *H. influenzae* (A, F, and nontypeable), *H. parainfluenzae*, *S. pneumoniae*, and *S. aureus*
  - There may also be viral etiologies

CLINICAL PRESENTATION

- Most common in children 2 to 7 years of age; may also occur in adolescents and adults
- Rapid onset of high fever, toxic appearance, muffled voice, and sore throat
- Symptoms progress over a few hours to dysphagia, drooling, and respiratory distress
- Respiratory failure secondary to airway obstruction can occur very rapidly after initial presentation
- Stridor is often a late finding and, when present, is indicative of near-complete airway obstruction
- Cough, if present, is minimal
- The child may sit in the "tripod" position, leaning forward with a hyperextended neck to promote airway opening

DIAGNOSIS AND EVALUATION

- Clinical diagnosis is critical because time is of the essence to maintain airway patency
- Lateral neck radiograph should be attempted only if the patient is stable and the diagnosis is in doubt
- Direct laryngoscopy confirms the diagnosis; however, this should be attempted only in a controlled setting by an experienced airway practitioner (ENT or anesthesiology)

TREATMENT

- Avoid causing the child to have anxiety or agitation because they can promote airway closure
- 100% oxygen should be provided via blow-by
- Intubation should be performed in the most controlled environment (operating room, if possible)
  - If unable to intubate, emergent tracheotomy should be performed
- Administration of IV antibiotics to cover both HIB and streptococcus (third-generation cephalosporins are most commonly used)

Bacterial Tracheitis (BT)

BASIC INFORMATION

- Also known as bacterial or membranous laryngotracheobronchitis and membranous or pseudomembranous croup
- Bacterial infection of the subglottic airway (most often *S. aureus*, rarely Gram-negative) that is often superimposed on a preceding viral laryngotracheobronchitis
- Mucosal inflammation, as well as purulent exudates and pseudomembranes in the trachea, can cause severe airway obstruction and respiratory failure
- The lower airways are often involved in cases of BT
- Most commonly occurs in children 6 months to 8 years of age (mean: 4 years of age)
- This is in contrast to tracheotomy-associated tracheitis, a condition characterized by Gram-positive and/or Gram-negative bacteria, in which patients present with indolent signs/symptoms of infection. These infections can be treated with antibiotics alone

CLINICAL PRESENTATION

- BT may be distinguished from viral croup by patient age (older in BT) and disease severity
- Children with BT are often toxic-appearing and have a high fever with rapidly progressing symptoms
- More insidious onset than epiglottitis
- Barking cough and hoarseness present
- Stridor may be biphasic depending on the level of tracheal involvement
- Dysphagia and orthopnea are often present, although the classic boards description will mention a child wanting to stay supine rather than sit upright or tripodding as in epiglottitis
- No response to nebulized epinephrine or corticosteroids

DIAGNOSIS AND EVALUATION

- Diagnosis is most often clinical
- White blood cell (WBC) count often shows leukocytosis with neutrophil predominance

Table 76.2. History and Physical Examination Findings in Children With Obstructive Sleep Apnea

History	Physical Examination
■ Frequent snoring (≥3 nights a week)	■ Tonsillar hypertrophy
■ Labored breathing during sleep	■ Overweight (more commonly) or underweight
■ Gasping or snorting during sleep	■ Adenoidal facies (intraorbital darkening, elongated face, mouth breathing)
■ Pauses in breathing with sleep (apneic pauses)	
■ Sleeping in a seated position or with the neck hyperextended	■ Micrognathia/retrognathia
■ Daytime sleepiness	■ High-arched palate
■ Headaches on awakening	■ Swollen nasal mucosa
■ Attention-deficit/hyperactivity disorder	■ Midface hypoplasia
■ Learning difficulties	■ Macroglossia

■ AP and lateral neck radiographs may show subglottic narrowing, haziness of the tracheal lumen, and a ragged edge to the tracheal air column (due to pseudomembranes and exudates on the tracheal wall)

■ Endoscopy confirms the diagnosis

TREATMENT

■ Endotracheal intubation to maintain airway patency
■ Endoscopy may be therapeutic to remove secretions and sloughed tissue from the airway lumen
■ Broad-spectrum antibiotics (with methicillin-resistant *S. aureus* [MRSA] coverage) should be administered
■ Patients may require intubation for 7 days or longer

Obstructive Sleep Apnea (OSA)

BASIC INFORMATION

■ Defined by the American Academy of Pediatrics (AAP) as a "disorder of breathing during sleep characterized by prolonged partial upper airway obstruction and/or intermittent complete obstruction (obstructive apnea) that disrupts normal ventilation during sleep and normal sleep patterns"
■ Occurs in 2% to 5% of children
■ Primary snoring occurs in 12% to 20% of children
■ Risk factors include adenotonsillar hypertrophy, obesity, craniofacial anomalies, and neuromuscular disorders

CLINICAL PRESENTATION

■ See Table 76.2 for signs and symptoms of OSA on history and physical examination

DIAGNOSIS AND EVALUATION

■ Providers should assess for snoring and signs/symptoms of OSA at each routine health supervision visit
■ If the child is having snoring or signs/symptoms of OSA, the provider should either obtain a polysomnogram or refer the patient to a sleep specialist or otolaryngologist for a more extensive evaluation

■ Children with high-risk conditions for OSA—craniofacial, metabolic, genetic, or neuromuscular disorders—should be referred to a specialist (pediatric pulmonologist, otolaryngologist, or sleep medicine specialist)
■ Polysomnography (performed overnight and in an attended sleep laboratory) is the gold standard for evaluating for the presence and degree of sleep disordered breathing
■ There is a shortage of sleep laboratories that perform pediatric polysomnography; thus alternative tests (nocturnal video recording, nocturnal oximetry, daytime nap polysomnography, or ambulatory polysomnography) may be considered. However, these tests have a high rate of false-negative and false-positive results, and results must be interpreted carefully

TREATMENT

■ Adenotonsillectomy (T&A) is the first line of treatment in children with OSA or with adenotonsillar hypertrophy on physical examination (with no surgical contraindications)
■ T&A is often performed on an outpatient basis; postoperative inpatient monitoring should be performed for children with risk factors for postoperative respiratory complications (i.e., obesity or failure to thrive, younger than 3 years of age, severe OSA, craniofacial abnormalities, neuromuscular disorders, or a current respiratory infection)
■ Providers should reassess OSA-related signs and symptoms 6 to 8 weeks postoperatively (to allow for healing of the operative site and recovery of the upper airway); in children with moderate-severe OSA, a repeat polysomnogram should be obtained 6 to 8 weeks postoperatively to evaluate for persistent OSA
■ Patients should be considered for referral for continuous positive airway pressure (CPAP) if OSA persists after T&A or if T&A is not performed
■ Weight loss therapy should be recommended if the child is overweight or obese
■ Watchful waiting with periodic retesting may be reasonable in select children with mild OSA and no significant sequelae, but T&A is recommended if there are significant symptoms or risk and in cases of moderate or severe OSA.

LOWER AIRWAY DISORDERS

The lower airways constitute the final leg of the journey from the atmosphere to the alveoli. The 23 divisions (or generations) of air conduits serve to subdivide the respiratory tract into microscopic units that optimize surface area per volume for gas exchange with the pulmonary capillaries. There are a number of processes that can obstruct or infect these small airways, interfering with their function and decreasing resultant airflow or gas exchange. Dysfunction of the lower airways will generally result in wheezing if there is obstruction and in crackles if there is decreased mucus clearance.

Bronchiolitis

BASIC INFORMATION

- Viral lower respiratory tract infection induces acute inflammation, edema, mucus production, and epithelial cell necrosis
  - Classically caused by RSV
    - Peak occurrence is during winter
    - First exposure occurs in 90% of children under 2 years of age
    - 40% of initial RSV infection manifests as bronchiolitis
    - Adaptive immunity does not prevent recurrent infection
  - Can be caused by most other respiratory viruses, including rhinovirus, influenza, human metapneumovirus, coronavirus, parainfluenza, and adenovirus
- Most commonly infects children <2 years old
- The most common cause of hospitalization in infants

CLINICAL PRESENTATION

- Begins with rhinorrhea and cough, but progresses to dyspnea and signs of increased work of breathing (tachypnea, retractions, nasal flaring, accessory muscle use, grunting)
- Adventitious lung sounds include wheeze, crackles, and rhonchi
- Due to increased respiratory effort, patients often have poor oral intake
- Young patients (<1 month old or <48 weeks postconception) are at risk for apnea; those with history of apnea are also at risk for apnea in the setting of bronchiolitis
- Natural history: peak symptoms occur in the first week, but may persist up to 3 weeks

DIAGNOSIS AND EVALUATION

- Diagnosed based on history and examination
  - <2 years old
  - Viral upper respiratory prodrome
  - Respiratory distress or signs of lower respiratory tract infection
- Factors portending more severe disease:
  - Moderate to severe respiratory distress with hypoxemia
  - Signs of dehydration
  - Change in mental status
  - Age <12 weeks or history of prematurity
  - Underlying cardiopulmonary disease or immunodeficiency
- Routine testing is not indicated; it is sought only if there is clinical suspicion for alternate diagnoses, severe distress, or pneumothorax

TREATMENT

- Supportive
  - Maintain hydration via oral intake (in mild respiratory distress) or IV/nasogastric (NG)/postpyloric administration (in more significant distress)
  - Hospitalization is often determined by need for aggressive nasal/oral suctioning, oxygen for hypoxia, or supplemental hydration (e.g., IV, NG)
  - Escalation of care may necessitate high-flow nasal cannula, noninvasive positive pressure ventilation, or mechanical ventilation
- No role for albuterol or steroids
  - These are only for children with underlying asthma or perhaps severe disease
- No role for antibiotics unless there is strong suspicion of concurrent bacterial infection
- Palivizumab is a monoclonal antibody targeting RSV used prophylactically in certain high-risk populations to prevent morbidity/mortality related to bronchiolitis (for details, see Chapter 45)
- Other prophylaxis
  - Screen for tobacco smoke exposure and counsel
  - Encourage exclusive breastfeeding for at least 6 months

Foreign Body Aspiration

BASIC INFORMATION

- Aspiration of foods or small objects into the airway is a leading cause of death in infants, toddlers, and preschoolers
  - Common foods include hot dogs, whole grapes, nuts, candies, seeds, popcorn, chewing gum, meat/cheese chunks, peanut butter, and raw vegetables
  - Common objects include coins, buttons, small toys, balloons, hair accessories, rubber bands, marbles, and pen caps. Of note, button batteries and magnets are especially problematic objects in aspirations/ingestions
  - For details regarding foreign body ingestions, see Chapter 19
- Risk factors for aspiration
  - Children under 3 years of age are at highest risk:
    - Narrow airways, natural curiosity, underdeveloped swallow, distractible
  - Children with developmental delay, altered level of consciousness, or dysphagia
- Certain foreign body characteristics lead to difficulty with clearance from the airway (e.g., similar to size of the airway, cylindrical, compressible)

CLINICAL PRESENTATION

- Signs and symptoms are highly variable
  - Usually witnessed aspiration or choking, but not always
  - Laryngotracheal foreign body: more likely to present with severe respiratory distress, stridor, and hoarseness
  - Bronchial foreign body: more likely to present with cough, tachypnea, and focal wheeze or decreased air entry. Can also be asymptomatic or have delayed presentation with fever
  - Foreign body aspirations can mimic other common illnesses: asthma, bronchiolitis, croup, pneumonia

- Natural history
  - Variable courses that depend on location and degree of obstruction. However, without intervention, outcomes carry significant morbidity. Spontaneous clearance with resolution is uncommon
  - Large laryngotracheal foreign bodies can result in asphyxiation and death
  - Undiagnosed cases of bronchial foreign bodies can lead to recurrent focal pneumonias, pulmonary abscesses, and bronchiectasis. Similarly, they may present as an "asthmatic with a persistent, focal wheeze"

DIAGNOSIS AND EVALUATION

- History and physical examination are critical for timely diagnosis. Focal pulmonary examination findings should prompt further investigation
- Role of testing
  - Posteroanterior (PA) and lateral chest radiographs
    - May detect radiopaque objects
    - Enlarged lung lobe may indicate object with ball valve effect
    - Atelectatic lung lobe may indicate complete airway obstruction
    - Findings may be nonspecific
  - Although historically performed for further evaluation, lateral decubitus chest radiographs may not add significant value
- Include neck and abdomen films for foreign body ingestions
- Early rigid bronchoscopy for reasonable concern, even if negative radiographs
- In cases with low acuity/low suspicion
  - Flexible bronchoscopy can rule out distal objects
    - Typically diagnostic, but not therapeutic

TREATMENT

- In life-threatening cases first, per basic life support guidelines
  - Abdominal thrusts (Heimlich maneuver) in older children
  - Back blows/chest thrusts in infants
- Supportive therapy: continuous monitoring, supplemental oxygen
- Emergent rigid bronchoscopy with foreign body removal may be necessary if compatible history, examination, or radiographic findings.
- May consider antibiotics if clinical presentation is consistent with concurrent infection
- Preventive policies
  - Educate parents: developmentally appropriate toys, safe infant/toddler foods
  - Federal legislation: warnings on packages with small parts, size regulations for toys for young children
  - AAP recommendations
    - <5 years, no gum or hard candy
    - Raw vegetables and fruit cut into small pieces
    - Supervise children when eating

- Children should sit when eating
- Caregivers should know rescue maneuvers

Chronic Pulmonary Aspiration

BASIC INFORMATION

- Chronic aspiration can occur in patients with any one or combination of the following predisposing conditions:
  - Dysphagia
    - Discoordinated swallow
    - Weakness of pharyngeal muscles
    - Developmental delay
    - Hypotonia
  - Anatomic abnormality with loss of airway protection
    - Vocal cord paresis/paralysis
    - Laryngeal cleft
    - TEF
    - Tracheostomy
      - Regardless of cuff or mental status
  - Chronically aspirated saliva, food particles, and/or stomach acid
    - Causes inflammation of small airways
    - Airway remodeling
    - Can cause bronchiectasis

CLINICAL PRESENTATION

- May present with chronic cough or wheeze, thus mimicking asthmatics
- May present with intermittent fevers, consistent with recurrent pneumonia
- Patients may also be asymptomatic
- Over time, patients can develop bronchiectasis and demonstrate a gradual decrease in pulmonary function

DIAGNOSIS AND EVALUATION

- History and physical examination are important for timely diagnosis
- Pulmonology referral may help determine the next best steps of evaluation:
  - Chest radiograph to identify inflammation and severity of disease
  - Modified barium swallow study with speech pathologist to diagnose dysphagia
  - Esophagram to identify fistulae or strictures
  - Flexible bronchoscopy with bronchoalveolar lavage
    - Can visualize airway erythema, edema, and secretions
    - Can culture pathogenic bacteria
    - Cytology can show lipid-laden macrophages
  - Pulmonary function testing in capable patients

TREATMENT

- Topical antiinflammatory such as inhaled corticosteroids (ICS)
- Trial of bronchodilators and other airway clearance therapies for respiratory symptoms, especially for patients with neuromuscular disease or scoliosis

Table 76.3. Causes of Bronchiectasis

Previous pneumonia	Airway tumor	Juvenile idiopathic arthritis
Primary immunodeficiency	Airway malformation	Inflammatory bowel disease
Chronic pulmonary aspiration	Primary ciliary dyskinesis	Celiac disease
Retained airway foreign body	Cystic fibrosis	Idiopathic

- Controversial therapies that may help decrease upper respiratory secretions include anticholinergic agents or salivary botulinum toxin injections
- Evaluate and treat comorbid GERD and dysphagia (e.g., speech/feeding therapy, feed thickening, percutaneous gastric feeds)
- Anatomic abnormalities of the upper airway may require surgical intervention
- Antibiotics during acute bacterial pneumonias, with consideration of anaerobic coverage

Bronchiectasis

BASIC INFORMATION

- Characterized by chronic/recurrent wet cough with bronchial dilatation
- Chronic bronchial inflammation and remodeling leads to destruction of the bronchial wall and distal small airway obstruction.
- Bronchiectasis comprises many different diseases (see Table 76.3 for differential diagnosis)
  - Primary ciliary dyskinesia (PCD) and cystic fibrosis (CF) are discussed more in Chapter 78
- Those with bronchiectasis are susceptible to recurrent infections
  - Most commonly nontypeable *H. influenzae*, *S. pneumoniae*, and *Moraxella catarrhalis*
  - Adults and CF with *Pseudomonas aeruginosa*, Aspergillus, and nontuberculous mycobacteria

CLINICAL PRESENTATION

- Symptoms
  - Chronic/recurrent wet cough
  - Frequent respiratory infections that are particularly unresponsive to usual treatments and supportive care
  - Adolescents and adults are likely to produce sputum
  - More severe disease has exertional dyspnea and may not respond to antibiotics
- Physical signs
  - Crackles, rhonchi, or perhaps wheeze
  - More severe disease with digital clubbing, cyanosis, low oxyhemoglobin saturation, or respiratory distress
- Natural history
  - Recurrent exacerbations and infections
  - Malnutrition or decreased growth
  - Decreased lung function
  - Hemoptysis

- Possible pulmonary hypertension
- Symptoms and examination/imaging findings may be reversible early on, especially if underlying cause is corrected/treated

DIAGNOSIS AND EVALUATION

- Pulmonology referral is necessary for workup after suspicion for bronchiectasis is raised by history and physical examination
- Diagnostic approach has two focuses: confirmation of bronchiectasis as a diagnosis and pursuit of a causal etiology. Although several possible testing modalities are available, the diagnostic approach should be tailored to the clinical scenario of the patient
  - Imaging is often necessary:
    - Chest radiograph: bronchial dilatation, other nonspecific findings
    - High-resolution CT chest (preferred imaging method)
      More sensitive than conventional chest radiograph
      Bronchial artery dilation indicates late disease and risk of hemoptysis
  - Spirometry and pulmonary function testing
  - Flexible bronchoscopy with bronchoalveolar lavage
    - Identify structural airway abnormalities and foreign bodies; provides opportunity to culture colonizing organisms (may reveal untreated indolent infection; also useful for future antibiotic choice)
  - Sputum culture in older patients
  - Common laboratory evaluation for other causes of bronchiectasis:
    - Evaluation for CF: sweat chloride test, consider genetic testing
    - Evaluate for PCD: brush biopsy from bronchoscopy, consider genetic testing
    - Studies for immune dysfunction:
      - Serum immunoglobulin levels
      - Vaccine antigen antibody response
      - Lymphocyte subsets and functional testing
      - Neutrophil function
      - HIV testing
    - Studies for autoimmune disease: inflammatory markers
    - Swallow study and speech pathology assessment for potential chronic dysphagia and aspiration

TREATMENT

- Provide etiology-specific therapy
- Improve airway clearance
  - Exercise, chest physiotherapy, chest vest, and/or oscillating positive expiratory pressure
  - Treat comorbid asthma
- Identify exacerbations and treat quickly
  - Increase frequency of airway clearance regimen
  - Antibiotics if indicated based on microbial results
  - Other therapies as indicated
- Provide adequate nutrition
- Surveillance imaging at regular intervals
- Surveillance of colonizing organisms with culture and sensitivity

- Consider surgical removal of severe, localized disease
- Anticipatory guidance
  - Education regarding symptoms and when to seek care
  - Tobacco smoke avoidance
  - Vaccinations for influenza and *S. pneumoniae*

Asthma

BASIC INFORMATION

- Bronchial hyperreactivity due to airway inflammation from various factors
  - Air pollution
  - Tobacco smoke exposure
  - Viral respiratory infections
  - Allergens
- These factors also trigger bronchoconstriction/airway hyperresponsiveness
  - Additional triggers include:
    - Exercise
    - Cold, dry air
    - Excessive heat or humidity
    - Aerosols
    - Aspirin
    - Beta-blockers
- Modulation of immune system responses
  - Hygiene hypothesis: lack of exposure to bacterial endotoxin early in life predisposes to asthma and allergy
- IgE-mediated allergens cause biphasic response
  - Early phase (within minutes)
    - Mast cell degranulation
      Histamine
    - Airway changes
      Edema from increased vascular permeability
      Contraction of smooth muscle
      Mucus secretion
    - Resulting in
      Reversible obstruction
      Air trapping
        Prolonged exhalation with incomplete emptying
        Less room for next inspired breath
  - Late phase (4–8 hours later)
    - Leukocyte tissue infiltration
    - Contributes to airway remodeling
- Bronchiolitis in infants may predispose to recurrent wheeze
- Epidemiology
  - Major cause of pediatric emergency room (ER) visits and hospital admissions
    - Prevalence varies, but the disease etiology appears to be multifactorial, including genetics, socioeconomic factors, environmental exposures, and intrauterine exposures (e.g., tobacco)

CLINICAL PRESENTATION

- Signs and symptoms
  - Patients have persistent coughing and complain of chest tightness and dyspnea

Table 76.4.   Asthma Predictive Index

Children <3 years with at least occasional wheezing, plus one major or two minor criteria ("stringent index")

Major Criteria	Minor Criteria
Physician-made diagnosis of eczema	Physician-made diagnosis of allergic rhinitis
Physician-made diagnosis of parental asthma	Wheezing apart from colds
	Eosinophilia ≥4%

Predicts chance of asthma/recurrent wheeze after 6 years of age

Positive index: 76% chance	Negative index: <5% chance

- On examination, they have visible increase in work of breathing (e.g., tachypnea, retractions), with diffuse polyphonic wheeze. In severe cases, patients may have significant decreased air movement, making wheeze inaudible
- Asthmatics characteristically demonstrate prolonged exhalation, indicative of lower airway obstruction, as they forcefully exhale
- Cyanosis and oxyhemoglobin desaturation also occur in severe cases
  - Decrease in respiratory effort and rate may predict respiratory failure
- Natural history
  - Different phenotypic patterns
    - Acute
    - Chronic
    - Acute on chronic
  - Asthma predictive index—see Table 76.4
  - Variable course
    - Some improve or resolve, usually during puberty
    - Some continue with occasional exacerbations
    - Some worsen
  - Factors that worsen course
    - Development of allergic triggers
    - Ongoing/new environmental exposures
    - Limited access to care
  - Increased risk of hospitalization or death
    - Poor perception of symptoms
    - Poor adherence
    - Psychosocial problems
    - Daily asthma symptoms or decreased pulmonary function
    - Daily use of oral steroids
    - Excessive use of bronchodilators

DIAGNOSIS AND EVALUATION

- Clinical
  - Typical symptoms brought on by triggers and generally relieved by bronchodilators
    - Classically wheezing, but not necessarily
  - Comorbid atopic conditions, allergic rhinitis, and eczema increase likelihood
  - Positive family history for asthma or allergy increases likelihood
- Role of testing
  - Spirometry
    - Evaluate flow and volume of forcefully exhaled air

Table 76.5. Red Flags and Differential Diagnosis of Asthma-Like Conditions

Red Flag	Differential Diagnosis
Two or more pneumonias	Immunodeficiency, cystic fibrosis, primary ciliary dyskinesia
Chronic wet/productive cough	Bronchiectasis, cystic fibrosis, primary ciliary dyskinesia
Digital clubbing	Bronchiectasis, cystic fibrosis, primary ciliary dyskinesia
Chronic rhinorrhea or sinus infections	Cystic fibrosis, primary ciliary dyskinesia
Family history of male sterility	Cystic fibrosis, primary ciliary dyskinesia
Poor growth and low body mass index	Cystic fibrosis, immunodeficiency
Coughing/choking while feeding	Chronic pulmonary aspiration
Sudden symptom onset	Foreign body aspiration
Teenage onset without prior asthma history	Vocal cord dysfunction
Symptoms since birth	Laryngomalacia, tracheomalacia, vascular rings, other upper airway abnormalities
History of intubation	Subglottic stenosis
History of prematurity	Chronic lung disease of prematurity/ bronchopulmonary dysplasia
Age <3 years	Virus-associated wheezing
Cough that is absent when asleep	Habit cough

- Establish presence of baseline obstruction or restriction
- Gauge response to albuterol
- Follow measurements over time to help make treatment decisions
- Normal values do not rule out asthma
  - Peak flow meters
    - Not routinely used
    - Can help patients with poor symptom perception
  - Environmental allergy testing may be useful for severe asthma
    - Detect/confirm allergic triggers when suspicious for allergies via skin or blood testing available
    - Interpret results in clinical context because clear clinical causal association supersedes test result
  - Advanced pulmonary function testing beyond scope of this chapter
- Red flags and differential diagnosis—see Table 76.5
- Common causes of poor asthma control
  - Nonadherence
  - Poor spacer/nebulizer technique
  - Incorrect diagnosis
  - Ongoing exposures
  - Comorbidities
    - Allergic rhinitis/sinusitis/postnasal drip
    - GERD
    - Obesity
    - Deconditioning to exercise
    - OSA
- Classification of asthma
  - Based on impairment and risk
    - Consider frequency and pattern of symptoms

- Evaluate impairment of activity
- ER visits and hospital admissions
- History of rapid decompensation
- Highest risk for future life-threatening exacerbation
  - Prior intensive care unit (ICU) admission due to asthma
  - Prior endotracheal intubation
  - Prior mechanical ventilation
- Assessment of asthma severity—see Table 76.6
- Exercise-induced asthma
  - Bronchoconstriction only with exercise
  - Wheeze or cough with dyspnea or chest tightness during physical exertion
  - Symptoms begin few minutes into exercise and last for at least 30 minutes
  - Diagnosis occasionally requires an exercise stress test with spirometry
  - Environmental factors can influence frequency and severity of symptoms
  - Treatment is with bronchodilator premedication 15 minutes before activity
    - Controller medication is second line

TREATMENT

- Medications
  - Inhaled bronchodilators
    - For quick symptom relief
    - Short-acting beta-2 adrenergic agonist (SABA), albuterol/salbutamol
      - Beta-2 adrenergic receptors present in bronchial smooth muscle induce relaxation of these small airways and allow easy flow of air and relief from wheezing
      - Toxic effects include:
        - Agitation and irritability
        - Tremor
        - Insomnia
        - Tachycardia
        - Arrhythmia
        - Hyperglycemia
        - Hypokalemia at high doses
  - Short-acting muscarinic antagonist (SAMA), ipratropium
    - Typically used in ER
  - Inhaled corticosteroids (ICS)
    - Antiinflammatory medications used for maintenance therapy
    - Slow-acting
      - 4 to 6 weeks to see full response
    - Available in low, medium, and high doses
    - Prolonged high dose may cause adrenal suppression; there is an association with prolonged steroid use and a very small decrease in final height
  - Leukotriene receptor antagonist (LTRA)
    - As an adjunctive to maintenance therapy
    - Treats allergies and asthma
    - Blocks inflammatory mediators

Table 76.6. Assessment of Asthma Severity

		CLASSIFICATION OF ASTHMA SEVERITY		
		PERSISTENT		
	Intermittent	Mild	Moderate	Severe
COMPONENTS OF SEVERITY				
IMPAIRMENT				
Daytime symptoms	≤2 days/week	>2 days/week but not daily	Daily	Throughout the day
Nighttime awakenings:				
Age 0–4 years	0	1–2×/month	3–4×/month	>1×/week
Age ≥5 years	≤2×/month	3–4×/month	>1×/week but not nightly	Often 7×/week
Short-acting β_2-agonist use for symptoms (not for prevention of exercise-induced bronchospasm)	≤2 days/week	>2 days/week but not daily, and not more than 1× on any day	Daily	Several times per day
Interference with normal activity	None	Minor limitation	Some limitation	Extreme limitation
LUNG FUNCTION:				
FEV_1 % predicted, age ≥5 years	Normal FEV_1 between exacerbations >80% predicted	≥80% predicted	60%–80% predicted	<60% predicted
FEV_1:FVC ratio:				
Age 5–11 years	>85%	>80%	75%–80%	<75%
Age ≥12 years	Normal	Normal	Reduced 5%	Reduced >5%
RISK				
Exacerbations requiring systemic corticosteroids:				
Age 0–4 years	0–1/year (see notes)	≥2 exacerbations in 6 months requiring systemic corticosteroids *or* ≥4 wheezing episodes/year lasting >1 day *and* risk factors for persistent asthma		
Age ≥5 years	0–1/year (see notes)	≥2/year (see notes)	≥2/year (see notes)	≥2/year (see notes)

Consider severity and interval since last exacerbation. Frequency and severity may fluctuate over time for patients in any severity category. Relative annual risk of exacerbations may be related to FEV_1.

RECOMMENDED STEP FOR INITIATING THERAPY				
All ages	Step 1	Step 2		
Age 0–4 years			Step 3	Step 3
Age 5–11 years			Step 3, medium-dose ICS option	Step 3, medium-dose ICS option *or* Step 4
Age ≥12 years			Consider a short course of systemic corticosteroids	Consider a short course of systemic corticosteroids

In 2 to 6 weeks, evaluate level of asthma control that is achieved and adjust therapy accordingly. If no clear benefit is observed within 4 to 6 weeks, consider adjusting therapy or alternative diagnoses.

FEV₁, Forced expiratory volume in 1 second; *FVC*, forced vital capacity; *ICS*, inhaled corticosteroids.

- Combination ICS and long-acting beta agonist (ICS/LABA)
  - For maintenance therapy in moderate to severe asthma
  - Available in low, medium, and high steroid doses
- Systemic steroids
  - For exacerbations not adequately treated with SABA alone
  - Oral, IM, or IV
  - If given early, may prevent/treat late-phase response
  - Prolonged or frequent use may cause adrenal suppression
- Exacerbation management
  - Outpatient management:

- SABAs are the mainstay of treatment and should be administered at first sign of symptoms (and may repeat two more times)
- If symptoms improve, then may manage as an outpatient with SABA every 4 hours if needed
- May administer systemic corticosteroids (e.g., oral prednisolone) if symptoms persist
- Inpatient management:
  - The appropriate location of care (e.g., wards, short-stay unit, ICU) should be based on severity of symptoms/signs
  - Supportive care as needed: oxygen, IV hydration
  - Advanced medication management beyond the scope of this book includes:

Table 76.7. Stepwise Approach for Asthma Therapy

AGE	THERAPY	INTER-MITTENT ASTHMA	PERSISTENT ASTHMA: DAILY MEDICATION					
		Step 1	Step 2	Step 3	Step 4	Step 5	Step 6	
0–4 years	Preferred	SABA prn	Low-dose ICS	Medium-dose ICS	Medium-dose ICS + *either* LABA *or* LTRA	High-dose ICS + *either* LABA *or* LTRA	High-dose ICS + *either* LABA *or* LTRA *and* oral corticosteroid	
	Alternative		Cromolyn or montelukast					
5–11 years	Preferred	SABA prn	Low-dose ICS	*Either* low-dose ICS ± LABA, LTRA, or theophylline *or* medium-dose ICS	Medium-dose ICS + LABA	High-dose ICS + LABA	High-dose ICS + LABA *and* oral corticosteroid	
	Alternative		Cromolyn, LTRA, nedo-cromil, or theophylline		Medium-dose ICS + *either* LTRA *or* theophylline	High-dose ICS + *either* LTRA *or* theophylline	High-dose ICS + *either* LTRA *or* theophylline *and* oral corticosteroid	
≥12 years	Preferred	SABA prn	Low-dose ICS	Low-dose ICS + LABA *or* Medium-dose ICS	Medium-dose ICS + LABA	High-dose ICS + LABA *and* consider omali-zumab for patients with allergies	High-dose ICS + LABA + oral corticosteroid *and* consider omalizumab for patients with allergies	
	Alternative		Cromolyn, LTRA, nedo-cromil, or theophylline	Low-dose ICS + LTRA, theophylline, or zileuton	Medium-dose ICS + LTRA, theophyl-line, or zileuton			

Each step: patient education, environmental control, and management of comorbidities. Age ≥5 years: Steps 2-4: Consider subcutaneous allergen immunotherapy for patients who have allergic asthma.

QUICK-RELIEF MEDICATION FOR ALL PATIENTS

SABA as needed for symptoms. Intensity of treatment depends on severity of symptoms: Up to three treatments at 20-min intervals as needed. Short course of oral systemic corticosteroids may be needed. *Caution:* Use of SABA >2 days/week for symptom relief (not prevention of exercise-induced bronchospasm) generally indicates inadequate control and the need to step up treatment. For ages 0–4 years: With viral respiratory infection: SABA q4–6h up to 24 h (longer with physician consult). Consider short course of systemic corticosteroids if exacerbation is severe or patient has history of previous severe exacerbations.

ICS, Inhaled corticosteroid; *LABA,* inhaled long-acting β₂-agonist; *LTRA,* leukotriene receptor antagonist; *prn,* as needed; *SABA,* inhaled short-acting β₂-agonist. Data from the National Asthma Education and Prevention Program: Expert Panel Report 3 (EPR 3): Guidelines for the diagnosis and management of asthma—summary report 2007. *J Allergy Clin Immunol* 2007;120(Suppl):S94–S138.

Continuous inhaled albuterol and inhaled ipratro-pium
IV/subcutaneous terbutaline
IV magnesium
- Chest radiography not usually indicated
  Except: severe or atypical presentation (or first-time wheeze), suspicion of foreign body, suspicion for pneumothorax
- Atelectasis is common in asthma exacerbations; therefore antibiotics, chest physiotherapy, and bronchoscopy are usually not indicated
- Chronic management
  - Confirm diagnosis
    - Clinically
    - Testing as indicated

- Determine severity (see previous assessment of asthma severity)
- Identify triggers
- Start medication
  - More severe disease requires more medication
  - Stepwise approach for asthma therapy (according to severity assessment)—see Table 76.7
- Follow-up visits
  - Assess control
  - Identify triggers
  - Step therapy up or down if needed
  - Review medication technique and indications
  - Review concerns and set goals
- Educate parent and patient
  - Goals of treatment

- Rationale for medications
  - Take controller medications consistently to prevent exacerbations
- Use of medications
- Spacer/nebulizer technique
- Elimination of triggers
- Establish an asthma action plan
  - Recognize signs of exacerbation
    - Cough, wheeze, chest tightness, dyspnea, activity limitation
    - Prolonged exhalation, tachypnea, retractions, grunting
    - Persistent signs or symptoms despite SABA are concerning
    - Severe exacerbation
      - Dyspnea prevents feeding, walking, or talking
      - Pallor or cyanosis
      - Irritability or lethargy
      - Severe retractions
      - Poor air movement
  - When and how to seek care
- Establish follow-up schedule
  - Every 2 to 6 weeks while establishing control
  - Every 3 months if step-down in therapy desired
- Assure adequate follow-up

Review Questions

For review questions, please go to ExpertConsult.com.

Suggested Readings

1. Balfour-Lynn IM, Davies JC. Acute infections that produce upper airway obstruction. In: Wilmott RW, et al., eds. *Kendig and Chernick's Disorders of the Respiratory Tract in Children.* 8th ed. Philadelphia: Elsevier Saunders; 2012:424–436.
2. Clemmens C, Piccione J. Airway evaluation: bronchoscopy, laryngoscopy, and tracheal aspirates. In: Goldsmith JP, ed. *Assisted Ventilation of the Neonate.* 6th ed. Philadelphia: Elsevier; 2017:118–123.
3. De Alarcon A, Cotton RT, Rutter MJ. Laryngeal and tracheal airway disorders. In: Wilmott RW, et al., eds. *Kendig and Chernick's Disorders of the Respiratory Tract in Children.* 8th ed. Philadelphia: Elsevier Saunders; 2012:424–436.
4. Goyal V, Grimwood K, Marchant J, Masters IB, Chang AB. Pediatric bronchiectasis: no longer an orphan disease. *Pediatr Pulmonol.* 2016;51(5):450–469.
5. Green SS. Ingested and aspirated foreign bodies. *Pediatr Rev.* 2015;36(10):430–436.
6. Licari A, Manca E, Rispoli GA, et al. Congenital vascular rings: a clinical challenge for the pediatrician. *Pediatr Pulmonol.* 2015;50:511–524.
7. Link HW. Pediatric asthma in a nutshell. *Pediatr Rev.* 2014;35(7):287–298.
8. Marcus CL, Brooks LJ, et al. Diagnosis and management of childhood obstructive sleep apnea syndrome. *Pediatr.* 2012;130(3):576–584.
9. O' Sullivan B, Kinane TB. Congenital lung anomalies. In: Light MJ, ed. *Pediatric Pulmonology.* 1st ed. American Academy of Pediatrics; 2011:277–307.
10. Ralston SL, Lieberthal AS, Meissner HC, et al. Clinical practice guideline: the diagnosis, management, and prevention of bronchiolitis. *Pediatrics.* 2014;134(5):e1474–e1502.
11. Schroeder JW, McColley S. Congenital abnormalities of the upper airway. In: Light MJ, ed. *Pediatric pulmonology.* 1st ed. American Academy of Pediatrics; 2011:263–276.
12. Sharma GD, Conrad C. Croup, epiglottitis, and bacterial tracheitis. In: Light MJ, ed. *Pediatric pulmonology.* 1st ed. American Academy of Pediatrics; 2011:347–363.
13. Vincencio AG, Parikh S. Laryngomalacia and tracheomalacia: common dynamic airway lesions. *Pediatr Rev.* 2006;27(4):33–35.
14. Virbalas J, Smith L. Upper airway obstruction. *Pediatr Rev.* 2015;36(2):62–74.

77 Parenchymal and Extrapulmonary Disorders

ELIZABETH GIBB, MD and KENSHO IWANAGA, MD, MS

Three important components of the respiratory system include the parenchyma (alveoli, interstitium, and pulmonary vasculature), the pleural space, and the thoracic cage (vertebrae, ribs, diaphragm, and accessory muscles of respiration). Disorders affecting these components of the respiratory system typically diminish lung compliance, which can manifest with tachypnea and use of the accessory muscles of breathing (retractions). A restrictive pattern with a decrease in forced vital capacity can be seen on spirometry and decreased lung volumes on body plethysmography. If extensive, it can also impair gas exchange, and initial symptoms can include exercise intolerance, dyspnea, and fatigue. Images of the chest (plain film and computed tomography) are the most helpful means to assess the degree and severity of involvement.

PARENCHYMAL DISORDERS

Pneumonia

BASIC INFORMATION

- Acute infection of the lung parenchyma
- Impacts on the population
  - Common cause of outpatient visits and hospitalization in children
  - Leading cause of childhood mortality worldwide
- Risk factors
  - Low socioeconomic status
  - Malnutrition
  - Air pollution
  - Cigarette smoke
  - Underlying cardiopulmonary disease
  - Immunodeficiency
  - Sickle cell disease
  - Neuromuscular weakness
  - Gastroesophageal reflux
  - Aspiration
- Etiologies can be divided into broad categories based on pathogens and host factors:
- Age
  - Neonatal (primarily vertical transmission)
    - Group B streptococcus
    - *Escherichia coli*
    - Listeria monocytogenes
    - Ureaplasma urealyticum
    - TORCH (*Toxoplasma gondii*, rubella, cytomegalovirus [CMV], herpes simplex virus [HSV])

- Infants (3 weeks to 3 months)
  - Vertical transmission
    - Includes neonatal infections (previous)
    - *Chlamydia trachomatis*
      - "Afebrile pneumonia of infancy"
      - Staccato cough
      - Diffuse inspiratory crackles
      - Possible conjunctivitis
      - Interstitial infiltrates on chest radiograph
  - Viruses
    - Respiratory syncytial virus (RSV)
    - Parainfluenza
    - Influenza
    - Adenovirus
    - Metapneumovirus
    - Rhinovirus
  - Bacteria
    - *Streptococcus pneumoniae* (most common bacterial cause of pneumonia in children)
    - *Bordetella pertussis* (afebrile, paroxysmal cough, apnea, and aspiration)
  - 3 months to <5 years
    - Viruses (same as infants, previous)
    - Bacteria
      - *S. pneumoniae*
      - *Haemophilus influenzae*
      - *Moraxella catarrhalis*
      - *Mycoplasma pneumoniae*
      - *Staphylococcus aureus*
      - *S. pyogenes*
  - 5 years to adolescence
    - Bacteria
      - *M. pneumoniae* (most common treatable cause in school-age children)
      - *Chlamydophila pneumoniae*
      - *S. pneumoniae*
    - Atypical Pneumoniae
      - Viral causes are still common
      - Depending on exposure and geography, consider
        - *Mycobacterium tuberculosis*
          - Homeless, incarcerated, or immigrants from Asia, Africa, Latin America, Eastern Europe
        - Endemic fungal infections
          - *Coccidioides immitis* (Southwest, Central, and Southern United States)
          - *Histoplasma capsulatum* (Mississippi, Missouri, and Ohio River Valley)
          - *Blastomyces dermatitidis* (Southeast and Great Lakes)

- Animal exposures
  - Birds (*Chlamydophila psittaci*)
  - Sheep, goats, cattle, cats (*Coxiella burnetii*)
- Host factors
  - Routine childhood pneumococcal vaccination has shifted the frequency of pneumococcal strains toward those not covered in the primary series
    - Whereas invasive pneumococcal disease has decreased after the introduction of pneumococcal vaccines, empyema has continued to increase
  - Immunocompromised status may increase the likelihood of certain infectious pathogens
    - Impaired cellular immunity (HIV, chemotherapy, systemic steroids)
      - Viruses (including rubeola, varicella-zoster virus [VZV], CMV, Epstein-Barr virus [EBV])
      - *Pneumocystis jirovecii*
      - Legionella
      - *S. aureus*
      - Opportunistic fungi, including *Aspergillus* and *Fusarium* spp.
    - Impaired humoral immunity (including functional asplenia seen in patients with sickle cell anemia)
      - Consider encapsulated organisms
      - *S. pneumoniae*
      - *H. influenzae*
      - *S. aureus*
  - Neurologic impairment
    - Increased risk for aspiration
    - Pathogens include anaerobic *Streptococci*, *Fusobacterium* spp., *Bacteroides* spp., and *Prevotella* spp.
  - Cystic fibrosis
    - *S. aureus*
    - *H. influenzae*
    - *Pseudomonas aeruginosa*
    - *Stenotrophomonas maltophilia*
    - *Burkholderia cepacia* complex
  - Health-care associated/nosocomial pneumonia
    - Gram-negative bacilli
    - *S. aureus*

CLINICAL PRESENTATION

- Symptoms consistent with a lower respiratory tract infection
  - Fever may be only sign, but presence is variable and nonspecific (may increase respiratory rate in children without pneumonia)
  - Cough (common)
  - May be associated with "rust"-colored sputum
- Presenting symptoms by pathogen
  - Viral
    - Low-grade/absent fever
    - Nasal congestion
    - Diffuse wheezes and/or crackles on auscultation
    - Diffuse interstitial infiltrates on chest imaging
  - Community-acquired bacterial pathogens
    - Abrupt onset
    - High fever
    - Ill appearance
    - Focal findings on chest examination
    - Focal infiltrate on chest imaging

- *S. pneumoniae* is the most common bacterial pathogen in all ages
- Prevalence of *S. aureus* is also increasing
  - Methicillin-resistant *S. aureus* (MRSA) can be hospital-acquired or community-acquired
  - Associated with rapid disease progression and complications including pneumatoceles, necrotizing pneumonia, empyema, and lung abscesses
- Mycoplasma and Chlamydophila
  - Prodrome of headache, fever, pharyngitis
  - Can also be associated with
    - Polyarthritis
    - Central nervous system involvement
    - Cardiac involvement
    - Gastrointestinal (GI) involvement (pancreatitis or hepatitis)
    - Rash (including Stevens-Johnson syndrome)
- Physical findings consistent with parenchymal involvement
  - Respiratory distress reflecting decreased pulmonary compliance
    - Tachypnea (most sensitive sign)
    - Retractions
    - Nasal flaring
    - Head bobbing
    - Grunting
  - Pulmonary examination
    - Airway involvement
      - Crackles
      - Wheezing (more common in atypical or viral pneumonia)
    - Findings seen with atelectasis and consolidation
      - Dullness to percussion
      - Tactile fremitus
      - Diminished breath sounds
      - Bronchial breath sounds
      - Egophony
      - Whispered pectoriloquy
  - Hypoxemia
    - More common in atypical or viral pneumonia
    - May not be seen even with large focal involvement
- Radiographic evidence of pulmonary infiltrates
- Complications
  - Local: pleural effusions, empyema, necrotizing pneumonia, abscess, pneumatocele
  - Systemic: respiratory failure, sepsis, hemolytic uremic syndrome
  - Metastatic: meningitis, osteomyelitis, septic arthritis
  - Other: hyponatremia, thought to be due to syndrome of inappropriate antidiuretic hormone secretion (SIADH)

DIAGNOSIS AND EVALUATION

- Imaging
  - Generally not indicated for most outpatients who are previously healthy, fully immunized, and well-appearing on examination
  - Indications for chest radiograph
    - Severe disease
    - Hospitalization
    - To exclude alternate explanations of respiratory distress
    - No improvement with initial therapy

- To assess for complications (pleural effusion)
- Radiographic findings
  - Typical bacteria: alveolar infiltrates, lobar consolidation
  - Atypical bacteria/virus: interstitial infiltrates
  - Tuberculosis (TB): mediastinal or hilar adenopathy, apical or interstitial infiltrates
- Repeat imaging after resolution of illness
  - Not routinely required in children who recover
  - Consider for patients with progressive symptoms or failure to improve within 48 to 72 hours of antibiotic therapy
  - Consider repeat imaging 4 to 6 weeks after recovery in patients with
    - Recurrent pneumonia in the same location
    - Suspicion for underlying anatomic abnormality
- Laboratory and microbiology
  - Generally not indicated for most outpatients who are previously healthy, fully immunized, and well-appearing on examination
  - Erythrocyte sedimentation rate (ESR) and C-reactive protein (CRP) may be helpful to monitor response to therapy for cases of complicated pneumonia
  - Culture
    - Blood
      - Although low yield in most pneumonia (e.g., outpatient, nontoxic in appearance), may be indicated in inpatients and those with moderate to severe pneumonia
    - Sputum
      - May be indicated in inpatients old enough to expectorate, those requiring intensive care, those with complicated pneumonia
      - An adequate sample is indicated by <10 epithelial cells and >25 neutrophils under low-power microscopy
    - Pleural fluid (see Parapneumonic Effusions and Empyema, below)
    - Other studies
      - Nasopharyngeal samples do not correlate well with lower-airway samples
      - Viral polymerase chain reaction (PCR) panel can be helpful to decrease need for further testing and avoid antibiotic therapy
      - Serologic testing is usually not recommended
        - PCR and serologic testing for Mycoplasma can be helpful, but false positives are common
      - Consider TB testing based on risk factors
        - Interferon gamma release assays are more specific than tuberculin skin tests, particularly if there is a history of Bacillus Calmette–Guérin (BCG) administration
      - Urine antigen testing for Legionella
      - Serum and urine testing for Histoplasmosis
      - Serum testing for *Cryptococcus* spp.
      - Beta-d-glucan and lactate dehydrogenase (LDH) for *P. jirovecii*
      - Galactomannan antigen from serum or bronchoalveolar lavage for *Aspergillus* spp.

TREATMENT

- Outpatient therapy (generally treated for 7–10 days)
  - 3 months to <5 years of age

- Initial: high-dose amoxicillin
- Consider addition of azithromycin if there is high suspicion for atypical pneumonia
  - >5 years of age
- Initial: azithromycin
- Consider addition of amoxicillin if there is high suspicion for bacterial pneumonia
- Indications for admission
  - Young age (<3-6 months)
  - Dehydration, inability to maintain hydration orally
  - Moderate to severe respiratory distress
  - Hypoxemia (SpO$_2$ <90%-92%) in room air
  - Ill or toxic appearance
  - Failed outpatient treatment (worsening or no response within 48–72 hours)
  - Complicated pneumonia (PNA)
  - Underlying medical conditions that may predispose patient to complicated pneumonia, may be worsened by pneumonia or affect patient's response to treatment
  - Inability of family to assure adherence to home therapy
- Inpatient therapy
  - Initial: ampicillin or penicillin G
    - If 0 to <3 months of age, add gentamicin or cefotaxime (and consider macrolide if there is concern for chlamydia or pertussis)
    - Consider azithromycin if there is high suspicion for atypical pneumonia
    - Alternative regimens include ceftriaxone or cefotaxime with or without vancomycin or clindamycin (especially for complicated pneumonia)
      - Consider vancomycin if patient is not fully immunized for *S. pneumoniae* or if there is a high prevalence of penicillin resistance in the community
      - Should consider vancomycin for MRSA coverage
  - Aspiration pneumonia
    - Initial: amoxicillin-clavulanic acid
    - Alternative regimens include ampicillin-sulbactam or clindamycin
  - Hospital-acquired pneumonia
    - Consider broader coverage, including Gram-negatives (gentamicin, piperacillin-tazobactam, meropenem, ceftazidime, cefepime) and Gram-positives (clindamycin, vancomycin)
  - Duration of therapy
    - Administer parenteral antibiotics until there is clinical improvement (afebrile for 24–48 hours, tolerating oral intake)
    - Complicated pneumonias often require regimens of at least 2 to 4 weeks

Acute Respiratory Distress Syndrome (ARDS)

BASIC INFORMATION

- Diffuse, progressive, inflammatory lung disease characterized by
  - Rapid onset of tachypnea, dyspnea, and hypoxemia
  - Diffuse alveolar opacities on chest radiographs
  - Noncardiogenic pulmonary edema

- Minimal or no response to supplemental oxygen therapy
- Etiology
  - Pulmonary (direct) causes
    - Pneumonia
    - Bronchiolitis
    - Near-drowning
    - Pulmonary contusion
    - Toxic inhalation injury
  - Nonpulmonary (indirect) causes
    - Sepsis
    - Nonthoracic trauma
    - Transfusion of blood products
    - Cardiopulmonary bypass
    - Acute pancreatitis

CLINICAL PRESENTATION

- Classically progresses through relatively discrete pathologic phases
  - Acute exudative
    - Diffuse but heterogeneous alveolar damage with pulmonary edema, cytokine release, and activated neutrophils
    - Increased intrapulmonary shunting
    - Reduced lung and chest wall compliance
  - Proliferative
    - Proliferation of type II alveolar cells
    - Interstitial infiltration by myofibroblasts
    - Early deposition of collagen
  - Fibrotic (progression to this phase is associated with worse outcomes)
    - Increased alveolar dead space
    - Hypoxemia
    - Reduced lung compliance

DIAGNOSIS AND EVALUATION

- Berlin definition of ARDS
  - Timing: respiratory symptoms occurring within 1 week of a known clinical insult, or new or worsening symptoms
  - Imaging: bilateral opacities not fully explained by pleural effusions, lobar collapse, lung collapse, or pulmonary nodules
  - Origin of pulmonary edema: respiratory failure not fully explained by cardiac failure or fluid overload
  - Impairment of oxygenation
    - Mild: 200 mm Hg < PaO_2/FiO_2 ≤300 mm Hg with positive end-expiratory pressure (PEEP) or continuous positive airway pressure (CPAP) ≥5 cm H_2O
    - Moderate: 100 mm Hg < PaO2/FiO2 ≤200 mm Hg with PEEP ≥5 cm H_2O
    - Severe: PaO_2/FiO_2 ≤100 mm Hg with PEEP ≥5 cm H_2O
- Pediatric Acute Lung Injury Consensus Conference (PALICC) definition of ARDS (2015)
  - Recently revised definition, with critical criteria similar to those of Berlin, except for measurement of oxygenation defect via calculation of oxygenation index (OI) or oxygen saturation index (OSI), which take into account the mean airway pressure delivered via ventilator

TREATMENT

- Ventilatory protective strategies
  - Low tidal volumes (~6–8 mL/kg)
  - Limiting peak inspiratory pressure to <30 cm H_2O
  - High PEEP (5–12 cm H_2O)
  - Limiting FiO_2 (accepting SpO_2 >mid-80%)
  - Permissive hypercapnia ($PaCO_2$ 60–80 mm Hg as long as pH is >7.2)
  - May consider high-frequency oscillatory ventilation
- Consider adjunctive therapies
  - Neuromuscular blockade
  - Prone positioning
  - Nitric oxide
  - Surfactant
- Most common cause of death is multiorgan system failure

Bronchopulmonary dysplasia (see Chapter 75)

Congenital diaphragmatic hernia (see Chapter 75)

Drowning (see Chapter 17)

EXTRAPULMONARY DISORDERS

Pleural Effusion

BASIC INFORMATION

- Normal pleural fluid volume reflects a complex interplay between pleural permeability and absorption (normally up to 0.3 mL/kg present)
  - Changes in hydrostatic and oncotic pressures, as well as lymphatic uptake, can lead to fluid accumulation in the potential space
- Exudative effusions
  - Causes
    - Pleural inflammation (secondary to infection, noninfectious inflammation, or malignancy) leading to endothelial barrier breakdown and leakage of proteins and plasma
    - Exacerbated by impaired lymphatic drainage of the pleural space
  - Diagnostic criteria (Light's Criteria Rule)
    - Pleural fluid protein/serum protein ratio greater than 0.5, or
    - Pleural fluid LDH/serum LDH ratio greater than 0.6, or
    - Pleural fluid LDH greater than two-thirds the upper limits of normal serum LDH
- Transudative effusions
  - Causes
    - Imbalances in hydrostatic and oncotic pressures in the chest
      Iatrogenic overhydration

Congestive heart failure

Nephrotic syndrome

Liver cirrhosis

- Special cases
  - Increased amylase in pleural fluid: esophageal rupture, pancreatitis, malignancy
  - Decreased glucose: systemic lupus erythematosus (SLE), rheumatoid arthritis, TB, malignancy, esophageal rupture
  - See also Nelson Textbook of Pediatrics, Chapter 410, Pleurisy, Pleural Effusions, and Empyema."

Parapneumonic Effusions and Empyema

BASIC INFORMATION

- Account for >95% of local complications of pneumonia
- Common pathogens
  - S. pneumoniae
  - Other streptococcal species (especially S. pyogenes)
  - S. aureus
- Simple parapneumonic effusion: not yet infected with bacteria
- Empyema: grossly purulent fluid in pleural cavity and infected with bacteria
  - Exudative stage
    - Pleura inflamed, leading to increased capillary permeability, which allows leakage of protein, leukocytes, and fluid
    - Fluid: normal glucose, normal pH, low cell count, sterile fluid
    - Pleural fluid normally layers out on chest imaging
  - Fibrinopurulent stage
    - Large numbers of polymorphonuclear leukocytes (PMNs) accumulate in pleural fluid
    - Bacteria invade
    - Fibrin deposition on pleural surfaces
    - Form loculations
    - Pleural fluid: low pH (<7.3) and glucose (<60), increased LDH, positive Gram stain and culture
  - Organizational stage
    - Fibroblasts grow on the pleural surfaces, forming an inelastic "peel"

CLINICAL PRESENTATION

- Failure to improve with appropriate antibiotic therapy should prompt suspicion for a parapneumonic effusion/empyema
- Symptoms
  - Dyspnea
  - Pleuritic chest pain
  - Referred pain to the back and/or shoulders
- Physical examination findings
  - Dullness to percussion
  - Decrease in tactile fremitus
  - Decreased breath sounds
  - Pleural friction rub

DIAGNOSIS AND EVALUATION

- Chest radiograph
  - Blunting of costophrenic angle
  - Layering on decubitus views suggests free-flowing fluid
  - Absence of layering suggests a loculated effusion or empyema
  - Air-fluid levels may be seen if infected with gas-forming organisms, or if there is communication with gas-filled cavities (e.g., pneumothorax, bronchopulmonary fistula)
- Ultrasound
  - Assess size of effusion
  - Assess for loculations that may preclude simple tube thoracostomy drainage
- Pleural fluid analysis (see previous)

TREATMENT

- Antimicrobial therapy
  - Coverage should be appropriate for S. pneumoniae and S. aureus
    - Length of therapy: no available data that have been derived from high-quality randomized controlled trials
  - Indications for a trial of oral antibiotics
    - Short duration of symptoms
    - Mild symptoms
    - No respiratory distress
    - Small effusion (measuring less than 10 mm on lateral decubitus view or occupying less than one-fourth of the hemithorax on upright view)
  - Indications for parenteral antibiotics include respiratory distress and expanding/large effusion
    - Continue parenteral antibiotics until the patient has been afebrile and is clinically improving overall (may use ESR and CRP to guide assessments)
    - Transition to enteral antibiotic, often for up to an additional 4 weeks
- Indications for needle or tube thoracostomy with parenteral antibiotics
  - Respiratory distress
  - Rapidly enlarging effusion
  - Large effusion (measuring more than 10 mm on lateral decubitus view or occupying more than one-fourth of the hemithorax on upright view)
- Indications for tube thoracostomy with possible fibrinolytic therapy or video-assisted thoracoscopic surgery (VATS), with parenteral antibiotics
  - Loculated parapneumonic effusion
  - Empyema
- Follow-up: repeat chest radiograph 1 to 2 months after recovery

Pneumothorax

BASIC INFORMATION

- Spontaneous pneumothorax occurs in the absence of trauma
  - Primary: no underlying lung disease that would predispose to air leak

- Secondary: associated with underlying disease
  - Connective tissue disease (Marfan, Ehlers-Danlos)
  - SLE
  - Smoking
  - Obstructive lung disease (distal air trapping and acinar dilation)
    - Cystic fibrosis
    - Asthma
  - Postinfectious with pneumatocele formation
    - *S. pneumoniae*
    - *M. tuberculosis*
    - *P. jirovecii*
- Spontaneous pneumomediastinum frequently occurs in the presence of acute asthma exacerbation
  - Due to alveolar rupture
    - Air tracks along vascular sheaths to the hilum
    - Air tracks cephalad to subcutaneous tissue of neck (crepitus on examination)
- Can also occur with esophageal rupture/perforation

CLINICAL PRESENTATION

- Symptoms
  - Acute-onset pleuritic chest pain
  - Dyspnea
  - Classic case: tall, thin males with history of smoking
- Physical examination
  - Tachypnea
  - Tachycardia
  - Cyanosis
  - Distant/muffled breath sounds
- Differential diagnosis of intrathoracic hyperlucency
  - Congenital diaphragmatic hernia with bowel herniation
  - Congenital lobar emphysema
  - Congenital pulmonary airway malformation

TREATMENT

- Initial
  - Small pneumothorax <25% of pleural space with no respiratory compromise
    - Observation: Patients can most often be observed
    - FiO_2 1.0 oxygen "washes out" ambient air (FiO_2 0.21) and favors resorption of extraalveolar air; this requires a nonrebreather (nasal cannula is insufficient to substantially increase FiO_2)
  - Large, persisting, and/or symptomatic pneumothorax
    - Thoracentesis: aiming towards the superior portion of the thorax (opposite of fluid drainage)
- Recurrent
  - VATS exploration
    - Removal of loculated areas
    - Removal or oversewing of blebs
  - Pleurodesis
    - Mechanical scraping of the pleural surface is thought to be more effective than application of a chemical irritant (talc, doxycycline)

Thoracic Deformities

BASIC INFORMATION

- Chest wall and spinal disorders can reduce respiratory system compliance and manifest with a restrictive pattern on objective pulmonary function testing
  - Decreased forced vital capacity (FVC) on spirometry
  - Decreased lung volumes including total lung capacity (TLC) on body plethysmography
  - Decreased maximal inspiratory pressures
  - Decreased maximal expiratory pressures
  - Decreased peak cough flow
- Scoliosis: lateral and/or rotational curvature of the spine
  - Idiopathic
    - Infantile (<3 years of age)
    - Juvenile (3–9 years of age)
    - Adolescent (10 years of age and older)
  - Congenital
    - Failure of vertebral formation
    - Failure of vertebral segmentation
  - Neuromuscular
    - Cerebral palsy
    - Muscular dystrophy
    - Syringomyelia
  - Associated with neurofibromatosis
  - Mesenchymal
  - Marfan syndrome
  - Mucopolysaccharidosis
  - Osteogenesis imperfecta
  - Traumatic
    - Fracture
    - Radiation
    - Surgery
    - Spinal cord tumor

CLINICAL PRESENTATION

- Exercise tolerance limited more by respiratory than cardiac factors
  - Increased dead space (Vd/Vt) with progressive scoliosis
  - Increased resting respiratory rate
  - Use of accessory muscles of inspiration
    - Sternocleidomastoid
    - External intercostals
  - Nocturnal hypoventilation/hypoxemia
    - Functional residual capacity is reduced in the supine position
    - Decreased muscle tone of the respiratory and upper airway muscles
  - Pain (based on spinal alignment)
    - Nerve root compression
    - Muscle strain

TREATMENT

- Bracing
  - Partial or temporary repair
  - May facilitate eventual surgical intervention needed later on

- Surgery
  - Goal is to avoid spine fusion or delay as long as possible to preserve spine growth
    - Adolescent idiopathic scoliosis
      - Can stabilize or improve lung volume to a variable amount
    - Congenital scoliosis
      - Can stabilize lung volume and attenuate progressive decline
    - Neuromuscular scoliosis
      - Can stabilize the chest and/or spine
      - No improvements in lung volume
      - May improve quality of life

Review Questions

For review questions, please go to ExpertConsult.com.

Suggested Readings

1. Bradley JS, Byington CL, Shah SS, Alverson B, Carter ER, Harrison C, Kaplan SL, Mace SE, McCracken Jr GH, Moore MR, St Peter SD, Stockwell JA, Swanson JT. The management of community-acquired pneumonia in infants and children older than 3 months of age: Clinical practice guidelines by the Pediatric Infectious Diseases Society and the Infectious Diseases Society of America. *Clin Infect Dis.* 2011;53(7):e25–e76.

2. Carter E, Waldhausen J, Zhang W, Hoffman L, Redding G. Management of children with empyema: Pleural drainage is not always necessary. *Pediatr Pulmonol.* 2010;45(5):475–480.

3. Ferguson ND, Fan E, Camporota L, Antonelli M, Anzueto A, Beale R, Brochard L, Brower R, Esteban A, Gattinoni L, Rhodes A, Slutsky AS, Vincent JL, Rubenfeld GD, Thompson BT, Ranieri VM. The Berlin definition of ARDS: an expanded rationale, justification, and supplementary material. *Intensive Care Med.* 2012;38(10):1573–1582.

4. Gereige RS, Laufer PM. Pneumonia. *Pediatr Rev.* 2013;34(10):438–456.

5. Idris AH, Berg RA, Bierens J, Bossaert L, Branche CM, Gabrielli A, Graves SA, Handley AJ, Hoelle R, Morley PT, Papa L, Pepe PE, Quan L, Szpilman D, Wigginton JG, Modell JH. American Heart Association. Recommended guidelines for uniform reporting of data from drowning: the "Utstein style." *Circulation.* 2003;108(20):2565–2574.

6. Kaplan SL, Barson WJ, Lin PL, Romero JR, Bradley JS, Tan TQ, Hoffman JA, Givner LB, Mason Jr EO. Early trends for invasive pneumococcal infections in children after the introduction of the 13-valent pneumococcal conjugate vaccine. *Pediatr Infect Dis J.* 2013;32(3):203–217.

7. Shah SS, DiCristina CM, Bell LM, Ten Have T, Metlay JP. Primary early thoracoscopy and reduction in length of hospital stay and additional procedures among children with complicated pneumonia: Results of a multicenter retrospective cohort study. *Arch Pediatr Adolesc Med.* 2008;162(7):675–681.

78 Systemic Diseases With Pulmonary Involvement

JAMIE DY, MD and GWYNNE CHURCH, MD

Cystic Fibrosis

Cystic fibrosis (CF) is the most common lethal genetic disease in the Caucasian population. It is caused by a mutation in the gene encoding the CF transmembrane regulatory protein (CFTR), a membrane glycoprotein that regulates ion transport at certain epithelial surfaces. Inherited in an autosomal recessive pattern, it causes a multisystem disorder that affects the sweat glands and respiratory, gastrointestinal, and reproductive tracts. Although historically a cause of early death in childhood, medical therapies and, more recently, genetically targeted therapies have extended life expectancy into middle age for many.

See also Nelson Textbook of Pediatrics, Chapter 403, "Cystic Fibrosis."

BASIC INFORMATION

- CFTR protein is a chloride channel of epithelial cells. Its functions include:
  - Downregulating active sodium transport by epithelial sodium channel (ENaC), an active sodium pump
  - Regulating calcium-activated chloride channels and potassium channels
  - Transporting or regulating bicarbonate transport through epithelial cell membranes
  - Regulating inflammatory responses and cell signaling
- CFTR dysfunction results in decreased chloride secretion and increased sodium absorption from the airway lumen, which leads to dehydrated and viscous mucus
  - In the sweat gland, decreased sodium and chloride absorption from the duct lumen leads to hypertonic sweat
- Although CF affects many parts of the body, the leading cause of morbidity and mortality is from the pulmonary manifestations
- Epidemiology
  - In the United States, the incidence of CF is most common in those of northern European ancestry (see Table 78.1)
  - Approximately 1 out of 25 people is an asymptomatic carrier (which also varies by race)
  - Median survival has increased to over 40 years of age
- Genetic mutations
  - *CFTR* is a large gene located on chromosome 7. Over 2000 *CFTR* mutations have been identified
  - There are five different classes of genetic mutations, which determine the amount of functioning CFTR at the surface and therefore the clinical severity (see Table 78.2)

- The most common mutation is $\Delta F508$; 85% of CF patients in the United States have at least one $\Delta F508$ mutation, and 50% are homozygous. Most of the non-$\Delta F508$ mutations are rare and occur in <1% of CF patients
- CF genotype predicts the severity of disease for the sweat duct, pancreas, and reproductive system
- CF genotype does not predict the severity of lung disease. Patients who are homozygous for $\Delta F508$ exhibit a wide spectrum in the rate of development and severity of lung disease
- 5% to 10% of functioning CFTR at the cell surface protects against severe disease

Lung Pathophysiology

- CFTR dysfunction induces pulmonary disease through a cascade of events that follow the initial formation of dehydrated secretions and results in chronic inflammation, bacterial infection, and eventually bronchiectasis, or dilated airways due to destruction of the muscular and elastic component of bronchial walls. Once the airways become bronchiectatic, the structure-function relationship is further distorted such that mucociliary clearance is even further impaired, resulting in a "vicious circle" and worsening of bronchiectasis
- Additional pathogenic factors include:
  - Impaired ciliary beating: the dehydrated airway surface liquid impairs normal ciliary beating, leading to mucus plaques adherent to the cell wall. The thick secretions become relatively impenetrable to the natural host defenses
  - Role of polymorphonuclear leukocytes (PMNs): PMNs become entrapped in the mucus. They release oxidants, elastase, and other proteases, which leads to destruction of the bronchial walls. As the PMNs die, their DNA is released into the mucus, which makes it even more viscous

Table 78.1. Incidence of Cystic Fibrosis in the United States by Race

Race	Incidence in the United States
Caucasian	1/3200
Hispanic	1/8450
Native American	1/11,000
African	1/15,000
Asian	1/31,000

Table 78.2. *CFTR* Mutation Classes

Mutation Class	Mutation Type	Defect	Phenotype	Common Mutation	*CFTR* Modulator
I	Nonsense; premature stop codon	*CFTR* is not produced	Severe	*G542X*	X
II	Defective protein processing	*CFTR* is improperly folded and is degraded in the endoplasmic reticulum	Severe	*ΔF508*	Lumacaftor/ivacaftor (improves misfolding and gating abnormality)
III	Defective regulation	Disordered regulation; for example, less ATP binding	Milder	*G551D*	Ivacaftor (improves gating abnormality)
IV	Defective conductance	Conduction defect	Milder	*R117H*	X
V	Reduced synthesis	Promotor or splicer abnormality leading to decreased synthesis	Milder	*3849+10kbC→T*	X

X = not yet developed.

- Oxidative gradients: the thick, sticky mucus gains in height as more secretions are formed and develops oxygen gradients, such that there is very low oxygen tension at the cell surface
- *Pseudomonas aeruginosa*: this bacteria is able to thrive in the mucus as a facultative anaerobe with a motile flagellum. Eventually the bacteria form macrocolonies, which produce an alginate gel that makes them practically invulnerable to the host defenses. At this point, the *P. aeruginosa* is referred to as mucoid, and a patient will most likely never be rid of it. Most CF patients acquire it by age 2 years, and eventually it is isolated from sputum cultures in 80% of patients
- Other microorganisms commonly associated with chronic infection and inflammation of the CF lung: *Staphylococcus aureus, Haemophilus influenzae,* Stenotrophomonas and other Gram-negative organisms, atypical mycobacteria, Aspergillus species

Gastrointestinal Pathophysiology

- Hepatobiliary disease: the thick secretions may lead to blocked bile ducts. Some patients will develop obstructive cirrhosis
- Pancreatic disease: the inspissated secretions block the pancreatic ducts, which begins in utero. The enzymes become activated, leading to autodigestion of the pancreas with exocrine dysfunction followed by endocrine dysfunction
- Exocrine dysfunction: Low or absent levels of pancreatic amylase, lipase, colipase, and phospholipases. Insufficient secretion of pancreatic enzymes into the gut results in malabsorption of fat, fat-soluble vitamins (ADEK), protein, and other nutrients
- Endocrine dysfunction: the development of insulin resistance and diabetes occurs in some patients during adolescence or young adulthood
- Intestinal disease: the dehydrated, thick secretions can lead to intestinal obstruction

Reproductive Pathophysiology

- More than 95% of men with CF are infertile secondary to congenital bilateral absence of the vas deferens (CBAVD). No spermatozoa are present in semen—obstructive azoospermia
- Female fertility can be reduced by viscous cervical mucus, advanced lung disease, or malnutrition

Table 78.3. Mnemonic for Clinical Presentations Associated With Cystic Fibrosis

I	Infertility
M	Meconium ileus
C	Cough
F	Failure to thrive
P	Pancreatic insufficiency
A	"Refractory asthma"
N	Nasal polyps
C	Clubbing
R	Rectal prolapse
E	Electrolyte abnormalities (hyponatremia, hypochloremia, hypokalemia, metabolic alkalosis)
A	Atypical organisms from sputum
S	"Sludge" (cholelithiasis/cholecystitis/pancreatitis), sinusitis

CLINICAL PRESENTATION

Historically, patients with CF had failure to thrive, steatorrhea, chronic productive cough, and recurrent severe respiratory infections. The advent of newborn screening and medical therapies has made the clinical presentation more varied. All of the symptoms listed later can be the presenting symptom of the disease (see Table 78.3 for a mnemonic for clinical presentations associated with CF).

- Pulmonary disease
  - Chronic productive cough, wheeze, tachypnea, or retractions
  - Recurrent/chronic pneumonia, bronchitis, bronchiolitis, atelectasis; may be initially described as "refractory asthma"
  - Bronchiectasis: suspected by chronic symptoms and the presence of coarse inspiratory rales in an otherwise well patient. The diagnosis is confirmed by imaging, typically by chest computed tomography (CT)
  - Growth of atypical organisms from a sputum culture or bronchoalveolar lavage without other explanation: methicillin-resistant *S. aureus* (MRSA), *P. aeruginosa, Stenotrophomonas maltophilia* or other Gram-negative organisms

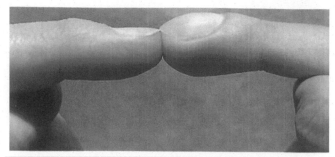

Fig. 78.1. Nail clubbing (right) and a normal nail (left). (From Zipes DP, et al, editors: Braunwald's heart disease: *a textbook of cardiovascular medicine*, ed 7, Philadelphia, 2005, Saunders. https://www.amazon.com/Diagnosis-Color-Physical-General-Medicine/dp/0723425876.)

- Pulmonary exacerbation: increased cough, mucus production, rales on examination, and often associated with weight loss
- Hemoptysis: typically presents only in patients with more advanced bronchiectasis. Can be life-threatening
- Nasal polyposis: because nasal polyps are otherwise very rare in children, all children with nasal polyps must have CF ruled out
- Chronic sinusitis: 90% to 100% of patients have panopacification of the sinuses
- Digital clubbing (hypertrophic pulmonary osteoarthropathy): obliteration of the normal angle of the base of the nail with the skin; the tips of the fingers enlarge, and the nails become extremely curved from front to back (see Fig. 78.1)
- Gastrointestinal disease
  - Pancreatic insufficiency: presents in two-thirds of newborns with CF. Pancreatic disease is progressive such that 85% of CF patients eventually are pancreatic insufficient
  - Failure to thrive (most common manifestation of CF)
  - Prolonged direct hyperbilirubinemia in the newborn period
  - Meconium ileus (obstruction of terminal ileum): 80% to 90% of newborns with meconium ileus have CF. Complications include fetal polyhydramnios, intestinal perforation, and meconium peritonitis
  - Rectal prolapse: related to constipation and malnutrition and is rare
  - Recurrent episodes of intussusception or intussusception beyond the usual age of presentation
  - Steatorrhea: bulky, fatty, and malodorous stools. Patients often have a protuberant abdomen and poor weight gain
  - Deficiency of the fat-soluble vitamins (ADEK)
  - Pancreatitis: seen in pancreatic-sufficient patients as adolescents or young adults
  - Advanced liver disease: occurs in 2% to 5%. Usually presents with asymptomatic elevations of liver function tests and hepatomegaly
  - Increased incidence of gallstones (12%)
  - Distal intestinal obstruction syndrome (DIOS), or meconium ileus equivalent in the older child or adolescent. Constipation associated with sausage-like mass in the right upper quadrant
  - CF-related diabetes: occurs in 25% by young adulthood and in 50% of adults

Table 78.4. Sweat Chloride Interpretation

Level	Normal mmol/L	Indeterminate mmol/L	Elevated mmol/L
Sweat chloride	≤29	30–59	≥60

- Reproductive
  - >95% of males are infertile due to CBAVD, although spermatogenesis is unaffected. May be the only symptom of CF for some patients. In vitro fertilization is possible
- Natural history
  - Patients with more severe mutations have more morbidity and a shorter life expectancy than those with milder mutations. With new therapies, patients with CF can now expect to live into adulthood. The median life expectancy is now over 40 years

DIAGNOSIS AND EVALUATION

- CF remains a clinical diagnosis. In the right clinical situation, an elevated sweat chloride and/or discovery of CF mutations is most often used to confirm the diagnosis
- Sweat test: collect sweat with pilocarpine iontophoresis to determine the chloride concentration; remains the primary method to diagnose CF (see Table 78.4). Intermediate sweat tests should be repeated and genetic analysis performed
- Diagnosing CF requires:
  - Presence of typical clinical features *or* CF in a sibling *or* positive newborn screen
  and
  - Elevated sweat chloride *or* abnormal nasal potential difference *or* identification of two disease-causing CF mutations
- *CFTR*-related metabolic syndrome: identification of one or two *CFTR* mutations in the absence of clinical symptoms or elevated sweat chloride, usually after newborn screening. Patients are monitored over time for the development of typical symptoms or elevated sweat chloride
- Newborn screening and CF:
  - Performed in every state, but technique varies by state. There is a balancing act between avoiding excessive false-negative and false-positive rates. Most states will screen with one assay, and if that is positive, screen with a second assay
    - Immunoreactive trypsinogen (IRT) assay: levels may be elevated in early years due to pancreatic dysfunction. Sensitivity is 80% for the diagnosis of CF (n.b., in later ages, after progressive fibrosis of the pancreas, serum trypsinogen may be normal or low in the majority of patients)
    - DNA assay: may be used as a primary screen or a secondary screen if the IRT is elevated. IRT + DNA analysis improves sensitivity to 96% in many states. Some states will test for only *ΔF508*, whereas others will test for 28 to 40 common mutations. To compensate for its racial diversity, California performs a full sequence panel if the initial mutations screen is negative. This has led to uncovering of *CFTR*

Table 78.5. Surveillance of Cystic Fibrosis Patients

Screening Test	Frequency	Function
Lung function	Quarterly	Changes in FEV1 can signal an exacerbation and are used to grade clinical severity as mild, moderate, or severe. FEV1 declines by 2% to 3% per year on average in cystic fibrosis.
Sputum or deep throat culture	Quarterly	Guides therapy for exacerbations and detects emergence of new pathogens
Chest computed tomography	Annually	Helps to determine clinical severity
Vitamin levels	Annually	Detects deficiencies
Liver function tests	Annually	Screen for cystic fibrosis–related liver disease
Hemoglobin A1C, oral glucose tolerance test	Annually after age 8 YEARS	Screens for glucose intolerance and diabetes

mutations of unknown clinical significance in many patients, which some feel is too high a false-positive rate
- Sweat test: performed after positive IRT and/or positive genetic screen to confirm the diagnosis; also performed if negative newborn screen result if there is history consistent with CF complications (e.g., meconium ileus)
- Nasal potential difference: airway is more negative in CF due to hyperabsorption of Na. Mainly a research tool
- Genotype: cannot rule CF in or out; needs to be combined with additional information (clinical symptoms and evidence of *CFTR* dysfunction); 1% of those with CF have no identifiable mutations; 18% with CF have only one abnormal gene identified
- Patients typically have quarterly visits at a CF center, where they are seen by a pulmonologist, nutritionist, respiratory therapist, and social worker. Screening tests are performed regularly (see Table 78.5)

TREATMENT

- Mucociliary clearance: typically done twice daily in most patients; usually takes 20 to 30 minutes to complete, sometimes longer
  - Different techniques and devices are used to dislodge mucus from the airway wall: manual chest physiotherapy, the external percussion vest, handheld oscillating devices, or intrapulmonary percussive ventilation (IPV). Superiority of one modality over the others has not been proven
  - Inhaled mucolytics help make the mucus thinner and more easily expectorated. DNase is recommended in all patients >6 years of age. *N*-acetylcysteine is often prescribed
  - Inhaled hypertonic saline: mechanism not quite well understood, but a clinically effective therapy
  - Bronchodilator (e.g. albuterol): use has never been proven beneficial in CF, but it is commonly used

- Suppressive antibiotic therapy: patients colonized with *P. aeruginosa* or those with more advanced lung disease will often be treated with regular antibiotic therapy, most commonly as an inhaled antibiotic alternating one month on and one month off to avoid the development of resistance. Commonly inhaled antibiotics include tobramycin, aztreonam, and colistin
- Antiinflammatory: both nonsteroidal antiinflammatory drugs (NSAIDs) and macrolides (azithromycin) are beneficial; the macrolides are the best tolerated and most often used, taken 3 days a week
- Optimization of nutrition
  - Pancreatic enzyme replacement: essential to the promotion of fat absorption and nutrition. Taken before every meal and snacks in increasing amounts with age
    - Excessive lipase administration (>2500 U/kg/meal) may result in fibrosing colonopathy
  - Vitamin supplements (especially fat-soluble vitamins, ADEK)
  - High-fat, high-protein diet. Sometimes tube feedings are needed (nasogastric [NG-tube], gastrostomy [G-tube])
  - Medium-chain triglycerides (MCT) are often added to the diet because they do not require micellar solubilization by bile salts (but they still need pancreatic lipase before absorption)
  - Insulin replacement may be required for CF-related diabetes
- Ursodeoxycholic acid: often used to prevent/treat liver disease
- Hospitalization
  - Required for patients with pulmonary exacerbations who fail outpatient antibiotics (can present with increasing respiratory symptoms, worsening pulmonary function testing, and/or subtle signs of infection)
  - Patients are treated with intravenous (IV) antibiotics and aggressive mucociliary clearance until the symptoms and forced expiratory volume in 1 second (FEV1) improve, typically for at least 2 weeks
  - Typical antibiotic regimens provide double coverage for pseudomonas:
    - Antipseudomonal cephalosporins: cefepime, ceftazidime
    - Aminoglycoside: amikacin, gentamicin
    - Others: carbapenem, fluoroquinolones, piperacillin-tazobactam, ticarcillin-clavulanate
    - Additional Gram-positive coverage may be warranted if there is history of MRSA colonization/infection
- CFTR modulators: new drugs directed toward improving the function of CFTR. The indications and efficacy depend on the mutations present. The results have been promising, and the potential for disease modification is still being discovered (see Table 78.1 for examples)
- Lung transplant: last-resort treatment for severe CF lung disease. The outcomes are poor, with approximately 50% survival at 5 years in children versus at 8 years in adults

Primary Ciliary Dyskinesia

Primary ciliary dyskinesia (PCD) is a genetic disorder in which either the function or the 9+2 microtubule ultrastructure of cilia is compromised. Inheritance is largely autosomal recessive, and around 34 genes have been identified to date. The disease is characterized by recurrent upper and lower respiratory tract infections, infertility, and aberrant organ laterality. Making the diagnosis of PCD involves appropriate recognition of the clinical phenotype and ruling out other immunodeficiencies and CF. Management of PCD is a multidisciplinary effort that includes surveillance of otosinopulmonary disease and providing appropriate hearing support, regular airway clearance, and antibiotic treatment of infections.

BASIC INFORMATION

- The prevalence of PCD has been difficult to estimate and varies widely in reports (1/4000 to <1/50,000), which reflects diagnostic complexities and varying access to centers with specialist testing
- PCD is characterized by chronic bronchitis, recurrent rhinosinusitis, frequent middle ear infections and associated hearing loss, and impaired fertility
- Frequent lower respiratory tract infections lead to structural lung damage and the development of bronchiectasis
- Kartagener syndrome describes a subgroup of PCD patients having the clinical triad of situs inversus, chronic sinusitis, and bronchiectasis
  - Only 40% to 50% of PCD patients have situs inversus; around 12% have situs ambiguous or heterotaxy
  - Heterotaxy is associated with higher morbidity due to congenital cardiovascular anomalies

CLINICAL PRESENTATION

- Perinatal events
  - 85% of infants have tachypnea, labored breathing, or atelectasis on chest x-ray despite term birth
  - They are usually diagnosed with transient tachypnea of the newborn, neonatal pneumonia, or meconium aspiration
  - There should be a high index of suspicion for PCD if a term infant presents with organ laterality defects and respiratory distress
- Respiratory symptoms
  - Persistent year-round cough—usually productive, but may be dry; partial improvement may be observed with antibiotics
  - Persistent year-round nasal congestion and chronic pansinusitis
    - Rhinitis may contribute to feeding difficulties and poor weight gain in infants
  - Recurrent upper and lower airway infections affect up to 80% of patients by preschool age
  - Bronchiectasis may develop in school-age children
  - Nasal polyposis affects 15% of patients
- Otitis media
  - 80% of patients with PCD have chronic otitis media
  - Many require tympanostomy tube placement and have conductive hearing loss by age 1 to 2 years
- Fertility
  - Men are infertile due to immotile spermatozoa or azoospermia
  - Women have decreased fertility due to defective ciliary function within fallopian tubes, leading to ectopic pregnancy or delayed ovum transport

- Physical examination
  - Growth may be normal, or patients can be underweight or have short stature
  - Ear examination may show otorrhea, glue ear, otitis media with effusion, tympanic membrane scarring, or cholesteatoma
  - Nasal examination may show turbinate hypertrophy, mucopurulent drainage, or polyposis
  - Lung auscultation may reveal wheezing, coarse rhonchi, and/or crackles
  - Pectus excavatum is reported in 10% of patients; there is a high prevalence of scoliosis
  - Dextrocardia or situs inversus of abdominal organs may be present

DIAGNOSIS AND EVALUATION

- More than one testing modality is often needed to confirm diagnosis of PCD
  - Ciliary biopsy is performed on nasal turbinates or bronchial walls (via bronchoscopy), and cilia ultrastructure is examined under transmission electron microscopy
    - This method may diagnose up to 70% of PCD cases
    - Yield is variable due to sampling or processing difficulties
  - Other testing includes: high-speed videomicroscopy (available only at specialized centers), exhaled nasal nitric oxide levels (as with CF, PCD is associated with low levels), saccharin/dye clearance time (currently less frequently used)
  - Genetic testing is commercially available for up to 34 genes, which to date account for up to 70% of PCD cases
- Chest x-ray, chest CT, sputum culture or bronchoalveolar lavage, pulmonary function tests, and hearing tests are indicated for baseline assessment and trending over time
  - Chest imaging may show peribronchial thickening, atelectasis, mosaic attenuation and air trapping, and bronchiectasis
  - Spirometry shows airflow obstruction as lung disease progresses
    - Normal forced vital capacity (FVC), reduced FEV1 <80% predicted, and reduced FEV1/FVC ratio <0.8
    - Response to bronchodilator is variable
  - *H. influenzae, Streptococcus pneumoniae, Moraxella catarrhalis, S. aureus,* and *P. aeruginosa* are commonly reported organisms in respiratory cultures
    - Appearance of *P. aeruginosa* tends to occur in adulthood, which is later than in CF patients

TREATMENT

- There are no validated therapies for PCD; management is extrapolated from patients with CF-related and non-CF-related bronchiectasis
- Management is multidisciplinary, involving pulmonary, otolaryngology, audiology, nutrition, and respiratory therapy
- Surveillance
  - Patients should undergo twice-yearly pulmonary assessment including spirometry and respiratory cultures

Table 78.6. Summary of Respiratory Muscle Weakness and Associated Complications

Muscle Group	Major Symptoms	Measure Function	Treatment
Expiratory muscles[1]	Weak cough	Maximal expiratory pressure, peak cough flow	Mucociliary clearance devices, insufflator-exsufflator
Inspiratory muscles[2]	Rapid shallow breathing, weak cough, sleep-disordered breathing	Forced vital capacity, maximal inspiratory pressure	Mucociliary clearance devices, insufflator-exsufflator, invasive or noninvasive ventilation
Bulbar dysfunction	Coughing on secretions, difficulty swallowing	Swallow study	Medical treatment to thicken secretions, enteral nutrition
Sleep-disordered breathing	Snoring, sleep disruption, daytime sleepiness, impaired attention	Overnight sleep study, overnight monitoring of SO_2 and CO_2 levels	Noninvasive or invasive ventilation

[1]Expiratory muscles: internal + external obliques, rectus abdominus, transverse abdominus, and intrathoracic intercostals.
[2]Inspiratory muscles: diaphragm and/or extrathoracic intercostal muscles, scalenes, sternocleidomastoids, and trapezii.

- Recommend vaccinations such as influenza and 23-valent pneumococcal polysaccharide vaccine (PPSV-23); encourage smoke avoidance
- Chest x-ray and nontuberculous mycobacterial cultures may be performed every 2 years and as needed with worsening respiratory status
- Repeat chest CT imaging, hearing tests, and bronchoalveolar lavage (for cultures); also sinus CT and screening for allergic bronchopulmonary aspergillosis are performed for cases of clinical worsening or for new symptoms
- Respiratory management
  - Airway clearance and acute/chronic antibiotic management are similar to respiratory management for CF (see previous)
  - Surgical lobe resection is reserved for cases of severe localized bronchiectasis, when it is thought to lend to frequent exacerbations and hemoptysis
  - Pulmonary angiography and bronchial artery collateral embolization are indicated for severe recurrent hemoptysis
- Otolaryngology management
  - 80% to 100% of children receive antibiotics and tympanostomy tube placement for recurrent otitis media, although benefit of the latter is debated
  - Hearing loss must be recognized early so that hearing aids and communication assistance can be provided
  - Chronic rhinosinusitis is managed with nasal steroids, irrigation, and antibiotics; functional endoscopic sinus surgery and nasal polyp removal may be required in patients refractory to medical management
- Prognosis
  - Patients may live a normal life span; decline in lung function is less rapid than with CF

Neuromuscular Diseases

BASIC INFORMATION

- Pulmonary complications of neuromuscular diseases are common and are often the cause of death
- They can be acute (e.g., Guillain-Barré syndrome), intermittent (e.g., myasthenia gravis), or gradually progressive (e.g., muscular dystrophy)

- The most common to cause respiratory insufficiency are cerebral palsy, muscular dystrophies (in particular, Duchenne and Becker), and spinal muscular atrophy
- Treating the respiratory insufficiency improves quality of life, decreases hospitalizations, and improves longevity
- Patients with respiratory muscle weakness who have reduced lung volumes on pulmonary function testing are diagnosed as having restrictive lung disease

CLINICAL PRESENTATION

- The manifestation of pulmonary complications depends on what respiratory muscles are involved and to what extent. The respiratory muscles include the diaphragm (the main muscle of inspiration), the chest wall muscles, abdominal wall muscles, and upper airway muscles (which are bulbar-innervated). Whereas a weak cough can arise from impairment of any of these muscles, other symptoms tend to occur due to impairment of the individual muscle groups (see Table 78.6)
- Impaired cough: weakness of several different muscle groups can cause a weak cough because the cough reflex requires use of inspiratory muscles (to generate a large vital capacity), upper airway adductor muscles (to close the glottis), and expiratory muscles (to expel air)
  - An impaired cough can give rise to symptoms such as prolonged cough with colds or recurrent bronchitis/pneumonia
- Impaired muscles of inspiration can lead to rapid shallow breathing and accessory muscle use (sternocleidomastoid and pectoral muscles)
  - Paradoxic breathing may be present in infants with weakness of intercostal muscles due to their compliant chest wall. During inspiration, instead of the chest wall and abdomen expanding, the chest wall caves inward
- Impairment of upper airway muscles can lead to dysphagia/aspiration, which increases the risk of chronic cough, recurrent bronchitis/pneumonia, and lung scarring/bronchiectasis
- Acute or chronic respiratory failure
  - Diseases with a more rapid onset such as Guillain-Barré syndrome can cause acute respiratory failure, whereas those with more gradual onset eventually cause chronic respiratory failure

- Patients with acute respiratory failure present with dyspnea and use of accessory muscles of respiration. If they progress without treatment, they may stop breathing and require urgent life support
- Chronic respiratory failure can be relatively asymptomatic, although patients will often have symptoms of nocturnal hypoventilation
- Nocturnal hypoventilation: often the first sign of pulmonary impairment in neuromuscular diseases
  - Patients are most at risk for hypercarbia during rapid eye movement (REM) sleep, when the inspiratory muscles of respiration are relatively atonic, except for the diaphragm
  - As muscle weakness progresses, patients develop hypercarbia in non-REM sleep and then eventually during the day. Symptoms can include daytime sleepiness, morning headaches, and problems with attention/concentration
- Scoliosis: common complication of muscle weakness in nonambulatory patients
  - Progression of scoliosis, which occurs most commonly during the adolescent growth spurt, aggravates restrictive lung disease
  - In Duchenne muscular dystrophy, surgical repair improves quality of life, but it has not been shown to increase longevity

DIAGNOSIS AND EVALUATION

- Pulmonary function testing is used to identify respiratory muscle weakness. Testing is done longitudinally to monitor for progression, usually beginning after age 6 years
  - Spirometry: pattern of lung restriction including FVC and FEV1 <80% predicted, and the FEV1/FVC >0.8
  - Full-body plethysmography: total lung capacity (TLC) <80% predicted
  - Maximal inspiratory pressure (MIP): reflects the strength of the inspiratory muscles
  - Maximal expiratory pressure (MEP): reflects the strength of the expiratory muscles
- Pulse oximetry detects oxygen desaturation that may be present due to the presence of atelectasis from retained secretions. End-tidal carbon dioxide ($ETCO_2$) measurements detect hypercarbia that may be present due to hypoventilation
- Overnight sleep studies (polysomnograms) are used to diagnose obstructive sleep apnea and/or nocturnal hypoventilation
- Barium swallow studies are often done to evaluate for dysphagia and aspiration
- Ideally, the pulmonologist sees the patient in a multidisciplinary clinic with a neurologist, respiratory therapist, gastroenterologist, social worker, and nutritionist, and for certain disorders (e.g., Duchenne muscular dystrophy), a cardiologist
- The frequency of visits and testing needed are dictated by lung function and muscular function
  - Ambulatory patients: annual visit
  - Wheelchair-bound with FVC >60%: biannual visit
  - FVC <60%: quarterly visits, annual polysomnogram

TREATMENT

- Pharmacotherapy
  - Novel medications have recently been developed that target the affected protein dysfunction in spinal muscular atrophy (SMA) and for certain genotypes of Duchenne Muscular dystrophy, and the long-term effects are not yet known
  - Glucocorticoid therapy in Duchenne muscular dystrophy delays time to loss of ambulation and development of scoliosis
- Enhancing mucociliary clearance via various methods of respiratory therapies (e.g., percussive vest, manual chest physiotherapy, insufflator-exsufflator) and inhaled medications (e.g., bronchodilator and hypertonic saline)
- Ventilation: patients with hypoventilation can be treated with noninvasive ventilation (e.g., continuous positive airway pressure [CPAP]/bilevel positive airway pressure [BiPAP]) via a mask interface or with invasive ventilation via a tracheostomy; this complex decision needs to take into account many factors, including patient wishes, goals of care, presence of bulbar dysfunction, severity of underlying problem, and number of hours a day ventilation will be needed
- Difficulty handling oral secretions/significant bulbar dysfunction is considered a relative contraindication to noninvasive ventilation
- The use of noninvasive ventilation has been shown to increase life expectancy in patients with Duchenne muscular dystrophy. It should be started once nocturnal hypercarbia is present
- Secretion and dysphagia management: important for patients who are chronically aspirating their oral secretions
  - Anticholinergic medications that thicken secretions
  - Botulinum toxin injection to the salivary glands to decrease saliva production
  - Enteral feeding with NG-tube or G-tube for supplemental hydration and nutrition to prevent aspiration
  - Occupational therapy to strengthen swallowing and feeding skills
- Immunizations
  - In addition to the routine immunizations (including the 13-valent conjugate pneumococcal vaccine), patients should be immunized with the 23-valent pneumococcal polysaccharide vaccine ≥2 years
  - Annual influenza vaccine
- Perioperative: patients with neuromuscular weakness are at high risk for postoperative respiratory failure, requiring coordination between multiple specialists (e.g., pulmonology, anesthesiology, critical care medicine, cardiology for Duchenne muscular dystrophy)

Primary Immunodeficiency

Primary immunodeficiencies are mostly inherited and comprise a varied and expanding group of diseases. Over 200 disorders now are recognized, covering defects in humoral and/or cellular immunity as well phagocytic and complement dysfunction. General details are provided in Section 9 (Immunology). In addition to manifesting with failure to thrive, recurrent fevers, and gastrointestinal and autoimmune disorders, these disorders often carry the burden of significant pulmonary disease, which contributes to significant morbidity and mortality.

BASIC INFORMATION

- Respiratory complications of immunodeficiency comprise acute or chronic infection, malignancy, and dysregulated inflammation, leading to structural lung damage
- Infections occurring throughout the respiratory tract include sinusitis, otitis media, bronchitis, and pneumonia
- Repeated cycles of inflammation and infection may cause bronchiectasis (dilated thickened airways) or bronchiolitis obliterans (concentric bronchiolar narrowing due to inflammation and fibrosis)
- Interstitial lung disease (ILD) occurs in various forms
  - Radiologic and histologic features are not specific to particular immunodeficiencies
  - IgG subclass deficiencies are most commonly associated with ILD
  - Granulomatous lymphocytic ILD (lymphoid interstitial pneumonia, follicular bronchitis, and non-necrotizing granuloma formation) affects 10% to 25% of patients with common variable immune deficiency (CVID); also linked to CTLA4 and LRBA deficiencies
  - Bronchiolitis obliterans organizing pneumonia has been linked to cases of CVID
    - Characterized by fever, dyspnea, and nonproductive cough
    - Fibroblast proliferation is present in peribronchiolar airspaces and alveolar ducts
- Pulmonary fibrosis with lymphocytic or lymphohistiocytic inflammation has been described in ataxia-telangiectasia
- Some conditions such as lymphocytic interstitial pneumonia can undergo malignant transformation
- Advanced-stage lung disease may feature chronic respiratory failure, pulmonary hypertension, and ultimately cor pulmonale

DIAGNOSIS AND EVALUATION

- Chest x-rays are generally insensitive for detecting pulmonary damage
- High-resolution chest CT is a better tool for assessing bronchiectasis and interstitial processes
- Bronchoscopy with bronchoalveolar lavage allows mucus sampling and broad microbial analysis to detect unusual infections
- Trending pulmonary function testing plays a role in tracking disease progression
- Lung biopsy is sometimes indicated to differentiate between infection, inflammation, and malignancy
- Video-assisted thoracoscopic surgery is generally preferred: it poses fewer complications than open lung biopsy and better sampling than transbronchial biopsy

TREATMENT

- Infection control involves routine daily precautions (such as proper hand hygiene), vaccination of the patient and close contacts, prophylactic antibiotics, and IV immunoglobulin replacement therapy
- Acute infections are treated with oral or IV antibiotics, depending on the source and severity of infection
- Immunomodulators and stem cell transplants can be therapeutic for certain immunodeficiencies
- Specific respiratory therapies
  - Bronchiectasis is managed with antibiotics and airway clearance therapies as described in previous sections
  - Surgical lobe resection, bronchial artery embolization, and lung transplantation are considered for advanced lung disease, as described in previous sections

Rheumatologic Disorders

Pulmonary complications are rare but contribute significant morbidity and mortality in certain rheumatologic disorders. Details of these disorders are presented in Section 20 (Rheumatology). Outlined later are common pulmonary manifestations in select rheumatologic diseases.

BASIC INFORMATION

- Common rheumatologic associations:
  - Systemic lupus erythematosus (SLE):
    - The most common respiratory complaint in SLE is pleuritis (affecting up to 80% of patients); association with pleural effusion (called serositis) is one diagnostic criterion for SLE
    - Pulmonary embolism may occur in the presence of antiphospholipid antibodies
    - Respiratory complications occur in 40% within first year of diagnosis of SLE; severity is widely variable
    - Late pulmonary complications of SLE include ILD, pulmonary hypertension, and shrinking lung syndrome
  - Systemic sclerosis
    - Over 50% of cases develop pulmonary disease, but presentation may be subclinical
    - The most common complications are ILD and pulmonary hypertension; pleurisy and aspiration pneumonia are possible
    - Histologic patterns seen in ILD are nonspecific interstitial pneumonia or usual interstitial pneumonia
    - Autoantibody expression predicts lung involvement, especially Scl-70
  - Juvenile dermatomyositis
    - Respiratory complications arise from ILD (typically affecting up to 50% of adults) and neuromuscular weakness (causing ineffective airway clearance and hypoventilation)
    - Histologic patterns seen in ILD are cryptogenic organizing pneumonia, diffuse alveolar damage, nonspecific interstitial pneumonia, or usual interstitial pneumonia
    - Lung disease may be subclinical and apparent only on lung function testing
    - Strongest predictive factor is presence of anti-Jo-1 autoantibodies
  - Mixed connective tissue disease
    - Respiratory complications occur in 35% to 60% of pediatric cases

- Up to two-thirds of adults demonstrate diffusion impairment, and half have restrictive lung disease on pulmonary function testing
- Pleural effusions, nonspecific interstitial pneumonia, pulmonary fibrosis, and pulmonary hypertension
- Granulomatosis with polyangiitis
  - Respiratory complications occur in up to 75% of pediatric cases
  - Upper respiratory tract involvement includes subglottic stenosis, rhinitis, sinusitis, and persistent otitis media with hearing loss
  - Lower respiratory tract involvement includes airway stenosis, alveolar hemorrhage, pleuritis, pneumothorax, mediastinal lymph nodes, pleural effusion, and nodular lung disease
- Juvenile idiopathic arthritis
  - Respiratory disease is uncommon but ranges from pleuritis, pleural effusion, pneumonitis, ILD, and pulmonary artery hypertension to alveolar proteinosis
- Sarcoidosis
  - Early form of sarcoidosis (in patients age <4) is manifest with skin rash, uveitis, and arthritis; respiratory disease is rare
  - Older children have disease similar to adults, in which noncaseating granulomas develop in lungs, lymph nodes, liver, skin, and eyes
    - 90% have abnormal chest x-ray with hilar adenopathy and/or parenchymal infiltrates
    - Late complications include development of bronchiectasis, recurrent pneumonia, and progression to pulmonary fibrosis
- Pulmonary hemosiderosis
  - The result of recurrent intraalveolar bleeding leading to the accumulation of iron in hemosiderin-laden macrophages
  - Pulmonary hemosiderosis may be a primary disorder (i.e., idiopathic pulmonary hemosiderosis) or secondary (often associated with rheumatologic diseases, but can be seen in other diseases capable of causing pulmonary hemorrhage)
    - Idiopathic pulmonary hemosiderosis is thought to be the result of complex immune-genetic-environment interactions
  - Classically presents as iron-deficient anemia, hemoptysis, and pulmonary infiltrates on chest radiographs
  - Steroids and immunosuppressants play a role in treating primary disease; control of the causative disease is critical in secondary pulmonary hemosiderosis

Oncologic Disorders

Advances in therapies for childhood cancers have led to overall improved survival. However, pulmonary complications are frequently seen as a result of both the primary disease and the treatments used.

BASIC INFORMATION

- Respiratory disease can range from subclinical to life-threatening, and may appear early or late in the course of treatment

- Chemotherapy, radiation, stem cell transplant, and surgery all exert adverse effects on the pulmonary system
- Complications of chemotherapeutic agents
  - Pulmonary edema is a significant early side effect of many chemotherapeutic agents, most commonly reported with cytarabine and bleomycin
  - Interstitial pneumonitis may develop early or after several months; common offending agents are methotrexate, bleomycin, and procarbazine
  - Immunosuppression caused by chemotherapeutic agents poses significant respiratory infection risks
  - Pulmonary fibrosis is a late complication of bleomycin and busulfan
- Complications of radiation therapy
  - Acute radiation pneumonitis (dyspnea, fever, cough, chest pain) may surface 1 to 3 months after completion of radiation therapy
  - Pulmonary fibrosis develops after 6 to 12 months
  - Lung injury is proportional to radiation dosage, volume of lung treated, and cotreatment with agents like bleomycin
- Complications of thoracic surgery
  - Pneumothorax and pneumomediastinum
  - Acquired chest wall deformities may predispose to scoliosis and cause restrictive lung disease
- Complications of hematopoietic stem cell transplant (HSCT)
  - Consider immune status, use of immunosuppressive agents and timing when evaluating for pulmonary complications
  - Preengraftment period (0–30 days after HSCT, absolute neutrophil count (ANC) <500)
    - Primary pulmonary complications related to risk of infection (due to neutropenia), fluid overload (due to the need for repeated blood transfusions), hyperacute graft-versus-host disease (GVHD), or adverse effects of conditioning agents
  - Engraftment syndrome occurs in 3% to 5% of autologous HSCT and in 7% to 10% of allogeneic HSCT
    - This is seen around the time of neutrophil recovery, when cytokine surge can cause capillary leak
    - Manifested as fever, hypoxemia, rash, noncardiogenic pulmonary edema, or acute respiratory distress syndrome
  - Hyperacute and acute GVHD is a concern in the first 2 weeks and first 3 months after allogeneic HSCT, respectively; due to HLA mismatch
    - Skin rash and noncardiogenic pulmonary edema
    - Pulmonary cytolytic thrombi may form and cause fever, cough, and respiratory distress
    - Chest CT findings consist of peripheral subpleural nodules and opacities
    - Diffuse alveolar hemorrhage may be caused by infectious or noninfectious processes; mortality is high
  - Postengraftment period (ANC >500, early and late)
    - Elevated infection risk is due to defective cellular and humoral immunity
      - Bacterial agents now include *Legionella* and *Nocardia* spp. or fungal species such as *Aspergillus* and *Pneumocystis jirovecii*; other causes include mycobacterial infections, cytomegalovirus (CMV), human herpesvirus 6 (HHV-6), and other respiratory viruses

- Idiopathic pneumonia syndrome affects up to 10% of allogeneic HSCT and 1% to 5% of autologous HSCT
    - Characterized by widespread alveolar injury causing cough, dyspnea, hypoxemia, and diffuse opacities on chest imaging, but without infectious cause
    - A more intense conditioning regimen (myeloablative regimen or high-dose radiotherapy) may predispose to development of idiopathic pneumonia syndrome (IPS)
    - Reported mortality is 50% to 75%
- Endothelial dysfunction is associated with transplant-associated thrombotic microangiopathy (TMA) or pulmonary venoocclusive disease (PVOD)
    - May be a consequence of infection, history of GVHD, radiation, or chemotherapy
    - TMA is diagnosed by the presence of thrombocytopenia, microangiopathic hemolytic anemia (decreased hemoglobin, negative Coombs testing, schistocytes on smear, increased lactate dehydrogenase, decreased serum haptoglobin), and increased creatinine
    - Both lead to vascular congestion, pulmonary hypertension, and heart failure
    - Mortality is >80%
- Diffuse alveolar hemorrhage is rare and may be caused by infection, acute GVHD, or diffuse alveolar damage; mortality is up to 80%
    - Patients develop cough, hypoxia, progressive respiratory failure, and sometimes hemoptysis
    - Usually occurring 1 to 4 weeks after transplant
- Autoimmune disease with pulmonary manifestations is a late complication (about 30 months after HSCT)
    - Antinuclear antibodies (ANA), antineutrophil cytoplasmic antibodies (ANCA), anti-Sm, and rheumatoid factor (RF) may be positive
    - History of GVHD and myeloablative conditioning regimen is common in affected patients
- Organizing pneumonia may present as mild illness or fulminant respiratory failure
    - This usually occurs in the first 100 days after transplant
    - May be cryptogenic, related to radiation therapy, history of GVHD, or CMV pneumonitis
    - Pattern of lung disease includes nonspecific interstitial pneumonia, lymphocytic pneumonia, or diffuse alveolar damage
    - Chest CT demonstrates patchy consolidation and nodular and ground-glass opacities
    - Lung biopsy may show plugging of bronchioles and alveoli, interstitial inflammation, and fibrosis
- Bronchiolitis obliterans causes cough, dyspnea, wheeze, and progressive respiratory failure
    - This is usually a later complication, surfacing a year or more after transplant
    - Chest CT shows hyperinflation, air trapping, and bronchiectasis
    - Progressive airway obstruction is caused by lymphocytic inflammation and fibrotic plugging of bronchioles

- Bronchiolitis obliterans syndrome is diagnosed when a patient demonstrates progressive airflow obstruction during spirometry without a confirmatory biopsy
- Patients can develop malignancy linked to relapse, development of second cancer, or secondary lymphoproliferative disease
    - Childhood cancer survivors have a sixfold increase in relative risk for developing second malignancies
    - Posttransplant lymphoproliferative disorder occurs when B lymphocytes infected with Epstein-Barr virus (EBV) proliferate in T-cell-deficient, seronegative transplant recipients

TREATMENT

- Discontinue medications that are implicated in respiratory pathology
- Most cases of respiratory involvement require oxygen and ventilator support; fluid restriction and diuresis in cases of pulmonary edema
- Bactrim prophylaxis for Pneumocystis
- Empiric broad-spectrum antibiotics should be provided with initial respiratory deteriorations; narrow to specific agents once infection is confirmed
- EBV-associated posttransplant lymphoproliferative disease is treated by reducing immunosuppression, use of EBV-specific cytotoxic lymphocytes, and rituximab
- Treatment of TMA is mainly supportive (treatment of infection, platelet transfusions, and dialysis for severe renal insufficiency), but plasma exchange may provide benefit (<50% response rate)
    - Eculizumab (humanized monoclonal antibody against complement C5) is a promising new therapy
- Treatment options for PVOD are limited, including vasodilators (calcium channel blockers, prostacyclins, sildenafil) and steroids; defibrotide (oligonucleotide with antithrombotic, fibrinolytic, and endothelial repair properties) is a promising therapy under investigation
- Systemic corticosteroid therapy is used for treating engraftment syndrome, cryptogenic organizing pneumonia, idiopathic pneumonia syndrome, bronchiolitis obliterans, and diffuse alveolar hemorrhage—after infection has been ruled out
    - Azithromycin, montelukast, and inhaled corticosteroids may offer steroid-sparing benefits to patients with bronchiolitis obliterans
    - Cyclosporine, azathioprine, antithymocyte globulin, and extracorporeal photopheresis have been used to treat bronchiolitis obliterans with variable results
- Lung transplantation is reserved for advanced respiratory failure in cases of bronchiolitis obliterans as well as for PVOD

Review Questions

For review questions, please go to ExpertConsult.com.

Suggested Readings

1. Farrell PM, White TB, Ren CL, et al. Diagnosis of cystic fibrosis: consensus guidelines from the cystic fibrosis foundation. *J Pediatr.* 2017;181(S):S4–S15.
2. Gibson RL, Burns JL, Ramsey BW. Pathophysiology and management of pulmonary infections in cystic fibrosis. *Am J Respir Crit Care Med.* 2003;168(8):918–951.
3. Josephson MB, Goldfarb SB. Pulmonary complications of childhood cancers. *Expert Rev Respir Med.* 2014;8(5):561–571.
4. Richardson AE, Warrier K, Vyas H. Respiratory complications of the rheumatological diseases in childhood. *Arch Dis Child.* 2016;101:752–758.
5. Turcios NL, Fink RJ. *Pulmonary manifestations of pediatric diseases.* Saunders; 2009.

Psychiatry

79 Selected Topics in Psychiatry

ANGELA T. ANDERSON, MD, GABRIELA ANDRADE, MD, PRADIPTA MAJUMDER, MD, BARBARA ROBLES-RAMAMURTHY, MD, ERIC SHUTE, MD, PREETI SOI, MD, CATHARYN A. TURNER II MEd, MD, JEEIN YOON, MD and AMY KIM, MD

Attention-Deficit/Hyperactivity Disorder

BASIC INFORMATION

- Epidemiology
  - Attention-deficit/hyperactivity disorder (ADHD) is the most common neurodevelopmental disorder
  - Estimated prevalence in childhood ADHD varies from 5.3% to 11%
  - Male:female = 2:1 in children
  - ADHD, combined type, is the most common subtype
- Common symptoms
  - Persistent pattern of inattention and/or hyperactivity-impulsivity that interferes with academic or social functioning or development that is not accounted for by another medical or psychiatric condition
- Natural history
  - Hyperactivity and impulsivity symptoms decrease with increasing age; 40% to 60% continue to be symptomatic in adulthood
  - Childhood predictors of adult ADHD symptom persistence: initial ADHD symptom severity, comorbidities, parental mental health problems
  - Teens and young adults with ADHD have higher rates of academic failure, delinquency, substance use, teen pregnancies, risky sexual behaviors, antisocial and criminal behavior, injuries, accidents, and employment and marital difficulties
- Comorbidities
  - More than 50% of ADHD patients also meet diagnostic criteria for oppositional defiant disorder (ODD)
  - A significant portion will develop conduct disorders (CDs) and substance abuse disorders
  - Approximately one-third of ADHD patients also have anxiety disorders
  - 25% to 35% of ADHD patients also have a learning or language disorder
- Etiology
  - The causes remain unknown, but research shows increasing evidence for strong genetic cause, twin studies estimating heritability to be 76%
  - Nongenetic risk factors: perinatal stress, traumatic brain injury, maternal alcohol, smoking exposure during pregnancy
  - See also Nelson Textbook of Pediatrics, Chapter 33, "Attention Deficit/Hyperactivity Disorder."

CLINICAL PRESENTATION

- Inattention and/or hyperactivity/impulsivity symptoms must present before 12 years of age and must meet the *Diagnostic and Statistical Manual of Mental Disorders, fifth edition (DSM-5)*, diagnostic criteria detailed in Table 79.1

DIAGNOSIS AND EVALUATION

- Clinical diagnosis is based on detailed history from parent and child; collateral information from teachers/school is also helpful
- Rating scales
  - Vanderbilt, Conners 3, ADHD Rating Scale-IV, and so forth
- Additional medical history
  - Include screening for syncope, cardiac history/symptoms/medications, and family history of sudden cardiac deaths or cardiac abnormalities to screen for underlying cardiac conditions that may be associated with increased risk of adverse cardiac effects from stimulant medications
  - Routine cardiac evaluation (i.e., electrocardiography, echocardiography) is unnecessary in otherwise healthy individuals with negative family history
- Laboratory and neurologic testing are not mandatory unless with specific concerns
- Differential diagnosis
  - Other psychiatric disorders: ODD, CD, anxiety disorders, mood disorders (depression, bipolar disorder), substance use disorders, learning and language disorders
  - Nonpsychiatric conditions: tics, sleep apnea, absence seizures, head trauma

TREATMENT

- Psychosocial interventions
  - Behavioral therapy
    - Key elements include psychoeducation and behavior modification strategies such as increased positive attention and selective ignoring
    - Can be used alone for mild impairment or, if family prefers, nonpharmacologic treatment
  - Academic accommodations
    - Advocacy to promote effective collaboration between families and schools

Table 79.1. Attention-Deficit/Hyperactivity Disorder

A	Inattentive symptoms (need ≥6)	Hyperactive/impulsive symptoms (need ≥6)	Combined type
	■ Fails to give close attention to details or makes careless mistakes	■ Fidgets, taps hands or feet, squirms in seat	Meets criteria for *both* Inattentive and Hyperactive/Impulsive types
	■ Difficulty sustaining attention	■ Leaves seat in situations when remaining in seat is expected	
	■ Does not seem to listen when spoken to directly	■ Runs or climbs when inappropriate, feeling restless for adolescents, adults	
	■ Difficulty following through on instructions	■ Unable to engage in leisure activities quietly	
	■ Difficulty organizing tasks	■ Is often "on the go," acting as if "driven by a motor"	
	■ Avoids or dislikes tasks that require sustained mental effort	■ Talks excessively	
	■ Often loses things	■ Often blurts out answers before a question has been completed	
	■ Easily distracted	■ Difficulty waiting his or her turn	
	■ Often forgetful in daily activities	■ Often interrupts or intrudes on others	

B	Symptoms present before age 12
C	Symptoms present ≥2 settings
D	Symptoms interfere with social, academic, or occupational functioning
E	Symptoms not better explained by another mental disorder

■ Consideration for psychoeducational assessment, 504 plan, or individualized education plans when indicated
■ Pharmacotherapy in ADHD
  ■ Stimulants: methylphenidates, amphetamines
    ■ Stimulants are first line among FDA-approved medication for ADHD with strongest evidence and effect size
    ■ More than 70% of children with ADHD respond to one stimulant medication at an optimal dose
    ■ Side effects: appetite suppression, weight loss, insomnia, headaches, tics, emotional lability/irritability
  ■ Atomoxetine (norepinephrine reuptake inhibitor)
    ■ Compared with stimulants, less strong but sufficient evidence for atomoxetine, extended-release guanfacine (later), and extended-release clonidine (later) in treatment of ADHD in order listed
    ■ May use if unable to tolerate stimulant side effects, or in ADHD with comorbid anxiety symptoms or substance abuse
    ■ Side effects: insomnia, gastrointestinal symptoms, appetite suppression, increase in suicidal thoughts (less common), hepatitis (rare)
  ■ Extended-release guanfacine, extended-release clonidine (α_2 agonist)
    ■ FDA approved for monotherapy or as adjunctive therapy with stimulants in ADHD
    ■ Side effects: somnolence, fatigue, nausea, lethargy, insomnia, dizziness, hypotension, bradycardia, constipation, dry mouth
■ Treatment monitoring
  ■ Monitor pulse, blood pressure, weight, and height at subsequent follow-up visits
  ■ Monitor for side effects while titrating to optimal dose targeting symptoms
  ■ Repeat ADHD rating scales to assess the degree of improvement on treatment
■ Age-specific considerations
  ■ Preschool-aged children (ages 4–5)

■ Start with evidence-based parent- or teacher-administered behavior therapy alone
■ Clinicians to weigh the risks and benefits of starting methylphenidate in younger children if symptoms cause moderate to severe dysfunction despite evidence-based behavior interventions
■ Most medications are not FDA approved for treatment of ADHD in preschool-aged children
■ Elementary school–aged children (ages 6–11)
  ■ Treat with FDA-approved medications for ADHD and/or behavioral therapy
  ■ Monotherapy with stimulants and/or combination of stimulant and behavioral therapy are proven to be more effective than behavioral therapy alone
■ Adolescents (ages 12–18)
  ■ Treat with FDA-approved medications for ADHD with assent of teen
  ■ Behavior therapy has weaker evidence in teens than in younger children

Disruptive Behavior Disorders and Aggression

BASIC INFORMATION

■ Behavioral disturbances fall on a spectrum, with symptoms of oppositionality, defiance, and temper tantrums being common among young children
■ These symptoms reach clinical significance when they are high in frequency or severity and/or cause functional impairment (i.e., child is suspended from day care or school, child cannot be left alone with siblings due to fear of aggression toward others)
■ Epidemiology
  ■ Disruptive behaviors are the most common cause for referral to behavioral health services across all ages
  ■ 5% to 10% of children between 5 and 15 years of age display clinically significant behavioral problems

- Natural history
  - Although aggression is considered to be a stable trait, not all children with ODD go on to develop the more severe forms of illness
  - Up to 50% of children who display aggressive behavior maintain these behaviors through adolescence. If left untreated, may develop conduct disorder (CD); 40% of youth with CD develop antisocial personality disorder (ASPD)
  - Long-term outcomes for untreated or treatment-resistant ODD, CD, and ASPD are negative and significantly affect social functioning, including high risk of school dropout, criminal behavior, psychiatric illness, and drug and alcohol use, with lower levels of academic achievement, employment, and family stability
- Risk factors
  - Internal risk factors: temperamental differences (irritable, quick to react), poor executive functioning, low verbal intelligence, deficits in processing social information
  - External risk factors: low socioeconomic status, parental unemployment and low educational status, parental mental illness, parental substance use, disrupted family life, exposure to violence (e.g., childhood abuse and neglect), deviant peer influence
    - Poor-quality parenting: characterized by the use of harsh and/or ineffective and inconsistent parenting skills, is one of the most significant predictors of early-onset conduct problems

CLINICAL PRESENTATION

- Aggressive and disruptive behaviors should be considered a symptom, and clinical presentation will vary based on underlying condition
- Diagnostic criteria
  - ODD
    - Angry/irritable mood, argumentative/defiant behavior or vindictiveness lasting at least 6 months
  - CD
    - A repetitive and persistent pattern of behavior in which the basic rights of others or major age-appropriate societal norms are violated
    - These violations may be displayed across different domains, including aggression to people and animals, destruction of property, deceitfulness or theft, and serious violations of rules (truancy, running away from home)
    - Behaviors cause significant impairment in social, academic, or occupational functioning
- Differential diagnosis
  - Other psychiatric disorders: ADHD, ODD, CD, mood disorder, anxiety disorders, obsessive compulsive disorder (OCD), post-traumatic stress disorder (PTSD), tic disorder, substance use disorder, learning disorder, autism spectrum disorder, psychotic disorder
  - Nonpsychiatric conditions: seizure disorders, acute metabolic syndromes that could result in delirium or confusion, exposure to toxins (lead), acute infections, head trauma, ingestions

DIAGNOSIS AND EVALUATION

- Clinical interview
  - It is recommended to interview the child and caregivers separately, if possible, because conflict can arise when behavioral difficulties are discussed
- Rating scales
  - Child Behavior Checklist (CBCL) and its companion the Teacher Report Form (TRF)
  - The Behavior Assessment System for Children, second edition (BASC-2)
- Consider psychoeducational testing if concerned about intellectual disability, learning disorder, or other cognitive dysfunction that may be impacting the child's behavior
- Assess for comorbid conditions, particularly ADHD, substance use, and mood and anxiety disorders
- Assess for common psychosocial stressors and factors that may be contributing to clinical presentation and may be addressed, such as food insecurity, parental mental illness or substance use, child abuse or neglect, bullying, and gang membership
- Physical examination should be used to screen for signs of abuse and for conditions associated with high-risk behaviors (e.g., sexually transmitted diseases [STDs], hepatitis, head trauma)

TREATMENT

- Aggressive and disruptive behavior should be considered a symptom of a condition until proven otherwise
- Management of underlying condition should result in improvement of behavioral disturbance (i.e., stimulant use in children with ADHD should result in reduction of impulsive and aggressive behavior)
- If behaviors are causing significant disruption in the home and/or school setting, consult clinical social worker and/or mental health provider
- Psychotherapeutic interventions
  - Positive data exist for the use of behavioral interventions for treatment of ODD and CD (e.g. behavioral parent training interventions, cognitive behavioral therapy)
  - For children in foster care or in the juvenile justice system, intensive outpatient therapies, such as multisystemic therapy, have been shown to decrease rates of recidivism, arrest, criminal offenses, and out-of-home placement
- Medication
  - The use of medication should be considered carefully and may require consultation with a mental health provider because medications are considered second-line treatment for ODD and CD after psychotherapeutic interventions have been tried and failed, or if symptoms are severe
  - Choice of medication will depend on underlying condition and will require medical monitoring for side effects
    - Stimulants (methylphenidate, amphetamine) and alpha agonists (clonidine) for children with ADHD

- Risperidone and aripiprazole for children with autism spectrum disorder, bipolar disorder, tic disorder, and schizophrenia

Anxiety Disorders

BASIC INFORMATION

- Important to distinguish between normative childhood worries/fears from anxiety disorders
  - Normal worries/fears are developmentally appropriate and transient, such as stranger anxiety in infants, separation anxiety in toddlers, and fear of monsters or the dark in preschoolers
  - Anxiety becomes clinically concerning when the content is no longer age appropriate, interferes with functioning, and/or causes distress for the child
- Common presenting complaints
  - Physical symptoms not otherwise explained by a medical cause: commonly headaches, abdominal complaints, difficulty sleeping
  - Avoidance behaviors: avoiding academic or social activities, such as school or parties
  - Oppositional behavior, angry outbursts, tantrums, or irritability
  - Changes in appetite: overeating or undereating that results in weight concerns or selective eating
- Natural history
  - Lifetime prevalence in children and teens is 15% to 32%
  - Anxiety disorders in childhood have a high comorbid rate with other anxiety disorders and are predictors of a range of psychiatric disorders in adolescence
  - Children affected are at higher risk of substance abuse, conduct problems, increased use of long-term psychiatric and medical services, and functional impairment
  - Anxious children are more likely to have lifelong health problems including gastrointestinal (GI) issues, asthma, and allergies
- Causes and etiology
  - Biologic influences: heredity, temperament, autonomic reactivity, anxious sensitivity
  - Environmental influences: attachment styles, parenting behaviors, peer/social problems, negative/stressful life events

CLINICAL PRESENTATION

Generalized Anxiety Disorder

- Characterized by excessive worry about many different situations or activities lasting more than 6 months
- Specific symptoms include feeling on edge or restlessness, fatigue, decreased concentration, irritability, muscle tension, or changes in sleep pattern

Separation Anxiety Disorder

- Characterized by inappropriate distress associated with separation from primary caretaker for >4 weeks and causing significant impairment related to functioning at home, school, and in social settings
- Specific symptoms: excessive distress in anticipation of separation from caretaker; persistent and excessive worry/anxiety about losing, or something bad happening to, the caretaker; reluctance to go to places secondary to fear of separation; reluctance to sleep away from home; nightmares of separation; can often be accompanied by physical symptoms
- Important to keep in mind that separation anxiety is considered normal and developmentally appropriate from ages 6 to 30 months

Social Anxiety Disorder

- Characterized by intense, excessive, and recurrent fear or anxiety in social situations lasting more than 6 months
- Specific symptoms: worries about looking anxious in front of others leading to humiliation, embarrassment, rejection, and avoidance of social situations. These must occur with peers, not just adults
- Can have a subtype of "performance-only social anxiety disorder" if the fear is restricted to public speaking or public performance

Panic Disorder

- Characterized by recurrent episodes of unexpected, intense fear
- These attacks typically are described as a surge of intense fear accompanied by physical symptoms, including:
  - Palpitations, sweating, trembling, shortness of breath, feeling of suffocation, chest pain, GI discomfort or nausea, fainting/dizziness, chills, paresthesias, derealization, fear of losing control, and fear of dying

Specific Phobia

- Characterized by intense and inappropriate fear of a particular object or situation, which results in functional impairment
- Specific symptoms: immediate fear when confronted with a specific object/situation and avoidance of object/situation. In children these symptoms can present as crying, tantrums, freezing, or increased clinging
- Typically occurs after a trauma to self or observed trauma to others

DIAGNOSIS AND EVALUATION

- Clinical interview
  - Beware that it is often difficult for children to communicate their anxiety symptoms, or they might not understand their symptoms
- Validated rating scales exist to further assess the presence, type, and severity of symptoms, including BASC-2, MASC-2, SCARED, and SCAS
- Laboratory considerations
  - No standard laboratory tests for children with anxiety disorders
  - Need to consider family history, medical illness, and physical symptoms in the patient
  - Thyroid panel should be considered, especially if positive history of family thyroid disease or comorbid depressive symptoms

- Differential diagnosis
  - Other psychiatric disorders: ADHD, autistic spectrum disorder, depression, bipolar disorder, learning disorders, psychotic disorders
  - Nonpsychiatric conditions: hyperthyroidism, caffeinism, migraine, asthma, seizure, lead intoxication, hypoglycemia, pheochromocytoma, central nervous system (CNS) disorders, chronic pain/illness
  - Medication side effects: antiasthmatics, sympathomimetics, steroids, selective serotonin reuptake inhibitors (SSRIs), antipsychotics, diet pills, cold medications, antihistamines

TREATMENT

- Determine treatment modality based on specific anxiety diagnosis, symptom severity, child and family choice, access, and affordability
  - Consider cognitive behavioral therapy (CBT) alone for mild symptoms, younger age, and absence of comorbid depression
  - Parent-child and family interventions, combined with CBT, can improve parent-child relationships, reduce parental anxiety, and bolster parenting skills that reinforce healthy coping
  - Consider combination, medications, or CBT alone for moderate to severe symptoms, older patients, and comorbid depression
- Pharmacologic treatments
  - SSRIs are considered first-line pharmacologic treatment, with fluoxetine and sertraline having the strongest evidence base
  - Other considerations: some serotonin norepinephrine reuptake inhibitors (SNRIs), tricyclic antidepressants (TCAs), benzodiazepines, and buspirone
  - Treatment guidelines recommend to treat for at least 1 year with medication before gradual trial of discontinuation

Obsessive-Compulsive Spectrum Disorders (OCD)

BASIC INFORMATION

- Though previously conceptualized and categorized as an anxiety disorders in the *DSM-IV-TR*, it is now a separate new category under Obsessive Compulsive Spectrum Disorders in the *DSM-5*
- OCD is defined by the presence of intense and recurrent obsessions (persistent thoughts, impulses, or images) or compulsions (repetitive behaviors or rituals). In a child with OCD, these obsessions or compulsions lead to significant distress and interference with everyday routines, school performance, social activities, or relationships
- Epidemiology
  - Prevalence rates of pediatric OCD: 1% to 2%
  - 3:2 male-to-female ratio (as opposed to adult OCD)

Table 79.2. Common Obsessive Thoughts

Superstitious fears that something bad will happen to self or others (e.g., death of a parent)
Contamination fears with everyday objects or certain people
Worrying excessively that the door is not locked, the lights are not turned off, and so forth
Worrying excessively about symmetrical arrangement
Superstitious fears of harming others, especially loved ones

Table 79.3. Common Compulsions

Avoidance of situations in which one thinks something bad might happen
Washing or bathing excessively
Ritualized behaviors such as touching a certain body part in a certain symmetric manner
Repeating prayers or certain words so that something bad will not happen
Excessive reassurance-seeking from loved ones about not having caused harm

- Childhood onset occurs in 30% to 50% of all OCD cases
- Two peaks of incidence across life span: in preadolescent children (9–10 years) and in early adult life (mean age 21 years)
- Natural history
  - Onset:
    - Typically a gradual onset without a history of precipitating stressors
    - Occasional dramatic onset after a psychosocial event such as physical or sexual assault or witnessing domestic violence, and so forth
  - Duration:
    - Predicting persistence risk factors: younger age of onset, inpatient treatment, comorbid psychiatric illness, poor initial treatment
    - Prognosis is better than in adult-onset OCD
- Causes and etiology
  - Multiple family and twin studies show evidence that there is likely a genetic factor involved in the expression and transmission of OCD; however, several "sporadic" cases of OCD suggest an important role for environmental factors as well
  - Role of family in pediatric OCD: the role of the family in children with OCD is now widely recognized as a possible perpetuating factor of the child's compulsive behavior. Parents may be trying to be helpful in providing constant verbal reassurance or in helping the child avoid certain "contaminated objects," but unfortunately this just reinforces the behavior
  - Autoimmunity: an immune response to group A beta-hemolytic streptococcus (GABHS) infections is believed by some to result in basal ganglia inflammation, leading to OCD, tics, and ADHD symptoms, a disorder called PANDAS (pediatric autoimmune neuropsychiatric disorders associated with streptococcal infections); this is a controversial topic

CLINICAL PRESENTATION

- The key symptoms of OCD are obsessions and/or compulsions that are recurrent, impair functioning, and cause significant distress
- Common obsessive thoughts and compulsions are listed in Tables 79.2 and 79.3
- Unlike adults with OCD, children with OCD may not have insight into the unreal nature of their obsessive thoughts

DIAGNOSIS AND EVALUATION

- Clinical evaluation
  - Clinical interview
    - Diagnosing pediatric OCD can be challenging because obsessions/compulsions are frequently hidden or poorly articulated, especially in younger children
    - Consider neuropsychological assessment if the child is struggling at school
    - If an abrupt onset of symptoms presents, consider screening for a GABHS infection, which can indicate a potential precipitant for PANDAS
- Assessment tools: reliable and validated scales can be used in conjunction with the history and examination
  - Children's Yale-Brown Obsessive Compulsive Scale (CY-BOCS) is the best studied and standardized scale for OCD
- Differential diagnosis
  - Normal behavior: repetitive and ritualistic behaviors can be part of the typical development at certain ages
  - Other psychiatric disorders: autistic spectrum disorder, tic disorder, psychotic disorder
  - Complex motor tics may resemble compulsions
    - The distinguishing feature is whether the action was preceded by an urge/uncomfortable feeling (indicative of tics) or by a specific anxious thought (such as a fear of something bad happening if the behavior is not done, indicative of OCD)

TREATMENT

- Psychotherapeutic treatments
  - There is strong evidence base for the efficacy of CBT
  - May consider supportive individual or family psychotherapy or insight-oriented therapy
- Pharmacologic treatments
  - Medications are reserved for moderate to severe cases of OCD or for CBT-resistant OCD
  - SSRIs are first-line medication treatment (e.g. FDA-approved agents include fluoxetine, fluvoxamine, sertraline, and clomipramine)

Post-Traumatic Stress Disorder (PTSD)

BASIC INFORMATION

- It is estimated that one in four children will experience a traumatic event before adulthood. Such an experience, which involves serious harm or threat of harm to others or oneself, can include (but is not limited to) the death of a loved one; a car accident; exposure to or being a victim of physical, emotional, or sexual trauma; natural disasters; or medical trauma. Although children are often resilient, there are times when children develop significant mental health sequelae after such a traumatic experience. Given the potential long-lasting impact of one such condition, PTSD, it is imperative for all medical professionals to be familiar with the clinical signs and symptoms of this disorder
- Natural history
  - There is some evidence that "natural recovery" occurs in children with PTSD, although this has not consistently been found across studies
  - Most children with PTSD symptoms that persist have a poor prognosis without effective intervention
  - Untreated PTSD is a significant risk factor for increased suicide attempts, major depression, dissociation, and impaired global emotional functioning
- Risk factors for developing PTSD: female gender, previous trauma exposure, multiple traumas, presence of a preexisting psychiatric disorder, parental psychopathology, lack of social support
- Protective factors: parental support, lower levels of parental PTSD, and resolution of other parental trauma–related symptoms
- Comorbidity: PTSD sufferers often present with psychiatric comorbidities including depression, anxiety behavioral issues, and substance use
- Causes and etiology
  - A required etiologic factor for developing PTSD is the experience of a traumatic event
  - The exact pathophysiology of PTSD is otherwise largely unknown
  - Other risk factors for developing PTSD include repeated media exposure after a disaster, delayed evacuation after a disaster, and the presence of a predisaster anxiety disorder

CLINICAL PRESENTATION

- Core symptoms
  - Intrusion symptoms: frequent intrusive memories, nightmares, flashbacks, intense distress on exposure to cues that recall the event
  - Avoidance symptoms: the child will actively avoid specific situations or anything that reminds them of the event
  - Negative changes in mood and cognition: increase in feeling such as guilt, anger, fear, and shame and decrease in positive emotions such as happiness and interest in things they enjoy
  - Excessive arousal: irritability, insomnia, angry outbursts, hypervigilance, exaggerated startle response, and concentration difficulty
- Special consideration of symptoms by age:
  - <5 years: fear of being separated from a parent, crying, whimpering, screaming, immobility and/or aimless motion, trembling, frightened facial expressions, excessive clinging, regression behaviors

- 6-11 years: withdrawal, disruptive behaviors, inability to focus, regressive behaviors, anxiety, nightmares, sleep problems, irrational fears, school refusal, somatic symptoms, mood dysregulation (irritability, anger outbursts, new-onset depression), feelings of guilt, emotional numbing
  - 12–17 years: may have responses similar to those of adults

DIAGNOSIS AND EVALUATION

- Clinical evaluation
  - Clinical interview
    - Children with this disorder are often trying to avoid thinking and talking about the trauma, so it can be difficult to diagnose
  - It is important to screen for other mental comorbidities, including depression and anxiety, because many symptoms can mimic or be comorbid with those of PTSD
  - A suicide safety screen should also be considered if appropriate
- Assessment tools: an evaluation should always include the use of parent/child rating scales for assessing PTSD. Scale type is dependent on age
  - Children >7 years of age can self-report and use measures, such as the UCLA PTSD Reaction Index or the Child PTSD Symptom Scale
  - Screening of children <7 years of age relies on caregiver rating scales, including the PTSD for Preschool-Age Children (PTSD-PAC) caregiver report measure
  - Other commonly used scales that screen for a wider range of trauma-related symptoms (depression, PT-DDS, anxiety) are the Trauma Symptom Checklist for Children (approved for children >8 years of age) and the Trauma Symptom Checklist for Younger Children (approved for children 3–12 years of age)
  - If a screening is positive, the child should be referred to a mental health specialist
- Differential diagnosis
  - Other psychiatric disorders: ADHD, ODD, panic disorder, social anxiety disorder, depressive disorders, bipolar disorder, substance use disorders, psychotic disorders

TREATMENT

- Psychotherapeutic treatments
  - Trauma-focused cognitive behavioral therapy (TF-CBT)
  - Cognitive-behavioral interventions for trauma in schools (CBITS)
  - Narrative exposure therapy for children (KidsNET)
  - Trauma grief component therapy for adolescents
  - Eye movement desensitization and reprocessing (EMDR): some evidence of improvement in intrusion symptoms but not in avoidance or hyperarousal symptoms
- Pharmacologic treatments
  - No RCTs showing efficacy of any medication treatment
  - Medications should be added to children *only* after they fail psychotherapy alone or if there is a comorbid psychiatric diagnosis, such as depression or anxiety

- Some trials suggest benefits of SSRIs (most evidence, approved for adults with PTSD), propranolol, and clonidine in children
- Prazosin (used often successfully in veterans with PTSD) has also shown to improve reexperiencing and hyperarousal symptoms in one published case report

Major Depressive Disorder and Persistent Depressive Disorder

BASIC INFORMATION

- Epidemiology
  - Estimated prevalence of major depessive disorder (MDD) is 2% in children and 4% to 8% in adolescents
  - Estimated prevalence of persistent depressive disorder (dysthymia) is 0.6% to 1.7% in children and 1.6% to 8% in adolescents
- Natural history
  - More commonly diagnosed after puberty but is possible at any age
- Comorbidities
  - Frequently coexist with other psychiatric disorders, including anxiety, ADHD, and substance abuse, as well as medical disorders such as hypothyroidism and anemia
- Causes and etiology
  - Combination of genetics and environmental

CLINICAL PRESENTATION

Major Depressive Disorder (MDD)

- Similar presentation to adults; however, differs depending on the developmental stage of the child
- Common feature is the presence of changes in mood, including sadness or irritability, as well as somatic and/or cognitive changes that disrupt daily function
- Symptoms last 2 or more weeks and must include either depressed or irritable mood and/or loss of interest or pleasure
- Other symptoms include changes in appetite and/or sleep, fatigue, inability to concentrate, wish to be dead, and increased guilt
- Consider this diagnosis when a child or teen who was previously doing well in school starts to perform poorly in school, begins to act withdrawn, and/or starts to act out
- Predominant mood may be irritability/aggression or hyperactivity, especially in children who are nonverbal

Persistent Depressive Disorder (Dysthymia)

- Depressed mood for most of the day that occurs most days and for at least 1 year (2 years in adults)
- Symptoms are not as severe as MDD but can cause the same level of impairment

DIAGNOSIS AND EVALUATION

- Clinical interview
- Current and past depressive symptoms can be obtained based on the following:
  - Diagnostic classification: *DSM-5* or *ICD-10*
  - Rating scales: BDI-II, CDI-II, CDRS-R, or PHQ-A and Severity Measure for Depression—Child
  - Structured diagnostic interviews: DISC, ChIPS, or MINI
  - Semistructured diagnostic interviews: Kiddie-SADS or ADIS
- Obtain current and past psychiatric review of systems to assess for comorbid disorders, including anxiety disorders, eating disorders, and autism spectrum disorders
- Family and mental health history, current/past psychosocial stressors, and a safety assessment including suicide risk assessment
- Medical history should be obtained, and consider laboratory work or referral to medical provider if indicated

TREATMENT

- Psychotherapy
  - Supportive therapy
  - CBT
  - Interpersonal psychotherapy for adolescents (IPT-A)
- Medication management
  - Not recommended when there is minor psychosocial impairment
  - Obtain informed consent before initiation
  - FDA-approved medications:
    - Fluoxetine (ages 8–17 years) or escitalopram (ages 12–17 years)
      After medication initiation, the child/adolescent should have follow-up weekly for one month, then biweekly for one month, then monthly
      Closely monitor child's response to medication by using a follow-up rating scale (use the same scale as initial evaluation) at weeks 2 and 4, and then monthly
        Dose can be increased after 4 weeks if there is no clinical change
        Adequate clinical response: 50 percent or more reduction of depressive symptoms within 8 to 12 weeks
    - Treatment goal: remission of symptoms within 12 weeks of initiation of antidepressant
      If child/adolescent is not responding to treatment within this time frame, refer to a child psychiatrist for further management

Bipolar Disorder

BASIC INFORMATION

- Phenomenology of pediatric bipolar disorder is relatively new, and there has been significant debate on the presentation of pediatric bipolar disorder

- Bipolar spectrum disorders have an estimated prevalence of 0% to 3% in community samples
- Prevalence of childhood-onset bipolar disorder is not well established because of the debate over and heterogeneity of the case definition of pediatric bipolar disorder
- Pediatric bipolar disorder increases the risk of several other significant mental health issues, including suicide, psychosis, and substance abuse disorder
- On average, it takes about 10 years to identify and begin treatment of bipolar disorder
- Genetic etiology for bipolar disorder with an estimated heritability at over 80%

CLINICAL PRESENTATION

- *DSM-5*–specified criteria for bipolar disorder are identical for adults and youth
- Criteria for mania:
  - Elevated or expansive or irritable mood and persistent goal-directed activity that lasts for at least 1 week, or less than that if hospitalization is necessary
  - Grandiosity, increased sexuality, racing thoughts, distractibility, reduced need for sleep, increased talkativeness, excessive involvement in activities that have a high potential for painful consequences
  - These symptoms must lead to significant dysfunction to amount to a diagnosis and must not occur exclusively in the context of any substance use, medication effect, or medical condition
- Criteria for depression:
  - Depressed mood nearly every day and/or reduced interest or feeling of no pleasure at all for at least 2 weeks
  - Insomnia or hypersomnia, increased or decreased appetite or significant weight loss when not dieting, weight gain or a change of more than 5% of body weight in a month, increased or decreased psychomotor activity, fatigue or loss of energy, feelings of worthlessness, inappropriate guilt, reduced ability to think or concentrate, recurrent thoughts of death or suicide
  - These symptoms must lead to significant dysfunction to amount to a diagnosis and must not occur exclusively in the context of any substance use, medication effect, or medical condition
- Bipolar type I requires a history of at least one manic episode
  - If there are psychotic features, the episode is considered manic
  - Most specific symptoms of mania: hypersexuality and grandiosity
- Bipolar type II requires at least one episode of depression and hypomania
  - Hypomanic episodes are not severe enough to cause marked impairment in social or occupational functioning or to necessitate hospitalization
- Bipolar disorder NOS (not otherwise specified): represents the largest group of patients with bipolar symptoms
  - This entity is for children who do not have clear-cut episodes of mood changes and who do not fulfill the full

DSM-5 criteria or meet the duration criteria. This also includes cases secondary to general medical condition

- Cyclothymia refers to episodic mood changes characterized by subtle hypomania and mild depression
- Phenomenology of pediatric bipolar disorder
  - Most common presenting symptom of mania: increased energy (89% of the sample)
  - Least common presenting symptom of mania: hypersexuality and flights of ideas
  - Prevalence of hallucination and delusion in mania: 42% of sample
  - More than 50% of bipolar disorder cases may present as depression
- Important to differentiate insomnia from reduced need for sleep. The latter is an important symptom of manic episodes

DIAGNOSIS AND EVALUATION

- Clinical interview
  - Assess whether mood and symptoms are abnormal and clearly different from the child's usual mood and behavior in the context of the child's level of development
- Assess for risk of suicide or homicide. Imminent danger to self and/or others warrants inpatient psychiatric hospitalization to ensure safety
- Assess for comorbid conditions. Bipolar disorder is associated with multiple comorbidities, ranging from 70% for ADHD to 8% for substance abuse
- It is important to distinguish bipolar disorder from ADHD; ADHD lacks distinct episodes of mania and depression, and clear-cut elevated mood and grandiosity are absent
- Rule out medical conditions and medication effects that may mimic manic episode:
  - Temporal lobe sclerosis
  - Hyperthyroidism
  - Closed or open head trauma
  - Multiple sclerosis
  - Systemic lupus erythematosus
  - Effects of TCAs, SSRIs, SNRIs, sympathomimetic amines, steroids, recreational drugs, and so forth

TREATMENT

- At any phase of treatment: psychoeducation, basic elements of support such as active listening, and restoration of hope are indicated
- Phases of treatment: acute, continuation, and maintenance phases

Pharmacotherapy

- The following drugs have received FDA approval for pediatric bipolar disorder with a minimum age range of 10 to 13 years, depending on the drug:
  - Mood stabilizer: lithium (≥12 years old)
  - Atypical antipsychotic: risperidone, olanzapine, quetiapine, aripiprazole, asenapine
  - Olanzapine-fluoxetine combination is approved for bipolar depression in ages 10 years and above

- Recent studies suggest atypical antipsychotics are equally efficacious compared with common mood stabilizers and appear to yield a quicker response
- In general, monotherapy with lithium or an atypical antipsychotic agent is preferable as the first line of treatment for acute manic/mixed episodes
- In cases of nonresponse or intolerable side effects to initial monotherapy, treatment with another mood stabilizer or an atypical antipsychotic not previously tried is recommended
- In cases of partial response, augmentation strategy is recommended. The choice of augmentation agent may be risperidone, aripiprazole, olanzapine, or quetiapine. The choice depends upon the side effect profile and previous treatment response
- For mania/mixed mania with psychotic features, a mood stabilizer combined with an atypical antipsychotic is the first choice. However, atypical antipsychotic monotherapy may serve as an alternative choice

Depression

- Youth with bipolar disorder spend substantial time with syndromal or subsyndromal depressive symptoms; there are limited available data regarding the treatment of pediatric bipolar depression. Most evidence is extrapolated from the adult literature
- Concerns that monotherapy with an SSRI may trigger a manic or hypomanic switch in pediatric bipolar disorder
- Often lamotrigine, lithium, valproate, or the atypical antipsychotics are used as first-line medications for bipolar depression. For partial responders or nonresponders, combinations of these medications with atypical antipsychotics, SSRIs, or bupropion are indicated
- For subjects with recurrent seasonal depression, light therapy is indicated

Continuation and maintenance treatments

- Limited research has been done on maintenance treatment of pediatric bipolar disorder. An 18-month naturalistic follow-up study involving bipolar adolescents discovered a relapse rate of 92% in adolescents who stopped lithium treatment compared with 38% who continued with lithium
- Because of the high relapse rate, the most current consensus recommendations suggest that medication taper may be considered once remission has been maintained for 12 to 24 months

Psychosocial treatment

- Psychosocial treatment options for bipolar disorder may be supportive psychotherapy, CBT, child- and family-focused CBT (CFF-CBT), multiple family group treatment, and family-focused therapy (FFT). Psychosocial treatments are also efficacious for the treatment of comorbid mental health issues such as ODD, substance use disorder, anxiety disorder, and so forth

Disruptive Mood Dysregulation Disorder (DMDD)

BASIC INFORMATION

- New entry in *DSM-5* under section on depressive disorders
- Characterized by frequent, severe, recurrent major temper outbursts and chronic irritable mood. Both of the symptoms must be present for at least 1 year and cannot be accounted for by another mood disorder
- The prevalence is unclear given the novelty of the diagnosis. One-year prevalence of DMDD is likely between 2% and 5% of the general pediatric and adolescent population
- Diagnosis of DMDD was included to reduce misdiagnosis of bipolar disorder in children with chronic irritability and temper outbursts but without any clear periodicity

CLINICAL PRESENTATION

- Central to the diagnosis of DMDD are:
  - Chronic, unremitting irritability and temper outbursts and rages that are clearly inconsistent with age/developmental stage
  - Occurring at least 3 times a week
  - Persistent irritable mood in between temper episodes
  - Symptoms must be present for more than a year and without any period lasting for more than 3 consecutive months when patient did not have these symptoms
  - Symptoms must be present in at least two settings (in comparison to ODD, which can be diagnosed even if symptoms are present in only one setting)
  - Diagnosis should not be made before 6 or after 18 years of age
- *Can* coexist with MDD, ADHD, CD, and substance use disorders
- *Cannot* coexist with ODD, intermittent explosive disorder, or bipolar disorder
  - Individuals whose symptoms meet criteria for both DMDD and ODD should only be given the diagnosis of DMDD
  - If an individual has ever experienced a manic or hypomanic episode, the diagnosis of DMDD should not be assigned

DIAGNOSIS AND EVALUATION

- Obtain a detailed clinical history from both the child (depending on age) and caregivers
- Assess severity of symptoms and psychosocial functioning
- Obtain current and past psychiatric review of systems to assess for comorbid disorders, including mood or anxiety disorders and ADHD
- Determine family and mental health history, current/past psychosocial stressors, and a safety assessment including suicide risk assessment

TREATMENT

- Nonpharmacologic intervention:
  - Parent management training
  - CBT
- Pharmacologic intervention:
  - Clear pharmacologic treatment guidelines have yet to be established
  - General recommendation is to follow established treatment protocol for comorbid conditions (e.g., stimulant for ADHD, CBT, and SSRI for MDD)
  - Treatment approach differs from that for pediatric bipolar disorder, which is treated by mood stabilizers and antipsychotics

Somatic Symptom and Related Disorders (Conversion Disorder)

- Conversion disorder (functional neurologic symptom disorder) and the related somatic symptom disorder, illness anxiety disorder, and factitious disorder are combined into one chapter in the *DSM-5* and have undergone significant criteria changes and simplification with the intention of making them more "user friendly" to nonpsychiatrists because these disorders generally present first in medical rather than in psychiatric settings
- Somatic symptom disorders should not be thought of as diagnoses of exclusion, but rather as a set of inclusive criteria and should be on the differential from the start when clinical findings provide evidence of incompatibility between the reported symptoms and any recognized neurologic or medical condition
- It is important to note that oftentimes somatic and conversion disorders will co-occur with, and frequently add complexity to the treatment and recovery of, organic medical problems and other psychiatric diagnoses such as depression

BASIC INFORMATION

- Epidemiology
  - 5% to 7% prevalence; these disorders tend to "run in families"
  - Females are 2 to 10 times more likely to be affected than males
  - Higher risk in patients with traumatic life events in late childhood or early adolescence (e.g., rape, death of parent or sibling, parent divorce)
  - Higher risk in patients who have had serious medical problems in the past
  - Often comorbid with depression, anxiety disorders, or PTSD

CLINICAL PRESENTATION

Conversion Disorder

- Criteria
  - One or more symptoms of altered voluntary motor or sensory function

- Clinical findings provide evidence of incompatibility between the symptom and recognized neurologic or medical conditions
- The symptom or deficit is not better explained by another medical or psychiatric diagnosis
- The symptom or deficit causes clinically significant distress or impairment or warrants a medical evaluation
- Historically these disorders have been called psychogenic or functional
  - "Functional blindness" or "psychogenic seizures"
- Common presentations of conversion disorder
  - "Pseudoseizures" (now called "nonepileptic" or psychogenic spells)
  - Arm/leg paresthesia
  - Tremors
  - Gait disturbances
  - Special sensory symptoms (e.g., vision, hearing, taste, smell abnormalities)

Somatic Symptom Disorder

- Criteria
  - One or more somatic symptoms (abdominal pain, headaches, fatigue, and nausea are most common in children and adolescents)
  - Excessive thoughts, feelings, or behaviors related to the symptoms that are out of proportion to the severity of the symptoms
  - 6+ months of symptom duration
- Common diagnoses under the somatic symptom disorder umbrella include abdominal pain, chronic fatigue, and functional stress headaches
- Symptoms often will worsen before or during school hours or during times of stress but will improve when family is attentive or when the patient is doing something fun/enjoyable
- Level of discomfort is generally out of proportion to the description of the symptoms and oftentimes will not be consistent and will not fit clinically with an organic diagnosis

DIAGNOSIS AND EVALUATION

- A medical evaluation should be completed on initial presentation, just as with any other diagnosis, but ongoing testing, repetitive imaging, trials of medications are not helpful and will serve to reinforce the use of the patient's somatic symptoms as a coping skill
- Somatic symptom disorder is not a diagnosis of exclusion, and criteria can be met without "ruling out" every diagnosis, regardless of how far down the differential it is
- Internal inconsistency at examination is one way to demonstrate incompatibility with organic neurologic disease and is helpful to find on examination. Examples of such findings are:
  - Hoover sign: weakness of hip extension returns to normal strength with contralateral hip flexion against resistance
  - Marked weakness of ankle plantar flexion when tested on the bed, when patient is able to walk on tiptoes
  - Tremor entrainment test: tremor changes when patient is distracted away from it

- The occurrence of closed eyes with resistance to opening or a normal electroencephalography (EEG) during a psychogenic nonepileptic attack
- La Belle indifference: lack of concern about the nature or implications of the symptoms (this is not specific to conversion disorder but is supportive)

TREATMENT

- Treat any comorbid psychiatric conditions (e.g., depression, anxiety)
- Parent and child education about role of psychological stress in functional symptoms
- Parent-child therapy and CBT can be helpful
- Schedule frequent follow-ups both for reassurance and for preventing excessive emergency department use or use of other physicians who may order unnecessary testing

Psychosis and Thought Disorders

BASIC INFORMATION

- Formal psychotic disorders are rare in children, but transient psychotic phenomena are more common in healthy, typically developing children (associated with anxiety or stress), as well as in those with other psychiatric or neurologic disturbances
- The most well known of the psychotic disorders are schizophrenia and bipolar disorder, which often appear in late adolescence or early young adulthood
- Psychotic symptoms can also can also be found in delirium, MDD with psychotic features, PTSD, anxiety disorders, depressive disorders, and other psychotic disorders, including schizoaffective disorder, delusional disorder, schizophreniform disorder, shared psychotic disorder, brief psychotic disorder, and substance-induced psychotic disorder, as well as a variety of medical illnesses
- Psychosis in children and adolescents can be a result of illness, delirium, intoxication, neurologic disorders, and other medical conditions
- Although psychosis is rare in children, lifetime outcomes are poorer with earlier onset; psychosis is associated with an increase in suicide risk and aggression, particularly when a patient is acutely ill

CLINICAL PRESENTATION

- Psychosis is defined by abnormalities in one or more of the following five domains: delusions, hallucinations, disorganized thinking (speech), grossly disorganized or abnormal motor behavior (including catatonia), and negative symptoms (see Tables 79.4 and 79.5)
- There may be a prodromal phase with changes in behavior and affect before an acute phase of psychotic illness
- In children and adolescents with developmental delay or autism, may present as changes in behavior
- May be precipitated by substance use

DIAGNOSIS AND EVALUATION

- Clinical interview

Table 79.4. Positive Symptoms of Psychosis

Hallucinations: false sensory perceptions in the absence of external stimuli	Auditory Visual olfactory Tactile Gustatory
Delusions: false, firmly held beliefs that persist despite conflicting evidence	Persecutory Referential Grandiose Religious Somatic
Disorganized thinking/speech	Tangentiality Derailment Loosening of associations Incoherent or incomprehensible Nonsensical, "word salad"
Disorganized or abnormal behavior	Inappropriate behavior for a given social situation Inappropriate laughter Unprovoked aggression or agitation Inability to engage in goal-directed behavior (e.g., unable to bathe, brush teeth, feed self, etc.) Catatonic behavior
Catatonic behavior	Marked decrease in reactions to surrounding environment Negativism: resistance to instruction Maintaining a rigid, inappropriate, or bizarre posture Complete lack of verbal response (mutism) Complete lack of motor response (stupor) Repetitive motions or speech including echolalia Purposeless/excessive motor activity (catatonic excitement)

Table 79.5. Negative Symptoms of Psychosis

Diminished emotional expression: reduced eye contact and facial expression, flat or blunted affect
Avolition: decrease in self-initiated purposeful activities
Alogia: marked decrease in speech output
Anhedonia: decreased ability to experience pleasure
Asociality: apparent lack of interest in social interactions, social withdrawal
Impaired cognitive performance in attention, concentration, memory, and planning
Reduced motivation

- Family and mental health history, current/past psychosocial stressors
- Mental status examination
  - Note thought content (e.g., delusions) and perceptual abnormalities (e.g., hallucinations)
  - Note thought form (e.g., pressured speech, internal preoccupation)
  - Assess insight
  - Assess safety, including risk of suicide, self-injury, and ability to care for self
- Comprehensive physical examination
- Laboratory, imaging, and other evaluations for early-onset psychosis (Table 79.6)

Table 79.6. Investigations Recommended at Baseline Assessment for Early-Onset Psychosis

Investigation	Rationale
Full blood count	- Detection of preexisting hematologic disorders such as anemia - Monitoring side effects of mood stabilizers
Urea, electrolytes, and liver function tests	- Exclusion of preexisting abnormalities (rare, but polydipsia can be seen in psychosis) - Monitoring for medication side effects (some antipsychotics and antidepressants can cause hypernatremia mood stabilizers can impair renal and liver function)
Fasting glucose, cholesterol, and triglycerides	- Detection of insulin resistance or lipid abnormalities; initial and 6-monthly monitoring because most antipsychotics can cause weight gain and insulin resistance
Thyroid function	- Thyroid abnormalities can cause mood elevation or depression and are a side effect of lithium treatment
Calcium levels	- Abnormalities are a rare cause of psychosis
Prolactin	- Exclusion of pretreatment hyperprolactinemia (e.g., due to pituitary tumor) - To monitor possible antipsychotic-induced hyperprolactinemia
Brain imaging (computerized axial tomography [CAT], magnetic resonance imaging [MRI])	- Exclusion of preexisting neuroanatomic lesions (injuries, malignancy) - MRI preferable because of higher-resolution image and less radiation exposure, but noise and claustrophobia may not be tolerated by patient
Electroencephalography (EEG)	- Exclusion of a seizure disorder
Urine drug screen	- To rule out recent drug use or identify illicit drugs taken recently

- Electrocardiogram (ECG) to evaluate for cardiac abnormalities, which may be affected by antipsychotic medication treatment
- Evaluation for medical causes of psychosis
  - Delirium
  - Autoimmune disorders (e.g., systemic lupus erythematosus, anti-NMDA receptor encephalitis)
  - Seizures
  - Thyrotoxicosis
  - Wilson disease
  - Vitamin B_{12} deficiency
  - Cushing disease
  - Substance intoxication or withdrawal
- Differential diagnosis:
  - Schizophrenia: symptoms last for at least 6 months and include at least 1 month of active-phase symptoms, with decline in functioning

- Brief psychotic disorder: symptoms present for at least 1 day but remit by 1 month
- Delusional disorder: at least 1 month of persistent delusions and no other psychotic symptoms
- Schizophreniform disorder: presentation similar to schizophrenia lasting for less than 6 months; patient does not have to have a decline in functioning
- Schizoaffective disorder: both a mood episode and the active-phase symptoms of schizophrenia occur together and are preceded or followed by at least a 2-week period of delusions or hallucinations without mood symptoms

TREATMENT

- Inpatient psychiatric hospitalization may be needed for an acute-phase illness when:
  - A patient represents a danger to self or others
  - A patient is unable to care for himself or herself
  - Illness is so severe that it cannot be managed as an outpatient
- Primary treatment for psychotic disorders is the use of antipsychotic medications
  - Atypical or second-generation antipsychotics (SGA), such as risperidone, quetiapine, or olanzapine, are preferable
    - Associated with risk of metabolic syndrome
    - Requires regular monitoring of weight, blood pressure, fasting glucose, and lipids
    - Lower risk of movement disorders (e.g., tardive dyskinesia) and extrapyramidal symptoms compared with first-generation antipsychotics (FGAs)
  - Typical or FGAs such as haloperidol
    - Associated with increased risk of extrapyramidal symptoms and neuroleptic malignant syndrome compared with SGAs
    - Less expensive and lower risk of metabolic syndrome compared with SGAs
- If depressive/anxiety symptoms are present with psychotic illness, may add an SSRI
- If fluctuating mood symptoms are present with psychotic illness, may add a mood stabilizer
- Comprehensive treatment involves other modalities in addition to medication
  - Psychoeducation
  - Cognitive behavioral therapy
  - Cognitive remediation therapy to promote improvement in cognitive deficits
  - Family therapy/intervention
  - Vocational/occupational services to facilitate return to school or work

Suicidal and Nonsuicidal Self-Injurious (NSSI) Behaviors

BASIC INFORMATION

- Definitions
  - Suicide attempt: self-directed, potentially injurious behavior with the intent to die
  - Suicidal ideation (SI): thinking, considering, or planning suicide without actually engaging in the behavior
    - *Passive SI*: the individual thinks about wanting to be dead
    - *Active SI*: the individual has thoughts about killing oneself
  - Nonsuicidal self-injurious behavior (NSSI): deliberate, self-inflicted destruction of one's body in an attempt to relieve distress or regulate emotions, without the intent to die
    - Common behaviors include cutting, scratching, biting, hitting, or burning oneself
- Epidemiology
  - Suicide
    - Third leading cause of death in youth aged 10 to 14 years
    - Second leading cause of death among persons aged 15 to 34 years
    - In 2013, a sample representing youth nationwide in grades 9 to 12 reported that in the 12 months before the survey:
      - 17.0% of students seriously considered attempting suicide
      - 13.6% of students made a plan about how they would attempt suicide
      - 8.0% of students attempted suicide one or more times
    - Age: the rate of suicide (ideation, attempts, and completion) increases with age after puberty
    - Sex: females report higher rates of suicide attempts than males. However, males have a higher rate of completed suicide compared with females. Males use more lethal means and have more associated risk factors—antisocial behaviors and substance use
    - Race/ethnicity: in the United States, the rate of suicide is higher among white youth compared with nonwhite youth. Of all ethnic groups in the United States, American Indians/Alaska Natives exhibit the highest suicide rate
  - NSSI
    - In the United States, one-third to one-half of adolescents have engaged in NSSI
- Risk factors
  - Suicide
    - Personal risk factors: history of suicidal behavior (strongest predictor of future suicidal behavior), engaging in NSSI, substance use, physical and/or sexual abuse, diagnosis of a psychiatric disorder (anxiety disorder, disruptive disorder, psychosis, highest risk with mood disorder)
    - Sexual orientation: youth who are lesbian, gay, bisexual, transgender, or questioning their sexual orientation have suicide rates two to three times higher than their heterosexual peers
    - Familial risk factors: family history of suicide, psychiatric disorders, substance abuse
    - Immediate risk factors: access to lethal means, agitation, intoxication, a recent stressful life event
    - Social risk factors: bullying, difficulties in school, social isolation, impaired parent-child relationship, homelessness, living in a corrections facility or group home, history of adoption

- Internet: excessive daily video gaming and Internet use (>5 hours/day) correlate with higher levels of suicidal ideation and attempts. Among youth, suicide-related internet search is associated with completed suicide
  - Rates of suicide often increase among adolescents with exposure to a peer suicide
- NSSI
  - Risk factors include depression, PTSD, generalized anxiety, disruptive disorders, eating disorders, and substance use
- Protective factors include effective coping strategies; absence of lethal means; religious engagement; strong connection with family, friends, and school; mental health access

CLINICAL PRESENTATION

- Suicide
  - Warning signs for youth include isolating self from others, talking about death more, expressing their suicidal intent or plan to peers (including through social media), or giving away belongings
  - Methods: in 2013, in youth aged 15 to 19 years, methods for suicide included suffocation (43%), discharge of firearms (42%), poisoning (6%), and falling (3%)
  - Mental status examination: assess level of current suicidal ideation/intent/plan, psychotic symptoms, mood and affect (withdrawn, dysphoric, apathetic, irritable, anxious), and level of insight and judgement
  - Physical examination: assess for physical signs of harming oneself (bruises or cuts) and signs of intoxication or delirium
- NSSI
  - Youth may deny engaging in NSSI
  - Physical examination: presence of old or new scars (possible areas include arms, wrists, thighs, legs, and trunk), lacerations (superficial or deep), scratch marks, burns, or contusions

DIAGNOSIS AND EVALUATION

- Adolescent should be interviewed separately from the parent
- Information gathering:
  - Suicidal ideation: evaluate for intent, frequency, intensity, specific plans, and access to lethal means
    - "Is the patient likely to commit suicide in the future? Is the patient likely to make a suicide attempt in the future? Will the patient follow through on a psychiatric referral on the basis of this evaluation?"
  - Suicide attempt: methods used; evaluate whether attempt was impulsive or planned
  - Assessment tools: youth who endorse suicidality on a scale should subsequently be evaluated clinically
- Columbia Suicide Severity Rating Scale: evaluates suicidality in youth >12 years of age

TREATMENT

- Acutely suicidal adolescents should be taken to the emergency department or to a psychiatric crisis center for psychiatric evaluation
  - Admit to appropriate level of care until the patient is medically stable
  - Consider 1:1 monitoring of patient for safety
  - Consult child and adolescent psychiatry and consider psychiatric medications
  - Consider for inpatient psychiatric care
- Patient stable for discharge
  - Appropriate for patients who exhibit low levels of suicidal behavior and who are prepared to participate in outpatient sessions with the support of their caregivers
  - Firearms should be removed from the home. Family must prevent access to medications, sharp objects, and alcohol to decrease risk
  - Contact patient's psychiatrist, therapist, or pediatrician before discharge. Instruct family to contact mental health provider or return to emergency department if they are concerned about their child's safety
  - Safety plans can be effective in preventing suicidal behavior (suicide contracts have not been)
  - Components of a safety plan include:
    - Recognizing warning signs
    - Using internal coping strategies
    - Naming people who can support and distract from suicidal thoughts/urges
    - Identifying adults who help during a crisis
    - Contacting mental health professionals or agencies (emergency department, suicide hotline)
    - Ensuring a safe environment (removal of lethal means)
    - Positive reasons to live identified by the patient

Review Questions

For review questions, please go to ExpertConsult.com.

Suggested Readings

1. American Academy of Child and Adolescent Psychiatry. Practice Parameters. https://www.aacap.org/aacap/Resources_for_Primary_Care/Practice_Parameters_and_Resource_Centers/Practice_Parameters.aspx
2. American Psychiatric Association. *Diagnostic and Statistical Manual of Mental Disorders.* 5th ed. Washington DC: American Psychiatric Publishing; 2013.
3. Dulcan M, ed. *Dulcan's Textbook of Child and Adolescent Psychiatry.* 2nd ed. Arlington, VA: American Psychiatric Publishing; 2016.
4. Rey JM, ed. *IACAPAP E-textbook of Child and Adolescent Mental Health.* Geneva: International Association for Child and Adolescent Psychiatry and Allied Professions; 2016.
5. Volkmar F, Martin A, eds. *Essentials of Lewis's Child and Adolescent Psychiatry.* Philadelphia: Lippincott Williams & Wilkins; 2011.

Rheumatology

80 Clinical Approach to Arthritis

JOYCE CHUN-LING CHANG, MD

When presented a patient with joint pain, your first task is to determine whether it is inflammatory (arthritis) or noninflammatory (arthralgia). Most often this can be established from several distinguishing features in the history alone. Morning stiffness and persistent joint swelling are more characteristic of arthritis. Ultimately arthritis is a clinical diagnosis made based on history and physical examination findings, although the diagnosis can be supported by imaging findings suggestive of joint effusions or synovitis. The differential diagnosis of arthritis in childhood is broad, ranging from infectious etiologies to post-infectious syndromes and chronic rheumatic diseases. There are also several mimics of inflammatory arthritis, including osteomyelitis and malignancy. Knowledge of the chronicity of symptoms, the number and distribution of joints involved, as well as the presence of other systemic findings, can help narrow the differential diagnosis and guide a targeted work-up.

See also Nelson Textbook of Pediatrics, Chapter 155, "Juvenile Idiopathic Arthritis."

History

- Symptoms of <u>inflammatory</u> joint pain:
  - Stiffness that is worse in the morning and improves with activity
    - May also occur on arising from a chair or after prolonged inactivity
    - Morning stiffness lasting >15 minutes is highly suggestive of inflammatory arthritis
    - Improves with activity and application of heat
    - A limp that improves throughout the day is characteristic of lower-extremity arthritis and may be the only abnormality observed by the parent in a young child
  - Persistent swelling
  - Warmth, ± erythema
  - Decreased range of motion
  - Pain may or may not be a prominent feature
  - Fever can accompany arthritis of infectious or systemic inflammatory causes
- Symptoms associated with noninflammatory musculoskeletal pain:
  - Pain that worsens toward the evening
  - Pain that is exacerbated by activity
  - Pain that is episodic and self-limited (e.g., growing pains)
  - If swelling is present, typically resolves within 1 to 2 weeks (e.g., trauma)
- Chronicity, severity, and pattern of joint involvement will help narrow the differential (Fig. 80.1):

- Is it acute (<72 hours), subacute, or chronic (>6 weeks)?
- Is there micromotion tenderness?
- Is it monoarticular (single joint), oligoarticular (few joints), or polyarticular (more than four joints)?
- Does it involve primarily large joints or small joints?
- Physical signs
  - Warmth, swelling, tenderness, and limited range of motion are characteristic of arthritis
    - In contrast, *arthralgia* refers only to joint pain
  - Knee and elbow arthritis: decreased extension occurs first
  - Hip arthritis: limited internal rotation
    - Note that any hip pathology can manifest with groin pain, as well as pain referred to the knee or thigh
  - Ankle (tibiotalar joint) arthritis: limited dorsiflexion
- A single red, hot joint is most concerning for septic arthritis
  - Overlying erythema is also seen with reactive arthritis and acute rheumatic fever, which typically involve more than one joint
- Skin findings can frequently make the diagnosis:
  - Vesiculopustular lesions on the extremities → disseminated gonococcal infection
  - Palpable purpura → vasculitis (e.g., Henoch-Schönlein purpura)
  - Erythema marginatum → acute rheumatic fever
  - Urticaria → serum sickness
  - Evanescent salmon-colored macules → systemic juvenile arthritis
- Warning signs (i.e., "red flags"):
  - Sudden refusal to weight bear
    - Consider trauma, osteomyelitis (fever, leukocytosis, increased inflammatory markers), or septic arthritis
  - Bone pain that occurs in the middle of the night
    - Leukemia, primary bone tumors

Diagnosis and Evaluation

- Arthritis is a clinical diagnosis based on joint swelling, warmth, tenderness, and limited range of motion
- Because arthritis is a key clinical feature in several syndromes, Table 80.1 provides a broad overview. Details for these diagnoses are included in Chapters 81 through 83
- Imaging can be used to support the clinical examination:
  - X-rays are useful for ruling out structural damage (e.g., fracture, slipped capital femoral epiphysis [SCFE], Legg-Calve-Perthes)

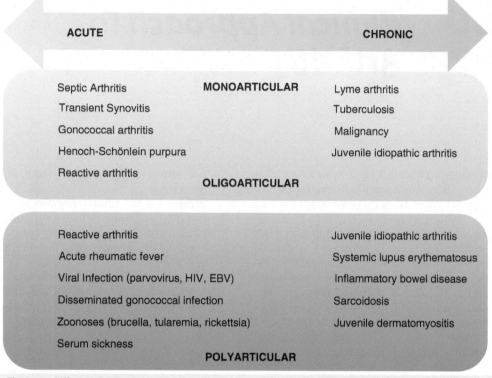

Fig. 80.1. Differential diagnosis of arthritis in children based on chronicity and pattern of joint involvement.

- Bone erosions are indicative of long-standing inflammatory arthritis
- Ultrasound is much better for evaluating effusions, particularly in the hip joints
  - Useful when toxic synovitis or septic hip arthritis is suspected
- Consider laboratory studies to screen for active infection, recent infection, or systemic illness:
  - Complete blood cell count with differential, C-reactive protein, and sedimentation rate to screen for systemic inflammation
  - Serum lactate dehydrogenase and peripheral smear if malignancy is on the differential
  - Testing for organisms associated with infectious arthritis:
    - Serologic testing for Lyme disease (if in an endemic area)
    - *Mycoplasma pneumoniae*
    - *Bartonella henselae*
    - Brucellosis
    - Tuberculosis
    - *Neisseria gonorrhoeae*
    - Viruses (parvovirus, Epstein-Barr virus [EBV], HIV)
  - Throat culture, antistreptolysin-O titers, and DNase B titers can all be used to document recent streptococcal infection
  - Renal function, liver enzymes, and urinalysis if systemic disease is suspected
  - Note: antinuclear antibody (ANA) and rheumatoid factor (RF) tests are *not* used to make a diagnosis of arthritis in children

- An ANA is useful as an initial screening test for systemic lupus erythematosus
- Synovial fluid analysis is most useful for determining whether joint fluid is inflammatory and for isolating infectious organisms (Table 80.2)
  - Gram stain and bacterial cultures should be sent with synovial fluid analysis
    - If the white blood cell (WBC) count is >50,000, the first priority is to rule out septic arthritis
      Gram-negative diplococci on Gram stain will almost always be gonorrhea

TREATMENT

- Nonsteroidal antiinflammatory drugs (NSAIDs) are frequently first line for symptomatic relief
- Treat the underlying cause:
  - Septic hip arthritis requires washout/drainage and antibiotics; other septic joints may be treated with antibiotics only (See Chapter 73)
    - Lyme arthritis is treated with antibiotics only
- Chronic inflammatory arthritis may require intraarticular steroid injections or systemic immunosuppression
- Transient postinfectious or viral arthritis: supportive care with NSAIDs

Review Questions

For review questions, please go to ExpertConsult.com

Table 80.1. Differential Diagnosis of Pediatric Arthritis Syndromes

Characteristic	Systemic Lupus Erythematosus	Juvenile Idiopathic Arthritis	Rheumatic Fever	Lyme Disease	Leukemia	Gonococcemia	Kawasaki Disease
Sex	F > M	Type-dependent	M = F	M = F	M = F	F > M	M = F
Age	10–20 years	1–16 years	5–15 years	>5–20 years	2–10 years	>12 years	<5 years
Pain	Yes	50%	Yes	Yes	Yes	Yes	Yes
Morning stiffness	Yes	Yes	No	Yes	No	Yes	No
Rash	Butterfly, discoid	Salmon-pink macules (systemic onset only)	Erythema marginatum	Erythema migrans (in early phase)	No	Palms/soles, papulopustules	Diffuse maculopapular (nonspecific), desquamation
Monoarticular	Yes	50%	No	Yes	Yes	Yes (second stage)	No
Polyarticular	Yes	Yes	Yes	No	Yes	Yes (early stage)	Yes
Small joints	Yes	Yes	No	Rare	Yes	Rare (early stage)	Yes
Temporomandibular joint	No	Yes	No	Rare	No	No	No
Eye disease	Uveitis/retinitis	Uveitis (not in systemic)	No	Conjunctivitis, keratitis	No	Conjunctivitis (early stage)	Conjunctivitis, uveitis
Total WBC count	↓	↑ (↓ in macrophage activation syndrome)	Normal to ↑	Normal	↑ or neutropenia ± blasts	↑	↑
ANA	Positive (>99%)	Positive (50%)	Negative	Negative	Negative	Negative	Negative
Rheumatoid factor	Positive or negative	Positive or negative (polyarticular only)	Negative	Negative	Negative	Negative	Negative
Other laboratory results	↓ Complement, + antibodies to double-stranded DNA	+ Anti-CCP antibody in adult-type RA	↑ASO, anti-DNase B	+ Lyme IgG	+ Bone marrow	+ Culture for *Neisseria gonorrhoeae*	↑Platelets
Erosive arthritis	Rare	Yes	Rare	Rare	No	Yes	No
Other clinical manifestations	Proteinuria, serositis, pancytopenia	Fever, serositis (systemic onset)	Carditis, nodules, chorea	Carditis, neuropathy, meningitis	Thrombocytopenia, anemia	Tenosynovitis, onset during menses	Fever, lymphadenopathy, swollen hands/feet, mouth lesions
Pathogenesis	Autoimmune	Autoimmune	Group A streptococcus	*Borrelia burgdorferi*	Acute lymphoblastic leukemia	*N. gonorrhoeae*	Unknown
Treatment	Corticosteroids, hydroxychloroquine, immunosuppressive agents	NSAIDs, methotrexate, TNF blockers for resistant disease	Penicillin prophylaxis, aspirin, corticosteroids	Penicillin, doxycycline, ceftriaxone	Corticosteroids, chemotherapy	Ceftriaxone	Intravenous immunoglobulin, aspirin

ANA, Antinuclear antibody; *ASO,* antistreptolysin-O titer; *CCP,* cyclic citrullinated protein; *NSAID,* nonsteroidal antiinflammatory drug; *RA,* rheumatoid arthritis; *TNF,* tumor necrosis factor; *WBC,* white blood cell.

Table 80.2.   Synovial Fluid Analysis

	While Blood Cell Count	% Neutrophils	Other
NONINFLAMMATORY			
Normal	<200	<25	Clear yellow
Traumatic	<2000	<25	Bloody/ xantho- chromic
INFLAMMATORY			
Rheumatic fever	5000	10–50	Cloudy yellow
Juvenile idiopathic arthritis	15,000–20,000	75	
Reactive arthritis	20,000	80	
PYOGENIC			
Tuberculous arthritis	25,000	50–60	Cloudy
Septic arthritis	>50,000	>75	Turbid; low glucose

Adapted from Petty R et al. *Textbook of Pediatric Rheumatology*, 7th ed. Philadelphia, Elsevier, 2016.

Suggested Readings

1. Berard R. Approach to the child with joint inflammation. *Pediatr Clin North Am.* 2012;59(2):245–262.
2. Tse SM, Laxer RM. Approach to Acute Limb Pain in Childhood. *Pediatr Rev.* 2006;27(5):170–179.

81 Inflammatory Arthritis

JOYCE CHUN-LING CHANG, MD

Inflammatory arthritis can be broadly separated into infectious, postinfectious, malignant, or chronic autoimmune causes (see Table 80.1 for a comparison of select diseases). In this chapter we will focus on a select group of postinfectious and autoimmune arthritides.

See also Nelson Textbook of Pediatrics, Chapter 155, "Juvenile Idiopathic Arthritis."

Reactive Arthritis

BASIC INFORMATION

- Classically occurs 1 to 4 weeks after genitourinary Chlamydia infection
  - "Can't see (conjunctivitis), can't pee (urethritis), can't climb a tree (arthritis)"
    - Previously known as Reiter syndrome
  - In children, most commonly occurs 1 to 4 weeks after bacterial gastroenteritis (Yersinia, Salmonella, Shigella, Campylobacter)
  - Symptoms are due to an immunologic response to preceding infection
    - Occurs most frequently in those who are human leukocyte antigen (HLA)-B27 positive and thus is considered to be a subset of the spondyloarthropathies

CLINICAL PRESENTATION

- History
  - Preceding diarrheal or genitourinary infection
  - Chlamydia infection is typically asymptomatic, so a history of dysuria and urethral or vaginal discharge may not be elicited
  - Low-grade fever can be present at onset of arthritis
- Physical signs
  - Asymmetric oligoarticular arthritis of the lower extremities, usually markedly painful
    - Unlike juvenile idiopathic arthritis (JIA), overlying erythema is common
  - Conjunctivitis in both Chlamydia and gastroenteritis-associated reactive arthritis may be purulent
  - Skin lesions are occasionally seen with Chlamydia-associated reactive arthritis:
    - *Keratoderma blenorrhagicum* (scaly psoriasis-like eruption on the feet)
    - Circinate balanitis (painless, shallow ulcers on the glans penis)
    - Erythema nodosum

DIAGNOSIS AND EVALUATION

- If reactive arthritis is suspected, documentation of a preceding infection is helpful but not always possible:
  - Stool cultures for enteric organisms
  - Urethral swab for polymerase chain reaction (PCR) to detect Chlamydia
- Synovial fluid is inflammatory (~20,000 white blood cells [WBCs]), but cultures are negative
  - Chlamydial antigens or nucleic acids may be detectable in synovial fluid
- Urethral and conjunctival cultures are sterile
- Other laboratory studies can support the diagnosis but are not specific:
  - Elevated erythrocyte sedimentation rate (ESR) and C-reactive protein (CRP) and mild leukocytosis with neutrophil predominance

TREATMENT

- Nonsteroidal antiinflammatory drugs (NSAIDs) are first line
  - Chlamydia should be treated, but symptoms may not improve with antibiotics alone
- Usually self-limited and resolves within 6 to 12 weeks, but may last up to 6 months
  - Referral to rheumatology is needed for persistent symptoms

Acute Rheumatic Fever (ARF)

BASIC INFORMATION

- Follows group A β-hemolytic streptococcal (GAS) pharyngitis
  - Triggered by an immune reaction to the streptococcal antigen
    - Possible cross-reactivity with heart, brain, and joint tissue
  - Does not occur after GAS skin infections
  - More common in developing countries and areas with more crowding

CLINICAL PRESENTATION

- Onset 2 to 3 weeks after streptococcal tonsillopharyngitis
  - Peak age 5 to 15 years old (school age)
- Fever and joint pain are the most common manifestations
- Migratory polyarthritis—may resolve spontaneously in one joint within 24 hours only to appear in another

Table 81.1.   Revised Jones Criteria for the Diagnosis of Acute Rheumatic Fever

Requirement	Documentation of recent group A β-hemolytic streptococcal infection with *at least one* of the following: positive rapid strep antigen test, throat culture, rising antistreptolysin-O or DNase B titer	
Diagnosis requires two major OR *one major plus two minor criteria:*		
Major	**Carditis** (can be subclinical)	
	Polyarthritis	Monoarthritis or polyarthralgias count in high-prevalence areas
	Erythema marginatum	
	Subcutaneous nodules	
	Chorea	
Minor	**Prolonged PR interval**	Only counts if there is no other evidence of carditis
	Fever ≥38.5°C	
	Arthralgia	Only counts if there is no arthritis
	Erythrocyte sedimentation rate ≥60 mm/hr or C-reactive protein ≥3.0 mg/dL	ESR ≥30 mm/hr counts in high-prevalence areas

- Carditis predominantly affects endocardium, especially valvular tissue
  - Present in >50% of cases, ranging from subclinical to severe
  - Mitral valve is the most commonly affected, followed by aortic valve
    - New-onset heart murmur is usually indicative of valvular insufficiency
    - Valvular disease may be present even in the absence of clinical signs
    - Heart failure due to severe valvular insufficiency occurs in 5% of children
- Erythema marginatum: nonpruritic macules with serpiginous pink borders on the trunk or inner thighs
- Subcutaneous nodules: firm and painless; present on the extensor surfaces of large joints (knees, elbows, and wrists)
- Sydenham chorea is a late finding, occurring 3 months later
  - Bilateral, involuntary, purposeless movements that disappear during sleep
    - Facial grimace, protruding tongue ("wormian tongue")
    - Irregular contractures of hand muscles on active grip ("milkmaid's grip")
  - Emotional lability and difficulty concentrating can persist for years

DIAGNOSIS AND EVALUATION

- Clinical diagnosis is made using the Jones Criteria (Table 81.1)
- Must document evidence of recent GAS infection:
  - Rapid streptococcal antigen test is often negative because of the 2- to 3-week latency period
  - Throat cultures have higher yield but are less specific due to carrier states
  - Antistreptolysin-O (ASO) titers are frequently positive in school-age children, but significant elevations (>1000) or rising titers are indicative of recent infection
  - Similarly, high or rising anti-DNase B titers can be used to document recent infection and do not necessarily correlate with ASO titers

- Echocardiogram should be performed on any child suspected of having ARF
  - May demonstrate valvular insufficiency, ventricular dysfunction/dilation, or pericardial effusions
- ECG can demonstrate conduction abnormalities, especially prolonged PR interval
- ESR and CRP should be elevated during acute disease

TREATMENT

- Eradicate streptococcal infection:
  - Single dose of IM penicillin G (preferred) *or* oral penicillin V × 10 days
  - For penicillin-allergic patients, use cefazolin, clindamycin, or a macrolide (e.g., azithromycin)
- High-dose aspirin for mild to moderate carditis
  - Oral prednisone is preferred for severe carditis
- The arthritis of ARF is uniquely sensitive to aspirin
  - Reconsider the diagnosis if arthritis fails to improve dramatically with aspirin
- All patients will warrant long-term secondary prophylaxis against recurrent GAS infection with monthly IM penicillin G or twice-daily oral penicillin V
  - Those with carditis require lifelong prophylaxis
  - Those without carditis receive prophylaxis until age 21 years or a minimum of 5 years

Poststreptococcal Reactive Arthritis (PSRA)

BASIC INFORMATION

- PSRA occurs after GAS pharyngitis but is a distinct entity from acute rheumatic fever
- Considered a specific type of postinfectious arthritis

CLINICAL PRESENTATION

- Onset is 7 to 10 days after streptococcal pharyngitis
  - Bimodal age distribution: peak at ages 8 to 14 years and young adulthood
- May be accompanied by low-grade fever

- Physical signs: nonmigratory, additive oligo- or polyarthritis of the lower extremities
  - Persistent rather than transient
    - No other major criteria for ARF

DIAGNOSIS AND EVALUATION

- In contrast to ARF, rapid streptococcal antigen tests and throat cultures are frequently positive due to the shorter latency period
  - ASO and DNase B titers may be elevated shortly thereafter
- ESR and CRP are only mildly to moderately elevated
- Baseline ECG and echocardiogram should be normal

TREATMENT

- Penicillin should be given at diagnosis to eradicate GAS infection
- Secondary penicillin prophylaxis and close clinical observation for carditis are recommended for up to 1 year
  - Generally, risk of late cardiac disease in PSRA is negligible; if carditis is discovered, the patient should be considered to have had ARF
- NSAIDs are first line for symptomatic relief
  - Compared with ARF, PSRA is poorly responsive to aspirin and NSAIDs

Juvenile Idiopathic Arthritis (JIA)

BASIC INFORMATION

- JIA is a chronic autoimmune condition affecting the joints and eyes
- By definition, age of onset is <16 years, and symptoms of arthritis must be present for at least 6 weeks
- Untreated arthritis leads to joint contractures and permanent joint damage
- Untreated uveitis (eye inflammation) leads to blindness
- There are six subtypes with varying prognosis and clinical manifestations:
  - Oligoarticular JIA
  - Polyarticular JIA with negative rheumatoid factor (RF)
  - Polyarticular JIA with positive RF
  - Psoriatic JIA
  - Enthesitis-related JIA
  - Systemic-onset JIA

CLINICAL PRESENTATION

- In all subtypes, stiffness and joint swelling are more prominent than joint pain
  - Decreased range of motion progresses over time
  - Leg length discrepancies or even growth retardation can result from chronic lower-extremity arthritis
  - Micrognathia and jaw asymmetry can result from temporomandibular joint arthritis

OLIGOARTICULAR JIA

- Most commonly occurs in toddler-age (3 years old) Caucasian females
- Four or more joints are involved initially
  - Large joints, knee > ankle > wrist (but almost never hip or shoulder)
  - Insidious onset
- Frequently antinuclear antibody (ANA) positive → highest risk of uveitis
  - Uveitis is usually asymptomatic; therefore all patients require regular ophthalmologic screening

POLYARTICULAR JIA

- Bimodal peak at age 1 to 3 years, and then adolescence, with female predominance
- More than five joints are involved
  - Symmetrically involves small joints of hands and feet, in addition to large joints
- RF positivity confers a worse prognosis:
  - Similar to adult rheumatoid arthritis; subcutaneous rheumatoid nodules may be present
- Asymptomatic uveitis is less common than in oligoarticular JIA

PSORIATIC JIA

- Arthritis and psoriasis or other features that overlap with psoriasis:
  - Dactylitis ("sausage digits"), nail pits or onycholysis, family history of psoriasis
- Asymmetrically involves small joints (especially distal interphalangeal [DIP]) and large joints
- Asymptomatic uveitis (especially if ANA positive)

ENTHESITIS-RELATED JIA/JUVENILE ANKYLOSING SPONDYLITIS

- Frequently HLA-B27 positive, and more common in adolescent boys
- Family history of other HLA-B27-positive spondyloarthropathies (ankylosing spondylitis, sacroiliitis with inflammatory bowel disease, reactive arthritis)
- Peripheral arthritis, enthesitis, or axial involvement:
  - Inflammatory back pain is associated with sacroiliitis
    - Back stiffness that is worse in the morning or with prolonged sitting and that improves with activity
      Difficulty with forward flexion and flattening of the natural lumbar lordosis
      Tenderness over the sacroiliac joints
    - Enthesitis is tenderness at insertion sites of tendons/ligaments into bone
    - Enthesitis-related JIA can progress to ankylosing spondylitis in adult years (fusion of lumbar vertebrae results in the classic "bamboo spine" radiographic finding)
- Uveitis presents as an acute, painful red eye rather than asymptomatic uveitis
- Significant overlap with inflammatory bowel disease–associated arthropathies, so close monitoring for gastrointestinal symptoms is necessary

SYSTEMIC-ONSET JIA

- Previously known as Still disease, it is a completely separate disease from other JIA subtypes
- Characterized by severe autoinflammation with peak onset at 1 to 5 years old:
  - High-spiking fevers for at least 2 weeks, classically in a quotidian (daily) pattern
  - Evanescent salmon-colored macules appear in conjunction with fever
    - May appear in linear streaks or look urticarial with surrounding pallor
  - Lymphadenopathy and hepatosplenomegaly
  - Serositis (pleural/pericardial effusions, ascites)
  - Polyarticular arthritis (especially hip and cervical spine)
- *Not* associated with a risk of uveitis
- Frequently complicated by macrophage activation syndrome (MAS), also known as secondary hemophagocytic lymphohistiocytosis, which is a severe, life-threatening state of dysregulated systemic inflammation and organ failure

DIAGNOSIS AND EVALUATION

- Laboratory testing can help characterize the type of JIA but is not used to make a diagnosis of JIA:
  - ANA determines risk of uveitis
    - A positive ANA at low titers (1:160) can be detected in up to 20% of healthy children, and therefore it is not useful for diagnosis
  - RF and HLA-B27 help determine JIA subtype
  - Lyme should be excluded as a cause of chronic arthritis
  - A mild leukocytosis, thrombocytosis, normocytic anemia, and mildly elevated ESR/CRP may be associated with active oligoarticular or polyarticular JIA
  - In contrast, systemic-onset JIA is characterized by prominent leukocytosis, thrombocytosis, anemia, and elevated acute-phase reactants, especially ferritin

  - ± Transaminitis, hypoalbuminemia, prolonged coagulation time
  - Cytopenias and dropping ESR (from fibrinogen consumption) in the setting of rising ferritin levels are indicators of MAS
- Synovial fluid analysis confirms that the effusion is inflammatory (WBC 5,000–20,000; up to 100,000 in systemic-onset JIA)
- Ultrasound can be used to demonstrate joint effusions if clinical examination is equivocal
- Demonstration of uveitis on slit-lamp examination can substantiate the diagnosis

TREATMENT

- All children suspected of having JIA should be referred to a rheumatologist
- Those diagnosed with JIA require ophthalmologic screening at regular intervals
- Mono- or oligoarticular arthritis is usually amenable to intraarticular corticosteroid injections
- Immunosuppressants such as low-dose methotrexate are usually needed for polyarticular arthritis
- NSAIDs can be helpful for pain and very mild arthritis
- Systemic-onset JIA is treated with systemic corticosteroids in combination with other antiinflammatory medications

Review Questions

For review questions, please go to ExpertConsult.com

Suggested Readings

1. Espinosa M, Gottlieb BS. Juvenile idiopathic arthritis. *Pediatr Rev.* 2012;33(7):303–313.
2. Hahn RG, Knox LM, Forman TA. Evaluation of poststreptococcal illness. *Am Fam Physician.* 2005;71(10):1949–1954.
3. John J, Chandran L. Arthritis in children and adolescents. *Pediatr Rev.* 2011;32(11):470–480.

82 Collagen Vascular Diseases

JOYCE CHUN-LING CHANG, MD

In this chapter we review the most common collagen vascular diseases in childhood, focusing on systemic lupus erythematosus and juvenile dermatomyositis. The goals are to recognize when to suspect a systemic inflammatory disease, to know the manifestations of the most common childhood collagen vascular diseases, and to plan an appropriate initial evaluation. Multiorgan involvement, prolonged constitutional symptoms, and unusual rashes should always prompt the inclusion of rheumatologic disease on the differential diagnosis.

See also Nelson Textbook of Pediatrics, Chapter 158, "Systemic Lupus Erythematosus."

Systemic Lupus Erythematosus

BASIC INFORMATION

- Systemic lupus erythematosus (SLE) is a chronic autoimmune condition with multiorgan involvement
  - Most commonly occurs in pubescent or postpubertal females
    - Younger age of onset or male sex may indicate a predisposing genetic cause
    - Greater frequency and severity of disease in African-Americans
  - Heterogeneous presentation
    - Renal and central nervous system (CNS) involvement: highest risk for poor outcomes
      ~40% of children with SLE develop nephritis, of which 20 to 50% go on to develop end-stage renal disease
    - Universally associated with positive ANA, but other serologic testing may vary
    - May overlap with other connective tissue diseases, such as dermatomyositis, Sjögren syndrome, and systemic sclerosis
  - Pathogenesis is complex and still poorly understood
    - Characterized by complement activation and immune-complex deposition in tissues
    - May result from impaired clearance of apoptotic cells
      Autoantibodies form against nuclear antigens such as double-stranded DNA

CLINICAL PRESENTATION

- Constitutional symptoms (fever, fatigue, weight loss, anorexia) with other multisystem complaints, such as joint pain, rash, chest pain, headache, and cognitive changes
- Signs and Symptoms by System:
  - Photosensitive rashes:
    - Malar rash that spares nasolabial folds (see Fig. 82.1)
      Light blush to intense erythema, which can be flat or raised; nonpruritic

Crosses the bridge of the nose, unlike "slapped cheek" appearance of parvovirus
- Discoid rash
  - Thick hyperpigmented plaques with adherent scale
  - Typically occurs on the face and scalp, especially around the eyes or ears
  - May lead to scarring and hair loss
- Subacute cutaneous lupus
  - Raised pink or hyperpigmented annular papules and plaques on sun-exposed areas
    UVA/UVB exposure can flare skin disease *and* systemic disease
- Oral/nasal mucosal erythema and ulcerations
  - Classically a painless ulcer on the hard palate
- Alopecia along the frontotemporal hair line
- Vascular skin changes
  - Raynaud phenomenon is common: cold-induced triphasic color changes of the fingertips or toes (white → blue → red)
  - Livedo reticularis, ischemic ulcerations
- Symmetric nonerosive polyarthritis, especially in the small joints of the hands
- Serositis
  - Pleuritic chest pain with pleural/pericardial rub
- Neuropsychiatric disease
  - Headache is the most common
  - Seizures and stroke are the most serious
  - New-onset psychiatric disease, school difficulties, other cognitive changes
    Chorea can be *unilateral*, in contrast to chorea in acute rheumatic fever, which is always bilateral
- Nephritis can present as nephritic, nephrotic, or mixed:
  - Nephrotic: extremity/periorbital edema, proteinuria, hypoalbuminemia, hyperlipidemia
  - Nephritic: hematuria, red cell casts, acute kidney injury, hypertension
- Cytopenias
  - SLE is always on the differential for pancytopenia
  - Leukopenia (specifically lymphopenia)
  - Coombs-positive hemolytic anemia or normocytic anemia of chronic disease
  - Immune-mediated thrombocytopenia (may be the presenting sign years before diagnosis)
- Hepatosplenomegaly and prominent lymphadenopathy may be present; must be distinguished from malignancy
- Gastrointestinal complaints: ascites, abdominal pain, peritonitis
- Drug-induced lupus can cause any of the previous clinical manifestations, but renal disease is rare
  - Antiepileptics, hydralazine, isoniazid, procainamide, minocycline

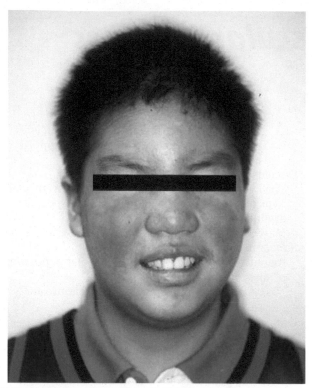

Fig. 82.1. Malar rash in a boy. (Marcdante KJ and RM Kleigman. Nelson Essentials of Pediatrics, 8th ed. Philadelphia, Elsevier; 2019; section 15 "Rheumatic Diseases of Childhood", p354.)

Table 82.1. American College of Rheumatology Revised Classification Criteria for Systemic Lupus Erythematosus (1997)

Criterion	Definition
1. Malar rash	Fixed erythema over malar eminences
2. Discoid rash	Erythematous plaques with keratotic scaling and follicular plugging
3. Photosensitivity	Skin rash as a result of unusual reaction to sunlight
4. Oral ulcers	Oral or nasal ulcers, usually painless
5. Arthritis	Nonerosive arthritis of ≥2 joints
6. Serositis	Pleuritis or pericarditis
7. Renal	Nephritis (proteinuria >0.5 g/day or cellular casts)
8. Neuropsychiatric	Seizure or psychosis
9. Hematologic	Hemolytic anemia *or* Leukopenia (white blood cells <4000/mm^3) × 2 *or* Lymphopenia (absolute lymphocyte count <1500) × 2 *or* Thrombocytopenia (platelet count <100,000/mm^3)
10. Immunologic	Positive anti-double-stranded DNA *or* positive anti-Smith antibody *or* presence of antiphospholipid antibodies
11. Antinuclear antibody	Positive antinuclear antibody

Must meet at least 4 of the 11 criteria to meet definition of SLE.

DIAGNOSIS AND EVALUATION

- Diagnosis traditionally requires 4 of 11 criteria from the American College of Rheumatology classification criteria (Table 82.1), although other criteria exist
- Laboratory testing
  - Antinuclear antibody (ANA) test is the initial screening test for suspected lupus
    - Negative ANA: excludes lupus
    - Positive ANA, low-titer (≤1:160): need further testing, but consider other diagnoses
    - Positive ANA, high-titer (>1:340): perform further testing to confirm lupus
      - Extractable nuclear antigen tests detect autoantibodies against specific nuclear antigens:
      - Anti-double-stranded DNA (dsDNA) is the most frequently positive and correlates with disease activity
      - Anti-Smith is less common but more specific
      - Antihistone antibodies are a marker of drug-induced lupus
      - Anti-Sjögren's-syndrome related antigen A (SSA/Ro), anti-Sjögren's-syndrome related antigen B (SSB/La) ribonucleoprotein (RNP), and centromere antibodies may be present in variable frequencies but are not diagnostic of SLE
  - Antiphospholipid antibodies may be present (anticardiolipin and anti-β_2 glycoprotein)
    - Results in false-positive rapid plasma reagin (RPR), prolonged activated partial thromboplastin time (aPTT), and abnormal dilute Russell venom viper test (DRVVT)
  - Always send a urinalysis and serum creatinine because the presence of renal disease is most likely to affect immediate management

- Complete blood count (CBC) frequently demonstrates cytopenias
  - Pancytopenia is especially characteristic of SLE; may be confused with malignancy
  - Positive Coombs seen with or without hemolytic anemia
- Liver enzymes may be elevated
- Complement levels C3 and C4 are both low in the setting of flares and can be used to track disease activity
  - High C3/C4 levels are indicative of infection
- Inflammatory Markers
  - Erythrocyte sedimentation rate is high with active disease
  - C-reactive protein is usually normal or low unless there is an infectious complication
- Chest radiograph
  - May demonstrate pleural effusions or cardiomegaly
- ECG
  - Diffuse ST elevation and PR depression are diagnostic of pericarditis
- Echocardiography
  - Pericardial effusions, rarely resulting in tamponade
  - Regional wall abnormalities and ventricular dysfunction due to myocarditis
  - Libman-Sacks endocarditis (sterile vegetations on mitral valve)
- Renal biopsy should be performed in all patients with hematuria, significant proteinuria, or an elevated serum creatinine
  - "Full house" pattern of immunofluorescence is diagnostic of lupus nephritis
    - C3, C4, C1q, IgG, IgA and IgM deposits

Histologic class of nephritis on biopsy determines aggressiveness of treatment
■ Lumbar puncture, electroencephalogram (EEG), brain magnetic resonance imaging (MRI), and angiography for suspected CNS lupus

TREATMENT

■ Induction therapy
  ■ High-dose glucocorticoids *and*:
    ■ Cyclophosphamide or mycophenolate for proliferative nephritis
      Consider adding Rituximab for refractory nephritis or cytopenias
    ■ Cyclophosphamide for CNS involvement
    ■ Other disease-modifying agents for mild disease (predominantly skin and joint manifestations), such as mycophenolate, methotrexate, or azathioprine
■ Maintenance therapy
  ■ Mycophenolate or azathioprine for nephritis and CNS disease
  ■ All patients receive lifelong maintenance with antimalarials (hydroxychloroquine)
  ■ Sun avoidance
■ For drug-induced lupus, treatment is to discontinue the offending agent
■ Complications of therapy
  ■ Early mortality from infectious complications due to immunosuppression
    ■ Pneumococcal and meningococcal infections due to low complement levels
    ■ Should receive 23-polyvalent pneumococcal vaccine
      No live vaccines while on immunosuppressive medications
    ■ Opportunistic infections: *Pneumocystis jirovecii*, cytomegalovirus (CMV) reactivation, fungal infection
  ■ Consequences of chronic glucocorticoid therapy: secondary adrenal insufficiency, bone demineralization, metabolic syndrome, Cushingoid features, and so forth
  ■ Hydroxychloroquine can cause retinal toxicity
    ■ Need annual screening ophthalmology examinations

Neonatal Lupus Erythematosus

BASIC INFORMATION

■ Passively acquired autoimmunity in the developing fetus and neonate due to anti-Ro (SSA) and anti-La (SSB) maternal autoantibodies
  ■ Congenital heart block due to injury to fetal cardiocytes is the most serious complication
  ■ Although mothers with known SLE or Sjögren syndrome have a higher risk of having a fetus with neonatal lupus, the majority of mothers of infants born with congenital heart block do not have known autoimmune disease at the time of delivery

CLINICAL PRESENTATION

■ Congenital heart block
  ■ Second- or third-degree heart block, usually detected in utero; clinical effects are related to the ventricular heart rate, with heart failure and hydrops fetalis developing with severe bradycardia
  ■ Can be associated with myocarditis or endocardial fibroelastosis
■ Cutaneous neonatal lupus
  ■ Scaly, annular plaques with central clearing on the face and scalp that can mimic ringworm
  ■ Resembles rash of subacute cutaneous lupus and is photosensitive
  ■ "Raccoon-like" distribution around the eyes; can also involve trunk and soles of feet
  ■ Appears within the first few weeks of life and resolves by 6 months without scarring
■ Other transient systemic findings
  ■ Hepatomegaly and transaminitis
  ■ Thrombocytopenia more common than anemia or neutropenia
  ■ Macrocephaly and hydrocephalus

DIAGNOSIS AND EVALUATION

■ Mothers test positive for high-titer anti-Ro (SSA) or anti-La (SSB) ribonucleoprotein antibodies
■ Anti-Ro antibodies are more commonly associated with heart block

TREATMENT

■ There are no treatments that can reverse complete (third degree) heart block once it is detected
  ■ Typically requires permanent pacemaker during childhood
■ Prenatal treatment with betamethasone/dexamethasone may prevent progression of incomplete (second degree) fetal heart block
  ■ Most primary prevention efforts have failed
■ Cutaneous manifestations and other systemic symptoms usually do not need to be treated

Juvenile Dermato-myositis

BASIC INFORMATION

■ A disease of skin ("dermato-") and muscle ("myo-") inflammation ("-itis")
  ■ Characterized by a vasculopathy preferentially affecting proximal muscles and sun-exposed skin, although internal organs can also be affected
  ■ Like SLE, it is a photosensitive disease and can flare with sun exposure
  ■ Unlike the adult form of the disease, juvenile dermatomyositis (JDM) is *not* associated with underlying malignancy
■ Bimodal age distribution, peaking at ages 4 to 9 years and again at ages 45 to 64 years
■ More common in females (2:1 ratio)

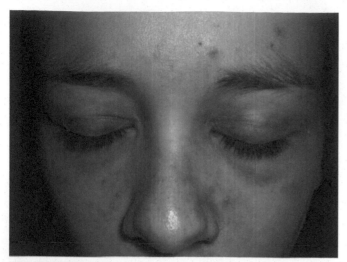

Fig. 82.2. Heliotrope rash involving upper and lower eyelids. (Courtesy Usatine RP. From Usatine R, Smith M, Mayeaux EJ, Chumley H. The Color Atlas of Family Medicine. 2nd ed. New York: McGraw-Hill; 2013.)

CLINICAL PRESENTATION

- History
  - Gradual onset proximal muscle weakness, fatigue, and photosensitive rash
  - Complaints of weakness include difficulty climbing stairs or rising from a chair (pelvic girdle weakness), difficulty brushing hair (shoulder weakness), and difficulty swallowing (oropharyngeal weakness); in children this can also manifest as an apparent delay or regression in milestones
  - May have arthralgias or myalgias
- Signs and Symptoms
  - Symmetric weakness of the proximal muscles
    - Unable to raise arms above head
    - Anterior neck weakness is a sensitive sign (head lag or inability to hold chin to chest while supine)
    - Gowers maneuver
    - Unlike in myasthenia, facial and ocular muscles are spared; furthermore, fatigability with repetition is *not* observed
  - Pathognomonic cutaneous findings:
    - Heliotrope rash: pink or violaceous lacy discoloration of eyelids (see Fig. 82.2)
      - May be accompanied by significant periorbital or facial edema
    - Gottron papules: shiny, scaly pink plaques and papules symmetrically distributed on extensor surfaces of finger joints, elbows, and knees (see Fig. 82.3)
  - Other cutaneous findings:
    - Unlike lupus, this malar rash does *not* spare the nasolabial folds
    - Shawl or V-sign: erythema over sun-exposed areas of the neck-line
    - Ulcerations can occur at sites of Gottron papules and corners of eyelids
    - Calcinosis results in firm, painful subcutaneous and deep nodules
  - May have true polyarticular arthritis or joint contractures resulting from muscle disease
  - Vascular changes
    - Raynaud phenomenon

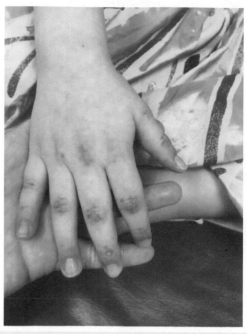

Fig. 82.3. Gottron papules on the extensor surface of nearly every metacarpophalangeal, proximal interphalangeal, and distal interphalangeal joint in a child with dermatomyositis. Note that some have a shiny papular appearance, whereas others have shallow central ulcerations and scale.

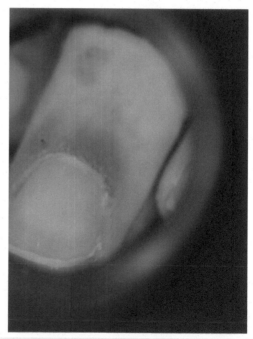

Fig. 82.4. Periungual erythema and dilated, tortuous capillary loops on the index finger of the same child with dermatomyositis.

- Dilated or tortuous nail fold capillaries with periungual erythema (Fig. 82.4)
- Interstitial lung disease is a poor prognostic sign

DIAGNOSIS AND EVALUATION

- To diagnose myositis, you need at least two of the following:
  - Proximal symmetric muscle weakness

- Elevated muscle enzyme: creatine kinase (CK), aspartate transaminase (AST), lactate dehydrogenase (LDH), or aldolase
- Electromyography (EMG) characteristics of myopathy and denervation
- Muscle biopsy documenting histologic evidence of myositis
- MRI showing proximal muscle inflammation has largely replaced muscle biopsy as a criterion for diagnosis
- Skin biopsy is rarely needed to confirm the characteristic cutaneous manifestations
- ANA test is usually positive, but lupus serologies (anti-dsDNA and anti-Smith) are negative

TREATMENT

- High-dose glucocorticoids
- Intravenous immune globulin (IVIG) is highly effective for both muscle and skin disease
- Methotrexate for milder disease
- Hydroxychloroquine for cutaneous disease

Scleroderma

BASIC INFORMATION

- Two distinct diseases:
  - Localized scleroderma (morphea): skin lesions only
  - Systemic sclerosis: diffuse multisystem connective tissue disease with poor prognosis
    - Includes the limited form previously known as CREST (*c*alcinosis, *R*aynaud phenomenon, *e*sophageal reflux, *s*clerodactyly, *t*elangiectasias)

CLINICAL PRESENTATION

- both types of scleroderma have very insidious onsets of sympyoms
- Localized scleroderma
  - Onset in school-age children
  - Slowly evolving oval or linear plaque, with erythematous or violaceous border and central white to yellow, waxy fibrosis
    - Followed by atrophy of the skin and subcutaneous tissue; can impair limb growth if it crosses joints or growth plates
  - *En coup de sabre* is a form involving the face that can be disfiguring and result in ipsilateral ocular or neurologic manifestations
  - Does *not* evolve into systemic sclerosis

- Systemic sclerosis
  - Extremely rare in children
  - Raynaud phenomenon is usually the first sign, often with digital ulcers
  - Symmetric fibrous thickening, hardening, or tightening of the skin (sclerosis)
  - Sclerodactyly: tightening skin over the fingers, resulting in finger contractures
  - Organ involvement: gastrointestinal dysmotility, pulmonary fibrosis/hypertension, cardiomyopathy (high risk of mortality)

DIAGNOSIS AND EVALUATION

- Localized scleroderma
  - Clinical diagnosis, requiring evaluation by a dermatologist or rheumatologist
  - Skin biopsy can be helpful if diagnosis is unclear, but not necessary
  - Ophthalmology examination and brain MRI should be performed in those with facial/scalp involvement
- Systemic sclerosis
  - Almost always ANA positive
  - Other associated autoantibodies include anti-SCL-70 and anticentromere
  - Pulmonary function testing, high-resolution chest computed tomography (CT), echocardiography, barium swallow, and manometry studies are used to characterize organ involvement

TREATMENT

- Localized scleroderma
  - Mild superficial disease: topical glucocorticoids or phototherapy (dermatology)
  - Moderate to severe disease: systemic therapy such as methotrexate (rheumatology)
- No effective treatments for systemic sclerosis

Review Questions

For review questions, please go to ExpertConsult.com.

Suggested Readings

1. Levy DM, Kamphuis S. Systemic lupus erythematosus in children and adolescents. *Pediatr Clin North Am.* 2012;59(2):345–364.
2. Robinson AB, Reed AM. Clinical features, pathogenesis and treatment of juvenile and adult dermatomyositis. *Nat Rev.* 2011;7:664–675.
3. Weiss JE. Pediatric systemic lupus erythematosus. *Pediatr Rev.* 2012;33(2):62–74.

83 Selected Topics in Rheumatology

JOYCE CHUN-LING CHANG, MD

Vasculitis refers to inflammation and injury of blood vessels, which can lead to hemorrhage, thrombosis, stenosis, or aneurysms, as well as end-organ damage associated with acute or chronic ischemia. The vasculitis syndromes are frequently classified according to the size of the vessels involved. HSP is a small vessel vasculitis, involving the capillaries of the skin, joints, renal glomeruli and gastrointestinal mucosa. In contrast, Kawasaki disease is a medium vessel vasculitis with a predilection for the coronary arteries. While both HSP and Kawasaki disease are typically self-limited, there can occasionally be serious long-term sequelae.

Lastly, we will briefly discuss conditions such as serum sickness that can mimic rheumatologic diseases, as well as several of the most common causes of noninflammatory musculoskeletal complaints in children. These include benign nocturnal musculoskeletal pains of childhood ("growing pains"), benign hypermobility, and functional joint complaints.

Henoch-Schönlein purpura (HSP)

BASIC INFORMATION

- Small-vessel leukocytoclastic vasculitis is characterized by IgA deposition in the skin, synovium, and glomeruli
- HSP is the most common childhood vasculitis
  - Peak onset in school-age years, more commonly in males
    - Seasonal variation with increased incidence in fall/winter
    - Many potential infectious triggers (e.g., β-hemolytic streptococcus)
- Usually self-limited, but can have long-term renal consequences

CLINICAL PRESENTATION

- All patients will have palpable purpura with a lower-extremity predominance
  - Two-thirds have gastrointestinal involvement
  - Two-thirds have joint involvement
  - One-third have renal involvement
- Skin manifestations:
  - Palpable purpura and petechiae (Fig. 83.1)
    - Affects Dependent areas, especially the lower extremities, buttocks, and behind the ears
      Pressure-exposed areas (e.g., sock line, blood pressure cuff)
      Early lesions may appear more pink and maculopapular

- Nonpitting acral edema and scrotal edema can be prominent
- Gastrointestinal manifestations:
  - Abdominal pain and vomiting: can precede purpura and mimic appendicitis, often delaying recognition of HSP until the development of skin manifestations
  - Gastrointestinal ulceration and bleeding with diarrhea, hematochezia, and melena
  - Ileoileal intussusception
- Joint manifestations:
  - Arthralgias or oligoarticular arthritis, especially in the knees and ankles
  - Periarticular soft tissue swelling
- Renal manifestations:
  - IgA glomerulonephritis: ranges from microscopic hematuria or mild proteinuria to crescentic glomerulonephritis and end-stage renal disease
  - Severe presentation with nephritic/nephrotic syndrome or acute kidney injury = worse prognosis
  - Late-onset renal disease can occur up to 6 months after initial disease onset

DIAGNOSIS AND EVALUATION

- HSP is a clinical diagnosis
  - Differential diagnosis includes infection (meningococcal and rickettsial disease), malignancy (leukemia, lymphoma), hemolytic uremic syndrome, immune thrombocytopenia purpura, and other autoimmune disorders featuring dermatologic manifestations and joint involvement (e.g., other vasculitides, systemic juvenile idiopathic arthritis [JIA], systemic lupus erythematosus [SLE])
- Laboratory testing
  - Inflammatory markers are normal or mildly elevated
  - Autoimmune antibody (e.g., antinuclear antibodies [ANA]) and complement testing are not necessary for diagnosis of HSP; they are sometimes sent if there is concern for other autoimmune diseases
  - Coagulation studies and platelet count are normal (in contrast to thrombotic thrombocytopenic purpura, hemolytic uremic syndrome, and rickettsial disease)
  - Serum IgA may be elevated, but this is *not* diagnostic
  - Urinalysis should always be sent to screen for renal disease
    - Proteinuria, hematuria, red cell casts
- Skin biopsy demonstrating leukocytoclastic vasculitis with IgA deposition is definitive but usually not necessary

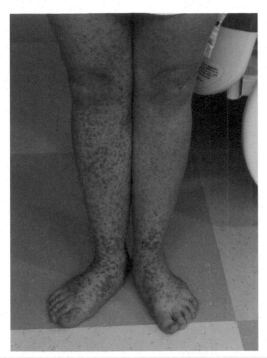

Fig. 83.1. Classic appearance of Henoch-Schönlein purpura with lower-extremity petechiae and palpable purpura. The lesions result from extravasation of red blood cells from injured capillaries and thus do not blanch.

- Renal biopsy is indicated for nephritic or nephrotic syndrome and acute renal failure
  - Demonstrates IgA nephropathy
- Imaging
  - Abdominal ultrasound is used to diagnose ileoileal intussusception
    - Barium enema is diagnostic and therapeutic for ileocolic intussusception, which is less common in HSP

TREATMENT

- Most cases resolve in 4 weeks, so supportive care is the mainstay of treatment:
  - Nonsteroidal antiinflammatory drugs (NSAIDs) or acetaminophen for pain (although in the presence of kidney involvement, some may choose to avoid NSAIDs)
- Glucocorticoids are effective for severe gastrointestinal and joint symptoms
  - Do *not* prevent development of nephritis, but may be used to treat severe renal disease
- Surgical or endoscopic intervention may be needed for severe gastrointestinal complications (e.g., hemorrhage, bowel perforation, bowel ischemia)
- Late-onset nephritis may develop up to 6 months after acute illness
  - Urinalysis and blood pressure should be checked weekly for the first 4 weeks, then monthly for 6 months
  - 1% to 2% of all children with HSP nephritis develop end-stage renal disease
  - Cases with severe renal involvement may necessitate empiric immune suppression or even renal transplant

Kawasaki Disease (KD)

BASIC INFORMATION

- Medium-vessel vasculitis with a predilection for the coronary arteries
  - Leading cause of acquired heart disease in children of developed countries
  - Although it is self-limited, treatment is warranted to prevent coronary artery aneurysms
- KD is the second most common childhood vasculitis, previously known as the "mucocutaneous lymph node syndrome"
- Peak onset is 2 to 5 years of age, more commonly in males
  - Highest incidence is in Asians/Pacific Islanders, especially Japanese
  - Global seasonal pattern with local epidemics suggests an infectious trigger, but none has been identified
  - There may also be a genetic predisposition because siblings of patients with KD are also at increased risk of developing KD
  - See also Nelson Textbook of Pediatrics, Chapter 166, "Kawasaki Disease."

CLINICAL PRESENTATION

- Classic clinical criteria ("CRASH and burn")
  - Fever for 5 days with at least 4 of the following:
    - *Conjunctivitis:* bilateral and nonpurulent, usually limbic sparing
    - *Rash:* polymorphous and nonspecific (but never vesicular or bullous), with a predilection for the perineum and trunk
    - *Adenopathy:* unilateral anterior cervical node >1.5 cm (usually nontender); the least common criterion of KD (~50% of cases)
    - *Strawberry tongue* (or other mucositis): swollen, red, cracked lips; erythema of the oropharynx without ulceration
    - *Hand/foot changes:* swelling over dorsum of hands and feet or erythema of the palms and soles followed by desquamation after 10 to 14 days
- Fever is the hallmark of the acute phase of illness
  - Persistent and above 38.5°C (often exceeding 40°C)
  - Poorly responsive to antipyretics
- Coronary artery aneurysms are the most characteristic manifestation
  - Occurs in 20% to 25% of untreated patients and in 5% of those treated with intravenous immunoglobulin (IVIG)
  - May lead to thrombosis, rupture, myocardial infarction, or sudden death
- Other manifestations not mentioned in the clinical criteria:
  - Myocarditis: frequently subclinical; tachycardia and S3 gallop
  - Gastrointestinal symptoms: diarrhea and abdominal pain are the most common
    - Hepatomegaly and liver enzyme elevation
    - Gallbladder hydrops
  - Arthralgia or arthritis
  - Scrotal pain and swelling (similar to HSP)

- Urethritis: results in sterile pyuria in the majority of KD patients
- Anterior uveitis: transient and asymptomatic; does not cause blindness
- Aseptic meningitis: manifests with extreme irritability
- Hematologic abnormalities: due to systemic inflammation
  - Normocytic anemia
  - Leukocytosis
  - Marked reactive thrombocytosis after the first week (can reach 1 million/mm^3)
  - Hemophagocytic lymphohistiocytosis is a rare but life-threatening complication

DIAGNOSIS AND EVALUATION

- All patients meeting classic clinical criteria require echocardiogram and treatment
- Echocardiographic findings
  - Coronary artery aneurysms as defined by:
    - Intraluminal diameter >3 mm in children younger than 5 years of age and >4 mm in children 5 years or older
    - Z-score ≥2.5 of the left anterior descending or right main coronary artery
  - Transient coronary artery dilation (ectasia) with perivascular brightness
  - Abnormal ventricular function, regional wall abnormalities, valvular regurgitation, pericardial effusions
- The differential diagnosis includes several viruses (e.g., adenovirus, enterovirus) and bacteria (e.g., scarlet fever, rickettsial disease); however, identification of an infectious organism does *not* rule out KD because concurrent or antecedent infections are documented in up to one-third of KD cases
- High suspicion is needed in infants (<1 year of age): often do not fulfill classic diagnostic criteria (incomplete/atypical KD)
- In patients with suspected incomplete KD who do not meet criteria for classical KD:
  - If C-reactive protein (CRP) ≥3.0 mg/dL or erythrocyte sedimentation rate (ESR) ≥40 mm/h, check supplemental laboratory criteria:
    - Albumin ≤3.0 g/dL
    - Anemia for age
    - Elevated alanine transaminase (ALT)
    - Platelet count ≥450,000/mm^3 after 7 days of illness
    - White blood cell count ≥15,000/mm^3
    - Sterile pyuria (urine ≥10 white blood cells/hpf)
- If ≥3 supplemental laboratory criteria → echocardiogram and treat
- If <3 supplemental laboratory criteria → echocardiogram and treat if coronaries are abnormal
  - If echocardiogram is normal, observe and reevaluate if fever persists

TREATMENT

- IVIG and aspirin should be administered as soon as the diagnosis is made:
  - IVIG 2 g/kg as a single dose

- Administration within 10 days of fever onset has been shown to reduce the risk of coronary artery aneurysms. The current trend is that earlier IVIG therapy may yield improved outcomes. Data on delayed treatment are more limited
- Aspirin 80 to 100 mg/kg/day divided in four doses per day while febrile, then 3 to 5 mg/kg/day in a single daily dose for antiplatelet effect until:
  - Platelets and inflammatory markers normalize, if no coronary abnormalities are detected
  - 2 years after coronary abnormalities resolve
  - Forever if coronary abnormalities persist
- Most patients defervesce quickly after IVIG
  - If fever recurs >24 hours after the first dose of IVIG, administer a second dose; some may consider trending CRP as adjunctive (although not definitive) laboratory data of disease response to IVIG, whereas ESR can be elevated by IVIG alone
- Use of corticosteroids remains controversial and is generally reserved for IVIG-resistant cases, but recent studies suggest they are beneficial when given early, especially for high-risk patients
- Follow-up echocardiograms at 2 and 6 weeks after illness, even if no abnormalities detected at baseline
  - Small to medium aneurysms usually appear to regress on echocardiogram, although fibrointimal proliferation and calcification remain risk factors for coronary artery disease and sudden death
  - Large aneurysms require chronic anticoagulation and may eventually necessitate angioplasty or bypass grafting

Other Vasculitides

BASIC INFORMATION

- Although HSP and KD are the most common childhood vasculitides, there are many other types of vasculitis affecting blood vessels of varying sizes
- Instances when you should suspect vasculitis:
  - Multisystem complaints with multiple organs involved
  - Prolonged constitutional symptoms and elevated inflammatory markers
  - Vasculitic-appearing rash (e.g., purpura, petechiae, ischemic ulcerations, digital gangrene)
  - An unusual presentation for age (e.g., claudication, myocardial infarction, or stroke in a child)
- Please refer to the suggested reading "Pediatric Vasculitis" at the end of the chapter for more details.

Sarcoidosis

BASIC INFORMATION

- Autoinflammatory disorder characterized by granulomatous inflammation
- Two rare pediatric subtypes:
  - Blau syndrome: familial form with classic triad of arthritis, uveitis, and rash
    - Onset before age 5

- "Adult-Type": more similar to adult sarcoidosis with lung involvement
  - Onset in adolescence

CLINICAL PRESENTATION

- Blau syndrome
  - Symmetric polyarticular arthritis with prominent cystlike swelling
  - Fine pink to tan maculopapular rash with fine desquamation or erythema nodosum
  - Severe, destructive panuveitis with high risk of vision loss
    - In contrast with JIA, which affects the anterior segment only
    - Characteristic iris and conjunctival nodules
- Adult-type pediatric sarcoidosis
  - Constitutional symptoms: fever, malaise, weight loss
  - Pulmonary nodules
  - Hilar adenopathy
  - Peripheral adenopathy and hepatosplenomegaly
  - Erythema nodosum
  - Uveitis, including keratic precipitates (clumpy white deposits on the cornea)
  - Neurologic manifestations: seizures, cranial nerve palsies

DIAGNOSIS AND EVALUATION

- Biopsy of affected tissues demonstrates noncaseating granulomas
- Supporting laboratory findings include elevated inflammatory markers, anemia, and elevated serum angiotensin-converting enzyme (ACE) levels
- Tuberculosis should be excluded

TREATMENT

- Glucocorticoids and other steroid-sparing immunosuppressive agents

Serum Sickness and Serum Sickness–Like Reactions

BASIC INFORMATION

- Classic serum sickness is a self-limited type III hypersensitivity reaction due to circulating immune complexes
  - Occurs 7 to 14 days after initial drug exposure
  - Classic serum sickness is usually caused by antitoxins and monoclonal antibodies
  - Characterized by constitutional symptoms, joint pain, and rash
- "Serum sickness–like reactions" result in similar symptoms, but there are *no* circulating immune complexes
  - More commonly caused by nonprotein drugs (e.g., penicillins, cefaclor, quinolones, NSAIDs, phenytoins)

CLINICAL PRESENTATION

- Classic serum sickness:
  - Fever, malaise, headache, abdominal pain
  - Often ill-appearing
  - Lymphadenopathy

- Arthralgias or polyarticular arthritis and myalgias
- Urticarial rash with areas that may appear ecchymotic—less commonly purpuric
  - Can also be morbilliform
  - Unlike HSP, predominantly involves the trunk and then spreads to extremities
  - Unlike Stevens-Johnson syndrome, there is *no* mucosal ulceration
- Renal involvement: proteinuria, microscopic hematuria, elevated creatinine, edema
- "Serum sickness–like reaction":
  - Fever less common; if present, it is low grade
  - Polycyclic or serpiginous urticarial rash and arthralgias
  - No renal involvement

DIAGNOSIS AND EVALUATION

- Laboratory studies
  - Reactive leukocytosis and thrombocytosis, with or without mild eosinophilia
  - Mildly elevated inflammatory markers
  - In classic serum sickness only:
    - Low C3 and C4 complement levels are seen due to immune complex deposition
    - Urinalysis may demonstrate proteinuria, microscopic hematuria, or casts
    - Serum creatinine may be elevated

TREATMENT

- Primary treatment is discontinuation of the offending agent
- Supportive therapy
  - Antihistamines for pruritus
  - NSAIDs for arthralgias or arthritis
  - Glucocorticoids for severe symptoms

Benign Nocturnal Pains of Childhood

BASIC INFORMATION

- Commonly referred to as "growing pains"
- Most common cause of episodic musculoskeletal pain in children
  - Peak onset at ages 3 to 12 years
  - Does not actually coincide with growth spurt; therefore the term "growing pains" is a misnomer

CLINICAL PRESENTATION

- Episodic, bilateral leg pain occurring primarily at night
  - Localized to the calf, shin, behind the knees, or sometimes thighs
  - Responds to massage or over-the-counter analgesics
  - Always disappears by morning
- Children are normally active and pain-free during the day in between episodes
  - Pain episodes may occur after days with increased physical activity
  - Motor development is normal
- Symptoms usually resolve by late childhood

DIAGNOSIS AND EVALUATION

- Physical examination is normal
- Children with flat feet (pes planus) or hypermobility may be predisposed
- Radiographs (if obtained) are also normal

TREATMENT

- Supportive care
- Warm baths before bedtime, massage, or over-the-counter analgesics as needed
- Education and reassurance that the pains are benign and self-limited

Benign Joint Hypermobility

BASIC INFORMATION

- Joint pain associated with generalized joint hypermobility in the absence of a connective tissue disorder or congenital syndrome
- More common in young girls

CLINICAL PRESENTATION

- Joint pain that is worse during activity or at the ends of days with increased physical activity
  - No associated swelling or stiffness
- Features of increased flexibility:
  - Able to passively touch elbows behind back
  - Able to put heel behind head
  - Beighton score ≥6 out of 9:
    - Touch thumb to forearm (1 point each)
    - Extend fifth metacarpophalangeal (MCP) joint to 90 degrees (1 point each)
    - >10 degrees of hyperextension of elbows (1 point each)
    - >10 degrees of hyperextension of knees (1 point each)
    - Touch palms to floor with knees straight (1 point)
- Absence of other findings is suggestive of underlying connective tissue disease:
  - Ehlers-Danlos syndromes (multiple types):
    - Skin fragility and hyperelasticity, easy bruising
    - Multiple joint dislocations
    - Hollow organ rupture or vascular aneurysms
    - Family history of the previous conditions
  - Marfan syndrome (autosomal dominant fibrillin mutation):
    - Arm span is greater than height
    - Characteristic elbow flexion contractures in contrast with hypermobility elsewhere
    - Aortic root dilation
    - Lens dislocation
    - Kyphoscoliosis and arachnodactyly
    - Pectus excavatum or carinatum

TREATMENT

- Supportive care
  - Over-the-counter analgesics as needed
  - Shoe inserts for children with symptomatic flat feet or hindfoot valgus
  - Physical therapy for older children
- Education and reassurance that the pain is benign

Functional Joint Complaints

BASIC INFORMATION

- There are a number of amplified pain syndromes in children that frequently cause unnecessary diagnostic testing and treatment
- Characterized by severe pain and functional limitation out of proportion to physical findings
  - Laboratory and imaging tests are all normal
- Exacerbated by psychosocial stressors
  - May occur only at school but not at home, or vice versa
    - May be a behavioral component if there is secondary gain
    - Frequently episodic

TREATMENT

- Limit secondary gain
- Avoid unnecessary diagnostic testing and medical intervention
- Physical therapy and psychological counseling

Review Questions

For review questions, please go to ExpertConsult.com.

Suggested Readings

1. Mathur AN, Mathes EF. Urticaria mimickers in children. *Dermatol Ther*. 2013;26(6):467–475.
2. Reid-Adam J. Henoch-Schönlein purpura. *Pediatr Rev*. 2014;35(10): 447–449.
3. Weiss PF. Pediatric vasculitis. *Pediatr Clin North Am*. 2012;59(2): 407–423.

Urology

84 | Disorders of the Collecting System, Kidney, Bladder, and Urethra

JASON P. VAN BATAVIA, MD, DIANA K. BOWEN and
DOUGLAS A. CANNING, MD

DISORDERS OF THE KIDNEY

Renal Tumors

BASIC INFORMATION

- Wilms Tumor is the most common primary pediatric malignant renal (and abdominal) neoplasm
  - See Chapter 63 for details regarding Wilms tumor
  - Most children receive multimodal therapy
    - Radical nephrectomy with lymph node sampling most common initial treatment in United States
    - Adjuvant chemotherapy based on staging (determined postsurgery)
    - Higher stages also get abdominal/flank radiation therapy
- Other renal tumors including congenital mesoblastic nephroma, clear-cell sarcoma of the kidney, rhabdoid tumor, renal cell carcinoma, and angiomyolipoma are covered in Chapter 63
- See also Nelson Textbook of Pediatrics, Chapter 499, "Neoplasms of the Kidney."

Renal Ectopia

BASIC INFORMATION

- Occurs when the mature kidney fails to reach normal location
- Location can be pelvic, iliac, abdominal, thoracic
- Incidence = 1/500 to 1/1000
- Horseshoe kidney is most common form
  - Both kidneys connected by parenchymal isthmus that crosses the midline
  - Gets trapped below inferior mesenteric artery (IMA)

CLINICAL PRESENTATION

- Vast majority asymptomatic; thus are found only incidentally on imaging
- Occasionally can have ureteropelvic junction obstruction (UPJO), urinary tract infections (UTIs), or stones
- Associated anomalies are very common (30%–60%)

- Genital:
  - Female (20%–60%) = bicornuate or unicornuate uterus, duplicated or septate vagina, Turner syndrome
  - Male (10%–20%) = cryptorchidism, duplicated urethra, hypospadias
  - Vesicoureteral reflux (VUR); up to 50%
  - Others anomalies: cardiac, skeletal, neural, anorectal

DIAGNOSIS AND EVALUATION

- Ultrasound (US) is primary imaging modality
  - US may miss ectopic kidney
  - Abdominal imaging in females should also evaluate for genital abnormalities

TREATMENT

- Majority of cases do not require treatment
- Intervention based on symptoms (e.g., obstruction, stone, mass, infection)
- Higher risk of Wilms tumor in horseshoe kidney

Solitary Kidney

BASIC INFORMATION

- Incidence: 1/450 to 1/1000 births
- Vast majority diagnosed incidentally on prenatal US screening
- Risk factors: maternal diabetes (3× increased risk), VACTERL association (30%)
- Solitary kidney undergoes compensatory hypertrophy
- In majority, kidney function is normal and maintains normal urine-concentrating abilities
- Associated with wolffian duct or müllerian duct abnormalities
- 30% will have VUR into solitary kidney
  - Voiding cystourethrogram (VCUG) recommended for all patients
- No increased risk of malignancy
- Management:
  - Avoid nephrotoxic medications
  - Annual blood pressure, serum creatinine and urinalysis (to check for proteinuria) given long-term risks of hypertension and progressive chronic kidney disease

Cystic Kidney Diseases

- See Chapter 54

DISORDERS OF THE COLLECTING SYSTEM

Antenatal Hydronephrosis (ANH)

BASIC INFORMATION

- Hydronephrosis is a dilation of collecting system (renal pelvis)
- In isolation, hydronephrosis is not indicative of obstruction, reflux or renal damage
- Incidence: 1 to 5 in every 100 pregnancies; the most common urologic anomaly
- There are many causes of ANH (see Table 84.1), although the majority of cases are mild and transient
- Severity based on in utero US measurement of renal pelvis diameter
  - "Severe" defined as >10 mm (second trimester) or >15 mm (third trimester)
  - Earlier fetal age at diagnosis portends a more severe condition

CLINICAL PRESENTATION

- Severe obstruction results in bilateral ANH, oligohydramnios, pulmonary hypoplasia, and often early/neonatal mortality

DIAGNOSIS AND EVALUATION

- Lower postnatal serum creatinine nadir in first year of life is associated with better prognosis
- Imaging
  - US:
    - Postnatal timing of imaging study depends on severity of ANH; often repeat US at 2 weeks
    - All US studies in first few days of life may underestimate the degree of hydronephrosis due to the relative dehydration of newborn
  - VCUG:
    - Controversy exists over when to obtain VCUG; more important if solitary kidney (higher incidence of VUR) or male with bilateral hydronephrosis (rule out posterior urethral valves)

Table 84.1.   Most Common Etiologies for Antenatal Hydronephrosis

Etiology	Percentage of Cases of Antenatal Hydronephrosis
Transient/physiologic	50%–70%
Ureteropelvic junction obstruction	10%–30%
Vesicoureteral reflux	10%–20%
Megaureter/ureterovesical junction obstruction	5%–15%
Multicystic dysplastic kidney	5%
Posterior urethral valves	1%–2%

- Nuclear renal scans:
  - No specific recommendations or guidelines
  - Helpful if suspect obstruction or concern of renal function

TREATMENT

- Fetal intervention (percutaneous vesicoamniotic drain placement) is controversial, with most studies not suggesting a benefit or long-term improved kidney function
- Postnatal treatment and/or need for surgery depends on severity of ANH and postnatal imaging findings
- Indications for antibiotic prophylaxis are controversial. Some consider amoxicillin during the first 2 months of life (n.b., trimethoprim/sulfamethoxazole in first 2 months of life associated with hyperbilirubinemia and kernicterus)

Ureteropelvic Junction Obstruction (UPJO)

BASIC INFORMATION

- Restriction or blockage of the flow of urine from the renal pelvis to the ureter
- Most common pathologic cause of ANH; a very common cause of an abdominal mass in a neonate (along with dysplastic kidney)
- Incidence: 1/500 to 1/1000 live births
- Increased risk if horseshoe or ectopic kidney
- Congenital is most common etiology
  - Infants = intrinsic narrowing or adynamic ureteral segment
  - Adolescents/adults = extrinsic compression from crossing vessel

CLINICAL PRESENTATION

- Typically asymptomatic if detected antenatally or incidentally; may have vague symptoms such as feeding difficulties or failure to thrive
- Older children/adolescents can present with episodes of flank pain, nausea and vomiting ("Dietl's crisis")
- Rarely presents with UTI or stones
- Physical examination
  - Palpable abdominal mass (depends on severity of dilation)
  - Costovertebral angle (CVA) tenderness if during acute episode
  - Hypertension due to increased renin-angiotensin-aldosterone activity

DIAGNOSIS AND EVALUATION

- Serum creatinine and blood urea nitrogen (BUN)
- Urinalysis is usually normal, but may detect microhematuria, proteinuria, or infection
- Imaging:
  - US = choice for initial screening
  - Computed tomography (CT) scan with intravenous (IV) contrast
  - MAG3 diuretic nuclear renal scan

- Can see split renal function between both kidneys and evaluate for obstruction
- Monitoring for reflux:
  - Risk of contralateral VUR 5% to 15%
  - VCUG not routinely obtained, but should be considered if distal ureter dilation or history of UTI

TREATMENT

- Antenatal or neonatal presentation may be observed and can resolve on own
- Often antibiotic prophylaxis will be given, but this is controversial
- Indications for surgical correction (pyeloplasty):
  - Solitary kidney
  - Bilateral obstruction
  - Progressively worsening of unilateral hydronephrosis
  - Progressive loss of renal function
  - Thinning of renal parenchyma
  - Infections or stones
  - Pain

Vesicoureteral Reflux (VUR)

BASIC INFORMATION

- Retrograde flow of urine from the bladder to the upper urinary tract (ureter and/or kidney)
- VUR is thought to increase risk of pyelonephritis from UTI, which can lead to renal scarring, hypertension, and eventual renal insufficiency or end-stage renal disease (ESRD). For details regarding UTI, see Chapter 54
- International classification of VUR: scale graded from 1 to 5 with 5 being the worst (Fig. 84.1)
- Incidence ~1% of pediatric population; found in up to 30% of children with febrile UTI

CLINICAL PRESENTATION

- Usually asymptomatic, but most commonly detected during workup for hydronephrosis, pyelonephritis, or febrile UTI
- History and physical examination should evaluate causes or sequelae of bladder or bowel dysfunction (e.g.,

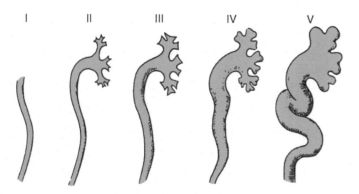

GRADES OF REFLUX

Fig. 84.1. International classification of vesicoureteral reflux. (From Khoury, Bagli. Chapter 137: Vesicoureteral reflux. In: Wein AJ, Kavoussi LR, Partin AW, Peters CA, eds. *Campbell-Walsh Urology.* 11th ed. Elsevier; 2016.)

spina bifida, palpable kidney, constipation) as well as renal injury (e.g., blood pressure)
- Risk factors: Caucasian, younger age, female, positive family history
- Associated anomalies: ureteral duplication, renal ectopia, multicystic dysplastic kidney, ureterocele, prune belly syndrome, bladder exstrophy, posterior urethral valves, neurogenic bladder (NGB)
- ~15% of pediatric ESRD cases are secondary to VUR nephropathy

DIAGNOSIS AND EVALUATION

- Urinalysis and urine culture if suspect UTI
- Serum laboratory tests (creatinine/BUN) not usually helpful unless other finding or concern
- Imaging:
  - Renal US: cannot be used to diagnosis VUR
    - Can detect dilation of ureter and/or renal pelvis, which may suggest VUR but does not definitely diagnose it
    - Good for assessing change in dilation or thinning of renal parenchyma
  - Voiding cystourethrogram (VCUG): gold standard to diagnose VUR
    - Urethral catheter placed into bladder and contrast instilled while periodic pelvic and abdominal plain x-rays are obtained
- Nuclear renal scan (DMSA): can determine if renal scarring has occurred
  - >50% of patients presenting with high-grade VUR (4 or 5) will have scar
- American Academy of Pediatrics (AAP) guidelines (2011) for first febrile UTI in children from 2 months to 2 years of age:
  - Renal/bladder US recommended in all cases
  - VCUG only if abnormality seen on US or if second febrile UTI

TREATMENT

- Aim of VUR treatment is to reduce febrile UTIs, pyelonephritis, and renal scarring
- Low-grade VUR (1–3) = majority will spontaneously resolve
- Use of antibiotic prophylaxis is controversial and depends on patient's age, gender, and VUR grade
  - AAP metaanalysis (2011) found no difference in UTI rates among children with VUR grades 1 to 4 taking antibiotic prophylaxis compared with children with VUR grades 1 to 4 who were not on antibiotic prophylaxis. Randomized Intervention for Children with Vesicoureteral Reflux (RIVUR) trial provided evidence for reduction in the risk of recurrent UTI by 50%, but without difference in renal scarring
  - Decision to use antibiotic prophylaxis is made on a case-by-case basis and may vary between providers
- Male circumcision significantly reduces UTI risk (especially in first year of life)
- Treat any bladder or bowel (i.e., constipation) dysfunction, which will decrease risk of future UTIs, increase spontaneous resolution rate, and increase success of future intervention

- Indications for surgical correction (controversial):
  - Persistent high-grade VUR, especially in females (concern for UTI/pyelonephritis during pregnancy)
  - Worsening renal function or new scarring
  - Recurrent UTIs/pyelonephritis
- Surgical options include:
  - Endoscopic injection of bulking agent via cystoscope
  - Open or robotic ureteral reimplantation

Megaureter/Ureterovesical junction (UVJ) obstruction

BASIC INFORMATION

- Ureter that is significantly dilated
- Most often due to UVJ obstruction and called primary obstructing megaureter (POM)
- VUR into megaureter can also occur (more commonly in females)
- Cause of up to 20% of ANH cases

CLINICAL PRESENTATION

- Majority (>80%) diagnosed based on prenatal imaging
- Occasionally presents with abdominal pain, UTI, stone, or hematuria

DIAGNOSIS AND EVALUATION

- Serum electrolytes, creatinine, and BUN
- Urinalysis and culture if UTI suspected
- Imaging:
  - US: evaluate ureter, kidney, and bladder
  - VCUG: rule out VUR and check for posterior urethral valves (PUV) in male
  - MAG3 diuretic renal scan: assess renal function and obstruction

TREATMENT

- Vast majority of megaureters will resolve on own
  - Obtain serial US to monitor
  - Consider antibiotic prophylaxis if obstructed or refluxing
- Indications for surgical intervention:
  - Breakthrough UTIs
  - Worsening renal function or new renal scarring
  - Renal stones
- Surgery involves excision of diseased distal ureteral segment and ureteral reimplant

Ureterocele

BASIC INFORMATION

- Cystic dilation of intravesical ureter (ureter in bladder wall at UVJ)
- Most (80%) associated with upper pole of duplicated collecting system
- Ureter opening into bladder often ectopic (lower in bladder)
- More common in females

CLINICAL PRESENTATION

- VUR in ipsilateral lower pole ureter if duplex system (50%–70%)
- Contralateral VUR seen in 10% to 30%
- Usually asymptomatic and discovered incidentally or during workup for ANH
- UTI and sepsis can occur
- Girls can have interlabial mass due to ureterocele prolapse

DIAGNOSIS AND EVALUATION

- Imaging:
  - US = "thin-walled cyst in bladder"
    - Check upper tracts for duplicated system and/or hydronephrosis
  - VCUG = "smooth, filling defect in bladder"
    - Also evaluate for VUR
  - Nuclear renal scan can be pursued if there is concern about renal function (often before surgery)

TREATMENT

- Goals include preserving renal function, minimizing infection, obstruction, and VUR
- Antibiotic prophylaxis usually given until surgical correction
- Surgery performed in majority of cases (e.g., endoscopic transurethral incision of ureterocele, open or minimally invasive correction)

Ectopic Ureter

BASIC INFORMATION

- Ureter does not insert into correct location in bladder, often inserting caudal to the usual location (location of insertion determines continence in females; males are always continent)
- Often associated with upper pole ureter of duplicated collecting system
- More common in females
- Assess renal parenchyma (US) and function (nuclear renal scan)
- Magnetic resonance (MR) urogram helpful in determining location of ureteral insertion and in guiding therapy
- Requires surgery (e.g., partial or total removal of affected kidney, ureteral reimplant)

Stone Disease

BASIC INFORMATION

- Details regarding stone diseases are provided in Chapter 54
- Clinical presentation can range from incidental detection on imaging study to vague symptoms (e.g., abdominal pain, poor feeding, nausea/vomiting), to focal flank pain and hematuria to UTI and sepsis

- Current recommendation from the American Urological Association (AUA) and European Society of Pediatric Radiology (ESPR) is renal/bladder US as first-line imaging in children and adolescents; CT imaging may be needed in ambiguous cases or for surgical planning
  - MR imaging (MRI) has no real role because stones not easily identified
- Treatment depends on clinical presentation and stone characteristics (size, number, and location)
  - Small, distal (closer to bladder) stone more likely to pass spontaneously
    - Increase fluid intake, pain control, strain urine for stone
  - Indications for acute emergency urinary decompression (ureteral stent or percutaneous nephrostomy tube):
    - Signs of infection or sepsis (hemodynamic instability, fever, elevated white blood cells (WBC), urinalysis suggestive of infection)
    - Obstruction of solitary kidney
    - Intractable pain, nausea, or emesis
  - If no indication for acute treatment, some may try medical expulsion therapy (e.g., off-label use of alpha-receptor blocker, tamsulosin)
  - Surgical interventions required in 22% to 60% of children with stones (e.g., shock wave lithotripsy, endoscopic/ureteroscopic intervention, percutaneous nephrolithotomy for larger and staghorn stones). Open or laparoscopic approaches are rare
  - All stones should be sent for stone analysis
- Follow-up depends on etiology of stone disease
  - Lifestyle modifications = increase fluid intake, minimize sodium and animal meat intake, increase citrate intake (lemonade or orange juice)
  - Monitoring with periodic US is preferred in almost all cases
  - Urine studies helpful to monitor effect of medical/lifestyle intervention

DISORDERS OF THE BLADDER

Prune Belly Syndrome

BASIC INFORMATION

- Also called Eagle Barrett Syndorme, Triad Syndrome
- Triad of:
  - Abdominal wall laxity from deficient musculature
  - Urinary tract dilation
  - Bilateral cryptorchidism (undescended testicles)
- Almost exclusively in boys (95%)
- Most cases sporadic; variable in severity
- Renal dysplasia in 50%

CLINICAL PRESENTATION

- Commonly prenatal diagnosis or suspicion based on US findings
  - Bilateral hydroureteronephrosis, tortuous dilated ureters, large distended bladder, occasionally oligohydramnios

- Can have urethral atresia or megalourethra (which may cause obstruction, poor urinary stream)
- Physical examination:
  - Wrinkled, redundant skin over lower abdomen with bulging flanks ("prune" like)
  - Undescended testes
- 75% have nonurologic manifestations:
  - Gastrointestinal (GI): intestinal malrotation, bowel atresia, omphalocele, gastroschisis, imperforate anus
  - Cardiac: patent ductus arteriosus (PDA), ventricular septal defect (VSD), atrial septal defect (ASD), tetralogy of Fallot
  - Pulmonary: pulmonary hypoplasia (>50%), pneumothorax
  - Orthopedics: pectus excavatum, scoliosis, sacral agenesis, congenital hip dislocation, clubfoot
- Associated with trisomy 13, 18, and 21
- Management generally focuses on UTI prophylaxis, potential surgical intervention to facilitate adequate bladder emptying, orchiopexies for cryptorchidism, and delayed abdominal wall reconstruction for cosmesis
- Progressive renal failure and ESRD will occur in 1/3 of patients

Neurogenic Bladder (NGB)

BASIC INFORMATION

- Normal bladder function (two phases):
  - Filling: store urine at low pressures (high compliance due to viscoelastic properties of bladder wall)
    - Estimated bladder capacity (EBC) can be calculated: If less than 2 years old: EBC (in mL) = weight (kg) × 7 If >2 years old: EBC (in mL) = (age [years] +2) × 30
  - Voiding: empty to completion via sustained bladder contraction
- NGB is a dysfunction of bladder due to disease of the central nervous system (CNS) or peripheral nerves that innervate the bladder
- Children with NGB cannot empty their bladders efficiently or completely
- Major concern is loss of bladder compliance (high bladder storage pressures due to bladder wall hypertrophy, fibrosis)
  - Increased bladder pressure is transmitted to upper tracts and kidney
  - Can result in hydroureteronephrosis, VUR, UTIs, and/or renal damage over time
- NGB is frequently seen in spina bifida (with no improvement in NGB rates with fetal surgery)
- Other etiologies include spinal cord injury, cerebral palsy, Guillain-Barré syndrome, stroke, multiple sclerosis

CLINICAL PRESENTATION

- Signs/symptoms:
  - UTIs
  - Urinary frequency or incontinence

- Abdominal voiding (Valsalva maneuver used to void)
- Stones
- Physical examination
  - Palpable distended bladder
  - Urine incontinence (overflow incontinence—leakage of urine from full bladder that cannot empty normally)
  - Sacral examination (dimple or hair tuft may suggest occult spinal dysraphism)

DIAGNOSIS AND EVALUATION

- Serum creatinine/BUN
- Urinalysis (proteinuria as result of renal dysfunction)
- Imaging:
  - Renal/bladder US at baseline and periodically (screen for calculus, hydroureteronephrosis)
  - DMSA = if concern about renal function or scarring after infection
  - Spinal MRI = to rule out spinal cord tethering
    - Consider if sudden change in lower urinary tract symptoms (LUTS)/dysfunction or imaging findings
- Urodynamic study (UDS) = assess function of bladder during storage (pressures, compliance) and voiding (bladder contraction and urine flow) via filling of bladder through catheter
  - Want low bladder pressures when bladder full to expected capacity
  - Can also detect neurogenic detrusor overactivity (NDO, unwanted bladder contractions that can lead to incontinence)

TREATMENT

- Main goal of NGB management: preserve the upper tracts
- Periodic UDS to ensure safe bladder filling/storage pressures
- If cannot empty completely on own, use CIC
  - CIC = catheter insertion and removal every 3 to 6 hours
  - Overnight bladder drainage with indwelling catheter helpful in some patients
- Medications:
  - Antimuscarinics (i.e., oxybutynin, tolterodine) = decrease storage pressure and minimize NDO
  - Alpha-adrenergic blockers (i.e., tamsulosin) = decrease internal sphincter resistance
- Surgical interventions include transuretrhal botulinum toxin A injection into the sphincter or bladder wall, catheterizable channel creation, and/or bladder augmentation

Nonneurogenic Lower Urinary Tract Dysfunction

BASIC INFORMATION

- LUTS without neurogenic or anatomic cause
- Also known as functional disorders of the lower urinary tract, voiding dysfunctions, or dysfunctional elimination syndromes

- 17% to 22% of "normal" school-age children will report at least one LUTS if questioned
- Most common reason for referral to pediatric urologist

CLINICAL PRESENTATION

- Common LUTS include:
  - Urinary frequency (≥ 8 voids per day)
  - Infrequent urination (≤ 3 voids per day)
  - Daytime incontinence = leakage of urine
  - Nocturnal enuresis = nighttime wetting
  - Urgency = sudden feeling of need to void ("running to bathroom")
  - Hesitancy = difficulty initiating voiding stream
  - Straining = using abdominal muscles as pressure to void
  - Intermittency = voiding in bursts ("starting and stopping" of stream)
  - Nocturia = awaking at night to void
- Signs:
  - Holding maneuvers = strategy to postpone void
    - Crossing legs
    - Standing on tiptoes
    - Squatting with heel pressed into perineum
- Can present with UTI (often recurrent and afebrile)
- Concomitant bowel dysfunction is common

DIAGNOSIS AND EVALUATION

- Urinalysis and culture if concern for UTI
- Differential diagnosis (specific conditions): see Table 84.2
- Evaluation:
  - First step: obtain voiding/elimination diary (patient/family records voids, bowel movements, and LUTS while at home)
  - Uroflowmetry = measure urinary stream to determine flow rates and curve/pattern
  - Check postvoid residual with US to ensure complete emptying
- Imaging/studies:
  - US—often reserved for severe cases or when concern of renal damage
    - Can assess bladder wall, which may find evidence of hypertrophy (wall thickening)
  - UDS—only in complicated cases resistant to standard therapy

TREATMENT

- Depends on specific diagnosis and condition
- General recommendations/treatment (called urotherapy):
  - Timed voiding (voiding every 2 to 3 hours daily)
  - Minimization of fluids with irritants (avoid caffeine, chocolate, carbonation/sodas) → water is best
  - Water bolus drinking (age +2 in oz TID taken over 10 min), which results in more rapid filling of the bladder and a better "signal" to the brain with resultant more frequent and effective voiding
  - Good posture during voiding

Table 84.2. Characteristics and Treatment Options for Specific Nonneurogenic Lower Urinary Tract Conditions in Children

Diagnosis	Definition/Symptoms	Epidemiology	Findings/Other	Treatment
Primary monosymptomatic nocturnal enuresis	Only nighttime wetting (no daytime symptoms); never had period of being dry at night	80% of all children with LUTS Affects: 15%–20% of children <5 years old, 5% of children at age 10, 0.5%–2% of adults	Family history is strong risk factor	Bed-wetting alarm—most effective long-term Desmopressin (DDAVP)—good initial response but high relapse rate (use only oral medication)
Overactive bladder	Urgency ± incontinence	Second most common cause of LUTS	Often due to bladder overactivity (idiopathic detrusor contraction) Associated with encopresis (bowel incontinence)	Antimuscarinics: Oxybutynin Tolterodine
Voiding postponement (aka willful retainer)	Infrequent voiding Voluntary holding of urine Often to avoid school or public bathrooms	>40% associated with behavioral or psychological issue (especially ADHD)	Large holding volumes Increased risk of UTIs (from urine stasis)	Timed voiding Treatment of behavioral (ADHD) or psychological issues
Dysfunctional voiding	Voluntary contracting of external sphincter during void	Much more common in girls (80%–90%) than boys	High risk of UTIs from large postvoid residuals Staccato voiding pattern of urinary stream	Biofeedback = method to teach child how to relax pelvic floor and external sphincter during voiding
Primary bladder neck dysfunction	Bladder neck does not open appropriately or completely during voiding, leading to urinary flow obstruction Hesitancy is most common LUTS	More common in boys than girls	Diagnosis often missed for years Weak urinary stream with decreased urinary flow rates/velocities	Alpha-blockers: Tamsulosin
Giggle incontinence	Involuntary large-volume incontinence during laughing	Almost exclusively in girls Starts at 4 to 8 years old and often improves during puberty		Methylphenidate is highly successful

ADHD, attention-deficit/hyperactivity disorder; *LUTS,* lower urinary tract symptoms; *UTI,* urinary tract infection.

- Treatment of bowel dysfunction (usually constipation) is critical
- Additional therapies (secondary measures) for specific conditions (see Table 84.2)

Bladder Exstrophy

BASIC INFORMATION

- Major anomaly with bladder open and exposed on the abdomen
- Occurs in 1/50,000 births. Twice as common in males
- Urethra and genitals also involved: glans penis in males is epispadiac and clitoris in females is bifid
- Often diagnosed prenatally (US demonstrates absence of bladder)
- Obvious on physical examination after birth
- Postnatal imaging includes renal US and pelvic x-ray (all have pubic diastasis)
- Immediate postnatal care:
  - Cover bladder plate with nonadherent dressing (e.g., plastic wrap), can keep moist with nonsaline irrigation with each diaper change
- Definitive treatment is surgical correction (single or staged procedure)
- All children will have VUR after bladder closure
  - Antibiotic prophylaxis can be used until surgical correction of VUR

Rhabdomyosarcoma

BASIC INFORMATION

- The most common soft tissue sarcoma in children and fourth most common solid tumor in children, with 25% to 33% involving the genitourinary (GU) tracts
- For details regarding rhabdomyosarcoma, see Chapter 63
- Signs/symptoms of GU rhabdomyosarcoma depend on site of origin but are generally a consequence of mass effect:
  - Bladder/prostate = LUTS, stranguria, urinary retention, hematuria
  - Paratesticular = scrotal pain or swelling
  - Vaginal/uterine = vaginal mass, discharge or bleeding
- Multimodal treatment most common, including chemotherapy, radiation, and surgery

Urachal Anomalies

BASIC INFORMATION

- Urachus is normally a fibrous remnant of the allantois (embryologic canal that drains the fetal bladder) with an obliterated lumen
- Runs from the apex/dome of the bladder to the umbilicus

CLINICAL PRESENTATION

- Failure of the urachal lumen to completely obliterate can lead to:
  - Patent urachus: opening from apex of bladder to umbilicus
    - Continuous or intermittent urine drainage from umbilicus in neonatal period
  - Urachal cyst: if only one part does not obliterate and fills with fluid
    - No communication with bladder or umbilicus
    - Can become infected and present as umbilical abscess
- Symptoms include:
  - Pain or palpable umbilical mass from abscess
  - UTI
- Physical examination:
  - Fluid/pus/urine draining from umbilicus
  - Palpable umbilical mass

DIAGNOSIS AND EVALUATION

- US best for imaging
- VCUG can be used if suspect patent urachus

TREATMENT

- Patent urachus requires surgical excision
- Urachal cyst:
  - If infection/abscess = incision and drainage, delayed complete excision after antibiotics management to reduce inflammation and minimize surgical risk

DISORDERS OF THE URETHRA

Posterior Urethral Valves (PUV)

BASIC INFORMATION

- Congenital obstructive folds (valve) in posterior (proximal) urethra, resulting in an obstructive uropathy exclusively in males
- Cause varying degrees of bladder outlet obstruction
- Incidence = 1/4000 to 1/8000 male births
- One-third of boys will progress to ESRD

CLINICAL PRESENTATION

- Antenatal diagnosis common, especially severe cases
  - Earlier diagnoses usually have worse severity
- Pulmonary distress at birth secondary to pulmonary hypoplasia
- Postnatal presentation:
  - Weak stream, straining with voiding
  - UTI or sepsis
  - Renal failure
  - Failure to thrive
- Physical examination:
  - Palpable, enlarged bladder

DIAGNOSIS AND EVALUATION

- Serum creatinine
  - Newborn creatinine will reflect mother's creatinine in first several days of life
  - Creatinine in neonate should never increase (any increase would be concerning for renal dysplasia or obstruction)
  - Nadir creatinine (<0.7–1) in first year of life predictive of better renal function and outcome
- Imaging:
  - Renal and bladder US:
    - Antenatal = bilateral hydroureteronephrosis, thickened bladder wall, dilation of posterior (proximal) urethra; can have oligohydramnios if significant obstruction
    - Postnatal = similar to above; also note renal parenchyma, presence of corticomedullary differentiation and renal echogenicity
  - VCUG (gold standard for diagnosis)
    - Dilated posterior urethra proximal to valve tissue
    - Can assess for VUR, bladder trabeculation, and diverticula if present
  - Nuclear renal scan (DMSA):
    - Evaluate renal function, extent of dysplasia

TREATMENT

- No clear benefit for prenatal intervention
- Urethral catheter should be placed immediately at birth
- Monitor electrolytes and treat as necessary
- Antibiotic prophylaxis recommended
- Surgery is performed immediately after diagnosis (e.g., transurethral incision, vesicostomy)
  - Consider circumcision to decrease UTI risk (risk of UTI in boy with PUV is as high as 60%)
- Long-term follow-up after surgical correction is critical:
  - Nephrologists will monitor for renal failure (even after correction!), urinary concentrating defects, and risk of renal dysplasia
  - Urologists will follow for bladder dysfunction

Imperforate Anus

BASIC INFORMATION

- Absence of anus that is most commonly with fistula between rectum and lower urinary tract:
  - Males = bladder, prostate, or urethra fistula
  - Females = vestibular fistula
- See Chapter 31 for details regarding imperforate anus
- Imperforate anus is associated with GU anomalies in up to 50%
  - VUR
  - Renal agenesis
  - Horseshoe kidney
  - Multicystic dysplastic kidney
- Diagnostic workup should include VCUG to detect VUR and possibly identify fistula to rectum
- Definitive surgical correction is complex and often completed before 2 years of life

Cloaca

BASIC INFORMATION

- Only in females; rare: 1/50,000 live births
- Common channel into which rectum, vagina, and urethra drain; common channel then goes to perineum, where one single opening is found
- Antenatal diagnosis: fetal ascites, cystic pelvic structures; bilateral hydroureteronephrosis
- Physical examination reveals one orifice in perineum ± abdominal mass (distended bladder or hydrometrocolpos)
- Evaluation includes abdominal US, spinal US or MRI (r/o tethered cord)
- Acute treatment may involve urethral or vaginal catheter—consult pediatric surgery and urology
- Complex surgical repair (often pediatric surgeon and urologist) around 6 months to 2 years

OTHER URETHRAL DISORDERS

Urethral Prolapse

BASIC INFORMATION

- Presents as circumferential herniation or eversion of urethral mucosa at meatus
- Prolapsed mucosa appears as donut-shaped beefy red mass and completely surrounds urethral meatus
- Symptoms may include bleeding, spotting in underwear/diaper, pain, or dysuria
- Most common in prepubertal girls (especially African-Americans)
- Treatment includes topical creams (estrogen or corticosteroids) and sitz baths
- Surgery may be required in some cases if pain or prolapsed mass persists

Spinning Top Urethral Deformity

BASIC INFORMATION

- Radiographic finding during VCUG or UDS
- During voiding, posterior urethra appears dilated and comes to a point at the level of the external sphincter, which is voluntarily contracted, leading to obstruction of urinary flow
- Mainly seen in females (80%–90%)
- Finding is indicative of dysfunctional voiding (see Table 84.2)
- Treatment is biofeedback

Urethral Duplication

BASIC INFORMATION

- Rare: several variants; can be complete or partial
- Presentation: incidental to dysuria or UTIs
- Physical examination: two distinct meatal openings
- Evaluation: retrograde urethrogram (inject contrast at each meatal opening and take intermittent x-ray images)
- Treatment varies from nothing if asymptomatic to complex surgery if severe

Urethrorrhagia

BASIC INFORMATION

- Irritation and bleeding of urethra
- Almost exclusively seen in boys and idiopathic in origin
- Usually spotting of blood in underwear or few drops at end of void
- Vast majority (>90%) have spontaneous resolution

Review Questions

For review questions, please go to ExpertConsult.com.

Suggested Readings

1. Bisceglia M, Galliani CA, Senger C, et al. Renal cystic diseases: a review. *Adv Anat Pathol.* 2006;13(1):26–56.
2. Gatti JM, Kirsch AJ. Posterior urethral valves: pre- and postnatal management. *Curr Urol Rep.* 2001;2(2):138–145.
3. Hernandez JD, Ellison JS, Lendvay TS. Current trends, evaluation, and management of pediatric nephrolithiasis. *JAMA Pediatr.* 2015;169(10):964–970.
4. Peters CA, Skoog SJ, Arant BS, et al. Summary of the AUA guideline on management of primary vesicoureteral reflux in children. *J Urol.* 2010;184(3):1134–1144.
5. Subcommittee on Urinary Tract Infection, Steering Committee on Quality Improvement and Management. Urinary tract infection: clinical practice guideline for the diagnosis and management of the initial UTI in febrile infants and children 2 to 24 months. *Pediatrics.* 2011;128(3):595–610.

85 Disorders of the Male Genital System

DIANA K. BOWEN, JASON VAN BATAVIA, MD and
DOUGLAS A. CANNING, MD

PENILE ANOMALIES

Phimosis, penile adhesions, and paraphimosis

BASIC INFORMATION

- Phimosis: narrowing of the opening of the prepuce, preventing it from being drawn back over the glans
  - It is normal for a newborn's foreskin to be adhered to the glans
  - Physiologic phimosis exists at birth—in 50% of newborns the foreskin cannot be retracted far enough to visualize the meatus
  - By teenage years, virtually all boys will have complete separation of foreskin; a urologic emergency!
- Paraphimosis: painful constriction of the glans by a foreskin that has been retracted behind the corona of the glans

CLINICAL PRESENTATION

- Phimosis:
  - Physiologic: as previous
  - Pathologic: history of recurrent infections (balanoposthitis) or ballooning of the foreskin causing a scarred foreskin (cicatrix)
- Paraphimosis: an uncircumcised male presenting with a painful, swollen head of the penis and "paraphimotic" constrictive ring proximal to the glans
- Penile adhesions: residual attachment of the glans to the foreskin, with or without circumcision; not inherently dangerous

DIAGNOSIS AND EVALUATION

- Phimosis: determine whether physiologic or pathologic; cicatrix, history of infections
- Paraphimosis: a clinical diagnosis
- Penile adhesions: determine whether simple or dense

TREATMENT

- Do not forcefully retract foreskin
- Phimosis
  - <3 years old: usually does not need intervention
  - Otherwise, may try topical corticosteroid cream (betamethasone) or surgical release in severe cases (cicatrix)

- Circumcision is most common surgical procedure in United States
  - Potential benefits: decreases risk of sexually transmitted diseases (STDs) and penile cancer; prevents balanoposthitis (superficial infection of the glans penis and foreskin); reduces risk of urinary tract infection (UTI) in males <1 year of age; prevents phimosis
  - Is indicated for recurrent balanitis
  - Risks: pain, procedural complications, irreversible removal of prepuce
  - Contraindications: hypospadias, webbed or concealed penis, micropenis, large hydrocele/hernia, penile curvature, bleeding diathesis (relative), prematurity (relative)
- Paraphimosis: Requires emergent treatment. Attempt manual reduction, but may require dorsal "slit" incision of the preputial ring if reduction fails
- Penile adhesions: usually resolve over time without treatment; if concerning to parents, may treat with topical steroids or surgically release
- See also *Nelson Textbook of Pediatrics*, Chapter 544, "Anomalies of the Penis and Urethra"

Priapism

BASIC INFORMATION

- Persistent penile erection lasting >4 hours
- Filling of the two corpora cavernosa with blood
- Three subtypes
  - Ischemic (low flow)—most common in children: sickle cell disease (>60% of cases), leukemia, drug/medication induced
  - Nonischemic (high flow)—follows perineal trauma lacerating artery
  - Stuttering (intermittent)

CLINICAL PRESENTATION

- Usually painful erection lasting >4 hours in patient with sickle cell disease (often with a history of prior episodes)
- Nonpainful priapism also possible but less common; associated with trauma

DIAGNOSIS AND EVALUATION

- Laboratory testing: consider evaluation for sickle cell disease and leukemia, and toxicology screen
- With urology, may consider cavernous aspiration with blood gas sampling (like an arterial blood gas test [ABG])

- Ultrasound: consider if unsure whether ischemic or nonischemic; may identify arteriovenous (AV) fistula in nonischemic (high flow) cases

TREATMENT

- Emergency therapy required (e.g., phenylephrine injection into corpora, surgery); therefore immediate urology consultation is needed
- For sickle cell disease, a trial of conservative management may be warranted at first (hydration, oxygen, alkalinization, analgesia)

Disorders of sexual differentiation (DSD)

BASIC INFORMATION

- See Chapter 21 for details
- Broad grouping of disorders that arise from abnormalities in chromosomes, gonadal development, or hormonal production/activity

CLINICAL PRESENTATION

- Newborn with ambiguous genitalia
- Inappropriate pubertal development or delayed puberty
- Infertility later in life

DIAGNOSIS AND EVALUATION

- Accurate diagnosis is challenging but imperative for future decision-making as well as for identifying life-threatening conditions such as salt-wasting with congenital adrenal hyperplasia (CAH)
  - Diagnosis is paramount to facilitate informed gender assignment in some cases and to manage future cancer risk associated with specific disorders
- Examination:
  - Abdomen and perineum; look for dehydration, failure to thrive, and hyperpigmentation of areola or labio-scrotal fold (CAH)
  - Genitalia: palpate for gonads—if palpable, will be a testis (ovaries do not descend)
    - Suspect any patients with bilateral undescended testes (UDT) or unilateral UDT with hypospadias of having a DSD
  - Symmetry versus asymmetry of gonadal examination
    - Symmetric examination implies hormonal cause (e.g., CAH, insufficient testosterone, deficiencies in androgen receptors or 5-alpha reductase)
    - Asymmetric examination implies discordant gonads on one side or the other with or without sex chromosomal anomalies (mixed gonadal dysgenesis or ovotesticular DSD)
  - Stretched penile length (tongue blade at the dorsal blade base of penis pushed down to pubic symphysis)
    - Micropenis = at least 2.5 standard deviations below the mean (<1.9 cm if full term); can be isolated hormonal abnormality after 14 weeks of gestation (Hypogonadotropic hypogonadism, hypergonadotropic

hypogonadism), idiopathic or chromosomal abnormalities (e.g., Prader-Willi, Kallman)
- Laboratory testing
  - Karyotype
  - Basic metabolic panel
  - Hormonal evaluation: luteinizing hormone (LH) and follicle-stimulating hormone (FSH), urinary steroids, human chorionic gonadotropin (hCG) stimulation test
  - Endocrine panel if there is asymmetry or absent gonad (17-OH progesterone)
- Ultrasound: abdominal ultrasound to identify müllerian structures; examine if adrenal glands are enlarged (suggestive, not diagnostic, of CAH) and to localize gonads if possible
- Genitography: if ultrasound is not clear; delineates the urogenital anatomy with contrast and x-ray
- Laparoscopy: occasionally necessary for gonadal biopsy to establish diagnosis. Never remove the gonad until confirmatory path (not frozen) is returned. Usually requires two surgical procedures

TREATMENT

- Dependent on ultimate type of DSD
- Surgical reconstruction is done on case-by-case basis with a multidisciplinary (geneticist, ethicist, pediatric urologist, etc.) approach to decision-making
- Timing of surgery is controversial

Hypospadias

BASIC INFORMATION

- Congenital defect of the penis: incomplete development of the anterior urethra, corpora cavernosa, and foreskin
- Accounts for 1 in 250 live male births; majority have no known cause
- Classified as distal or proximal based on location of meatus on penile shaft

CLINICAL PRESENTATION

- Often asymptomatic and noticed in infancy
- Symptoms can include a downward-deflected urinary stream
- Usually associated with penile curvature
- No increased risk of UTI
- Often associated with UDT and hernia
- Proximal hypospadias associated with additional genitourinary malformations and can be associated with other genetic abnormalities (e.g., Russell-Silver, Beckwith-Wiedemann)

DIAGNOSIS AND EVALUATION

- Severe hypospadias (very proximal) or if associated with bilateral nonpalpable testes: undergo evaluation for potential DSD
- If hypospadias are not associated with unilateral hernia or UDT, no further workup is needed
- No laboratory testing or imaging is necessary otherwise in straightforward cases

TREATMENT

- Do not perform newborn clamp circumcision (penile foreskin used for repair)
- Surgical correction between ages 6 months and 18 years, before toilet training
- May require several stages of repair if severe

Epispadias

BASIC INFORMATION

- Dorsal opening of urethra
- Variant of bladder exstrophy spectrum
- May have wider pubic diastasis (obtain pelvic x-ray)
- Will usually have incontinence, particularly if proximal (at bladder neck)
- Females have bifid clitoris
- Requires complex surgical repair in most cases

SCROTUM/TESTES

Cryptorchidism/UDT

BASIC INFORMATION

- Definition: testis that is not in the scrotum or cannot be brought down to the scrotum and stay there without tension on physical examination
- Most common surgical condition in pediatric urology
  - 3% to 5% of full-term males
    - 5% to 15% of that population will have bilateral UDT
  - 75% will descend by 3 months → 1% rate at 1 year old
  - Uncommon to descend after 3 months
- Associated with prematurity (30%), low birth weight, and some genetic abnormalities (trisomy 21, Prader-Willi, prune belly syndrome)
- Paternity rates are compromised in bilateral UDT
- Risks: slight increased risk of testis tumor later (seminoma), which is decreased if orchiopexy is performed before puberty; increased risk of torsion and hernia

CLINICAL PRESENTATION

- Asymptomatic; found on physical examination by parent or primary care provider (PCP)

DIAGNOSIS AND EVALUATION

- Physical examination of the scrotum and inguinal region
  - Determine whether palpable or nonpalpable testis—palpable means in the high scrotum or the inguinal canal; if nonpalpable, this indicates the testis is either in the abdomen or is absent/atrophic
  - Hypertrophy of a descended testis may indicate atrophy of the contralateral testis
  - Retractile testis: not truly undescended; can be brought into scrotum on physical examination, then retracts due to overactive cremasteric reflex
  - Identify other anomalies: hypospadias (see previous)

- Laboratory testing: none (unless bilateral UDT with hypospadias or ambiguous genitalia, which would require DSD workup)
- Ultrasound: not routinely indicated in diagnosis of cryptorchidism

TREATMENT

- Retractile testes require only annual follow-up
- Management: surgery to release the testis and spermatic cord and to fix the testis in the scrotum (orchiopexy) at 6 to 18 months of life

Hydrocele/hernia

BASIC INFORMATION

- Hydrocele: accumulation of fluid around the testis
  - Communicating: persistence or delayed closure of processus vaginalis; same pathophysiology as an indirect hernia (see later), but smaller and not associated with herniation of abdominal contents. The fluid in the hydrocele commonly changes in volume from examination to examination
  - Noncommunicating: no connection to the peritoneum; occurs commonly in the newborn, and rarely in children older than 1 year. The fluid in the hydrocele is constant and usually resolves in the first year
- Hernia: a protrusion of an organ or tissue through an abnormal opening
  - Indirect inguinal hernia: congenital; persistence of processus vaginalis; allows abdominal contents (often small bowel) through internal ring and sometimes to scrotum; can become incarcerated (cannot reduce) and strangulated (reduced or absence of blood flow)
- 1% to 3% of children have a hernia; rate 3× higher with prematurity (depending on degree); M > F

CLINICAL PRESENTATION

- Bulge in scrotum or groin

DIAGNOSIS AND EVALUATION

- Physical examination: differentiate between hydrocele and hernia by palpation for bowel versus simple fluid; illuminate with light source (if light transilluminates, this suggests hydrocele); listen for bowel sounds in sac; examine for bulge in groin
- Ultrasound: can identify whether testis is present and normal if nonpalpable secondary to large hydrocele/hernia; can detect bowel and peristalsis; can determine extent of hydrocele

TREATMENT

- Communicating hydroceles: if truly changing in volume, can be corrected in the first year. If persistent, but fluid volume is constant after 1 year, correct at age 1 year

- Inguinal hernia with bowel
  - If reducible, proceed with surgical repair (usually within a few weeks)
  - If incarcerated: surgical emergency

Varicocele

BASIC INFORMATION

- Tortuous veins of pampiniform plexus
- Epidemiology: 15% of male adolescents; left-sided predominance (90%)
- Presents with painless scrotal swelling (or a dull ache), with some having palpable/visible veins on examination (often more prominent with Valsalva)
- Classically described as "bag of worms"
- May be associated with adverse effect on spermatogenesis and infertility (20% of adults with infertility are found to have varicocele)
- Treatment: observation is most common
  - Indications for surgery or embolization (controversial): >20% difference in testicular volume, persistent pain, or abnormal semen parameters (most reliable in Tanner V or >18-year-old males)

Spermatocele

BASIC INFORMATION

- Painless, mobile testicular mass that is posterior and superior to testes
- Transilluminates
- No treatment necessary

Testicular torsion

BASIC INFORMATION

- True surgical emergency and a *clinical* diagnosis
- Mechanism: twisting of the spermatic cord
- Torsion is either intravaginal (typically outside the newborn period) or extravaginal (neonatal)
- Predisposition to intravaginal torsion: "bell-clapper" deformity—incomplete attachment of the epididymis/testis to the scrotum from partial or complete fusion of tunica vaginalis along the epididymis
- Extravaginal/neonatal torsion is the most common scrotal mass in infants

CLINICAL PRESENTATION

- Intravaginal: peak age is 12 to 16 years old, but can occur outside this age range
  - Acute-onset pain with nausea/vomiting, referred abdominal pain, high-riding testis with horizontal lie, and absent cremasteric reflex
  - Elevation of the testicle does not relieve pain
- Extravaginal: incidental discovery in newborn with firm, swollen scrotum

DIAGNOSIS AND EVALUATION

- Clinical diagnosis! If suspicion is present, take to operating room
- No laboratory testing needed
- Ultrasound: use only for equivocal cases or >6 hours
  - Absent blood flow within testis; ± swirl of cord itself

TREATMENT

- Surgical correction ideally within 6 hours (ischemic injury)
  - If viable, fixation of testis (and contralateral testis for prevention) into the scrotum
  - If not viable, perform orchiectomy and contralateral fixation
  - Neonatal torsion: timing is controversial
    - Torsion usually begins before birth, and rarely is salvage of testis viable; thus surgery is mainly to fix the other testis in place (scrotal orchiopexy) to prevent asynchronous torsion

Testicular appendage or epididymal appendage torsion

BASIC INFORMATION

- Twisting of the vestigial müllerian (testicular appendage) or wolffian (epididymal appendage) remnant; often misdiagnosed as epididymitis
  - Very common cause of scrotal pain and often confused with testicular torsion

CLINICAL PRESENTATION

- Pain in scrotum with no change in position of testis, no nausea/vomiting, and no UTI symptoms

DIAGNOSIS AND EVALUATION

- Physical examination: swollen, "blue dot" sign on scrotum
- Ultrasound: appendage is often enlarged; blood flow intact to testis

TREATMENT

- Conservative—nonsteroidal antiinflammatory drugs (NSAIDs), scrotal supporter, limitation of activity

Epididymitis/orchitis

BASIC INFORMATION

- Inflammation of the epididymis and/or the testis that is bacterial, viral, or chemical in origin
  - Classic associations:
    - Sexually transmitted: gonorrhea, chlamydia, enteric organisms

- Nonsexually transmitted: *Escherichia coli* or pseudomonas
- Infants and young children: almost never bacterial, rather viral, voiding dysfunction and chemical epididymo-orchitis

CLINICAL PRESENTATION

- Gradual onset of pain and swelling; may be associated with voiding symptoms (UTI) or urethral discharge (STD)
  - Unlike testicular torsion, skin may have an orange-peel appearance, and cremaster reflex should be maintained
  - Testicle has normal lie
  - Pain may improve with elevation
  - Classically, dysuria is a feature of epididymitis rather than orchitis

DIAGNOSIS AND EVALUATION

- Laboratory testing
  - Urinalysis ± urine culture—rule out urinary source
  - Neisseria gonorrhoeae/chlamydia if history or examination is suspicious
- Ultrasound: increased blood flow and perfusion are observed (usually performed to rule out torsion)

TREATMENT

- If bacterial sources are identified, treat with antibiotics (e.g., intramuscular [IM] ceftriaxone and per os [PO] doxycycline)
- If noninfectious, conservative management with NSAIDs and scrotal support

Testicular tumors

BASIC INFORMATION

- Rare among children and usually benign
- Neonates: usually teratomas, but other tumors are possible

- Older children more likely to have yolk sac tumor—potential for metastasis

CLINICAL PRESENTATION

- Usually asymptomatic; painless mass

DIAGNOSIS AND EVALUATION

- Laboratory testing: CBC, basic metabolic panel, liver enzymes
  - Tumor markers: alpha fetoprotein (AFP), beta-hCG, lactate dehydrogenase (LDH) (AFP elevated in newborns but useful for comparisons later)
- Ultrasound (both sides, even if mass is unilateral)
- Further imaging: abdominal imaging with computed tomography (CT) or magnetic resonance imaging (MRI) may be needed depending on the pathology of the tumor

TREATMENT

- Excision by partial orchiectomy or radical orchiectomy is usually curative
- Depending on pathology, may need further therapy with chemotherapy, radiation, or retroperitoneal lymph node dissection (RPLND)
- See Chapter 63 for details regarding gonadal tumors

Review Questions

For review questions, please go to ExpertConsult.com.

Suggested Readings

1. Bowlin PR, Gatti JM, Murphy JP. Pediatric testicular torsion. *Surg Clin North Am.* 2017;97(1):161–172.
2. Kolon TF, Herndon CD, Baker LA, et al. Evaluation and treatment of cryptorchidism: AUA guideline. *J Urol.* 2014;192(2):337–345.
3. McGregor TB, PIke JG, Leonard MP. Pathologic and physiologic phimosis: approach to the phimotic foreskin. *Can Fam Physician.* 2007;53(3):445–448.

Ambulatory Pediatrics

86 Nutrition

ERIN R. LANE, MD, KIM BRALY, MD and DALE YOUNG LEE, MD, MSCE

Evaluation of nutritional status and adequate growth is essential to the clinical evaluation of the pediatric patient. Age-appropriate growth is a hallmark of adequate nutritional status in children. Alternatively, poor weight gain or linear growth is often the first clue to systemic disease. Adequate nutritional status is critical to the maintenance of health and the achievement of developmental milestones. This chapter aims to summarize nutritional evaluation of the infant and child, including micro- and macronutrient requirements, modes of delivery of nutrition (including enteral and parenteral nutrition), and consideration of nutritional requirements in specific disease states.

See also Nelson Textbook of Pediatrics, Chapter 44, "Nutritional Requirements."

Nutritional Assessment

BASIC INFORMATION

- Components of comprehensive nutritional assessment:
  - Clinical history
    - Birth history, past diagnoses and surgical history, medications, dietary allergies, neurologic function with attention to patient's ability to chew and/or swallow
    - Social history
  - Nutrition-focused physical examination
    - Review height, weight, head circumference, weight for length or body mass index (BMI; kg/m^2) and compare with age- and sex-based reference norms (i.e., World Health Organization [WHO] and Centers for Disease Control and Prevention [CDC] growth charts); review of micronutrient deficiencies through skin, hair, eyes, and fingernails; review presence of edema and bony abnormalities
    - Recognize loss of subcutaneous fat
    - Anthropometric measurements: skinfold (triceps, mm) and mid-upper arm circumference (MUAC)
  - Detailed diet history:
    - Types of foods
    - Frequency of intake
    - Mixing recipe if patient is an infant on formula
    - Volume of juice/milk consumption
    - Caregivers involved in feedings
  - Biochemical analyses
    - Complete blood count
    - Iron panel
    - Albumin: half-life is 20 days and is not an ideal marker of nutritional status because serum levels are affected by chronic protein energy malnutrition, hepatic synthetic disease, protein-losing enteropathy or nephrotic syndrome, and negative acute-phase reactant in presence of inflammation
    - Prealbumin: half-life is 2 days; acceptable indicator of short-term nutritional status but is also a negative acute-phase reactant like albumin
    - C-reactive protein (CRP), erythrocyte sedimentation rate (ESR)
    - Disease-specific nutrition laboratory testing if indicated
- Normal growth
  - "Normal" growth is defined based on the individual patient. Care should be taken to ensure growth is plotted on the appropriate growth curve. Several syndrome-specific growth charts are available
  - WHO growth charts should be used for infants and children <24 months of age
    - The reference population for these charts was infants who were still breastfed at 12 months and predominantly breastfed for at least 4 months. Clinicians should be aware that (1) fewer U.S. children will be identified as underweight using the WHO charts, (2) slower growth among breastfed infants during ages 3 to 18 months is normal, and (3) gaining weight more rapidly than indicated on the WHO charts may raise concerns for developing obesity
  - CDC growth charts should be utilized for patients ages 2 to 20 years
  - For premature infants, plot growth on premature growth charts (Fenton gender-based reference charts) according to gestational age until 50 weeks; then correct for prematurity (corrected gestational age) on standard growth charts until 24 months
  - Infants and children who are "tracking" along their individual growth curves may have normal growth, regardless of percentile
  - Age-appropriate weight gain
    - Goal weight gain for preterm infants: 15 to 20 g/day
    - Goal weight gain for full-term infants, birth to 3 months: 20 to 30 g/day
    - Goal weight gain for 3- to 6-month-old patients: 15 to 25 g/day
    - Goal weight gain for 6- to 12-month-old patients: 10 g/day
    - Goal weight gain for 2-year-old to prepubertal patients (approximate age of 9–10 years): boys, ranges 5.7–7.8 g/day; girls, ranges 6.0–9.9 g/day, depending on age

Malnutrition and Failure to Thrive

BASIC INFORMATION

- WHO Z-scores (standard deviation from median) versus percentile on growth charts
- Z-scores are useful to assess age-specific associations
- Z-scores to consider for malnutrition include weight for length, BMI, and height

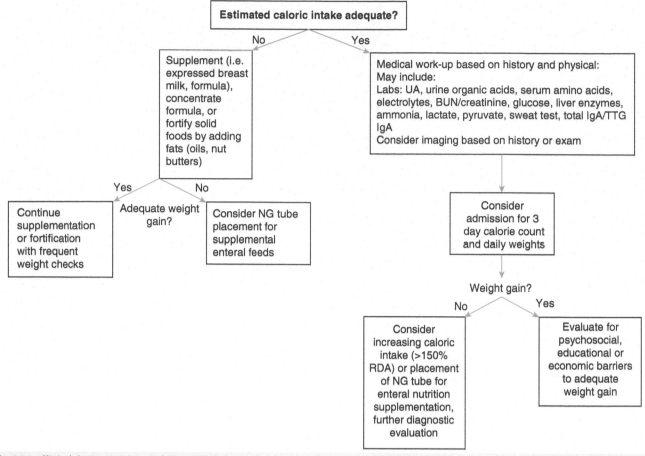

Fig. 86.1. Clinical decision making in failure to thrive.

- At risk of malnutrition: −1.0 < Z-score <0
- Mild malnutrition: −2.0 < Z-score < −1.0
- Moderate malnutrition: −3.0 < Z-score < −2.0
- Severe malnutrition: Z-score < −3.0
- Change in growth Z-score ≥0.67 = significant change in growth velocity
- Duration of nutritional abnormalities:
    ≤3 months = acute
    ≥3 months = chronic (hallmark is linear growth stunting; may include pubertal delay)
- Growth failure/failure to thrive: inability to maintain adequate growth (weight gain, linear growth, or weight for length)
    - Weight crossing >2 percentile lines on growth chart, Z-score indicating greater than mild malnutrition, or <80% ideal body weight

CLINICAL PRESENTATION

- Marasmus: protein-calorie malnutrition presents without edema
- Kwashiorkor: protein-calorie malnutrition presents with edema

DIAGNOSIS AND EVALUATION

- Failure to thrive (see Fig. 86.1): evaluation of etiology/pathogenesis of nutritional abnormalities should focus on:
    1. Inadequate caloric intake

2. Increased metabolic demand or altered utilization of nutrients (i.e., endocrine disorder, chronic inflammatory disease, neoplasm, etc.)
3. Increased losses (i.e., malabsorption, vomiting, diarrhea, etc.)

- Organic etiologies are uncommon because the most common cause is inadequate caloric intake
- After history and physical examination, biochemical/laboratory evaluation and imaging and/or endoscopic evaluation may be considered if there is no improvement in growth with increased caloric provision
- Laboratory investigations are included in Fig. 86.1

TREATMENT

- Growth changes may be reversible or irreversible, depending on age of onset, duration of malnutrition, ongoing presence of disease, completion of puberty, and genetic and psychosocial factors
- Complications of chronic malnutrition include poor wound healing, developmental delays or decreased IQ, behavioral changes, relative immunodeficiency, and prolonged hospitalization
- Refeeding syndrome (RFS): starvation is characterized by total body and intracellular deficit of potassium, magnesium, and phosphorus, as well as vitamin deficiencies (thiamine)
    - Risk factors for RFS: underfeeding >14 days, weight <80% of ideal body weight, rapid weight loss of >5%

to 10% weight in <2 months; patients with hypothermia or bradycardia secondary to malnutrition
- Hypophosphatemia may occur within the first 1 to 7 days of refeeding; this is due to shift to carbohydrate (rather than fatty acid) metabolism and increased intracellular utilization of phosphate, as well as increased insulin secretion (causes intracellular shift of K, Mg, and P)
- Additional clinical manifestations include heart failure and pulmonary edema, arrhythmias, encephalopathy, rhabdomyolysis, seizures, ileus, diarrhea or vomiting, and death
- Treatment includes gradual introduction of calories (start at 25%–75% resting energy expenditure and increase by 10%–25% daily), monitoring serum electrolytes daily, following daily weights (fluid status), and providing adequate protein and vitamin supplementation (i.e., thiamine)

Obesity

BASIC INFORMATION

- Overweight: BMI ≥85% to 95% for age- and sex-based norms
- Obesity: BMI ≥95% for age- and sex-based norms
- Age ≥18 years:
  - Overweight: BMI ≥25 kg/m^2
  - Obesity: BMI ≥30 kg/m^2
  - Severe obesity: BMI ≥35 kg/m^2

CLINICAL PRESENTATION

- Dyslipidemia, insulin resistance/diabetes, hypertension, obstructive sleep apnea, polycystic ovary syndrome, pseudotumor cerebri, slipped capital femoral epiphysis, depression, and reduced quality of life
- Gastrointestinal (GI) manifestations: nonalcoholic fatty liver disease (NAFLD) and nonalcoholic steatohepatitis (NASH), gastroesophageal reflux, cholelithiasis, pancreatitis

DIAGNOSIS AND EVALUATION

- Family history of obesity, cardiovascular disease, dyslipidemia, hypertension, and diabetes
- Physical examination: weight, BMI, blood pressure, evidence of acanthosis nigricans (insulin resistance), pubertal staging, hirsutism, abdominal striae
- Laboratory evaluation: hemoglobin A1C, fasting glucose, alanine aminotransferase (ALT), thyroid-stimulating hormone (TSH), lipid panel

TREATMENT

- Multidisciplinary, intensive approach with focus on wellness of entire family
  - Referral to dietitian
  - Frequent follow-up
  - Goal setting with motivational interviewing: encourage >5 servings of fruit and vegetables daily, <2 hours

of screen time daily, >1 hour of exercise daily, complete elimination of sugary foods/beverages
- Ineffective intervention: lack of sensitivity to racial/ethnic, cultural, and socioeconomic factors; lack of focus on the entire family unit; benefit of artificially sweetened beverages remains an area of active research
- Bariatric or weight loss surgery recommendations for adolescents: when the following criteria are met: BMI is >35 kg/m^2 and type 2 diabetes, pseudotumor cerebri, severe NASH, or obstructive sleep apnea is present or if BMI is >40 kg/m^2

Nutritional Requirements

BASIC INFORMATION

- U.S. Department of Agriculture (USDA) recommendations have shifted from traditional "food pyramid" to new dietary guidelines based on healthy portion size and percentage of the surface area of a plate occupied by grains, fruits/vegetables, protein, and dairy
- Dietary Reference Intakes (DRI) is a set of reference values used to assess nutrient intake; vary by age and sex and include:
  - Recommended Dietary Allowance (RDA): average daily level of intake sufficient to meet the nutrient requirements of nearly all (98%) healthy people
  - Reference values are available at: https://ods.od.nih.gov/Health_Information/Dietary_Reference_Intakes.aspx
- Macronutrients
  - Fats
    - Dietary fat requirements differ for patients of various ages, including those born prematurely, and those requirements may change in certain circumstances
    - Essential fatty acid deficiency: human body cannot synthesize linolenic (omega-3) and linoleic (omega-6) fatty acids. Preterm infants and those on prolonged total parenteral nutrition (TPN) are at risk as well as children on a very low-fat formula
      Clinical symptoms include hair loss, poor growth, poor wound healing, xerosis, rash, anemia, and developmental delays
      Monitor essential fatty acid profile (includes serum linoleic and linolenic acid levels or measuring triene-to-tetraene ratio)
    - Table 86.1 demonstrates daily fat requirements when starting TPN
  - Protein
    - Dietary protein requirement differs according to the patient's age (see Table 86.2). Premature infants have higher needs—up to 4 g/kg/day. Protein requirements decline over time into adulthood. In the setting of acute illness such as burns or another inflammatory process, protein requirements are elevated
    - Protein-losing enteropathy is a condition in which serum protein is lost into the intestines. This may present as low serum albumin and require greater protein intake
  - Carbohydrates
    - Caloric requirements vary by age, among other factors

Table 86.1.   Daily Fat Needs (g/kg/day):** General Guidelines for Parenteral Nutrition

Age	Begin at:	Advance by:	Usual Maximum:
Preterm	0.5	0.5	2.5–3
Term <6 months	0.5	0.5	2–3
6 to 12 months	1	0.5	2–3
Toddlers	1	0.5–1	2–3
Children	1	0.5–1	2–3
Teens	1	0.5–1	1.5–2

**In general, about 0.5 g/kg/day of fat is enough to prevent essential fatty acid deficiency.

Table 86.2.   Daily Protein Needs (g/kg/day)

Age	Proteins
Preterm	3–4
Term <6 months	2–3
6 to 12 months	2–3
Toddlers	1–2
Children	1–2
Teens	0.8–1.5

Table 86.3.   Estimate of Caloric Needs

Age	kcal/kg/day
Preterm	90–120
Term <6 months	85–105
6 to 12 months	80–100
1 to 7 years	75–90
7 to 12 years	50–75
12 to 18 years	30–50

- Estimated daily energy requirements are based upon calculations using age, sex, weight, height, and a "stress factor." These are estimations only and require evaluation of growth trends over time to fine-tune (see Table 86.3)
- Micronutrients
  - Vitamins and minerals are organic and inorganic compounds, respectively, that play key roles in several different functions in the body. They are sourced from a variety of foods, and deficiencies or excesses can be problematic (see Tables 86.4 and 86.5 for summary)
    - Vitamins:
      Fat-soluble: require fat to be absorbed and stored in adipose tissue; deficiency often occurs with fat malabsorption, such as pancreatic exocrine insufficiency and cholestasis
      Vitamins A, D, E, and K
      Water-soluble: generally not toxic because they are primarily excreted by kidneys, not stored in large amounts in the body

Restriction Diets

- Specialized diets such as vegetarian, vegan, multiple food allergies, and other restriction diets require close follow-up with pediatric dietitian to ensure nutritional adequacy (meeting macronutrient and micronutrient requirements; see Table 86.6)

Infant Feeding

BASIC INFORMATION

- Breastfeeding:
  - Human milk is dynamic and changes in content from colostrum to late lactation, varies between mothers and between feeds

- Colostrum is secreted within first few days after birth and is higher in protein content than mature breast milk and is rich in secretory IgA, lactoferrin, leukocytes, lysozyme, and developmental factors that are important for the development of the infant's immune system and defenses
- Mature breast milk produced 10 to 14 days postpartum (in mothers of term infants)
  - Has higher concentration of lactose; foremilk is thinner and lower in fat than hind milk
  - Protein content: approximately 70% whey and 30% casein
  - Lipids account for approximately 50% of calories from breast milk
  - Carbohydrate is lactose plus bioactive oligosaccharides that act as prebiotics
  - Mineral content of breast milk is lower than that of formulas; however, it has higher bioavailability. Mature breast milk generally has 0.3 to 0.9 mg iron/L compared with 10 to 12.2 mg/L in formula
  - Vitamin D is inadequate for nutritional requirements and must be supplemented to meet RDA of 400 IU/day in infants primarily receiving breast milk
  - Vitamin K: exclusively breastfed infants do not achieve adequate levels until approximately 6 weeks of life; subcutaneous or intramuscular vitamin K (phytonadione, 0.5–1 mg) at birth prevents hemorrhagic disease of the newborn
- There are many benefits from breastfeeding as well as misconceptions (see Table 86.7). There is also risk from breastfeeding because some medications and communicable diseases can be transmitted to babies (see Table 86.8 and Chapter 43)
- Formula feeding:
  - Multiple formulas exist, which fulfill different clinical needs (see Table 86.9).
  - Commonly, trials of soy and protein hydrolysate formulae are performed if there is high clinical suspicion for milk protein allergy

Table 86.4. Overview of Required Vitamins

Vitamin	Absorption	Dietary Source	Function	Deficiency	Toxicity	Serum Measure
Vitamin A (retinol and β-carotene)	Small bowel	Carrots, sweet potatoes, dairy products, leafy greens, liver	Important for vision, epithelium	Night blindness, keratomalacia, Bitot spots, xerophthalmia	Hepatotoxicity, hyperlipidemia, alopecia, ataxia, cheilitis, headache, and pseudotumor cerebri	Retinol and retinol binding protein
Vitamin D (cholecalciferol)	Small bowel and skin synthesis	Sunlight, fortified dairy, egg yolk, liver	Regulates serum levels of calcium and phosphate	Rickets, hypocalcemia/hypophosphatemia (see Chapter 24 for details)	Hypercalcemia, exacerbates milk-alkali syndrome	25-OH vitamin D level, parathyroid hormone
Vitamin E	Small bowel	Nuts, seeds, vegetable oils	Cell membrane antioxidant	Prolonged prothrombin time (PT), abnormal bone development	Coagulopathy/hemorrhage	α-tocopherol
Vitamin K (phytonadione)	Small bowel	Liver, leafy vegetables, soybean oil	Activation of clotting factors	Increased PT (coagulopathy)	Hemolysis	International normalized ratio (Vitamin K–dependent clotting factors: II, VII, IX, and X)
Vitamin B₁ (Thiamine)	Small bowel (jejunum)	Grains, fish, poultry, meat, dairy, leafy greens (similar for all B vitamins)	Synthesis of ATP, co-factor for pyruvate dehydrogenase	Can occur with refeeding syndrome and alcoholism. Wet beriberi results in dilated cardiomyopathy, Wernicke encephalopathy, and refractory lactic acidosis. Dry beriberi results in ophthalmoplegia and Korsakoff psychosis (confabulation, amnesia)	No systemic toxicity	Erythrocyte transketolase activity, characteristic brain MRI changes to thalami and mammillary bodies
Vitamin B₂ (riboflavin)	Small bowel	—	Macronutrient metabolism, iron absorption	Angular stomatitis, cheilosis glossitis, seborrheic dermatitis	No systemic toxicity	Erythrocyte glutathione reductase activity, or 24-hr urine riboflavin (<30 mcg/day)
Vitamin B₃ (niacin)	Stomach and small bowel	—	Precursor of NAD⁺/NADP⁺ critical for DNA repair and hormone synthesis	Pellagra (dermatitis, diarrhea, dementia, death)	Vasodilation, pruritus, myopathy, headache	Urine excretion of niacin-methylated metabolites
Vitamin B₆ (pyridoxine)	Small bowel (jejunum)	—	Hemoglobin synthesis, nerve cell function, glucose homeostasis	Dermatitis, glossitis, seizures, anemia	Ataxia, sensory neuropathy	Pyridoxal phosphate and 24-hr urine excretion
Vitamin B₇ (biotin)	Small bowel	—	Coenzyme	Dermatitis, alopecia, seizures, ataxia	No systemic toxicity	Biotin level, 24-hr urine collection
Vitamin B₉ (folic acid)	Small bowel	—	DNA synthesis and repair, red blood cell production, neural tube formation	Neural tube defects, anemia, delayed growth, diarrhea, weakness	Rare	Folate level
Vitamin B₁₂ (cyanocobalamin)	Terminal ileum, requires intrinsic factor	—	Hemoglobin synthesis	Macrocytic anemia, weakness, paresthesia. At risk for deficiency with chronic gastritis, Crohn disease, bariatric surgery, or ileal resections	None	Low or normal B₁₂ levels with increased serum methylmalonic acid or homocysteine levels
Vitamin C (ascorbic acid)	Small bowel (ileum)	Citrus, tomatoes, strawberries	Collagen synthesis (wound healing)	Scurvy, anemia, gingival bleeding, perifollicular hemorrhage, poor wound healing	Rare, but avoid supplementation in renal failure, iron overload (increases absorption of iron), or if taking anticoagulants (warfarin)	Ascorbic acid level

Table 86.5. Overview of Required Minerals

Mineral	Absorption	Dietary Source	Function	Deficiency	Toxicity	Serum Measure
Iron	Small bowel, improved by vitamin C and acidic environment	Meat, poultry, fish	Heme synthesis	Microcytic anemia	Chronic and acute overdose (gastritis, small bowel obstruction)	Iron, ferritin, hemoglobin, total iron-binding capacity, % saturation of transferrin receptor
Iodide	Stomach and small bowel	Eggs, fish, iodized salt, sea vegetables	Building block of thyroid hormone	Goiter, hypothyroidism	Hyperthyroidism	TSH/free T4, 24-hr urine excretion
Zinc	Small bowel	Pork, beef, shellfish	Enzyme function, immune function, wound healing, antioxidant	Acrodermatitis enteropathica, poor growth, diarrhea, hair loss	Nausea/vomiting	Zinc level, low alkaline phosphatase, red blood cell zinc concentration
Calcium	Duodenum and mobilized from bone	Dairy, calcium-fortified beverages	Bone homeostasis	Low bone density, fatigue, depression, seizures, tetany	Renal stones, headache, ataxia, bone pain	Bone density or serum ionized calcium
Copper	Stomach, small bowel, bound to ceruloplasmin	Liver, shellfish	Antioxidant, connective tissue maturation	Neutropenia, myelopathy, neuropathy prothrombin time (coagulopathy)	Coagulopathy, thrombocytopenia	Copper level
Chromium	Small bowel	Whole grain cereals	Glucose homeostasis	Weight loss, peripheral neuropathy, impaired glucose utilization	Rhabdomyolysis, liver dysfunction, renal failure	Erythrocyte and urine chromium levels
Manganese	Small bowel	Green leafy vegetables	Cholesterol synthesis, cartilage/bone synthesis	Dermatitis, poor hair/nail growth, poor growth, abnormal bone/cartilage growth	Parkinson-like syndrome	Serum level, brain MRI (basal ganglia changes)
Selenium	Small bowel	Nuts, meats	Thyroid function, immune function, free radical scavenger	Arrhythmias, cardiomyopathy, muscle weakness, hypothyroidism	Diarrhea, muscle cramps, vomiting	Selenium level, glutathione peroxidase activity

Table 86.6. Deficiencies Associated With Restriction Diets

Restriction Diet	Risk for Deficiency
Vegan	Vitamins B_{12} and D, calcium, iron
Consuming goat's milk instead of cow's milk	Folic acid
Rice milk instead of cow's milk	Protein
Gluten-free	B vitamins, iron

Table 86.7. Benefits and Misconceptions about Breastfeeding

Benefits	Misconceptions
Breast milk is more easily digested than infant formula	Switching between breast and bottle creates confusion for the baby
Contains antibodies that can help prevent infection	Frequent breastfeeding leads to poor milk production
Decreased risk of asthma and allergies	All babies must be weaned from the breast before 12 months of age
Decreased risk of acute otitis media	Breastfeeding is certain to prevent conception
Mother-infant bonding	

Table 86.8. Medications Contraindicated in Breastfeeding Mothers

Cyclophosphamide	Methotrexate
Cyclosporine	Amiodarone
Doxorubicin	Chloramphenicol

From online NIH resource: https://toxnet.nlm.nih.gov/newtoxnet/lactmed.htm

- Term infant formula:
  - Standard cow's milk–based infant formulas are 19 to 20 kcal/oz
  - Protein content: whey-to-casein ratio ranges from 18:82 (similar to whole cow's milk) to 100:0
  - Fat content is similar to human breast milk
  - Carbohydrate is generally lactose, but some brands use glucose, corn syrup solids, rice starch, or maltodextrin
  - Vitamin D is adequate to meet nutritional requirements if intake is sufficient
- Preterm infant formula:
  - Standard concentration is 22 to 30 kcal/oz
  - Increased protein (whey-to-casein ratio is 60:40, or more closely resembles human milk), vitamins, and minerals (calcium and phosphorus) compared with term infant formulas

Table 86.9. Infant and Pediatric Formulas

Type of Formula	Indication for Use	Contraindications/ Drawbacks	Carbohydrate Content	Fat Content	Protein Content
Soy formula	Galactosemia, cow's milk protein allergy (however, high >50% cross-reactivity), religious or cultural objections to use of animal products Taste preference	Prematurity, renal disease, fructose intolerance	Corn syrup solids, sucrose, maltodextrin	Blend of long-chain triglyceride (LCT) and medium-chain triglyceride (MCT)	Soy-protein isolate, must be supplemented with methionine and taurine, contains higher amounts of less bioavailable protein
Protein hydrolysate (semi-elemental)	Food protein allergy, auto-immune enteropathy, malabsorption	Higher osmolality than some intact protein formulas (260–370 mOsm/kg water) Poor palatability	Lactose-free: corn syrup solids, sucrose, dextrose, or maltodextrin	High MCT	Casein or whey heat-treated and hydro-lyzed to short chains of peptide and some free amino acids, still requires pancreatic peptidases for digestion
Amino acid-based formula (elemental)	Cow's milk protein allergy, short bowel syndrome, allergic enteropathy, or eosinophilic esophagitis "Hypoallergenic" formula	Higher osmolality (350–375 mOsm/kg water) Poor palatability	Lactose-free (corn syrup solids)	Blend of LCT and MCT	Free amino acids
Home-blenderized diet	Desire to use "whole foods," often higher fiber	May require large volumes to achieve caloric requirements	Varies/personalized	Varies/personalized	Varies

Table 86.10. Modular Additive Products

Product	Indications	Carbohydrate Source	Fat Source	Protein Source
Human milk fortifiers	Increase caloric density of breast milk	Corn syrup solids	Medium-chain triglycerides (MCT), soy	Whey
Long-chain triglyceride	More soluble in formula than MCT, better for continuous tube feeds	n/a	Safflower oil, soy	n/a
Medium-chain triglyceride	Does not require micellar solubilization for intestinal absorption and is absorbed directly into portal venous system (use in cholestasis, lymphangiectasia, pancreatic insufficiency)	n/a	Coconut or palm oil	n/a
Soluble fiber supplements	Slows gastric emptying, fermented into short-chain fatty acids in colon	n/a	n/a	n/a
Protein supplements	Increased protein requirements	n/a	n/a	Concentrated protein, mixed soy, and whey
High-calorie supplements	Formula fortification	Cornstarch	MCT, corn, coconut oils	n/a

- Carbohydrates: blend of glucose polymers (corn syrup solids) and lactose
  - Lipids: blends with increased medium-chain triglyc-erides (MCT) to optimize absorption
- Lactose intolerance
  - Extremely rare in infancy
- Modular additive products can be utilized to supplement total calories or a particular macronutrient component (Table 86.10)
- Introduction of solid foods
  - Breastfeeding or bottle-feeding only until ages 0 to 4 months
  - Purees by spoon for ages 4 to 6 months, working on variety from all food groups
  - Choose foods that provide key nutrients, such as iron and calcium
  - Early introduction of peanut (peanut butter) between 4 and 6 months can reduce risk of subsequent peanut allergy
  - Withhold cow's milk (and other milk substitutes not formulated for infants, such as goat's milk) until after 1 year of life
  - Exclude juice
  - Avoid choking hazards: raw vegetables, whole grapes, hot dogs, raisins, nuts, hard candies

Nutritional Support

BASIC INFORMATION

- Indications for supplemental enteral feeding (either oral or via enteral tube):
  - Inability to support required fluid, energy, and macro- or micronutrient needs by mouth
  - Nutritional rehabilitation is critical to avoid irrevers-ible growth stunting and permanent neurocognitive delays

- Considerations in enteral feeding:
  - Can this child support growth by oral feeds, and is he/she safe for oral feeding, or is support with nasogastric (NG) tube or gastrostomy (G-tube) required?
  - Preferred over intravenous (IV) nutrition due to decreased risk of bloodstream infection, electrolyte abnormalities including hypo- or hyperglycemia, thrombosis or vascular injury, and liver disease
  - Promotes intestinal maturation and growth
  - Decreases cholestasis and risk of intestinal bacterial translocation
- Contraindications and potential drawbacks for enteral feeding:
  - Mechanical or functional bowel obstruction
  - Intestinal ischemia (necrotizing enterocolitis)
  - Risk of aspiration (if feeding into stomach) and potential development of oral aversion or delayed oral motor skills
  - Tube-related complications
- Indications for parenteral nutrition (PN): primary, adjunctive, or supportive role in nutritional therapy
  - More than 5 to 7 days nil per os (NPO)
  - Inability to utilize enteral feeds or inability to absorb or tolerate enteral nutrition
  - May use peripheral PN for short durations; maximum dextrose solution is 10% to 12.5% to avoid phlebitis
  - Central PN allows for hypertonic solutions
  - PN caloric requirements are often approximately 85% of enteral requirements

TREATMENT

- Tube feeding: choose feeding modality and type of enteral nutrition
  - Types of feeding tubes:
    - Nasoenteric tubes (i.e., NG tubes)
    - G-tubes: percutaneous endoscopic gastrostomy tubes (PEG tubes) or low-profile "button" G-tubes
    - Postpyloric tubes: nasoduodenal or nasojejunal versus gastrojejunal tubes
  - Feeding regimen:
    - Bolus feedings are more physiologic but can be done only with gastric feedings
    - Continuous feeds should be considered for recurrent vomiting (i.e., inability to tolerate large gastric volumes)
  - Discontinuing enteral feeds: after demonstration of maintenance of adequate hydration and nutritional status for some period of time without utilization of tube. Generally, G-tubes will not be removed until demonstration of these parameters for at least 6 months without accessing tube
- Parenteral nutrition
  - Protein source:
    - Crystalline amino acids (caloric density = 4 kcal/g)
    - Daily protein needs are presented in Table 86.2
    - Increased protein requirements are seen in states of increased metabolic demand (critical illness) or with increased protein losses
  - Carbohydrate:
    - Dextrose (caloric density = 3.4 kcal/g) is the primary carbohydrate

- Maximal glucose infusion rate (GIR) is approximately 15 mg/kg/min but can be exceeded in certain clinical circumstances and depending on age
- May require addition of insulin to maintain adequate calories in setting of hyperglycemia
- In infants, care must be taken during even short periods off PN, given high risk of hypoglycemia
- Lipids:
  - Different IV fat emulsions, sources may be soy, omega-6 or omega-3 fatty acid, MCT, olive oil, and fish oil. Newer formulations include mixture of soy, MCT, olive oil, and fish oil
  - Caloric density = 9 kcal/g
  - Minimum requirement estimated to prevent essential fatty acid deficiency is approximately 0.5 g/kg/day; goals are presented in Table 86.1
  - In infants and children in whom long-term TPN is anticipated, lipid minimization to less than 1 g/kg/day is indicated to prevent development of PN-associated liver disease (PNALD)
- Electrolytes are added based on serum levels and normal requirements
- Trace elements (iron, zinc, copper, chromium, manganese, selenium, molybdenum) are added
- Complications: hyper- or hypoglycemia, central line–associated bloodstream infections, thrombosis, air embolus, electrolyte abnormalities, PNALD, essential fatty acid deficiency, vitamin or mineral deficiency, metabolic bone disease

NUTRITIONAL CONSIDERATIONS FOR SPECIFIC DISEASES

Inflammatory Bowel Disease

- Nutritional deficiency is common in inflammatory bowel disease (IBD) secondary to poor enteral intake, increased losses (malabsorption), and increased metabolic demand (chronic inflammatory state); some patients may struggle to take in adequate calories by mouth to support adequate nutrition, prompting early consideration of NG tube placement
- Common micronutrient deficiencies include vitamin D, B_{12}, folate, zinc, and iron
- Nutrition is a key component of improved outcomes and may even be utilized as a primary therapy for IBD
  - Exclusive enteral nutrition (EEN), a type of restriction diet that utilizes nutrition with selected formulas (exclusion of table foods), results in induction of remission and maintenance in pediatric Crohn disease

Short Bowel Syndrome

- Often occurs in infants secondary to bowel loss from necrotizing enterocolitis, intestinal atresias, gastroschisis, or volvulus
- Intestinal failure results when an infant or child has insufficient bowel to support normal growth and nutritional status when fed via enteral route; consequently, children require PN support with upward titration of

enteral feeds and slow weaning of PN support over a variable amount of time

- Children requiring PN are at greater risk for micronutrient and essential fatty acid deficiencies and need close monitoring
- Tolerance of enteral feeds is assessed by vomiting, abdominal distention, and frequency and consistency of stools
- All patients who cannot be weaned from PN support should be referred to a pediatric gastroenterologist specializing in intestinal rehabilitation/intestinal failure

Renal Disease

- Special considerations may include fluid restriction, reduced mineral content, reduced-sodium and reduced-potassium diet, ensuring adequate vitamin D intake, and whey-to-casein ratio of 60:40

Cardiac Disease

- Special considerations may include fluid restrictions (for heart failure), increased protein requirements (protein-losing enteropathy, or postsurgical for wound healing), and use of high-MCT-content formulas in setting of chylothorax
- With increased metabolic demand (increased myocardial and respiratory work), with fluid restriction (occasionally to 80–100 mL/kg/day), this may require concentration of enteral feeds to 30 kcal/oz

Cystic Fibrosis

- Poor nutritional status is multifactorial in cystic fibrosis:
  - Increased metabolic demand: frequent infections, respiratory distress
  - Pancreatic insufficiency (endocrine and exocrine)
  - Malabsorption
  - Liver/biliary disease
- High-calorie diets (120%–150% RDA) recommended
- Pancreatic enzyme replacements and supplementation of fat-soluble vitamins are necessary to treat exocrine deficiency and malabsorption
- Dietary sodium supplementation is required to avoid hyponatremia

Critical Illness

- There is increased metabolic demand/stress during periods of critical illness
- Failure to provide optimal nutritional support results in energy imbalances and potentially malnutrition and nutrient deficiencies that influence outcome from critical illness
- Upon admission to critical care, infants and children should undergo nutritional evaluation to determine energy requirements; in critically ill infants and children with functioning GI tract, enteral nutrition is the preferred mode of nutritional support

Neurologic Impairment

- Ketogenic diets: diets rich in fat content and limited carbohydrates to shift metabolism to produce ketone bodies. Increase in serum ketone bodies may decrease seizures in some forms of epilepsy
- Ratios of fat to protein+carbohydrates of 1.5:1 to 4:1 require specialized dietitian support
- Formulas generally are not palatable or ideal for children with enteral feeding tubes
- Drawbacks: worsening reflux or constipation, water-soluble vitamin deficiency, bone demineralization, kidney stones

Review Questions

For review questions, please go to ExpertConsult.com.

Suggested Readings

1. Daniels SR, Hassink SG. Committee on nutrition. The role of the pediatrician in primary prevention of obesity. *Pediatrics*. 2015;136:e275–e292.
2. Du Toit G, Roberts G, Sayre PH, et al. Randomized trial of peanut consumption in infants at risk for peanut allergy. *N Engl J Med*. 2015;372:803–813.
3. Grummer-Strawn LM, Reinold C, Krebs NF, et al. Use of World Health Organization and CDC growth charts for children aged 0-59 months in the United States. *MMWR Recomm Rep*. 2010;59:1–15.
4. Hall JG, Allanson JE, Gripp KW, et al. Special section. Syndrome-specific growth charts. *Am J Med Genet A*. 2012;158A:2645–2646.
5. Lucendo AJ, De Rezende LC. Importance of nutrition in inflammatory bowel disease. *World J Gastroenterol*. 2009;15:2081–2088.
6. Mehta NM, Compher C, A.S.P.E.N. Board of Directors. A.S.P.E.N. clinical guide nutrition support of the critically ill child. *J Parenter Enteral Nutr*. 2009;33:260–276.
7. Mehta NM, Corkins MR, Lyman B, et al. Defining pediatric malnutri a paradigm shift toward etiology-related definitions. *J ParEnteral Nutr*. 2013;37:460–481.
8. Speiser PW, Rudolf MC, Anhalt H, et al. Childhood obesity. *J Clin EndoMetab*. 2005;90:1871–1887.

87 Immunizations

GRACE KIM, MD, FAAP

Immunizations are a cornerstone of effective preventive medicine and have significantly reduced the morbidity and mortality related to infectious diseases. Vaccines stimulate the immune system to produce humoral and cellular immunity to a specific antigen. This type of protection is long-term, often for a lifetime. Pediatricians should know vaccine indications and schedules, and must also be familiar with contraindications to certain vaccines to avoid any adverse events (Table 87.1). The information in this chapter is for the purposes of board review; the most up-to-date recommendations and additional details are available on the Centers for Disease Control and Prevention website (https://www.cdc.gov/vaccines/schedules/).

See also Nelson Textbook of Pediatrics, Chapter 172, "Immunization Practices."

Hepatitis B (HepB) Vaccine

INDICATIONS AND SCHEDULES

- All newborns within 24 hours of birth (Fig. 87.1 and Table 87.2)
- If the series was interrupted, it does not need to be restarted. The remaining doses should be given as soon as possible (Fig. 87.2)
- Unvaccinated patients should complete three doses. Routine vaccination is recommended through 18 years of age

ADVERSE REACTIONS AND EVENTS

- There are few adverse effects

Rotavirus (RV) Vaccine

- Live, attenuated oral vaccine

INDICATIONS AND SCHEDULES

- All infants (Fig. 87.1)
- If the series was interrupted, it does not need to be restarted (Fig. 87.2)
- Maximum age for the first dose in the series is 14 weeks and 6 days of age
- Maximum age for any dose in the series is 8 months and 0 days of age
- Can be administered to a preterm infant who meets the following criteria:
  - Chronologic age is at least 6 weeks
  - Clinically stable
  - Vaccine is given at the time of discharge or after discharge from the hospital

Attenuated Human Rotavirus Vaccine (RV1, HRV)

- Two-dose series: at 2 and 4 months of age

Pentavalent Human-Bovine Rotavirus Reassortant Vaccine (RV5, PRV)

- Three-dose series: at 2, 4, and 6 months of age

ADVERSE REACTIONS AND EVENTS

- Rare and potential increased risk of intussusception

Diphtheria, Tetanus, and Pertussis Vaccines

INDICATIONS AND SCHEDULES

Diphtheria-Tetanus

- Diphtheria and tetanus toxoid vaccine (DT): children <7 years of age who have a contraindication to pertussis vaccine
  - Four-dose series if the first dose is given at <12 months of age
  - Three-dose series if the first dose is given at ≥12 months of age
- Reduced diphtheria toxoid and tetanus toxoid vaccine (dT): used as a booster dose in adolescents

Diphtheria, Tetanus, and Acellular Pertussis

- Amount of diphtheria and tetanus toxoids and pertussis antigens vary depending on the vaccine
  - Diphtheria, tetanus, and acellular pertussis vaccine (DTaP) contains more diphtheria toxoid and pertussis antigens and may contain more tetanus toxoid than the vaccine for older children and adolescents
- If the series was interrupted, it does not need to be restarted (Fig. 87.2)
- DTaP vaccine
  - Use in children <7 years of age
  - Five-dose series: at 2, 4, 6, and 15 to 18 months, and at 4–6 years of age (Fig. 87.1). Fifth dose is unnecessary if the fourth dose was given at ≥4 years of age
  - Catch-up immunizations for underimmunized individuals
- Pertussis vaccine
  - Lower risk of adverse reactions with acellular compared with whole-cell pertussis vaccine (which is no longer used in the United States)
  - Immunity after pertussis is not permanent. There is also waning immunity to pertussis in contacts of infected patients

Table 87.1. Contraindications to Vaccines

Vaccines	Specific Vaccine Contraindications* and Ingredients With Potential for Reaction
Hepatitis B and human papillomavirus	■ Contains yeast
Rotavirus	■ Severe allergic reaction to latex (RV1 only) ■ Infants with severe combined immunodeficiency ■ History of intussusception ■ In infants with known or suspected altered immunocompetence, consultation with an immunologist or infectious diseases specialist is recommended before administration of the vaccine
Diphtheria, tetanus, pertussis	■ Some DTaP, Tdap, and Td vaccines contain latex ■ DTaP and Tdap may contain casein (a concern for severely milk-allergic individuals) ■ Encephalopathy (not just seizures) without another identifiable cause within 7 days of vaccine administration (contraindication to future use of pertussis-containing vaccines) ■ Individuals with a progressive neurologic disorder (e.g., uncontrolled epilepsy); pertussis-containing vaccines should be deferred and vaccination reassessed
Haemophilus influenzae type b	■ Infants <6 weeks of age
Poliovirus	■ Contains trace amounts of streptomycin, neomycin, and polymyxin B
Inactivated influenza	■ Some contain gelatin
Live attenuated influenza	■ History of anaphylaxis to gentamicin, gelatin, or arginine ■ <2 years of age ■ Children 2–4 years of age with recurrent wheezing ■ Chronic pulmonary (including asthma), cardiovascular, renal, hepatic, neurologic, hematologic, or metabolic disorders ■ Immunodeficiency or those on immunosuppressive therapy ■ Pregnancy ■ Long-term aspirin or salicylate therapy ■ Receipt of a live virus vaccine within the previous 4 weeks ■ Egg allergy per the U.S. Food and Drug Administration. However, the Centers for Disease Control and Prevention's Advisory Committee on Immunization Practices suggests that individuals with egg allergy may receive any age-appropriate influenza vaccine. The amount of egg protein in the vaccines has significantly decreased over time. There were no serious reactions reported in studies of individuals with egg allergy who received inactivated influenza vaccine and live attenuated influenza vaccine. Individuals with reactions to egg that involve symptoms other than hives should receive the vaccine in a medical setting supervised by a health care provider.
Measles, mumps, rubella	■ Contains small amounts of neomycin, sorbitol, and gelatin. Egg allergy is not a contraindication. ■ Pregnancy or intending to become pregnant ■ Immunosuppression—congenital immunodeficiency, HIV infection (<15% of total CD4 cell count), malignancy, iatrogenic (e.g., high-dose corticosteroids)
Varicella-zoster virus	■ Contains minute amounts of neomycin and hydrolyzed gelatin ■ Pregnancy or intending to become pregnant ■ Immunosuppression—congenital immunodeficiency, HIV infection (<15% of total CD4 cell count), malignancy, iatrogenic (e.g., high-dose corticosteroids) ■ Untreated active tuberculosis
Meningococcus	(A history of Guillain-Barré syndrome as a precaution for vaccination was removed in 2010. However, this remains listed as a precaution in the package insert for MenACWY)

*Each vaccine is contraindicated if there is a *severe* reaction to a vaccine component or after a prior dose of the vaccine. This includes those mentioned in this table as well as those not included (e.g., pneumococcal, hepatitis A).

■ Tetanus, diphtheria, and acellular pertussis vaccine (Tdap)
  ■ Use in children ≥7 years of age (Fig. 87.1)
  ■ Children 7 to 10 years of age
    ■ Children not fully vaccinated against pertussis: one dose of Tdap and additional doses of Td as necessary
    ■ Children with an unknown vaccination status or not vaccinated against tetanus, diphtheria, or pertussis: three doses (one dose of Tdap followed by two doses of Td)
  ■ Children ≥10 years of age
    ■ 11 to 12 years of age: one booster dose of Tdap
  ■ Use in pregnant adolescents as early as possible in the 27- to 36-week gestational period

ADVERSE REACTIONS AND EVENTS

■ Exaggerated local reactions are occasionally reported
■ May have an increased risk of febrile seizures after pertussis-containing vaccines

Haemophilus influenzae type b (Hib) Vaccine

INDICATIONS AND SCHEDULES

■ All infants
■ Three- or four-dose series, depending on the vaccine formulation (Fig. 87.1):
  ■ At 2 and 4 months of age (for PRP-OMP) or at 2, 4, and 6 months of age (for PRP-T)
  ■ Booster dose at 12 to 15 months of age
■ Catch-up schedule for children <5 years of age depends on the age when vaccination was initiated and the number of doses received (Fig. 87.2). Catch-up is generally not recommended for children ≥5 years of age. However, for unimmunized individuals ≥5 years of age with anatomic or functional asplenia and HIV infection, one dose should be administered

(FOR THOSE WHO FALL BEHIND OR START LATE, SEE THE CATCH-UP SCHEDULE [FIGURE 2]).
These recommendations must be read with the footnotes that follow. For those who fall behind or start late, provide catch-up vaccination at the earliest opportunity as indicated by the green bars in Figure 1. To determine minimum intervals between doses, see the catch-up schedule (Figure 2). School entry and adolescent vaccine age groups are shaded in gray.

Vaccine	Birth	1 mo	2 mos	4 mos	6 mos	9 mos	12 mos	15 mos	18 mos	19-23 mos	2-3 yrs	4-6 yrs	7-10 yrs	11-12 yrs	13-15 yrs	16 yrs	17-18 yrs
Hepatitis B[1] (HepB)	1st dose	←2nd dose→			←—————————————— 3rd dose ——————————————→												
Rotavirus[2] (RV) RV1 (2-dose series); RV5 (3-dose series)			1st dose	2nd dose	See footnote 2												
Diphtheria, tetanus, & acellular pertussis[3] (DTaP: <7 yrs)			1st dose	2nd dose	3rd dose		←————4th dose————→					5th dose					
Haemophilus influenzae type b[4] (Hib)			1st dose	2nd dose	See footnote 4		←—3rd or 4th dose,— See footnote 4										
Pneumococcal conjugate[5] (PCV13)			1st dose	2nd dose	3rd dose		←——4th dose——→										
Inactivated poliovirus[6] (IPV: <18 yrs)			1st dose	2nd dose	←————————— 3rd dose —————————→							4th dose					
Influenza[7] (IIV)					←——————— Annual vaccination (IIV) 1 or 2 doses ———————→									←—— Annual vaccination (IIV) 1 dose only ——→			
Measles, mumps, rubella[8] (MMR)					See footnote 8	←——1st dose——→						2nd dose					
Varicella[9] (VAR)						←——1st dose——→						2nd dose					
Hepatitis A[10] (HepA)						←—————2-dose series, See footnote 10—————→											
Meningococcal[11] (MenACWY-D ≥9 mos; MenACWY-CRM ≥2 mos)			←——————————————— See footnote 11 ———————————————→											1st dose		2nd dose	
Tetanus, diphtheria, & acellular pertussis[13] (Tdap: ≥7 yrs)														Tdap			
Human papillomavirus[14] (HPV)														See footnote 14			
Meningococcal B[12]														←——————— See footnote 12 ———————→			
Pneumococcal polysaccharide[5] (PPSV23)												←——————————— See footnote 5 ———————————→					

☐ Range of recommended ages for all children	☐ Range of recommended ages for catch-up immunization	☐ Range of recommended ages for certain high-risk groups	☐ Range of recommended ages for non-high-risk groups that may receive vaccine, subject to individual clinical decision making	☐ No recommendation

NOTE: The above recommendations must be read along with the footnotes of this schedule.

Fig. 87.1. Recommended immunization schedule for children and adolescents through 18 years of age—United States, 2017 (accompanying footnotes may be accessed at https://www.cdc.gov/vaccines/schedules/downloads/child/0-18yrs-child-combined-schedule.pdf).

Table 87.2. Indications and Schedules for Hepatitis B (HepB) Vaccine and Hepatitis B Immune Globulin (HBIG)

	HBsAg-Positive Mother	HBsAg-Negative Mother	HBsAg Unknown Mother
Birth weight ≥2 kg	▪ HepB vaccine and HBIG as soon as possible after delivery (within 12 hours) ▪ HepB vaccine at 1–2 and 6 months of age	▪ HepB vaccine at birth, 1–2, and 6–18 months of age	▪ HepB vaccine at birth (within 12 hours); the remainder of the schedule and need for HBIG depend on the mother's HBsAg status once determined
Birth weight <2 kg	▪ HepB vaccine and HBIG as soon as possible after delivery (within 12 hours) ▪ HepB vaccine at 1, 2–3, and 6 months of age	▪ HepB vaccine at 30 days of age or at hospital discharge; then at 2 and 6–18 months of age	▪ HepB vaccine and HBIG at birth (within 12 hours) if the maternal status remains unknown or is positive; then three additional doses of HepB vaccine at 1, 2–3, and 6 months of age

▪ For individuals at increased risk of invasive Hib disease, the schedule depends on the individual's age, prior doses, and medical condition (Fig. 87.3)
▪ Preterm infants should be vaccinated according to their chronologic age

ADVERSE REACTIONS AND EVENTS

▪ Serious adverse events are rare

Pneumococcal Vaccine

▪ Conjugated vaccine: 13-valent vaccine (PCV13) that is used in the United States and includes 13 serotypes. It replaced the 7-valent vaccine (PCV7) for routine immunizations
▪ Unconjugated vaccine: 23-valent polysaccharide vaccine (PPSV23) that includes 23 serotypes; not immunogenic in children <2 years of age; used in children at high risk of invasive pneumococcal disease

The figure below provides catch-up schedules and minimum intervals between doses for children whose vaccinations have been delayed. A vaccine series does not need to be restarted, regardless of the time that has elapsed between doses. Use the section appropriate for the child's age. Always use this table in conjunction with Figure 1 and the footnotes that follow.

Vaccine	Minimum Age for Dose 1	Minimum Interval Between Doses			
		Dose 1 to Dose 2	Dose 2 to Dose 3	Dose 3 to Dose 4	Dose 4 to Dose 5
Children age 4 months through 6 years					
Hepatitis B[1]	Birth	4 weeks	8 weeks **and** at least 16 weeks after first dose. Minimum age for the final dose is 24 weeks.		
Rotavirus[2]	6 weeks Maximum age for first dose is 14 weeks, 6 days	4 weeks	4 weeks[2] Maximum age for final dose is 8 months, 0 days.		
Diphtheria, tetanus, and acellular pertussis[3]	6 weeks	4 weeks	4 weeks	6 months	6 months[3]
Haemophilus influenzae type b[4]	6 weeks	4 weeks if first dose was administered before the 1st birthday. 8 weeks (as final dose) if first dose was administered at age 12 through 14 months. No further doses needed if first dose was administered at age 15 months or older.	4 weeks[4] if current age is younger than 12 months **and** first dose was administered at younger than age 7 months, **and** at least 1 previous dose was PRP-T (ActHib, Pentacel, Hiberix) or unknown. 8 weeks **and** age 12 through 59 months (as final dose)[4] • if current age is younger than 12 months **and** first dose was administered at age 7 through 11 months; OR • if current age is 12 through 59 months **and** first dose was administered before the 1st birthday, **and** second dose administered at younger than age 15 months; OR • if both doses were PRP-OMP (PedvaxHIB; Comvax) **and** were administered before the 1st birthday. No further doses needed if previous dose was administered at age 15 months or older.	8 weeks (as final dose) This dose only necessary for children age 12 through 59 months who received 3 doses before the 1st birthday.	
Pneumococcal conjugate[5]	6 weeks	4 weeks if first dose administered before the 1st birthday. 8 weeks (as final dose for healthy children) if first dose was administered at the 1st birthday or after. No further doses needed for healthy children if first dose was administered at age 24 months or older.	4 weeks if current age is younger than 12 months and previous dose given at <7 months old. 8 weeks (as final dose for healthy children) if previous dose given between 7-11 months (wait until at least 12 months old); OR if current age is 12 months or older and at least 1 dose was given before age 12 months. No further doses needed for healthy children if previous dose administered at age 24 months or older.	8 weeks (as final dose) This dose only necessary for children aged 12 through 59 months who received 3 doses before age 12 months or for children at high risk who received 3 doses at any age.	
Inactivated poliovirus[6]	6 weeks	4 weeks[6]	4 weeks[6] if current age is < 4 years 6 months (as final dose) if current age is 4 years or older	6 months[6] (minimum age 4 years for final dose).	
Measles, mumps, rubella[8]	12 months	4 weeks			
Varicella[9]	12 months	3 months			
Hepatitis A[10]	12 months	6 months			
Meningococcal[11] (MenACWY-D ≥9 mos; MenACWY-CRM ≥2 mos)	6 weeks	8 weeks[11]	See footnote 11	See footnote 11	
Children and adolescents age 7 through 18 years					
Meningococcal[11] (MenACWY-D ≥9 mos; MenACWY-CRM ≥2 mos)	Not Applicable (N/A)	8 weeks[11]			
Tetanus, diphtheria; tetanus, diphtheria, and acellular pertussis[13]	7 years[13]	4 weeks	4 weeks if first dose of DTaP/DT was administered before the 1st birthday. 6 months (as final dose) if first dose of DTaP/DT or Tdap/Td was administered at or after the 1st birthday.	6 months if first dose of DTaP/DT was administered before the 1st birthday.	
Human papillomavirus[14]	9 years	Routine dosing intervals are recommended.[14]			
Hepatitis A[10]	N/A	6 months			
Hepatitis B[1]	N/A	4 weeks	8 weeks **and** at least 16 weeks after first dose.		
Inactivated poliovirus[6]	N/A	4 weeks	6 months[6] A fourth dose is not necessary if the third dose was administered at age 4 years or older and at least 6 months after the previous dose.	A fourth dose of IPV is indicated if all previous doses were administered at <4 years or if the third dose was administered <6 months after the second dose.	
Measles, mumps, rubella[8]	N/A	4 weeks			
Varicella[9]	N/A	3 months if younger than age 13 years. 4 weeks if age 13 years or older.			

NOTE: The above recommendations must be read along with the footnotes of this schedule.

Fig. 87.2. Catch-up immunization schedule for children and adolescents through 18 years of age—United States, 2017 (accompanying footnotes may be accessed at https://www.cdc.gov/vaccines/schedules/downloads/child/0-18yrs-child-combined-schedule.pdf).

INDICATIONS AND SCHEDULES

- All infants and children 2 to 23 months of age (Fig. 87.1)
- Incompletely immunized children 24 to 59 months of age (Fig. 87.2)
- Children 6 to 18 years of age who have not received PCV13 and have the following conditions:
  - Anatomic or functional asplenia
  - Cerebrospinal fluid leak
  - Chronic renal failure
  - Cochlear implant
  - Immunocompromised status
  - Nephrotic syndrome
- Healthy children
  - Four-dose series: at 2, 4, 6, and 12 to 15 months of age
  - Catch-up schedule depends on the individual's current age and age when the first dose was received
  - Preterm infants should be vaccinated according to their chronologic age

- High risk for invasive pneumococcal disease (Fig. 87.3)
  - <2 years of age: follow the schedule for healthy children
  - ≥2 years of age: receive PPSV23 after completing immunization with PCV13
  - Catch-up schedule depends on the patient's age, number of prior doses, and the high-risk condition

ADVERSE REACTIONS AND EVENTS

- Serious adverse events are rare

Poliovirus Vaccine

- Inactivated poliovirus vaccine (IPV) is the only vaccine used in the United States. It does not cause vaccine-associated paralytic poliomyelitis, which can be associated with the oral poliovirus vaccine (OPV)
- Highly effective in producing immunity
  - After two doses, ≥90% of recipients are immune
  - After three doses, ≥99% of recipients are immune

VACCINE ▼ INDICATION ▶	Pregnancy	Immunocompromised status (excluding HIV infection)	HIV infection CD4+ count[†] <15% or total CD4 cell count of <200/mm³	HIV infection CD4+ count[†] ≥15% or total CD4 cell count of ≥200/mm³	Kidney failure, end-stage renal disease, on hemodialysis	Heart disease, chronic lung disease	CSF leaks/ cochlear implants	Asplenia and persistent complement component deficiencies	Chronic liver disease	Diabetes
Hepatitis B[1]										
Rotavirus[2]		SCID*								
Diphtheria, tetanus, & acellular pertussis[3] (DTaP)										
Haemophilus influenzae type b[4]		▨						▨		
Pneumococcal conjugate[5]		▨								▨
Inactivated poliovirus[6]										
Influenza[7]										
Measles, mumps, rubella[8]										
Varicella[9]										
Hepatitis A[10]									▨	
Meningococcal ACWY[11]			▨					▨		
Tetanus, diphtheria, & acellular pertussis[13] (Tdap)	▨									
Human papillomavirus[14]		▨								
Meningococcal B[12]								▨		
Pneumococcal polysaccharide[5]		▨								

Vaccination according to the routine schedule recommended | Recommended for persons with an additional risk factor for which the vaccine would be indicated | Vaccination is recommended, and additional doses may be necessary based on medical condition. See footnotes. | No recommendation | Contraindicated | Precaution for vaccination

*Severe Combined Immunodeficiency
[†]For additional information regarding HIV laboratory parameters and use of live vaccines; see the General Best Practice Guidelines for Immunization "Altered Immunocompetence" at: www.cdc.gov/vaccines/hcp/acip-recs/general-al-recs/immunocompetence.html; and Table 4-1 (footnote D) at: www.cdc.gov/vaccines/hcp/acip-recs/general-recs/contraindications.html.
NOTE: The above recommendations must be read along with the footnotes of this schedule.

Fig. 87.3. Vaccines that might be indicated for children and adolescents through 18 years of age based on medical indications (accompanying footnotes may be accessed at https://www.cdc.gov/vaccines/schedules/downloads/child/0-18yrs-child-combined-schedule.pdf).

INDICATIONS AND SCHEDULES

- Four-dose series: at 2, 4, and 6 to 18 months of age, and at 4 to 6 years of age (Fig. 87.1)
- Final dose should be administered at ≥4 years of age (Fig. 87.2)
- Fourth dose is not required if the third dose was administered after 4 years of age
- Routine vaccination of adult residents in the United States is not recommended. Unvaccinated adults at increased risk of exposure to poliomyelitis should be immunized with IPV

ADVERSE REACTIONS AND EVENTS

- No serious adverse events

Influenza Vaccine

- Inactivated influenza vaccine (IIV)
  - Trivalent or quadrivalent
  - For individuals ≥6 months of age
- Live attenuated influenza vaccine (LAIV)
  - Quadrivalent
  - For individuals ≥2 years of age
- Strains of influenza A and B used in the vaccine are updated annually to cover the strains that are anticipated to be circulating in the upcoming influenza season
- For the 2016 to 2017 influenza season, only IIV was recommended for all patients because of the poor efficacy of LAIV in previous influenza seasons. The impact on future influenza vaccine routes of administration has not yet been decided at the time of this publication

INDICATIONS AND SCHEDULES

- All individuals ≥6 months of age (Figs. 87.1 and 87.3)
- Annually (Fig. 87.2)
  - 6 months to 8 years of age: two doses during the first season of vaccination; the number of doses required for subsequent seasons depends on the recommendations for the current season
  - ≥9 years of age: one dose only
- All health care personnel

Table 87.3. Recommended Individuals to Receive IIV Instead of LAIV (During Seasons When Both Vaccines Are Available)

- ≥6 months to 23 months of age
- Children 2–4 years of age with a history of recurrent wheezing
- Individuals with asthma
- Individuals who are close contacts of severely immunocompromised individuals
- Individuals at high risk for severe or complicated influenza infection
  - Chronic pulmonary, cardiovascular, renal, hepatic, neurologic, hematologic, or metabolic disorders
  - Immunosuppression
  - Pregnancy or intending to become pregnant
  - Receiving long-term aspirin therapy
  - Residents of chronic care facilities
  - Extremely obese

IIV, Inactivated influenza vaccine; *LAIV,* live attenuated influenza vaccine.

- Certain individuals are recommended to receive IIV instead of LAIV (during seasons when both vaccines are available); see Table 87.3

ADVERSE REACTIONS AND EVENTS

- Serious adverse events are rare

Measles, Mumps, Rubella (MMR) Vaccine

- Live, attenuated vaccine

INDICATIONS AND SCHEDULES

- Two-dose series: at 12 to 15 months of age and 4 to 6 years of age (Fig. 87.1)
- Catch-up immunizations to ensure that all school-age children and adolescents have had two doses (Fig. 87.2)
- Immunization is not initiated in children younger than 12 months of age to allow the decline of passively acquired maternal antibody. Children vaccinated before 12 months of age should be revaccinated with two doses when the child is at least 12 months of age
- During a measles outbreak:
  - Infants 6 to 11 months of age receive one dose and are revaccinated with two additional doses starting at 12 to 15 months of age
  - Children ≥12 months of age receive two doses
- During a mumps outbreak:
  - Children who are incompletely immunized should be immunized. Also, a third dose may be warranted
- Delay immunizations in individuals who recently received immune globulin or blood products. The vaccine may also transiently reduce tuberculin skin test sensitivity
- Pregnancy should be avoided for 4 weeks after receiving the vaccine

ADVERSE REACTIONS AND EVENTS

- Arthralgias or joint symptoms in up to 25% of susceptible individuals
- Individuals with a history of thrombocytopenia or thrombocytopenic purpura may have an increased risk of thrombocytopenia after vaccination

Varicella-Zoster Virus (VAR) Vaccine

- Live, attenuated vaccine

INDICATIONS AND SCHEDULES

- Two-dose series: at 12 to 15 months of age and 4 to 6 years of age (Fig. 87.1)
- Individuals 7 to 18 years of age without evidence of immunity should receive two doses (Fig. 87.2)
- Delay immunizations in individuals who recently received immune globulin, blood products, salicylate therapy, or antiviral therapy against herpesvirus (e.g., acyclovir, famciclovir)
- For individuals who are exposed to varicella and do not have evidence of immunity, vaccination within 3 days (possibly up to 5 days) is recommended. Postexposure prophylaxis decreases the risk and severity of illness

ADVERSE REACTIONS AND EVENTS

- Serious adverse events are rare

Hepatitis A (HepA) Vaccine

INDICATIONS AND SCHEDULES

- All children 12 to 23 months of age (Fig. 87.1)
- Two-dose series: given at least 6 months apart
- If the series was interrupted, it does not need to be restarted (Fig. 87.2)

ADVERSE REACTIONS AND EVENTS

- No serious adverse reactions have been reported

Meningococcal Vaccine

INDICATIONS AND SCHEDULES

- Quadrivalent meningococcal conjugate vaccine (Menactra, MenACWY-D; Menveo, MenACWY-CRM)
  - Vaccine against serogroups A, C, W, and Y
  - All children and adolescents between 11 and 18 years of age (Fig. 87.1)
    - Two-dose series: at 11 to 12 years of age and a booster dose at 16 years of age
    - If the first dose is administered at ≥16 years of age, a booster dose is not needed unless the individual becomes at increased risk for meningococcal disease (Fig. 87.2)
  - Individuals who are at increased risk for meningococcal disease (Fig. 87.3):
    - Menactra or Menveo for children 2 to 10 years of age

- Menactra for infants and children ≥9 months of age
- Menveo for infants ≥2 months of age
- Combination meningococcal and *Haemophilus influenzae* type B conjugate vaccine (Hib-MenCY)
  - Vaccine against meningococcus serogroups C and Y, as well as Hib
  - Certain infants and toddlers 6 weeks to 18 months of age who are at increased risk for meningococcal disease (Fig. 87.3)
  - Discontinued use in the United States in 2017

ADVERSE REACTIONS AND EVENTS

- Serious events are rare

Human Papillomavirus (HPV) Vaccine

INDICATIONS AND SCHEDULES

- Recommended for both females and males
- All children at 11 to 12 years of age
  - Series may be started as young as 9 years of age. Children with a history of sexual abuse or assault should be vaccinated starting at this age
- Two-dose series for children <15 years of age and three-dose series for adolescents ≥15 years of age (Fig. 87.1)
  - Immunocompromised individuals should receive three doses
- Catch-up immunizations for adolescents ≥13 years of age; if the schedule was interrupted, the series does not need to be restarted (Fig. 87.2)
- Use in pregnant women is not recommended, although there is no evidence that it poses harm

ADVERSE REACTIONS AND EVENTS

- No serious adverse events

Immunizations for Travel

- Individuals should seek advice from a travel clinic or a provider with expertise in travel medicine. Information is also available through the Centers for Disease Control and Prevention and Global TravEpiNet (GTEN), a network of travel clinics across the United States

Special Populations

- Recommended vaccines for individuals with the conditions described in (Fig. 87.3)

IMMUNOCOMPROMISED STATUS (EXCLUDING HIV INFECTION)

- HepB, DTaP, Hib, pneumococcal conjugate and polysaccharide, IPV, IIV, HepA, meningococcal ACWY, Tdap, and HPV vaccines
  - Hib vaccine should be administered 6 to 12 months after receiving a hematopoietic cell transplant

- Pneumococcal conjugate and/or polysaccharide vaccine should be administered at least 2 weeks before starting immunosuppressive therapy
- Precaution for RV vaccine; contraindicated in individuals with severe combined immunodeficiency (SCID). Close contacts can receive RV vaccine
- Close contacts should receive IIV and MMR vaccines

HIV INFECTION

- HepB, DTaP, Hib, pneumococcal conjugate and polysaccharide, IPV, IIV, MMR (if ≥15% of total CD4 cell count), VAR (if ≥15% of total CD4 cell count), HepA, meningococcal ACWY, Tdap, and HPV vaccines
  - Pneumococcal conjugate and/or polysaccharide vaccine should be administered at least 2 weeks before starting immunosuppressive therapy
- Precaution for RV vaccine. Close contacts can be vaccinated
- Close contacts should receive IIV and MMR vaccines

ASPLENIA

- HepB, RV, DTaP, Hib, pneumococcal conjugate and polysaccharide, IPV, IIV, MMR, VAR, HepA, meningococcal ACWY and B, Tdap, and HPV vaccines
  - Hib vaccine should be administered in unimmunized individuals before an elective splenectomy
  - Pneumococcal conjugate and/or polysaccharide vaccine should be administered at least 2 weeks before an elective splenectomy
- Close contacts should receive IIV and MMR vaccines. Close contacts can receive RV vaccine

PREGNANCY

- HepB, IIV, and Tdap vaccines
  - Influenza vaccine may be administered at any time during pregnancy
  - Tdap may be administered at any time during pregnancy, but ideally between 27 and 36 weeks' gestation
- Precaution for IPV vaccine
- Close contacts should receive influenza vaccine. Close contacts can receive RV and MMR vaccines

Adverse Reactions to Vaccine Constituents

ANTIMICROBIALS

- Neomycin, polymyxin B, and streptomycin are common
- May be present in vaccines in trace amounts
- Individuals with anaphylactic reactions due to these drugs should be evaluated by an allergist before receiving vaccines containing them

COW'S MILK

- Casein can cause anaphylaxis to DTaP or Tdap vaccines in severely milk-allergic individuals

EGG

- Egg protein is present in yellow fever, MMR, and some influenza and rabies vaccines
- Clinically significant only in the yellow fever vaccine. Individuals with an egg allergy should be evaluated by an allergist before yellow fever vaccine administration

GELATIN

- Used in many vaccines as a stabilizer
- Responsible for many anaphylactic reactions to MMR and varicella vaccines. There are also reports of anaphylaxis from gelatin in influenza vaccine
- Individuals with a gelatin allergy should be evaluated by an allergist before administration of gelatin-containing vaccines

NATURAL RUBBER LATEX

- Vaccine vial stopper or syringe plunger may be natural rubber latex or synthetic rubber
- Individuals with latex-induced anaphylaxis: if the vaccine has a natural rubber latex stopper, the vaccine should be drawn up from the vial without passing the needle through the stopper

PRESERVATIVES

- Thimerosal, aluminum, and phenoxyethanol are added to some vaccines
- Can cause delayed-type hypersensitivity reactions and contact dermatitis. Individuals with known contact sensitivity should receive a preservative-free vaccine, if available. If such a vaccine is not available, this should not preclude vaccination

YEAST

- Yeast protein is present in some vaccines, including HepB and HPV vaccines
- Individuals with a yeast allergy should undergo skin testing before vaccine administration

Vaccine-Hesitant Family

- Individually acknowledge and address specific parental concerns about vaccines, and correct any misconceptions
  - Address questions about the production and composition of vaccines by directly providing the information
- Discuss the development and safety testing of vaccines, and communicate that vaccines are safe and effective
  - Personalizing the message about the safety and necessity of vaccines can be powerful
- Discuss the reasons for immunizing and the risks of not immunizing, and articulate that serious disease can occur if the child is not immunized
- Support the current vaccine schedule as the only evidence-based schedule. Deviation from this schedule may be considered as a last resort if it is the only way to immunize the child
- Establish a positive and nonconfrontational dialogue, and maintain a respectful and trusting relationship

Review Questions

For review questions, please go to ExpertConsult.com.

Suggested Readings

1. Allergic reactions to vaccines. Retrieved from: https://www.uptodate.com/contents/allergic-reactions-to-vaccines; 2017.
2. Centers for Disease Control and Prevention. *Epidemiology and Prevention of Vaccine-Preventable Diseases.* 13th ed. 2015. Retrieved from: https://www.cdc.gov/vaccines/pubs/pinkbook/index.html.
3. Edwards KM, Hackell JM, The Committee on Infectious Diseases, The Committee on Practice and Ambulatory Medicine. Countering Vaccine Hesitancy. *Pediatrics.* 2016:e20162146. https://doi.org/10.1542/peds.2016-2146.
4. Global TravEpiNet. Retrieved from; http://www.massgeneral.org/infectiousdisease/services/treatmentprograms.aspx?id=1939; 2017.
5. Recommended Immunization Schedule for Children and Adolescents Aged 18 Years or Younger: United States. Retrieved from: https://www.cdc.gov/vaccines/schedules/downloads/child/0-18yrs-child-combined-schedule.pdf; 2017.
6. Travelers' Health. Retrieved from; https://wwwnc.cdc.gov/travel/; 2017.

88 Preventive Pediatrics

MARIA ESTHER RIVERA, MD, MPH, FAAP

Preventive care and well-child visits are the cornerstone of pediatrics. Although addressing parental concerns and identifying illnesses are important elements of the office visit, a substantial amount of effort is also aimed at keeping a child healthy. During each visit, attention will be directed toward assessing growth, nutrition, and development; addressing social concerns; providing anticipatory guidance; and completing a full physical examination. Finally, visits should also include scheduling appropriate screening tests and providing recommended immunizations (see Chapter 87).

Screening Tests

BLOOD PRESSURE SCREENING

- The American Academy of Pediatrics (AAP) most recently revised its hypertension guidelines in 2017
- Routine blood pressure (BP) screening is recommended yearly in all children starting at age 3 years during preventive care visits
  - Appropriate cuff size is important for accurate measurement and should cover approximately two-thirds of the child's upper arm
- Hypertension in children is defined as systolic BP and/or diastolic BP that on repeated measurement is greater than 95th percentile
  - Appropriate blood pressure in children is determined by age and height of child
  - Refer to the normative tables included in the Suggested Readings (Tables 4 and 5 in Flynn et al.) for specific definitions of hypertension per height and age
- See Chapter 5 for details regarding hypertension

HEARING SCREENING

Newborn Hearing Screening

- All newborns should receive a hearing test before discharge from the newborn nursery
- One of two methods is typically used: otoacoustic emissions (OAE) and auditory brainstem response (ABR)
  - OAE: small earphones are placed inside the baby's ears, sounds are transmitted, and response to sound is measured
  - ABR: sticky electrodes are placed on an infant's scalp, sounds are transmitted to the ear, and transmission of impulse to the brain is measured
- Any baby who fails a newborn hearing test should have further hearing testing within the first 3 months of life

- If hearing loss is found, the AAP's Early Hearing Detection and Intervention (EHDI) initiative aims for entry into early intervention services by 6 months of age
- See Chapter 69 for details regarding hearing tests and hearing loss

Hearing Screening for Older Children

- Parental concern about hearing should be assessed in all children
- All children should have audiologic testing of sounds by their fourth birthday
  - Head Start requires testing to start at age 3 years
- Screening should then be done yearly until age 10 years and periodically during adolescence
- Speech sound and quality should be followed in children because abnormalities may signal hearing difficulties
- Speech delay should prompt hearing evaluation
- See Chapter 69 for details regarding hearing tests and hearing loss

VISION SCREENING

- Parental concern about vision should be assessed in all children
  - Concern about vision in infants should be referred to pediatric ophthalmology
- Vision screening should start in all children at age 3 years if developmentally appropriate
- Screening should be done yearly during childhood and follow Bright Futures guidelines
- Children with gross motor delays such as failure to reach for objects should be assessed for vision problems
- Clinical findings in vision impairment: nystagmus, failure to react to stimuli, wandering eye movements, inability to reach for objects, delayed smiling
- Retinopathy of prematurity is the most common cause of severe visual impairment. Other causes include congenital cataracts, severe refractive errors, albinism, hydrocephalus, congenital cytomegalovirus (CMV), and birth asphyxia

ANEMIA SCREENING

- Premature or low-birth-weight infants are screened for anemia at birth
- Healthy term infants should be screened for anemia at 12 months of age and have a risk assessment done every year

LEAD SCREENING

- Lead intoxication may cause developmental delays, behavioral problems, and other hematologic and metabolic complications (see Chapter 36)
- Main risk factors for lead intoxication: living in an older home with cracked or peeling lead-based paint, industrial exposure, use of foreign remedies that contain lead, use of pottery with lead paint glaze
- Standardized screening questions on risk for lead intoxication should be asked of all children between ages 6 months and 6 years
- Blood lead screening is recommended at 12 and 24 months
  - Capillary blood sampling may produce false-positive results
  - Venous sample is preferred
- There is no safe level of lead in blood. However, any level above 5 µg/dL warrants further investigation and repeat testing

CHOLESTEROL AND LIPIDS

- All children between ages 9 and 11 years should receive one screening fasting lipid profile
  - A second screen should be done between the ages of 18 and 20 years
- See the section on heart disease prevention for screening for high-risk children
- See Chapter 8 for details regarding hyperlipidemias

TUBERCULOSIS SCREENING

- Risk assessment for tuberculosis (TB) should be done at every well-child visit, especially after the age of 12 months
- Universal screening of children with purified protein derivative (PPD) is not recommended; instead, only children at higher risk for TB are recommended to have a PPD
- Children at high risk for TB include:
  - Foreign-born children from areas with high TB rates (Asia, Africa, Latin America, Eastern Europe, and Russia)
  - Those in close contact with persons known to have TB, with those who are suspected to have TB, or with those who have a positive TB test
  - Those exposed to high-risk adults including those who are homeless, incarcerated, IV drug users, or HIV positive

Disease Prevention

HEART DISEASE

- According to the National Heart, Lung, and Blood Institute (NHLBI), there is growing evidence that atherosclerosis begins in childhood and progresses in adulthood, and therefore recommendations have been made by the AAP and the National Cholesterol Education Program for Children

- Children with the following risk factors are at higher risk of hypercholesterolemia, and hyperlipidemia should be screened with a fasting lipid panel at ages 2, 4, 6, 8, and 10 years, and annually in adolescence:
  - At least one parent with high cholesterol or heart disease
  - Unknown family history
  - Children with obesity (body mass index [BMI] >95th percentile), high blood pressure, or diabetes

OBESITY

- BMI is a tool used to screen for obesity; it correlates with body fat proportion in children and adults
- There are BMI-specific and gender-specific curves that should be used
  - BMI <5th percentile is considered underweight, between 85th and 95th percentile is considered overweight, and >95th percentile is considered obese
- Important activities for overweight/obesity prevention:
  - Limiting screen time to less than 1 to 2 hours a day, and no screen time for children <2 years of age
  - Minimize consumption of sugar-sweetened beverages
  - Daily healthy breakfast
  - Family dinners at the table
- Healthy eating and activity patterns should be encouraged before children develop obesity. These include:
  - Incorporating exercise into daily life—for example, walking or biking to school
  - Introducing regularly scheduled meals and snacks to infants

RESPIRATORY DISEASE

- There are several common environmental irritants that increase respiratory disease in children; those on which parents should be cautioned include the following:
  - Dust mites and mold
  - Animal dander, particularly from cats and dogs
  - Cockroaches and rodents
  - Use of gas stoves and appliances
  - Tobacco smoke
  - Household chemicals from air fresheners and other cleaners

DENTAL DISEASE

- Dental caries are the most common chronic disease of childhood
- Annual dental health care visits are recommended for all children starting at age 1 year as well as dental cleaning every 6 months
- Pediatricians should provide the following anticipatory guidance related to caries:
  - Limit sugary foods and drinks
  - Discourage putting a child to bed with a bottle, and wean the bottle by 1 year of age
  - Begin brushing child's teeth twice a day as soon as first tooth erupts, and supervise tooth brushing until child is 8 years old
  - Drink tap water if in an area where water has been fluorinated

- Use fluoride toothpaste to brush teeth in all children
- The U.S. Preventive Services Task Force recommends that primary care physicians apply fluoride varnish to teeth of children every 3 to 6 months after first tooth eruption
- Over-the-counter fluoride supplements are not necessary in children less than 6 years of age

Anticipatory Guidance

SAFETY

Beyond the first few months of life, the most common causes of death in childhood and adolescence are injuries including traffic accidents, drownings, and other unintentional injuries. Because of this, safety counseling should be a significant part of anticipatory guidance for all well-child visits and should be age appropriate.

Car Safety

- According to the Centers for Disease Control and Prevention (CDC), motor vehicle accidents are the leading cause of unintentional injury in those 0 to 19 years old
- Seat belt recommendations:
  - Infants and toddlers: rear-facing safety seat until they are 2 years of age or reach the highest weight or height on the car seat
  - Children >2 years old: forward-facing car seat for as long as possible, until the highest weight or height recommended by the manufacturer is reached
  - Once forward-facing car seat is outgrown, children should use a belt-positioning booster seat until the seat belt fits properly, usually when height is about 4 feet 9 inches and children are between ages 8 and 12 years
  - All older children should always wear lap and shoulder seat belts
  - Children should sit in back seat until age 13 years to protect them from airbags, which can cause injury in children
- Drivers 15 to 17 years of age have twice the risk of collision compared with those 18 years or older. Causes for increased crashes in teen drivers include:
  - Driving with other young riders in the car
  - Inexperience while driving at night
  - Drunk driving or driving under the influence of another substance
  - Distracted driving from texting or talking on the phone

Stairways

- Stair-related injuries are common in children less than 5 years of age, either on their own or while being carried by a parent on the stairs
- Stairway safety tips include:
  - Installing stair gates at both the top and bottom of stairs
  - Installing and using stair rails
  - Keeping stairs clean and clutter free

Bicycles

- All children should wear helmets while riding a bicycle, regardless of how short the bike ride is

- Bicycle helmets dramatically decrease incidence of traumatic brain injury and death
- Helmets must be appropriately sized to cover the forehead and fit snugly on the head
- Children should obey traffic laws if biking on roads and should always be supervised by an adult

Recreational Equipment

- Children should always be supervised on playgrounds
- Playgrounds should have safety-tested mats or loose fill material (such as wood chips) around the equipment in case of falls
- Home trampolines are not recommended for children
  - Trampoline nets do not protect children from injury
  - If children do play on a trampoline, it is recommended that only one child at a time be on it because injuries are more likely to occur when more than one child is on a trampoline

Burns

- More than 90% of burns occur in the home
- Prevention is possible and recommended through the following:
  - Reducing temperature on the hot water heater to 49°C
  - Having smoke and carbon monoxide detectors in every room of the house
  - Avoiding any use of fireworks, including sparklers. The AAP recommends prohibiting the public sale of fireworks

Bites and Stings

- Preventions of stings and bites by insects is essential, particularly in children prone to anaphylactic reactions
- Children who have had systemic reactions to bites or stings should have access to self-injectable epinephrine at all times
- Prevention measures include:
  - Avoiding perfumes, fragrant soaps, or hair spray
  - Avoiding bright-colored clothing
  - Wearing long pants and shoes with socks when walking in the grass or through fields
  - DEET is the insect repellent of choice and may be used in children above age of 2 months. DEET in concentrations of 10% to 30% should be used
  - An alternative to DEET is picaridin in concentrations of 5% to 10%
  - Hats should be worn in areas with ticks
- Ticks should be removed by applying a soapy cotton ball on the tick for 30 seconds. Usually the tick will be stuck on the cotton ball when lifted away
  - Tweezers should be second line if cotton ball does not work. Tick should be grasped close to skin and pulled straight upward without twisting or crushing
    - If part of tick head remains, clean skin with rubbing alcohol and use a sterile needle to lift it out. If a large amount remains, a doctor should be called
- All tick bites should then be covered with antibiotic ointment
- Covering the tick with petroleum jelly, nail polish, or alcohol is an ineffective treatment

Water Safety

- According to the CDC, fatal drowning remains the second leading cause of unintentional injury after motor vehicle accidents in children ages 1 to 14 years
- Children ages 1 to 4 years are at the highest risk and most often drown in home swimming pools
- Home swimming pool safety
  - Children should always be supervised by a responsible adult. An adult should be in the water at arm's length for children less than 4 years of age
  - Fences at least 4 feet high should be installed around all four sides of the pool without any openings. Water alarms can add a layer of protection but do not substitute for a fence
  - Clear the pool area and deck of toys after swimming so children are not tempted to enter the pool
  - Swimming lessons help but do not prevent drowning deaths. Research shows they may help prevent deaths only in children over age 1 year
- Boating safety
  - Children should wear life jackets of the correct size at all times when on a boat or a deck or when near any large body of water

Sun Exposure

- Sunscreens
  - Babies under 6 months of age should be dressed in protective clothing and protective hats to prevent sun exposure. A small amount of sunscreen with minimum SPF 15 can be applied to small areas
  - All children over 6 months of age should be covered up and wear sunscreen of SPF 15 or greater daily
- Sun exposure should be limited in children during peak hours between 10 a.m. and 4 p.m.
- Clothing should be light-colored and lightweight, and drinking water should be readily available if playing in the sun

Firearms

- The AAP recommends that firearms not be kept in a home where children or teenagers live
- If guns are kept in the home, safe gun storage is recommended. This includes:
  - Guns unloaded and locked
  - Ammunition locked separately

Screen Time

- Screen media other than video-chatting is discouraged by the AAP in all children less than 18 months of age
- Children 18 to 24 months of age may have high-quality programming or apps for use with their parents. They should not have unsupervised screen time
- Children older than 2 years should have media limits of no more than 1 hour per day

Sleep Hygiene

- Sleep disorders can be treated and prevented with appropriate sleep hygiene
- Consistent and appropriate-for-age bedtimes and wake-up times are recommended
- Consistent bedtime routines promote healthy sleep

- No television or other electronics in the bedroom
- Naps should be avoided unless developmentally appropriate—usually for children younger than 3 years old
- Infants should be placed to sleep on their backs. Cribs should be clear of any loose blankets, pillows, or bumpers. Only a flat sheet should be on the crib with a firm mattress and child dressed in temperature-appropriate clothing

COMMON BEHAVIORAL COMPLAINTS

In addition to clinical complaints, pediatricians are often asked about different childhood behaviors. These are well represented on the boards. Some of the most common behaviors are characterized and discussed later, but the list is by no means complete

Sleep Training

- Infants should be placed down drowsy but still awake after their needs have been met (fed, diapered, comforted)
- It is expected that there will be some level of crying that must be tolerated for children to achieve self-regulation of sleep
- Several methods of sleep training exist for infants to learn how to self-soothe and go to sleep, including the unmodified extinction method (cry it out), graduated extinction method (allowing to cry but checking in periodically), and others, until child is comforted but allowed to go to sleep on his or her own

Picky Eaters

- Picky eating is very common for toddlers and other young children, who may eat only one or two preferred foods for weeks
- Healthy food choices should be made available to the toddler, and his or her appetite or food preference changes should be acknowledged
- Offer healthy finger foods so they can feed themselves
- Sit your child at the dinner table
- Children's eating habits usually improve with time, and if weight is normal, supplements are not encouraged

Toilet Training

- Child must be developmentally ready to be toilet trained. This means being able to sense the urge to go, understanding that feeling, and being able to verbalize the need to use the toilet
- Tools that encourage toilet training once child is ready include:
  - Creating a toilet training plan, including appropriate location to use
  - Being positive and consistent
  - Staying involved
- Bed-wetting is very common and does not need medical intervention until ages 8 through 10 years old

Temper Tantrums

- Temper tantrums are normal developmentally in children 18 months to 4 years of age
- The main goal for families is to identify the typical antecedents of the child's tantrums in order to intervene—for example, identifying that a child is more likely to throw a tantrum if a nap is missed

- Pediatricians should identify problems related to hunger, fatigue, inadequate physical activity, or overstimulation that could be causing aggression, acting out, or tantrums
- The majority of children do not have underlying medical problems
- Medical conditions that can be related to bad behavior and tantrums include:
  - Iron deficiency anemia
  - Lead exposure
  - Genetic conditions
  - Brain injury and other brain disorders
  - Hearing loss and language delay
- Treatment:
  - Parental education, including stressing that tantrums are developmentally normal
  - Parents should be consistent with the child and discipline with what is allowed and what isn't
  - Not giving in to demands
  - Using distractions to control the behavior

Infant Crying

- Normal infant crying typically follows the following pattern:
  - Little crying during the first 2 weeks of life
  - Increase in crying peaks around 6 weeks of life to an average of 3 hours per day
  - Decrease to about 1 hour per day by 12 weeks of life
- Increased crying in the evening and late afternoon is common
- Fussing or crying for 10 episodes in a 24-hour period is normal

Colic

- Colic is typically diagnosed using Wessel's "rule of threes": crying for more than 3 hours a day, at least 3 days per week, for more than 3 weeks
- Colic is a diagnosis of exclusion. Less than 5% of infants are found to have an organic etiology
- Symptoms such as facial grimacing, leg flexion, reddening of face, and passing gas are common
- Treatment
  - Colic usually resolves on its own by 3 months of age in about 85% of infants
  - Use of the five S's is helpful in soothing infants that are crying. These include swaddling, swinging, side-lying or stomach (while awake), shushing, and sucking (using pacifier or breast)

- Medications should be avoided
- In most circumstances dietary changes are not helpful. In some specific cases, infants may be diagnosed with milk protein intolerance

Lying in School-Age Children

- Lying is usually due to the child wanting to cover up something they do not want to accept
- Habitual lying can be due to poor adult modeling
- Chronic lying may be a signal of underlying psychopathology or family dysfunction
- Intervention is warranted when it becomes a common way of the child communicating. Intervention is recommended by showing the child what is acceptable and limit setting. Professional help may be needed in some circumstances

Stealing in School-Age Children

- It is common for children to steal something at some point in their lives
- Stealing is typically a response to anger, frustration, stressful environment, or modeling of parental behavior
- The parent must help the child undo the theft
- Mental health evaluation is warranted if stealing becomes a habit

Review Questions

For review questions, please go to ExpertConsult.com

Suggested Readings

1. Bright Futures. Recommendations for Preventive Pediatric Care. https://www.aap.org/en-us/documents/periodicity_schedule.pdf.
2. Flynn JT, Kaelber DC, Baker-Smith CM, et al. Clinical practice guideline for screening and management of high blood pressure in children and adolescents. *Pediatrics.* 2007:140(3).
3. Hagan J, Duncan P. Maximizing Children's Health: Screening, Anticipatory Guidance, and Counseling. In: Kliegman R, Stanton B, St Geme J, Schor N, eds. *Nelson Textbook of Pediatrics.* 20th ed. Philadelphia: Elsevier; 2016:37–47.
4. Marcdante K, Kliegman R. Evaluation of the Well Child. In: *Nelson Essentials of Pediatrics.* 7th ed. Philadelphia: Elsevier; 2015:20–25.

89 Normal Development and Disorders of Cognition, Language, and Learning

EILEEN M. EVERLY, MD

Normal Development

The first five years of a child's life is a time of intense, rapid learning and growth. Pediatricians are in a prime position to monitor the development of the child, to screen for delays, and to refer for intervention when delays are suspected. Early identification of possible delays allows for early referral for further assessment and treatment.

See also *Nelson Textbook of Pediatrics*, Chapter 12, "The Preschool Years," and Chapter 13, "Middle Childhood."

BASIC INFORMATION

- Five major domains of development:
  - Cognitive: reasoning, memory, problem-solving
  - Social-emotional and behavioral: interaction with others, self-care (dressing, feeding, etc.), playing, attachment
  - Language: expressive and receptive, facial expressions, gestures, body language, vocalizations, verbal comprehension
  - Physical:
    - Gross motor: large muscle groups, overall muscle tone, head and body balance, sitting, crawling, walking, and so forth
    - Fine motor: small muscle groups, use of hand and fingers in grasping/manipulating, used often in activities of daily living
- Adaptive: hand-eye coordination, object permanence, symbolic thought
- Developmental delays
  - Global delay: delayed in two or more domains
  - Specific delay: delay in only one area of development
- A delay in one domain may affect skills in another domain; a child who is speech delayed may have trouble communicating with playmates, affecting his or her social development as well
- "Delay" refers to a delay in exhibition of the particular developmental milestone outside of the normal range of expected ages in which that milestone is customarily achieved
- Preterm birth is a leading cause of developmental delay and of neurodevelopmental disabilities in children, and delays associated with preterm birth can be manifest in all domains
  - Incidence of vision and hearing problems is higher in preterm infants than in term infants (preterm infants are at risk for retinopathy of prematurity, cortical hemorrhages, hyperbilirubinemia and jaundice, serious bacterial infections, etc.)

- Preterm child's increased risk for intraventricular hemorrhage also puts him or her at higher risk for motor impairments, such as those found with cerebral palsy
- Language delays are also more common in preterm infants
- When comparing preterm infants with their term peers in developmental surveillance and screening, the preterm child's "corrected age" (age from due date rather than birth date) is usually used
- Currently the general practice is to use corrected age for the first 24 months after birth, though there is no consensus at this time among experts
- Developmental milestones (see Tables 89.1 and 89.2)

DIAGNOSIS AND EVALUATION

- Surveillance: geared toward population trends in disease/disorders;
  - Developmental surveillance should occur at all well-child visits from birth to school age
- Screening: the administration of specific tools or tests to detect disease or disorder (these are not intended to provide a diagnosis; rather, to identify those children who would benefit from further evaluation)
  - Developmental screening (examples later) using validated, age-appropriate tools at 9 months, 18 months, 24 months, and 30 months; they may also be used whenever a parent raises a serious concern about his or her child's development or when the pediatrician notes a possible delay during the course of an office visit
  - If the child fails the screening, he or she should be referred immediately for full developmental evaluation
- Evaluation: more detailed history, comprehensive physical examination, psychosocial and family history, hearing and vision testing, and further tests of development and/or cognition

Commonly Used Developmental Screening Tools

- Survey of Well-being of Young Children (SWYC):
  - Completed by parents
  - Set of questions assessing developmental milestones in children aged 2 to 60 months at different intervals (e.g. 2 months 4 months, 6 months, 9 months)
- Ages and Stages Questionnaire:
  - Completed by the parents
  - For use in children ages 4 to 48 months
  - Gives domain-specific results indicating pass or fail

Table 89.1.   Developmental Milestones

Age	Gross Motor	Fine Motor–Adaptive	Personal-Social	Language	Other
2 weeks	Moves head side to side		Regards face	Alerts to bell	
2 months	Able to lie with head midline; lifts shoulder while prone	Tracks past midline; hands unfist 50% of the time	Smiles responsively	Cooing ("ooh," "aah"); searches for sound with eyes	Still has primitive reflexes
4 months	Rolls front to back (then back to front); if pulled to sit from supine, no head lag	Reaches for object; brings hands to midline; can bring object to mouth	Looks at hand; smiles spontaneously	Laughs and squeals	Primitive reflexes extinguish (Moro, grasp, Gallant)
6 months	Sits without support; can bear weight if stood up and held	Transfers object hand to hand; can hold two objects simultaneously; holds bottle; raking grasp	Feeds self	Babbles (e.g., "ba," "ma," "da")	Begins to develop object permanence
9 months	Crawls; pulls to stand and cruising; gets into sitting position	Starting to pincer grasp (thumb and index finger); bangs two blocks together	Waves bye-bye; plays pat-a-cake	Says "dada" and "mama" nonspecifically; imitates sounds; two-syllable sounds	Turns to his or her name; has object permanence; begins to have separation anxiety
12 months	Walks; stoops and stands	Fine pincer grasp; voluntarily releases object from grasp; puts block in cup; rolls a ball	Drinks from a cup; imitates others	Says "mama" and "dada" specifically; says one to two other words; begins jargon (pretend speech, sounds that mimic speech in pattern and intonation)	Understands "no"; may begin following simple commands without gestures
15 months	Walks backward; stoops to pick up toy; creeps up stairs	Scribbles; stacks two to three blocks	Uses spoon and fork; helps with housework	Says three to six words; follows commands	May know 1–2 body parts
18 months	Runs; walks up stairs with one hand held; climbs into a chair	Uses spoon; stacks four blocks; copies vertical lines	Removes garment; "feeds" doll	Says at least six words (usually 10–25 words)	Can point to 2–3 objects when named; understands when they have done something wrong and can start to feel shame, guilt, remorse
2 years	Walks up and down stairs (although not alternating feet)	Kicks a ball; throws overhand; stacks six blocks; copies circles and horizontal lines	Washes and dries hands; brushes teeth; puts on clothes; able to parallel play (plays near other children but not with them)	Puts two words together using noun and verb; points to pictures; knows body parts	Can follow 2-step command; understands concept of *today*
3 years	Walks up steps alternating feet; balances on one foot for 3 seconds; broad jumps; pedals tricycle	Stacks eight blocks; wiggles thumb; spontaneously draws a circle	Uses spoon well, spilling little; puts on T-shirt; engages in pretend/imaginative play	Names pictures; speech understandable to stranger 75%; says three-word sentences; has over 200 words; participates in conversations	Understands concepts of *tomorrow* and *yesterday*; can draw a 2- to 3-part person; fears imaginary things (e.g., monsters under the bed)
4 years	Balances well on each foot 5–8 seconds; hops on one foot	Copies circle; maybe + ; draws person with three parts	Brushes teeth without help; dresses without help	Names colors; understands adjectives; 100% speech intelligible with multiple sentences	
5 years	Skips; heel-to-toe walks	Copies square		Counts; understands opposites	
6 years	Balances on each foot 6 seconds	Copies triangle; draws person with six parts		Defines words	Begins to understand *right* and *left*

- Denver Developmental Screening Test II:
  - Administered by the pediatrician
  - Can be used from birth to 6 years
  - Contains 125 items in four domains and gives a global result
- Modified Checklist for Autism in Toddlers (MCHAT):

- Can be completed by the parents or administered by the pediatrician
- Indicated for toddlers between 16 and 30 months
- identifies children who may benefit from a more thorough developmental and autism evaluation

Table 89.2. Developmental Red Flags in the First Three Years

No fixing on objects by 2 months	No protoimperative pointing by 15 months
No cooing or smiling by 4 months	No words by 15 months
No laughing by 6 months	No walking independently by 18 months
No turning toward objects by 6 months	No protodeclarative pointing by 18 months
No transferring objects by 6 months	No two-word sentences by 2 years
No babbling by 9 months	No imitation of parent or caregiver by 2 years
No sitting by 9 months	No pretend play by 3 years
No weight-bearing/standing by 12 months	No three-word sentences by 3 years
No looking where parent points by 12 months	

TREATMENT

- If a child fails any screening tests, the child should be immediately referred for further evaluation
- Studies show that beginning intervention earlier in the child's development leads directly to better outcomes
- Interventions include but are not limited to: physical therapy, occupational therapy, speech therapy, special instruction

Speech Delay

BASIC INFORMATION

- Language delays are the most common form of developmental delay in toddlers/preschool children
- The earlier the diagnosis, the earlier the therapy can begin and the better the final outcome

CLINICAL PRESENTATION

- Not meeting speech/language milestones at a normal rate or at all
- Using gestures rather than words
- Displaying any of the red flags noted previously
- Displaying difficulties initiating words or conversation

EVALUATION AND DIAGNOSIS

Referral for Developmental/Speech Evaluation

- Children who have no words by 18 months, no phrases by 2 years; children whose speech is unintelligible or does not meet milestones for intelligibility at ages 2, 3, and 4 years
- Children who have echolalia persisting after age 3
- Children whose parents express reasonable concern or worry about their child's language delay
- Children who have failed developmental or screening tests

- Evaluate for disorders on the differential: hearing loss, intellectual disability, autism spectrum disorder, and environmental deprivation
- All children with suspected speech delay should have a full audiologic evaluation

TREATMENT

- Once identified as having a speech delay, children proceed to speech therapy as well as occupational therapy, if indicated
- Speech delays are characterized as expressive, receptive, or mixed expressive/receptive language delay

Learning Disabilities

BASIC INFORMATION

- Neurologically based processing problems that interfere with learning of both basic skills (reading, writing, math) and higher-level skills (abstract thinking, attention, organization)
- Can have consequences outside the classroom and affect a child's relationships
- Most often recognized during school years
- Most children are of average or above average intelligence
- Categories:
  - Auditory processing disorder: problem with how sound that travels uninterrupted from the ear is processed by the brain
    - May have difficulty in distinguishing between subtle differences in sounds or in localizing where a sound is coming from
  - Dyslexia: problem with reading and language-based processing skills
    - May have difficulty with fluency, decoding, and spelling
  - Dysgraphia: problem with handwriting and fine-motor skills
    - May have difficulty thinking and writing at the same time
  - Dyscalculia: problem with understanding numbers and learning math facts
    - May have poor comprehension of math symbols or difficulty telling time or counting
  - Language processing disorder: a specific type of auditory processing disorder
    - May have difficulty attaching meaning to sound groups that form words, sentences, and stories
  - Nonverbal learning disabilities: characterized by a discrepancy between higher verbal skills and weaker motor, visual-spatial, and social skills
    - May have difficulty interpreting nonverbal cues like facial expressions or body language
  - Visual perceptual/visual motor deficits: problem understanding information that a person sees, or impaired ability to draw or copy; can be seen in other disabilities such as dysgraphia or nonverbal learning disability
    - May lead to missing subtle differences in shapes or printed letters, losing place frequently, struggles with cutting, holding pencil too tightly, or poor eye-hand coordination

CLINICAL PRESENTATION

- Child may present with difficulty in a particular subject
- Child may have grades that do not match natural ability
- Child may have difficulty in one area or a large discrepancy between grades/scores in different subjects
- Child may avoid schoolwork, neglect homework, not finish seatwork

DIAGNOSIS AND EVALUATION

- Rule out hearing or vision problems, intellectual disability, motor deficits, emotional/behavioral difficulties, and environmental disadvantages
- Child undergoes testing, history taking, and observation by a trained psychologist, occupational therapist, speech and language therapist
- Usually begins with the child's school, which may have a multidisciplinary team to review cognitive test results, classroom performance, teacher input, and grades to arrive at a diagnosis together

TREATMENT

- No cure: goal is to manage the disability to achieve success academically, socially, and personally
- Special education services; speech-language therapy when indicated
- IEP: individualized education program to provide the child with accommodations to maximize his potential
- Environmental support: sitting closer to the board, untimed tests, tests given orally rather than written, and so forth

Intellectual Disability

BASIC INFORMATION

- Neurodevelopmental disorder with multiple etiologies, characterized by deficits in intellectual and adaptive functioning
- Presents before 18 years of age
- Children with global developmental delay at younger ages are more likely to be diagnosed with intellectual disability at an older age, when more reliable IQ testing can be performed

EVALUATION AND DIAGNOSIS

- Comprehensive medical history, prenatal and birth histories
- Full family history of at least three or more generations
- Full physical and neurologic examinations, paying attention to dysmorphic features and neurologic or behavioral signs that may point to a specific recognizable syndrome or diagnosis
- IQ/cognitive testing
- Clinical genetic evaluation, including chromosomal microarray, screening for inborn errors of metabolism: serum total homocysteine, acyl-carnitine profile, amino acids; and urine organic acids, glycosaminoglycans, oligosaccharides, purines, pyrimidines, GAA/creatine metabolites; fragile X testing

- Brain magnetic resonance imaging (MRI) is not a routine part of evaluation but is done if workup described previously reveals microcephaly, macrocephaly, or abnormal findings on neurologic examination

TREATMENT

- Keystone of management for intellectual disability is a multidisciplinary comprehensive plan developed by the child's special educators, language therapists, behavioral therapists, occupational therapists, teachers, parents, and medical professionals
- Early identification of children with developmental delays is fundamental
- Start early intervention services for children from birth to 3 years of age, and start early childhood education services for children aged 3 to 5 years
- Adaptive equipment, individualized education programs, extra time, family or other support persons
- Treatment of pain (constipation, neuropathic pain, dental caries), emotional distress, maladaptive behaviors (kicking, rocking, screaming)
- Written, verbal, and/or picture communication
- Attention to dosing of anesthetics to avoid adverse effects common in children with intellectual disability
- Protection from and close surveillance for sexual abuse/assault

Autism Spectrum Disorders (ASD)

BASIC INFORMATION

- The autism spectrum refers to a continuum of neurodevelopmental disorders characterized by delays/difficulties in social communication and by persistent restrictive and/or repetitive behaviors
- Symptoms may vary within and among individual children, over time, and in severity
- Symptoms start in early childhood, even infancy, and are lifelong
- There is no cure for autism, but treatment can improve symptoms and increase functionality

CLINICAL PRESENTATION

- Symptoms best described by the DSM V criteria (see Table 89.3); symptoms must present in early childhood and impair everyday functioning

EVALUATION AND DIAGNOSIS

Screening

- Autism is a clinical diagnosis, made after a comprehensive history and physical, full developmental history and assessment, family and social history, and evaluation for possible comorbidities (there is no blood test or imaging study to diagnose autism)
- Children should be evaluated for ASD whenever there is a parental or physician concern
- Children should also be screened for developmental delay with validated developmental screening tools at 9

Table 89.3.   DSM V Criteria for Autism Spectrum Disorders

PERSISTENT DEFECTS IN SOCIAL COMMUNICATION AND INTERACTION (REQUIRES 3 OF 3 CRITERIA)

Criteria	Example Symptoms	Example Parental Concerns
Deficits in social-emotional reciprocity	■ Lack of back-and-forth conversation	■ Not answering a parent asking questions about a book being read
	■ Abnormal social approach	■ Not respecting personal space of others
	■ Reduced sharing of interests, emotions, or affect	■ Not pointing to show parent something the child sees
	■ Failure to initiate or respond to social interactions	■ Not playing with other children
Deficits in nonverbal communicative behaviors used in social interaction	■ Poorly integrated verbal and nonverbal communication	■ Paucity of speech
	■ Abnormal eye contact and/or body language	■ Not making eye contact with parents, not looking where parent is pointing
	■ Lack of facial expression or gestures	■ Not smiling, not frowning
	■ Trouble understanding and using nonverbal communication	■ Not recognizing the meaning of parents' or siblings' smiles and/or frowns
Deficits in developing, maintaining, and understanding relationships	■ Difficulties adjusting behavior to suit various social contexts	■ Not being quiet in a library, being inappropriately cheerful or nonchalant when a friend is crying or sad
	■ Difficulties in sharing imaginative play	■ Not playing house or tea party
	■ Difficulties in making friends	■ Having trouble connecting with peers or playmates
	■ Absence of interest in peers	■ Not joining in games or play when invited

RESTRICTED, REPETITIVE PATTERNS OF BEHAVIOR, INTERESTS, OR ACTIVITIES (REQUIRES 2 OF 4 CRITERIA)

Criteria	Example Symptoms
Stereotyped or repetitive motor movements, use of objects, or speech	■ Simple motor stereotypies: hand-flapping, twirling ■ Lining up toys ■ Echolalia ■ Idiosyncratic phrases
Insistence on sameness, inflexible adherence to routines, or ritualized patterns of verbal or nonverbal behavior	■ Extreme distress at small changes ■ Difficulty with transitions ■ Need to take same route or eat same food every day ■ Rigid thinking patterns ■ Greeting or taking leave rituals
Highly restricted, fixated interests that are abnormal in intensity or focus	■ Strong attachment to or preoccupation with unusual objects: spinning the wheels on a truck for hours ■ Excessively circumscribed or perseverative interests: being obsessed with dinosaurs, trains, Minecraft
Hyper- or hyporeactivity to sensory input or unusual interest in sensory aspects of the environment	■ Apparent indifference to pain or temperature ■ Adverse response to specific sounds or textures ■ Excessive touching or smelling of objects ■ Visual fascination with lights or movement

months, 18 months, 24 months, and 30 months, and screened with an autism spectrum disorder screening tool at 18 and 24 months

■ Special attention should be paid to groups at risk for developing ASD: siblings of a child with ASD, children with a positive family history of ASD, children with a history of delay or regression in language/social skills, children with syndromes associated with ASD, and children with sensory issues such as hyperacusis, texture issue, or food aversions

■ If screening yields a high level of concern, the child should be referred for diagnostic evaluation

Diagnostic Evaluation

■ The DSM V criteria are those most often used in the diagnosis of ASD; symptoms must begin in early childhood, occur across more than one milieu (home, school, extracurricular activities, etc.), and cause impairment in functioning; they cannot be better explained by intellectual disability or global developmental delay

■ Referrals should be made to audiology, a qualified autism diagnostician, and community resources (e.g., early intervention, school/preschool services, private speech/ behavioral therapy)

■ Consider referral to family support organization

■ Consider and treat potential comorbidities: sleep disorders, constipation, seizure disorders, hearing impairments, attention-deficit hyperactivity disorder (ADHD), anxiety

■ Consider other medical conditions that can cause ASD (e.g., trisomy 21, fragile X, tuberous sclerosis, velocardial facial syndromes)

■ Consider referral to genetics (up to 20% of children with ASD have genetic abnormalities on genetic microarray)

TREATMENT

- There is no cure for autism spectrum disorders
- Therapies are designed to improve quality of life, decrease impairments, improve relationships, and minimize dysfunction
- The most commonly used therapy in the management of autism is applied behavior analysis, or ABA
  - ABA is the application of the principles of behavioral analysis; i.e., increasing useful behaviors and reducing those that may cause harm or interfere with learning, to bring about meaningful and positive change in behavior
- Many children with autism may also benefit from speech therapy, physical or occupational therapy, or special instruction, as well as from specific medication/therapy to treat any comorbid conditions or to improve quality of life
- The child with autism should also have consistent and frequent follow-up for nutritional deficiencies if selective diet is a concern; pediatricians taking care of children with selective diets often refer these patients to pediatric gastrointestinal (GI) specialists and/or pediatric nutritionists who are board certified and well trained in treatment of vitamin and mineral deficiencies that may occur in the child with restrictive diets and food refusals
- Communication issues may be managed with augmented communication devices

Rett Syndrome

BASIC INFORMATION

- Classic Rett syndrome is a rare, X-linked neurodevelopmental disorder seen in females
- Atypical Rett syndrome is much less commonly seen and is described as a neonatal encephalopathy with intellectual disability, seen in males
- Rett syndrome has no cure and can be particularly upsetting because babies are healthy and meeting developmental milestones for the first 6 to 9 months before rapidly losing milestones; these specific milestones are coordination, speech, and use of hands, after which symptoms can either continue to worsen or can be followed by a period of stabilization
  - Girls with classic Rett syndrome never regain the skills they have lost

CLINICAL PRESENTATION

- Clinical features of the classic form of Rett syndrome include loss of milestones after a period of normalcy, culminating in acquired microcephaly, stereotypical hand-washing or hand-wringing behaviors, paucity of speech, and onset of seizures by 3 years of age in 90% of patients
- Dysfunctional hand movements typically present at age 2 to 3 years
- Autistic-like features typically are seen between 2 and 3 years also, with loss of language, speech, and social interaction

- There often can be a plateau at age 5 to 7 years, followed by progressive deterioration of autonomic function leading to scoliosis, growth delay, and cold extremities (hands and feet), which are often smaller than expected for age

DIAGNOSIS AND EVALUATION

- Five criteria are necessary to make a clinical diagnosis of Rett syndrome:
  - A pattern of development, regression, then recovery or stabilization
  - Partial or complete loss of purposeful hand skills such as grasping with fingers, reaching for things, or touching things on purpose
  - Partial or complete loss of spoken language
  - Repetitive hand movements, such as hand-wringing, washing, squeezing, clapping, or rubbing
  - Gait abnormalities, including walking on toes or with an unsteady, wide-based, stiff-legged gait
- In addition, there is a genetic test that can be done, which identifies mutations in 80% of classic females

TREATMENT

- There is no cure for Rett syndrome
- Treatment is geared toward management of symptoms and preservation of as much normal development as possible, and is performed by a multidisciplinary team
- As with other disorders of development, the earlier the intervention, the better the outcome
- Physical therapy: aids in balance, mobility, and weight-bearing training
- Occupational therapy: reduces stereotypic hand movements, improves or maintains use of hands
- Speech-language therapy: teaching of nonverbal communication, improvement of social interaction
- Nutrition therapy: maintains adequate weight and nutritional status via proper supplementation of calcium and essential minerals; also monitors for aspiration risk and recommends tube feeds, if necessary
- Splints and braces as needed for scoliosis/hand movements
- Medication as needed to treat respiratory difficulties, seizures, and/or long QT syndrome

Review Questions

For review questions, please go to ExpertConsult.com.

Suggested Readings

1. Moeschler JB, Shevell M, Committee on Genetics. Comprehensive evaluation of the child with intellectual disability or global developmental delays. *Pediatrics*. 2014;134(3):e903–918. https://doi.org/10.1542/peds.2014-1839.
2. Scharf RJ, Scharf GJ, Stoustrup A. Developmental milestones. *Pediatr Rev*. 2016;37(1):25–38.
3. Simms MD, Jin XM. Autism, language disorder and social (pragmatic) communication disorder: DSM-V and differential diagnoses. *Pediatr Rev*. 2015;36(8):355–362.

Child Abuse and Neglect

RICKI STEPHANIE CARROLL, MD, MBE

The mistreatment of children is a pervasive problem worldwide with short- and long-term physical, emotional, mental, and social consequences. Over 900,000 children are substantiated victims of abuse or neglect annually in the United States, and it's likely that this is a gross underestimate of the true number of child victims. It's extremely important that providers consider abuse and/or neglect in the differential diagnosis for injuries without obvious accidental etiology or with a story that is inconsistent with a child's presentation. There are multiple types of child maltreatment, including physical abuse, sexual abuse, psychological abuse, and neglect, and children victims can present in all different ways, many of which are not obviously detected on physical examination. Therefore it is always important for a physician to have a high index of suspicion and to know the red flags to watch for during each pediatric encounter.

See also Nelson Textbook of Pediatrics, Chapter 40, "Abused and Neglected Children."

Obligations and Duties

- Mandated reporting
  - Physicians have a legal and ethical obligation to report suspected child abuse and neglect
  - Mandated reporter: one who is required by law to report to Child Protective Services (CPS) any child one suspects is the victim of abuse or neglect
  - State regulations vary, but medical providers are mandated reporters in all 50 states
  - The suspected maltreatment can result from the acts or omissions of a parent, stepparent, or other caretaker
  - For it to be reportable, one must have only reasonable grounds for suspicion, not clinical certainty
  - There are no penalties for reporting in good faith, but there can be severe penalties for failure to report
- Addressing and supporting the family
  - Child health care professionals should supportively inform the family of the report. Concerns of maltreatment should be conveyed to the parents, kindly but forthrightly, without blame or accusation
  - Be empathetic and state an interest in helping. The report can be explained as being an effort to clarify the situation and provide help, as well as being a professional and legal obligation
  - Establish specific objectives, and help the family come up with a concrete plan
  - Help address contributing factors, such as accessing nutritional services and obtaining health insurance. Encourage both formal (community resources, appropriate referrals) and informal (family, friends, religious affiliates) supports

- Recognize that maltreatment often requires long-term management with ongoing support for the child and family

Physical Abuse

BASIC INFORMATION

- Definition
  - Infliction of bodily injury that causes significant or severe pain, leaves physical evidence, impairs physical functioning, or significantly jeopardizes the child's safety
- Epidemiology
  - A phenomenon found in all socioeconomic, cultural, racial, ethnic, and religious subsets of society
  - Incidence is greatest in lower socioeconomic groups
- Risk factors: see Tables 90.1 and 90.2
  - Most common trigger events: incessant crying, toilet training
  - *Not* important risk factors
    - Gender of the child
    - Parental education
    - Parental employment status

CLINICAL PRESENTATION

- Common history red flags
  - No explanation or vague/implausible explanation for a significant injury, or a history that is incompatible with the type or degree of injury (e.g., the child or sibling reportedly did something that is inconsistent with the child's developmental or physical capabilities)
  - History changes with time, or different caregivers provide contradictory histories
  - Caregivers show lack of appropriate concern
  - Injury occurred as a result of inadequate supervision
  - Unexplained or unexpected delay in seeking care
  - Children with injuries as a result of family/domestic violence
  - Repeated visits for "accidents" or "injuries," often to different facilities
  - Ingestion of illegal substance or history of repeated ingestions
  - Poor compliance with well-child care (e.g., missed visits, immunization delay)
- Signs and Symptoms
  - There are various signs of physical abuse, which will be covered below. One must also be wary of imitators, which include (but are not limited to) medical disorders that cause or increase susceptibility to findings, natural accidents, congenital conditions, and physiologic conditions (see Table 90.3)

Table 90.1. Risk Factors for Abuse

External	Parental	Child Vulnerabilities
Poor housing	Past history of abuse or neglect as a child	Age <3 years old
Multiple young children	Unwanted or unexpected parenthood	Congenital disabilities, intellectual disabilities, or chronic illness
Social isolation/lack of social support	Limited ability to handle stress and negative emotions	Prematurity or small weight for gestational age
Family discord	Alcoholism/substance abuse	Children in a foster home or adopted
Acute life stressors (e.g., loss of job, financial insecurity, loss of home, loss of parent, loss of sibling)	Domestic violence in parental relationship	Children with hyperactivity or attention-deficit/hyperactivity disorder
	Mental illness	Children who are oppositional or defiant
	Unrealistic expectations of child	

Table 90.2. Risk Factors for Neglect

External	Parental	Child Vulnerabilities
Poverty, lack of resources, homelessness, lack of utilities	Father abandonment after learning of pregnancy	Being born last of many children or of multiple children in succession
Limitations in knowledge and understanding of the importance of nutrition in child growth and development	Teenage mother (2× risk)	

- Bruises
  - Most common manifestation of physical abuse
  - Features suggestive of inflicted bruises:
    - Bruising in preambulatory infant
    - Bruising of padded and less-exposed areas (ears, cheeks, mouth/frenulum, torso, buttocks, under chin, genitalia)
    - Patterned (in the shape of an object or ligatures around extremities—loop, hand print, bite mark, subgaleal hematoma from hair pulling)
    - Multiple, especially if in different stages
- Burns
  - May be inflicted or due to inadequate supervision
  - Features suggestive of inflicted burns:
    - Delineation between the burned and healthy skin and uniform depth
    - Sock and glove distribution
    - Absence of splash marks
    - Symmetric burns
    - Burns of the buttocks and perineum
    - Patterned (curling iron, radiator, steam iron, metal grid, hot knife, cigarette, lighter)
    - Extensive, deep burns that are unlikely to be caused by fleeting contact with a hot object
- Fractures
  - Features and types of fractures suggestive of abuse:
    - Multiple fractures, especially if in various stages of healing
    - Multiple rib fractures, especially if posterior
    - Metaphyseal fracture—for example, bucket-handle fracture or corner fracture (from pulling an extremity)
    - Long-bone fracture in child <6 months of age

- Any fracture in preambulatory child
- Skull fracture, especially if multiple
- Spinous process and vertebral body fractures
- Scapular fractures
- Sternal fractures (these rarely result from home resuscitation efforts and should raise concern)
- Fractures unlikely to be abuse:
  - Bucket fracture of the distal radius
  - Single nondisplaced linear skull fracture
  - Clavicular fractures
  - Supracondylar elbow fracture
  - Subluxation of the radial head (nursemaid's elbow)
- Intracranial injuries
  - Results in the most significant morbidity and mortality
  - Can be caused by direct impact, asphyxia, or shaking
  - Features suggestive of abusive head trauma, especially when co-occurring:
    - Subdural hematomas
    - Retinal hemorrhages, especially when extensive and involving multiple layers
    - Diffuse axonal injury
- Intraabdominal injuries
  - Young children are especially vulnerable because of their relatively large abdomens and lax abdominal muscles
  - A forceful blow can cause hematoma of solid organs or rupture of hollow organs
  - Features suggestive of abusive intraabdominal trauma:
    - Liver hematoma
    - Spleen hematoma
    - Kidney hematoma
    - Duodenal hematoma
    - Stomach rupture

EVALUATION AND MANAGEMENT

- If concern for abuse is low, consider a social worker consult and primary doctor follow-up
- If there is significant concern for abuse:
  - Screen for occult injury
    - 0 to 12 months old: skeletal survey, laboratory testing (complete blood count [CBC], prothrombin time/partial thromboplastin time [PT/PTT], basic metabolic panel [BMP], hepatic function test [HFP], amylase, lipase, urinalysis [UA]), head computed tomography (CT) if symptomatic, abdominal CT if symptomatic

Table 90.3. Imitators of Physical and Sexual Abuse

Bruises	Burns	Fractures	Intracranial Injuries	Intraabdominal Injuries	Sexual Molestation
Ink, paint, dye	Accidental burns due to car seat or brushing against radiator	Osteogenesis imperfecta	Arteriovenous malformations	Sports injuries, especially in the setting of mononucleosis	Genital irritation from nonspecific vulvovaginitis, eczema
Birthmarks (e.g., congenital dermal melanocytosis [Mongolian spots])	Skin lesions (e.g., hemangiomas, impetigo, severe diaper dermatitis)	Hypophosphatasia	Coagulopathies, inherited or acquired	Bicycle accidents	Nonsexually transmitted infection (e.g., staphylococcus, group A streptococcus, Haemophilus, Neisseria, yeast, Salmonella, Shigella, Yersinia)
Blood dyscrasias (e.g., hemophilia, idiopathic thrombocytopenic purpura, leukemia, vitamin K deficiency, inherited coagulopathies)	Skin conditions (e.g., Stevens-Johnson syndrome, erythema multiforme, epidermolysis bullosa)	Infantile cortical hyperostosis (Caffey disease)	Hemorrhagic disease of the newborn		Foreign body (e.g., toilet paper)
Connective tissue disorders (e.g., Ehlers-Danlos)	Cultural practices, such as coining, cupping, moxibustion (will likely mention Asian/Vietnamese/Cambodian background)*	Osteopenia of prematurity	Birth trauma—can cause subdural hematomas and retinal hemorrhages**		Physiologic leukorrhea
Vasculitides (e.g., Henoch-Schönlein purpura)		Metabolic and nutritional disorders (e.g., scurvy, severe rickets)	Metabolic disorders (e.g., glutaric aciduria type 1)		Nonsexually transmitted genital ulcers (e.g., Epstein-Barr virus, varicella-zoster virus, Crohn disease, Behçet disease, human papilloma virus***)
Inflammatory conditions (e.g., erythema nodosum, phytophotodermatitis)		Osteomyelitis	Carbon monoxide poisoning—can cause retinal hemorrhages		Vaginal bleeding due to urethral prolapse, vaginal foreign body, accidental trauma, vaginal tumor
Neuroblastoma causing periorbital bruising		Neoplasia (e.g., osteosarcoma, Ewing sarcoma)	Tumors		Hymenal damage due to accidental trauma (e.g., bicycle seat injury)

Note: There are many imitators of abuse that cause similar physical examination findings. Some of these are listed here under their most commonly mistaken physical examination concerning for abuse.
*These are cultural norms and technically not abuse.
**These should resolve in 2 to 6 weeks.
***Commonly transmitted nonsexually and not necessarily indicative of sexual abuse, but if restricted to the hymen, sexual abuse is more likely.

- 12 to 24 months old: skeletal survey, laboratory testing
- 2 to 6 years old: laboratory testing (the patient should be able to indicate pain during physical examination if fractures are present)
- Consider photo documentation and/or forensic evidence collection
- Social work consult and consider filing CPS report and/or police report
- Consider inpatient admission for safety and treatment

Sexual Abuse

BASIC INFORMATION

- Definition
  - The involvement of dependent, developmentally immature children and adolescents in sexual activities that they do not fully comprehend, to which they are unable to give consent, or that violate the social taboos of family roles
  - Any sexual behavior or action toward a child that is unwanted or exploitative

- Epidemiology
  - Approximately 25% of girls and 10% of boys are sexually abused at some point during childhood
  - 40% are abused by parent or stepparent, 25% by other relative, 25% by a trusted acquaintance such as a teacher or coach, and 10% by a stranger

CLINICAL PRESENTATION

- Disclosure
  - May provide a clear spontaneous disclosure to a trusted adult
  - Barriers
    - Fear
    - Shame
    - Threats of harm or death
- Common history red flags
  - Child displaying sexually explicit behaviors outside of the norm for child's developmental age
    - Preschool/school age: compulsive masturbation, attempting to perform sex acts on other adults or children, asking adults or children to perform sex acts on them

- Teenagers: sexual promiscuity, prostitution, sexually abusing younger children
  - Abrupt behavior changes
    - Preschool/school age: social withdrawal, acting out, clinginess, fearfulness, learning difficulties
    - Teenagers: depression, use of alcohol or drugs, truancy, running away from home
  - Regression in developmental milestones
  - Bed-wetting or encopresis
- Signs and Symptoms
  - 95% of children who undergo a medical evaluation after sexual abuse have normal examinations
  - Physical examination findings that indicate sexual abuse
    - Lacerations or bruising of the labia, penis, scrotum, perianal tissue, or perineum
    - Hymenal bruising and lacerations
    - Perianal lacerations extending deep to the external anal sphincter
    - Complete transection of the hymen to the base between the 4 and 8 o'clock position—that is, absence of hymenal tissue in the posterior rim
    - Vaginal discharge due to *Neisseria gonorrhoeae* (chlamydia can be vertically transmitted and persist for up to 3 years)
    - Pregnancy
      - Imitators are presented in Table 90.3

EVALUATION AND MANAGEMENT

- If abuse is suspected, report immediately to CPS and police
- Abuse within 72 hours (may be useful up to within 120 hours of event for postpubescent females)
  - Refer immediately to closest referral center
  - Referral center will obtain forensic evidence, including external, genital, vaginal, anal, and oral swabs (i.e., a "rape kit")
- Abuse greater than 72 hours ago (or 120 hours in postpubescent females)
  - Likelihood of recovering forensic evidence is extremely low
  - Refer to outpatient referral site
- The interview
  - The team should interview parent/guardian alone and interview child alone
  - Identify patient's "body part" language
  - Ask open-ended questions
  - Document direct quotes as much as possible
- General examination
  - Examiner wears gloves during examination
  - Patient removes clothing one piece at a time, placing each article in separate bag
  - Complete head-to-toe examination, looking specifically for evidence of trauma
  - Inspect hands, fingernails, and oropharynx
  - Genital examination
    - Use analgesia as necessary
    - Inspect introitus and anus
    - Pelvic examination if postmenarchal
    - Colposcopy
  - Use Bluemaxx forensic light to identify areas to be swabbed and sent for semen analysis
  - Photo documentation as necessary

- Laboratory evaluation
  - Sexually transmitted infection (STI) testing for all victims of acute assault, all postpubertal patients, and any prepubertal patients with indication of, or concern for, genital, oral, or anal penetration
    - *N. gonorrhoeae* and *Chlamydia trachomatis* testing
      - "Dirty urine" for cervical, vaginal, and male urethral testing
      - Swab for rectal and pharyngeal testing
    - Trichomonas culture swab
    - Herpes simplex virus (HSV) culture swab
    - HIV serum testing
    - Rapid plasma reagin (RPR) for syphilis serum testing
    - Hepatitis B serum testing if not fully immunized
  - Pregnancy testing for all patients >12 years old or with history of menarche
  - CBC, BMP, liver function tests (LFTs)
  - Other tests to consider:
    - Trauma laboratory testing and radiographic studies
    - Urine/serum toxicology if clinically indicated
    - Hepatitis C polymerase chain reaction (PCR)
- Prophylaxis medication considerations
  - Prophylaxis for STIs for all postpubertal patients and any prepubertal patient with symptoms or any evidence of penetration on examination
  - First dose of hepatitis B vaccine if not immunized
  - HIV prophylaxis is indicated if <72 hours from a high-risk exposure
  - Pregnancy prophylaxis is indicated for all postpubertal females presenting within 120 hours of an assault
- Outpatient support services
  - Follow up with pediatrician and psychiatrist
  - Continued aftercare contact with Children and Youth Services and the police
  - Facilitate social work and crisis support systems

Psychological (Emotional) Abuse

BASIC INFORMATION

- Definition
  - Verbal abuse, humiliation, or any other acts that scare or terrorize a child
  - Can range from inattentiveness to frank rejection, threats, or scapegoating
- Epidemiology
  - Emotional abuse accompanies all other forms of abuse but can also occur in isolation
  - Because it is difficult to document and leaves no visible stigmata, it accounts for the smallest proportion of reported cases

CLINICAL PRESENTATION

- Common psychological symptoms include anxiety, depression, agitation, hyperactivity, and psychosis
- Common social symptoms include low self-esteem, social isolation, difficulty relating to peers, poor school performance, and lack of empathy

EVALUATION AND MANAGEMENT

- Child health care providers must have a high index of suspicion for this type of maltreatment
- If suspected, psychological testing and psychiatric examination may prove helpful in confirming its existence and directing treatment
- Many children experience more than one kind of maltreatment; if suspected, it must be reported
- Refer to outpatient support services
  - Child and family counseling
  - Behavioral, educational, and mental health services

Neglect

BASIC INFORMATION

- Definition
  - Omissions in care (resulting in actual or potential harm) or the failure to meet a basic need of a child (adequate food, clothing, shelter, health care, education, nurturance)
  - Four subtypes
    - Medical: a child's health is jeopardized or harmed by not receiving necessary medical, dental, or vision care
    - Supervisional: caregiver fails to ensure a child's safety within and outside the home, given the child's emotional and developmental needs
    - Physical: caregiver fails to provide adequate nutrition, hygiene, or shelter, or when a caregiver fails to provide clothing that is adequately clean, appropriate size, or adequate for the weather
    - Educational: caregiver fails to provide access to adequate education
- Epidemiology
  - Neglect is the most commonly reported type of child abuse (>50%)
  - Risk factors: see Tables 90.1 and 90.2

CLINICAL PRESENTATION

- Common history red flags
  - Mother sought little or no prenatal care
  - Maternal depression
  - Lack of interest in physician encounter
  - Little knowledge of infant's feeding schedule or child's typical per os (PO) intake
  - Report of bottle propping
  - Report that the infant sleeps well and/or doesn't "need" feeds overnight
  - Report of many unrelated caregivers
  - Many missed well-child visits and delayed immunizations
  - Lack of follow-up with referrals to subspecialists
- Signs and Symptoms
  - Observations during the encounter
    - Lack of attachment/bonding with infant
    - Lack of appropriate bundling or clothing
    - Lack of concern or attentiveness with infant's cry
  - Physical examination findings
    - Irritability
    - Poor weight gain or weight loss
    - Infrequent smile
    - Infant/child appears apathetic and withdrawn

- Delayed milestones
- Poor eye contact
- Poor hygiene and dirty clothes
- Severe diaper rash
- Severe baby-bottle dental carries

EVALUATION AND MANAGEMENT

- Inquire into mother's and/or family's support system
- Consult social work, and report to CPS
- If there is severe weight loss/malnutrition, please refer to Failure to Thrive section
- Refer to Women, Infant, and Children (WIC) program when needed
- Frequent physician visits

Caregiver-Fabricated Illness (Formerly Munchausen Syndrome by Proxy)

BASIC INFORMATION

- Definition
  - When a parent or guardian falsely presents a child for medical attention, either via fabricating a story or directly causing a child's illness
  - Diagnosis rests on clear evidence of a child repeatedly being subjected to unnecessary medical tests and treatment, primarily stemming from a parent's actions
- Epidemiology
  - Parent commonly in the medical field or with a high degree of education
  - Preverbal child is usually the victim
  - If child is older, he or she may be convinced by the parent that he or she has a particular problem

CLINICAL PRESENTATION

- Common history red flags
  - Parent has knowledge and comfort with medical terms that is unjustified by her profession
  - Many emergency room (ER) visits
  - History of "doctor shopping"
  - Reported symptoms are noted by only one parent
  - Appropriate testing has failed to confirm diagnoses in the past and/or seemingly appropriate treatment has been ineffective
- Signs and Symptoms
  - Observations during the encounter
    - Parent typically shows great concern for the child
    - Parent typically appears as a devoted, model parent
    - Parent forms close relationships with the health care team
    - Symptoms of child are mostly associated with proximity of the offending caregiver to child
  - Common chief complaints
    - Bleeding: adding dye to samples, adding parent's or child's blood to samples, giving child an anticoagulant
    - Seizures: fabricated history or symptoms induced by toxins; medications such as insulin, water, or salt

- Apnea: observation falsified or created by partial suffocation
- Gastrointestinal signs/symptoms: forced ingestion of medications such as ipecac to induce chronic vomiting, or laxatives for diarrhea
- Skin manifestations: burned, dyed, tattooed, lacerated, or punctured skin to simulate acute or chronic skin conditions
- Recurrent infection and/or sepsis: infectious agent such as feces administered via intravenous (IV) or long-term central venous catheter; urine or blood samples could be contaminated with foreign blood or stool
- Imitators
  - Parental anxiety and true concern about a potential medical problem due to history of a chronically ill or deceased child, their own mental illness, things read on the Internet, or something told to them by a trusted physician
  - Exaggeration of true events to evoke concern from the physician and/or justify an ER visit

EVALUATION AND MANAGEMENT

- Once suspected, first step is gathering and reviewing all of child's medical records and speaking with all involved physicians
- Ensure all specimens are collected carefully, with no opportunity for tampering, and that all vital signs are collected by medical professionals
- Hospitalization may be necessary for close observation to help make the diagnosis
- Consult social work and report to CPS
- Once the diagnosis is made, treatment plan should be worked out by the medical team and CPS
- Treatment may include out-of-home placement and should include mental health care for the offending parent and affected child

Failure to Thrive

- See Chapter 86 for details

BASIC INFORMATION

- Failure to thrive is generally the result of inadequate usable calories necessary for a child's metabolic and growth demands, resulting in physical growth that is significantly less than that of peers
- A detailed history with a high index of suspicion is necessary for prompt diagnosis
- Table 90.4 depicts a differential diagnosis for causes of failure to thrive that must be considered, in addition to child abuse and/or neglect

Table 90.4.   Differential Diagnosis for Failure to Thrive by Etiology, Which Are Also Imitators of Neglect

	Common Causes	Common History Findings	Signs and Symptoms	Laboratory Findings
Psychosocial	Poverty, limitations in knowledge, food insecurity	Inconsistent or unknown diet history, improper formula mixing	Vitamin deficiencies, poor socialization, delayed milestones	None
Gastrointestinal	Gastroesophageal reflux disease, celiac disease, food allergies, inflammatory bowel disease, constipation	Chronic vomiting, chronic diarrhea, crying with feeds	Often none, possibly abdominal distention	Abnormal pH probe, abnormal stool studies
Cardiac	Congenital heart lesion, congestive heart failure (CHF), vascular ring or sling	Dyspnea and diaphoresis with feeds	Cyanosis, hypoxia, signs of CHF	Abnormal electrocardiogram, echocardiogram
Neurologic	Cerebral palsy, neuromuscular disorders, neurodegenerative disorders	Poor feeding, gross developmental delay	Grossly abnormal neurologic findings	Abnormal electroencephalography, magnetic resonance imaging, or neuromuscular function tests
Genetic/ metabolic/ congenital	Inborn errors of metabolism, chromosomal disorders, TORCH infections	May have positive family history, developmental delay	Syndromic facies, skeletal abnormalities, visceromegaly, microcephaly	Abnormal chromosome testing, abnormal metabolic screen
Pulmonary	Cystic fibrosis, bronchopulmonary dysplasia, obstructive sleep apnea, severe asthma	Dyspnea with feeds, tachypnea, chronic cough, frequent lung infections	Grossly abnormal lung examination findings	Abnormal chest x-ray (CXR)
Renal	Recurrent urinary tract infections, renal tubular acidosis, chronic renal failure	Possible history of polyuria	Often negative	Abnormal urinalysis, abnormal blood urea nitrogen/ creatinine, renal osteodystrophy on x-ray
Endocrine	Diabetes mellitus, diabetes insipidus, thyroid dysfunction, growth hormone deficiency, adrenal insufficiency	Constipation, decreased activity, history of shock, polyuria, polydipsia	Short stature with normal weight, dehydration, ketotic breath, hyperpnea, delayed tooth eruption, umbilical hernia, open fontanelles	Abnormal thyroid function tests, elevated blood glucose, abnormal pituitary function study tests
Infectious	HIV, Tuberculosis, parasitic infection	Fevers, recurrent illnesses, chronic cough, may have a history of travel or visitors from another country or born in another country	Often negative	Abnormal complete blood count, eosinophil elevation, abnormal CXR

Review Questions

For review questions, please go to ExpertConsult.com.

Suggested Readings

1. Christian SW. Committee on Child Abuse and Neglect. Evaluation of suspected child physical abuse. *Pediatrics*. 2015;135:e1337–e1354.

2. Davis HW, Carrasco MM. Child Abuse and Neglect. In: Zitelli BJ, McIntire SC, Nowalk AJ, eds. *Atlas of pediatric physical diagnosis*. 6th ed. Philadelphia: Saunders; 2012:181–257.

3. Leeb RT, Paulozzi L, Melanson C, Simon T, Arias I. *Child maltreatment surveillance: uniform definitions for public health and recommended data elements, Version 1.0*. Atlanta (GA): Centers for Disease Control and Prevention, National Center for Injury Prevention and Control; 2008.

4. Mollen CJ, Goyal MK, Frioux SM. Acute sexual assault: a review. *Pediatr Emerg Care*. 2012;28(6):584–590.

Adolescent Medicine

91 Menstrual Disorders and Hormonal Contraception

BROCK D. LIBBY, MD and JENNIFER H. CHUANG, MD, MS

Menstrual Disorders

NORMAL MENSTRUATION

- Cycle length 21 to 35 days (during first 3 years after menarche, can be 21–45 days)
- Duration of menses is 7 or fewer days
- Blood flow is six or fewer soaked pads/tampons per day
- Age of menarche is 12.5 years (varies by racial/ethnic background); often close concordance between mother and daughter
- Generally takes place in sexual maturity rating (SMR) 4 and 2.5 years after thelarche (formation of breast buds)

MENSTRUAL IRREGULARITIES

- The terms menorrhagia and metrorrhagia are no longer used because they were too nonspecific; practitioners now use abnormal uterine bleeding (AUB) and categorize menstrual irregularities by O (anovulatory), C (coagulopathy), or N (not yet classified)

Abnormal Uterine Bleeding

BASIC INFORMATION/CLINICAL PRESENTATION

- Two general categories:
  - Irregular menstrual bleeding
    - Anovulation: immaturity of hypothalamic-pituitary ovarian axis, absence of midcycle luteinizing hormone (LH) surge to stimulate ovulation, no corpus luteum production of progesterone (n.b., progesterone's key function is providing stabilization of the endometrial lining), no stabilization, and thus increased risk of irregular bleeding
  - Heavy and prolonged menstrual bleeding
    - Regular, cyclic menses long/heavy: hematologic cause should be considered (heavy from menarche)
    - Von Willebrand disease and platelet function disorders can range from 36% to 44% in this population
    - Flooding (changing tampon/pad more than hourly) and passing clots larger than 1 inch in diameter are other clues

DIAGNOSIS AND EVALUATION

- Complete blood count (CBC) with platelets, urine pregnancy, sexually transmitted infection (STI) testing, prothrombin time (PT) and partial thromboplastin time (PTT), ferritin, von Willebrand testing, liver function tests (LFTs), kidney function, thyroid function tests (TFTs)
- Pelvic ultrasound (US) (to assess anatomy) if diagnosis is elusive
- Treatment:
  - Mild bleeding (hemoglobin >10 g/dL):
    - Iron supplementation/menstrual calendar
    - Nonsteroidal antiinflammatory drugs (NSAIDs) (naproxen) to treat heavy bleeding
    - Active bleeding responds well to combined oral contraceptives (COCs) starting with twice-daily dosing, if needed, until bleeding stops and then spacing to daily (norethindrone if contraindications to estrogen; see list in the second half of this chapter)
  - Moderate bleeding (hemoglobin 8–10 g/dL):
    - May be necessary to start with three to four COCs per day and then taper to daily dosing over next two weeks
    - Can become mildly symptomatic in this category (symptoms include those of anemia: dizziness with standing, decreased capillary refill time, etc.), but if symptomatic, have a low threshold to hospitalize
  - Severe bleeding (hemoglobin <8 g/dL)
    - May need intravenous (IV) estrogen and then transition to per os (PO) COC; can add fluids/blood products as is recommended

Amenorrhea

BASIC INFORMATION/CLINICAL PRESENTATION

- See Table 91.1 for causes of primary and secondary amenorrhea:
  - Primary amenorrhea: no menses 4 years after thelarche, or if no menstruation by 15
  - Secondary amenorrhea: no menses for the length of three cycles in a postmenarchal patient
- Lack of pubertal signs by age 13: needs evaluation for pubertal delay (see Chapter 21)

DIAGNOSIS AND EVALUATION

- Physical examination: careful attention to growth chart trajectories, clues to eating disorder, thyroid disease, or hyperandrogenism should be sought
- Body mass index (BMI), SMR stage, skin and genital examination important as well (rarely requires an internal pelvic examination)
- Laboratory testing: urine pregnancy test, prolactin, thyroid-stimulating hormone (TSH) and follicle-stimulating hormone (FSH) should be considered in *all* patients
- Brain magnetic resonance imaging (MRI): limited to those with neurologic symptoms *or* galactorrhea *or* elevated prolactin level

Table 91.1. Major Causes of Primary and Secondary Amenorrhea

Abnormality	Causes
PREGNANCY	
ANATOMIC ABNORMALITIES	
Congenital abnormality in müllerian development	Isolated defect
	Androgen insensitivity syndrome
	5-alpha-reductase deficiency
Congenital defect of urogenital sinus development	Agenesis of lower vagina
	Imperforate hymen
Intrauterine adhesions	Asherman syndrome
	Tuberculous endometritis
DISORDERS OF THE HYPOTHALAMIC-PITUITARY-OVARIAN AXIS	
Hypothalamic dysfunction	
Pituitary dysfunction	
Ovarian dysfunction	Gonadal dysgenesis (Turner syndrome, 46,XY)
	Other causes of primary ovarian insufficiency

- Karyotype and pelvic US often indicated if FSH greater than 30 mIU/mL plus amenorrhea (confirmed with repeat); Turner syndrome is most likely
- Treatment:
  - Treatment varies depending on underlying cause. Sample treatments described later:
  - Primary:
    - Eating disorders or other conditions that render one hypoestrogenic: normalizing weight and improving nutritional status
    - Ovarian insufficiency: exogenous hormones required; start at age 10 to 12 with low-dose estrogen transdermal patch and then slowly work up to increased doses of estrogen and cyclic progestin
  - Secondary:
    - Patients with normal postpubertal levels of estrogen: progesterone can be used periodically to induce shedding of endometrial lining (e.g., medroxyprogesterone 10 mg daily for first 12 days of the month)

Polycystic Ovary Syndrome (PCOS)

BASIC INFORMATION

- PCOS is an anovulatory state affecting approximately 5% of premenopausal females
- Clinical presentation:
  - Patient will present with one or two of the following (likely both at the same time) and complaint of irregular periods:
    - Signs of androgen excess:
      - Severe acne, hirsutism (Ferriman-Gallwey hirsutism scoring system frequently quoted)
    - Physical stigmata associated with PCOS:
      - Rapid pubertal weight gain, acanthosis nigricans

DIAGNOSIS AND EVALUATION:

- Diagnosis quite controversial
  - Variations in menstrual irregularity (amenorrhea to dysfunctional uterine bleeding [DUB])
  - Physical/biochemical evidence of androgen excess
  - Absence of other androgen disorders
  - Polycystic ovarian morphology noted on pelvic US, elevated LH and FSH levels (3:1), increased body weight; these three not required but help to supplement the diagnosis
- Evaluation:
  - 17-hydroxyprogesterone, free and total testosterone, dehydroepiandrosterone sulfate (DHEAS), and androstenedione
- Treatment:
  - Lifestyle modifications and suppression of ovarian androgens (with COCs)
  - Many benefit from addition of metformin and spironolactone (androgen receptor blocker)
  - Ongoing monitoring of lipids, also monitor for future risk of diabetes mellitus

Dysmenorrhea

BASIC INFORMATION

- Pain with menstruation
- Occurs in up to 93% of adolescent females; 10% have functional disability from it
- Primary dysmenorrhea: absence of pelvic pathology, accounts for 90% of cases
  - After ovulation, withdrawal of progesterone → synthesis of prostaglandins by endometrium → local vasoconstriction, uterine ischemia, and smooth muscle contraction
- Secondary dysmenorrhea: underlying pathology
  - Most common is endometriosis – implants of endometrial tissue found outside uterus (severe pain at time of menses, can also have noncyclic pain)
  - Increasingly severe pain despite adequate therapy
- Can also have müllerian anomalies with partial outflow obstruction; pain begins at or shortly after menarche, presence of known renal tract anomaly (the two often coexist); hematocolpos with imperforate hymen usually presents as pelvic pain
- Mittelschmerz: brief severe pain at the time of ovulation (midcycle)
- Treatment:
  - NSAIDs: first line; start day before menstruation (if possible) and continue (can be up to 5 days)
  - Hormonal contraception (COCs) is second line (pathophysiology not fully delineated)

Premenstrual Syndrome/ Premenstrual Dysphoric Disorder

BASIC INFORMATION

- Premenstrual syndrome (PMS) found in up to 30% of adolescent females

- Symptoms of anxiety/depression begin in luteal phase of cycle and improve within few days after the onset of menses
- PMS has similar timing but much less severe presentation
- Has to occur in the majority of cycles; present in final week before onset of menses and starts to improve a few days after onset
- Treatment:
  - PMS: stress management techniques, including exercise
  - Premenstrual dysphoric disorder (PMDD): selective serotonin reuptake inhibitors (SSRIs), can be continuous versus intermittent
    - Can also supplement diet with 1200 mg calcium

CONTRACEPTION

It is paramount for general pediatricians to have a working knowledge of hormonal contraception because the United States is the leading country in the industrialized Western world in terms of birth rates between the ages of 15 and 19 years. Although these numbers have been dropping, the United States remains at the top of the list. Furthermore, the United States remains at the bottom of the list of adolescent females (in the same cohort) who utilize hormonal forms of contraception. The data are clear: if a physician discusses this prophylactically with his or her patients, the usage rate increases. Table 91.2 outlines the broad categories of contraceptives available, including long-acting reversible contraceptives, other progestin-only methods, COCs, emergency contraception, dual protection, and other barrier methods.

Fig. 91.1 shows the rationale behind hormonal contraception: the hormonal control it provides allows one to determine when ovulation occurs, making the time frame for possible pregnancy more predictable.

Long-Acting Reversible Contraception

INTRAUTERINE DEVICES

- Copper IUD: inhibition of sperm transport and prevention of implantation
- Progesterone: thickens cervical mucus and inhibits sperm survival
- Common IUD misconceptions: IUDs cause infections and infertility and are unsafe for teenagers or nulliparous women
  - Initial data showed an increase in risk of upper genital tract infection with placement, but no further data has supported this, despite multiple studies
  - Can place if current chlamydia or gonorrhea; cannot place if current pelvic inflammatory disease (PID) diagnosis
  - Very few contraindications to IUD placement: active pregnancy, active PID, and anatomic abnormalities
- Advantages: progesterone IUDs decrease dysmenorrhea, menorrhagia, and endometriosis (copper does not share these benefits)

IMPLANTS

- Etonogestrel implant: small rod that goes in the anterior upper arm; Nexplanon is the name most commonly heard for this
- Released at a steady state for roughly 3 years; works primarily to inhibit ovulation
- Atrophic endometrium is induced, and cervical mucus is thickened
- No pelvic examination is required
- Common side effects: amenorrhea, irregular bleeding, infrequent bleeding, or (rarely) prolonged or frequent bleeding
- Advantage: decreases dysmenorrhea

Other Progestin-Only Methods

MEDROXYPROGESTERONE ACETATE

- Depo-Provera, deep intramuscular (IM) injection
- Particularly good for patients who are intellectually or physically impaired or chronically ill
- 50% will develop amenorrhea after 12 months of use
- Decrease in bone mineral density is cited as a side effect, but this returns after discontinuation; no increased risk of fractures
  - Not recommended in patients on chronic corticosteroids
- Weight gain: systematic review article found that early weight gain is predictive of progressive gain, so those who gain weight in the first 3 to 6 months may want to consider another method

Progestin-Only Pills

- Amenorrhea and breakthrough bleeding are commonly seen
- Pill-taking must be punctual; if the pill is more than 3 hours late, an unintended pregnancy may occur
- Frequently called the "mini-pill"
- This is used when patients cannot tolerate estrogen (see contraindications) and do not want any of the longer-acting options (Depo, Nexplanon, IUD)

Combined Hormonal Contraceptives

- Includes COCs, a transdermal patch, and a vaginal ring
- Prevents surge of LH so no ovulation occurs; thickens cervical mucus and thins endometrial lining
- Decreases risk of endometrial and ovarian cancer; decreases risk of colorectal cancers
- Contraindications to estrogen-containing compounds are listed in Table 91.3

COMBINED ORAL CONTRACEPTIVES

- Start immediately: as soon as the pill is dispensed, can take first pill
- Usually 28 pills/pack: 21 containing hormones, 7 placebo
- Also supply patient with concomitant emergency contraception

Table 91.2. Contraceptive Methods

Method	FAILURE RATE (%) Typical Use	Perfect Use	Dosing	Mechanism of Action	Potential Side Effects	Advantages
HORMONAL CONTRACEPTIVES						
Implant (Implanon or Nexplanon)	0.05	0.05	Insertion of implant into upper arm once every 3 years	Progestin effects: thickening of cervical mucus, inhibition of ovulation, endometrial atrophy	Rare insertion complications, possible weight gain, uterine bleeding changes including amenorrhea	High efficacy, discreetness, relief of dysmenorrhea, reduced risk of ectopic pregnancy, reversibility, high acceptability and continuation rates; no estrogen
Progestin-releasing IUD (Skyla and Mirena)	0.2	0.2	3 or 5 years Releases 14 or 20 μg/day levonorgestrel	Progestin effects (see above) and IUD effect of preventing sperm from fertilizing ovum	Breakthrough bleeding in first 3 to 6 months, then hypomenorrhea or amenorrhea	High efficacy, easy to use, long-acting; no estrogen; decrease in: menstrual blood loss, dysmenorrhea, endometriosis pain, PID risk
Progestin-only injection (Depo-Provera)	6	0.2	3 months (13 weeks) 150 mg depot medroxyprogesterone IM	Progestin effects (see above)	Irregular bleeding or amenorrhea, weight gain, breast tenderness, acne, depression, possible decrease in bone density	No estrogen; decrease in menstrual blood loss, dysmenorrhea, PID risk
The patch	9	0.3	Weekly for 3 weeks (off on fourth wk) 20 μg ethinyl estradiol 150 μg norelgestromin released daily	Combined hormonal method: thickens cervical mucus, inhibits ovulation, inhibits sperm's ability to fertilize egg, slows tubal mobility, disrupts ovum transport, induces endometrial atrophy	Breakthrough bleeding, nausea, headaches, breast tenderness, skin site reaction; less effective if patient weighs >90 kg (198 lb)	Similar to OCPs but less-frequent dosing
Vaginal ring (NuvaRing)	9	0.3	Monthly (insert for 3 weeks of each month) Serum levels of 15 μg ethinyl estradiol Releases 150 μg norelgestromin daily	Combined hormonal method (see above)	Vaginal irritation, vaginal discharge, headache	Similar to OCPs but less-frequent dosing
Combined OCPs	9	0.3	Daily Varies 20–50 μg estrogen Varies 0.15–1 μg progestogen	Combined hormonal method (see above)	Breakthrough bleeding, nausea, headaches, breast tenderness	Decrease in PID risk, ectopic pregnancy risk, menstrual blood loss, dysmenorrhea, acne
Progestin-only pills	9	0.3	Daily (within 3-hr period) 0.35 mg norethindrone or 0.075 mg norgestrel	Progestin-only hormonal method: inhibits ovulation, thickens and decreases cervical mucus, atrophies endometrium	Irregular bleeding, breast tenderness, depression	No estrogen; effective after 2 days of use
NONHORMONAL CONTRACEPTIVES						
IUD copper-containing (ParaGard)	0.8	0.6	10 years 36 × 22 mm, copper wire wound around vertical stem of T	IUD: prevents sperm from fertilizing ova, and copper ions may act as spermicide	Heavier menses	Easy to use, long-acting nonhormonal
Male condom	18	2	Every act of intercourse	Barrier method: blocks passage of semen	Latex allergy	Recommended to be used in addition to another contraceptive; only method that decreased STD, HIV risk
Female condom	21	5	Every act of intercourse	Barrier method: lines the vagina fully and perineum partially	Vaginal discomfort, partner penile irritation	Provides some protection against STD, HIV; polyurethane can be used with latex allergy
Spermicides	28	18	Every act of intercourse nonoxynol-9 (in United States). Dose varies by formulation; e.g., gel, suppository from 52.5 to 150 mg	Kills sperm by destroying sperm cell membrane	Allergy or sensitivity to ingredients, recurrent urinary tract infections	Recommended to be used in addition to another barrier contraceptive

IM, intramuscular; *IUD*, intrauterine device; *OCP*, oral contraceptive pills; *PID*, pelvic inflammatory disease; *STD*, sexually transmitted disease.

Data from Trussell J. Contraceptive failure in the United States, *Contraception.* 2011;83:397–404; Hatcher RA, Trussell J, et al, eds. *Contraceptive technology,* New York, 2011, Ardent Media; and As-Sanie S, Gantt A, Rosenthal MS. Pregnancy prevention in adolescents, *Am Fam Physician* 2004;70:1517–1524.

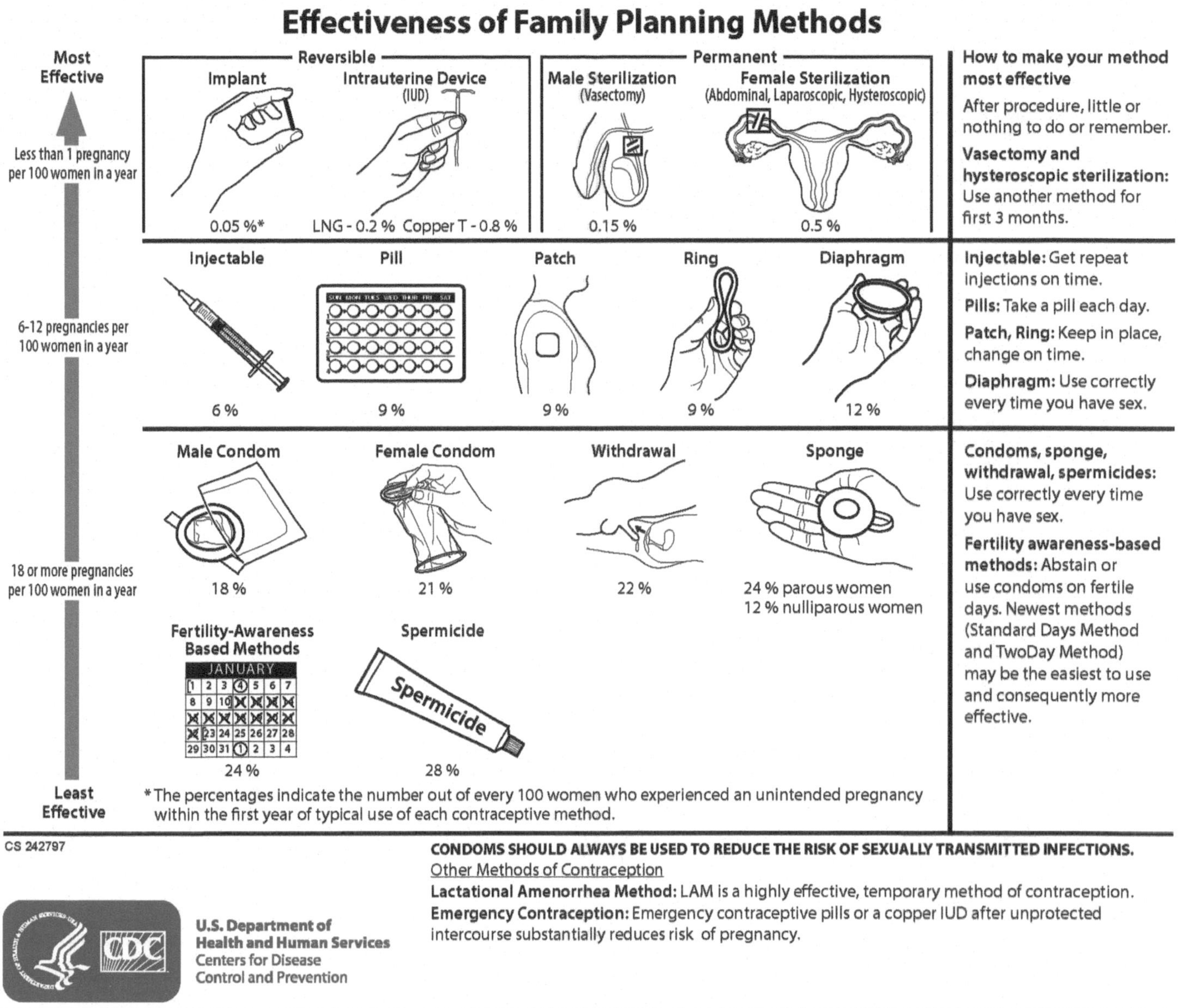

Effectiveness of Family Planning Methods

Fig. 91.1. Effectiveness of family planning methods. (From: Centers for Disease Control and Prevention, 2011.)

- If miss one day, can take two together on the next; if miss more than two days of pills, must use emergency contraception (if intercourse within the last 5 days) *and* should avoid sexual intercourse until 7 days of pills have been taken
- *Extended 91-day cycles* are available: have four periods/year, increase risk of intermenstrual bleeding and/or spotting
- *Multiphasic pills* are available as well: have differing levels of hormones depending on the week; more complicated and used less in adolescent patients
- Side effects: nausea and weight gain (mild and outweigh risk); this is why people will use lower doses of estrogen in their pills, cannot tolerate the nausea or other side effects; some women also prefer the lowest amount of estrogen possible to minimize the side effects
- Inhibition of ovulation or suppressant effect of estrogens on prostaglandin production by the endometrium helps decrease dysmenorrhea

- Interactions: phenobarbital, phenytoin, griseofulvin, rifampin (all will have decreased efficacy when taken with an estrogen-containing compound)

TRANSDERMAL PATCH

- Leave in place for one week, change × 3 weeks, and then one week with no patch
- Apply to lower abdomen, buttocks, or upper body

VAGINAL RING

- Placed inside vagina and remains in place for 3 weeks, then removed
- If removed for longer than 48 hours, a backup method is needed (condoms, emergency contraception if sex within the past 5 days)

Table 91.3. Conditions Classified as U.S. MEC Category 3 and 4 for Combined Hormonal Contraceptive Use

CATEGORY 4

Complicated valvular heart disease
Current breast cancer
Severe decompensated cirrhosis
Deep venous thrombosis/pulmonary embolism (acute; history, not on anticoagulation, or on established therapy for at least 3 months with higher risk of recurrence; major surgery with prolonged immobilization)
Complicated diabetes with nephropathy, retinopathy, neuropathy, or other vascular disease, or duration of diabetes >20 years
Migraine with aura
Hypertension (blood pressure above 160/100 mm Hg) or hypertension with vascular disease
Ischemic heart disease (history of or current)
Hepatocellular adenoma
Malignant liver tumor
Peripartum cardiomyopathy (diagnosed <6 months prior or with moderately or severely impaired cardiac function)
Postpartum <21 days
History of cerebrovascular accident
Systemic lupus erythematosus with positive antiphospholipid antibodies
Thrombogenic mutations
Viral hepatitis (acute or flare)

CATEGORY 3

Past breast cancer with no evidence of disease for 5 years
Breastfeeding and <1 month postpartum
Deep venous thrombosis/pulmonary embolism (history of deep venous thrombosis/pulmonary embolism with lower risk of recurrence)
Gallbladder disease (current, medically treated)
Migraine without aura (if worsens or first starts while using combined hormonal contraceptives)
History of malabsorptive bariatric surgery
History of cholestasis and related to past combined oral contraceptive
Hypertension (adequately controlled or blood pressure less than 160/100 mm Hg)
Peripartum cardiomyopathy with mild impairment or >6 months
Postpartum 21 to 42 days with other risk factors for venous thromboembolism
Drug interactions (ritonavir-boosted protease inhibitors, certain anticonvulsants, rifampin or rifabutin)

From: Centers for Disease Control and Prevention: U.S medical eligibility criteria for contraceptive use, 2010, *MMWR Recomm Rep* 59(RR-4):1–86, 2010.

Emergency Contraception

BASIC INFORMATION

- Can be effective up to 120 hours after unprotected sexual intercourse (all methods can work up to 120 hours; levonorgestrel most effective first 72 hours but can be used up to 12)

- All work to delay ovulation by thickening cervical mucus, which prevents fertilization
- Copper IUD: role in emergency contraception is unclear
- Ulipristal acetate: selective progesterone receptor modulator
- Levonorgestrel: available over the counter as an option; nausea and vomiting are rare
- Yuzpe method: COCs at home; take a total of 200 µg ethinyl estradiol and 2.0 mg norgestrel or 1.0 mg levonorgestrel; nausea and vomiting are common

Additional Contraception

BARRIER METHODS

- Condoms are needed with all forms of birth control for prevention of STIs (called "dual protection")
- Other barrier methods include diaphragm, cervical cap, and sponge; rarely used by adolescents

OTHER METHODS

- Spermicides: nonoxynol-9; must be inserted into vaginal cavity shortly before intercourse and then after; some concern about the effect on epithelial layer and increased risk of HIV, not substantiated in the literature
- Withdrawal: failure rate of 22%, but likely higher in adolescents
- Fertility awareness–based methods: basal body temperature method; should be used with extreme caution in adolescents; requires a regular cycle
- Lactational amenorrhea method: use only if no return of menses after delivery, infant is less than 6 months old and exclusively breastfeeding

Review Questions

For review questions, please go to ExpertConsult.com.

Suggested Readings

1. Neinstein LS, ed. *Neinstein's Adolescent and Young Adult Health Care: A Practical Guide.* 5th ed. Philadelphia: Lippincott Williams & Wilkins; 2010.
2. Emans J, Laufer M. *Goldstein's Pediatric and Adolescent Gynecology.* 6th ed. Philadelphia: Lippincott Williams & Wilkins; 2011.
3. Sucato G, Burstein G. Menstrual problems and contraception. In: *Nelson Textbook of Pediatrics.* 20th ed. Philadelphia: Elsevier; 2016.

Infectious Diseases of the Genital Tract

ROSHEEN GRADY, MD and JENNIFER H. CHUANG, MD, MS

Overview

- Sexually transmitted diseases (STDs) occur most frequently among sexually experienced adolescents and young adults
- Centers for Disease Control and Prevention (CDC) estimates that youth ages 15 to 24 account for half of the 20 million new sexually transmitted infections (STIs) that occur in the United States annually
- Adolescents identified as at higher risk for STDs include those who have sex at a younger age, attend STD clinics, or are youth in detention, young men having sex with men (MSM), and youth who use injection drugs
- Additional factors contributing to adolescents' increased risk include: failing to use barrier protection consistently, having multiple sexual partners, having increased biologic susceptibility to infection, and facing barriers in accessing reproductive health care
- Although each state and the District of Columbia allow minors to provide consent for their sexual health services, each jurisdiction can place unique restrictions on the basis of age or type of service (i.e., prevention, diagnosis, or treatment only)

Screening and Prevention

- Although many STDs present with specific symptom patterns, most are asymptomatic and identified only through laboratory investigation. Table 92.1 details recommended screening tests as part of routine health care maintenance
- Prevention and control of STDs rely on education, screening, early diagnosis and treatment
- Health care providers should educate adolescents about risk reduction strategies (e.g., correct condom use, decreasing number of sexual partners)
  - Discussions between adolescents, young adults, and health care providers regarding sexual behavior should be appropriate for a patient's developmental level, confidential, aimed at identifying risk behaviors and free from judgment
- The CDC provides a framework to assist health care providers with sexual history taking, emphasizing the five p's: partners, practices, protection from pregnancy, protection from STDs, and past history of STDs

STDS PRESENTING WITH GENITAL, ANAL, OR PERIANAL ULCERS

OVERVIEW

- In the United States, the most likely diagnoses for young, sexually active patients with genital, anal, or perianal ulcers are genital herpes or syphilis. Less common infections include chancroid and Granuloma inguinale (Donovanosis), which are more prevalent in other parts of the world. Table 92.2 provides an overview of the presentations of diseases causing genital ulcers
- Diagnosis of a genital ulcer disease (herpes simplex virus [HSV], syphilis, and chancroid) has been associated with an increased risk of human immunodeficiency virus (HIV)
- 2015 CDC STD guidelines state that diagnosis of ulcers based on history and physical examination is inaccurate and recommend that evaluation of any patient with a genital, anal, or perianal ulcer have consideration for specific investigations, including:
  1. Syphilis serology (typically nontreponemal first as a screening test, with treponemal to confirm), dark-field examination, or polymerase chain reaction (PCR) testing (for *Treponema pallidum* DNA) of ulcer exudate
  2. Viral culture or PCR testing of the ulcer with type specificity (HSV-1 or HSV-2) for genital herpes
  3. Serologic testing for type-specific HSV antibody
  4. All patients presenting with evaluation for anogenital ulcers should receive HIV testing

Herpes Simplex Virus

BASIC INFORMATION

- Genital herpes is a recurrent, lifelong infection
- There are two types of HSV: HSV-1 and HSV-2
  - HSV-1 most commonly causes orolabial herpes ("cold sores")
  - HSV-2 is the most common cause of recurrent genital herpes; however, HSV-1 has become an increasingly prominent cause of anogenital herpetic infections in young women and MSM
- Most people infected with HSV-2 (up to 70%) have mild or unrecognized infection but can still shed the virus intermittently
- Incubation period: 2 to 7 days

Table 92.1. Routine Laboratory Screening Recommendations for Sexually Transmitted Infections in Sexually Active Adolescents and Young Adults

CHLAMYDIA TRACHOMATIS AND NEISSERIA GONORRHOEAE

- Routine annual screening for *C. trachomatis* in all sexually active females aged ≤25 years is recommended
- Consider screening annually for *C. trachomatis* in sexually active adolescent and young adult males who have a history of multiple partners in settings with high prevalence rates, such as jails or juvenile corrections facilities, national job training programs, STD clinics, high school clinics, or adolescent clinics
- Routine annual screening for *N. gonorrhoeae* in all sexually active females aged ≤25 years is recommended
- Routine annual screening of sexually active adolescent and young adult MSM for rectal and urethral chlamydia and gonorrhea is recommended if they engage in receptive anal or insertive intercourse, respectively, and for routine gonorrhea if they engage in receptive oral sex. More frequent STD screening (i.e., at 3- to 6-month intervals) is indicated for MSM who have multiple or anonymous partners or who have sex in conjunction with illicit drug use

HIV

- HIV screening should be discussed and offered to all adolescents ≥13 years in health care settings, unless identified at an earlier age with HIV risk factors
- Persons who test positive should receive prevention counseling and referral to care before leaving testing site

SYPHILIS

- Syphilis screening should be offered to sexually active adolescents reporting risk factors
- The majority of U.S. syphilis cases occurring among young MSM and many early syphilis cases are identified from correctional facilities
- Providers should consult with their local health department regarding local syphilis prevalence and risk factors associated with syphilis acquisition

HEPATITIS C VIRUS

- Screen adolescents for hepatitis C virus who report risk factors, i.e., injection drug use, MSM, received blood products or organ donation before 1992, long-term hemodialysis, being born to a mother with HCV infection, intranasal drug use, receipt of an unregulated tattoo, or high- prevalence setting, i.e., correctional facilities

HCV, hepatitis C virus; HIV, human immunodeficiency virus; MSM, men who have sex with men; STD, sexually transmitted diseases.
Adapted from Centers for Disease Control and Prevention: Sexually transmitted diseases treatment guidelines, 2015, MMWR 64 (No. RR03):1-137, 2015. https://www.cdc.gov/std/tg2015/

CLINICAL PRESENTATION

- Primary genital herpes classically presents with painful, itchy lesions and multiple vesicles (see Fig. 92.1); however, it also is commonly asymptomatic
  - Primary infection may also present with constitutional symptoms (low-grade fever, headache, malaise), myalgias, inguinal lymphadenopathy, watery vaginal discharge, or mucoid urethral discharge
- Recurrent disease is less severe than primary infection, but may be severe in immunosuppressed individuals
- The average initial infection lasts 12 days; recurrent infections have an average duration of 4 to 5 days
- Complications include central nervous system (CNS) involvement (e.g., meningitis or encephalitis) and urinary retention, which can be due to severe urethritis and dysuria

DIAGNOSIS

- Clinical diagnosis can be confirmed through preferred HSV tests: cell culture and PCR
  - Viral culture has low sensitivity, and false negatives can occur during viral shedding
  - Nucleic acid amplification tests (NAATs), including PCR assays for HSV DNA, are more sensitive and becoming more widely available; PCR is the preferred method for diagnosis of CNS and systemic infections
  - Tzanck preparation (uses cytologic detection of cellular changes associated with HSV infection) has very low sensitivity and should not be used
- Type-specific HSV serologic assays also exist. Although the presence of IgG antibodies to HSV-2 implies anogenital infection, IgG antibodies to HSV-1 are more difficult to interpret and could reflect either orolabial infection or genital infection
- A combination of history, physical examination, and laboratory test results is needed to assess whether an adolescent's ulcer is attributable to HSV

TREATMENT

- Systemic antiviral therapy (acyclovir, famciclovir, or valacyclovir) is the mainstay of treatment and should be offered as episodic or suppressive therapy for all patients suspected of having anogenital HSV
  - Antiviral medications offer most benefit if initiated within 24 hours of symptom onset
- Suppressive therapy reduces the frequency of genital herpes by 70% to 80% in patients who have frequent recurrences
  - Even with suppressive antiviral therapy, subclinical viral shedding still occurs, so counseling on appropriate condom use is essential
  - Once-daily valacyclovir in the infected partner, in addition to consistent condom use, may help decrease transmission to an uninfected partner by approximately 55%
- For those with severe disease or disseminated infection, admission to hospital and use of parenteral acyclovir is necessary

HSV IN PREGNANCY

- Risk of transmission of HSV to neonates from an infected mother with initial, primary HSV near the time of delivery is very high, estimated between 25% and 60%
- More than 75% of neonates who contract HSV are born to women who are asymptomatic and had no history of HSV at delivery
- Women who have no signs or symptoms of herpes at delivery may deliver vaginally
- Cesarean section should be performed if lesions are present at the time of delivery
- Neonatal herpes infection is associated with high mortality rates; many survivors have severe ocular and neurologic sequelae

Table 92.2. Differential Diagnosis of Genital Ulcers

Infection	Clinical Presentation	Associated Symptoms	Diagnosis
Chancroid Cause: *Haemophilus ducreyi*	*Painful* Shallow, friable, nonindurated with *ragged* margins, granulomatous base, yellow or gray, necrotic purulent exudate	Painful inguinal adenopathy called "buboes" present	Culture of lesion (not widely available) CDC criteria for diagnosis: 1. >1 painful genital ulcer 2. No evidence of syphilis on dark-field or serologic test performed 7 days after onset of ulcer 3. Typical clinical presentation 4. Negative HSV test of ulcer
Lymphogranuloma venereum Cause: L1, L2, or L3 forms of *C. trachomatis*	*Painless* ulcer, small pustule at site of inoculation, can disappear rapidly	▪ First stage: small, painless ulcer ▪ Second stage: constitutional illness, painful, lymphadenopathy, "groove" sign pathognomonic ▪ Third stage: proctocolitis	Genital lesion swab or lymph node aspirate tested using nucleic acid amplification tests
Granuloma inguinale Cause: *Klebsiella granulomatis*	*Painless*, slowly progressive ulcerative lesion on genitals or perineum; bleeds easily on contact	Regional lymphadenopathy is *uncommon*	Identification of Donovan bodies within histiocytes of granulation tissue smears or biopsy specimens
Syphilis Cause: *Treponema pallidum*	*Painless* ulcer with indurated hard, raised border and "punched-out" appearance	Regional lymphadenopathy may occur	▪ Screen: Nontreponemal tests (RPR, VDRL) ▪ Confirm: treponemal tests (FTA-ABS or TPPA) ▪ Dark-field microscopy showing spirochetes
Genital Herpes Cause: HSV-1 or HSV-2	*Painful* vesicular lesions developing into ulcers	Constitutional symptoms present in primary infection	Viral culture or PCR for HSV DNA (from lesion)

FTA-ABS, fluorescent treponemal antibody-absorbed; *HSV,* herpes simplex virus; *PCR,* polymerase chain reaction; *RPR,* rapid plasma reagin; *TPPA, Treponema pallidum* particle agglutination; *VDRL,* Venereal Disease Research Laboratory.
Adapted from Centers for Disease Control and Prevention: Sexually transmitted diseases treatment guidelines, 2015, MMWR 64 (No. RR03):1-137, 2015. Available from: https://www.cdc.gov/std/default.htm

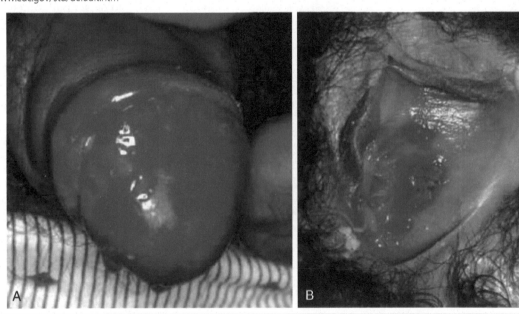

Fig. 92.1. (A) Initial herpes infection showing multiple erosions with polycyclic outlines surrounded by an erythematous halo and associated with intense pain. (B) Erosions surrounded by an erythematous halo. Clinical signs and symptoms of recurrences are usually less intense than those of initial infection. (From Martín JM, Villalón G, Jordá E. Update on treatment of genital herpes. *Actas Dermosifiliogr,* 2009; 100:22–32;, Figs. 1 and 2.) (Kliegman RM, Stanton BF, St. Geme III JW, Schor NF, Behrman R, eds. *Nelson Textbook of Pediatrics.* 20th ed. Philadelphia: Elsevier; 2016.)

Syphilis

BASIC INFORMATION

- Syphilis is a systemic illness due to the spirochete *T. pallidum.* There are three well-described stages of syphilis (primary, secondary, and tertiary). Patients may present at any stage
- Major routes of transmission are via sexual intercourse or vertical transmission from mother to fetus

CLINICAL PRESENTATION

Primary Syphilis

- Begins as a chancre (single painless ulcer) at the site of inoculation 2 to 3 weeks after exposure; is often not recognized
  - Chancre appears flat with raised, rolled border with sharp, firm, slightly elevated borders. Lesions are associated with firm, nontender bilateral regional lymphadenopathy. They spontaneously resolve

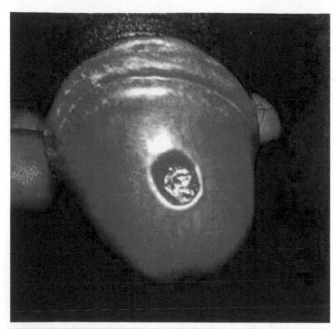

Fig. 92.2. Primary syphilis infection: chancre at glans penis. (Available from website https://www.cdc.gov/std/syphilis/images/chancre-penile.htm)

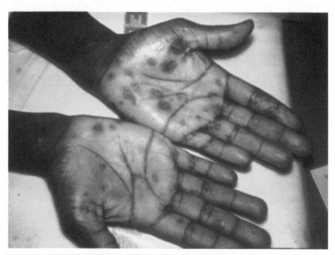

Fig. 92.3. Secondary syphilis on palms of hand. (Available from website https://www.cdc.gov/std/training/clinicalslides/slides-dl.htm)

- Common sites include penis, vagina, perianal region, lip, tongue (see Fig. 92.2)

Secondary or Disseminated Syphilis

- Begins 2 to 6 weeks after appearance of chancre
- May occur with constitutional symptoms: mild fever, sore throat, headache, arthralgia
- Skin lesions include rashes of the whole body or of the palms and soles, as well as alopecia (see Fig. 92.3)
- Also present with condylomata lata—raised, painless gray-white lesions appearing in intertriginous areas and mucous membranes that are highly infectious

Tertiary Syphilis

- Late manifestations of syphilis characterized by gummatous (soft, rubbery noncancerous tumor) lesions of skin, bone, muscle, eyes, cardiac, viscera

- Average onset is 4 to 12 years after initial infection

Neurosyphilis

- Can present at any syphilis stage; more common among HIV-infected persons
- Can manifest as meningitis, neurologic symptoms such as personality changes, hallucinations, stroke symptoms, or hearing loss

Latent Syphilis

- Term that describes situation of positive serology tests accompanied by lack of clinical manifestations
- Latent syphilis acquired within the preceding year is called "early latent." "Late latent" generally occurs after the first year of infection

DIAGNOSIS

- If lesions are present, dark-field examination or direct fluorescent antibody testing of exudate or tissue is diagnostic of syphilis
- A presumptive diagnosis of syphilis requires two types of serologic tests:
  1. Nontreponemal tests (Venereal Disease Research Laboratory [VDRL] and rapid plasma reagin [RPR])
  2. Treponemal tests (fluorescent treponemal antibody absorbed [FTA-ABS] and *T. pallidum* particle agglutination [TP-PA]) and newer automated tests (enzyme immunoassays [EIA] or chemiluminescent immunoassay [CIA])
- Use of only one type of test is not sufficient for diagnosis with the potential for false-positive and false-negative results
  - False-positive nontreponemal tests can be due to medical conditions such as HIV, autoimmune disease, immunizations, pregnancy, and intravenous (IV) drug use
- Although traditionally nontreponemal testing has been used as a first-pass screening test, many clinical laboratories now use "reverse sequence" screening where a treponemal EIA/CIA is performed first
- A treponemal EIA or CIA test that is positive can indicate a previously treated, untreated, or incompletely treated syphilis infection
- If EIA/CIA and nontreponemal (e.g., RPR or VDRL) test results are discordant, a follow-up treponemal test is necessary to confirm the diagnosis
- Diagnosis of neurosyphilis is based on a combination of serologic tests, cerebrospinal fluid (CSF) abnormalities (greater than five white blood cells [WBCs]/mm³ ± abnormal protein), and/or a reactive CSF VDRL (specific, but only 50% sensitive)

TREATMENT

- Penicillin G or benzathine penicillin G, administered through IV or intramuscular (IM) injection, is the first-line agent for all stages of syphilis. Treatment regimens are detailed in Table 92.3
  - Penicillin G is the only accepted therapy for syphilis during pregnancy and neurosyphilis, requiring patients with penicillin allergy to undergo desensitization
- Response to therapy is monitored by change in titer of a nontreponemal test (e.g., RPR) over 12 to 24 months

Table 92.3. Recommended Treatment Regimens for Syphilis

Clinical Stage	Treatment
Primary, secondary, and early latent syphilis	Benzathine penicillin G: 50,000 units/kg IM up to the adult dose of 2.4 million units in a single dose (if penicillin allergic: doxycycline 100 mg PO BID for 2 weeks, except pregnant patients, who should be desensitized and treated with penicillin)
Late latent syphilis, syphilis of unknown duration, or tertiary syphilis (gummatous and cardiovascular syphilis)	Benzathine penicillin G: 50,000 units/kg IM up to the adult dose of 2.4 million units, administered as three doses at 1-week intervals (total 150,000 units/kg up to the total adult dose of 7.2 million units)
Neurosyphilis	Aqueous crystalline penicillin G: 18 to 24 million units per day for 10 to 14 days

BID, twice daily; *IM,* intramuscularly; *PO,* orally.
From Centers for Disease Control and Prevention: Sexually transmitted diseases treatment guidelines, 2015, MMWR. Available from: https://www.cdc.gov/std/default.htm

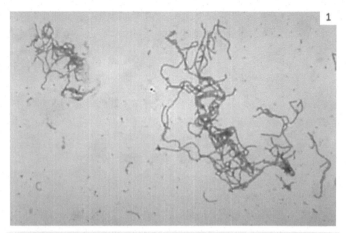

Fig. 92.4. Chancroid. (Available from website **https://www.cdc.gov/std/training/clinicalslides/slides-dl.htm**)

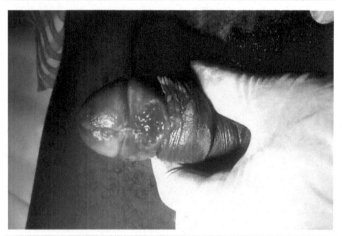

Fig. 92.5. Granuloma inguinale. (Available from website **https://phil.cdc.gov/phil/details.asp?pid=5363**)

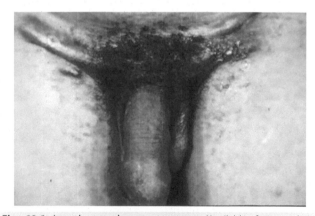

Fig. 92.6. Lymphogranuloma venereum. (Available from website https://www.cdc.gov/std/training/clinicalslides/slides-dl.htm)

(at least a fourfold decrease in titer must be achieved to indicate cure)
- Treponemal test titers do not correlate with disease activity or cure (and will remain positive for life)
- The Jarisch-Herxheimer reaction is an acute febrile response with headache, myalgia occurring within the first 24 hours after beginning treatment for syphilis, believed to be due to activation of inflammatory cascade associated with lysis of spirochetes. Treatment is supportive

Chancroid

BASIC INFORMATION

- Chancroid is much rarer than herpes or syphilis and is declining in incidence worldwide, but it can occur in the United States. The infection is due to *Haemophilus ducreyi,* which must be cultured on special media
- Classically presents with painful, friable, superficial (nonindurated) genital ulcers (unlike syphilis) surrounded by erythema and with a foul-smelling yellow-gray exudate; ulcers may self-resolve
- Also associated with bubo, a unilateral swollen, ruptured inguinal lymphadenopathy
- Diagnosed clinically after excluding syphilis and HSV; cultures lack sensitivity, but Gram stain may demonstrate a "school of fish" (see Fig. 92.4)
- Treated with azithromycin 1 gram orally in a single dose; or ceftriaxone 250 mg IM in a single dose; or ciprofloxacin 500 mg orally twice daily for three days; or erythromycin 500 mg orally three times daily for 7 days

Granuloma Inguinale (Donovanosis)

BASIC INFORMATION

- Genital ulcerative disease caused by Gram-negative *Klebsiella granulomatis* (formally known as *Calymmato-*

bacterium granulomatis). Rarely occurs in United States, endemic in tropical and developing areas
- Classically presents with painless, slowly progressive ulcerative lesion on the genitals or perineum without regional lymphadenopathy (see Figs. 92.5 and 92.6)
  - Lesions are extremely vascular and can easily bleed on contact
  - Can also have extension of infection to pelvis, disseminate to intraabdominal organs, bones, or mouth

- Can also occur with subcutaneous granulomas (called pseudobuboes—not swelling of lymph node, but rather granulation tissue)
- Diagnosis: difficult to culture. Diagnosed by dark staining Donovan bodies (intracytoplasmic inclusion bodies) on tissue-crush preparation or biopsy
- Treatment: azithromycin 1 gram orally once per week or 500 mg daily for at least 3 weeks until all lesions have completely healed; relapse can occur frequently

Lymphogranuloma Venereum

BASIC INFORMATION

- Due to *Chlamydia trachomatis* serovars L1, L2, or L3
- Patients present with painless genital ulcer at the site of inoculation, followed by unilateral tender inguinal and/or femoral lymphadenopathy. Ulcer usually disappears before the patient presents for treatment. May also develop severe proctocolitis
- Diagnosis: anorectal specimens and lymph node specimens (i.e., lesion swab or bubo aspirate) can be tested for *C. trachomatis* by culture, direct immunofluorescence, or NAAT
- Treatment: doxycycline 100 mg orally twice a day for 21 days

STDS PRESENTING WITH URETHRITIS AND CERVICITIS

- Urethritis may present with urethral discharge, dysuria, urethral irritation, or meatal pruritus. Classic finding is mucoid or purulent discharge
- Approximately 30% to 50% of males are asymptomatic but may have signs of discharge at the time of diagnosis
- *C. trachomatis* and *Neisseria gonorrhoeae* are the most commonly identified pathogens for both urethritis and cervicitis
- *Mycoplasma genitalium* and *Ureaplasma urealyticum* may also be associated with urethritis
  - Males very rarely contract urinary tract infections. If dysuria and urethral discharge are described in a sexually active adolescent male with no known genitourinary abnormalities, consider STD until proven otherwise
  - Cervicitis involves inflammation of the deeper structures in the mucous membrane of the cervix. Can present with vaginal discharge, but is frequently asymptomatic. Can also present with complaints of irregular, vaginal, or postcoital bleeding

Gonococcal Infections

BASIC INFORMATION

- STDs caused by *N. gonorrhoeae* (small intracellular Gram-negative cocci)
- Requires mucosal surface contact; can involve genital tract, rectum, oropharynx, or be disseminated

- Incubation period is 3 to 7 days; symptoms manifest within 10 to 14 days after exposure

CLINICAL PRESENTATION

- Approximately 30% to 50% of males are asymptomatic. In those with symptoms, most present with purulent urethral discharge or dysuria
- Women with cervicitis may have vaginal discharge or vaginal bleeding; 50% may be asymptomatic
- Other presentations in adolescent women include urethritis, Bartholin gland abscess, or pelvic inflammatory disease (PID)
- Gonorrheal infections in women can cause the same complications as chlamydia infections, including PID, increased risk of ectopic pregnancy, and infertility

DIAGNOSIS

- Specific testing for *N. gonorrhoeae* is recommended using culture, nucleic acid hybridization tests, or NAATs
  - NAATs provide quicker results and higher sensitivity
  - NAATs can be used with endocervical swabs, vaginal swabs, male urethral swabs, oropharynx, rectum, and urine
  - In persistent infections, culture and susceptibility testing should be performed

TREATMENT

- Treatment of *N. gonorrhea* is complicated by developing resistance to antimicrobials; recommendations for managing uncomplicated STIs in adolescents and adults are detailed in Table 92.4
- Combination therapy using two antimicrobials with different mechanisms of action (ceftriaxone 250 mg IM and azithromycin 1 gram PO or doxycycline 100 mg PO twice daily for 7 days) is recommended to potentially slow resistance as well as address frequent coinfection with *C. trachomatis*
- Medication for gonococcal infection should be provided on-site and directly observed
- Patients should be instructed to abstain from sexual activity for 7 days after treatment and until all partners are adequately treated
- Test-of-cure is not needed for patients with uncomplicated genital or rectal gonococcal disease who are treated with recommended or alternative regimens. Anyone with an oropharyngeal infection should return 2 weeks after treatment using culture of NAAT. If NAAT is positive, culture should be obtained before retreatment
- Retest all patients 3 months after completing therapy because reinfection rates are high

Disseminated Gonococcal Infection

BASIC INFORMATION

- Occurs in 1% to 3% of all gonococcal infections through hematogenous spread

Table 92.4. Management Guidelines for Uncomplicated Bacterial Sexually Transmitted Infections in Adolescents and Adults

Pathogen	Recommended Regimens	Alternative Regimens and Special Considerations
Chlamydia trachomatis	Azithromycin 1 g orally once *or* doxycycline 100 mg orally twice daily for 7 days	For pregnancy: azithromycin 1 g orally once Alternative regimens: erythromycin base 500 mg orally four times a day for 7 days *or* Erythromycin ethylsuccinate 800 mg orally four times a day for 7 days *or* levofloxacin 500 mg orally once daily for 7 days *or* ofloxacin 300 mg orally twice a day for 7 days
Neisseria gonorrhoeae (cervix, urethra, and rectum)	Ceftriaxone 250 mg IM in a single dose *or* Single-dose injectable cephalosporin *plus* azithromycin 1 g orally once	Alternative if unable to offer IM: cefixime 400 mg orally in a single dose *plus* azithromycin 1 g orally once If azithromycin is not available or if patient is allergic to azithromycin, doxycycline 100 mg orally twice daily for 7 days may be substituted for azithromycin as the second antimicrobial Severe cephalosporin allergy: contact infectious disease specialist
N. gonorrhoeae (pharynx)	Ceftriaxone 250 mg IM in a single dose *plus* azithromycin 1 g orally once	No alternative therapy available Patients treated with an alternative regimen should return 14 days after treatment for a test of cure using either culture or NAAT. If the NAAT is positive, every effort should be made to perform a confirmatory culture
Treponema pallidum (primary and secondary syphilis or early latent syphilis, i.e., infection <12 months)	Benzathine penicillin G 2.4 million units IM in 1 dose	Penicillin allergy: doxycycline 100 mg orally twice daily for 14 days. Limited data suggest ceftriaxone 1–2 g daily either IM or IV for 10–14 days
Treponema pallidum (late latent syphilis or syphilis of unknown duration)	Benzathine penicillin G 7.2 million units total, administered as three doses of 2.4 million units IM each at 1-week intervals	Penicillin allergy: doxycycline 100 mg orally twice daily for 28 days with close serologic and clinical follow-up
Haemophilus ducreyi (chancroid: genital ulcers, lymphadenopathy)	Azithromycin 1 g orally in a single dose *or* ceftriaxone 250 mg IM in a single dose *or* ciprofloxacin 500 mg orally twice a day for 3 days *or* erythromycin base 500 mg orally 3 times a day for 7 days	
C. trachomatis serovars L1, L2, or L3 (lymphogranuloma venereum)	Doxycycline 100 mg orally twice daily for 21 days	Alternative: erythromycin base 500 mg orally four times a day for 21 days *or* azithromycin 1 g orally once a week for 3 weeks

IM, intramuscular; *IV*, intravenous; *NAAT*, nucleic acid amplification test.
Modified from Centers for Disease Control and Prevention: *Sexually transmitted diseases treatment guidelines, 2014 MMWR* http://www.cdc.gov/std/treatment/update.htm.
From Nelson Pediatrics Twentieth Edition: Elsevier; 2016.

CLINICAL PRESENTATION

- Most common presentations:
  - Tenosynovitis/dermatitis syndrome with fever, chills, skin lesions, polyarthralgia (hands, wrists, fingers), positive blood cultures (30%–40%), and negative synovial cultures
  - Monoarticular arthritis (commonly the knee), associated with positive synovial culture and negative blood culture. Polyarthralgia may precede monoarticular infection

DIAGNOSIS

- NAAT or culture specimens from urogenital and extragenital sites should be collected with specimens from disseminated sites of infection (e.g., skin, synovial fluid, blood, and the CNS)

TREATMENT

- Inpatient hospitalization and consultation with an infectious disease specialist are recommended for initial IV therapy

- There is no agreed-upon duration of treatment for all types of disseminated gonococcal infection
- When treating for arthritis dermatitis syndromes, IV therapy is initially started with change to oral agent guided by antimicrobial susceptibility 24 to 48 hours after substantial improvement, with recommended duration of at least 7 days
- Examination for clinical evidence of endocarditis and meningitis should be performed because those diagnoses require longer duration of therapy

Chlamydial Infections

BASIC INFORMATION

- *C. trachomatis* is the most common bacterial STD in the United States (D through K serotypes). Lymphogranuloma venereum is caused by L1–L3 serotypes
- Young age (adolescents and young adults) most at risk for *C. trachomatis*

CLINICAL PRESENTATION

- Most patients asymptomatic!
- Females may present as urethritis or cervicitis; can also have vaginal discharge, lower- abdominal pain, or dysuria
- Males may develop urethritis with dysuria, mucopurulent discharge, or epididymitis

DIAGNOSIS

- Method of choice is NAAT
- Annual screening of all sexually active young women is recommended to prevent complications because asymptomatic infection is common
- Untreated chlamydial infection in women is a major cause of PID, ectopic pregnancy, and infertility

TREATMENT

- Azithromycin or doxycycline first line; see Table 92.4
- As in gonococcal infections, repeat testing is warranted 3 months after therapy. Sexual partners in the preceding 2 months should be referred for treatment

Epididymitis

BASIC INFORMATION

- Inflammation of the epididymis in males most often associated with STD in adolescents, typically *C. trachomatis* or *N. gonorrhoeae*

CLINICAL PRESENTATION

- Presentation of unilateral scrotal swelling and tenderness; can often be accompanied by hydrocele and palpable swelling of epididymis with urethral discharge

- Relief of pain with elevation of the testicle is present with epididymitis (positive Prehn sign); pain worsens upon elevation with diagnosis of testicular torsion
- Most commonly gradual onset; can be sudden. Always consider testicular torsion in your differential diagnosis, also the need for urgent surgical consultation
- Males who have insertive anal intercourse are also vulnerable to *Escherichia coli* epididymitis

EVALUATION

- Obtain objective evidence of urethral inflammation by Gram stain of secretions, positive leukocyte esterase, or >10 WBC per high-power field on first void urine sample
- All suspected cases should have urine NAAT for *C. trachomatis* and *N. gonorrhoeae*. Urine culture is not typically recommended (insensitive for chlamydia and gonococcal infection). Could be helpful for men with sexually transmitted enteric infections
- Always test for other STDs including HIV

TREATMENT

- Empiric therapy before availability of any laboratory test results is recommended to prevent complications and further transmission
- For infections most likely caused by STDs, ceftriaxone 250 mg IM plus doxycycline 100 mg orally twice daily for 10 days. Consider use of levofloxacin 500 mg orally once a day for 10 days or ofloxacin in the setting of males who practice insertive anal sex at risk of enteric organisms
- Advise return to care if symptoms fail to improve in 72 hours
- Bed rest, scrotal elevation, and pain relief

EXPEDITED PARTNER THERAPY

- Patient delivers medication or prescription to partner for treatment without a medical assessment
- Strategy shown to reduce further transmission; endorsed by American Academy of Pediatrics and Society of Adolescent Health and Medicine, but not all states permit this practice

INFECTIONS WITH VAGINAL DISCHARGE

- Combination of history, examination, and laboratory testing is important to determine cause of vaginal discharge
- Physiologic leukorrhea is a common reason for presentation to a primary care provider or gynecologist in early adolescence. Three to six months before menarche, vaginal lubrication increases and a clear vaginal discharge appears (physiologic leukorrhea). Aside from discharge, other symptoms are absent
- See Table 92.5 and Fig. 92.7 for common infectious causes of vaginal discharge
- Obtaining gender of sex partners, menstrual history, vaginal hygiene practices (e.g., douching), and self-treatment with over-the-counter medications can guide diagnosis

Table 92.5. Summary Diagnosis and Management of Vaginal Discharge

Disease	Organism	Type of Organism	Discharge	Diagnostic Features
Bacterial vaginosis	Replacement of normal vaginal flora (*Lactobacillus* sp.) with anaerobes	Bacteria	Thin, gray-white, foul-smelling; adheres to vaginal walls	"Clue cells" on wet prep; vaginal pH >4.5, + whiff test (KOH reveals "fishy odor")
Trichomoniasis	*Trichomonas vaginalis*	Protozoan	Green-yellow, malodorous, frothy	Motile trichomonads on wet mount, culture, PCR; can also cause cervicitis with red, punctate "strawberry" cervix
Vulvovaginal Candidiasis	Candida	Fungus (yeast)	White "cottage cheese" discharge	Fungal elements on wet prep; vaginal <4.5

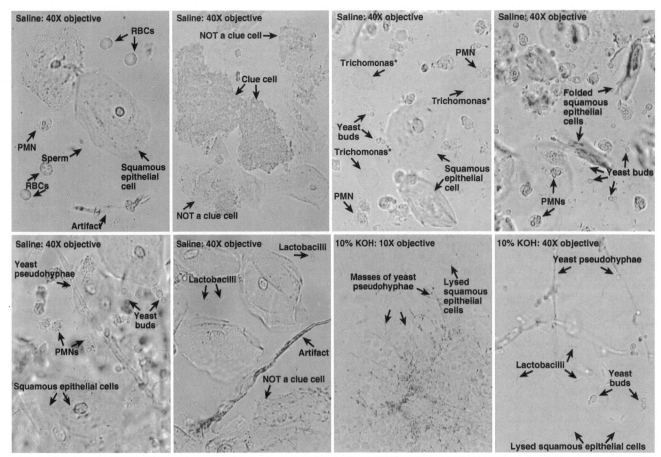

Fig. 92.7. Common microscopic findings on examination of vaginal fluid. (*KOH*, potassium hydroxide solution; *PMN*, polymorphonuclear leukocyte; *RBC*, red blood cell. From Kliegman RM, Stanton BF, St. Geme III JW, Schor NF, Behrman R, eds. ***Nelson Textbook of Pediatrics***. 20th ed. Philadelphia: Elsevier; 2016. Fig. 120-8. (From Adolescent medicine: state of the art reviews, vol 14, no 2, Philadelphia, 2003, Hanley & Belfus, pp 350–351.)

Bacterial Vaginosis (BV)

BASIC INFORMATION

- BV is the most common cause of vaginal discharge seeking medical attention
- Most women are asymptomatic (50%–75%)
- Not always considered an STD. Associated with new sex partner, multiple male or female partners, douching, lack of condom use
- Presence of BV increases risk of acquiring some STDs (HIV, *N. gonorrhoeae*, *C. trachomatis*, HSV-2), complications in pregnancy

- Diagnosed through clinical criteria or Gram stain (gold standard laboratory method)
  - Clinical diagnostic criteria (Amsel criteria) for diagnosis require 3/4 of the following:
    1. Homogeneous, thin, white discharge that smoothly coats vaginal walls
    2. Clue cells on microscopic examination
    3. Vaginal discharge pH >4.5
    4. Fishy odor of vaginal discharge before or after addition of KOH 10% (i.e., positive whiff test)
- Treatment is recommended for all women with symptoms
  - Treatment of <u>asymptomatic</u> pregnant women is controversial. Current evidence is not sufficient to

recommend treating asymptomatic women with positive BV testing at high or low risk of preterm delivery
- Recommended: metronidazole 500 mg orally twice a day for 7 days or metronidazole gel 0.75% intravaginally once daily for 5 days or clindamycin cream 2%, one full applicator intravaginally at bedtime for 7 days
- Treatment of male sex partners not shown to be beneficial in preventing recurrence of BV

Trichomoniasis

BASIC INFORMATION

- Most prevalent nonviral STD in the United States due to protozoa/parasite *Trichomonas vaginalis*
- Associated with two- to threefold increase of HIV acquisition, preterm birth, adverse pregnancy outcomes
- Occurs more commonly in women. Most men are asymptomatic
- In addition to discharge (see Table 92.5), presents with dysuria, pruritus, and vulvar irritation. Cervicitis, "strawberry cervix," is common
- Diagnosis via NAAT is highly sensitive; wet mount can be used (poor sensitivity)
- Treatment: metronidazole 2 grams orally in a single dose or tinidazole 2 grams orally in a single dose
  - Treatment of sexual partners is recommended
  - Due to high rate of reinfection, recommend that all women treated are retested 3 months after initial treatment, regardless of whether they believe their sex partner was treated
  - Retesting of males is not recommended due to insufficient evidence

Vulvovaginal Candidiasis

BASIC INFORMATION

- Vulvovaginal candidiasis (VVC) is usually due to *Candida albicans*, but other candida species can cause infection
- Most women will have at least one episode of uncomplicated VVC; complicated occurs in patients with recurrent infection, uncontrolled diabetes, immunosuppression (e.g., HIV), or pregnancy. May also see VVC after an antibiotic course
- In addition to discharge (see Table 92.5), symptoms include intense itching, burning, and soreness
- Diagnosis: can be made via wet prep vaginal mount or Gram stain of vaginal discharge (budding yeasts, hyphae, or pseudohyphae). Use of 10% KOH is very helpful because it disrupts cell material that may obscure visualization of yeast
  - Candida vaginitis is associated with a normal pH (<4.5)
- If a negative wet prep is obtained and a patient has signs or symptoms of VVC, a culture for yeast should be obtained
- Treatment:
  - Uncomplicated VVC: short courses of topical formulations (single dose or 1–3 days). Topical "azole" drugs

(i.e., clotrimazole cream, miconazole cream) are more effective than nystatin
- Alternative: oral agent is fluconazole 150 mg oral tablet × 1 dose
- Complicated VVC (non–*Candida albicans*, immunocompromised host): longer duration of initial therapy with oral fluconazole course weekly
- Only topical azole therapies × 7 days are recommended for pregnant women
- Treatment of sexual partners unnecessary

Pelvic Inflammatory Disease

BASIC INFORMATION

- PID is a broad term to describe a variety of inflammatory disorders of the upper female genital tract
- Includes any combination or single diagnosis of endometritis, salpingitis, tubo-ovarian abscess, pelvic peritonitis
- Most commonly *N. gonorrhoeae* and *C. trachomatis* cause PID, but it is usually polymicrobial—involving anaerobes, *Gardnerella vaginalis*, Gram-negative rods, cytomegalovirus (CMV), *M. genitalium*

CLINICAL PRESENTATION AND DIAGNOSIS

- PID can be difficult to diagnose due to varied symptom presentation and signs. Can be subtle or mild symptoms, resulting in potential for many unrecognized cases
  - Commonly, patients complain of dull, steady, unilateral or bilateral lower abdominal pain and or/pelvic pain, which can be indolent or excruciating
  - Additional symptoms can include fever, right upper quadrant pain, vomiting, and irregular vaginal bleeding
- PID should be considered in any young sexually active female presenting with vaginal discharge or abdominal pain
- Patients can also present with right upper quadrant pain and sometimes elevated transaminases, which can indicate perihepatitis (Fitz-Hugh–Curtis) syndrome. This results from dissemination of PID-causing bacteria from the fallopian tubes through the peritoneum to the liver capsule

DIAGNOSIS

- See Table 92.6 for CDC diagnostic criteria for PID
- Most females with PID have either mucopurulent cervical discharge or WBC on microscopic evaluation of a vaginal fluid saline preparation
- It is essential that criteria are very sensitive so as not to miss a diagnosis of PID due to potential devastating long-term adverse outcomes (sterility, abscess)

TREATMENT

- Reasons to hospitalize young women with PID include:
  - Surgical emergencies (e.g., ectopic pregnancy, appendicitis)
  - Pregnancy
  - Inadequate response to therapy

Table 92.6. Diagnosis of Pelvic Inflammatory Disease

2015 CDC DIAGNOSTIC CRITERIA

Minimal Criteria

- Cervical motion tenderness *or*
- Uterine tenderness *or*
- Adnexal tenderness

Additional Criteria to Enhance Specificity of the Minimal Criteria

- Oral temperature >101°F (>38.3°C)
- Abnormal cervical mucopurulent discharge or friable cervix
- Presence of abundant numbers of WBCs on saline microscopy of vaginal secretions*
- Elevated ESR or C-reactive protein
- Laboratory documentation of cervical *Neisseria gonorrhoeae* or *Chlamydia trachomatis* infection

Most Specific Criteria for Diagnosing PID (rarely used clinically)

- Transvaginal sonography or MRI techniques showing thickened, fluid-filled tubes, with or without free pelvic fluid or tubo-ovarian complex; or Doppler studies suggesting pelvic infection (e.g., tubal hyperemia)
- Endometrial biopsy with histopathologic evidence of endometritis
- Laparoscopic abnormalities consistent with PID

ESR, erythrocyte sedimentation rate; MRI, magnetic resonance imaging; PID, pelvic inflammatory disease; WBC, white blood cell.
*If the cervical discharge appears normal and no WBCs are observed on the wet prep of vaginal fluid, the diagnosis of PID is unlikely, and alternative causes of pain should be investigated.
Diagnosis of Pelvic Inflammatory Disease Disease Control and Prevention: Sexually transmitted diseases treatment guidelines, 2015, MMWR 64 (No. RR03):1-137, 2015.

Table 92.7. Treatment of Pelvic Inflammatory Disease

2015 CDC RECOMMENDATIONS

IV Antibiotic Treatment

- Cefotetan 2 g IV every 12 hr *or* cefoxitin 2 g IV every 6 hr *plus* doxycycline 100 mg PO (PO is preferred) or IV every 12 hr (classic option)
- Other option:
  - Clindamycin 900 mg IV every 8 hr plus gentamicin IV or IM loading dose (2 mg/kg of body weight) followed by maintenance dose (1.5 mg/kg) every 8 hours
IV therapy can be discontinued 24 hr after clinical improvement
Therapy should be continued with doxycycline 100 mg PO twice per day or clindamycin 450 mg PO four times per day to complete 14 days of treatment

IM/PO Antibiotic Treatment

- Ceftriaxone 250 mg IM in a single dose or cefoxitin 2 g IM and probenecid 1 g PO concurrently in a single dose *or* IV third-generation cephalosporin *plus* doxycycline 200 mg PO twice per day for 14 days *with* or *without* metronidazole PO twice per day for 14 days

IV, intravenous; *IM*, intramuscular; *PO*, by mouth.
Adapted from Centers for Disease Control and Prevention: Sexually transmitted diseases treatment guidelines, 2015, MMWR 64 (No. RR03):1-137, 2015.

- Patient unable to follow or tolerate outpatient oral regimen
- Severe illness, nausea, vomiting, or high fever present
- Tubo-ovarian abscess
- See Table 92.7 for treatment regimens for PID
- In any treatment setting, important things to consider:
  - All patients should be educated about the importance of completing the full 14-day course of antibiotics
  - IV therapy should be discontinued after 24 hours of clinical improvement. Therapy should continue with oral doxycycline to complete 14 days total of therapy.

- IV doxycycline should be avoided due to side effect of pain and venous sclerosis
- When treating severe PID or PID with tubo-ovarian abscess, clindamycin or metronidazole can be added to optimize anaerobic coverage
- All sex partners within 2 months of women diagnosed with PID require treatment for chlamydia and gonorrhea, regardless of patient's or partner's test results
- Male partners are often asymptomatic
- Nonsteroidal antiinflammatory drugs are recommended for abdominal pain or cramping during treatment
- Single dose of azithromycin (used for chlamydial cervicitis or urethritis) is not effective for treatment of PID
- Intrauterine devices have an increased risk of PID in the first 3 weeks after insertion. IUD does not need to be removed if PID diagnosed. Consideration can be given if no clinical improvement occurs within 48 to 72 hours of treatment
- Patients and partners should refrain from sexual intercourse until they have completed treatment and symptoms have resolved
- If baseline gonorrhea and chlamydia tests are positive, repeated screening for reinfection 3 to 6 months after treatment is recommended
- If symptoms of PID persist beyond 72 hours despite adequate treatment, consider evaluation for tubal-ovarian abscess (pelvic ultrasound)
- Treatment of Fitz-Hugh–Curtis is the same as for PID because right upper quadrant pain should resolve within 2 days of starting treatment

SEQUELAE

- Recurrence rates vary widely; at least one in five women will experience another episode
- PID is the most common cause of tubal factor infertility. Risk is higher in severe PID and with recurrence. Caution should be exercised when counseling an adolescent with PID because they may incorrectly assume they are unable to conceive after an episode of PID and not use effective contraception
- Ectopic pregnancy and chronic pelvic pain are risks after an episode of PID

Human Papillomavirus Infection (HPV)

BASIC INFORMATION

- Most common viral STD in the United States
- Most HPV infections are subclinical and asymptomatic
- HPV-6 and -11 cause 90% of warts (can be genital, nasal, oral, conjunctival, laryngeal)
- High-risk HPV types 16, 18, 31, 33, and 35 are most strongly associated with cervical neoplasia
- Same types also associated with anal neoplasia. Cause most cervical, penile, vulvar, vaginal, anal, and oropharyngeal cancers and precancers

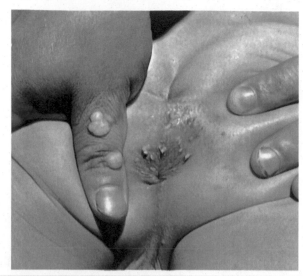

Fig. 92.8. Common warts of the hand in a mother and perianal condylomata acuminata in her son. (From Meneghini CL, Bonifaz E: *An atlas of pediatric dermatology*, Chicago, 1986, Year Book Medical Publishers, p. 44)

- Several HPV vaccines are available in the United States; a quadrivalent vaccine prevents infection with types 6, 11, 16, 18. A new 9-valent vaccine is available

CLINICAL PRESENTATION

- Most HPV infections are subclinical and asymptomatic
- Anogenital warts can be found on the penis, urethra, or rectum in males and on any genital mucosal surface in females. Lesions are painless (see Fig. 92.8)

DIAGNOSIS

- Based on visual inspection. Can use colposcopy, biopsy, acetic acid application (whitens lesions, making them easier to visualize), or laboratory tests
- Subclinical genital HPV infection tests (DNA, RNA) are not recommended for adolescents and women under age 30 due to the transient nature of the virus at younger ages

TREATMENT

- Treatment is not recommended for subclinical DNA, RNA detected infection
- Several HPV vaccines are available in the United States
    - Bivalent vaccine (Cervarix): prevents infections with HPV 16 and 18
    - Quadrivalent vaccine (Gardasil 4): protects against types 6, 11, 16, adn 18
    - A new 9-valent vaccine is available (Gardasil 9)
- Quadrivalent vaccine is approved for boys and girls aged 9 to 26. Bivalent vaccine is approved only for young women aged 9 to 26
- Cervical cancer screening remains necessary because not all cancer-causing HPV types are included in available vaccines

CERVICAL CANCER SCREENING

- Current guidelines from the American Cancer Society, U.S. Preventative Services Taskforce, and American College of Obstetrics and Gynecology recommend that cervical screening begin at age 21 years
    - This is because most HPV infections resolve in healthy adolescents
    - Screening in ages 21 to 29 should occur every 3 years. In certain circumstances (HIV, immunocompromised), Pap smears may be indicated in younger women
    - HPV DNA testing is not recommended as an adjunctive to Pap test—and **not** recommended for primary screening
    - All women, regardless of sexual orientation, should obtain cervical cancer screening

PROCTITIS

- Proctitis is inflammation limited to the rectum (distal 10–12 cm) and is associated with rectal pain, tenesmus, or rectal discharge. *N. gonorrhoeae, C. trachomatis, T. pallidum*, and HSV are most common sexually transmitted agents
    - Occurs most commonly among persons who participate in receptive anal intercourse. Treatment is ceftriaxone 250 mg IM in a single dose *plus* doxycycline 100 mg orally twice per day for 7 days

ECTOPARASITIC INFECTIONS

Pediculosis Pubis (Pubic Lice)

BASIC INFORMATION

- Presents with itching, or patient notes nits (eggs) in pubic hair
- Nits are yellow-white, shiny particles attached to hair shafts; lice are tan or grayish-white
- Transmitted by sexual contact
- Treatment with permethrin 1% cream rinse applied to affected areas and washed off after 10 minutes
    - Lindane 1% shampoo is no longer recommended

Scabies

BASIC INFORMATION

- Organism is Sarcoptes scabiei
- The main symptom of scabies is severe pruritus-Initially, the first time a person is infested it may take weeks to develop severe itching
- With subsequent exposures, symptoms typically begin more quickly, as early as 24 hours
- Scabies in adults is typically sexually acquired, while in children it is not

- Treatment for scabies is permethrin 5% cream to all areas of the body from the neck down, and wash off after 8 to 14 hours
- Sexual partners and close personal contacts within the last month should be examined and treated
- Decontamination of bedding and clothing recommended
- Itching and rash can persist up to 2 weeks after treatment

Review Questions

For review questions, please go to ExpertConsult.com.

Suggested Readings

1. Burstein G. Sexually transmitted infections. In: Kliegman RM, Stanton BF, St. Geme III JW, Schor N, Behrman R, eds. *Nelson Textbook of Pediatrics*. 20th ed. Philadelphia: Elsevier; 2016:985–995.e.
2. Centers for Disease Control and Prevention. *Sexually Transmitted Diseases Treatment Guidelines*; 2015. Available from: https://www.cdc.gov /std/tg2015/.
3. Kimberlin D, Baley J. Guidance on management of asymptomatic neonates born to women with active genital herpes lesions. *Pediatrics*. 2013;131(2):e635–e646.
4. Neinstein L, Katzman D, Callahan T. *Neinstein's Adolescent and Young Adult Health Care: A Practical Guide*. 6th ed. Philadelphia: Wolters Kluwer; 2016.
5. Soren K, Teplow-Phipps R, Potter J, Romo D. Adolescent Medicine. In: Polin R, Ditmar M, eds. *Pediatric Secrets*. 6th ed. Philadelphia: Elsevier; 2016.

Clinical Exam of Female Genital Tract

- Adolescent females may present with complaints in the pelvic or genital area which may or may not be related sexual activity. Most times, taking a thorough history including sexual history, menstrual history, vaginal hygiene practices, and performing an external genitourinary exam are sufficient for diagnosis.
- There are few times when a speculum or bimanual exam will be needed for diagnostic purposes.
  - A speculum exam is needed to place an IUD or to perform a Pap smear.
  - A bimanual exam is performed if evaluating for pelvic inflammatory disease to look for for signs of cervical motion tenderness, adnexal tenderness, or uterine tenderness.
- Patients do not need a pelvic exam to begin most forms of birth control, including combined oral contraceptive pills, the contraceptive patch, the vaginal ring, depot medroxyprogesterone, or a long-acting reversible contraceptive implant.

DISORDERS OF THE EXTERNAL GENITALIA

Vulvar Ulcers

BASIC INFORMATION

- Only *nonsexually* acquired genital ulcers will be covered here; see chapter 92 for clinical presentation, diagnosis, and treatment of sexually acquired acute genital ulcers
- Etiology and differential diagnosis
  - Sexually acquired
    - Genital herpes from herpes simplex virus (HSV) 1 or 2
    - Syphilis chancre from *Treponema pallidum*
    - Chancroid ulcer from *Haemophilus ducreyi*
    - Lymphogranuloma venereum from *Chlamydia trachomatis* serovars L1, L2, and L3
    - Donovanosis (also known as granuloma inguinale) caused by *Klebsiella granulomatis*
  - Nonsexually acquired
    - Aphthous ulcers ("Lipschütz ulcers")
    - Crohn disease
    - Behçet syndrome

- Epstein-Barr virus (EBV)
- Cytomegalovirus (CMV)
- Mycoplasma species

CLINICAL PRESENTATION

- Aphthous ulcers: may present on the vagina, labia minora, or labia majora. The patient may experience a viral-like illness in the days preceding the appearance of the ulcers, which develop a purple appearance before the surface begins to denude. This is a diagnosis of exclusion
- Genital ulcers associated with viral etiology including HSV (although HSV is usually sexually transmitted), EBV, or CMV:
  - Symptoms: prodromal symptoms with fever, vulvar pain, myalgias, lymphadenopathy, and headache
  - Physical signs: painful red or white lesions with sharply demarcated rims; base may be necrotic or eschar-appearing
- Ulcers associated with Crohn disease may present with asymmetric labial swelling and ulcers in the vagina or on the labia; ulcers may also be found inside the mouth
- Ulcers associated with Behçet syndrome may present with recurrent oral and genital ulcers; patients may also present with uveitis and arthritis

DIAGNOSIS AND EVALUATION

- Noninfectious ulcers are usually diagnosed by clinical presentation and physical examination (Fig. 93.1)
- Consider testing for causes of sexually acquired genital ulcers. May also consider CBC, EBV serology, CMV serology, mycoplasma testing, or HSV testing

TREATMENT

- Nonsexually acquired acute genital ulcers may be a single incident or they may be recurrent; symptoms usually resolve in 10 to 14 days per episode, although they may take up to 6 weeks to resolve
- Symptomatic treatment with sitz baths, acetaminophen, ibuprofen, or topical anesthetics
- Antibiotics may be considered for cellulitis or superinfection; also used in the treatment of sexually acquired ulcers
- Information regarding the use of topical steroids is lacking

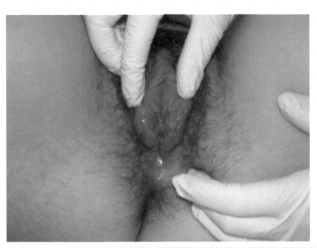

Fig. 93.1. Aphthous vulvar ulcer. (From Garcia, J. G., Pavon, B. M., Martin, L. M., Martinez, B. F., Norniella, C. M., & Caro F. A. Lipschütz ulcer: a cause of misdiagnosis when suspecting child abuse. *American Journal of Emergency Medicine, 34*(7), 1326.e1–1326.e2, Fig 2.)

Labial Adhesions

BASIC INFORMATION

- Can occur in up to 5% of prepubertal girls
- Labia minora fuses over the vaginal vestibule
- Related to lack of estrogen in prepubertal girls, may also be exacerbated by poor hygiene or diaper rash

CLINICAL PRESENTATION

- Usually asymptomatic
- Parent or patient may note that the vaginal opening appears covered
- If symptomatic, patient may experience vulvar irritation or urinary complaints

DIAGNOSIS AND EVALUATION

- Physical examination is sufficient for diagnosis; examiner should see a flat plane of labial tissue with a central vertical line at the area of adhesion; introitus may be partially or completely obstructed by the adhesion
- Manual separation of labial adhesions by the examiner should be avoided

TREATMENT

- Treatment is not necessary in asymptomatic cases; most labial adhesions will resolve spontaneously by puberty as a result of increased endogenous estrogen
- A small amount of estrogen cream may be used on the adhesions once or twice a day for 2 to 4 weeks

Imperforate Hymen

BASIC INFORMATION

- Most common obstructive anomaly of female reproductive tract
- Present at birth but may not be diagnosed until menarche

CLINICAL PRESENTATION

- May be present in the newborn period as a bulging introitus
- If not diagnosed in newborn period, may present at menarche with the following:
  - Hematocolpos (bulging blue-black membrane)
  - Pelvic or abdominal pain, which may be reported as cyclic
  - Amenorrhea
  - Normal secondary sex characteristics
  - Pelvic or abdominal distension

DIAGNOSIS AND EVALUATION

- Diagnosis usually made by physical examination on finding of hematocolpos
- Ultrasound or magnetic resonance imaging (MRI) may be helpful

TREATMENT

- Hematocolpos caused by imperforate hymen requires surgery to relieve the obstruction

Bartholin Gland Cysts

BASIC INFORMATION

- Bartholin glands are located bilaterally at the lower opening of the vagina; their function is to produce mucus and lubrication
- Bartholin gland ducts may become obstructed and form abscesses
- Infection may be caused by mixed vaginal flora or sexually transmitted bacteria

CLINICAL PRESENTATION

- Patients typically present with vulvar or vaginal pain from abscess formation at the Bartholin glands
- Abscesses present in the lower opening of the vagina at the 5 o'clock or 7 o'clock positions

DIAGNOSIS AND EVALUATION

- Diagnosis made by clinical examination
- Testing should be sent for chlamydia and gonorrhea

TREATMENT

- If small, may be treated with sitz baths, antibiotics, and hot compresses
- If large, needs to be drained with a Word catheter placed by a gynecologist

Sebaceous Glands

BASIC INFORMATION

- May be incidental finding along labia minora and labia majora; their function is to secrete lubrication in the genital skin

- May present as white, cream-colored, pink, yellow, or pigmented spots on the medial and lateral aspects of labia minora; may have "cobblestone" appearance
- Normal finding does not need treatment

Lichen Sclerosis

BASIC INFORMATION

- A chronic inflammatory skin disease; etiology is unknown, although thought to be autoimmune in nature
- Manifests in vulvar and perianal area
- Can occur at any age

CLINICAL PRESENTATION

- Itching, vulvar discomfort, dysuria
- Vulvar lesions with atrophic, light-colored, thickened skin; skin may appear shiny, smooth, or crinkled (Fig. 93.2)
- Symmetric fashion often with an hourglass configuration appearance

DIAGNOSIS AND EVALUATION

- Diagnosis made by visualization
- Occasionally by biopsy

TREATMENT

- Potent topical corticosteroids with close follow-up
- Occasionally surgery is needed to repair vulva and adhesions around the clitoris

Irritant Vulvovaginitis

BASIC INFORMATION

- Common in females
- May involve normal vaginal flora, enteric flora, *Streptococcus pyogenes* or other bacteria, or pinworms
- May be predisposed by poor hygiene, hot weather, or tight nonbreathable clothing

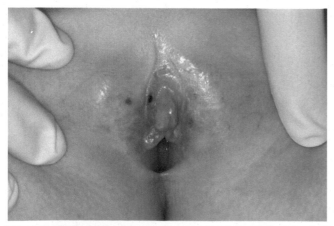

Fig. 93.2. Lichen sclerosis. (From Kliegman, R. M., Stanton, B. F., St Geme, J. W., & Schor, N. F. (Eds.), (2016). *Nelson textbook of pediatrics.* (20th ed.). Philadelphia: Elsevier, Fig 659-5.)

CLINICAL PRESENTATION

- Symptoms: pruritus, vulvar pain, dysuria
- Physical examination may reveal erythematous vulva or labial adhesions
- Vulva and perianal areas may have a "beefy red" appearance

DIAGNOSIS AND EVALUATION

- Usually a clinical diagnosis
- May evaluate for candida and pinworms
- Consider vaginal culture for *S. pyogenes* or other bacteria

TREATMENT

- Improvement with hygiene, sitz baths, and removal of tight clothing
- Occasionally can be treated with topical steroids
- Treat with antibiotics if *S. pyogenes* or other bacteria isolated
- Treat for pinworms if isolated

Infectious Vulvovaginitis

BASIC INFORMATION

- Most commonly caused by vulvovaginal candidiasis, trichomoniasis, and bacterial vaginosis (see Chapter 92)

DISORDERS OF THE UPPER GENITAL TRACT

Ovarian cysts

BASIC INFORMATION

- Etiology and differential diagnosis
  - Functional ovarian cysts are most common; they are benign and usually self-limited
    - Simple follicular cysts
    - Hemorrhagic corpus luteum cysts
    - Theca-lutein cyst
  - Ovarian tumors (benign or malignant):
    - Teratoma: mature and immature
    - Common "epithelial" tumors: mucinous, serous, mixed
    - Sex cord-stromal tumors: granulosa cell, thecoma, fibroma, Sertoli-Leydig
    - Endodermal sinus tumor
    - Dysgerminoma
    - Choriocarcinoma

CLINICAL PRESENTATION

- Functional ovarian cysts may be asymptomatic or may cause menstrual irregularities, pelvic pain, or urinary frequency
- Cysts may rupture; corpus luteum cysts in particular may cause intraabdominal hemorrhage
- Concern for torsion if in acute pain, nausea, and vomiting

DIAGNOSIS AND EVALUATION

- Pelvic ultrasound may determine size and nature of cyst (simple, complex, presence of septations, or hyperechoic)
- MRI of the pelvis may be considered
- Tumor markers may be sent if cyst does not appear to be a benign functional ovarian cyst (i.e., imaging appears to have complex nature to cyst): alpha-fetoprotein (AFP), CA-125, human chorionic gonadotropin (HCG), lactate dehydrogenase (LDH), and inhibin

TREATMENT

- Most functional ovarian cysts resolve spontaneously
- If cyst >6 cm in asymptomatic patient, may observe for resolution
- If >6 cm and symptomatic, then consultation to gynecology or pediatric surgery for cyst aspiration or cystectomy
- Consider starting a hormonal contraceptive to suppress ovulation to reduce future cysts from forming; examples include combined estrogen-progestin oral contraceptive pill, patch, vaginal ring, or depot medroxyprogesterone

Ovarian Torsion

BASIC INFORMATION

- Twisting of the ovary and/or fallopian tube with risk of occluding venous and arterial blood supply
- Often, but not always, associated with ovarian cyst

CLINICAL PRESENTATION

- Acute pelvic pain, nausea, and vomiting; pain may come in waves if having intermittent torsion
- Occurs more in ages 7 to 11
- More common on right side than left; may mimic acute appendicitis

DIAGNOSIS AND EVALUATION

- Pelvic ultrasound may show echogenic mass within the ovary
- "String of pearls" appearance caused by peripheral ovarian follicles (note that the term string of pearls is also used to describe polycystic ovarian syndrome (PCOS), which is unrelated to torsion)
- Doppler studies may show reduced blood flow

TREATMENT

- Urgent involvement of gynecology or pediatric surgery to detorse ovary with focus on conservation of the ovary
- Ovarian cystectomy if cyst involvement
- Prophylactic oophoropexy of the contralateral ovary should be considered to reduce risk of future ovarian torsion

Ectopic Pregnancy

BASIC INFORMATION

- Pregnancy implants outside of the uterus, usually in the fallopian tube
- Rupture can be life-threatening
- Risk factors: history of sexually transmitted diseases (STDs), pelvic inflammatory disease, endometriosis, prior ectopic pregnancy, previous pelvic surgery, and congenital pelvic abnormalities
- Past or current IUD are no longer considered increased risk for ectopic pregnancy

CLINICAL PRESENTATION

- Abdominal or pelvic pain
- Vaginal bleeding or spotting
- Nausea and vomiting
- Shock

DIAGNOSIS AND EVALUATION

- Serial serum β-HCG testing and transvaginal ultrasound
- Absence of intrauterine gestational sac on ultrasound at serum β-HCG above 1500 mIU/mL is highly suggestive of ectopic pregnancy
- A normal uterine pregnancy has mean doubling time of β-HCG of 1.4 to 2.1 days until day 41 of gestation; ectopic pregnancies and other nonviable pregnancies have slower rates of increase of β-HCG
- Evaluate for hemodynamic instability because a patient with a ruptured ectopic pregnancy can go into shock

TREATMENT

- Most women with ectopic pregnancies require surgery to remove the ectopic pregnancy and repair the fallopian tube
- An ectopic pregnancy detected early may be treated with methotrexate

Polycystic Ovarian Syndrome

BASIC INFORMATION

- Common among females
- Characterized by hyperandrogenism, irregular menstrual cycles, acne, hirsutism, and insulin resistance
- Patients have higher risk of developing type 2 diabetes mellitus and infertility than the general population
- Abnormal uterine bleeding is usually related to anovulatory state
- Irregular periods are also common in the normal child or adolescent in the first 2 years postmenarche

CLINICAL PRESENTATION

- Abnormal uterine bleeding: irregular periods, abnormally heavy or infrequent periods

Table 93.1.   Diagnostic Criteria for Polycystic Ovary Syndrome

National Institutes of Health Criteria	Rotterdam Criteria	Androgen Excess Society
■ Oligoovulation or anovulation *and* ■ Clinical or biochemical hyperandrogenism	Two of three of the following: ■ Oligoovulation or anovulation ■ Polycystic ovaries on ultrasonography (12 or more follicles in a single ovary or ovarian volume of >10 mm³ in one ovary) ■ Clinical and/or biochemical hyperandrogenism	Clinical or biochemical hyperandrogenism and at least one of the following: ■ Polycystic ovaries *or* ■ Oligoovulation or anovulation

From Kliegman, R. M., Stanton, B. F., St Geme, J. W., & Schor, N. F. (Eds.), (2016). *Nelson textbook of pediatrics*. (20th ed.). Philadelphia: Elsevier, Table 522-1.

- Skin: acne, hirsutism, acanthosis nigricans (sign of insulin resistance)
- A higher body mass index (BMI) is often characteristic, but PCOS may also present in patients with normal BMI

EVALUATION AND DIAGNOSIS

- Diagnosis is often made by clinical presentation based on history and physical examination findings
- Laboratory studies and ultrasound may be helpful in diagnosis
- Ultrasound may show characteristic string of pearls appearance around the ovaries
- See Table 93.1 regarding diagnostic guidelines according to National Institutes of Health (NIH), Rotterdam Criteria, and Androgen Excess Society
- Androgenic studies that may be helpful include free testosterone, dehydroepiandrosterone sulfate (DHEAS), and androstenedione
- Luteinizing hormone (LH)/follicle-stimulating hormone (FSH) is typically described as elevated with a >3:1 ratio, although clinically a normal midcycle LH surge may also manifest with an elevated LH/FSH ratio

TREATMENT

- First-line treatment would typically be a combined estrogen-progestin method (combined oral contraceptive pill, patch, or vaginal ring)
- Combined estrogen-progestin methods lower androgen levels and allow for more regularity of periods

- Must ensure no contraindications for estrogen use (history of venous thromboembolism, migraine with aura, lupus with antiphospholipid antibodies present, systolic blood pressure (SBP) ≥ 160 or diastolic blood pressure (DBP) ≥ 100)
- Exercise and improved nutrition can help with PCOS if patient is at a higher BMI
- Metformin may be added to improve insulin sensitivity and reduce hyperinsulinemia
- Spironolactone may be added for antiandrogenic effects
- Insulin sensitivity does not improve with combined oral contraceptive

Review Questions

For review questions, please go to ExpertConsult.com.

Suggested Readings

1. Berlan ED, Emans SJ, O'Brien RF. *"Vulvovaginal Complaints in the Adolescent."* Emans, Laufer: Pediatric and Adolescent Gynecology. 6th ed. Philadelphia: Lippincott Williams & Wilkins; 2012:305–324.
2. Emans SJ. *"Vulvovaginal Problems in the Prepubertal Child."* Emans, Laufer: Pediatric and Adolescent Gynecology. 6th ed. Philadelphia: Lippincott Williams & Wilkins; 2012:42–59.
3. Hoefgen HR, Merritt DF. *"Vulvovaginitis."* Kliegman, Stanton, St Geme, Schor: Nelson Textbook of Pediatrics. 20th ed. Philadelphia: Elsevier; 2016:2607–2613. e1.
4. Wolff M, Chuang JH, Mollen CJ. *"Gynecology Emergencies."* Fleisher and Ludwig's Textbook of Pediatric Emergency Medicine. 7th ed. Philadelphia: Lippincott Williams & Wilkins; 2016:784–803.

94 Selected Topics in Adolescent Medicine

JENNIFER H. CHUANG, MD, MS

In addition to progressing through the physical stages of puberty, adolescence is a time of maturation in cognition from concrete to abstract thinking. As adolescents begin to identify more with their peer group and establish independence from their parents, they also engage in increased experimentation, impulsivity, and risk taking behaviors. Thus caring for adolescents requires additional focused attention on the behavioral, social, and psychologic aspects of their well-being because these are likely to play a larger role in their overall health than organic diseases such as cancer or heart disease.

See also *Nelson Textbook of Pediatrics*, Part XIII, "Adolescent Medicine."

Causes of Adolescent Mortality

BASIC INFORMATION

- Unintentional injuries, suicide, and homicide comprise the top three causes of death in adolescents ages 15 to 19 years, accounting for more than two-thirds of deaths at this age
1. Unintentional injuries
   - Motor vehicle accidents
   - Poisonings including overdoses
   - Drowning
2. Suicide
   - Suffocation: hanging, asphyxiation
   - Firearms
   - Poisonings including overdoses
   - Females attempt suicide more than males, but males are more likely than females to die from suicide
3. Homicide
   - Majority by firearm
   - Although homicide is the third leading cause of death among teenagers 15 to 19 years, homicide is the leading cause of death for non-Hispanic black male teenagers

Psychologic Growth and Development

BASIC INFORMATION

- Generally divided into early, middle, and late phase (Table 94.1)
  - Each phase with biologic, cognitive, and psychosocial general characteristics
- Brain maturation and "pruning" of synaptic connections continues into the mid-20s

- The prefrontal cortex, the decision-making center of the brain, is among the last areas of the brain to mature
- Separation from parents is a hallmark of adolescent development
  - Increased importance of peer group
  - May seek other adult role models such as coaches, teachers, or friends' parents

Minors' Rights and Emancipation

BASIC INFORMATION

- In most cases, a parent or legal guardian must consent to medical care for the child; there are a few emergency exceptions to consent to treatment including the following:
  - Child is suffering from an emergent condition that places their life or health in danger
  - Treatment or transport cannot be safely delayed until consent from the legal guardian can be obtained
- In the United States, the details of a minor's right to consent varies state by state
- In many states, an emancipated minor may consent to their own medical treatment; a minor may be considered emancipated if they have met any of the following (details will vary by state):
  - Ever been married
  - On active-duty status in the military
  - Is a parent or is pregnant
  - Not living at home and is self-supporting themselves financially
  - In some states, a court needs to declare the minor emancipated
- Most states recognize that a minor may consent for certain medical services confidentially; ages and details will vary by state, but most include:
  - Testing and treatment for sexually transmitted infection, including HIV testing
  - Contraceptive services
  - Prenatal care
  - Mental health services
  - Substance abuse treatment
- Abortion laws vary state by state and include variability of the following:
  - Whether a minor requires parental consent or notification for abortion
  - Whether there is a mandatory waiting period for abortion
  - Fetal gestational age on which an abortion may be performed

Table 94.1.   Milestones in Early, Middle, and Late Adolescent Development

	Early Adolescence	**Middle Adolescence**	**Late Adolescence**
Approximate age range	10–13 years	14–17 years	18–21 years
Sexual maturity rating	1–2	3–5	5
Cognitive features	■ Concrete thinking ■ Egocentricity ■ Unable to perceive long-term outcome of current decisions ■ Follow rules to avoid punishment	■ Emergence of abstract thought ■ Sense of invulnerability ■ Growing ability to see others' perspectives	■ Abstract thinking ■ Future-oriented with sense of perspective ■ Improved impulse control ■ Able to distinguish law from morality
Self-concept/ identity formation	■ Self-consciousness about appearance and attractiveness	■ Concern with attractiveness ■ Increasing introspection	■ More stable body image ■ Consolidation of identity
Family	■ Increased need for privacy ■ Exploration of independence and boundaries	■ Conflicts over control and independence ■ Increased separation from the parents	■ Emotional and physical separation from family ■ Increased autonomy
Peers	■ Same-sex peer affiliations	■ Intense peer group Involvement ■ Conformity	■ Peer group recedes in intensity and importance
Sexual	■ Increased interest in sexual anatomy ■ Anxieties and questions about pubertal changes	■ Initiation of relationships and sexual activity ■ Questions of sexual orientation	■ Consolidation of sexual identity ■ Focus on intimacy and formation of stable relationships

Modified from Kliegman, R. M., Stanton, B. F., St Geme, J. W., & Schor, N.F. (Eds.). (2016). *Nelson textbook of pediatrics* (20th ed.). Philadelphia: Elsevier, p. 926–936. e1, Table 110-1.

Eating Disorders

BASIC INFORMATION

- Onset of eating disorders most commonly occurs during adolescence
- No single cause of eating disorders has been identified, although there are genetic predispositions
- Although most cases are diagnosed in females, eating disorders are underdiagnosed in males; most studies state that males account for 10% of eating disorders in the adolescent population, although some studies suggest that males account for a higher number
- Eating disorders are increasingly recognized in patients with a prior history of obesity
- With appropriate care, most adolescents diagnosed with an eating disorder have a good prognosis

Anorexia Nervosa

- Diagnostic and Statistical Manual of Mental Disorders (DSM)-5 criteria:
  - Restriction of energy intake relative to requirements
  - Intense fear of gaining weight, becoming fat, or persistent behavior that prevents weight gain
  - Distorted perception of body weight and shape
  - *There are no longer any absolute weight or amenorrhea criteria in DSM-5 for the diagnosis of anorexia nervosa*
- Subtypes
  - Anorexia nervosa restricting type
  - Anorexia nervosa binge-purge type
    - Typically the amount of calories in a binge in the anorexia nervosa binge-purge type is less than in bulimia nervosa because the amount of intake may appear to be a normal amount to an average person who does not have an eating disorder

- Lifetime prevalence of 0.5% to 2%, with a peak age of onset of 13 to 18 years
- Mortality rate at least 5% to 6% (some estimates say up to 10%), which is the highest mortality rate of any psychiatric illness
  - Approximately half of deaths are by suicide
- May begin as restriction of food groups and development of food rituals before restriction of calories is apparent to others

Bulimia Nervosa

- Recurrent episodes of binge eating; these episodes include eating more food in a period of time than most people would eat
- Episodes are coupled with a sense of loss of control and followed by compensatory purging behaviors such as self-induced vomiting, excessive exercise, or misuse of laxatives, diuretics, or other medication
- May be of any weight, often are normal weight or overweight
- DSM-5 criteria: objective binge episodes and subsequent compensatory behaviors at least once a week for 3 months

Binge-Eating Disorder

- Binge-eating disorder is distinguished from bulimia nervosa in that episodes of binge eating are not associated with inappropriate compensatory behaviors (purging)

Avoidant Restrictive Food Intake Disorder

- Comprises of restrictive eating behaviors that lead to physical and emotional impairment, but do not involve a fear of weight gain or distorted body image; they may start with a choking event, a swallowing phobia, or a textural aversion

CLINICAL PRESENTATION

- Weight loss, poor growth, not meeting pubertal milestones, amenorrhea, decreased libido, cold intolerance, lightheadedness, syncope, constipation
- Patients are frequently asymptomatic, even if weight loss has been profound
- Patients with severe purging may present with hematemesis, Mallory-Weiss tears, esophageal rupture, or pneumomediastinum
- Vital signs:
  - Bradycardia
  - Low blood pressure
  - Orthostatic heart rate (jump >20 beats/min from supine to standing) or orthostatic by blood pressure (drop in systolic or diastolic >10 mm Hg from supine to standing)
- Physical examination:
  - Skin: dry skin, thinning hair, lanugo, calluses on knuckles if self-induced vomiting
  - Head, eyes, ears, nose, and throat (HEENT): temporal wasting
    - If purging: parotic enlargement, dental enamel erosion, abrasion in posterior oropharynx
  - Musculoskeletal: prominent spinous processes, cold extremities, discolored toes
  - Refeeding syndrome may present with edema (e.g., face, extremities, sacral area); severe cases may have pulmonary edema or pericardial effusion
- Severe weight loss can cause superior mesenteric artery syndrome
- Gastroparesis is often seen in the setting of weight loss with disordered eating patterns, although it is not always clear whether the gastroparesis precedes the weight loss or is a result of it

DIAGNOSIS AND EVALUATION

- Differential diagnosis for workup of weight loss should include the following: hyperthyroidism, hypercortisolism, inflammatory bowel disease, celiac disease, HIV, malignancy
- Electrocardiogram (ECG) if profound weight loss and bradycardia; severe eating disorders may lead to arrhythmia from malnutrition or purging
- Electrolytes including potassium, magnesium, and phosphorus:
  - Hypokalemia, hypophosphatemia, and hypochloremia may be present if frequent self-induced vomiting
  - Refeeding syndrome may result in hypophosphatemia, hypokalemia, and hypomagnesemia (see later)
- Amylase levels may be elevated if purging from release of amylase from salivary glands; lipase levels are often, but not always, normal
- Endocrinopathies:
  - Thyroid studies may show a "sick euthyroid" picture with slightly elevated thyroid-stimulating hormone (TSH) and normal thyroxine or free thyroxine levels; treatment with levothyroxine is not indicated, and thyroid function tests normalize when patients return to normal weight

- Follicle-stimulating hormone (FSH), luteinizing hormone (LH), estrogen (females), and testosterone (males) levels may be low because of suppression of the hypothalamic-pituitary-gonadal axis; levels normalize when patients return to normal weight
  - Estrogen levels may be falsely reassuring in females on combined oral contraceptives that contain estrogen
- Risk of reduced bone mineral density
  - Recommend dual-energy x-ray absorptiometry (DEXA) bone density scan if amenorrhea × 6 months or long-standing poor growth
- Complete blood count (CBC):
  - Iron and B_{12} deficiencies may lead to anemia
  - Long-standing malnutrition may lead to bone marrow suppression

TREATMENT

- May need admission to hospital if patient has severe bradycardia (<45 beats/min), low blood pressure (systolic blood pressure [SBP] <90 mm Hg), syncope, electrolyte abnormalities, arrhythmias, intractable vomiting, hematemesis, suicide risk, or <75% ideal body weight (IBW) (for an adolescent, IBW is typically mBMI which would be the 50th percentile of BMI for age on the growth chart)
- Most adolescents diagnosed with an eating disorder are able to be treated in an outpatient setting
- The majority of children and adolescents with anorexia nervosa have a good outcome with family-based treatment (FBT) (also known as the Maudsley Method) in which the parent(s) oversees the meal planning and supervision; the parent is empowered to refeed their child back to health
  - The focus of FBT is not on the etiology of the disorder because there is no known one cause of eating disorders
- Other treatment models are individual therapy, cognitive behavioral therapy, and residential or inpatient eating disorder treatment
- No pharmacotherapies have been approved by the Food and Drug Administration (FDA) for the treatment of anorexia nervosa
- Some selective serotonin reuptake inhibitors (SSRIs) have been approved by the FDA for the treatment of bulimia nervosa

Refeeding Syndrome

BASIC INFORMATION

- Occurs after a prolonged period of starvation (at least 5–7 days) when the patient is reintroduced to food
- Body shifts metabolism from catabolic to anabolic state
- Reintroduction of calories leads to insulin release because the body uses phosphorus stores to make adenosine triphosphate (ATP)
- Hypophosphatemia is the hallmark laboratory abnormality, although hypokalemia and hypomagnesemia may also occur

- Fluid shifts may occur, causing edema in the face, lower back, and extremities
  - When refeeding syndrome is severe, it may cause pulmonary edema, pericardial effusion, congestive heart failure, and death
- To prevent refeeding syndrome, it is prudent to start calories low and increase calories slowly
- Electrolyte abnormalities, including hypophosphatemia, should be corrected with repletion

Substance Abuse

BASIC INFORMATION

- Initiation of drug use at an early age is a greater risk factor for addiction
- Drug use in adolescents may substitute for coping strategies and enhance vulnerability to poor decision-making
- First use of most drugs occur before age 18
- Many teens may experiment for months or years, but their drug use may not become recognized by a parent, teacher, or physician until they have negative consequences
- Protective factors include:
  - Emotionally supportive parents with open communication styles
  - Involvement in organized school activities
  - Having mentors or role models outside of the home
  - Recognizing the importance of academic achievement

Alcohol

BASIC INFORMATION

- Alcohol is the most popular drug among teenagers in the United States
- Binge drinking is associated with higher incidences of risky behaviors, academic problems, and assault
- Alcohol acts as a central nervous system (CNS) depressant by binding to gamma-aminobutyric acid (GABA) receptors in the brain
- Adolescents and young adults often drink alcohol mixed with caffeine in energy drinks; caffeine and other stimulants may mask the CNS depressant effects of the alcohol
- Inhibition of release of antidiuretic hormone from pituitary causes diuretic effect
- Rapidly absorbed in stomach and transported to liver
- Binge drinking (some variability with different surveys)
  - Males ≥5 drinks single occasion
  - Female ≥4 drinks single occasion

CLINICAL PRESENTATION

- Euphoria, impaired short-term memory
- Vasodilation, hypothermia
- Respiratory depression at high blood alcohol levels
- May also present as acute erosive gastritis or acute alcoholic pancreatitis
- Blood alcohol level
  - <0.01 to 0.1%: euphoria, mild deficits in coordination, attention, and cognition

- 0.1 to 0.2%: slurred speech, impaired judgment, ataxia
- 0.2 to 0.3%: confusion, nausea/vomiting, incoherent thoughts, lack of coordination
- 0.3 to 0.4%: stupor, loss of consciousness
- >0.4%: coma, respiratory depression, death

DIAGNOSIS AND EVALUATION

- May cause transaminitis with higher aspartate transaminase (AST) to alanine transaminase (ALT) ratio; with chronic use may progress to alcoholic fatty liver disease and cirrhosis
- Screening tools validated for use in adolescents
  - CRAFFT Questionnaire
    - Have you ever ridden in a CAR driven by someone (including yourself) who was "high" or had been using alcohol or drugs?
    - Do you ever use alcohol or drugs to RELAX, feel better about yourself, or fit in?
    - Do you ever use alcohol or drugs while you are by yourself, or ALONE?
    - Do you ever FORGET things you did while using alcohol or drugs?
    - Does your FAMILY or FRIENDS ever tell you that you should cut down on your drinking or drug use?
    - Have you ever gotten into TROUBLE while you were using alcohol or drugs?
  - AUDIT: Alcohol Use Disorders Identification Test
    - Ten-item questionnaire

TREATMENT

- Ventilation and supportive care
- Monitor for withdrawal if chronic alcohol use
  - Minor symptoms: insomnia, tremors, anxiety, gastrointestinal (GI) upset, loss of appetite, diaphoresis, palpitations
  - Severe withdrawal: seizures, hallucinations, delirium tremens, death
- Treat symptoms of withdrawal with benzodiazepines
- Referral for treatment of alcohol abuse

Tobacco

BASIC INFORMATION

- Average smoker in United States starts at age 12
- 90% of adolescent smokers become adult smokers
- Actions of nicotine, the addictive component of tobacco:
  - Acts through nicotinic acetylcholine receptors in the brain leading to increased levels of dopamine
  - Stimulates epinephrine release from the adrenal glands, causing elevations in heart rate and blood pressure
  - Cotinine, the major metabolite of nicotine, can be detected in urine, serum, and saliva
- Electronic cigarettes (e-cigarettes)
  - Battery-operated delivery system that heats and vaporizes nicotine
  - Vary in shapes and sizes, easy to disguise

- Nicotine in e-cigarettes may come in different flavors, which may be tempting to adolescents
- Has not been shown to be effective in smoking cessation among adolescents
- Smokeless tobacco
  - Increases risk for oral cancers of the mouth, pharynx, larynx, and esophagus, as well as gum disease and nicotine addiction

CLINICAL PRESENTATION

- Increased prevalence of chronic cough, sputum production, and wheezing
- Withdrawal symptoms: irritability, poor concentration, increased appetite, strong cravings
- Subtle scent or aroma of fruit, chemical, or perfume may be a sign of e-cigarette use
- Smoking during pregnancy is associated with a decreased fetal weight and increased perinatal morbidity and mortality

DIAGNOSIS AND EVALUATION

- Laboratory and imaging investigation for acute tobacco use are usually not clinically indicated

TREATMENT

- Nicotine replacement therapy may be considered (e.g., nicotine patch)
- Other medications, such as bupropion and varenicline, have not been FDA approved for use in adolescents for smoking cessation
  - Although varenicline has been used in adults, it may have side effects such as agitation, depressed mood, and suicidal ideation
  - Bupropion is contraindicated in patients with seizures because it lowers the seizure threshold

Marijuana

BASIC INFORMATION

- Most commonly abused illicit drug among adolescents
- Tetrahydrocannabinol (THC) is the main active chemical and is responsible for hallucinogenic properties
- Absorbed rapidly by smoking or vaping (peak 10 minutes)
- Oral ingestion has slower onset of absorption (peak 1 hour)
- Lipid soluble, accumulates in fatty tissues
  - Reaches peak concentrations in 4 to 5 days in fatty tissues
  - Half-life about 7 days
  - Complete elimination may take up to 30 days

CLINICAL PRESENTATION

- Euphoria, relaxation, increased appetite, impairment of short-term memory, poor coordination, distortion of time perception, visual hallucinations, "flashbacks" of hallucinations, dry mouth, anxiety symptoms

- Antiemetic effect for some
- Cannabis hyperemesis syndrome: typically seen with chronic use and includes nausea, vomiting, and abdominal pain; patients often say these improve with hot showers
- Vital signs: tachycardia, increased SBP, orthostatic hypotension
- Physical examination: conjunctival injection, dry mouth, ataxia

DIAGNOSIS AND EVALUATION

- THC may be present in urine drug screens for up to 2 weeks
- Urine drug screens do not quantify the level of intoxication and are of limited clinical value

TREATMENT

- Behavioral interventions, including cognitive-behavioral therapy and motivational incentives

Synthetic Marijuana

BASIC INFORMATION

- Names: "Spice", "K2", "crazy clown", "aroma", "black mamba", "blaze", "dream", "funky monkey"
- Second most common illicit drug used by high school seniors
- Mixture of herbs or plant materials that have been sprayed with artificial chemicals similar to THC
- Mainly used by smoking, mixed with marijuana, or brewed as a tea for drinking

CLINICAL PRESENTATION

- Euphoria, relaxation, altered perception
- Tachycardia, hypertension, mydriasis, diaphoresis, anxiety, seizures, delusions, aggression, vomiting, hyperthermia
- Rhabdomyolysis, acute kidney injury, and myocardial ischemia have been described

DIAGNOSIS AND EVALUATION

- Synthetic cannabinoids will not be detected in currently commercially available rapid urine drug screens
- Specialty laboratory tests are available to test for synthetic cannabinoids, but they do not return in a timely manner
- Clinical index of suspicion is needed to differentiate whether patient's symptoms are caused by synthetic cannabinoids and whether they were mixed with or without other substances

TREATMENT

- Acute intoxication
  - Agitation and psychosis may respond to a quiet dimly lit room
  - Benzodiazepines may be needed if severely agitated

Inhalants

BASIC INFORMATION

- "Huffing," "sniffing," "bagging"
- Group of volatile vapors that can be inhaled
- Popular among younger adolescents
- Examples: paint thinners, glue, spray paint, hair spray, propane tanks, lighter fluid, nitrous oxide, nitrites "poppers," propellers in whipped cream dispensers, computer cleaning aerosol cans

CLINICAL PRESENTATION

- Euphoria, slurred speech, decreased coordination, dizziness, headache, syncope
- Coma may result from prolonged or rapid inhalation
- Vital signs: hypotension, tachycardia
- Physical examination:
  - Chemical odors on breath, skin, or clothes
  - Cutaneous flushing, "glue-sniffer's rash" around perioral area

DIAGNOSIS AND EVALUATION

- Diagnosis may be difficult because of common availability of products
- Toluene, which is present in some inhalants, may be detectable as hippuric acid in urine in specialized laboratory tests
- Toluene may cause hypokalemia and metabolic acidosis
- Halogenated inhalants may cause liver or renal impairment
- ECG to evaluate for arrhythmias

TREATMENT

- Supportive care
- Withdrawal symptoms do not usually occur

Hallucinogens

BASIC INFORMATION

- Lysergic acid diethylamide (LSD) and methylenedioxymethamphetamine (MDMA) are the most common (see section regarding phencyclidine [PCP])
  - Exact mechanisms of action are unclear, but hallucinogens have serotonergic activity
  - LSD and MDMA have been implicated in serotonin syndrome
- LSD
  - Made from lysergic acid found in ergot, a fungus that grows on grains
  - May be ingested as a liquid or tablet or licked from absorbent paper
- MDMA: 'X', 'Ecstasy', 'Molly'
  - Ingested as tablets

CLINICAL PRESENTATION

- LSD
  - Distortions in vision, time, and perception
  - Anxiety, panic, flashbacks
  - Tachycardia, hypertension, mydriasis, diaphoresis
- MDMA
  - Euphoria, heightened sensual awareness
  - Jaw clenching, teeth grinding
  - Anxiety, psychosis
  - Hyperthermia
  - Confusion, seizures from hyponatremia by drinking large amounts of water at "raves"

DIAGNOSIS AND EVALUATION

- Electrolytes to evaluate for hyponatremia
- Liver function tests (LFTs) to evaluate for hepatic injury
- Creatine kinase (CK) and urine myoglobin if suspect rhabdomyolysis

TREATMENT

- Usually supportive care in a calm environment is sufficient in mild intoxication
- Manage complications of hyponatremia if present

Phencyclidine

BASIC INFORMATION

- Synthetic hallucinogen with properties similar to ketamine
- Tablet, liquid, powder: "angel dust," "dust," "peace pill," "whack," "hot," "sherm"
- When mixed with marijuana, may be called "wet," "fry," "super weed," "killer weed"
- Mechanism of action
  - Acts on N-methyl-D-aspartate (NMDA) receptors: produces acute psychosis, agitation, seizures
  - Inhibits reuptake of dopamine, norepinephrine, and serotonin
    - Causes adrenergic effects: tachycardia, hypertension
    - Causes dopaminergic effects: dystonia, choreoathetosis, anticholinergic findings
  - Binds to sigma receptor, causing psychotic, anticholinergic, and movement abnormalities

CLINICAL PRESENTATION

- Aggressive behavior, staring spells, altered mental status, agitation
- Muscle rigidity, seizures, rhabdomyolysis
- Vital signs: irregular breathing, tachycardia
- Eye findings: horizontal, vertical, or rotary nystagmus
- Duration of action typically brief (resolved within 4–8 hours)

DIAGNOSIS AND EVALUATION

- Laboratory evaluation:
  - Serum CK and urine myoglobin to evaluate for rhabdomyolysis
  - LFTs may be elevated
- Urine toxicology
  - PCP may remain positive for several weeks
  - The following drugs may give a false positive for PCP in the urine drug screen:
    - Ketamine, dextromethorphan, diphenhydramine, venlafaxine, lamotrigine, and tramadol

TREATMENT

- Place in a dark quiet room, remove dangerous objects from room
- Supportive care is the usual treatment, although benzodiazepines may be helpful if patient is very agitated

Cocaine

BASIC INFORMATION

- Extracted from coca plant
- May be smoked, snorted, injected, or ingested
- Crack is crystallized rock form of cocaine that is smoked
- Stimulates alpha-1, alpha-2, beta-1, and beta-2 adrenergic receptors through increased levels of norepinephrine (and to some extent epinephrine)

CLINICAL PRESENTATION

- Euphoria, increased alertness
- Loss of sense of smell if chronic snorting of cocaine
- Nosebleeds, chronic rhinorrhea
- Vital signs: hyperthermia, hypertension, tachycardia
- Physical examination:
  - Pupillary dilation
  - Pharyngeal edema and angioedema may occur when smoking crack cocaine
  - Track marks on arms if intravenous (IV) drug use
- Severe intoxication may cause coronary ischemia and/or stroke
- Pregnant patients who use cocaine are at risk of premature delivery, low birthweight, and developmental disorders

DIAGNOSIS AND EVALUATION

- ECG and troponins may show signs of ischemia caused by coronary vasoconstriction
- Cocaine is detectable in rapid urine drug screens

TREATMENT

- Beta-blockers should be avoided because of concerns of unopposed alpha-adrenergic stimulation, thus exacerbating coronary artery vasoconstriction and hypertension

Methamphetamine, Amphetamines

BASIC INFORMATION

- "Crystal meth," "meth," "ice"
- Injected, ingested, inhaled, smoked, absorbed through mucous membranes
- Stimulates dopamine, norepinephrine, epinephrine, and serotonin

CLINICAL PRESENTATION

- Agitation, psychosis
- Tachycardia, arrhythmia, hypertension, hyperthermia
- Seizures
- Mydriasis, diaphoresis
- Metabolic acidosis, hyperkalemia

DIAGNOSIS AND EVALUATION

- Although urine drug screen may be positive, specialized laboratory screens may be time intensive; treatment should not be delayed while waiting for results
- CK if suspect rhabdomyolysis
- Electrolytes to evaluate for metabolic acidosis, hyperkalemia, and kidney injury

TREATMENT

- Benzodiazepines may be used for aggression

Opiates

BASIC INFORMATION

- Heroin, morphine, fentanyl, methadone, oxycodone
- Originally derived from poppy plant
- Activates mu receptors
- Injected, snorted/sniffed, ingested, smoked

CLINICAL PRESENTATION

- Acute intoxication:
  - Sedated ("nodding")
  - Slurred speech
  - Miosis
  - Track marks on arms if IV drug use
  - Constipation
  - Respiratory depression, coma, death
- Withdrawal (typically >8 hours after use)
  - Yawning, mydriasis, diarrhea, tachycardia, hypertension, lacrimation

DIAGNOSIS AND EVALUATION

- Opioids may be positive in urine drug screens but do not measure level of intoxication

TREATMENT

- Acute intoxication: naloxone (opioid antagonist)
- Treatment for opioid addiction
  - Methadone
  - Buprenorphine ± naloxone
- Acute opioid withdrawal
  - Tachycardia, hypertension, diarrhea, vomiting
  - Clonidine may be used in acute opioid withdrawal

Bath Salts

BASIC INFORMATION

- "Ivory wave," "cloud nine," "vanilla sky"
- White or brown crystalline powder that can be inhaled, ingested, or injected
- Contain cathinone, an amphetamine analog
- Raises dopamine, norepinephrine, and serotonin levels

CLINICAL PRESENTATION

- Euphoria, aggressive behavior, panic attacks, psychosis, hallucinations
- Tachycardia, hyperthermia, hypertension, chest pain, diaphoresis

DIAGNOSIS AND EVALUATION

- Bath salts do not show up in standard urine drug screens
- Specialized laboratory may be available, but results do not return rapidly
- Treatment should be based on clinical index of suspicion that the patient has used bath salts

TREATMENT

- Supportive care
- Benzodiazepines may be helpful in the event of seizures

Suggested Readings

1. Burstein GR. Delivery of healthcare to adolescents. In: Kliegman RM, Stanton BF, St Geme JW, Schor NF, eds. *Nelson Textbook of Pediatrics.* 20th ed. Philadelphia: Elsevier; 2016:939–944.e2.
2. Campbell K, Peebles R. Eating disorders in children and adolescents: state of the art review. *Pediatrics.* 2014;134:582–592.
3. Kliegman RM, Stanton BF, St. Geme JW, Schor NF. Adolescent development. In: Kliegman RM, Stanton BF, St Geme JW, Schor NF, eds. *Nelson Textbook of Pediatrics.* 20th ed. Philadelphia: Elsevier; 2016:9260936.e1.
4. Kreipe RE. Eating disorders. In: Kliegman RM, Stanton BF, St Geme JW, Schor NF, eds. *Nelson Textbook of Pediatrics.* 20th ed. Philadelphia: Elsevier; 2016:162–170.e1.
5. Stager MM. Substance abuse. In: Kliegman RM, Stanton BF, St Geme JW, Schor NF, eds. *Nelson Textbook of Pediatrics.* 20th ed. Philadelphia: Elsevier; 2016:947–962.e2.
6. **The Alan Guttmacher Institute: An Overview of Minors' Consent Laws. Updated June 1, 2018.** https://www.guttmacher.org/state-policy/explore/overview-minors-consent-law

95 Selected Topics in Prenatal Medicine and Obstetrics

ADAM BONNINGTON

PREGNANCY

Screening Tests

- Pregnant patients are routinely screened for several infections (or history of infections) throughout pregnancy; the most commonly screened agents include:
  - HIV, syphilis, gonorrhea, chlamydia
  - Hepatitis B
  - Rubella immunity (i.e. serologies)
  - Varicella immunity (i.e. serologies)
  - Group B *Streptococcus* (GBS)
    - Screened for in third trimester
    - Determines whether mothers are provided with intrapartum antibiotics to decrease the risk of early-onset sepsis in newborns
- Pregnant patients are also tested for blood type and Rhesus (Rh) factor because these help determine the risk for maternal alloimmunization and/or ABO incompatibility in the newborn
- Pregnant patients undergo routine screenings for certain fetal chromosomal abnormalities and throughout pregnancy by using serum markers and ultrasound measurements (Table 95.1)
  - First trimester screening
    - Collected at 10 to 13 weeks' gestation
    - Includes plasma protein A (PAPP-A), β-human chorionic gonadotropin (hCG), and ultrasound assessment of nuchal translucency (NT)
  - Second trimester screening (i.e., "Quad Screen")
    - Collected at 15 to 20 weeks' gestation
    - Includes maternal serum alpha-fetoprotein (MSAFP), estriol, hCG, and inhibin
  - Noninvasive prenatal screening (i.e., "cell-free DNA" [cfDNA])
    - Collected at >10 weeks' gestation from mothers with specific indications (e.g., advanced maternal age)
    - Circulating cfDNA from fetus or placenta is isolated from maternal blood
    - Screens for trisomy 21 (Down syndrome), trisomy 18, trisomy 13, and sex chromosome aneuploidies

Genetic Diagnostic Procedures

- For certain indications (e.g., positive genetic screens), pregnant mothers may undergo additional diagnostic testing that offers increased specificity for genetic abnormalities

- Chorionic villus sampling (CVS)
  - Performed at 10+ week's gestation
  - Sample of chorionic villi (immature placenta) transcervically or transabdominally under ultrasound guidance
- Amniocentesis
  - Performed at 15 to 20 week's gestation
  - Sample of amniotic fluid transabdominally under ultrasound guidance

Ultrasounds in Pregnancy

- Pregnant mothers undergo multiple ultrasounds throughout pregnancy, each with a specific purpose
- Dating ultrasound
  - Performed at the first prenatal visit to confirm viability and establish estimated date of delivery
- NT
  - Performed between 10 and 13 weeks' gestation
  - Measures thickness of the lucent area behind the head in the nuchal region
  - Used as a screening marker for some genetic disorders
- Second and third trimester ultrasounds
  - Basic examination includes assessment of fetal number, fetal biometry, fetal presentation, placenta appearance and location, amniotic fluid volume, survey of fetal anatomy, and maternal anatomy
  - Limited examination used to address specific focused questions (e.g., fetal cardiac activity, fetal position, fetal biometry, cervical length, amniotic fluid volume)
  - Detailed examination assesses fetal anatomy

Assessment of Fetal Well-Being

- Nonstress test (NST)
  - Monitoring of fetal heart rate for a 20-minute period
  - Reactive tests have two or more fetal heart rate accelerations and provide evidence of normal fetal oxygenation
  - Nonreactive tests may be a sign of poor fetal oxygenation and metabolic acidemia
- Contraction stress test (CST)
  - Assessment of fetal heart rate in the setting of uterine contractions at a frequency of three per 10 minutes
  - Positive tests (nonreassuring) have late decelerations after >50% of contractions and may indicate fetal hypoxemia
  - Negative tests have no late decelerations or significant variable decelerations

Table 95.1. Maternal Serum Marker Screening Patterns

Genetic Disorder	First Trimester Screening			Second Trimester Screening			
	NT	PAPP-A	β-hCG	AFP	Estriol	hCG	Inhibin A
Trisomy 21	↑↑	↓↓	↑	↓	↓	↑	↑
Trisomy 18	↑↑	↓↓	↓↓	↓↓	↓↓	↓↓	↔
Trisomy 13	↑	↓↓	↓	↔	↔	↔	↔

AFP, Alpha-fetoprotein; *hCG*, human chorionic gonadotropin; *NT*, nuchal translucency; *PAPP-A*, plasma protein A.

- Biophysical profile (BPP)
  - Assesses five parameters over a 30-minute period, each given a score of 0 points or 2 points
    - Fetal movement: 2 points for 3+ discrete body or limb movements
    - Fetal tone: 2 points for one episode of fetal extremity or spine extension and flexion
    - Fetal breathing: 2 points for rhythmic breathing >30 seconds
    - Amniotic fluid volume: 2 points for deepest vertical pocket >2 cm
    - NST: 2 points if reactive
  - Normal result is 10/10 or 8/10 (−2 points for fetal movement, tone, or breathing)
    - Risk of fetal death within 1 week is low
  - Abnormal result is 0 to 4/10
    - Risk of fetal asphyxia within 1 week is elevated and delivery usually indicated
- Doppler ultrasound of umbilical artery
  - Provides noninvasive measure of fetoplacental hemodynamic state
  - Abnormal Dopplers (i.e., elevated ratio of peak systolic frequency shift to end-diastolic frequency shift) associated with fetal hypoxia, fetal acidosis, and adverse perinatal outcomes

Ultrasound Diagnosis of Fetal Conditions

- Pediatricians should be aware of certain ultrasound diagnoses because they are associated with certain fetal and maternal risk factors that may complicate the pregnancy, delivery, and postnatal course
- Intrauterine growth restriction (IUGR)
  - Estimated fetal weight <10th percentile
  - Fetal risk factors include genetic abnormalities, structural anomalies, infection, multiple gestation, single umbilical artery, velamentous umbilical cord insertion
  - Maternal risk factors include conception via assisted reproductive technologies, poor weight gain, short interpregnancy interval, extremes of maternal age, abnormal serum analytes, preeclampsia, placenta abruption, medical comorbidities, and exposure to teratogens
  - Complications for neonate include preterm delivery, perinatal asphyxia, impaired thermoregulation, hypoglycemia, polycythemia, impaired immune function, death

- Macrosomia
  - Estimated fetal weight >4500 g (9 pounds 15 ounces)
  - Risk factors include obesity, multiparity, advanced maternal age, postterm pregnancy, previous macrosomic infant, excessive weight gain, male infant sex
  - Complications for neonate include birth trauma from shoulder dystocia, hypoglycemia, respiratory problems, polycythemia
- Single umbilical artery
  - Risk factors include fetal genetic anomalies, maternal smoking, diabetes, hypertension, and seizure disorder
  - Complications may include preterm delivery, growth restriction, perinatal mortality, neonatal intensive care unit admission
- Oligohydramnios
  - Amniotic fluid index <5 cm or deepest vertical pocket <2 cm
  - Risk factors include preeclampsia, placenta abruption, twin-to-twin transfusion syndrome (TTTS), fetal chromosomal and congenital abnormalities, growth restriction, intrauterine fetal demise (IUFD), postterm pregnancy, rupture of membranes
  - Timing of delivery based on etiology
- Polyhydramnios
  - Amniotic fluid index >25 cm or deepest vertical pocket >8cm
  - Risk factors include fetal chromosomal and congenital abnormalities, maternal diabetes, multiple gestation, TTTS, fetal anemia, fetal infection
  - Timing of delivery variable by institution
- IUFD
  - Incidence approximately 6/1000 births
  - Typically caused by decreased fetal swallowing or increased fetal urination
  - Risk factors include maternal medical disorders, nulliparity, cigarette smoking, obesity, advanced maternal age, black race, previous stillbirth, recreational drug use, conception via assisted reproductive technology

Multifetal Gestation

BASIC INFORMATION

- There are several types of multifetal gestations determined by the relationship of the amniotic sac(s) and placenta(s):
  - Diamniotic/dichorionic
    - Separate amniotic sacs and placentas
  - Diamniotic/monochorionic
    - Separate amniotic sacs but shared placenta
  - Monoamniotic/monochorionic
    - Shared placenta and amniotic sac
  - Conjoined twins
    - Shared placenta and amniotic sac with incomplete separation during embryo formation
- Risks associated with multifetal gestation
  - Growth restriction
  - Congenital anomalies
  - Preterm delivery
- TTTS
  - Occurs in monochorionic pregnancies

- Caused by imbalanced fetoplacental blood flow in the shared placental circulation
- Leads to hypovolemia in the donor twin and hypervolemia in the recipient twin, which can cause cardiovascular changes in response to volume changes
- Complications include severe cardiac, neurologic, and developmental disorders and high risk of fetal/neonatal mortality

Fetal Exposures during Pregnancy

- Some medications may cause harmful effects on the fetus and should be avoided
  - The quality of available evidence of the fetal effects of specific drugs allows for categorization of risk factor as A, B, C, D, or X (Table 95.2)
  - Table 95.3 provides an overview of commonly prescribed drugs and their teratogenic effects

Table 95.2. US Food and Drug Administration Classification for Medications in Pregnancy and Breastfeeding

Risk Factor Category	Description
A	Controlled human studies show no evidence of risk
B	Animal studies show no evidence of risk, but no adequate and controlled human studies have been conducted *or* Animal studies do show adverse effect, but no evidence of risk in adequate and controlled human studies
C	Animal studies do show adverse effect and there are no adequate or controlled human studies *or* No animal studies have been conducted and no adequate and human studies have been conducted
D	Human studies have demonstrated risk, although benefits of therapy may outweigh the potential risk
X	Human studies have demonstrated risk; the risk of the product is contraindicated in women who are or may become pregnant

Table 95.3. Teratogenicity of Various Medications

Drug	Effect	Timing of Exposure
ACE inhibitors	Fetal hypotension resulting in fetal kidney hypoperfusion and anuria, oligohydramnios, pulmonary hypoplasia, cranial bone hypoplasia, and fetal growth restriction and demise Neonatal oliguria, anuria, hypotension, and renal tubular dysgenesis	Second and third trimester
Androgens	Full masculinization, including labial fusion Partial masculinization, including clitoral hypertrophy	7–12 weeks >12 weeks
Beta-blockers	Fetal growth restriction, neonatal hypoglycemia, transient mild hypotension	Second and third trimester
Carbamazepine	Facial dysmorphology, neural tube defects, cardiovascular defects, urinary tract defects	First trimester
Cyclophosphamide	Missing or hypoplastic digits of the hands and feet	First trimester
Danazol	Clitoromegaly, urogenital sinus malformation, labioscrotal fusion, vaginal atresia, ambiguous genitalis	Throughout pregnancy
Isotretinoin	Spontaneous abortion, premature birth, birth defects (facial, eye, ear, skull, central nervous system, cardiovascular, thymus, and parathyroid gland), intellectual disability, fetal death	Throughout pregnancy
Lithium	Cardiovascular malformations (e.g., Ebstein anomaly)	First trimester
Methotrexate	Growth restriction, severe limb abnormalities, posteriorly rotated ears, micrognathia, hypoplastic supraorbital ridges, intellectual disability	First trimester
Nitrofurantoin	Hemolytic anemia in women with G6PD deficiency	Third trimester
Phenobarbital	Neonatal withdrawal with seizures, hyperirritability, respiratory depression	Third trimester
Phenytoin	Orofacial clefts, cardiac defects, dysmorphic facial features, nail/digit hypoplasia, microcephaly, mental deficiency	Throughout pregnancy
Pseudoephedrine	Gastroschisis	First trimester
Quinolones	Arthropathies and cartilage erosion	Evidence in animal studies only
Radiation	Microcephaly, growth retardation, intellectual disability (at higher doses)	Fust trimester
SSRIs	Neonatal behavioral syndrome with increased muscle tone, irritability, jitteriness, and respiratory distress	Third trimester
Paroxetine	Ventral and atrial septal cardiac defects	First trimester
Sulfonamides	Hyperbilirubinemia	Second and third trimester
Testosterone and anabolic steroids	Virilization (labioscrotal fusion, phallic enlargement)	Throughout pregnancy
Tetracyclines	Bone and teeth staining	Second and third trimester
Thiazide diuretics	Thrombocytopenia with associated bleeding and electrolyte disturbances	Close to delivery
Valproic acid	Spina bifida, facial dysmorphology, autism, atrial septal defect, cleft palate, hypospadias, polydactyly, craniosynostosis, limb abnormalities	First trimester
Warfarin	Warfarin embryopathy with nasal and midface hypoplasia with stippled vertebral and femoral epiphyses Hemorrhage-related abnormalities (e.g., hydrocephalus), growth restriction	6–9 weeks Second and third trimester

ACE, Angiotensin-converting enzyme; *SSRI,* selective serotonin reuptake inhibitor.

Table 95.4.   Pregnancy Complications Associated with Selected Substances

Substance	Effect on Pregnancy
Opioids	Placenta abruption, IUFD, intraamniotic infection, IUGR, preeclampsia, PPROM, placental insufficiency, postpartum hemorrhage, septic thrombophlebitis
Cocaine	Preterm birth, low birthweight, small for gestational age, shorter gestational age, reduced birth weight
Amphetamines	Growth restriction, gestational hypertension, preeclampsia, abruption, preterm birth, IUFD, neonatal death, infant death
Tobacco	Miscarriage, IUFD, neonatal death, PPROM, reduced birth weight, placental abruption, placenta previa, preterm birth, congenital malformations (cleft lip, gastroschisis, anal atresia, transverse limb reduction defects, cardiac defects, digital anomalies, bilateral renal agenesis or hypoplasia), preeclampsia
Alcohol	IUFD, fetal alcohol spectrum disorder (hypoplastic midface, epicanthal folds, decreased interpupillary distance, flat nasal bridge, altered palmar crease, fifth finger clinodactyly, long philtrum)

IUFD, Intrauterine fetal demise; *IUGR,* intrauterine growth restriction; *PPROM,* preterm, premature rupture of membranes.

Table 95.5.   Embryonic and Fetal Infections

Infection	Effect	Timing of Exposure
Cytomegalovirus	Retinopathy, CNS calcification, microcephaly, intellectual disability	First 6 months
Herpes simplex	Fetal infection, liver disease, death	Throughout pregnancy
HIV	Perinatal HIV infection	Throughout pregnancy
Parvovirus infection, B19	IUFD, hydrops	Up to 20 weeks
Rubella	Deafness, congenital heart disease, microcephaly, cataracts, intellectual disability	Up to 16 weeks
Syphilis	Maculopapular rash, hepatosplenomegaly, deformed nails, osteochondritis at joints of extremities, congenital neurosyphilis, abnormal epiphyses, chorioretinitis	Throughout pregnancy
Toxoplasmosis	Hydrocephaly, microphthalmia, chorioretinitis, intellectual disability	Throughout pregnancy
Varicella zoster	Skin and muscle defects, IUGR, limb reduction defects, CNS damage	First trimester

CNS, Central nervous system; *HIV,* human immunodeficiency virus; *IUFD,* intrauterine fetal demise; *IUGR,* intrauterine growth restriction.

- Similarly, some drugs of abuse may also affect the fetus (Table 95.4)
- Maternal infections may produce untoward effects on the fetus (Table 95.5)
- Maternal medical history may also have significant effects on the fetus (Table 95.6)

Table 95.6.   Teratogenicity of Maternal Diseases

Disease	Effect
Iodine deficiency	Goiter, intellectual disability
Diabetes	Spontaneous abortion, congenital anomalies (cardiac, CNS, renal, limb, sacral agenesis), macrosomia, polyhydramnios, neonatal hypoglycemia
Folic acid deficiency	Neural tube defects
Malnutrition	Spontaneous abortion, neural tube defects, IUGR
Hyperthyroidism	Spontaneous abortion, preterm labor, low birth weight, IUFD, preeclampsia, heart failure (maternal)
Hypothyroidism	Gestational hypertension/preeclampsia, placental abruption, preterm delivery, low birth weight, postpartum hemorrhage, neuropsychological and cognitive impairment in the child
Systemic lupus erythematosus	Preeclampsia, preterm birth, fetal death, IUGR, neonatal lupus

CNS, Central nervous system; *IUFD,* Intrauterine fetal demise; *IUGR,* intrauterine growth restriction.

Neonatal Abstinence Syndrome

BASIC INFORMATION

- Associated primarily with opioid use, but also nicotine; effects can be worsened by concurrent use of cigarettes, benzodiazepines, and selective serotonin reuptake inhibitors (SSRIs)
- Thought to be caused by altered levels of neurotransmitters (e.g., norepinephrine, dopamine, serotonin)
- Clinical manifestations include high-pitched cry/irritability, sleep/wake disturbances, alterations in tone or movement, feeding difficulties, gastrointestinal disturbances, autonomic dysfunction, failure to thrive
- Treatment regimens generally require establishing an effective opiate dose to prevent withdrawal after birth, followed by a prolonged taper

Alloimmunization

BASIC INFORMATION

- Rh D-negative pregnant woman who are exposed to fetal D-positive red cells are at risk for developing anti-D antibodies
- Risk factors include spontaneous or induced abortion, invasive prenatal diagnostic or therapeutic procedures (e.g., CVS, amniocentesis, fetal blood sampling, fetoscopy/fetoscopic surgery, multifetal reduction), abdominal trauma, external cephalic version, ectopic pregnancy, threatened abortion, IUFD, antepartum hemorrhage
- Risk of alloimmunization decreased with administration of anti-D immune globulin
- Can cause hemolytic disease leading to severe fetal anemia in Rh-positive fetuses and hydrops fetalis
- Severe fetal anemia is monitored with monthly indirect Coombs titers; once critical titer is reached, Doppler velocimetry is used to assess for fetal anemia; fetuses with evidence of severe anemia can be managed with intrauterine fetal transfusions (<35 weeks) or delivery (>35 weeks)

Postterm Pregnancy

BASIC INFORMATION

- Pregnancy lasting 42 weeks' gestation or beyond
- Effects include:
  - Macrosomia: associated with increased risk of birth trauma
    - Shoulder dystocia
    - Clavicle fracture
    - Brachial plexus injury
      - Erb-Duchenne palsy: injury to C5 and C6 causes limb to hang limply close to the side, with forearm extended and internally rotated
      - Klumpke paralysis: injury to C8 and T1 causes paralysis of the hand
  - Meconium aspiration syndrome (see Chapter 75)
  - Dysmaturity syndrome
  - Oligohydramnios

LABOR AND DELIVERY

Fetal Heart Rate Monitoring

- Baseline
  - Normal 110 to 160 beats/min, assessed over a 10-minute interval
  - Tachycardia is >160 beats/min
    - Can be caused by chorioamnionitis, maternal fever, thyrotoxicosis, medication, fetal cardiac arrhythmias
  - Bradycardia is <110 beats/min
- Variability
  - Fluctuations in the baseline
  - Minimal (<5 beats/min), moderate (5–25 beats/min), marked (25 beats/min)
  - Moderate variability reflects adequate fetal oxygenation and normal brain function
- Accelerations
  - Abrupt increase in fetal heart rate
  - Should be 15 beats above baseline and last for 15 seconds for gestational age (GA) >32 weeks
- Decelerations
  - Early decelerations: nadir coincides with peak of contraction; this is thought to be caused by pressure on the fetal head; physiologic, not a cause of concern
  - Late decelerations: nadir occurs after peak of contraction; this is thought to be caused by placental insufficiency; considered "nonreassuring," especially when repetitive
  - Variable decelerations: abrupt and not associated with contractions; this is thought to be caused by cord compression
- Sinusoidal pattern
  - Smooth, sine wave-like undulating pattern with a cyclic frequency of three to five per minute

Neonatal Cranial Injuries

- Extracranial injuries
  - Caput succedaneum

    - Edema and swelling of the scalp above the periosteum, sometimes hemorrhagic
    - Generally benign, caused by prolonged engagement of the fetal head in the birth canal or after vacuum extraction
    - Extends over suture lines
  - Cephalohematoma
    - Subperiosteal collection of blood cause by rupture of vessels beneath the periosteum
    - Usually self-resolving, more common with forceps or vacuum deliveries
    - Does not extend over suture lines
  - Subgaleal hemorrhage
    - Blood accumulates in the loose areolar tissue in the space between the periosteum of the skull and the aponeurosis
    - Caused by traction on the scalp during delivery, which causes the emissary veins between the scalp and dural sinuses to be sheared or severed
    - High chance of mortality because of the potential for massive blood loss
- Intracranial hemorrhage
  - Subdural hemorrhage
    - Bleeding between the dura mater and arachnoid membrane
    - Most common type of intracranial hemorrhage, increased risk with operative deliveries
    - Can cause neonatal seizures, respiratory depression, apnea, irritability, altered tone, altered level of consciousness
  - Subarachnoid hemorrhage
    - Rupture of bridging veins in the subarachnoid space or small leptomeningeal vessels
    - Second most common type of intracranial hemorrhage, increased risk with operative deliveries
    - Can cause apnea, respiratory depression, seizures, posthemorrhagic hydrocephalus
  - Epidural hemorrhage
    - Bleeding between the dura and inner table of the skull, usually caused by injury to the middle meningeal artery
  - Intraventricular hemorrhage
    - Associated with preterm delivery and birth injury in term infants
    - Usually resolves spontaneously

Postdelivery Care

- Assessment of babies after birth is commonly performed at 1 and 5 minutes via the Apgar scoring system (Table 95.7)
- In the event of clinical concern, umbilical artery blood gases may provide some indication of the perfusion and acid-base balance of the baby at birth (Table 95.8)

Infant Mortality

BASIC INFORMATION

- Definitions
  - Infant death and mortality rate: number of infant deaths less than 1 year of age during a year, divided

Table 95.7. Apgar Scoring System

Sign	0	1	2
Color	Blue or pale	Acrocyanotic	Completely pink
Heart rate	Absent	<100 beats/min	>100 beats/min
Reflex activity response to stimulation	No response	Grimace	Cry or active withdrawal
Muscle tone	Limp	Some flexion	Active motion
Respirations	Absent	Weak cry; hypoventilation	Good, crying

Table 95.8. Umbilical Artery Blood Gas Values

Umbilical Arterial Blood	Term Newborn Average	Preterm Newborn Average
pH	7.27	7.28
PCO$_2$ (mmHg)	50.3	50.2
HCO$_3$ (mEq/L)	22	22.4
Base excess (mEq/L)	−2.7	−2.5

Table 95.9. Infant Mortality Rates per 100 Live Births by Maternal Race in the United States (2005 and 2013)

Race and Hispanic Origin	2005	2013
Asian or Pacific Islander	4.89	4.07
Non-Hispanic white	5.76	5.06
All Hispanic groups	5.62	5.00
American Indian or Alaska native	8.06	7.61
Non-Hispanic black	13.63	11.11
Total	6.86	5.96

Data from Centers for Disease Control and Prevention, National Vital Statistics System.

by the number of live births reported during the same year, expressed per 1000 live births
- Neonatal mortality rate: number of neonatal deaths (before 28 days of age) during a year, divided by the number of live births during the same year, expressed per 1000 live births
- Postnatal death: infant death occurring between 28 and 365 days of age
- Perinatal deaths: combination of fetal deaths and live births with only brief survival (days or weeks)
- Top five causes of infant death (Table 95.9)
  - Congenital malformations or chromosomal abnormalities
  - Low birth rate or prematurity
  - Sudden infant death syndrome
  - Neonatal death caused by maternal complications
  - Unintentional injuries

Adolescent Pregnancy

BASIC INFORMATION

- Birth rates among teenagers aged 10 to 14 years and 15 to 19 years were 0.2 and 20.3/1000, respectively, in 2016

- Birth rate in Hispanic teens and non-Hispanic black teens was approximately twice that as in non-Hispanic white teens
- In the United States: 26% terminated electively, 14% result in miscarriage, 60% result in a birth
- Risk factors
  - Adolescents with mental health symptoms or major mental illness appear to be at increased risk of pregnancy
  - Risk factors for repeat teenage pregnancy include depression, history of abortion, and living with a partner or increased partner support
  - Protective factors include higher levels of education and use of contraception

CLINICAL PRESENTATION

- Adolescent patients may present with missing or irregular periods or other vague complaints
- Detailed menstrual and sexual history should be elicited routinely
- Ask teenage patients what they would do with a positive pregnancy test before it is performed

OUTCOMES

- Adolescents appear to be at increased risk for preeclampsia, preterm birth, fetal growth restriction, infant deaths, and postpartum depression
  - Unclear if outcomes are caused by biologic immaturity or sociodemographic factors related to adolescent pregnancy
- Additional association with adolescent pregnancies:
  - Maternal associations
    - Less likely to receive a high school diploma
    - More likely to live in in poverty and receive public assistance for long periods
    - Increased risk for intimate partner violence
  - Paternal associations
    - Finish fewer years of school
    - Earn less income
    - Less likely to be employed
  - Child associations
    - More likely to have health and cognitive disorders
    - More likely to have poor academic performance and repeat a grade or drop out of high school
    - More likely to be neglected or abused
    - Females more likely to have an adolescent pregnancy; males are more likely to be incarcerated

PREVENTION

- Successful programs include a combination of interventions that provide comprehensive sexuality education, focus on delay of sexual activity in young teens, and promoted consistent and correct use of effective contraceptives
- Infant simulator programs are not effective in reducing teen pregnancy, despite their popularity

Review Questions

For review questions, please go to ExpertConsult.com.

Suggested Readings

1. American College of Obstetricians and Gynecologists.
2. Committee Opinion Number 699. *Adolescent Pregnancy, Contraception, and Sexual Activity*; 2017.
3. Committee Opinion Number 711. *Opioid Use and Opioid Use Disorder in Pregnancy*; 2017.
4. Practice Bulletin Number 116. *Management of Intrapartum Fetal Heart Rate Tracings*; 2010. Reaffirmed 2017.
5. Practice Bulletin Number 151. *Cytomegalovirus, Parvovirus B19, Varicella Zoster, and Toxoplasmosis in Pregnancy*; 2015. Reaffirmed 2017.
6. Practice Bulletin Number 175. *Ultrasound in Pregnancy*; 2016. Reaffirmed 2018.

Research and Statistics

96 *Clinical Epidemiology*

CRAIG POLLACK and TERRY DEAN JR, MD, PhD

Common Terms and Concepts in Research

- Standard deviation: measure of the spread of data points about the mean of a data set
- Standard error: also called "standard error of the mean" and "standard deviation of the mean"; a measure of the precision of the data about a mean (see later)
  - Standard error provides an indication of how close the mean of a data set is to the true mean of a population
  - Unlike standard deviation, standard error will decrease with increasing number of observations (e.g., increasing sample size)
- Confidence interval: a range of values within which the true value of a parameter lies, as calculated from a data set and a prespecified probability
  - Example: a 95% confidence interval suggests that based on the observed data, there is a 95% likelihood that the true value lies in the calculated range
- Many common terms and concepts derive from the 2 × 2 table (Fig. 96.1)
- Prevalence: the number of existing cases of a disease at any given time divided by the total population at that time
- Incidence: the number of new cases of a disease that develop over a specific time divided by the population at risk for developing the disease
  - Prevalence and incidence are related to each other via the duration of disease: prevalence = incidence × duration of disease
    - Example: before 1972, the prevalence of end-stage renal disease (ESRD) was very low (the duration of disease was very short because ESRD patients died quickly without dialysis). After the Medicare dialysis program, the prevalence of ESRD soared (the duration of disease was extended, so prevalence increased)

Validity and Reliability of Diagnostic and Screening Tests

- Sensitivity and specificity: characteristics of the test that reflect the test's ability to correctly identify disease in any population (see Fig. 96.1)
  - Sensitivity (positive in disease): the ability of the test to correctly identify persons who have the disease of interest; screening tests should have a high sensitivity to identify all people who potentially have the disease
    - Example: if a test is able to correctly identify 80 persons as having diabetes out of 100 who have diabetes, the sensitivity of the test is 80/100 (80%)
  - Specificity (negative in health): the ability of the test to correctly identify persons as disease-free; confirmatory tests should have a high specificity to exclude people who do not have the disease
    - Example: if a test is able to correctly identify 95 persons as not having diabetes out of 100 who do not have diabetes, the specificity of the test is 95/100 (95%)
- Positive and negative predictive values: the test result's likelihood of reflecting disease presence or absence in a specific population. These values are affected by the disease prevalence in the population being studied (see Fig. 96.1)
  - Positive predictive value: the probability that a positive test in a patient reflects disease. The positive predictive value increases as prevalence increases
    - Example: if 200 people test positive for diabetes but only 80 of those people have diabetes, the positive predictive value of a positive test is 80/200 (40%)
  - Negative predictive value: the probability that a negative test in a patient reflects health (no disease). The negative predictive value increases as prevalence decreases
    - Example: if 200 persons test negative for diabetes but only 40 do not have diabetes, the negative predictive value of the negative test is 40/200 (20%)

Sources of Error in Measurement, Interpretation, or Analysis

- Precision: on repeated measurement of the same sample, how closely do the results *cluster together*?
  - Precision does not consider how close a result is to the truth
  - Precision depends on random error. Greater random error results in lower precision; increasing sample size decreases the effect of random error
- Accuracy: how close are the results to the truth?
  - Bias: systematic error, resulting in decreased accuracy (Table 96.1)
  - Bias is reduced by careful study design
  - Randomization and blinding are powerful tools used in clinical trials to reduce selection and information bias
- Confounding (Fig. 96.2)
  - Confounding describes a relationship between an exposure and an outcome of interest that is distorted by a second exposure that is related to both the outcome and the exposure of interest

		Disease: Present (or develops)	Disease: Absent (or does not develop)
Test Result (or exposure)	Present	a	b
	Absent	c	d

Sensitivity: Of those with disease, what percent test positive? ("sensitivity is positive in disease, or PID")

$$\text{Sensitivity} = a/(a + c)$$

Specificity: Of those without disease, what percent test negative? ("specificity is negative in health, or NIH")

$$\text{Specificity} = d/(b + d)$$

Prevalence: The percentage of a population that has a disease

$$\text{Prevalence} = (a + c)/(a + b + c + d)$$

Positive predictive value: If the test is positive, what percent will have disease? Markedly increases with increasing prevalence

$$\text{PPV} = a/(a + b)$$

Negative predictive value: If the test is negative, what percent will not have the disease? Markedly increases with decreasing prevalence

$$\text{NPV} = d/(c + d)$$

Relative risk: Risk of developing disease in those exposed, divided by the risk of developing disease in those not exposed

$$\text{RR} = \text{Risk(exp)/Risk(unexp)} = (a/[a + b])/(c/[c + d])$$

Attributable risk (AR): The absolute increase in risk of developing disease in those exposed compared to those not exposed. Absolute risk reduction (ARR) is the absolute decrease in risk among those taking a medication compared to those not taking it

$$\text{AR} = \text{Risk(exp)} - \text{Risk(unexp)} = a/(a + b) - c/(c + d)$$
$$\text{ARR} = \text{Risk(not taking)} - \text{Risk(taking)} = c/(c + d) - a/(a + b)$$

Number needed to treat: How many individuals will need to be treated to prevent a single event?

$$\text{NNT} = 1/\text{ARR}$$

Odds ratio: In individuals with disease, what are the odds of having been exposed compared to those who were exposed who do not have disease?

$$\text{OR} = \text{Odds (exposure in those with disease)/odds (exposure in those without disease)}$$
$$\text{OR} = (a/c)/(b/d)$$

Fig. 96.1. The 2 × 2 table.

- Simply termed, confounding is guilt by association
- Confounding is a particular problem in observational studies
- Internal and external validity
  - Internal validity in a study refers to whether the results accurately reflect the connection between exposure and disease within the population being studied
  - Randomized clinical trials maximize internal validity through randomization, blinding, and placebo control
- External validity (i.e., generalizability)
  - Ability of a study to produce results that can be applied to a broader population (beyond the study participants)

Table 96.1. Types of Bias

Type of Bias	Example
Selection bias: when those chosen for a study (or those leaving a study) systematically differ from those not chosen (or those not leaving) with respect to characteristics important to the study question	In a case-control study of pancreatic cancer, control subjects are chosen from a gastrointestinal (GI) clinic. If the control subjects are avoiding coffee because of GI side effects, this will tend to create a false association between coffee drinking and pancreatic cancer.
Information bias: occurs when individuals with a particular exposure or outcome are systematically (and erroneously) classified as having a different exposure or outcome. For instance, recall bias occurs when individuals try to remember an exposure. Their memory may be influenced by their later outcomes.	Mothers of infants with a birth defect are more likely to remember taking a medication than other mothers. This will tend to create a false association between the medication use and birth defects.
Lead-time bias: seen in studies of screening tests, in which identification of disease at an earlier stage will "lengthen" apparent survival, even if prognosis is not improved.	A new test for detecting pancreatic cancer is associated with a doubling of survival time. However, the test merely detected the cancer at an earlier, untreatable stage.
Length bias: seen in studies of screening tests when screening a population will detect those with longer survival times (i.e., less severe disease) rather than those with shorter survival times (i.e., more severe disease). This creates the illusion that the screening test prolongs survival when in fact it does not.	A new screening test for renal cell cancer is performed every 5 years. Survival rates in the screened group are 7 years, compared with 4 years in an unscreened group. Those with more aggressive disease die before the screening interval so that those screened have less aggressive disease.

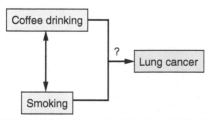

Fig. 96.2. Smoking as a confounder in the relationship between coffee and lung cancer.

- To be externally valid, a study must also be internally valid. A study with restrictive inclusion criteria enhances internal validity at the expense of external validity
- Analyzing "crossovers" in clinical trials: intention to treat
  - Intention to treat is a conservative approach to the analysis of a clinical trial, in which analysis is based on the original assignment of a participant regardless of what treatment the participant actually received in the study
    - Example: in a randomized clinical trial of medical versus surgical treatment of mild carotid stenosis, some patients assigned to the medical treatment may cross over into the surgical arm (e.g., end up getting surgery). Why not analyze them in the

surgical group? People may have crossed over for a particular reason that could bias the results. If all patients in the medical treatment group had transient ischemic attacks and are then counted in the surgical group, it will make surgery look worse than it really is.
  - When performing analyses using intention to treat, crossover will bias study results toward the null, meaning that the study will find fewer differences between study groups. It will never bias the association away from the null (i.e., results demonstrating more differences between study groups)

Statistical Hypotheses, Significance, and Power

- When designing an experiment, researchers must distinguish between the null hypothesis and alternative hypothesis
  - Null hypothesis (H_0): hypothesis in which there is no difference to be detected between two (or more) measured phenomena. In other words, any differences are due to chance alone
    - Example: there is no relationship between caloric intake and BMI
  - Alternative hypothesis (H_A): hypothesis in which the difference between measured phenomena is attributable to some nonrandom cause. For researchers, this is often the driving hypothesis of the research question
    - Example: there is a relationship between caloric intake and BMI
  - Thus statistical analysis will help quantitatively assess the likelihood that the null hypothesis is true
- P-value: in a statistical test, the p-value is a calculable metric between 0 and 1 describing the probability of observing data that is at least as different as the recorded data set. In other words, it answers, "If the null hypothesis is true, how likely was it to have provided the recorded observations?"
  - If the p-value is high (closer to 1), the likelihood of the data being consistent with the null hypothesis is high
  - If the p-value is low (closer to 0), the likelihood of the data being consistent with the null hypothesis is low. This supports the alternative hypothesis
- Type I errors and "significance":
  - Type I errors are errors of rejecting the null hypothesis, even if it is true. This is commonly referred to as a "false-positive" result
    - Example: concluding that there is a relationship between caloric intake and BMI, although the truth is that there was none
  - Type I error rate is also considered "a significance level," denoted α
    - It is common for the significance level to be set at 0.05
  - If the p-value from a statistical test is less than α, the difference is deemed "statistically significant," suggesting that it was unlikely that the observed differences were due to chance alone

Table 96.2. Types of Observational Studies

Name	Design/Example	Strengths	Weaknesses
Case report/series	Observations from clinical practice *Example:* case report of seizure associated with cat-scratch disease	Useful for generating hypotheses	Limited use in clinical decision-making; no control group; selection bias
Ecologic study	Compare average exposure with average outcome between populations *Example:* comparison of mean salt intake and mean blood pressure in the United States and Japan	Useful for generating hypotheses; can be used to compare prevalence of disease or exposures in various populations	No individual data; not useful for demonstrating causation
Cross-sectional study	Determine exposure and disease status simultaneously in a representative sample of a population *Example:* prevalence of *Chlamydia* antibodies in patients with coronary artery disease	Good initial step in evaluating associations; useful for public health surveys	Causation cannot be determined; temporal relationship not defined; cannot evaluate prognosis
Case-control study (retrospective study)	Identify cases (with disease) and select controls (without disease). Determine exposure status retrospectively in both groups *Example:* is history of head trauma greater in Alzheimer disease patients than in control subjects?	Lower cost than cohort studies; useful for studying uncommon diseases	Susceptible to recall bias and selection bias; cannot evaluate prevalence, incidence, prognosis; can only determine odds ratio
Cohort study (prospective study)	Prospective study of subgroup in a population that shares a particular characteristic; determine exposure at beginning and ascertain outcomes with follow-up over time *Example:* incidence of mesothelioma in steel mill workers who smoke	Studies incidence and prognosis; establishes temporal relationships; strong external validity	Long and costly; limited in studying treatment effects

- It should be noted that even if a difference between two groups is noted to be statistically significant, it does not necessarily entail clinical importance. One should also consider the degree of difference versus the recorded values
  - Example: finding that increased caloric intake is associated with a statistically significant increase in BMI of 1.0 might not be clinically important if the average BMIs of the test groups are 32.0 and 33.0
- Type II errors and "power":
  - Type II errors are errors of not rejecting the null hypothesis, even if it is false. Commonly referred to as a "false-negative" result
    - Example: concluding that there is no relationship between caloric intake and BMI, even if the truth is that there was one
  - Type II error rate is denoted β and is related to the "power" of a statistical test $(1-\beta)$
    - Example: a power of 80% indicates that a true difference will be missed 20% of the time
  - One common use of the concepts β and power is in the planning of the recruitment size for a study. To ensure that a study has enrolled enough subjects to detect a significant difference, researchers will use a predicted effect size (relative to the predicted average and standard deviation for a population), a set α, and a set β to calculate an appropriate sample size

Study Design

- Observational studies: no intervention performed; observations made between exposures and outcomes (Table 96.2)

- Strengths
  - Only way possible to study a number of important research questions
  - May reflect real-world situations (external generalizability)
  - Less expensive and generally faster to perform than randomized controlled trials (RCTs)
- Limitations
  - Lower validity
  - More subject to bias and confounding
- Experimental studies: the randomized clinical trial
  - RCTs are a true experiment, the purpose of which is to test interventions
  - Strengths
    - The gold standard study designed to evaluate therapeutic interventions without bias or confounding; patients with different characteristics (even characteristics that you may not observe) are randomly assigned to the study arms
    - Stronger internal validity than cohort studies
  - Limitations
    - Limited to questions of clinical equipoise and clinical benefit
    - The study is run under ideal conditions and therefore most often measures efficacy, not effectiveness: efficacy refers to how the intervention performs under ideal conditions. Effectiveness refers to how the intervention performs in the real world
    - Generalizability often can be questioned
- Data synthesis studies
  - Qualitative review article: no explicit methods; must trust author's judgment
  - Practice guidelines: consensus statements; quality varies

- Decision analysis
  - Create a decision analysis tree; assign probabilities and utilities
  - Calculate the expected value of various decisions
- Systematic review and metaanalysis
  - Explicit methods to review and possibly pool or combine (metaanalysis) data from multiple studies
  - Metaanalysis of observational studies may reflect bias or confounding within pooled results
  - Publication bias: positive studies are published more frequently than negative studies and are most often included in systematic reviews and metaanalyses

Measures of Risk Reduction (See Also Fig. 96.1)

- Example: results of a recently performed RCT demonstrating patients' 5-year risk of death from breast cancer on treatment A versus treatment B is 50% versus 40%, respectively
- Absolute risk reduction: absolute improvement provided by treatment B versus treatment A is 50% − 40% = 10%
- Relative risk reduction: improvement provided by treatment B versus treatment A is (50% − 40%)/50% = 20%

- Number needed to treat (NNT): number of patients needed to treat with treatment B to prevent one additional death over 5 years compared with what would happen with treatment A (NNT = 1/absolute risk reduction) is 1/0.1 = 10. Similarly, number needed to harm (NNH) reflects how many people would need to be exposed to a treatment or risk factor to cause harm in one patient (NNH = 1/absolute risk)

Acknowledgment

The author would like to thank L. Ebony Boulware, MD, MPH, for her work on previous editions of this chapter.

Review Questions

For review questions, please go to ExpertConsult.com.

Suggested Readings

1. Gordis L. *Epidemiology*. Philadelphia: WB Saunders; 1996.
2. Last JM. *A Dictionary of Epidemiology*. New York: Oxford Press; 1995.
3. Sackett DL, Haynes RB, Guyatt GH, et al. *Clinical Epidemiology: A Basic Science for Clinical Medicine*. Boston: Little Brown; 1991.

Ethics

97 *Ethics*

SARA TAUB, MD, MBE and MATTHEW DRAGO, MD, MBE

Ethical Theories

- Medical ethics concerns itself with the moral issues that arise in the field of medicine, particularly, though not exclusively, surrounding patient care. Over time, several approaches have emerged to help guide clinicians toward acceptable resolution of the ethical quandaries that can arise for medical professionals. Among the most often cited and applied in the clinical setting are principlism and the Four Box Method.

PRINCIPLISM

- Principlism, which arose from the work of Beauchamp and Childress, relies on four principles—autonomy, beneficence, nonmaleficence, and justice—to help resolve issues in clinical medicine. Briefly summarized, the four principles stand for the following concepts:
  - Autonomy: the notion of self-determination, from which derives a patient's right to provide informed consent
  - Beneficence: the pursuit of the patient's best interest
  - Nonmaleficence: the notion of "do no harm"
  - Justice: construed broadly as fairness in distribution of resources and treating like cases alike
- The framework sometimes has been critiqued for giving little direction as to how to proceed when the principles compete with each other. There is no hierarchy offered to suggest that one would clearly trump the other.

FOUR BOX METHOD

- In the Four Box Method, developed by Jonsen, Siegler, and Winslade, clinicians are encouraged to analyze a case by looking at it from four discrete angles:
  - Medical indications
  - Patient preferences
  - Quality of life
  - Contextual features (including social, economic, legal, and administrative)
- The method is intended to be user-friendly at the bedside and to shed light on challenging questions by helping to elucidate the most pertinent information about a case.
- As with principlism, though, it has been faulted for not offering more guidance about how to proceed when closer analysis of a case still does not help identify an obvious path of resolution.

Mediation

- In clinical bioethics, theoretic principles can be applied to real-life dilemmas and disputes through bioethical mediation. Mediation is a private, voluntary, informal process to resolve disputes between parties through a third-party facilitator.
- Liebman and Dubler have described a stepwise approach to the mediation process:
  - Assessment and preparation
    - Identify key players in decision-making
    - Collect needed background information, medical and social, to fully understand situation
  - Starting the mediation
    - Set up time and space to openly discuss conflict with all parties
    - Introduce participants, present and refine each participant's interests/goals
  - Gather information
    - Ensure all parties have had an equal voice
  - Problem-solve
    - Focus on establishing common interests, not on conflicting positions
  - Resolution and follow-up
    - Solutions should seek to provide consensus that is in keeping with bioethical principles

ETHICS AND THE LAW

- Though ethics and the law are two areas that are often conflated, it helps to recognize that the law spells out what individuals may or may not do, whereas ethics aspires to identify what people should do.

Professionalism

- As professionals, physicians have entered into a contract with society. Though it is seldom spelled out anymore, other than through oaths taken at the time of medical school graduation, this contract remains fundamental to what it means to be a medical professional.
- Physicians are afforded:
  - The reputation and financial rewards of the profession
  - The privilege to self-regulate
  - The trust of patients who make themselves vulnerable by sharing personal information and permitting physical examination and procedures
- In exchange for these, physicians agree to take on certain obligations, including:
  - The acquisition of a specialized body of knowledge that must be maintained current
  - The duty to develop and uphold professional standards of behavior
  - The commitment to serve the medical needs of individual patients, first and foremost, as well as those of society at large

- Physicians have a fiduciary duty to their patients. Fidelity, which is central to it, encompasses some of the roles and responsibilities outlined previously, including trust, dedication, and loyalty, as well as others addressed elsewhere in this chapter, such as fairness and veracity.

Selected Ethical Issues

- One of the unique features of pediatric medicine is that the physician routinely enters into a relationship with a patient who is a child, as well as with the patient's parent(s) or guardian(s).
  - Depending on the age of the child and his or her cognitive development, the child may be able to participate at varying levels in decisions regarding his or her overall health and medical care
  - Personal preferences and family mores/values will also help define how this triangular dynamic is managed

INFORMED CONSENT

- To provide informed consent, an individual must have decision-making capacity (which assumes competence, an all-or-nothing concept, or the ability to arrive at a rational decision). Traditionally, the law has made it a requirement that a person reach the age of majority (age 18) to be able to provide binding consent for most medical decisions.
- Elements of informed consent include:
  - An understanding of the proposed decision, intervention, or procedure
  - An honest appraisal of pertinent risks, benefits, and uncertainties associated with the decision, intervention, or procedure
  - An understanding of the reasonable alternatives to said intervention or procedure, including the option not to proceed
  - The capacity to make a decision that is reasoned and rational, which assumes competence, an all-or-nothing legal concept, and decision-making capacity, an aptitude that may vary with the complexity and ramifications of the decision at hand
  - The opportunity to make a voluntary decision, free of coercion or duress
- Exceptions to usual informed consent practice:
  - Minors may provide consent independently to care for certain issues considered particularly sensitive and stigmatizing and to which they might not seek access if the involvement of a parent or guardian were required. These include reproductive health, mental health, care surrounding substance use and abuse, care for crime-related injuries
  - For adolescents, a group nearing adulthood, certain unique categories have been defined for granting them complete autonomy, such as:
    - Mature minors: individuals usually 14 or older and below the age of 18 who are felt to possess the maturity to make medical decisions (this exception should take into consideration the complexity of the decision and its implications)
    - Emancipated minors: individuals whose life circumstances (be it marriage, enlistment in the military, or emancipation by court permission in the setting, for instance, of financial self-sufficiency or alternative living arrangements separate from family) require them to assume adult responsibilities and grant them independence from their parents for decision-making purposes

THE "BEST INTEREST STANDARD"

- Unlike in adult medicine where the patient might decide for himself/herself, parents/guardians are often in the situation of making decisions on behalf of their children
- The principle that should guide these decisions is that of best interest—what would most promote the well-being of the child?
- Although adults are granted the autonomy to decide for children then, this privilege is not unbounded and requires a certain degree of selflessness in placing the interests of another person first
- Parents/guardians are afforded much discretion in the health care decisions they make for their children. Where limitations on their authority come into question is when there is concern that a decision is not being made in the child's best interest and particularly if said decision begins to resemble abuse or neglect

PARENTAL PERMISSION/ASSENT/DISSENT

- Irrespective of who the recognized primary decision-maker is (parent/guardian or child), there are instances in which input from the other party (parent/guardian or child) still will be sought and respected
- For instance, children may be able to make a particular health care decision but are required nonetheless to receive parental permission to proceed (e.g., proceed with pregnancy termination in certain states)
- Assent requires that a pediatric patient agree to the decision, intervention, or procedure at hand before it can be performed, even after their parent or guardian has decided to proceed
- Dissent gives them the opportunity to decline, even after the parent or guardian has elected to move forward

PRIVACY AND CONFIDENTIALITY

- Privacy refers to the right of an individual to be free from intrusion into their personal matters and information, including health information. Several laws protect the privacy of health information, including The Health Insurance Portability and Accountability Act, state privacy laws, state minor consent laws, and the Family Educational Rights and Privacy Act.
- Confidentiality is the protection of information disclosed in confidence. Conflict over confidentiality may arise in pediatrics, particularly when working with adolescents.
  - Adolescents are on a trajectory toward adulthood—in terms of usually having increasing decision-making capacity and becoming more accountable for their health

- Pediatricians often will spend one-on-one time with their adolescent patients, both to empower them to assume some of these growing responsibilities and to offer them a private space to discuss health-related matters with their clinician
- During adolescent patient visits, physicians should:
  - Explain explicitly the meaning of privacy and confidentiality
  - Encourage patients to discuss their health with parents or trusted adult support figures
  - Clearly list reasons that would require a breach of confidentiality
    - Actions that would result in direct harm to patient or another person
    - Disclosure of abuse
  - If confidentiality must be breached, seek to partner with patient in disclosing difficult information to parents or other necessary parties

TRUTH-TELLING/VERACITY

- Issues of truth-telling may arise in pediatrics, particularly when a child receives a serious diagnosis or experiences a significant change in prognosis for the worse. There are some parents who think it would be in the best interest of their child to shield him or her from the difficult news and who therefore ask clinic or hospital staff not to disclose the information to the child.
  - This practice is intended to protect children. However, for health care professionals who are asked to withhold key information, it is often perceived as problematic and uncomfortable
  - Indeed, veracity, the principle of truth-telling, which is intricately linked to notions of respect and self-determination, has become widely accepted as a guiding principle in medicine over the past 50 years
- One important approach is to enter into a constructive dialogue with parents so that they may understand the value of honesty. Some important concepts to communicate include:
  - Although health care professionals may be willing to adhere to the preferences of parents, they may not be willing to lie to the child if the child poses a direct question. How these situations will be handled should be discussed up front
  - Children often understand far more than they are told directly, even if information is being withheld. By avoiding an open dialogue around the details of their circumstances, we sometimes deny children the opportunity to voice their fears, concerns, and questions, which could lead to them imagining scenarios that are worse than reality or feeling isolated in their suffering
  - There are often additional support staff available who can help parents decide how best to communicate difficult information to a child in a sensitive and developmentally appropriate fashion

CULTURAL COMPETENCY

- In our diverse, pluralistic society, patients' and families' cultural background(s) may inform their medical decisions. It is important that, as health care professionals, we make it a priority to better understand the cultural beliefs that influence the decisions of people from the various populations for whom we care. Asking about preferences with a genuine curiosity and using open-ended questions will avoid making inaccurate assumptions.

MANDATED REPORTING

- Pediatricians, by working with children in a professional capacity, are required by law to report when there is *reasonable suspicion* of child abuse. Mandated reporters are protected from prosecution in civil and criminal courts as long as they have reported possible abuse cases in good faith.

PERIVIABILITY

- Consensus on the edge of viability remains a gray zone in neonatal care. Review of international guidelines shows that although most neonatologists recommend noninitiation of care at 22 weeks 0 days to 22 weeks 6 days, and trial of resuscitation at and above 25 weeks and 0 days, there remain large variations in recommendations between these gestational ages.
- The guidelines of the American Academy of Pediatrics' Committee on Fetus and Newborn acknowledge this gray zone and support shared decision-making with families. Beyond gestational age, factors such as expected birth weight, sex, antenatal steroid administration, and singleton versus multiples have been shown to strongly affect outcome.

FUTILITY

- Medical futility refers to the concept that a treatment is ineffective in achieving its medical goal and is therefore futile.
  - Quantitative futility: failure to achieve a physiologic goal, i.e., giving antibiotics to treat a viral infection
  - Qualitative futility: judgment that even if a treatment has a reasonable potential for medical benefit, it is not worthwhile due to other concerns such as patient suffering, quality of life, or cost
- Determining when to withhold or provide treatment should be based on the patient's best interest and preferences, above claims of futility. Considerations in helping to determine when withholding or withdrawing life-sustaining therapies may be appropriate include that:
  - Life-sustaining medical treatment encompasses any and all interventions that prolong life, such as respirators, organ transplantation, dialysis, insulin, nutrition, and hydration
  - Withholding versus withdrawing life-sustaining interventions is considered to be morally and legally equivalent, despite some care providers expressing greater distress over withdrawing interventions after they have been started

BRAIN DEATH

- Brain death is defined as the absence of neurologic function with a known irreversible cause of coma and is an accepted criterion to recognize death.

- This recognition is in response to advances in cardiopulmonary support that mask the recognition of cardiorespiratory death, or the cessation of the heart and breathing.
- For details, see Chapter 56.

ADVANCE CARE PLANNING

- In addition to taking into consideration what options are available, feasible, and recommended from a medical standpoint, health care professionals and families should take time to understand how the unique values and preferences of the child and his/her family play a role in informing decisions surrounding the extremes of health care and death.

LIMITATIONS ON MEDICAL INTERVENTION

- There may come a point at which parents/guardians/ children themselves decide that certain medical interventions should not be attempted for the simple reason that more harms than benefits are likely to ensue from them. There are mechanisms that exist to put in place protections to shield children from such interventions, be they in the health care setting or in the community.
- It is key that children and their families be made to understand that, irrespective of whether limitations are put into place, the care of the child will not cease.

CODE STATUS

- In the hospital setting, code status helps define which resuscitative interventions should be attempted on a person who is in respiratory failure or in cardiac arrest.
  - No limitations assumes that every attempt should be made, however invasive and aggressive, to restart a patient's heart (with compressions, electricity, and/or medications) or respirations (including intubation and mechanical ventilation)
  - Do Not Resuscitate (DNR)—also sometimes referred to as Do Not Attempt Resuscitation (DNAR) or Allow Natural Death (AND)—assumes that no aggressive, invasive interventions will be pursued to resuscitate a person whose heart or respirations have ceased
  - Do Not Intubate (DNI) specifically limits the step of providing an artificial airway through intubation and mechanical ventilation, though it does not speak to cardiac resuscitation and other modalities, such as bagging or noninvasive positive-pressure ventilation though continuous positive airway pressure (CPAP) or bilevel positive airway pressure (BiPAP), to try to restore respirations
  - Limited Code, which requires additional specifications, may allow a health care team and family to outline a more individually tailored approach to resuscitation
  - Physician Orders for Life-Sustaining Treatment (POLST) is a form that can be used in the field to place limitations on what aspects of resuscitation will be initiated on an individual in the home, school, or other community setting in the event or cardiac arrest or respiratory failure. Where there is no POLST form available to document limitations, first responders are currently mandated by law to perform all attempts to restore an individual to life upon arriving at a scene in the field. It is a good idea to keep an individual's POLST form in a medical folder that travels with them everywhere or to have original forms on file in the various settings they frequent regularly

ORGAN DONATION AND AUTOPSY

- If a child dies in the hospital, families should be offered the opportunity, as feasible, to gift the child's organs to the regional organ procurement organization. It is worth noting that specific procedures have been outlined at many institutions surrounding who should approach the family regarding this topic, how, and when.
- It is important for families to understand also that there are some circumstances under which autopsies are legally mandated and nonoptional. Physicians are encouraged to become familiar with the policies in place at the institution(s) where they practice.

EUTHANASIA

- Euthanasia, the active killing of a patient suffering from an incurable disease, is not legally permitted in the United States.
- Physician-assisted suicide, the act of supplying a method, such as a cocktail of medications, that enables a patient to end his or her own life, is allowed in some U.S. states, but it is not legally permitted for minors in any U.S. state.
- These terms ought to be distinguished from palliative sedation, a state that may be reached in trying to achieve adequate pain management near the end of life through progressive increases in medications that may be sedating, with the intent not of hastening death, but rather of relieving distress from inadequately managed symptoms by titrating to comfort.

RELIGIOUS AND PHILOSOPHICAL OBJECTIONS

- The importance of religion and spirituality spans virtually every culture, and in the United States the free exercise of religion is a fundamental societal value. Society grants parents wide latitude in this process: parents may choose to raise a child in a strict religious tradition or entirely devoid of religion.
- Although this choice is a personal one, its importance becomes prominent when parental religious beliefs come into conflict with recommended medical care of a child.
  - Medical providers must work to respect parental authority to raise their child in a particular religious tradition and to make decisions in line with that tradition while upholding their duty to protect the best interest of a child
  - Parental latitude is narrowed in medical decision-making for a child because the best interest of the child and the child's future autonomy take precedent over a parent's right to raise religious objections to care that may pose harm to the child

- In instances where religious objection to medical care puts a child at direct potential for harm, providers must work with parents to understand the nature of their objections, possibly consulting with religious leaders close to the family, and be clear about what medical treatments may be optional, versus which are felt to be necessary to avoid harm to a child
- Legal means should be pursued to protect a child if an acceptable compromise cannot be achieved

VACCINATIONS

- The argument for mandating vaccination stems from the principle of best interest, which creates a professional duty for physicians to ensure early childhood vaccination for their patients. Recommendations to clinicians when facing objection(s) to vaccination reinforce the need for communication with parents around the reasons for their refusal, with the aim of educating parents about how vaccination promotes their child's physical best interest and of correcting any misconceptions.
  - Religious exemptions to vaccination exist in 48 states and the District of Columbia, with several states also allowing philosophical exemptions; the appropriateness of these exemptions is contested
  - Inclusion of religious objection in child neglect laws and the interpretation of what constitutes adequate religious conviction to allow for objection vary from state to state. When cases of vaccine refusal on religious grounds have gone before a court to decide whether a parent is neglectful, court opinions have been mixed
  - More policy work is needed to clarify this matter for providers and state health officials given the importance and complexity of this issue on both a personal and public health level

Research

- Modern bioethics was born out of the historical development of protections for human subjects in research after World War II, starting with the Nuremberg Code, written in response to Nazi physician experimentations during the war. The Declaration of Helsinki, the Belmont Report, and finally the Department of Health and Human Services' Code of Federal Regulations for Protection of Human Subjects built off the Nuremberg Code in refining protection for human research subjects.
- Children represent a vulnerable population as research subjects because they may lack fully developed decision-making capacity and usually do not have the authority to provide autonomous informed consent for participating in pediatric research. Several regulations, based on minimizing risk and maximizing potential benefit, have been developed to protect children from improper use in research (Table 97.1).
- Similar to informed consent for medical procedures (previous), informed consent for research is a pivotal protection for potential human subjects and consists of three central pillars:
  - Disclosing risks and benefits of research

Table 97.1. Requirements for Child Participation in Research Based on Potential Risks and Benefits of Participation

Risk Benefit Category	Requirements for Participation
No greater than minimal risk research	1. Institutional Review Board approval 2. Child assent 3. Informed consent of at least one parent
Greater than minimal risk and prospect of direct benefit to subject	1–3 and: 4. Risk justified by anticipated benefit to subject 5. Anticipated benefit at least as favorable as alternative approaches
Greater than a minimal risk and without prospect of direct benefit to subject	1–3 and: 4. Only minor increase over minimal risk 5. Study likely to yield generalizable, vital knowledge about child's condition 6. Research intervention presents experiences to the child that are reasonably commensurate with the child's actual or expected medical/psychological/social situations
Research not otherwise advisable	1–3 and: 4. Institutional Review Board approves research as reasonable opportunity to further the understanding of a serious problem affecting children 5. Approval of the Secretary of the Department of Health and Human Services after consultation with a panel of experts in pertinent fields, and after opportunity for public review and comment

Modified from Burns J. Research in children. *Crit Care Med*, 2003;3(31):S131–S136.

- Ensuring comprehension of these disclosures and research protocols
- Voluntary decision-making free of coercion of potential subject to participate or not
- Informed consent stems from the principle of autonomy or "self-rule." Children's capacity to participate in informed consent depends upon their developmental level and should be assessed individually as they approach the teenage years.
- Assent refers to affirmative agreement and should be sought when enrolling children in a research study:
  - Assent is not equivalent to informed consent
  - Lack of objection is not equivalent to affirmed agreement
  - Obtaining assent should focus on engaging the child as a person and on providing information that is developmentally appropriate and targeted to their areas of concern
- Therapeutic misperception is the incorrect belief by a research participant that taking part in a research study offers direct therapeutic benefit to them as a patient. Institutional Review Board (IRB) review, informed consent, and assent all serve as protections to prevent parents and children from participating in research for incorrect reasons.

New Frontiers

- Advances in science and technology will further push ethical discussions as new and unforeseen challenges arise.

- For instance, with increasing ubiquity of genetic testing/sequencing, dilemmas arise concerning proper consent for and disclosure of incidental findings or inherited diseases with adult onset (e.g., breast/ovarian cancer). The American College of Medical Genetics and Genomics (ACMG) and the AAP have provided guidelines regarding preconsent discussions and disclosure of results.
- Special ethical considerations must be taken into account when contemplating future enhancements (therapies seeking to improve upon something already within the normal range) and novel therapies (interventions that may lack high-level evidence demonstrating benefits and risks). In all, similar questions should be addressed:
  - What is the goal of the intervention?
  - What are the risks of the intervention?
  - If parents request the intervention, is the request in the child's best interest?
  - Is the intervention part of a research trial that is being conducted appropriately? (e.g., monitoring of outcomes, informed consent)
  - If so, do the parent and child understand that participating in research for a therapy may not carry a direct benefit.

Review Questions

For review questions, please go to ExpertConsult.com.

Suggested Readings:

1. American Medical Association. *Code of Medical Ethics.* Available from: http://www.ama-assn.org/ama/pub/physician-resources/medical-ethics/code-medical-ethics.page.
2. Diekema DS, Mercurio MR, Adam MB, eds. *Clinical Ethics in Pediatrics: A Case-Based Textbook.* New York: Cambridge University Press; 2011.
3. Fleishman A. *Pediatric Ethics: Protecting the Interests of Children.* New York: Oxford University Press; 2016.
4. Forman EN, Ladd RE. *Ethical Dilemmas in Pediatrics: A Case Study Approach.* New York: Springer-Verlag; 1991.
5. Frankel LR, Goldworth A, Rorty MV, Silverman WA, eds. *Ethical Dilemmas in Pediatrics: Cases and Commentaries.* New York: Cambridge University Press; 2009.
6. Jonsen AR, Siegler M, Winslade WJ. *Clinical Ethics: A Practical Approach to Ethical Decisions in Clinical Medicine.* 8th ed. New York: McGraw-Hill Education; 2015.

Patient Safety and Quality Improvement

98 Patient Safety and Quality Improvement

JESSICA HART, MD and ERIN PETE DEVON, MD

INTRODUCTION TO PATIENT SAFETY

- Terminology: see Table 98.1

EPIDEMIOLOGY

- In 1999, the Institute of Medicine (IOM) released *To Err Is Human: Building a Safer Health System*, which revealed that between 44,000 and 98,000 people died each year in hospitals in the United States due to medical errors and adverse events
- Preventable medical errors have been estimated to result in total costs between $17 billion and $29 billion
- Great efforts have been undertaken to improve standards and expectations for patient safety. The Joint Commission developed the National Patient Safety Goals program to help organizations address patient safety (https://www.jointcommission.org/standards_information/npsgs.aspx)
- The Children's Hospitals' Solutions for Patient Safety is a large national effort of over 100 hospitals to collaborate on goals to improve patient safety

PATIENT SAFETY IN PEDIATRICS

- Pediatric patients are at high risk for adverse events due to:
  - Changing physiology
  - Reliance on the family for medical information
  - Normal developmental milestones that prevent cooperation and participation with examinations and procedures
  - Lack of pediatric-specific information in adult-focused computerized physician ordering entry systems
- Patient and family participation is becoming increasingly recognized as a key component to improving patient safety
  - Example: patient and family participation in hand hygiene promotion to prevent health care–associated infections
- See also Nelson Textbook of Pediatrics, Chapter 2, "Quality and Safety in Healthcare for Children."

REPORTING AND DISCLOSURE

- Error reporting refers to the exchange of information among providers and regulators
  - Voluntary incident-reporting systems are used in health care to report the occurrence of errors

- Trigger tools (clues found on review of the medical record to identify an adverse event) can complement error-reporting systems
- State law may require reporting of sentinel events and adverse events leading to patient harm
- Learning from errors:
  - Morbidity and mortality conferences are important local efforts for sharing and learning from adverse events
  - National efforts to learn from safety events and share between institutions occur through patient safety organizations
- Disclosure is communication with patients and families after events
  - Disclosure of a medical error is a fundamental ethical responsibility of the physician
  - Patients generally favor disclosure of all harmful errors, accompanied by an explanation of why the error occurred, how the error's impact will be minimized (in their own care), and what steps the physician and organization will take to prevent its recurrence
  - The patient's medical record should contain accurate, factual documentation of the event and of conversations surrounding the event, without subjective opinion
- Second victim syndrome
  - Emotional and psychological effects that a health care provider experiences when involved in a medical error that results in patient harm
  - Formal and informal peer support systems and employee assistance programs can offer guidance and support

SYSTEMS APPROACH TO MEDICAL ERROR

- Model for patient safety
  - Shift from a system of "blame and shame" to a systems analysis approach
  - James Reason's Swiss cheese model: harm is caused by a series of systemic failures. The Swiss cheese slices represent the layers of defense in an organization's safety system. When the systems fail, the holes line up, and the trigger causes harm
    - Active failures: errors whose effects are felt almost immediately and almost always involve a front-line provider
      - Example: ignoring an alarm on a monitor for what turns out to be a real event
    - Latent conditions: defect in the design and organization of processes and systems. "Accidents waiting to happen"
      - Example: alarm fatigue or inadequate staffing

Table 98.1. Terminology

Term	Definition	Notes	Example
Medical error	Failure to complete a planned action as intended (error of execution) or the use of a wrong plan to achieve an aim (error planning).	Medical errors can result in serious harm, mild and temporary harm, or no harm. Medical errors can be diagnostic, treatment, or preventative.	A patient received an incorrect dose of amoxicillin but had no known side effects. This is a medical error not causing harm.
Near miss	Any process variation that did not affect the outcome but for which a recurrence carries a significant chance of serious outcome.	Reviewing a near miss is an important learning opportunity.	A patient with Kawasaki disease is prescribed an incorrect dose of intravenous immunoglobulin that is discovered by the reviewing pharmacist and corrected by the ordering provider. This is a near miss.
Adverse event	Management plan or intervention that leads to patient injury. Adverse events can be preventable or nonpreventable (see Fig. 98.1).	Harm can occur without a medical error being committed.	A patient with a known allergy to penicillin was prescribed amoxicillin and developed anaphylaxis and required intubation. This is a preventable adverse event.
Sentinel event	A patient safety event that reaches a patient and results in death, permanent harm, or severe temporary harm and that requires intervention to sustain life.	This information is reported to the Joint Commission, and an investigation as to the root causes must be undertaken.	Infant is discharged from the well-baby nursery to the wrong family.

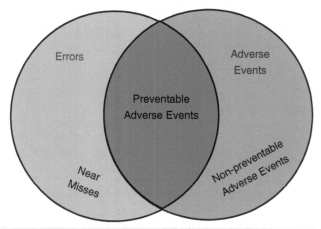

Fig. 98.1. Adverse events and medical errors. (From Rolston JD, Bernstein M. Errors in neurosurgery. *Neurosurg Clin N Am*, 2015;26(2):149–155, Fig 1.)

- Event analysis
  - A root cause analysis is a process that focuses on a systems analysis, not individual performance, for identifying the root causes of an event and then develops an action plan to reduce the risk of similar events occurring in the future
- Human factors engineering is a discipline that studies all the factors that make it easier to do the work in the right way
  - Example: how physical demands, skill demands, mental workload, team dynamics, and the work environment can be optimized for successful completion of a task

REDUCING MEDICAL ADVERSE EVENTS

- Pediatric medication management
  - Medication errors are a frequent cause of adverse events in pediatrics
  - Pediatric medication management is complex due to weight-based dosing, off-label use of medications, and the need to compound and dilute medications
  - Giving simple instructions both verbally and in writing, using visual aids, using interpreter services, collaborating with pharmacists, and electronic prescribing can reduce medication errors
- Teamwork and communication
  - Communication is frequently cited as a root cause in sentinel events
  - Critical times of information exchange occur during handoffs, when there is a change in clinical status, and whenever a team member has a concern
  - Communication errors can be reduced by:
    - Practicing closed-loop communication and using a formal handoff tool (e.g., IPASS)
    - Promoting situational awareness with the use of huddles and debriefs
    - Creating shared mental models (e.g., using an acuity scoring system)
    - Using a checklist
- Cognition and decision-making
  - Diagnostic errors are defined as a delayed, missed, or incorrect diagnosis
  - Approaches to decision-making:
    - Fast (type I): application of patterns of disease recognition that allows for rapid diagnosis and treatment. This is helpful in a fast-paced environment that thrives on efficiency
    - Slow (type II): requires purposeful dissection of a case and often involves a thoughtful and deliberate approach
  - Efforts to reduce diagnostic errors involve learning about heuristics (diagnostic shortcuts) and being thoughtful about their presence in your daily practice and taking "diagnostic time-outs" when something doesn't fit
- Technology
  - Computerized physician/provider order entry reduces error by:
    - The elimination of handwritten orders
    - Avoidance of "do not use" abbreviations published by The Joint Commission
    - Avoidance of errors caused by trailing or leading zeros

- Decision support regarding drug formulation and dosing
- Links to clinical pathways for correct drug prescribing decision support and links to drug-drug interactions
- Be wary of content-importing technology (copy forward) and macros (commands that insert preset text) and of selecting the wrong diagnostic test, medication, or dose from a drop-down menu. Information overload can lead to overlooking important information

Core Principles of Quality Improvement

- Background: the science of improvement is an applied science that emphasizes innovative changes, rapid-cycle testing, and spread of ideas to generate learning about what changes, in which contexts, produce improvements. It is characterized by the combination of evidence-based medicine with improvement methods and tools. Quality improvement efforts generally attempt to avoid attributing blame and instead focus on creating systems that prevent problems from occurring in the first place
  - Definition of quality: care that has the greatest potential for returning a patient to health in the shortest amount of time for the lowest possible cost with the lowest risk to the patient
  - In 2001, IOM published *Crossing the Quality Chasm: A New Health System for the 21st Century*, which outlined the following six aims for the health care system:
    - Safe: avoiding harm to patients from the care that is intended to help them
    - Effective: providing services based on scientific knowledge to all who could benefit and refraining from providing services to those not likely to benefit (avoiding underuse and misuse, respectively)
    - Patient-centered: providing care that is respectful of and responsive to individual patient preferences, needs, and values and ensuring that patient values guide all clinical decisions
    - Timely: reducing waits and sometimes harmful delays for both those who receive and those who give care
    - Efficient: avoiding waste, including waste of equipment, supplies, ideas, and energy
    - Equitable: providing care that does not vary in quality because of personal characteristics such as gender, ethnicity, geographic location, and socioeconomic status
  - Value equation: value is defined as the health outcomes achieved per dollar spent
    Value = Quality/Cost
- Improvement methodologies
  - Fundamental principles of improvement:
    - Knowing why you need to improve
    - Having a feedback mechanism to tell you whether the improvement is happening
    - Developing an effective change that will result in improvement

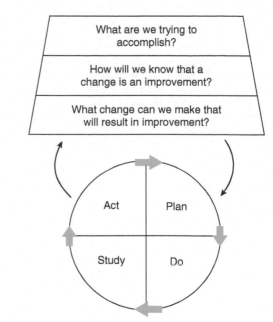

Fig. 98.2. Model for Improvement. (From Institute for Healthcare Improvement.http://www.ihi.org/resources/Pages/HowtoImprove/ScienceofImprovementHowtoImprove.aspx)

    - Testing a change before attempting to implement it
    - Knowing when and how to make the change permanent (implementing and sustaining the change)
  - W. Edwards Deming's "System of Profound Knowledge": insight into how to make changes that will result in improvement
    - Appreciation for a system: a system is an interdependent group of items, people, or processes working together toward a common purpose
    - Understanding variation: data will always show variation. One of the key questions is whether the variation is normal for the process or is unexpected, indicating that something special or out of the ordinary is happening
    - Building knowledge: the more knowledge one has about how a particular system functions or could function, the better one can predict that a change will result in improvement
    - Human side of change: understanding how people interact with each other and with a system to predict how people will react to a specific change and how to gain commitment
- Improvement frameworks
  - Model for improvement:
    - Framework for applying the five fundamental principles of improvement based on three questions:
      What are we trying to accomplish?
      How will we know that a change is an improvement?
      What changes can we make that will result in improvement?
    - The questions define the end point—any effort to improve should result in answers to these questions
  - Plan-do-study-act (PDSA) cycle (see Fig. 98.2)
    - Framework for efficient trial and learning methodology

- Multiple plan-do-study-act cycles are often needed to make successful changes
- Develop a change, test it on a small scale, and observe how the system responds
- Measurement
  - Types of variation:
    - Common cause (chance, routine)
      Causes that are inherent in the system all the time
    - Special cause (assignable)
      Causes that are not part of the system all the time
      Arise out of specific circumstances
  - Run chart: plots data over time to study trend
  - Statistical control charts/Shewhart chart: used to study how a process changes over time, using an upper control limit and a lower control limit, with limits of the mean ± sigma. By comparing current data to these lines, you can draw conclusions about whether the process variation is consistent (in control) or is unpredictable (out of control, affected by special causes of variation)
  - Types of measures:
    - Structural measure: presence or absence of a trait—is everything necessary to implement the change in place?
    - Process measure: reliability of carrying out an action—how will you demonstrate that the change has been implemented?
    - Outcome measure: results of carrying out an action—how will you demonstrate that the change has resulted in improvement?
    - Balancing measure: how will you demonstrate any unintended consequences?
- Improvement tools:
  - Aim statement: specific, measurable, achievable, realistic, and timely (SMART) statement that clarifies the question, "What are we trying to accomplish?"
    - Example aim statement: "decrease adverse drug events in the pediatric intensive care unit by 75% within 1 year"

- Process map: develop a picture of the process to communicate and standardize processes
- Driver diagrams and fishbone diagrams: cause and effect diagrams; organizes current knowledge regarding a problem or issue
- Effort/impact diagram: method of prioritization for the purpose of deciding which of many suggested solutions to implement based on which solutions seem easiest to achieve with the most effects
- Pareto chart: used to determine which interventions would solve 80% of the problem

Review Questions

For review questions, please go to ExpertConsult.com

Suggested Readings

1. Disclosure of adverse events in pediatrics. policy statement. *Pediatrics.* 2016;138(6):e20163215.
2. Kohn LT, Corrigan JM, Donaldson MS, et al. *To Err is Human: building a safer health system.* Washington, DC: National Academies Press; 1999.
3. Landrigan CP. The safety of inpatient pediatrics: preventing medical errors and injuries among hospitalized children. *Pediatr Clin North Am.* 2005;52(4):979–993.
4. Langley GL, Moen R, Nolan KM, Nolan TW, Norman CL, Provost LP. *The improvement guide: a practical approach to enhancing organizational performance.* 2nd ed. Jossey-Bass; 2009.
5. Leonard MS. Patient safety and quality improvement: medical errors and adverse events. *Pediatr Rev.* 2010;31(4):151–158.
6. Pereira-Argenziano L, Levy F. Patient safety and quality improvement: terminology. *Pediatr Rev.* 2015;36(9):403–413.
7. Principles of pediatric patient safety. reducing harm due to medical care. *Pediatrics.* 2011;127(6):1199–1210.
8. Provost LP, Murray SK. *The Healthcare Data Guide: Learning from Data for Improvement.* Jossey-Bass; 2011.
9. Sharek PJ, Classen D. The incidence of adverse events and medical error in pediatrics. *Pediatric Clin North Am.* 2006;53(6):1067–1077.
10. The Joint Commission. *National Patient Safety Goals.* 2017. Available at https://www.jointcommission.org/standards_information/npsgs.aspx.
11. Wachter R. *Understanding Patient Safety.* 2nd ed. McGraw Hill; 2012.

Index

Note: Page numbers followed by "f" indicate figures and "t" indicate tables.